# Nursing Outcomes Classification (NOC)

# Iowa Outcomes Project

# Nursing Outcomes Classification (NOC)

## Third Edition

### Editors

Sue Moorhead, PhD, RN
Marion Johnson, PhD, RN
Meridean Maas, PhD, RN, FAAN

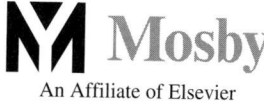

Mosby
An Affiliate of Elsevier

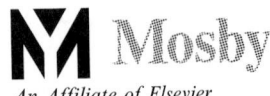

*An Affiliate of Elsevier*

11830 Westline Industrial Drive
St. Louis, Missouri 63146

NURSING OUTCOMES CLASSIFICATION (NOC), THIRD EDITION ISBN 0-323-02391-6

**Library of Congress Cataloging-in-Publication Data**

Nursing outcomes classification (NOC) / Iowa Outcomes Project ; editors, Sue Moorhead, Marion Johnson, Meridean Maas.–3rd ed.
   p. ; cm.
  Includes bibliographical references and index.
  ISBN 0-323-02391-6
   1. Nursing audit. 2. Outcomes assessment (Medical care) I. Moorhead, Sue. II. Johnson, Marion, 1936- III. Maas, Meridean. IV. Iowa Outcomes Project.
  [DNLM: 1. Nursing Process–standards. 2. Outcome Assessment (Health Care)–standards. WY 100 N9734 2003]
RT85.5.N864 2003
610.73–dc21

2003056216

*Executive Publisher:* Barbara Nelson Cullen
*Developmental Editor:* Julie Vitale
*Publishing Services Manager:* Deborah Vogel
*Senior Project Manager:* Mary Drone
*Design Manager:* Bill Drone

Printed in the United States of America

Last digit is the print number: 9 8 7 6 5 4 3 2

# Members of the NOC Research Team

## CO-PRINCIPAL INVESTIGATORS

**Marion Johnson, PhD, RN**
Professor Emerita
College of Nursing
The University of Iowa
Iowa City, IA

**Sue Moorhead, PhD, RN**
Associate Professor
College of Nursing
The University of Iowa
Iowa City, IA

**Meridean Maas, PhD, FAAN, RN**
Professor
College of Nursing
The University of Iowa
Iowa City, IA

## MEMBERS OF THE IOWA OUTCOMES PROJECT RESEARCH TEAM

### TEAM MEMBERS

**Mary Ann Anderson, PhD, RN**
Associate Professor
The University of Illinois at Chicago
College of Nursing
Quad Cities Regional Program
Moline, IL

**Mary Lober Aquilino, PhD, RN, FNP**
Clinical Assistant Professor
The University of Iowa
Department of Community and Behavioral
   Health
College of Public Health
Iowa City, IA

**Sandra Bellinger, EdD, RN**
Retired Academic Dean
Trinity College of Nursing
Moline, IL

**Veronica Brighton, MA, ARNP, CS**
Clinical Assistant Professor
The University of Iowa
College of Nursing
Iowa City, IA

**Carol L. Caldwell, MS, ARNP, CS**
Nurse Educator
Eastern Iowa Community College District
Bettendorf, IA

**Mary Clarke, MA, RN**
Informatics Nurse Specialist
Genesis Medical Center
Davenport, IA

**Sister Ruth Cox, OSF, PhD, RN**
President & CEO
The Alverno Health Care Facility
Clinton, IA

**Lois Dixon, MSN, RN**
Clinical Nurse Educator
Genesis Medical Center
Davenport, IA

**Linda Guebert, MS, RN**
Nurse Educator
Trinity Medical Center
Education Department
Rock Island, IL

**Barbara J. Head, PhD, RN**
Assistant Professor
UNMC College of Nursing—Omaha
   Division
Omaha, NE

**Cathy Konrad, PhD, RNC**
Associate Professor
Trinity College of Nursing
Moline, IL

**Jan Levsen, MA, RN**
CHF Program Coordinator
Genesis Medical Center, East
Davenport, IA

**Lisa Payden, MSN, RN**
Clinical Coordinator-Emergency Medicine
  School
Trinity Medical Center
Moline, IL

**Shelley-Rae Pehler, MSN, RN**
Maternal/Child Clinical Nurse Specialist
Genesis Medical Center
Davenport, IA

**Aleta Porcella, MSN, RN**
Advanced Practice Nurse
University of Iowa Hospitals & Clinics
Iowa City, IA

**Cindy Scherb, RN, PhD**
Associate Professor
Winona State University
Rochester, MN

**Deborah Perry Schoenfelder, PhD, RN**
Clinical Associate Professor
The University of Iowa
College of Nursing
Iowa City, IA

**Jo Ellen Sharer, PhD, RN**
President
Trinity College of Nursing & Health Sciences
Moline, IL

**Janet Specht, PhD, RN**
Associate Professor
The University of Iowa
College of Nursing
Iowa City, IA

**Elizabeth A. Swanson, PhD, RN**
Associate Professor
The University of Iowa
College of Nursing
Iowa City, IA

**Jill Valde, PhD, RN**
Assistant Professor
Nursing Grand View College
Des Moines, IA

**Cheryl Wagner, MSN, MBA, OCN, RNC**
Parish Nurse
Our Lady of Victory Parish
Davenport, IA

**Bonnie Wakefield, PhD, RN**
Associate Chief, Nursing Research
VA Medical Center
Iowa City, IA

**Dianne Wasson, MSN, RN, CDE**
Advanced Practice Nurse
University of Iowa Hospitals & Clinics
Iowa City, IA

**Marilyn Willits, MS, RN, CPHQ**
Standards Nurse Specialist
Genesis Medical Center, East
Davenport, IA

**Karen Wilson, MSN, RN**
Assistant Professor
Trinity College of Nursing
Moline, IL

**STUDENTS**

**Raeda Al Ad Rub**
Doctoral Student, Research Assistant

**Jenny Castle**
BSN Student, Honors Practicum

**Peg Kerr**
Doctoral Student, Research Assistant

**K. M. Reeder**
Doctoral Student, Research Assistant

**Maneewan Sanubol**
Doctoral Student, Research Practicum

**Debra Schutte**
Doctoral Student

**Wannee Tapaneeyakorn**
Doctoral Student

**Michelle Umbarger**
Master's Student, Research Assistant

**VISITING PROFESSOR**

**Tania Couto Machado Chianca, PhD, RN,
  MSN**
Researcher & Associate Professor
College of Nursing Federal University of
  Minas Gerais
Belo Horizonte Minas Gerais State, Brazil

**STAFF**

**Lori J. Penaluna Jarmon, BS, MA**
Project Manager
The University of Iowa
College of Nursing
Iowa City, IA

**David Reed, PhD**
Data Manager & Statistical Consultant
The University of Iowa
College of Nursing
Iowa City, IA

**Sharon Sweeney**
Data Coordinator
The University of Iowa
College of Nursing
Iowa City, IA

## UNIVERSITY OF MICHIGAN SUBCONTRACT

**PRINCIPAL INVESTIGATOR**

**Gail Keenan, PhD, RN**
Associate Professor
The University of Michigan
Ann Arbor, MI

**RESEARCH TEAM MEMBERS**

**Vi Barkauskas, PhD, RN, FAAN**
Associate Professor
The University of Michigan
Ann Arbor, MI

**Joanne Pohl, PhD, RN**
Associate Professor
The University of Michigan
Ann Arbor, MI

**Jan Lee, PhD, RN**
Director of Undergraduate Programs
Associate Professor
The University of Michigan
Ann Arbor, MI

**STAFF**

**Evelyn Clingerman, MS, RN**
Research Associate
The University of Michigan
Ann Arbor, MI

**Crystal Health, RN, BSN**
Research Associate
The University of Michigan
Ann Arbor, MI

**Julie Stocker, MS, RN**
Research Associate
The University of Michigan
Ann Arbor, MI

**Marcy Treder, RN**
Research Associate
The University of Michigan
Ann Arbor, MI

We wish to thank the following individuals who have shared their expertise by reviewing or developing specific outcomes, or contributing examples for this edition.

**Carolyn Kay Bauer, RN, BSN**
VA Central Iowa Healthcare System
Knoxville Division
Knoxville, IA

**Lisa Burkhart, MPH, PhD, RN**
Assistant Professor
Loyola University
Marcella Niehoff School of Nursing
Chicago, IL

**Mary Kathleen Clark, PhD, ARNP, FNP**
Associate Professor
The University of Iowa
College of Nursing
Iowa City, IA

**Perle Slavik Cowen, PhD, RN**
Associate Professor
The University of Iowa
College of Nursing
Iowa City, IA

**Martha Craft-Rosenberg, PhD, RN, FAAN**
Professor
The University of Iowa
College of Nursing
Iowa City, IA

**Ken Culp, PhD, RN, CS**
Associate Professor
The University of Iowa
College of Nursing
Iowa City, IA

**Janice Denehy, PhD, RN**
Associate Professor Emerita
The University of Iowa
College of Nursing
Iowa City, IA

**Cynthia Finesilver, RN, MSN, CNRN**
Assistant Professor of Nursing
Bellin College of Nursing
Green Bay, WI

**Lynette Hartsock, MSN, RN**
Nurse Manager
Medical Surgical II Nursing Division
University of Iowa Hospitals and Clinics
Iowa City, IA

**Elaine D. Hernandez**
Post Anesthesia Care Unit
Veteran Administration Medical Center
Iowa City, IA

**Peg Kerr, MS, RN**
Staff Development Coordinator
Mercy Hospital
Iowa City, IA

**Maryanne Krenz, RN**
Brookdale Community College of Nursing
Lincroft, NJ

**Scott Chisholm Lamont, BSN, RN, CCRN, CFRN, ENC(C)**
Specialty Nurse III, UNM Children's Hospital
University of New Mexico Health Sciences Center
Albuquerque, NM
PhD Student
University of California
San Francisco, CA

**Leslie Marshall, PhD, RN**
Associate Professor
The University of Iowa
College of Nursing
Iowa City, IA

**Debbie Metzler, RN, C, MSN**
Assistant Professor of Nursing
Bellin College of Nursing
Green Bay, WI

**Margaret Rankin, PhD, RN**
Retired Faculty Member
The University of Iowa
College of Nursing
Iowa City, IA

**K.M. Reeder, RN, MSE, MSN, CNS**
Assistant Professor Nursing
Grand View College
Des Moines, IA

**Cindy Scherb, RN, PhD**
Associate Professor
Winona State University
Rochester, MN

**Deborah Perry Schoenfelder, PhD, RN**
Clinical Associate Professor
The University of Iowa
College of Nursing
Iowa City, IA

**Barbara Van de Castle, APRN, BC**
Instructor
Johns Hopkins University, School of Nursing
Baltimore, MD

**Rosalind R. Willis, RN, C**
Staff Nurse
Good Samaritan Hospital
Puyallup, WA

## FORMER MEMBERS

**Rojann Alper**
Team Member, 1st edition

**Anne Bodensteiner**
Team Member, 1st edition

**Kristine Bonnett**
Master's Student, 1st edition

**Katie Brady-Schluttner**
Team Member, 1st edition

**Helga Bragdottir**
Master's Student 2nd edition

**Jane Brokel**
Doctoral Student, Research Practicum
2nd edition

**John Brooks**
Advisory Board, 2nd edition

**Ginette Budreau**
Co-Investigator, 1st edition

**Gloria Bulecheck**
Consultant, 1st edition

**Linda Chlan**
Post Doctoral Fellow, 2nd edition

**Christopher Chute**
Advisory Board, 2nd edition

**Judy Collins**
Team Member, 1st edition

**Sandy Daack-Hirsch**
Master's Student, 2nd edition

**Kala Minnick Dahns**
Team Member, 1st edition

**Jeannette Daly**
Co-Investigator, 1st edition

**Diane Davidson**
Master's Student, 1st edition

**Kris Davis**
Team Member, 1st & 2nd edition

**Connie Delaney**
Consultant, 1st edition

**Joanne McCloskey Dochterman**
Consultant, 1st edition

**Kerri Doeden-Gores**
Master's Student, 1st edition

**Pat Donahue**
Co-Investigator, 1st & 2nd edition

**Joyce Eland**
Co-Investigator, 1st & 2nd edition

**Susan Ellenbecker**
Team Member, 1st edition

**Paula Forte**
Postdoctoral Fellow, Team Member
2nd edition

**Vicky Fraser**
Team Member, 1st edition

**Linda Garand**
Doctoral Student, Team Member
1st & 2nd edition

**Rose Gebhart**
Team Member, 1st edition

**LaRonda Giles**
Office Assistant, 2nd edition

**Mee Ock Gu**
Visiting Professor, 2nd edition

**Sheila Haas**
Advisory Board, 1st edition

**Cheryl Hardison**
Team Member, 1st & 2nd edition

**Jane Hartsock**
Team Member, 1st & 2nd edition

**Pam Harvey**
Team Member, 1st edition

**Yaseen Ahmed Hayajneh**
Doctoral Student, 1st & 2nd edition

**Brenda Hollingsworth**
Master's Student, Research Assistant
2nd edition

**Mary Ann Hovda**
Master's Student, 1st edition

**Marna Jacobi**
Team Member, 1st & 2nd edition

**Ada Jacox**
Advisory Board, 1st edition

**Lisa James**
Team Member, 1st edition

**Roxanne Joens-Martre**
Team Member, 2nd edition

**Shayna J. Johnson**
Team Member, 1st edition

**Katherine Jones**
Advisory Board, 2nd edition

**Julie Katseres**
Team Member, 1st & 2nd edition

**Kathleen Kelly**
Co-Investigator, 1st edition

**John Knapp**
Master's Student, Research Assistant
2nd edition

**Vicki Kraus**
Team Member, 1st & 2nd edition

**Tom Kruckeberg**
Co-Investigator, 1st edition

**Edith Lassengard**
Doctoral Student, Research Assistant
1st & 2nd edition

**Donna Laube**
BSN Student, Office Assistant
1st & 2nd edition

**Eunjoo Lee**
Research Assistant, 2nd edition

**Melissa Lehan**
Baccalaureate Student, Research Assistant,
1st & 2nd edition

**Anne Lewis**
Co-Investigator, 1st edition

**Leslie Marshall**
Co-Investigator, 1st & 2nd edition

**Tom Martz**
Team Member, 1st edition

**Becki Maxson**
Team Member, 1st edition

**Linda McCabe**
Master's Student, 1st edition

**Kathleen A. McCormick**
Advisory Board, 1st edition

**Jeanette Miller-Criswell**
Team Member, 1st edition

**Heidi Nobiling**
Team Member, 1st edition

**Colleen Prophet**
Co-Investigator, 1st & 2nd edition

**Cheryl Ramler**
Doctoral Student, Team Member
1st & 2nd edition

**Margaret Rankin**
Co-Investigator, 1st & 2nd edition

**Polly Ryan**
Advisory Board, 1st edition

**Sharon Schneider**
Master's Student, Research Assistant
1st & 2nd edition

**Bev Soukup-Platz**
Team Member, 1st edition

**Janice L. Stone**
Team Member, 1st edition

**Ora Strickland**
Advisory Board, 2nd edition

**Toni Tripp-Reimer**
Consultant, 1st edition

**Jill Valde**
Team Member, 2nd edition

**Donna Valiga**
Secretary, 1st & 2nd edition

**Sonia Van De Keift**
Master's Student, 1st edition

**Joyce Verran**
Advisory Board, 1st & 2nd edition

**Fran Vlasses**
Postdoctoral Fellow, 2nd edition

**JoAnne Wedig**
Team Member, 2nd edition

**Bonnie L. Westra**
Co-Investigator, 1st edition

**George Woodworth**
Co-Investigator, 1st & 2nd edition

**Liwei Wu**
Doctoral Student, Research Assistant
2nd edition

## TEST SITES

**The Alverno Health Care Facility, Clinton, IA**
Sister Ruth Cox OSF, PhD, RN
Kim Zickau-Quick, BA
Theresa Bickford, LPN

**Genesis Medical Center, Davenport, IA**
Mary Clarke, MA, RN
Marilyn Willits, MS, RN, CPHQ
Monica Youngblut, BSN, RN

**International Parish Nurse Resource Center**
Advocate Health Care
Lisa Burkhart, RN, PhD
Kay Guptail, RN, BSN

**Mayo Clinic, Rochester, MN**
Julia Behrenbeck, RN, MS, MPH
Jane Timm, RN, MS
Linda Griebenow, RN, MS
Kathy Demmer, RN, MS

**Mayo Health System, Immanuel St. Joseph, Mankato, MN**
Cindy Scherb, RN, PhD
Kathie Foreman, RN, MS
Carol Busman, RN, MS
Shawna Mueller, RN, BSN
Heidi Riehl, RN, BSN

**Austin Medical Center, Austin, MN**
Janet Wagenaar, RN, BA
Sue Bos, RN

**Michigan Subcontract**
Gail Keenan, PhD, RN
Marcy Treder, RN

**University of Iowa Hospitals & Clinics, Iowa City, IA**
Aleta Porcella, MSN, RN
Michelle Umbarger, BSN, RN

# Preface

The third edition of the Nursing Outcomes Classification (NOC) contains 330 outcomes. Each outcome includes a label name, a definition, a set of indicators that describe specific patient, caregiver, family, or community states related to the outcome, a five-point Likert-type measurement scale, and selected references used in the development of the outcome. The classification standardizes the outcome name and definitions. The research team has refined the indicators and measurement scale(s) associated with the outcome in this edition. The outcomes assist nurses and other health care providers to evaluate and quantify the status of the patient, caregiver, family, or community outcome. Since the publication of the last edition of the classification, the reliability and validity of the outcomes and measurement scales have been tested in 10 clinical sites from four midwest states. Feedback from clinicians using the outcome measures in clinical settings has been positive, and their suggestions have helped improve the classification.

Seventy-six new outcomes have been added to the classification in this edition, and six have been retired. A complete list of changes in the outcomes can be found in Appendix A. Changes in this edition reflect the results of testing in clinical practice in a variety of practice sites. This research helped us improve the format of the outcomes and refine definitions, measurement scales, and indicators. Additions to this edition include the identification of core outcomes by specialty organizations and the placement of NOC outcomes in the taxonomy of Nursing Practice. Minor changes were made in the NOC Taxonomy for this edition.

This edition provides more guidance on how to use NOC in clinical practice. Chapter 1 remains essentially the same and provides an overview of outcome research in health care and nursing. This chapter is helpful for nurses who are beginning to consider the use of outcome measures in their practice. Chapter 2 describes the current classification presented in this edition. Definition of terms, frequently asked questions, and a detailed summary of measurement scale changes, as well as overall changes to the classification, are described. Chapter 3 provides research results from Phase III of our research testing the reliability and validity of the outcomes. Chapter 4 discusses how to use NOC in clinical practice and has useful suggestions and updated examples of forms used in a variety of settings. Chapter 5 discusses the use of NOC in education and research.

Linkages between the NANDA diagnoses and the NOC outcomes are included in Part IV of the book. The reader will note that the NANDA diagnoses are listed by key concept in alphabetical order and are consistent with the terminology used in the 2003-2004 edition of the NANDA International Classification. Also included in this section are linkages with Gordon's Functional Health Patterns. It is important to note that these linkages are not prescriptive and have not been validated with clinical data. They are suggested to assist nurses with identifying possible outcomes when a diagnosis is made or to develop a framework for clinical information systems. *The nurse's clinical judgment remains the most important factor in selecting outcomes.*

The need for nursing to define the patient outcomes that are responsive to nursing care has continued to increase since the first edition of this book was published. The growth of managed care and the emphasis on cost containment continue to bring concerns about outcomes effectiveness and health care quality to the fore. Nursing plays a key role in the delivery of cost-effective care in every health care setting; therefore it is imperative that nursing data be included in the evaluation of health care effectiveness. The NOC completes the nursing process elements of the Nursing Minimum Data Set (NMDS). NOC is a companion language to the NIC interventions and the NANDA diagnoses. Standardized nursing languages are required to ensure that the nursing elements identified in the NMDS are included in electronic patient databases. They also facilitate the study and teaching of diagnostic reasoning and the development of mid-range theory as linkages between patient characteristics, nursing diagnoses, nursing interventions, and nursing-sensitive outcomes are tested.

The editors of this book thank the many nurses who have contributed to the development of NOC. The research team has worked diligently to continue to expand and evaluate the NOC outcomes. The past and current members of the research team are identified in the front part of the book. Many individuals have shared their knowledge and work with us or have agreed to review an outcome related to their specialty. Without them, this edition would not be possible.

*Sue Moorhead*
*Marion Johnson*
*Meridean Maas*

# Strengths of the Nursing-Sensitive Outcomes Classification

*Comprehensive.* The NOC contains outcomes for individuals, family caregivers, the family, and the community that can be used in all settings and clinical specialties. Although all possible outcomes are not yet developed, there are outcomes that are useful for the entire scope of nursing practice, and plans are to develop others as they are identified. Because each is comprehensive, the NANDA International Classification, NIC, and NOC provide standardized languages for the nursing process elements of the Nursing Minimum Data Set

*Research-based.* The research, conducted by a large team of University of Iowa College of Nursing faculty and students in conjunction with clinicians from a variety of settings, began in 1991. Both qualitative and quantitative strategies were used to develop the classification. Methods included content analysis, concept analysis, survey of experts, similarity analysis, hierarchical clustering analysis, multidimensional scaling, and clinical field site testing. The outcomes were evaluated for inter-rater reliability, validity, and usefulness in 10 clinical sites representing the care continuum.

*Developed inductively and deductively.* Sources of data for initial development of the outcomes and indicators were nursing textbooks, care plan guides, nursing clinical information systems, standards of practice, and research instruments. Research team focus groups reviewed outcomes in eight broad categories that were drawn from the Medical Outcomes Study and nursing literature. Based on a review of literature, outcomes subsumed by the broad categories were identified and refined through concept analysis.

*Grounded in clinical practice and research.* Developed initially from nursing texts, care plan guides, and clinical information systems, the outcomes were reviewed by clinical experts, and many were tested in clinical field sites. Feedback from clinicians and educators is solicited through a defined feedback process. Beginning work on core NOC outcomes for specialty practice is included in the third edition.

*Uses clear, clinically useful language.* Throughout the development of the NOC, clarity and usefulness of the language has been emphasized. Care has been taken to ensure that the language distinguishes NOC outcomes from nursing interventions and diagnoses. The outcomes are developed for patients, caregivers, families, and communities.

*Has easy to use organizing structure.* The taxonomy has five levels: domains, classes, outcomes, indicators, and measurement scales. All five levels have been coded for use in practice. New outcomes are added to the taxonomy as the classification is further developed. This structure aids nurses in identifying outcomes to use in their clinical practice and provides a framework for teaching NOC to students in educational settings.

*Outcomes can be shared by all disciplines.* Although the NOC emphasizes outcomes that are most responsive to nursing interventions, the outcomes describe patient, family, or community states at a conceptual level. Thus the NOC provides a classification of patient outcomes that are potentially influenced by all health care disciplines. The NOC contains indicators for the outcomes that are expected to be most responsive to nursing interventions. Use of the outcomes by all members of the interdisciplinary team provides standardization, yet allows the selection of indicators that are most responsive to each discipline. Field testing demonstrated that the outcomes were useful to interdisciplinary teams in practice.

*Optimizes information for the evaluation of effectiveness.* The outcomes and indicators are variable concepts. They allow for measurement of the patient, family, or community outcome at any point on a continuum from most negative to most positive and at different points in time. Rather than the limited information provided by the measurement of whether a goal is met or unmet, NOC outcomes can be used to monitor the extent of progress, or lack of progress, throughout an episode of care and across different care settings. Change in outcome ratings can be reported as a result of nursing interventions and monitored across time and care setting.

*Funded by extramural grants.* To date, the NOC research has received 9 years of peer-reviewed grant funding: 1 year from Sigma Theta Tau International and 8 years from the National Institute of Nursing Research (NINR).

*Tested in clinical field sites.* Testing of the NOC has been conducted in a variety of clinical field sites, including tertiary care hospitals, intermediate care hospitals, a nursing home, home health care settings, nurse managed clinics, and through a parish nursing organization. The field tests have provided important information about the clinical usefulness of the outcomes and indicators; linkages between nursing diagnoses, interventions, and outcomes; and the process of implementing the outcomes in clinical nursing information systems.

*Dissemination emphasized.* Information about the classification, its development, and use is available in this book *Nursing Outcomes Classification (NOC)*, Third Edition, published by Mosby and in numerous journal articles and book chapters. The NOC research is described on a University of Iowa College of Nursing World Wide Web home page (http://www.nursing.uiowa.edu/noc/), and a *LISTSERV* is maintained to share information about the NOC and for dialogue with interested users. The NOC work has been disseminated in a number of national and international presentations. Although developed in the United States, nurses in other countries are finding the classification useful. Translations are complete or in process for the following languages: Chinese, Dutch, French, German, Japanese, Korean, and Spanish.

*Linked to other nursing languages.* Linkages have been developed by the NIC and NOC research teams to assist nurses with the use of the classifications and to facilitate use in clinical information systems. NANDA-NOC linkages and links to Gordon's Functional Health Care Patterns are included in the book. NIC-NOC linkages have been developed by the NIC team and are available through the Center for Nursing Classification and Clinical Effectiveness. NOC has been linked with the Omaha System Problems and the Resident Assessment Protocols (RAPs) for long-term care; these linkages are also available from the Center for Nursing Classification and Clinical Effectiveness. Linkages with OASIS assessment categories are in development. Linkages among NANDA diagnoses, NOC outcomes, and NIC interventions have been completed and are available in the book *Nursing Diagnoses, Outcomes, & Interventions: NANDA, NIC, and NOC Linkages* published by Mosby.

*Included in the NNN taxonomy.* NOC is included in the combined taxonomy under development that includes NANDA Diagnoses, NIC interventions, and NOC outcomes. This initiative focuses on the development of a taxonomic structure that includes all three languages for use in practice and educational settings. This is a project of the NANDA-NIC-NOC Alliance.

*Included in initiatives for electronic clinical record.* Concepts for NOC will be included in SNOMED Clinical Terms, a reference terminology for use in clinical information systems. NOC has been registered with Health Level 7, a U.S. standards organization dedicated to simplifying the exchange, management, and integration of clinical and administrative data in health records. Several vendors have licensed NOC for inclusion in their software development initiatives for a nursing component of an electronic clinical record.

*Developed as companion to the NIC.* Experience with the NIC at Iowa has aided the NOC research. Both classifications are comprehensive, research-based, and reflect current clinical nursing practice. They are both housed in the Center for Nursing Classification and Clinical Effectiveness.

*Recipient of national recognition.* NOC is recognized by the American Nurses Association (ANA), included in the Metathesaurus for a Unified Medical Language at the National Library of Medicine, included in the CINAHL index, and listed as one of the languages that meets the standards set by ANA's Nursing Information and Data Set Evaluation Center (NIDSEC).

*Structure for continued development and refinement.* The classification continues to be evaluated, developed, and refined by the NOC research team. Continued refinement will be facilitated through the Center for Nursing Classification and Clinical Effectiveness, the College of Nursing, and the University of Iowa. In addition to seeking continued grant support, a $1 million endowment is being raised to ensure a solid financial foundation for supporting further development of both NIC and NOC.

# Definition of Terms

## NURSING-SENSITIVE PATIENT OUTCOME

An individual, family, or community state, behavior, or perception that is measured along a continuum in response to a nursing intervention(s). Each outcome has an associated group of indicators that are used to determine patient status in relation to the outcome. In order to be measured, the outcome requires identification of a series of more specific indicators.

## OUTCOME INDICATOR

A more concrete individual, family, or community state, behavior or perception that serves as a cue for measuring an outcome. Nursing-sensitive patient outcome indicators characterize a patient, family, or community state at the concrete level. Some examples of indicators include "Describes strategies to maximize health," "Maintains usual family routines," "Intake of adequate fluid."

## MEASURE

A five-point Likert-type scale that quantifies a patient outcome or indicator status on a continuum from least to most desirable and provides a rating at a point in time. Measurement will reflect a continuum, such as 1 = Severely compromised; 2 = Substantially compromised; 3 = Moderately compromised; 4 = Mildly compromised; 5 = Not compromised.

## CHANGE IN RATING SCORE

The difference between a baseline rating of the outcome and the postintervention rating(s) of the outcome. This change score can be positive (the outcome rating increased), negative (the outcome rating decreased), or there can be no change (the outcome rating stayed the same). This change in rating score represents the outcome achieved following a health care intervention(s).

## NOC TAXONOMY

A systematic organization of outcomes into groups or categories based on similarities, dissimilarities, and relationships among the outcomes. The NOC taxonomy structure has five levels: domains, classes, outcomes, indicators, and measures.

# Acknowledgments

Continual development of the Nursing Outcomes Classification (NOC) and this publication would not have been possible without the work and support of numerous individuals and organizations that we would like to acknowledge and thank for their efforts:

- *Sigma Theta Tau International* for a one year grant (1992-1993) and the Office of Nursing Research, University of Iowa, for seed grants (1992-1993). These grants partially funded the pilot work and beginning development of the NOC.
- *The National Institute of Nursing Research, National Institutes of Health*, for a 4-year grant (1993-1997) to continue the development of the classification, construct the taxonomy, and field test the outcomes and for a 4-year continuation grant (1998-2001) entitled "Evaluation of Nursing-Sensitive Patient Outcome Measures" to pilot the outcomes and evaluate the measurement scales in clinical sites.
- The support from the *College of Nursing* at the *University of Iowa* for initial support of this work by *past Dean Geraldene Felton* and the continued support by *Dean Melanie Dreher*. Dean Dreher's support for the Center for Nursing Classification and Effectiveness since it was founded in 1995 has been instrumental in the continuing development and refinement of both NIC and NOC.
- The *team members, clinicians, and students* who have devoted hours of work to develop, review, and refine the outcomes, associated indicators, and measurement scales that appear in the NOC.
- The *American Nurses' Association* for supporting the validation survey and the *ANA's Congress of Nursing Practice Steering Committee on Databases to Support Clinical Nursing Practice* for recognizing NOC as a classification system useful for clinical nursing practice.
- The *NANDA International* organization for its partnership through the Alliance that links NANDA, NIC and NOC in efforts such as the NNN taxonomy structure development and NANDA, NIC and NOC national conferences.
- The *field test sites and their staff* who have worked diligently to include the NOC outcomes and measurement scales in their clinical sites: Alverno Health Care Facility-Clinton, IA; Mayo Clinic-Rochester, MN; Genesis Medical Center-Davenport, IA; University of Michigan Community Family Health Center-Ann Arbor, MI; North Campus Nursing Center-Ann Arbor, MI; Huron Valley Visiting Nurse Association-Ann Arbor, MI; Pontiac-Oakland Visiting Nurse Association-Waterford, MI; University of Iowa Hospitals and Clinics-Iowa City, IA, Mayo Health System, Mankato and Austin, MN.
- *Nurses from a variety of nursing specialty organizations* who shared their expertise by completing validation surveys and core surveys to further this effort.
- The many *patients and their families* who were willing to participate in our research and complete both outcome ratings and criterion tool measures as we tested our outcomes in clinical settings.
- Our very competent staff, *Lori Penaluna Jarmon, David Reed, and Sharon Sweeney*, who believed in this work, shared in our vision, and managed the data and details of this classification to make this edition possible.

# Organizations That Have Contributed to the Development of NOC

Nurses from a variety of specialty organizations have participated in the development and validation of NOC. These organizations are:

Academy of Medical Surgical Nurses
Air and Surface Transport Nurses Association
American Academy of Ambulatory Care Nursing
American Association Occupational Health Nurses
American Association of Critical-Care Nurses
American Association of Neuroscience Nurses
American Association of Nurse Anesthetists
American Association of Spinal Cord Injury Nurses
American College of Nurse Practitioners
American Holistic Nurses' Association
American Nephrology Nurses Association
American Nurses Credentialing Center–Cardiac Rehabilitation
American Nurses Credentialing Center–Clinical Specialist in Medical Surgical Nursing
American Nurses Credentialing Center–Community Health
American Nurses Credentialing Center–Family Nurse Practitioner
American Nurses Credentialing Center–Gerontological
American Nurses Credentialing Center–Home Health
American Nurses Credentialing Center–Pediatric
American Nurses Credentialing Center–Psychiatric/Mental Health
American Nurses Credentialing Center–School Nurse
American Nurses Credentialing Center–Medical-Surgical
American Psychiatric Nurses Association
American Radiological Nurses Association
American Society for Parenteral & Enteral Nutrition
American Society of Ophthalmic Registered Nurses, Inc.
American Society of Pain Management Nurses
American Society of PeriAnesthesia Nurses
ANA: Community Public Health
ANA: General Practice
ANA: Gerontology
ANA: Medical Surgical Nurses
ANA: Pediatrics
ANA: Psychiatric/Mental Health
Association of Community Health Nursing Educators
Association of Nurses in AIDS Care
Association of Operating Room Nurses, Inc.
Association of Pediatric Oncology Nurses

Association of Perioperative Registered Nurses
Association of Rehabilitation Nurses
AWHONN: Association of Women's Health Obstetric and Neonatal Nurses
Dermatology Nurses Association
Developmental Disabilities Nurses Association
Drug & Alcohol Nursing Association, Inc.
Emergency Nurses Association
Home Healthcare Nurses Association
Hospice and Palliative Nurses Association
International Society of Nurses in Genetics
Intravenous Nurses Society
Midwest Nursing Research Society
NANDA International
NAPNAP: National Association of Pediatric Nurse Associates & Practitioners
National Association of Neonatal Nurses
National Association of Orthopaedic Nurses
National Association of School Nurses
National Consortium of Chemical Dependency Nurses
National Gerontological Nursing Association
Oncology Nursing Society
Respiratory Nursing Society
Society for Education and Research in Psychiatric-Mental Health Nursing
Society for Vascular Nursing
Society of Gastroenterology Nurses and Associates, Inc.
Society of Otorhinolaryngology and Head-Neck Nurses, Inc.
Society of Pediatric Nurses
Society of Urologic Nurses & Associates, Inc.
Wound Ostomy and Continence Nurses Society

# Contents

# Detailed Contents

# PART ONE

# Nursing Outcomes Classification: Background, Testing, and Use in Clinical and Educational Settings

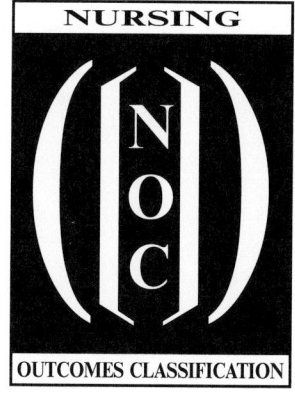

# CHAPTER ONE

# Outcome Development
# and Significance

The restructuring of the U.S. health care system to increase economic efficiency has resulted in an emphasis on health care costs and patient outcomes as measures of system effectiveness. As health care costs stabilize, consumers and payers have turned their attention to patient satisfaction and patient outcomes as criteria for selecting health care providers. The result has been the creation of a variety of evaluation tools designed to measure the outcomes of health care delivery systems. Although these measures have the potential to improve care delivery and to provide information about physician practice and organizational outcomes, the interventions and outcomes of nursing care are not readily apparent in most evaluation systems. As the nursing profession struggles to retain its identity in a health care system being restructured for greater efficiency, the need for nursing to define its interventions and outcomes has never been greater.

This book documents the development of standardized outcomes for the evaluation of nursing care. Part One provides background information for the standardized outcomes, which appear in Part Three. In Chapter 1, outcome development in health care with an emphasis on nursing is described, and the need for a standardized outcome language for nursing is discussed. The current Classification is discussed in Chapter 2. Results of testing the outcomes at 10 clinical sites are reported in Chapter 3. Chapter 4 describes implementation of the outcomes in clinical practice, and Chapter 5, use of the Nursing Outcomes Classification (NOC) in education and research. The taxonomy and its development are described in Part Two, and the appendices contain a number of implementation examples from practice and educational settings.

## OUTCOME DEVELOPMENT IN HEALTH CARE

The systematic use of patient outcomes to evaluate health care began when Florence Nightingale recorded and analyzed health care conditions and patient outcomes during the Crimean War.[48,87] Since that time, attempts to identify, measure, and use patient outcomes in the evaluation of health care delivery have been sporadic, often discipline-specific, and commonly focused on physician practice.[39] Efforts to evaluate physician practice began in the early 1900s when Codman, a Boston surgeon, proposed the use of outcome-based measures as indicators of medical care quality.[85] His work is considered the precursor of modern outcomes research. However, it wasn't until the mid-1960s that a model for assessing the quality of physician practice was proposed by Donabedian.[17] The model, which emphasized structure, process, and outcome, was adopted by other health care disciplines and gained wide use as the preferred method of evaluating the quality of health care services. However, the complexity of problems inherent in identifying and measuring patient outcomes resulted in measures of structure and process developing more rapidly than measures of patient outcomes. Until the 1980s, mortality, morbidity, and clinical signs served as traditional outcome measures. With the emphasis on effectiveness in the mid-1980s, fueled by political pressure and the availability of large data sets because of advances in information technology, attention again turned to measures of patient outcomes to evaluate physician practice.

An important study of physician practice, the Medical Outcomes Study (MOS), used a conceptual framework based on structure, process, and outcome elements to evaluate medical care effectiveness.[91] Outcome measures in the MOS were defined in the following broad categories: clinical end points, which included signs and symptoms, laboratory values, and death; functional

3

status, which included physical, mental, social, and role statuses; general well-being, which included health perceptions, energy/fatigue, pain, and life satisfaction; and satisfaction with care, which included access, convenience, financial coverage, quality, and general satisfaction. The study is significant for nursing because it was one of the first large national studies in which patient outcomes attributed to physician practice moved beyond the realm of disease-specific clinical outcomes to dimensions such as functional status, general well-being, and satisfaction. The study also has significance for health care in general because shortened versions of the form used to evaluate patient outcomes, such as the Medical Outcomes Study Short Form-36 (MOS-SF-36),[94] have gained wide acceptance as a general measure of health care delivery effectiveness.

In addition to the MOS-SF-36, other standardized performance measures, often referred to as *report cards*, have been developed in an attempt to quantify the quality and effectiveness of health care delivery systems and organizations. Examples are the Outcome Concept System and the Health Plan Employer Data and Information Set (HEDIS).[70,71] An analysis of report cards in current use showed that while some contain outcomes sensitive to nursing interventions, many have no nursing content.[7]

Accrediting organizations have assumed a major role in fostering the use of outcomes to evaluate organizational effectiveness and care quality. The Joint Commission on Accreditation of Healthcare Organizations (JCAHO) initiated a requirement that all hospitals and long-term care organizations seeking JCAHO accreditation use a performance measurement system to provide data about patient outcomes and other indicators of care effective January 1, 1998.[95] Organizations can select the JCAHO's Indicator Measurement System (IMSystem), one of the commercial systems approved by the commission, or can develop their own system for approval.[69,95] The IMSystem contains 31 measures for perioperative, obstetric, trauma, oncology, and cardiovascular patients, as well as 11 measures of medication use and infection control.[69] It is anticipated that other organizations, such as home care agencies, will be required to implement similar requirements for JACHO accreditation. The National Committee on Quality Assurance (NCQA) monitors outcomes as part of its evaluation and accreditation of managed care plans. The data set used to measure performance, HEDIS 3.0, includes measures of care effectiveness, access and availability of care, patient satisfaction, and cost of care, as well as measures that describe the health care plan.[62]

The federal government has assumed an active role in outcomes research and management, primarily through the Agency for Health Care Policy and Research (AHCPR) and the Health Care Financing Administration (HCFA). Between 1992 and 1996, AHCPR sponsored the development and dissemination of 20 clinical practice guidelines. The agency has initiated a new program called *the Clinical Improvement Program* with three new initiatives: the creation of evidence-based practice centers, a national guideline clearinghouse, and product research and evaluation.[62] HCFA has used the work of the AHCPR to develop and test national quality indicator modules[62] and to set requirements for standardized data collection for nursing homes and home care agencies.

## OUTCOME DEVELOPMENT IN NURSING

The use of patient outcomes to evaluate nursing care quality began in the mid-1960s, when Aydelotte[6] used changes in behavioral and physical characteristics of patients to evaluate the effectiveness of nursing care delivery systems. Since that time, additional outcome measures have been developed and tested for nursing,[26] and a variety of patient outcomes have been used to evaluate the quality of nursing care and the effects of nursing interventions.[47,72,90]

In addition to the development and testing of outcome measures, nurses have expended considerable effort to categorize outcomes, and more recently, to identify "core" outcome measures. Early work to classify nursing-sensitive patient outcomes took place in the late 1970s. Hover and Zimmer[30] identified the following five general outcome measures focused on the patient's knowledge: knowledge of illness and its treatments, knowledge of medications, self-care skills, adaptive behaviors, and health status. These broad outcome categories were based on a review of patient outcomes used by nurses at that time.

Horn and Swain[29] conducted a major research effort to identify outcome measures useful for nursing research and categorized more than 300 indicators in the broad categories of universal demands and health deviation. Daubert[14] proposed the following five categories to measure rehabilitation potential in home care: (1) recovery, (2) self-care, (3) rehabilitation, (4) maintenance, and (5) terminal care. Lalonde[46] developed and tested the following measures for home health evaluation: taking prescribed medications as instructed, general symptom distress, discharge status, caregiver status, functional status, knowledge of major health problems and diagnosis, and physiologic indicators.

In the 1980s two outcome categorizations, based on extensive reviews of outcomes used in nursing research, were formulated. Lang and Clinton[47] identified the following six outcome categories: (1) physical health status; (2) mental health status; (3) social and physical functioning; (4) health attitudes, knowledge, and behavior; (5) use of professional health resources; and (6) patient perceptions of the quality of nursing care. Marek[54] identified 15 outcome categories describing patient status and resource use based on a review of outcomes used to evaluate nursing care. Table 1-1 lists these categories. This work by Marek was the foundation on which outcomes research was based.

The increased importance placed on health care effectiveness in the 1990s resulted in a renewed emphasis on outcome development in nursing, including efforts to identify "core" patient outcomes for evaluation of nursing care effectiveness. McCormick[61] proposed a list of measurable outcomes that included process and patient outcomes as a means of evaluating nursing effectiveness, primarily in acute-care settings. Patient outcomes identified as salient for nursing were normal fluid hydration, continence, mobility, and the absence of decubitus and mucous membrane ulcers. The American Nurses Association (ANA) developed a Nursing Care Report Card for Acute Care.[3] The report card identifies a core set of nursing quality indicators, including structure, process, and outcome indicators. Outcome indicators include mortality rate, length of stay, adverse incidents, complications such as nosocomial infections and decubitus ulcers, and patient satisfaction with nursing care. The ANA outcome indicators are aggregated measures that characterize the hospital or patient care unit rather than individual patients.

In addition to the identification of core outcome measures sensitive to nursing interventions, there has been increased emphasis on the development of conceptual models or frameworks to describe the patient outcomes relevant for nursing and the relationships among patient outcomes, structure and process elements, and patient characteristics. A framework generated for use in hospital settings suggested the measurement of outcomes that evaluate patient/family education, facilitation of self-care, symptom distress management, provisions for patient safety, and enhancement of patient satisfaction.[22] Brown[10] proposed a conceptual framework for quality evaluation that included physiological condition, psychological status, health knowledge,

| Table 1-1   OUTCOME CATEGORIES DEVELOPED BY MAREK[54] | |
| --- | --- |
| Physiological measures | Goal attainment |
| Psychosocial measures | Patient satisfaction |
| Functional measures | Safety |
| Client behaviors | Frequency of service |
| Client knowledge | Cost |
| Symptom control | Rehospitalization |
| Home maintenance | Resolution of nursing diagnoses |
| Well-being | |

and satisfaction. Naylor and associates[72] have suggested functional status, mental status, stress level, satisfaction with care, burden of care, and cost of care as appropriate outcomes for the evaluation of nursing care effectiveness. Most recently, the Quality Health Outcomes Model has been developed by an American Academy of Nursing expert panel.[66] The model incorporates structure and process elements as system characteristics and proposes a reciprocal relationship among system characteristics, interventions, outcomes, and client characteristics.

Efforts have also focused on the development of nursing vocabularies and taxonomies. In addition to the classification described in this book, there are other classifications that contain patient outcome systems recognized by the ANA. Two of these were developed for use in home care. The Omaha System[57] includes a problem classification scheme, an intervention scheme, and the Problem Rating Scale for Outcomes (PRSO). The rating scale is a five-point ordinal scale measuring patient progress in relation to knowledge, behavior, and status. The scale can be applied to any of the problems identified in the classification. An initial assessment of the content validity and inter-rater reliability of the scale has been published.[58] The Home Health Care Classification uses three discharge status measures—improved, stabilized, and deteriorated.[86] The measures can be assigned to any problem identified in the classification. The Patient Care Data Set[78] was developed for use in hospital settings. It provides a range of possible outcomes for specific patient problems common in acute-care settings.

Two other outcome systems important for nursing are in use or being tested. The Outcome Assessment Information Set (OASIS) was developed at the Center for Health Policy Research at the University of Colorado.[88] The system contains core measures that apply to all client groups and specific measures for client groups with a particular diagnosis or problem. Each outcome is measured on a scale specific for the outcome to determine whether the patient has improved, stabilized, or deteriorated. This is the only system that has reported testing of risk adjustment factors. Beginning in 1998 the HCFA's Conditions of Participation required all Medicare-accredited home health organizations to incorporate the OASIS data set into their processes of care.[13] The OASIS data set includes information about the sensory, integumentary, respiratory, elimination, neurologic, emotional, behavioral, and functional status of the patient in addition to demographic and other information. The other classification of importance to nursing is the International Classification for Nursing Practice (ICNP). The ICNP is a multi-axial classification of nursing phenomena in which an outcome classification is replaced by nursing diagnostic judgments of patient status made at different points in time.[73] The diagnostic judgments include terms such as *altered*; *disturbed*; *enhanced*; and *dysfunctional applied to a focus of nursing practice, for example, body nutrition or sleep.* A range of five measures—extremely, substantially, moderately, mildly, or not—is applied to the diagnostic judgment, for example, "mildly altered" or "extremely disturbed." In the examples provided, degree of patient dependency is the only nursing judgment in which the five terms identified previously are not used; rather, terms similar to those in the NOC dependency scale are used.

Patient outcomes used to evaluate nursing practice are at varied levels of abstraction. A number of broad outcome categories without specific measures have been identified. At the other extreme, a multitude of specific outcome measures are used in clinical practice and clinical studies to evaluate patient outcomes for a particular nursing diagnosis or intervention. There are also increasing numbers of outcomes at a middle level of abstraction in nursing care plans, critical paths, quality assurance programs, and nursing information systems. Unfortunately, many of the specific and intermediate level outcomes used in clinical practice are developed for a particular setting with little or no evaluation or relevancy to other settings. Thus there is a pressing need for nursing to continue to identify and standardize outcomes sensitive to nursing practice.

## A CONCEPTUAL MODEL OF OUTCOMES

Political interest in patient outcomes and health care costs initiated a revolution in health care in the late 1980s, which has been labeled the "era of assessment and accountability."[32,83] This has put pressure on health care providers to justify their practice and its effects on patients and national health and has created a distinct area of study that Wennberg has labeled "clinical evaluation science."[9,15] Basic questions being raised are: Is the care provided by one organization or agency worth the cost relative to the care provided by other organizations or agencies? What are the benefits patients receive from health care? What is the quality, and is it adequate in light of what is being paid?[88] What are the benefits to the health of the general population and individuals?[32] What outcomes can be expected, given various patient characteristics and states of health? If outcomes are not adequate, what changes are needed for improvement? If outcomes are adequate, can improvements still be achieved?[11] A variety of outcome measures, shown in Fig. 1-1, have been developed in the last decade to answer these questions.

Patient, system, and provider factors in Figure 1-1 are the heath care delivery and individual patient factors that influence outcome achievement. Although much has been written about the effect of these factors on outcomes, only recently has the influence of these factors been empirically investigated in a systematic manner. The nursing literature emphasizes the need to consider these factors when evaluating patient outcomes and determining quality.[37,55,67] The core represents the global or end outcomes, such as health status. Global, multidisciplinary outcomes measure general health status and patients' satisfaction with their health and with the health care provided. These measures provide useful information for payers evaluating alternative health plans but are not specific enough to determine accountability for changes to improve outcomes and are not suitable for monitoring the health and treatment status of individual patients, particularly those with chronic diseases.[64]

The outer circle represents intermediate outcome measures currently available: outcomes specific to a particular medical diagnosis, system, or type of provider. The outcomes in each of these areas are often intermediate outcomes that must be realized to achieve the more global long-term outcomes related to health status and satisfaction with care. Intermediate outcomes

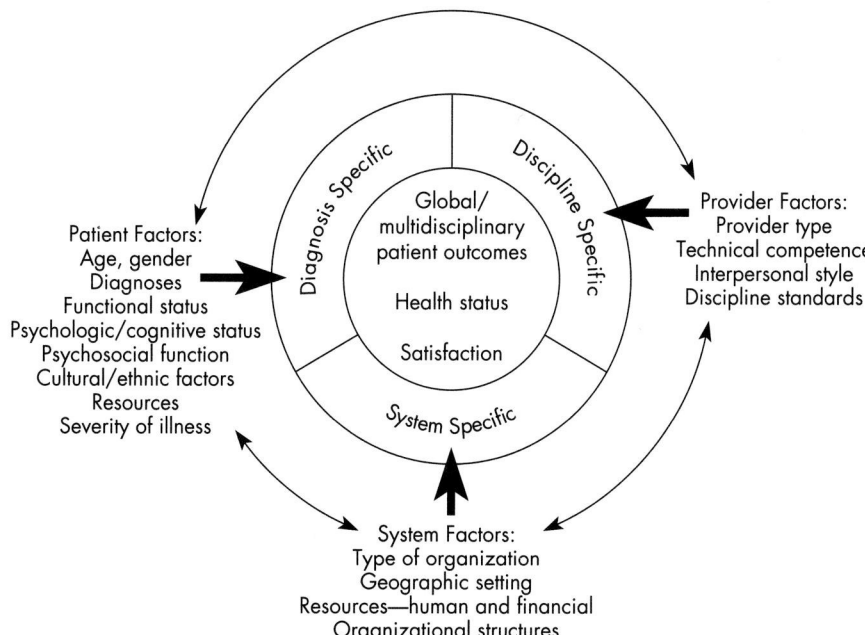

**Fig. 1-1** Conceptual model of outcomes research.

may include measures that evaluate the effect of intervention on client knowledge, attitudes, and behaviors that affect health status and satisfaction.[12]

1. *System-specific outcomes* include adverse factors such as medication errors, infection rates, and patient falls and measures of organizational effectiveness such as cost and productivity. These measures are commonly found in benchmarking or total quality management systems and emphasize multidisciplinary, system-wide outcomes.

2. *Diagnosis-specific outcomes* are used in critical paths and standardized evaluation instruments such as those developed by the Health Outcomes Institute. Outcomes in critical paths are often organization-specific and stated as multidisciplinary patient goals that are met or not met. Standardized instruments have primarily captured indicators of physician practice; some may include multidisciplinary outcomes.

3. *Discipline-specific outcomes* reflect the practice and standards of a health care discipline and are important for evaluating the performance and quality of that practice. To date, the focus of effectiveness research in which discipline-specific outcomes are used has primarily been on physician practices or processes of care.[82] Each health care discipline must identify and measure patient outcomes most influenced by their practice to foster the development of knowledge and ensure that standards of care evolve as knowledge increases. Nursing must have validated outcome measures for use in clinical settings, as well as for research, to ensure that outcome data necessary for the elaboration of nursing knowledge and maintenance of the highest standards are available.

### Reasons for Standardized Outcomes for Nursing

For the nursing profession to become a full participant in clinical evaluation research, policy development, and interdisciplinary work, it is essential that patient outcomes influenced by nursing care be identified and measured.[38,42,50,54] Although it is recognized that the majority of patient outcomes, including those traditionally used to evaluate physician practice, are not influenced by any one discipline alone, it is essential for each discipline to identify the patient outcomes influenced by its practice to ensure that these discipline-specific outcomes are included in the evaluation of health care effectiveness. If nursing relies on physician-centered information only, "the impact of nursing care will remain largely unmeasured and therefore invisible."[53] For nurses to work effectively with managed care organizations to improve quality and reduce costs, nurses must be able to measure and document patient outcomes influenced by nursing care.[80] For example, the costs of decubitus ulcers are well documented, and prevention is largely a function of nursing[63]; however, information about tissue integrity is not readily available in most clinical evaluation systems. The challenge facing the nursing profession is to create a common language that can be used to organize the phenomena of nursing practice without depersonalizing the patient.[45]

## CREATION OF A COMMON NURSING LANGUAGE

Creation of a common language for the nursing profession requires the identification, testing, and application of common terms and measures for nursing diagnoses, nursing interventions, nursing care delivery structures and processes, and patient outcomes. Standardized nursing diagnoses have been under development since 1973, when the first invitational meeting of the National Conference Group for the Classification of Nursing Diagnoses was convened in St. Louis.[96] Development of nursing diagnoses was formalized by the North American Nursing Diagnosis Association (NANDA) in 1982.[16] In addition to the development of new diagnoses, current diagnoses are being revised by a research team at the University of Iowa, the Nursing Diagnosis Extension and Classification research team, in conjunction with NANDA members.[75] A comprehensive classification of nursing interventions, Nursing Interventions Classification (NIC), was developed by a research team at the University of Iowa.[35] This classification is coded for use in nursing information systems and is being included in the reimbursement system by

Alternative Link.[2] This system provides codes for interventions used by multiple health care disciplines as a means for reimbursing complementary and holistic care. Work to standardize administrative data, including information about nursing care delivery systems, has been conducted under the auspices of a research team at the University of Iowa and the American Organization of Nurse Executives.[21] This work provides the information necessary to study the effects of administrative variables on patient outcomes.

The outcomes presented in this text represent the work of a research team at the University of Iowa committed to creating outcomes and related measures at the individual, family, and community levels, which can be used to evaluate nursing care across the patient care continuum. Individual patient outcome data can be aggregated in a number of ways to assess nursing care effectiveness within an organization and across various settings. The Classification is not specific to a patient diagnosis or clinical setting, although some outcomes and related indicators will be used more frequently with a particular patient population or in a particular setting.

Preliminary work to develop and classify nursing interventions laid the foundation for the NOC research, specifically, the conceptualization of outcomes responsive to nursing interventions and the qualitative and quantitative methods used to develop the outcomes and to assess the content validity of the outcomes and indicators. In phase I of the research, conceptual and methodological issues were identified and resolved; and outcome statements used by nurses were gathered, organized in common referent clusters, and given conceptual outcome labels. Phase II included the refinement and content validation of each outcome through concept analysis and surveys of nurse experts. Preliminary field testing of the nursing-sensitive patient outcomes was accomplished; and the outcomes and indicators were organized in a classification structure, supported by hierarchical analysis, with defined rules and principles determining the structure. Phase III focused on testing the psychometric integrity and practicality of measurement scales and procedures with clinical data from 10 field sites representing the continuum of care settings. The validity of the NOC structure was evaluated, and clinical field data were used to describe the use of the outcomes and linkages among nursing diagnoses, interventions, and outcomes in specific populations and health care settings. Four years of funding for this phase of the research was provided by the National Institute of Nursing Research (RO1-NR03437). This edition of the Classification is based on refinements identified through this phase of the research. Detailed descriptions of phases I and II of this research are provided in the previous edition of the NOC.

Professional practice languages and classification systems are the fundamental vocabularies and categories of thought that define the profession and its scope of practice. The nursing profession has made considerable progress in the last decades in labeling and categorizing the phenomena of nursing. The languages and categories discussed previously attest to the efforts expended toward development of a professional practice language that facilitates the efforts of nursing in the areas described in the following paragraphs.

## Computerized Nursing Information Systems

The growth of electronic nursing information systems creates a compelling need for a standardized language for nursing that includes, but is not limited to, patient outcomes influenced by nursing care. Nursing information systems have the potential for improving nursing performance, increasing nursing knowledge, and providing data and information necessary for nursing to participate in the formulation of health care policy.[31] However, realization of the potential of such information systems requires turning currently invisible nursing data into visible, productive data[89] that are standardized and can be aggregated and used to answer the pressing questions faced by the nursing profession. Unfortunately, few attempts have been made to standardize nursing data in clinical information systems, but rather, current setting-specific terminologies and documentation systems have been automated.[34,61] As a consequence, software companies have tended to develop shells that can be individualized for each organization, rather than producing software that creates comparable data across organizations.

To move nursing forward, the ANA has developed a set of standards for nursing data sets in information systems. The Nursing Information and Data Set Evaluation Center (NIDSEC) is charged with reviewing and evaluating information systems that support nursing practice.[4,5] Standards used to review the systems include standards related to the nomenclatures, the clinical content linkages, the clinical data repository, and general system requirements. In relation to the nomenclatures, terms from ANA-recognized languages are to be used as the core nursing vocabulary.[4,5] Through this process, the ANA hopes that NIDSEC approval of information system data sets will provide large, retrievable pools of patient data (uniform nursing data sets) that can be used to determine the nature, costs, and effects of nursing practice.[5]

## Uniform Nursing Data Sets

A uniform data set "defines the central core of data needed on a routine basis by the majority of decision-makers about a given facet or dimension of the health care delivery system, and it establishes standard measurements, definitions, and classifications for this core."[68] Database development requires a common language and a standard way to organize data.[38] The essential first step in organizing and standardizing nursing information is to develop meaningful categories of data and establish uniform terminology. This can be accomplished with the use of one standard terminology, the use of synonyms linked to current terminologies, and the mapping of current terminologies to each other.[23]

A core set of data, referred to as the *Nursing Minimum Data Set (NMDS)*, was identified in the 1980s under the leadership of Harriet Werley.[98] Consensus was reached on 16 core elements, which were grouped under the categories of nursing care, patient demographics, and service characteristics. Patient demographics and service characteristics are not unique to nursing and can be obtained from other health care databases. The four elements in the nursing care category—nursing diagnosis, nursing intervention, nursing outcome, and intensity of nursing care—are not available in a standardized data set because of the lack of agreement on a standardized language for each nursing care element.[16,56]

The National Association for Home Care has developed a uniform data set for home care and hospice. The data set is structured around organizational- and individual-level data items.[79] Items at the organizational level include service type and use and financial and personnel resources. Items at the individual level include patient demographics, medical diagnoses, surgical procedures, and patient use of services. The data set does not contain nursing diagnoses, interventions, or outcomes because these are areas without national consensus[79] and thus represent items that need to be developed.

A number of nursing minimum data sets have been or are being developed in countries other than the United States, including Australia, Canada, and Belgium and other European countries. The European TELENURSE project includes the development of a nursing vocabulary and minimum data set among its objectives.[23] In some instances, nursing data sets are included in multidisciplinary databases and health information systems.

Standardized data sets facilitate the linkage of information in one data set to other data sets. This allows data in clinical information systems to be linked with administrative and other data sets for analysis. The use of logically linked data sets also decreases documentation work by reducing the need for repetitive documentation of information used for multiple purposes in an organization.[99]

## National Data Sets

Physicians, health care organizations, and policy makers are extracting and analyzing data from national data sets to compare effectiveness and costs of care by provider and geographic area. "Results of such analyses increasingly form the basis of institutional, regulatory, and reimbursement policy decisions."[78] However, most of these data sets contain little information that reflects nursing practice, resulting in a lack of data supporting the effectiveness of nursing practice and its contributions to patient outcomes. The absence of nursing data is not the result of discrimination, but rather the result of the profession's failure to agree on and offer a set of clearly defined, valid, reliable, and standardized nursing data elements for inclusion in national data sets.[77] Therefore the establishment of a set of standardized nursing data elements would allow data collected at the individual patient level to be coded and included in national data sets. This requires agreement on the data elements that are important and relevant for nursing; the terms, measures, or indicators to be used; a uniform coding system; and a cost-effective way to gather the data and input it into a computerized system.[74] The ideal solution for data input is the electronic clinical record that allows for data input at the point of service. The outcomes presented in Part Two have been coded for use in the electronic record and clinical information systems.

## Evaluation of Nursing Care Quality

The need for information about patient outcomes influenced by nursing has increased as organizations have restructured to achieve greater efficiency. Without these data, organizations have little information on which to base decisions about adjusting staff mix, determining cost-effectiveness of various structural or process changes in the nursing care delivery system, or providing information about the quality of nursing care available in the organization.

Although quality of care can be examined from the perspectives of structure, process, and outcome, outcomes are essential components of any quality assurance or quality improvement program. "Outcomes are the changes, either favorable or adverse, in the actual or potential health status of persons, groups, or communities that can be attributed to prior or concurrent care."[18] Outcomes are the trigger for quality assurance programs, since they answer the question, "Did the patient benefit or not benefit from the care provided?"[88] Information about patient outcomes should identify not only inadequate outcomes but also those that are marginal, adequate, and superior to facilitate continual quality improvement. Given that nursing care represents a majority of the hours of care provided in most settings,[1,20] it is essential that health care organizations and nursing practice settings be able to evaluate the quality of care provided by nursing staff. For this to be accomplished, the identification and documentation of patient outcomes influenced by nursing practice are necessary, as well as the application of outcomes influenced by multiple health care providers. However, the Institute of Medicine[33] found, in a review of nurse staffing and quality of care, that existing work in outcome measurement typically has not focused on isolating the contribution of nursing to overall hospital quality.

The NOC described in this book is a comprehensive list of standardized outcomes, definitions, and measures to describe patient outcomes influenced by nursing practice. The outcomes are presented as variable concepts that reflect patient states (e.g., mobility, hydration, coping) that can be measured on a continuum rather than as discrete goals that are met or not met. This variablity of concepts will facilitate the identification and analysis of current outcome status for specific patient populations and also facilitate the identification of realistic standards of care for specific populations.[51] For example, patients can be aggregated in a number of ways, such as by nursing or medical diagnosis, by service unit, or by severity of illness; and differences in outcome achievement can be analyzed by patient characteristics such as age, gender, or functional status, as sell as by the interventions used. This type of information will assist nurses in developing realistic standards that reflect currently achieved outcomes if the outcomes are satisfactory or can reflect desired, higher standards of achievement.[51] Such standards reflect variations in outcomes that occur within a patient population because of patient characteristics that cannot be changed. This is quite different from the usual practice of setting one standard or selecting one goal for all patients, regardless of individual patient characteristics, which may constitute considerable risk in relation to outcome achievement. "From a quality improvement perspective, it is important to be able to identify a realistic outcome to be achieved. Unrealistic outcome expectations are inefficient in that resources may be expended to no good effect."[65] For comparison of quality across organizations, it is necessary to ensure that the effects of structure and process on patient outcomes are being measured, and not the effects of patient characteristics that differ among the organizations.[93]

Quality patient care requires the collaboration of all health care providers and is measured at the organizational level by using outcomes that reflect an interdisciplinary approach to patient care. Illness-related measures have been the traditional measures of quality but are now being expanded to include wellness-related measures and patient satisfaction. The addition of nursing-sensitive patient outcomes related to wellness and satisfaction will contribute to organizational data used to evaluate health care quality. In addition, knowledge of intermediate outcomes that may be influenced primarily by one discipline is necessary to identify and change structures and processes that inhibit the achievement of quality patient care. For example, functional status may be hindered by decubitus ulcers or inadequate patient knowledge; these are intermediate outcomes of concern, primarily to nurses, that will not be available for outcome analysis if they are not measured by nurses.

## Evaluation of Nursing Effectiveness

Outcomes management and effectiveness research has become an imperative in nursing practice in this era of managed care and integrated health care systems,[76] but the evaluation of nursing effectiveness is hindered by a number of factors, including the inability to quantify nursing outcomes in most clinical settings. Outcomes used to evaluate nursing care commonly appear as goal statements designed for use with either a particular patient or specific patient population and are frequently developed for use in one organization. Because they serve different purposes, goal statements vary in their degree of specificity. Statements may be quite specific and designed to reflect a discrete patient status or population (e.g., walks 10 feet without assistance, lists three expected effects of digitalis, and systolic blood pressure is between 100 and 150). Goal statements may also be more generic, applicable to a wide range of patients, and require a nursing judgment to determine whether a goal has been met (e.g., anxiety level is decreased, understands activity limitations, and blood pressure in desired range).

One problem created by goal statements is that if the goal is not met, the health care professional has no way of knowing how close or how far the patient was from achieving the goal. Another problem is that information about patient status may be lost, since patients may move from one health care setting to another over time and goal accomplishment is often not transferred. However, the major deficit is that goal statements developed in each organization create nonstandardized data that cannot be easily aggregated with data from other settings and populations. The use of a nationally standardized language and classification system with accepted coding enables the aggregation of data internally for organization reports and externally to add more comprehensive data to community and national databases.[19]

Effectiveness research depends on information obtained from large data sets to evaluate the effects of interventions provided by multiple providers in noncontrolled practice situations in which patients are receiving routine care. Because of the multiple factors that influence patient outcomes, large data sets are needed to identify the nursing contribution and to determine patient outcomes sensitive to nursing interventions.[55] Effectiveness research also requires the ability to quantify data, including patient outcomes. Although nursing effectiveness research is still in its infancy, the extent to which nursing is moving forward in effectiveness research is illustrated by the inclusion of the topic in nursing literature and the initiation of a journal, *Outcomes Management for Nursing Practice*, devoted to outcomes management and effectiveness research for nursing.

Models for the aggregation of data for evaluating effectiveness of nursing interventions have also been developed. One model provides an example of how atomic-level or patient-specific data can be collected once and aggregated to provide agency, community, national, and worldwide data for decision makers from administrators to world health officials.[100] A more recent model illustrates how patient data collected at the individual level can be aggregated and correlated with other data sets to provide information about cost and quality at the unit or organizational level.[36] This model also illustrates aggregation of individual level data for use in networks and regional and national data sets.

In the current health care climate, nurses do not have the luxury of waiting for the future, because it is here. The nursing profession must be able to analyze the effectiveness of its interventions and practice and provide information about its role in patient welfare to ensure its role in health care and to influence health care policy. As the electronic patient care record develops, it is essential that nursing languages be included in the efforts to capture heath care data. If nursing's data needs are not addressed, the efforts of nurses and the outcomes of nursing care for patients will remain invisible.

## Evaluation of Nursing Innovations

Innovations are new ideas or techniques used to solve a problem.[41] They are necessary for the development and refinement of basic and applied knowledge. Nursing innovations may consist of new interventions, revised interventions, or the use of interventions in a new way to solve clinical problems. They may also be strategies, structures, or processes used to solve management problems.[59] In each instance, patient outcomes are desirable criteria for evaluating innovation effectiveness. In the case of clinical innovations, improved patient outcomes may be the only evaluation criterion. In the case of management innovations, patient outcomes need to be evaluated in conjunction with other outcomes, such as cost reduction or staff mix, to ensure that the management innovation did not adversely affect patient outcomes.

Clinical innovations are initially evaluated through controlled clinical studies, with attention given to the measurement of desired or expected outcomes. Many clinical studies in nursing are conducted at one or a few sites and with relatively small samples. Generalizability of such studies can be increased by using meta-analysis if study variables are similar. The use of standardized patient outcomes as one of the study variables would increase the ease with which findings could be compared across settings.

Management innovations may be initiated without an evaluation plan, and when such a plan is used, it may not include patient outcomes. The result is a paucity of empirical data about the relationships between structural measures, such as nurse staffing ratios, and quality of care in terms of patient outcomes[33] and the relationship between processes, such as the type of nursing care delivery system, and quality of care. This is particularly bothersome in an era of restructuring and rapid change in health care organizations. Although managers may be forced to make decisions about structural and process changes without empirical data, potential problems can be alleviated if adequate outcome data, including patient outcome data, are identified and routinely collected. The use of standardized outcomes will allow for the comparison of patient outcomes across sites and increase understanding of the effects of structural and process changes on patient outcomes and quality of care.

## Participation in Interdisciplinary Care

The use of interdisciplinary teams and collaborative strategies is being promoted as a means of maintaining quality and controlling costs in an increasingly complex health care system. Interdisciplinary teams function when the different disciplines pool their knowledge to jointly evaluate or develop a plan of care to accomplish something that is too complex for one discipline.[97,60] For interdisciplinary teams to be effective, each discipline must contribute its unique perspective and knowledge.[52,60] This requires that nurses have information about their interventions and outcomes to share with other disciplines. Professional languages supply the vocabulary for communication and systematic data collection; and analysis, research, and professional literature supply information about the effectiveness of nursing interventions.

Collaboration is the hallmark of interdisciplinary practice and differentiates it from multi-disciplinary practice in which various disciplines contribute to patient care but do not necessarily plan together. Collaboration requires the sharing of each discipline's unique perspective and is characterized by mutual trust and respect for the contribution of each discipline.[97] To be colleagues with members of other disciplines, nurses need a language that allows them to articulate their unique perspective[81] and to continue the advancement of nursing knowledge.[60] Without the continual advancement of professional knowledge, the unique contributions of the nursing discipline to interdisciplinary practice will be minimal and decrease the individual member's ability to function in a collegial capacity.

The NOC provides one professional language that nurses can use to identify and evaluate the effects of nursing interventions. Outcome data will allow nurses to participate in a collegial relationship in an interdisciplinary team, as well as to develop the knowledge base necessary for advancing nursing practice.

## CONTRIBUTION TO KNOWLEDGE DEVELOPMENT

The development of nursing knowledge requires the use of patient outcome measures. The effectiveness of a nursing intervention and the appropriateness of the decision-making process in selecting an intervention for a patient are determined by the resulting patient outcomes. Expanding this knowledge beyond the individual patient to patient populations requires massive amounts of clinical data that describe linkages between and among diagnoses, patient characteristics, interventions, and outcomes.[34] Use of standardized databases with common languages is the most feasible method of obtaining information necessary for analysis of these linkages. Large databases can provide information to a discipline about the effectiveness of current practices and assist in the development of performance goals and practice parameters. Practice parameters, such as the guidelines developed by the AHCPR, provide strategies for patient management and assist clinicians in clinical decision making.[28]

Classifications of nursing diagnoses, nursing interventions, and patient outcomes contain lexical elements for the development of middle-range theories that delineate the substantive structure or the aspects of health care that nurses address,[92] as illustrated in Fig. 1-2. Classifications that define the pattern of nursing diagnoses, interventions, and outcomes provide the vertical shafts for the development of middle-range theories used to create the substantive structure of nursing.[92] Use of these classifications enables middle-range theory development to build on elements unique to nursing, as well as the "borrowed knowledge" and theories from other disciplines.[84,92] The usefulness of each classification depends on research that links the processes of care to outcomes and the development of explanatory theory.[8,43] Lexical and taxonomic development that provides standardized terms in a constructed classification fosters inductive theory formulation and the empirical testing of deductive theories. Although these classifications provide the basic elements that are important for the development of substantive nursing theory, they will be expanded or complemented by other knowledge and theories as nursing knowledge develops.

A classification of nursing-sensitive patient outcomes may be the first, but not the only, step for the use of outcomes in the study of nursing practice. Issues related to outcome measurement have been well documented in the literature,[8,24,27,40,44,49] but some of these issues will be best resolved with the use of standardized languages and clinical databases that can be used to study relationships between outcomes, between outcomes and patient characteristics, and between outcomes and nursing interventions.

For example, attributing a change in health status to nursing practice requires an understanding of factors that influence patient outcomes and the appropriate timing for data collection. The identification of patient characteristics or risk factors that influence outcome achievement has been used in the study of physician outcomes, but its use has been rare in nursing research. Identification of such factors is a prerequisite for the study of nursing care effectiveness when the

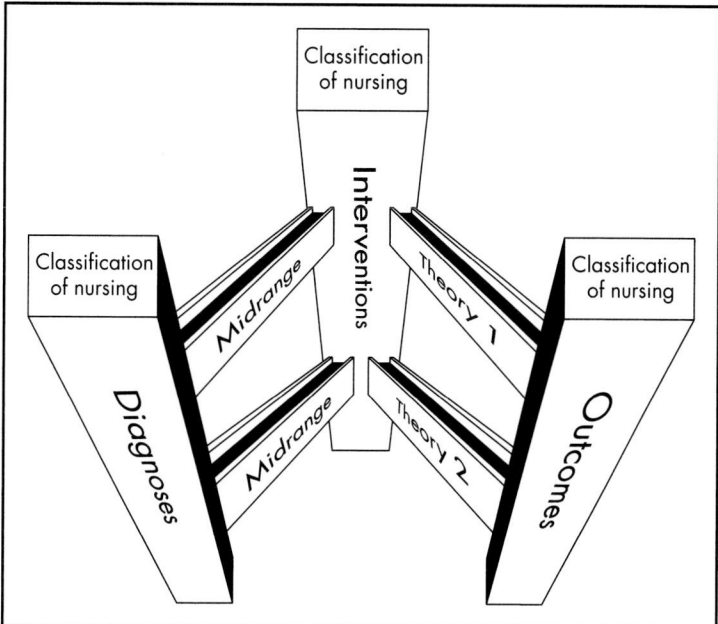

**Fig. 1-2** Relationships of nursing diagnoses, interventions, and outcomes of mid-range theories. *(From Tripp-Reimer, T., Woodworth, G., McCloskey, J., & Bulechek, G. M. (1996). The dimensional structure of nursing interventions.* Nursing Research, 45 [1].)

controls used in efficacy research are not in place. Identification of risk factors is also necessary in comparison of outcomes across settings. While it is recognized that the anticipated change in patient health status may not occur immediately after a nursing intervention, the ideal time for evaluation of clinical outcomes, that is, when treatment outcomes are sufficiently robust to be significant,[34] is often not known. These are only two examples of the questions that must be addressed for nursing to participate fully in outcomes research that focuses on the effectiveness, rather than the efficacy, of health care processes.

## SUMMARY

There is a need for standardized language and database development in nursing if nursing is to become a full participant in health care restructuring and effectiveness research. Policy decision makers will not be responsive to a discipline that cannot provide data supporting its effectiveness. Nursing-sensitive patient outcomes provide one of the data elements for the Nursing Minimum Data Set. Development and use of such a data set will provide nurses with the information needed for the determination of nursing practice effectiveness.

## References

1. Aiken, L. A., Smith, H. L., & Lake, E. T. (1994). Lower Medicare mortality among a set of hospitals known for good nursing care. *Medical Care, 32,* 771-787.
2. Alternative Link ABC codes to include NIC. (1998). *NIC/NOC Newsletter, 6,* 1.
3. American Nurses Association. (1995). *Nursing care report card for acute care.* Washington, D.C.: Author.
4. American Nurses Association. (1997). *Nursing Informatics & Data Set Evaluation Center (NIDSEC) standards and scoring guidelines.* Washington, D.C.: Author.

5. Averill, C. B., Marek, K. D., Zielstorff, R., Kneedler, J., Delaney, C., & Milholland, D. K. (1998). ANA standards for nursing data sets in information systems. *Computers in Nursing, 16,* 157-161.

6. Aydelotte, M. (1962). The use of patient welfare as a criterion measure. *Nursing Research, 11,* 10-14.

7. Badger, K. A. (1998). Patient care report cards: An analysis. *Outcomes Management for Nursing Practice, 2,* 29-36.

8. Bond, S., & Thomas, L. H. (1991). Issues in measuring outcomes of nursing. *Journal of Advanced Nursing, 16,* 1492-1502.

9. Brook, H. L. (1989). Practice guidelines and practicing: Are they compatible? *Journal of the American Medical Association, 262,* 3027-3030.

10. Brown, D. S. (1992). A conceptual framework for the evaluation of service quality. *Journal of Nursing Care Quality, 6,* 66-74.

11. Carey, R. G., & Lloyd, R. C. (1995). *Measuring quality improvement in healthcare: A guide to statistical process control applications.* New York: Quality Resources, a Division of the Kraus Organization Limited.

12. Centers for Disease Control and Prevention. (1992). *The planned approach to community health: A guide for the local PATCH coordinator.* Atlanta, GA: U.S. Department of Health and Human Services, Public Health Service.

13. Clark, L. C. (1998). Incorporating OASIS into the Visiting Nurses Association. *Outcomes Management for Nursing Practice, 2,* 24-28.

14. Daubert, E. A. (1979). Patient classification and outcome criteria. *Nursing Outlook, 27,* 450-454.

15. DeFriese, G. H. (1990). Measuring the effectiveness of medical interventions: New expectations of health services research. *Health Services Research, 25,* 697-708.

16. Delaney, C., Mehmert, P. A., Prophet, C. Bellinger, S. L., Huber, D. H., & Ellerbe, S. (1992). Standardized nursing language for healthcare information systems. *Journal of Medical Systems, 16,* 145-159.

17. Donabedian, A. (1966). Evaluating the quality of medical care. *Milbank Memorial Fund Quarterly, 44,* 166-206.

18. Donabedian, A. (1985). *The methods and findings of quality assessment and monitoring: An illustrated analysis* (Vol. 3). Ann Arbor, MI: Health Administration Press.

19. Donaldson, M. S., & Lohr, K. N. (Eds.). (1994). *Health data in the information age: Use, disclosure, and privacy.* Washington, DC: National Academy Press.

20. Flarey, D. L., & Blancett, S. S. (1995). Management and organizational restructuring: Reforming the corporate system. In S. S. Blancett & D. Flarey (Eds.), *Reengineering nursing and health care.* Gaithersburg, MD: Aspen.

21. Gardner, D. L., Delaney, C., Crossley, J., Mehmert, P., & Ellerbe, S. (1992). A nursing management minimum data set: Significance and development. *Journal of Nursing Administration, 22,* 35-40.

22. Gillette, B., & Jenko, M. (1991). Major clinical functions: A unifying framework for measuring outcomes. *Journal of Nursing Care Quality, 6,* 20-24.

23. Goossen, W., Epping, P., Feuth, T., Dassen, T., Hasman, A., & van den Heuvel, W. (1998). A comparison of nursing minimal data sets. *Journal of the American Medical Informatics Association: JAMIA, 5,* 152-163.

24. Harris, M. R., & Warren, J. J. (1995). Patient outcomes: Assessment issues for the CNS. *Clinical Nurse Specialist, 9,* 82-86.

25. Health Outcomes Institute. (1993). *Condition-specific type specifications.* Bloomington, MN: Author.

26. Heater, B. S., Becker, A. M., & Olson, R. K. (1988). Nursing interventions and patient outcomes: A meta-analysis of studies. *Nursing Research, 37,* 303-307.

27. Hegyvary, S. (1991). Issues in outcomes research. *Journal of Nursing Quality Assurance, 5,* 1-6.

28. Hirshfeld, E. B. (1994). Practice parameters versus outcome measurements: How will prospective and retrospective approaches to quality management fit together? *Nutrition in Clinical Practice, 9,* 207-215.

29. Horn, B. J., & Swain, M. A. (1978). *Criterion measures of nursing care* (DHEW Publication No. PHS 78-3187). Hyattsville, MD: National Center for Health Services Research.

30. Hover, J., & Zimmer, M. (1978). Nursing quality assurance: The Wisconsin system. *Nursing Outlook, 26,* 242-248.

31. Huber, D., Schumacher, L., & Delaney, C. (1997). Nursing management minimum data set (NMMDS). *Journal of Nursing Administration, 27,* 42-48.

32. Iezzoni, L. I. (1994). Risk and outcomes. In L. I. Iezzoni (Ed.), *Risk adjustment for measuring health care outcomes* (pp. 1-28). Ann Arbor, MI: Health Administration Press.

33. Institute of Medicine. Wunderlich, G. S., Sloan, F. A., & Davis, C. K. (Eds.). (1996). *Nursing staff in hospitals and nursing homes: Is it adequate?* Washington, DC: National Academy Press.

34. Iowa Intervention Project. (1992). *Nursing Interventions Classification (NIC).* St. Louis, MO: Mosby.

35. Iowa Intervention Project. (1996). *Nursing Interventions Classification (NIC)* (2nd ed.). St. Louis, MO: Mosby.

36. Iowa Intervention Project. (1997). Proposal to bring nursing into the information age. *Image, 29,* 275-281.

37. Irvine, D., Sidani, S., & Hall, L. M. (1998). Linking outcomes to nurses' roles in health care. *Nursing Economics, 16,* 58-64.
38. Jennings, B. M. (1991). Patient outcomes research: Seizing the opportunity. *Advances in Nursing Science, 14,* 59-72.
39. Johnson, M., & Maas, M. (1994). Nursing-focused patient outcomes: Challenge for the nineties. In J. McCloskey & H. Grace (Eds.), *Current issues in nursing* (4th ed., pp. 643-649). St. Louis, MO: Mosby.
40. Jones, K. R. (1993). Outcomes analysis: Methods and issues. *Nursing Economics, 11,* 145-152.
41. Kanter, R. M. (1983). *The change masters: Innovation for productivity in the American corporation.* New York: Simon & Schuster.
42. Keenan, G., & Aquilino, M. L. ((1998). Standardized nomenclatures: Keys to continuity of care, nursing accountability and nursing effectiveness. *Outcomes Management for Nursing Practice, 2,* 81-85.
43. Keith, R. A. (1995). Conceptual basis of outcome measures. *American Journal of Physical Medicine & Rehabilitation, 74,* 73-80.
44. Kelsey, A. (1995). Outcome measures: Problems and opportunities for public health nursing. *Journal of Nursing Management, 3,* 183-187.
45. Kritek, P. V. (1989). An introduction to the science and art of taxonomy. In American Nurses Association (Ed.), *Classification systems for describing nursing practice: Working papers* (pp. 6-12). Kansas City, KS: American Nurses Association.
46. Lalonde, B. (1988). Assuring the quality of home care via the assessment of client outcomes. *Caring, 12,* 20-24.
47. Lang, N. M., & Clinton, J. F. (1984). Assessment of quality of nursing care. *Annual Review of Nursing Research, 2,* 135-163.
48. Lang, N. M., & Marek, K. D. (1990). The classification of patient outcomes. *Journal of Professional Nursing, 6,* 153-163.
49. Lohr, K. N. (1988). Outcome measurement: Concepts and questions. *Inquiry, 25,* 37-50.
50. Lower, M. S., & Burton, S. (1989). Measuring the impact of nursing interventions on patient outcomes: The challenge of the 1990s. *Journal of Nursing Quality Assurance, 4,* 27-34.
51. Maas, M. L., Johnson, M. R., & Kraus, V. L. (1996). In K. Kelly (Ed.), *Outcomes of effective management practice, SONA 8* (pp. 20-35). Thousand Oaks, CA: Sage.
52. Maas, M. (1998). Nursing's role in interdisciplinary accountability for patient outcomes. *Outcomes Management for Nursing Practice, 2,* 92-94.
53. Mallison, M. B. (1990). Access to invisible expressways [Editorial]. *American Journal of Nursing, 90,* 7.
54. Marek, K. D. (1989). Outcomes measurement in nursing. *Journal of Nursing Quality Assurance, 4,* 1-9.
55. Marek, K. D. (1997). Measuring the effectiveness of nursing care. *Outcomes Management for Nursing Practice, 1,* 8-12.
56. Mark, B. A., & Burleson, D. L. (1995). Measurement of patient outcomes: Data availability and consistency across hospitals. *Journal of Nursing Administration, 25,* 52-59.
57. Martin, K. S., Norris, J., & Leak, G. K. (1999). Psychometric analysis of the problem rating scale for outcomes. *Outcomes Management for Nursing Practice, 3,* 20-25.
58. Martin, K. S., & Scheet, N. J. (1992). *The Omaha System: Applications for community health nursing.* Philadelphia: W. B. Saunders.
59. McCloskey, J. C., Maas, M. L., Huber, D. G., Kasparek, A., Specht, J. P., Ramler, C. L., et al. (1996). Nursing management innovations: A need for systematic evaluation. In K. Kelly (Ed.), *Outcomes of effective management practice, SONA 8,* (pp. 3-19). Thousand Oaks, CA: Sage.
60. McCloskey, J. C., & Maas, M. (1998). Interdisciplinary team: The nursing perspective is essential. *Nursing Outlook, 46,* 157-163.
61. McCormick, K. (1991). Future data needs for quality care monitoring, DRG considerations, reimbursement and outcome measurement. *Image, 23,* 29-32.
62. McCormick, K. A., Cummings, M. A., & Kovner, C. (1997). The role of the Agency for Health Care Policy and Research (AHCPR) in improving outcomes of care. *The Nursing Clinics of North America, 32,* 521-542.
63. McFarland, G. K., & McFarlane, E. A. (1993). *Nursing diagnosis and intervention: A model for clinical practice.* St. Louis, MO: Mosby.
64. McHorney, C. A., & Tarlov, A. R. (1995). Individual-patient monitoring in clinical practice: Are available health status surveys adequate? *Quality of Life Research, 4,* 293-307.
65. Mills, W. C. (1994). Tacking through troubled waters: Toward desired outcomes. In R. M. Carroll-Johnson & M. Paquette (Eds.), *Classification of nursing diagnosis: Proceedings of the tenth conference* (pp. 126-130). Philadelphia: J. B. Lippincott.
66. Mitchell, P. H., Ferketich, S., & Jennings, B. M. (1998). Quality health outcomes model. *Image, 30,* 43-46.
67. Mitchell, P. H., Heinrich, J., Moritz, P., & Hinshaw, A. S. (Eds.). (1997). Outcome measures and care delivery systems conference. *Medical Care, 35*(11, Suppl.), NS1-5.
68. Murnaghan, H. (1978). Uniform basic data sets for health statistical systems. *International Journal of Epidemiology, 7,* 263-269.

69. Nadzam, D. M., & Nelson, M. (1997). The benefits of continuous performance measurement. *The Nursing Clinics of North America, 32,* 543-559
70. National Committee for Quality Assurance. (1993). *Health Plan Employer Data and Information Set 2.0 (HEDIS 2.0).* Washington, DC: Author.
71. National Committee for Quality Assurance. (1995). *Health Plan Employer Data and Information Set 2.1 (HEDIS 2.1).* Washington, DC: Author.
72. Naylor, M. D., Munro, B. H., & Brooten, D. A. (1991). Measuring the effectiveness of nursing practice. *Clinical Nurse Specialist, 5,* 210-215.
73. Nielsen, G. H., & Mortensen, R. A. (1998). The architecture of ICNP: Time for outcomes—part II. *International Nursing Review, 45,* 27-31.
74. Niemeyer, L. O., & Foto, M. (1995, April/May). Using outcomes data. *REHAB Management,* 105-106.
75. NANDA International. (2003). *Nursing diagnoses: Definitions and classification 2003-2004.* Philadelphia: Author.
76. Oermann, M., & Huber, D. (1997). New horizons. *Outcomes Management for Nursing Practice, 1,* 1-2.
77. Ozbolt, J. (1991, September 11-13). *Strategies for building nursing databases for effectiveness research.* Invited paper presented to National Center for Nursing Research, Rockville, MD.
78. Ozbolt, J. G., Fruchtnight, J. N., & Hayden, J. R. (1994). Toward data standards for clinical nursing information. *Journal of the American Medical Informatics Association: JAMIA, 1,* 175-185.
79. Pace, K. B. (1995). Data sets for home care organizations. *Caring, 14,* 38-42.
80. Phoon, J., Corder, K., & Barter, M. (1996). Managed care and total quality management: A necessary integration. *Journal of Nursing Care Quality, 10,* 25-32.
81. Pike, A. W. (1994). Entering collegial relationships: The demise of nurse as victim. In J. C. McCloskey & H. K. Grace (Eds.), *Current issues in nursing* (4th ed., pp. 643-649). St. Louis, MO: Mosby.
82. Prescott, P. A. (1993). Nursing: An important component of hospital survival under a reformed health care system. *Nursing Economics, 11,* 192-199.
83. Relman, A. S. (1988). Assessment and accountability: The third revolution in medical care. *New England Journal of Medicine, 319,* 1220-1222.
84. Retsas, A. (1995). Knowledge and practice development: Toward an ontology of nursing. *The Australian Journal of Advanced Nursing, 12,* 20-25.
85. Reverby, S. (1981). Stealing the golden eggs: Ernest Amory Codman and the science and management of medicine. *Bulletin of the History of Medicine, 55,* 156-171.
86. Saba, V. (1992). The classification of home health care nursing: Diagnoses and interventions. *Caring, 11,* 50-57.
87. Salive, M. E., Mayfield, J. A., & Weissman, N. W. (1990). Patient outcomes research teams and the Agency for Health Care Policy and Research. *Health Services Research, 25,* 697-708.
88. Shaughnessy, P.,W. & Crisler, K. S. (1995). *Outcome-based quality improvement: A manual for home care agencies on how to use outcomes.* Washington, DC: National Association for Home Care.
89. Simpson, R. (1991). Adopting a nursing minimum data set. *Nursing Management, 22,* 20-21.
90. Sovie, M. D. (1989). Clinical nursing practices and patient outcomes: Evaluation, evolution, and revolution. *Nursing Economics, 7,* 79-85.
91. Tarlov, A. R., Ware, J. E., Greenfield, S., Nelson, E. C., Perrin, E., & Zubkoff, M. (1989). The Medical Outcomes Study: An application of methods for monitoring the results of medical care. *Journal of the American Medical Association, 262,* 925-930.
92. Tripp-Reimer, T., Woodworth, G., McCloskey, J. C., & Bulechek, G. M. (1996). The dimensional structure of nursing interventions. *Nursing Research, 45,* 10-17.
93. United States General Accounting Office. (1994). *Health care reform "report cards" are useful but significant issues need to be addressed* (Publication No. GAO/HEHS 94-219). Gaithersburg, MD: Author.
94. Ware, J. E. & Sherbourne, C. D. (1992). The MOS 36-item short-form health survey (SF-36). I. Conceptual framework and item selection. *Medical Care, 30,* 473-481.
95. Warren, A. (1997). JCAHO's measurement mandate. *The IHS Primary Care Provider, 22,* 1-3.
96. Warren, J. J. & Hoskins, L. M. (1991). The development of NANDA's nursing diagnosis taxonomy. *Nursing Diagnosis, 1,* 162-168.
97. Warren, M. L., Houston, S., & Luquire, R. (1998). Collaborative practice teams: From multidisciplinary to interdisciplinary. *Outcomes Management for Nursing Practice, 2,* 95-98.
98. Werley, H., & Lang, N. (1988). *Identification of the Nursing Minimum Data Set.* New York: Springer.
99. Westra, B., & Raup, G. (1995). Computerized charting: An essential tool for survival. *Caring, 14,* 57-61.
100. Zielstorff, R., Hudgings, C., & Grobe, S. (1993). *Next-generation nursing information systems: Essential characteristics for professional practice.* Washington, DC: American Nurses Association.

# CHAPTER TWO

# The Current Classification

Identifying outcomes responsive to nursing care is important work for nursing with today's emphasis on cost and effectiveness in the health care system. Efforts to measure outcomes and capture changes in the status of patients over time allow nurses to improve the quality of patient care and add to the knowledge base of nursing. In the past, we have been dependent on the use of interdisciplinary outcomes developed mostly for physician practice. Consensus among nurses on standardized nursing-sensitive patient outcomes allows nurses to study the effects of nursing interventions over time and across care settings. Measurement of outcomes validates whether the patient is responding to the nursing interventions provided and helps determine whether changes in care need to be made. The use of standardized outcomes provides the data needed to (1) elucidate nursing knowledge, (2) advance theory development, and (3) determine the effectiveness of nursing care for health care policy formulation. Nurses have been documenting the outcomes of their interventions for decades, but the lack of a common language and associated measures for outcomes has impeded data aggregation, analysis, and synthesis of information about the effects of nursing interventions and practice.

Outcome evaluation in health care has expanded to include not only the efficacy of health care interventions but also the effectiveness of interventions. In efficacy research, the outcomes of interventions are studied under controlled conditions,[9] whereas in effectiveness research, outcomes are studied in an uncontrolled practice situation. In a sense, efficacy research illustrates what outcomes are possible, given ideal conditions and without consideration of cost; and effectiveness research demonstrates what outcomes are achieved in practice and at what cost. An important result of the emphasis put on the evaluation of health care effectiveness has been the recognition that all initiatives to evaluate effectiveness require the identification, standardization, and use of valid measurement tools for patient outcomes.[12]

The Nursing Outcomes Classification (NOC) is complementary to taxonomies of the North American Nursing Diagnosis Association (NANDA)[14,15] (recently renamed NANDA International) and the Nursing Interventions Classification (NIC).[6] The NOC provides the language for the evaluation step of the nursing process and the content for the outcomes element of the Nursing Minimum Data Set (NMDS). The documentation of the outcomes has been encouraged by the work of NANDA International,[14] the advancement of the NMDS,[19,20] the NIC work,[4,6,16] the development of computerized information systems in health care and the associated large uniform databases, and the emphasis on demonstrating health care effectiveness. However, the definition and classification of clinically useful nursing-sensitive patient outcomes was not accomplished before the NOC. Further, there are few conceptual frameworks of nursing-sensitive patient outcomes, and existing ones tend to describe broad categories of outcomes that are not validated. The NOC is especially significant because standardized languages for computerized nursing diagnoses, interventions, and outcomes are needed for the study of linkages among these patient phenomena with actual patient data. Further, the standardized languages represent concepts that describe the basic phenomena for which the nursing discipline is accountable, and together with the linkages among the concepts, represent an important stage of nursing theory development.

## THE CLASSIFICATION

This book presents one way to standardize terminology for nursing-sensitive outcomes. Each outcome presented in Part Three represents a concept that can be used to assess the state of a patient, family caregiver, family, or community/population to evaluate the effects of nursing interventions. Each outcome has a definition, a measurement scale, and associated indicators and measures. The NOC taxonomy, described and presented in Part Two, facilitates the identification of outcomes in the classification for use in practice. An alphabetical listing of the outcomes and the page numbers of their locations are provided in the table of contents in the beginning of the text.

## The Classification—What It Is

The current classification is a list of 330 outcomes with definitions, indicators, and measurement scales. Outcomes in the classification are for use at individual, family, and community levels. The term *patient* is used in the classification to denote an individual who is the recipient of nursing care. It is recognized that the term *client* is used in many community and health maintenance settings and that *resident* is used in many long-term care settings. For purposes of brevity, the terms *patient* and *client* are used, since they are commonly used in nursing and health care literature. Likewise, the term *family caregiver* is used to denote a family member, a significant other, a friend, or another person who cares for or acts on behalf of the patient.

A family is two or more people who are related biologically, legally, or by choice that has a societal expectation to socialize, enculturate, and care for its members. A population is generally understood as a collection of individuals who have one or more personal (e.g., gender, age, illness) or environmental (e.g., country, worksite) characteristics in common.[17] A community is an interactive population with relationships that emerge as members develop and use, in common, some agencies and institutions. The American Nurses Association Division on Community Health Nursing[1] defines community health nursing as a synthesis of nursing practice and public health practice applied to promoting and preserving the health of populations, with the dominant responsibility to the population as a whole.

However, *community* and *population* are terms that suffer from lack of conceptual clarity. When individuals speak of communities, they are ordinarily referring to the social context within which persons reside. Interaction among members is inherent in the notion of community but is not so for a population.[7] Sociologists refer to a community as the immediate social context of an individual's life, the natural area or human landscape that is personally experienced or encountered by an individual in everyday life. Thus the community is the natural area into which a child moves as he or she leaves the immediate circle of the family. In the more common vernacular, *community* may refer to a neighborhood; a town, small to very large, rural or urban; a country; or any interacting population and the relationships that emerge as members develop and use, in common, some agencies and institutions. Thus one may speak of the "international community" or the "community of nurses." For NOC, a community level outcome characterizes the immediate social context of persons and the relationships that emerge as members (individuals, families, groups) interact, develop, and use, in common, agencies and institutions. Community level NOC outcomes also characterize populations of individuals who share an attribute or belong to particular groups, families, neighborhoods, or communities but do not necessarily interact with one another.

We have modified our definition of an outcome for this edition. A nursing-sensitive outcome is an individual, family, or community state, behavior, or perception that is measured along a continuum in response to nursing intervention(s). The outcomes are variable concepts that can be measured along a continuum, which means the outcomes are stated as concepts that reflect a patient, family caregiver, family, or community actual state rather than expected goals. It also means that the outcomes are neutral; that is, they don't specify the desired state, although they can be used to set goals. This retains the variability of the outcome and allows measurement of the patient condition at any point in time. For example, the outcome Cognition is measured on a five-point scale from "Severely compromised" to "Not compromised," and Caregiver Performance: Direct Care is measured on a five-point scale from "Not adequate" to "Totally adequate." This allows nurses to follow changes in or maintenance of outcome states over time and across settings. The true outcome is the change seen in the outcome rating after nursing interventions.

Outcomes in the classification are at a higher level of abstraction than goal statements typically are. In other instances, the indicators used to determine patient condition in relation to an outcome represent the more specific outcomes often reflected in goal statements. For example, a few of the indicators used to determine the outcome Cognition are "demonstrates immediate memory," "demonstrates remote memory," "communicates clearly and appropriately for age and ability," and "processes information." Although these may serve as intermediate outcomes or indicators of cognition, when used alone, they do not measure the multidimensional aspects of the concept Cognition. The use of midlevel concepts facilitates the use of outcomes in computerized systems and the aggregation of data for effectiveness research and policy formulation, which for individuals tend to focus on patient conditions that influence functional and health status. The midlevel concept may also be useful in efficacy research. For example, a researcher evaluating an intervention to improve memory can use outcome indicators to determine the effects of the intervention not only on memory but also on other factors that determine cognition. Although the outcomes currently do not provide tested measures for assessing the effects of an intervention on memory, they do suggest other factors to consider and can be used in conjunction with tested measures to arrive at a determination of how improvement of memory influences cognition. Further, if outcomes are found to be psychometrically sound, there is potential for the use of outcomes to measure impact variables in efficacy research. Development and testing of outcome measures that have practical use in clinical settings and are valid for use in research have important implications for documenting the nursing profession's contributions to health care and providing data to influence health care policy. These advantages also apply to family and community level outcomes.

Although the outcomes are representative of broad, midlevel concepts, they are at varied levels of specificity. For example, Risk Control is a broad outcome defined as "personal actions to prevent, eliminate, or reduce modifiable health threats," which can be used with any nursing intervention directed toward assisting patients to identify and control risks. However, more specific outcomes for risks of common concern to nurses (e.g., Risk Control: Alcohol Use and Risk Control: Drug Use) are also in the Classification. Community Health Status versus Community Health Status: Immunity is another example of the variability in level of abstraction among the outcomes in the current Classification and taxonomy. As additional outcomes are developed and refined, we expect that greater homogeneity of level of abstraction among outcomes will evolve. Decisions regarding the inclusion of outcomes that are relatively broad versus those that are more specific, however, will depend on what is shown to be useful to nurses. In the taxonomic structure, level of abstraction is also reflected in domain, class, and outcome categories, which facilitate the ease with which the Classification is used.

The language used in the outcomes reflects the language used by nurses in nursing literature. Language used most consistently by nurses, rather than by those in other disciplines, was selected for the outcomes whenever possible. However, there are exceptions when terminology most familiar to nurses is too specific to reflect a broad patient state or is stated as a negative outcome. For example, *decubitus ulcer*, or skin breakdown, is a common term used by nurses, but the term used in the Classification to describe the condition of the skin is Tissue Integrity: Skin & Mucous Membranes. The wording allows the outcome to be stated as a neutral term and as a midlevel concept that is addressed by nursing interventions. In some instances, undesirable or negative patient conditions are used as the outcome when the concept cannot be captured adequately with a neutral term. For example, the classification contains the outcomes Pain Level and Infection Severity, both undesirable patient states that represent important outcomes that need to be monitored but cannot be adequately described by terms such as *comfort level* or *immune status*. Undesirable patient conditions are also used as outcomes when the language is commonly accepted and used by both health care providers and policy makers. For example, the Agency for Health Care Policy and Research uses Pain Level in published guidelines, as do researchers and practitioners when they are evaluating the effects of interventions on pain.

The classification structure uses colons to separate broad outcome terms from terms that make the outcomes more specific. As much as possible, the first term in the outcome reflects the term that the practitioner might select when looking for the outcome. For example, recovery from abuse is found under the broad category Abuse Recovery but is further specified by Abuse Recovery: Emotional, Abuse Recovery: Financial, Abuse Recovery: Physical, and Abuse Recovery: Sexual. For the current edition of the Classification, a more global outcome called *Abuse Recovery Status* was added.

Each concept represents a patient, family caregiver, family, or community/population state, sensitive in varying degrees to nursing interventions. Although the research team assessed sensitivity to nursing interventions by (1) selecting the concepts from outcomes in nursing literature and clinical information systems, (2) determining that the outcomes have been used to measure the effects of nursing interventions, and (3) surveying expert nurses about the importance of the outcomes as measures of the effects of nursing interventions, it is recognized that the ultimate test of sensitivity will be the widespread selection and use of outcomes in practice and research with analyses that isolate the effects of the interventions on the outcomes. Because the outcomes have been developed for use in all settings where nurses provide care, some of the outcome indicators may be more applicable in one setting than another. For example, blood values and other diagnostic results used as indicators may be pertinent in an intensive care or acute care setting but may be less useful in a home or nursing home care setting. More obviously, community level outcomes are most likely useful in community health settings.

Many of the nursing-sensitive outcomes are not specific for nursing interventions only and thus could be used to evaluate the care provided by other health care disciplines. For example, physical therapists may greatly influence a patient's overall outcome rating for Mobility. In this case this outcome measures the collaborative results of nursing care and physical therapy. While the outcomes may be used in other disciplines, the indicators used to assess patient condition in relation to the outcome may vary from discipline to discipline. For example, physical therapists may use indicators that measure progress with the use of equipment not routinely used by nurses. The Classification also contains outcomes most often associated with nursing interventions such as Breastfeeding Establishment: Infant, Bowel Elimination, Health Promoting Behavior, and Knowledge: Treatment Procedure(s).

As standardized NOC outcomes are selected and used in practice, more information will be available to determine their frequency of use and the conditions under which they are selected. Because most NOC outcomes are shared by several disciplines, large clinical databases will be needed to assess the effectiveness of nursing interventions. Variables indicating the contributions of other disciplines; attributes of the individual, family, or community; and variables describing the environmental context of care can be controlled to reveal the effects of nursing. For efficacy research, randomized clinical trials (RCTs) are the gold standard. Randomization helps control for factors other than nursing interventions that are competing explanations for outcome effects. This type of research, however, is often very difficult to implement and maintain in nursing clinical practice, underscoring the need to build large nursing databases to enable nursing effectiveness research.

## The Classification—What It Is Not

Although the classification of outcomes presented in this text contains outcomes frequently used by nurses, at this stage of development, the text does not include all outcomes that might be important for nursing. As nurses review the outcomes and use them in practice and research, other outcomes will be identified and current outcomes may require modification. The project investigators anticipate that any classification of outcomes will undergo modification to reflect changes in nursing practice and health care delivery, and therefore, the classification will be continually evolving. The testing of the outcomes in clinical sites resulted in many revisions to the current edition based on feedback from nurses in practice. Efforts of this type enhance the Classification, build nursing knowledge, and improve the care nurses provide to patients, families, and communities.

The outcomes published in this volume do not include all outcomes for individuals, groups, families, and communities for which nurses provide interventions. Family and community level outcomes are included in this edition, building on our previous work, but more outcomes are needed in this area. However, many individual level outcomes can be aggregated to characterize families, communities, and populations (e.g., by a nursing or medical diagnosis, by a diagnosis-related group [DRG], by the unit or geographical location in which care is provided, or by the nurse providing the care). Additional family and community outcomes will be developed to assess the effectiveness of nursing interventions aimed at these units. It is possible that some of the individual level outcomes can be modified for use with aggregates, and feedback about such modifications from users will be extremely helpful to the investigators. The outcome classification also does not contain outcomes of organizational performance or the cost of health care. These outcomes are important in effectiveness research but do not reflect the effects of interventions on a patient. Rather, organizational and cost outcomes are more often useful for evaluating the effectiveness of nursing management or health services delivery interventions.

The outcomes are not prescriptive. They are not goals for individual patients or patient populations, although they can be translated into goals by identifying the desired state on the measurement scale. Individual level outcomes are not prescribed for a particular nursing diagnosis or nursing intervention. They can be selected for a diagnosis or intervention based on the judgment of the nurse responsible for the care of an individual patient or based on the collective judgment of the health care providers responsible for developing a critical path for a patient population. Possible linkages to NANDA nursing diagnoses are suggested and can be found in Part Four. These linkages are presented in this text to assist the user in the selection of outcomes and to stimulate study of the suggested linkages.

The outcomes are not nursing diagnoses, although many of them assess the same states addressed by nursing diagnoses. A diagnosis identifies a state that is altered, has the potential to be altered, or has the potential to be improved; whereas an outcome assesses the actual state at a given point in time by means of a five-point measurement scale. Table 2-1 illustrates some of the differences in diagnostic and outcome language by using NANDA diagnoses and NOC outcomes.

The comparisons in Table 2-1 illustrate the difference between the language used to identify a state for which a diagnosis is made and the state that is measured as an outcome. They also illustrate that some outcomes are more specific than a related diagnosis (e.g., Knowledge Outcomes), while some diagnoses are more specific than the related outcome (e.g., Diagnoses of Bowel Function). There are also some global outcomes for which similar language is not used in the NANDA diagnoses; however, these outcomes might be selected for a number of the diagnoses.

Outcomes are not assessments, although indicators may represent patient states, behaviors, or perceptions evaluated during a patient assessment. No outcome represents the total range of individual, family, or community states that comprise a comprehensive assessment. An assessment provides the database for clinical reasoning and decisions, including the selection of nursing diagnoses, outcomes, and interventions. Although the defining assessment data for a diagnosis should correspond with outcome indicators that refer to the same patient state, the validation of nursing diagnoses and nursing-sensitive patient outcomes needed to achieve complete correspondence has not yet been done. When an outcome is selected, the individual, family, or community state, behavior, or perception needs to be evaluated and rated on the measurement scale to provide a baseline measure for comparison with postintervention measures. The baseline measure of a variable outcome state should correspond to the diagnosis.

| Table 2-1 | COMPARISONS OF NANDA DIAGNOSES AND NOC OUTCOMES |
|---|---|
| **NANDA Diagnosis** | **NOC Outcome** |
| Impaired Physical Mobility | Mobility |
| Hopelessness | Hope |
| Deficient Knowledge | Knowledge: Disease Process |
| | Knowledge: Medication |
| | Knowledge: Health Behavior |
| | Knowledge: Treatment Regimen |
| Constipation | Bowel Continence |
| Diarrhea | Bowel Elimination |
| Stress Urinary Incontinence | Urinary Elimination |
| Reflex Urinary Incontinence | Urinary Continence |
| | Tissue Integrity: Skin & Mucous Membranes |
| | Personal Well-Being |
| Interrupted Family Processes | Family Functioning |
| | Family Coping |
| | Family Social Climate |

## Commonly Asked Questions

Initial work on the NOC identified conceptual questions that have formed the foundation on which this work is built. The research team reviewed the literature on patient outcomes, information systems, taxonomic classification science, effectiveness research, and relevant qualitative and quantitative methods to address these issues. Team members reviewed multiple sources of patient outcomes used by nurses (textbooks, nursing information systems, critical pathways and care plans, outcome studies, standards of practice, conceptual frameworks, and outcome classifications). As nurses begin to use standardized outcomes rather than goals in their practice, many of these initial issues and other questions arise about the NOC. We have included the most commonly asked questions about the Classification here and briefly address each question.

### Who Is the Patient?

Patient outcomes focus on the recipient of care; however, the traditional use of the term *patient* is too limiting for evaluation of all nursing practice purposes. *Patient* is traditionally defined as an individual recipient of care; however, because family caregivers and significant others are often integrally involved with patients and their care, they are also recipients of nursing care. The term *patient* is used in many of the outcomes, even though the team recognizes that the care recipient may be called *client* or *resident* in some settings. In the previous editions, we have used the term *patient* consistently. When the satisfaction outcomes were added to this edition, the term *patient satisfaction* as the label name was considered by the research team to be too limiting so the term *client satisfaction* was used to describe these outcomes. This issue has continued in nursing, with some health care organizations wanting to use the term *consumers* for their patients. Regardless of what they are called, individuals are the focus of most of the outcomes in this classification.

Data are ordinarily collected on individuals and aggregated to characterize other units of analysis (e.g., patient groups, organizations, communities), but some outcomes require data to be collected at a group level.[5] The research team decided to use individuals as the focal unit for the initial development of the NOC, with family caregivers included to assess the impact of nursing on the family members as individuals. The development and testing of outcomes for other units, such as family, community, and organization, are included in the current and previous editions.

This work focuses on developing outcomes that characterize family and community units as a whole.

## What Do Patient Outcomes Describe?

Like nursing diagnoses, the phenomena of concern with nursing-sensitive patient outcomes are individual patient or family caregiver states or behaviors, including perceptions or subjective states.[3,6] These phenomena are in contrast to nursing interventions that describe nurse behaviors.[6] The phenomena of concern for nursing-sensitive patient outcomes are also in contrast to nursing diagnoses where the phenomena of concern are patient states identified because an improvement is desired. Outcomes, on the other hand, define a patient status at a particular point in time and may indicate improvement or deterioration of the state compared with a previous assessment. The defining data for a diagnosis typically correspond to outcomes and indicators at an undesirable point on the status continuum. Patient states that are assessed but do not follow an intervention are not outcomes. Outcomes describe patient states that follow and are expected to be influenced by an intervention. For the team's research, a *nursing-sensitive patient outcome* is defined as an individual, family, or community state, behavior, or perception that is measured along a continuum in response to nursing intervention(s). Each outcome has an associated group of indicators that are used to determine patient status in relation to the outcome. A *nursing-sensitive patient outcome indicator* is defined as a more concrete individual, family, or community state, behavior, or perception that serves as a cue for measuring an outcome. The definitions and indicators acknowledge that nurses, family caregivers, and patients supply outcome data and that both the patient and the family caregiver are the focus of outcomes. Definitions of terms used in the research are listed in Box 2-1.

In contrast to the Joint Commission on Accreditation of Healthcare Organizations' use of the term *indicator* as a quantitative measure,[13] the team uses the term *nursing-sensitive outcome indicator* to describe a specific patient state that is most sensitive to nursing interventions and for which measurement procedures can be defined. For the purpose of facilitating measurement of change, outcomes are conceptualized as nonevaluative, variable patient states influenced by nursing intervention. Thus patient outcomes represent patient states that vary and can be measured and compared with a baseline over time. As Bond and Thomas[2] note, the requirement of predetermined outcomes that call for a specific change is unnecessary. Unintended consequences of nursing interventions and maintenance of steady states are also valid and may be desirable outcomes. Therefore nursing-sensitive patient outcomes are not viewed as goals, although the outcomes and indicators can be used to set goals for specific patients, with baseline status and change in status being assessed over time.

The testing of the NOC in clinical practice indicated that the change in rating after intervention is important information for nursing to collect. This creates a *change in rating score* when the baseline measurement score before intervention is compared with the measurement after intervention. This *difference in scores* captures the effects of the intervention on the outcome and is one of the main benefits of using variable outcomes rather than goals. The change score can be positive when the second outcome score increases and negative when the outcome score decreases, or the score can be zero if no change occurs.

## At What Levels of Abstraction Should Outcomes Be Developed?

The nursing-sensitive patient outcomes classification contains patient outcomes and indicators at four general levels of abstraction with measurement procedures at the empirical level (Table 2-2). At the highest levels, outcome categories and classes were derived from the results of hierarchical clustering and qualitative strategies used in the research. These were compared with the outcome categories promulgated by the Medical Outcomes Study[18] and with current nursing outcome categories.[8,11] The least abstract level contains indicator statements for each outcome label. Outcomes are at middle levels of abstraction, and in some instances, indicators for more

## Terms and Definitions

**Nursing-Sensitive Patient Outcome**

An individual, family, or community state, behavior, or perception that is measured along a continuum in response to a nursing intervention(s). Each outcome has an associated group of indicators that are used to determine patient status in relation to the outcome.

**Patient Outcome Indicator**

A more concrete individual, family, or community state, behavior, or perception that serves as a cue for measuring an outcome.

**Measure**

A five-point Likert-type scale that quantifies a patient outcome or indicator status on a continuum from least to most desirable and provides a rating at a point in time.

**Change in Rating Score**

The difference between a baseline rating of the outcome and the postintervention rating(s) of the outcome. This change score can be positive (the outcome rating increased) or negative (the outcome rating decreased), or there can be no change (the outcome rating stayed the same). This change in rating score represents the outcome achieved following a health care intervention(s).

**NOC Taxonomy**

A systematic organization of outcomes into groups or categories based on similarities, dissimilarities, and relationships among the outcomes. The NOC taxonomy structure has five levels: domains, classes, outcomes, indicators, and measures.

**Family**

A family is two or more people who are related biologically, legally, or by choice that has a societal expectation to socialize, enculturate, and care for its members.

**Population**

A collection of individuals who have one or more personal (e.g., gender, age, illness) or environmental (e.g., country, worksite) characteristics in common.

**Community**

A community is an interactive population with relationships that emerge as members develop and use, in common, some agencies and institutions.

**Care Recipient**

Patient, Caregiver (specify), Parent (specify), Family Unit, Community (specify).

**Data Source**

Patient, family member, caregiver, direct observation by health care provider, clinical record, other.

**Health Care Providers**

Professional and assistive personnel who are reimbursed for providing health care services.

**Health Care Professionals**

Individuals with advanced education and licensure who are reimbursed for providing health care services.

**Family Caregiver**

A family member, a significant other, a friend, or another person who cares for or acts on behalf of the patient.

*Continued*

| Box 2-1 |
|---|

### Terms and Definitions—Cont'd

**Childcare Provider**

Family caregiver or an individual who is paid to provide childcare.

**Normal**

What is expected and accepted as normal for a population according to their race, age and gender.

**Child**

Overall term for childhood from 1 year through 17 years old.

**Newborn**

The term used for a baby for the first 28 days of life.

**Infant**

The term used for a baby from birth to first birthday.

**Toddler**

The term used for a child from 1 year through 2 years.

**Preschool**

The term used for a child from 3 years through 5 years.

**Early Childhood**

The period in a child's life from 1 year through 5 years (includes Toddler and Preschool).

**Middle Childhood**

The period in a child's life from 6 years through 11 years.

**Adolescence**

The period in a child's life from 12 years through 17 years.

**Health**

Physical, psychological, social, and spiritual functioning.

**Well-Being**

Extent of positive perception of health and life circumstances.

---

abstract, global outcomes are developed as more specific, less abstract outcomes. For example, an indicator for the outcome Mobility is joint movement, whereas "flexion" is an indicator for the outcome Joint Movement: Neck. The empirical level includes measurement activities for each outcome and its indicators.

For the development of manageable computerized databases that are optimally useful for assessing the efficacy and effectiveness of nursing interventions it is important that all outcome measures be quantifiable and psychometrically sound. Phase III of the research (RO1-NR03437) tested the measurement scales. Chapter 3 discusses this research.

### How Should the Outcomes Be Stated?

Because the outcomes and indicators are conceptualized as variable patient, family, or community states, behaviors, or perceptions, they are given labels representing concepts that can be measured along a continuum as negative or positive states. Whenever possible, the team avoids

| Table 2-2 | LEVELS OF OUTCOMES IN THE TAXONOMY |
|---|---|
| Most Abstract | Nursing-Sensitive Outcome Domain |
| High Middle Level Abstraction | Nursing-Sensitive Outcome Classes |
| Middle Level Abstraction | Nursing-Sensitive Outcome |
| Low Level Abstraction | Nursing-Sensitive Outcome Indicators |
| Empirical Level | Measurement Activities for Outcomes |

using labels that describe an undesirable state. However, because of the common use of some labels or difficulty in identifying an antonym, some do describe an undesirable state. Examples are Infection Severity and Pain Level. Conceptualization of the outcomes as variables allows measurement of negative or positive changes, as well as no change, resulting from nursing interventions.[3] To assist in conceptualization of the outcomes and writing nursing-sensitive outcome labels, the research team defined the set of rules listed in Box 2-2.

### Why Are the Outcomes Not Stated As Goals?

The research team developed the outcomes as variable concepts for several reasons. First, NOC outcomes are developed as variable concepts so that the response of the patient, family, or community to nursing interventions can be documented and monitored over time and across settings and compared. A goal developed for each patient does not allow for this cross-comparison. Second, variable outcomes yield more information than just whether a goal has been met. For clinical and research purposes, either/or type data provide a very limited amount of information and constrain nurses' abilities to adequately evaluate the effectiveness of their interventions. If goals are not met, it is important to know whether any progress was made or the extent that the outcome status deteriorated, if at all. Third, with current short lengths of stay in acute care settings, it has become very important to be able to document even slight increases in outcome scores at discharge. Goals for short time frames become meaningless for monitoring progress across time. NOC outcomes can be used to state a goal for a patient, family, or community; but this should be in addition to measurement of status on the variable outcome at baseline and over time. Fourth, in many cases, the goal of nursing care may be to maintain a patient at a particular outcome rating when improvement in status is not possible. For example, the goal for a patient with self-care issues may be to maintain their outcome status at a "3" for the outcome Self-Care: Bathing. Finally, the strength of using outcomes rather than goals is that a change in rating score can be determined after nursing care is provided. This change in rating score is not possible with

---

**Box 2-2**

#### Rules for Standardization of Nursing-Sensitive Outcomes

Outcome labels should be concise (stated in five words or less).
Outcome labels should be stated in nonevaluative terms rather than as a decreased, increased, or improved state.
Outcome labels should *not* describe a nurse behavior or interventions.
Outcome labels should *not* be stated as a nursing diagnosis.
Outcome labels should describe a state, behavior, or perception that is inherently variable and can be measured and quantified.
Outcome labels should be conceptualized and stated at a middle level of abstraction.
Colons should be used to make broader concept labels more specific; however, the broader label is stated first, with the colon and more specific label following (e.g., Nutritional Status: Nutrient Intake, Nutritional Status: Energy).

goals and is important for evaluating the effectiveness of nursing treatments and comparing outcomes for specific patient populations over time.

## What Are Nursing-Sensitive Patient Outcomes?

To be useful for assessing the effectiveness of nursing, outcomes and indicators that are influenced by nursing and comprehensive enough to assess all aspects of nursing practice must be identified. The team recognized that the majority of patient outcomes, including those traditionally used to evaluate physician care, are not influenced by any one discipline alone. However, for nursing to monitor and improve its practice, it is important to identify the outcomes that are responsive to nursing care.

The more abstract and global the outcome, the more likely its achievement will be the result of interventions from several health care disciplines. Specific disciplines will have more influence on certain intermediate outcomes than others. For example, at different times, nursing, medicine, and physical therapy have the most impact on Mobility, although, overall, all share influence on the outcome. Specific indicators of outcomes are more likely to be sensitive to the interventions of a single discipline. Therefore it is essential to identify the indicators most sensitive to nursing interventions to enable nurses to document the effects of their interventions and to hold them individually and collectively accountable for care delivered to patients. To develop and refine the list of nursing-sensitive outcomes and indicators, the team defined a set of criteria for evaluating evidence of nursing sensitivity or responsiveness to nursing interventions. These criteria are listed in Box 2-3.

## Are Nursing-Sensitive Patient Outcomes the Resolution of Nursing Diagnoses?

The majority of nursing-sensitive patient outcomes represent the resolution of nursing diagnoses, although some outcomes are more generic and not necessarily related to specific diagnoses. Clearly, patient satisfaction and the financial charges to patients that are attributable to nursing care are not diagnosis specific and cannot be conceived as the resolution of a diagnosis. At this time, it appears that the more general (abstract) the outcome, such as quality of life, the less likely it will be diagnosis specific; and conversely, the less abstract the outcome concept, such as Self-Care: Toileting, the more likely it will be nursing diagnosis specific.

## How Are the Outcomes Different from Nursing Diagnoses?

NOC outcomes describe a variable state, behavior, or perception. The outcome state at a particular time can be at any point on a negative to positive continuum. The outcomes can be used to measure nursing diagnoses stated as problems, risk states, or potential for enhancement diagnoses with the same measure. Nursing diagnoses, on the other hand, for the most part describe

---

**Box 2-3**

### Criteria for Evaluating Nursing Sensitivity

A nursing intervention produced a positive outcome.
A nursing intervention influenced a positive outcome.
A nursing intervention was carried out with the intent to produce or influence the outcome.
A nursing intervention produced improvement or maintenance of the outcome or prevented deterioration or occurrence of a negative outcome.
The nursing intervention occurred before observation of the outcome.
A failure to provide nursing intervention resulted in failure to achieve a positive outcome or to prevent a negative outcome.
The interventions that produced or influenced the outcome are within nursing's scope of practice.

states that are in some way less positive than what is desired. Nursing diagnoses describe problems, actual or potential, that the nurse seeks to resolve through intervention.

### When Should Patient Outcomes Be Measured?

The appropriate time to measure patient outcomes will vary. This is because some outcomes respond very quickly to intervention and others respond over a longer period. For example, the outcomes of health promotion interventions are likely to occur over a considerable period, whereas the response to interventions to improve nutritional intake could be immediate. There also are outcomes, such as Transfer Performance, where the full response may take several weeks. One problem is selecting a time for measurement close enough to the intervention to be assured that change is due to the intervention, but far enough removed to be able to measure a change. This is why medicine has begun to place more emphasis on intermediate outcomes.

### At What Intervals Should the Outcomes Be Assessed and Documented?

More research is needed to definitively answer this question. At present, the nurse will determine the intervals for measurement and documentation of the outcome based on clinical judgment as to when the effects of interventions need to be assessed. Setting organizational policies will also determine the intervals for measurement and documentation in some situations. However, at minimum, the outcomes selected should be rated and documented when (1) the patient or family is admitted to a care setting or makes an initial visit to a nurse for care; (2) the patient or family is discharged, transferred, or referred to another setting or clinician for care; or (3) there is a significant change in status for an outcome. Time intervals for measurement of outcomes should vary based on the characteristics of the concept. For example, the nurse might want to measure Pain Level every 4 hours but would not measure the patient's Quality of Life on the same time frames. The nurse and/or interdisciplinary health care team will determine the measurement time frames for family and community level outcomes.

### How Are the Outcomes Used in Standardized Care Plans/Critical Paths?

NOC outcomes are very useful in clinical pathways because they allow quantification of the patient state, behavior, or perception that is expected to occur at specific points in time for a desired pathway of an episode of care. Examples of use of the NOC in care plans are included in Appendix E. Major advantages of their use are the ability to monitor variance from the pathway and the ability to compare the achievement of specific states across settings and providers. Use of the standardized outcomes will greatly facilitate the development of large databases across settings and providers, rather than the more limited, unique setting or provider databases that result when setting-specific or provider-specific outcomes are used in critical pathways and care planning.

### Why Is It Necessary for Nurses to Have Their Own List of Outcomes?

The NOC includes patient, family, and community level outcomes that are responsive to nursing interventions. These outcomes are not intended to be unique to nursing. Clearly, most, if not all, patient outcomes are influenced by multiple health care providers, as well as by other patient, family, and community/population characteristics and by environmental factors. However, it is critically important for nurses to measure the effects of their interventions on patient outcomes. The NOC provides a set of indicators for each outcome that is considered to be sensitive to nursing interventions. When used with interdisciplinary teams, different indicators may be the focus of interventions for various disciplines. Without discipline-specific indicators for shared outcomes, it will be impossible to monitor the accountability of each discipline for its contribution to outcome improvement or deterioration. To ensure that the contributions of nursing interventions to patient, family, and community level outcomes are not credited to other health care providers, standardized nursing data elements must be included in clinical databases. Large data sets that include these data along with other salient system, patient, family, or community level characteristics, as well as provider characteristics, are necessary to isolate the independent effects of nursing interventions on patient outcomes.[10]

### Why Is It Important to Assess Outcomes across Care Settings?

Continuity of care is always an important value for the nursing profession. Yet communication among settings and nurse providers is constrained. A major obstacle is the lack of standardized nomenclatures to describe the problems that nurses treat, the interventions used, and the resulting outcome states. The inability to optimize continuity of care is costly to patients, families, and the health care system. In the current resource-constrained environment, more emphasis is placed on continuity of care to reduce costs. Further, networks that include providers and settings across the continuum of care are being developed to enhance continuity and optimize care in the most cost-efficient environment. The effort to reduce costs has prompted a corresponding emphasis on the demonstration of outcomes effectiveness. The NOC provides a standardized language for outcomes that can be measured across the entire continuum of care, providing essential information that clinicians need to achieve continuity and to assess the cost-effectiveness of care.

### Why Is It Necessary To Use the Outcome Labels When the Indicators May Be More Useful?

Along with medicine, the nursing profession is a key member of the interdisciplinary health care team. The profession's contribution to interdisciplinary outcomes must be documented and the effectiveness of nursing interventions must be evaluated. Large standardized databases contain outcomes such as those provided by NOC, but likely not discipline-specific indicators in all cases because of space limitations. Therefore it is essential that the nursing profession use the standardized outcome labels and that these be included in large databases so that the profession's influence on outcomes will be assessed to determine nursing effectiveness and to influence health policy.

### Why Is the Standardization of Outcomes Advocated When Each Patient, Family, or Community/Population Is Unique?

Standardizing the language used to describe outcomes in no way interferes with assessing the unique response of each patient, family, or community/population. Rather, use of the NOC outcomes will enable nurses to measure each outcome state for each individual, family, and community and will provide more information for monitoring the progress of each. Further, specific quantified goals can be set for each and the extent to which the goals are or are not met can be documented over time and across settings and compared. In other words, standardized nursing diagnoses, interventions, and outcomes actually increase the ability of nurses to identify and document the diagnoses that are unique for each patient, prescribe interventions that are specific for the patient, and document the patient outcomes in response to the interventions for each individual across time and settings.

### How Do I Identify Outcomes for Use in My Practice?

With 330 outcomes in the third edition of NOC, this task may seem difficult at first. The scope of the classification is to identify all outcomes needed by nurses to evaluate the outcomes of nursing interventions, whereas most nurses will focus on a limited set of outcomes based on their specialty and practice setting. Beginning efforts to identify core outcomes for specialty practice have supported this belief that nurses can identify a list of outcomes they use daily with their patients. The easiest way to begin to identify outcomes for use in clinical practice is to review the NOC Taxonomy where similar outcomes are grouped under key concepts in nursing. A second way to identify outcomes is to review the list of outcomes identified by various specialty organizations to determine whether the outcomes identified match the outcomes you need to evaluate the effectiveness of your interventions.

### When Is a New Outcome Developed and How Is It Done?

New outcomes are identified by the research team, nurses from our test sites and in clinical practice, and through the linkage work with NANDA diagnoses and NIC interventions. The team maintains a list of potential concepts for development and these are addressed as we work on new outcomes. A nurse or group of nurses conducts a concept analysis, defines the outcome, identifies indicators, and chooses a measurement scale(s) for use with the outcome. The NOC focus groups have been primarily responsible for the development of new outcomes. The entire research team reviews the potential outcomes, and revisions are made based on this expert review. Part of this review process involves ensuring that the outcome is useful and clinically accurate for patients across the life span. If it is not, then a target population is identified in the concept label. Many outcomes are sent to additional experts for further review. Once the outcome is accepted for inclusion in the NOC, the outcome is placed in the taxonomy and coded. Instructions on how to submit an outcome can be found in Appendix G.

### NOC Measurement Scales

The second edition of the Classification contains 17 measurement scales for use with the NOC outcomes. Because the outcomes are variable concepts representing patient, family, or community states, behaviors, and perceptions, a method of measuring the concepts is essential. The original scales were created based on the advice of practitioners in our field sites and measurement experts. A five-point Likert-type scale is used with all outcomes and indicators. The five-point scoring format provides an adequate number of options with which to demonstrate variability in the state, behavior, or perception described by the outcome. This scale structure does not demand the degree of precision required for a 10-point scoring format. Each scale is constructed so that 1 reflects the worst possible score for the outcome and 5 reflects the most desirable score for the outcome. As previously indicated, the most desirable condition will not be achievable in all patients or patient groups, and the optimal outcome for an intervention in a given situation may be less than the most desirable patient condition. For example, in some situations a 5 is not a realistic outcome, given the patient's physiological condition. Patient's with end-stage kidney disease will not achieve a rating of 5 for the outcome Kidney Function without a kidney transplant. As nursing knowledge increases and more effective interventions are developed, improvement in the outcomes achieved may be expected. Lack of change in the outcome score after nursing intervention may indicate that another approach to the problem is required. What is important is that outcomes are measured reliably and validly so that the effectiveness of nursing interventions can be examined.

Although the outcome scales had been used in pilot studies and field testing before the publication of the second edition, additional statistical analysis was needed to estimate reliability, validity, and sensitivity of the measurement scales in a variety of clinical settings. Testing these psychometric properties of the outcome measures was the principal purpose of the second 4-year grant funded by the National Institutes of Health Funding, which was completed in 2002 (NR #RO1 NR03437). This testing has identified important changes needed in the scales and helped enhance and refine this current edition of the NOC. Input from practicing nurses has been very helpful in improving the measurement scales and making them easier to use with patients, families, and communities. Results of this research are highlighted in Chapter 3, and the major changes in the measurement scales are highlighted here.

### Modifications in Measurement Scales Based on Use in Clinical Practice

Testing the outcomes in 10 clinical sites allowed the research team to evaluate the 17 measurement scales used in the NOC. The goals of the measurement scale review were to (1) reduce, if possible, the number of scales used in the Classification to make it easier to use in practice; (2) ensure that the scales are capable of capturing change in outcome status following nursing treatments; (3) identify indicators that were difficult for the nurses to measure; (4) refine the terms used as anchors on the scales; and (5) evaluate the utility of the "other" indicator in each outcome. The review process involved examining each scale by using the data from our clinical sites, reviewing nurses' comments concerning use of the scales in practice, and examining the data comparing NOC scales with criterion tools selected for each outcome. On the basis of this review, several scales were deleted from this edition.

## Changes Facilitating the Elimination of Scales

Perhaps the most problematic of the scales evaluated in the clinical testing of the NOC was the scale "Dependent, does not participate" to "Completely independent." The issues about this scale came from nurses in a variety of settings trying to use the Self-Care outcomes. Although the anchors had clear terms that were very concrete, the scale did not work very well in practice. The primary reason for this was that the scale captured two components of the outcome: degree of assistance/participation and the use of an assistive device. Concerns about this scale also included the fact that some patients could do an activity independently if they were cued but did not do the activity without the reminder by nursing personnel. Nurses did not know whether to count this mental cueing as "assistance," and most commented that "it seemed different than physical assistance." Ironically, before testing, this scale was considered one of the best in the Classification by the research team because the anchors on the scale were concrete and easy to differentiate.

The second major problem with this scale was that it did not allow for a change in score after nursing interventions. Most patients who needed an assistive device still needed to use it after intervention. The nurses could not rate a patient as a "5" if a device was used by the patient, even when the patient was completely independent while using that device. Although interventions were completed, the structure of the scale did not allow for many patients to receive a change in rating. The deletion of this scale affected 17 outcomes, the largest group being the Self-Care outcomes. In this edition of the Classification, the scale used for these outcomes was changed to "Severely compromised" to "Not compromised."

Several scales were eliminated because they were infrequently used in the NOC and other scales could be substituted. The scale "Not at all" to "To a very great extent" had only seven outcomes that used this scale in the second edition, and many of the revisions to these outcomes resulted in a need for a different scale. For example, Blood Glucose Control was changed to Blood Glucose Level, and the scale "Severe deviation from normal range" to "No deviation from normal range" is used for this outcome. This was considered a better match with the definition. The third scale eliminated based on a review was the scale "No motion" to "Full motion." Only two outcomes used this scale in the second edition—Joint Movement: Active and Joint Movement: Passive. After revision of the outcomes, the scale "Severe deviation from normal range" to "No deviation from normal range" was used for the revised Joint Movement outcomes. The scale "None" to "Complete" was used with only three outcomes and was eliminated. The Child Development outcomes had previously used the scale "Extreme delay from expected range" to "No delay from expected range" in the second edition of the NOC. This scale was the fifth scale eliminated. These outcomes focus on behaviors, and the scale "Never demonstrated" to "Consistently demonstrated" is used in the current edition. The final scale eliminated from the NOC is the scale "No evidence" to "Extensive evidence." Only two outcomes used this scale. The outcome indicators were modified to add the term *evidence* to the indicators, and the scale was changed to "None" to "Extensive." A total of six scales were eliminated from the NOC classification in the third edition based on the results of our research and extensive review. Table 2-3 summarizes the scales with all five anchors that have been eliminated to date from the classification.

## Changes in Measurement Based on Difficulty Measuring the Indicators

Another issue identified from the testing of the NOC in clinical sites was the problem that some indicators were difficult to use. An example of this type of indicator is "dizziness not present"

| **Table 2-3** | SUMMARY OF MEASUREMENT SCALES ELIMINATED FROM THE NOC (THIRD EDITION) | | | | |

| Code | 1 | 2 | 3 | 4 | 5 |
| --- | --- | --- | --- | --- | --- |
| c | Dependent, does not participate | Requires assistive person & device | Requires assistive person | Independent with assistive device | Completely independent |
| d | No motion | Limited motion | Moderate motion | Substantial motion | Full motion |
| e | Not at all | To a slight extent | To a moderate extent | To a great extent | To a very great extent |
| j | None | Slight | Moderate | Substantial | Complete |
| o | No evidence | Limited evidence | Moderate evidence | Substantial evidence | Extensive evidence |
| p | Extreme delay from expected range | Substantial delay from expected range | Moderate delay from expected range | Mild delay from expected range | No delay from expected range |

from the outcome Sensory Function: Vision. This outcome uses the scale "Extremely compromised to "Not compromised" in the second edition. Nurses found it difficult to rate this indicator with this scale. Part of the problem was this indicator really was a "yes or no" situation but needed to be measured on the compromised scale. Nurses believed the indicators in this format were important indicators because they focus on symptoms indicating complications of the patient's condition and are frequently monitored by nurses in practice. As a solution to this type of problem, a second scale, for measuring the negative indicators, was added in this edition to this outcome. The outcome Sensory Function: Vision now uses two scales—"Severe deviation from normal range" to "No deviation from normal range" and "Severe" to "None"—for the indicators. The overall outcome rating is based on the Deviation scale, considered the primary measurement scale for this outcome. We believe this is an important revision to the Classification because it allows for better documentation of complications associated with the outcome. To better match the two scales, the rating of "1" was changed from "Extreme" to "Severe" on the Deviation scale.

A second problem that made the indicators hard to use was wording of indicators as "free of" (e.g., "free of bleeding"). The addition of a second scale allows the nurse to rate the severity of the bleeding in the outcome Oral Hygiene. This allows the nurse to rate the severity of bleeding experienced by the patient, rather than whether bleeding is present or absent. This provides better data and more information on a change in the patient's status. As a result of these changes, 72 outcomes use two scales to measure the indicators in this edition.

## Evaluation of the Utility of the "Other" Indicator

The final revision made to this edition of the Classification focused on the general inclusion of an "Other" as an indicator to allow for the addition of more indicators. Evaluation of the data for the indicator "Other" identified few additional outcomes for the current edition and created issues with the measurement of the outcome. In many cases, nurses rated the indicator without specifying what concept they were rating. The decision was made by the research team to retire this indicator from all outcomes.

## Outcome Measurement Scales Used in the Third Edition

Each outcome in the classification has the scale identified by an alphabetical code. This is the code used within the outcomes and appears in the heading section of each outcome along with its domain and class in the taxonomy. The codes have no meaning themselves and are mainly important for computerization of NOC in electronic patient records and databases. With the inclusion of two measurement scales to measure indicators, some outcomes will have two scales identified, each with an alphabetical code. Table 2-4 provides a list of the scales used in this edition as primary measurement scales for the 330 outcomes in this edition. *Primary scales* are those that are used to measure the outcome globally. Eleven scales are used as primary measures in this edition. When additional scales are used to measure indicators for one outcome, we call them *secondary scales*. Some of the primary scales are used as secondary scales in some outcomes. Two scales are used as secondary scales in this edition. In future editions of this work, these scales could be used as primary scales, but at present, they are used only with indicators. Table 2-4 contains the outcomes that use each scale. A brief description of the 11 primary scales follows.

## Primary Outcome Measurement Scales

- *Scale a* provides a measure for the degree of compromise seen in an outcome with the scale "Severely compromised" to "Not compromised." This scale is used to measure a wide variety of outcomes such as Activity Tolerance, Concentration, Self-Care Status, and Spiritual Health. A total of 37 outcomes use this scale as the only measurement scale for the outcome.
- *Scale b* measures the amount of deviation with the scale "Extreme deviation from normal range" to "No deviation from normal range." This scale is used with physiological states with known ranges for normal such as Blood Glucose Level, Growth, Vital Signs, and Joint Movement: Knee. This scale had a change in the reference point for this edition. The word *normal* was substituted for *expected*, used in the previous edition. This was done to establish the reference person for the outcome as a normal individual for the race, age, and gender of the patient. The term *expected* did not work well in practice, since some patients have "expected" laboratory values that are outside the normal range because of their disease. For comparison purposes, nurses need to use the same reference person when measuring outcomes to allow for comparisons across populations, settings, and time. Testing of the measurement scales in practice reinforced this as an important change. A total of 24 outcomes use this scale as the only measurement scale for the outcome.
- *Scale f* measures the level of adequacy for outcomes related to patient performance and safety and has a range from "Not adequate" to "Totally adequate." Examples of outcomes that use this scale are Abuse Protection, Family Physical Environment, and Social Support. Sixteen outcomes use this scale as the only measurement scale for the outcome.
- *Scale g* is a numerical scale used to measure the extent of falls. The anchor for "1" was changed in this edition to "10 and over," since the previous version of this scale had 9 in both the rating for "1" and "2." Only one outcome, Falls Occurrence, uses this scale as the only measurement scale for the outcome.
- *Scale i* measures the extent of patient states, behaviors, and knowledge with the scale "None" to "Extensive." All of the knowledge outcomes use this scale, as well as several outcomes related to abuse and neglect. A total of 35 outcomes use this scale as the only measurement scale for the outcome.
- *Scale k* with anchors from "Never positive" to "Consistently positive" is used with two outcomes: Body Image and Self-Esteem. This scale was retained because it was a good match with these concepts and other scales did not work as well. This scale measures an individual's perception.

*Text continued on p. 40*

| Table 2-4 | PRIMARY MEASUREMENT SCALES USED IN NOC | | |
|---|---|---|---|

| Scale Letter | Scales and Associated Outcomes | | |
|---|---|---|---|
| a | *Severely compromised* | *Substantially compromised* | *Moderately compromised* |
| | Activity Tolerance | | Coordinated Movement |
| | Ambulation | | Decision-Making |
| | Ambulation: Wheelchair | | Electrolyte & Acid/Base Balance |
| | Appetite | | Information Processing |
| | Body Positioning: Self-Initiated | | Memory |
| | Caregiver-Patient Relationship | | Mobility |
| | Caregiver Physical Health | | Personal Well-Being |
| | Cognition | | Physical Fitness |
| | Cognitive Orientation | | Preterm Infant Organization |
| | Communication | | Rest |
| | Communication: Expressive | | Self-Care: Activities of Daily Living (ADL) |
| | Communication: Receptive | | Self-Care: Bathing |
| | Concentration | | Self-Care: Dressing |
| b | *Severe deviation from normal range* | *Substantial deviation from normal range* | *Moderate deviation from normal range* |
| | Blood Glucose Level | | Joint Movement: Knee |
| | Fetal Status: Antepartum | | Joint Movement: Neck |
| | Fetal Status: Intrapartum | | Joint Movement: Passive |
| | Growth | | Joint Movement: Shoulder |
| | Joint Movement: Ankle | | Joint Movement: Spine |
| | Joint Movement: Elbow | | Joint Movement: Wrist |
| | Joint Movement: Fingers | | Newborn Adaptation |
| | Joint Movement: Hip | | Nutritional Status |
| f | *Not adequate* | *Slightly adequate* | *Moderately adequate* |
| | Abuse Protection | | Caregiver Performance: Direct Care |
| | Breastfeeding Establishment: Infant | | Caregiver Performance: Indirect Care |
| | Breastfeeding Establishment: Maternal | | Caregiving Endurance Potential |
| | Breastfeeding Maintenance | | Community Disaster Readiness |
| | Breastfeeding Weaning | | Family Physical Environment |
| | Caregiver Home Care Readiness | | |
| g | *10 and over* | *7-9* | *4-6* |
| | Falls Occurrence | | |
| i | *None* | *Limited* | *Moderate* |
| | Abuse Cessation | | Knowledge: Energy Conservation |
| | Abuse Recovery: Financial | | Knowledge: Fall Prevention |
| | Abuse Recovery: Physical | | Knowledge: Fertility Promotion |
| | Abuse Recovery Status | | Knowledge: Health Behavior |
| | Knowledge: Body Mechanics | | Knowledge: Health Promotion |
| | Knowledge: Breastfeeding | | Knowledge: Health Resources |
| | Knowledge: Cardiac Disease Management | | Knowledge: Illness Care |
| | Knowledge: Child Physical Safety | | Knowledge: Infant Care |
| | Knowledge: Conception Prevention | | Knowledge: Infection Control |
| | Knowledge: Diabetes Management | | Knowledge: Labor & Delivery |
| | Knowledge: Diet | | Knowledge: Medication |
| | Knowledge: Disease Process | | Knowledge: Ostomy Care |

| *Mildly compromised* | *Not compromised* |
|---|---|

Self-Care: Eating
Self-Care: Hygiene
Self-Care: Instrumental Activities of Daily Living (IADL)
Self-Care: Non-Parenteral Medication
Self-Care: Oral Hygiene
Self-Care: Parenteral Medication
Self-Care: Toileting
Self-Care Status
Skeletal Function
Spiritual Health
Transfer Performance

| *Mild deviation from normal range* | *No deviation from normal range* |
|---|---|

Nutritional Status: Biochemical Measures
Nutritional Status: Energy
Physical Aging
Physical Maturation: Female
Physical Maturation: Male
Sensory Function Status
Vital Signs
Weight: Body Mass

| *Substantially adequate* | *Totally adequate* |
|---|---|

Nutritional Status: Food & Fluid Intake
Nutritional Status: Nutrient Intake
Role Performance
Safe Home Environment
Social Support

| *1-3* | *None* |
|---|---|

| *Substantial* | *Extensive* |
|---|---|

Knowledge: Parenting
Knowledge: Personal Safety
Knowledge: Postpartum Maternal Health
Knowledge: Preconception Maternal Health
Knowledge: Pregnancy
Knowledge: Prescribed Activity
Knowledge: Sexual Functioning
Knowledge: Substance Use Control
Knowledge: Treatment Procedure(s)
Knowledge: Treatment Regimen
Neglect Cessation

*Continued*

| **Table 2-4** | PRIMARY MEASUREMENT SCALES USED IN NOC—CONT'D | | |
|---|---|---|---|

| k | *Never positive* | *Rarely positive* | *Sometimes positive* |
|---|---|---|---|
| | Body Image | | |
| | Self-Esteem | | |

| l | *Very weak* | *Weak* | *Moderate* |
|---|---|---|---|
| | Health Beliefs | | Health Beliefs: Perceived Control |
| | Health Beliefs: Perceived Ability to Perform | | Health Beliefs: Perceived Resources |

| m | *Never demonstrated* | *Rarely demonstrated* | *Sometimes demonstrated* |
|---|---|---|---|
| | Abusive Behavior Self-Restraint | | Fall Prevention Behavior |
| | Acceptance: Health Status | | Family Coping |
| | Adaptation to Physical Disability | | Family Functioning |
| | Adherence Behavior | | Family Integrity |
| | Aggression Self-Control | | Family Normalization |
| | Anxiety Self-Control | | Family Participation in Professional Care |
| | Aspiration Prevention | | Family Resiliency |
| | Body Mechanics Performance | | Family Social Climate |
| | Cardiac Disease Self-Management | | Family Support During Treatment |
| | Caregiver Adaptation to Patient | | Fear Self-Control |
| |   Institutionalization | | Grief Resolution |
| | Child Development: 1 Month | | Health Promoting Behavior |
| | Child Development: 2 Months | | Health Seeking Behavior |
| | Child Development: 4 Months | | Hearing Compensation Behavior |
| | Child Development: 6 Months | | Hope |
| | Child Development: 12 Months | | Identity |
| | Child Development: 2 Years | | Immunization Behavior |
| | Child Development: 3 Years | | Impulse Self-Control |
| | Child Development: 4 Years | | Leisure Participation |
| | Child Development: Preschool | | Motivation |
| | Child Development: Middle Childhood | | Nausea & Vomiting Control |
| | Child Development: Adolescence | | Ostomy Self-Care |
| | Compliance Behavior | | Pain Control |
| | Coping | | Parent-Infant Attachment |
| | Depression Self-Control | | Parenting: Infant/ Toddler |
| | Diabetes Self-Management | |   Physical Safety |
| | Dignified Life Closure | | Parenting: Early/Middle Childhood |
| | Discharge Readiness: Supported Living | |   Physical Safety |
| | Distorted Thought Self-Control | | Parenting: Adolescent Physical Safety |
| | Energy Conservation | | Parenting Performance |
| | | | Parenting: Psychosocial Safety |

| n | *Severe* | *Substantial* | *Moderate* |
|---|---|---|---|
| | Allergic Response: Localized | | Fear Level: Child |
| | Allergic Response: Systemic | | Fluid Overload Severity |
| | Anxiety Level | | Hyperactivity Level |
| | Blood Loss Severity | | Infection Severity |
| | Blood Transfusion Reaction | | Infection Severity: Newborn |
| | Caregiver Stressors | | Loneliness Severity |
| | Depression Level | | Nausea & Vomiting: Disruptive Effects |
| | Fear Level | | Nausea & Vomiting: Severity |

| r | *Poor* | *Fair* | *Good* |
|---|---|---|---|
| | Community Competence | | Community Risk Control: Chronic Disease |
| | Community Health Status | | Community Risk Control: Communicable |
| | Community Health Status: Immunity | |   Disease |

| *Often positive* | *Consistently positive* |
|---|---|

| *Strong* | *Very strong* |
|---|---|

Health Beliefs: Perceived Threat
Health Orientation

| *Often demonstrated* | *Consistently demonstrated* |
|---|---|

Participation in Health Care Decisions
Personal Autonomy
Personal Safety Behavior
Play Participation
Prenatal Health Behavior
Psychosocial Adjustment: Life Change
Risk Control
Risk Control: Alcohol Use
Risk Control: Cancer
Risk Control: Cardiovascular Health
Risk Control: Drug Use
Risk Control: Hearing Impairment
Risk Control: Sexually Transmitted Diseases (STD)
Risk Control: Tobacco Use
Risk Control: Unintended Pregnancy
Risk Control: Visual Impairment
Risk Detection
Seizure Control
Self-Direction of Care
Self-Mutilation Restraint
Sexual Functioning
Sexual Identity
Social Interaction Skills
Social Involvement
Suicide Self-Restraint
Symptom Control
Treatment Behavior: Illness or Injury
Vision Compensation Behavior
Weight Control

| *Mild* | *None* |
|---|---|

Pain: Adverse Psychological Response
Physical Injury Severity
Stress Level
Substance Addiction Consequences
Suffering Severity
Symptom Severity
Symptom Severity: Perimenopause
Symptom Severity: Premenstrual Syndrome (PMS)

| *Very good* | *Excellent* |
|---|---|

Community Risk Control: Lead Exposure
Community Risk Control: Violence
Community Violence Level

*Continued*

| Table 2-4 | Primary Measurement Scales Used in NOC—cont'd | |
|---|---|---|

| s | Not at all satisfied | Somewhat satisfied | Moderately satisfied |
|---|---|---|---|
| | Caregiver Well-Being | | Client Satisfaction: Functional Assistance |
| | Client Satisfaction: Access to Care Resources | | Client Satisfaction: Physical Care |
| | Client Satisfaction: Caring | | Client Satisfaction: Physical Environment |
| | Client Satisfaction: Communication | | Client Satisfaction: Protection of Rights |
| | Client Satisfaction: Continuity of Care | | Client Satisfaction: Psychological Care |
| | Client Satisfaction: Cultural Needs Fulfillment | | Client Satisfaction: Safety |

- *Scale l* is used primarily with the Health Belief outcomes to measure the strength of personal beliefs or values. Six outcomes use this scale as the only measurement scale for the outcome.
- *Scale m* is used to measure outcomes for a number of behaviors in which consistency of behavior is important. The anchors range from "Never demonstrated" to "Consistently demonstrated." A total of 87 outcomes use this scale as the only measurement scale for the outcome. Examples of outcomes that use this measurement scale are the Child Development outcomes, the Risk Control outcomes, and many of the Family and Parenting outcomes.
- *Scale n* measures the severity of a concept from "Severe" to "None." This scale is frequently used to measure the intensity of symptoms or psychological states. A total of 24 scales use this measurement scale as the only measurement scale for the outcome. Examples of outcomes that use this scale are Fear Level, Nausea & Vomiting Severity, and Substance Addiction Consequences.
- *Scale r* measures the quality of the concept from "Poor" to "Excellent." This scale is currently used to measure the Community outcomes in the Classification. Eight outcomes use this scale to measure the outcome and indicators.
- *Scale s* is a new scale to this edition. It is used to rate the patient's satisfaction with various concepts. The anchors range from "Not at all satisfied" to "Completely satisfied." Eighteen outcomes use this scale to measure the outcome and indicators.

## Scale Combinations Used in the Third Edition

The following section describes pairs of measurement scales used together for the first time in this edition. When two scales are used to measure the indicators, the outcomes have a primary scale listed first and a secondary scale added to assist in measuring specific indicators that do not fit the primary scale well. Table 2-5 lists the scales with the anchors and outcomes that use each combination of scales. A brief description of each of these combined scales is provided in the following section.

- *Combination of Scales a and n* is used frequently in this edition. This combines the compromise scale with the severity scale. A total of 43 outcomes use the scales in combination. The overall outcome rating uses the Severely compromised scale as the primary scale. This allows for rating of the degree of compromise while rating the severity of important complications or symptoms.
- *Combination of Scales i and h* is used with six outcomes. This combines the two mirror image scales of "None" to "Extensive" and "Extensive" to "None." The overall rating of the outcomes uses the anchor "extensive " for the best rating "5." Scale *h* is the reverse of Scale *i* and has the anchors "Extensive" to "None." In the present edition it is only used in combination with Scale i as a secondary scale.
- *Combination of Scales m and t* is used with seven outcomes. This combines the two demonstrated scales for use within one outcome. The overall rating uses "Never demonstrated"

| *Very satisfied* | *Completely satisfied* |
| --- | --- |

Client Satisfaction: Symptom Control
Client Satisfaction: Teaching
Client Satisfaction: Technical Aspects of Care
Comfort Level
Personal Well-Being
Quality of Life

to "Consistently demonstrated" as the primary scale. Examples of outcomes that use this pair of scales are Asthma Self-Management, Mood Equilibrium, and Urinary Continence. Scale t is a new scale to this edition and is only used as a secondary scale to measure indicators.

- *Combination of Scales n and a* is used in six outcomes. Examples of outcomes that use this combination of scales are Pain Level and Caregiver Lifestyle Disruption. The overall outcome rating uses "Severe" to "None" as the primary scale.

In summary, the results of testing in 10 clinical sites have allowed for many refinements in the measurement scales used in the NOC. The current edition has 11 primary measurement scales for rating each outcome, 6 fewer than the previous edition. The indicators are measured by using 13 scales, with some outcomes using 2 scales to better measure the indicators. This has been changed to make it easier for nurses to measure the indicators. Some minor changes have been made to the anchors of some of the scales. Table 2-6 summarizes the changes and deletions of scales as a result of revisions made in this edition. The two most frequently used scales in the Classification are the Compromised scale, used in 80 outcomes as a primary scale, and the Demonstrated scale, used in 94 of the outcomes as a primary scale. These two scales are used in more than half of the outcomes in this edition.

## Changes in Format of the Outcomes

Testing NOC in a variety of settings provided us with valuable information for the refinement of this classification. Several key changes were made in the format of the outcomes. The addition of a second scale is discussed in the previous sections and has had a major impact on the layout of the outcomes. The area devoted to the overall score for the outcome was increased to make it more prominent in the outcome format. A second header was added for the additional scale as needed. Both of these headers help the nurse focus on the scale needed for documenting the outcome.

As a result of revisions to the indicators, the numerical sequence of the indicators may have changed. Some of these changes resulted from moving indicators to a second scale within the outcome. Others were moved to organize the indicators in a more logical way based on feedback from practicing nurses. The numbers attached to the indicators were retained as they were moved, so many do not appear in numerical order if they were published in the previous edition. In all outcomes the "Other" indicator was deleted and the code retired as discussed previously in this chapter. The use of abbreviations in the indicators is greatly reduced in this edition of the Classification.

Another major addition to the format of the outcomes is an area for Outcome Target Ratings. Testing of the Classification in a variety of settings and populations revealed the need to identify the goal of nursing interventions in terms of the numerical scale. We have added *Maintain at* and *Increase to* so nurses can identify the expected outcome rating they hope to achieve with an

*Text continued on p. 46*

| Table 2-5 | COMBINATION MEASUREMENT SCALES USED IN NOC |

| | *Severely compromised* | *Substantially compromised* | *Moderately compromised* |
|---|---|---|---|
| *a and n* | *Severe* | *Substantial* | *Moderate* |
| | Balance | | Medication Response |
| | Bowel Elimination | | Neurological Status |
| | Cardiac Pump Effectiveness | | Neurological Status: Autonomic |
| | Caregiver Emotional Health | | Neurological Status: Central Motor Control |
| | Circulation Status | | Neurological Status: Consciousness |
| | Comfortable Death | | Neurological Status: Cranial Sensory/ Motor Function |
| | Endurance | | Neurological Status: Spinal Sensory/ Motor Function |
| | Family Health Status | | |
| | Fluid Balance | | Oral Hygiene |
| | Hemodialysis Access | | Respiratory Status: Airway Patency |
| | Hydration | | Respiratory Status: Gas Exchange |
| | Immune Status | | Respiratory Status: Ventilation |
| | Kidney Function | | Sleep |
| | Mechanical Ventilation Response: Adult | | Student Health Status |
| | Mechanical Ventilation Weaning Response: Adult | | Swallowing Status |

| | *Severe deviation from normal range* | *Substantial deviation from normal range* | *Moderate deviation from normal range* |
|---|---|---|---|
| *b and n* | *Severe* | *Substantial* | *Moderate* |
| | Blood Coagulation | | Post Procedure Recovery Status |
| | Maternal Status: Antepartum | | Sensory Function: Cutaneous |
| | Maternal Status: Intrapartum | | Sensory Function: Hearing |
| | Maternal Status: Postpartum | | |

| | *None* | *Limited* | *Moderate* |
|---|---|---|---|
| *i and h* | *Extensive* | *Substantial* | *Moderate* |
| | Abuse Recovery: Emotional | | Bone Healing |
| | Abuse Recovery: Sexual | | Neglect Recovery |

| | *Never demonstrated* | *Rarely demonstrated* | *Sometimes demonstrated* |
|---|---|---|---|
| *m and t* | *Consistently demonstrated* | *Often demonstrated* | *Sometimes demonstrated* |
| | Asthma Self-Management | | Discharge Readiness: Independent Living |
| | Bowel Continence | | Mood Equilibrium |
| | Child Adaptation to Hospitalization | | |

| | *Severe* | *Substantial* | *Moderate* |
|---|---|---|---|
| *n and a* | *Severely compromised* | *Substantially compromised* | *Moderately compromised* |
| | Caregiver Lifestyle Disruption | | Immobility Consequences: Psycho-Cognitive |
| | Immobility Consequences: Physiological | | Immune Hypersensitivity Response |

|  *Mildly*<br>*compromised* | *Not*<br>*compromised* |
|---|---|
| *Mild* | *None* |

Swallowing Status: Esophageal Phase
Swallowing Status: Oral Phase
Swallowing Status: Pharyngeal Phase
Systemic Toxin Clearance: Dialysis
Thermoregulation
Thermoregulation: Newborn
Tissue Integrity: Skin & Mucous Membranes
Tissue Perfusion: Abdominal Organs
Tissue Perfusion: Cardiac
Tissue Perfusion: Cerebral
Tissue Perfusion: Peripheral
Tissue Perfusion: Pulmonary

Urinary Elimination
Will to Live

|  *Mild deviation*<br>*from normal range* | *No deviation*<br>*from normal range* |
|---|---|
| *Mild* | *None* |

Sensory Function: Proprioception
Sensory Function: Taste & Smell
Sensory Function: Vision

|  *Substantial* | *Extensive* |
|---|---|
| *Limited* | *None* |

Wound Healing: Primary Intention
Wound Healing: Secondary Intention

|  *Often demonstrated* | *Consistently demonstrated* |
|---|---|
| *Rarely*<br>*demonstrated* | *Never*<br>*demonstrated* |

Psychomotor Energy
Urinary Continence

|  *Mild* | *None* |
|---|---|
| *Mildly*<br>*compromised* | *Not*<br>*compromised* |

Pain: Disruptive Effects
Pain Level

**Table 2-6**  SUMMARY OF CHANGES IN SCALES (CHANGES ARE MARKED IN BOLD)

| Scale Number | NOC Scales | | |
|---|---|---|---|
| a | **Severely** compromised | Substantially compromised | Moderately compromised |
| b | **Severe** deviation from **normal** range | Substantial deviation from **normal** range | Moderate deviation from **normal** range |
| c | Dependent, does not participate | Requires assistive person & device | Requires assistive person |
| d | No Motion | Limited Motion | Moderate Motion |
| e | Not at all | To a slight extent | To a moderate extent |
| f | Not adequate | Slightly adequate | Moderately adequate |
| g | **10 and over** | 7-9 | 4-6 |
| h | Extensive | Substantial | Moderate |
| i | None | Limited | Moderate |
| j | None | Slight | Moderate |
| k | Never positive | Rarely positive | Sometimes positive |
| l | Very weak | Weak | Moderate |
| m | Never demonstrated | Rarely demonstrated | Sometimes demonstrated |
| n | Severe | Substantial | Moderate |
| o | No evidence | Limited evidence | Moderate evidence |
| p | Extreme delay from expected range | Substantial delay from expected range | Moderate delay from expected range |
| r | Poor | Fair | **Good** |
| s | Not at all satisfied | Somewhat satisfied | Moderately satisfied |
| t | Consistently demonstrated | Often demonstrated | Sometimes demonstrated |

| | | |
|---|---|---|
| Mildly compromised | Not compromised | |
| Mild deviation from **normal** range | No deviation from **normal** range | |
| Independent with assistive device | Completely independent | RETIRED |
| Substantial motion | Full motion | RETIRED |
| To a great extent | To a very great extent | RETIRED |
| Substantially adequate | Totally adequate | |
| 1-3 | None | |
| Limited | None | |
| Substantial | Extensive | |
| Substantial | Complete | RETIRED |
| Often positive | Consistently positive | |
| Strong | Very strong | |
| Often demonstrated | Consistently demonstrated | |
| **Mild** | None | |
| Substantial evidence | Extensive evidence | RETIRED |
| Mild delay from expected range | No delay from expected range | RETIRED |
| **Very** good | Excellent | |
| Very satisfied | Completely satisfied | ADDED |
| Rarely demonstrated | Never demonstrated | ADDED |

individual, family, or community after intervention. As *change in rating scores* were examined in our clinical sites, it was clear that nurses needed a way to document that the goal of interventions might be to maintain a rating at the current state. This was especially true for nursing home personnel working with the elderly and nurses in settings that provided care for terminally ill patients. In these cases it may be a major accomplishment to maintain a patient at a chosen rating, thus preventing a decline in that outcome. We hope this change is helpful to nurses in clinical sites using the Classification.

Two additional areas for documentation were added to the top of the outcome. *Care Recipient* specified as a Patient, Caregiver (specify), Parent (specify), Family Unit, or Community (specify) was added to allow for the documentation of who is receiving the care. This is useful when nurses are working with caregivers and parents and may be maintaining a family record with interventions being used with a variety of family members. *Data Source* deals with the source of the information used in the rating; for example, the nurse obtained information from the patient, family member, or caregiver; by direct observation; or from a clinical record. Health care agencies can determine whether these areas are useful to them. We believe the source of the data may be more than one of these categories and may become important to document in an electronic patient record.

Testing the outcomes in clinical sites also pointed out the need to document the location of fractures and wounds within the outcomes. Two diagrams have been added to the classification to meet this need. One is a skeleton with the bones of the body coded for the outcome Bone Healing. An area called *Site of fracture* allows addition of this code to the outcome. If more than one fracture is present, the nurse can create an outcome for each fracture and measure the outcome of each fracture separately. The second diagram added is a diagram of the body divided into sites for use with the two wound outcomes, Wound Healing: Primary Intention and Wound Healing: Secondary Intention. Again, the outcome provides a means to specify the site and follow more than one wound by identifying separate outcomes for each site. In several places the opportunity to specify exact data about an outcome has been added. For example, in the outcome Blood Loss Severity, the estimated blood loss can be included in the outcome.

The final addition to the format of the outcomes is documentation at the end of each outcome as to when the outcome was first published in the classification and the editions in which revisions were made. Most of the outcomes have "Revised 3rd edition" in this area if they had been published in previous editions because of the extensive work we have done in the last 4 years to test and refine the outcomes in the Classification. Documenting the history of each outcome is important ongoing work. We believe the inclusion of this information will help in our efforts to maintain a very current classification of nursing-sensitive patient outcomes. As part of the revisions of the outcomes in this edition, references were updated and definitions were modified to better fit the measurement scales attached to the outcomes. These changes are minor in most cases but have added to the quality of the work and the consistency across outcomes. We believe these changes will make the Classification easier to use in practice and educational settings.

## The Classification—Ongoing and Future Work

The current classification represents the completion of more than 8 years of research to develop and test a classification and taxonomy of nursing-sensitive patient outcomes. The Classification contains 330 outcomes for measuring the impact of nursing treatments on individual, family, and community outcomes. The 330 outcomes are classified in the taxonomy, which has 7 domains and 29 classes. All elements of the taxonomy are coded, including the measurement scales. Outcomes for individual patients continue to be identified for development by members of the team and clinician users. Currently, there are 35 outcomes on a list "for development." The research team performs the concept analyses that are needed to develop and evaluate the outcomes to be added to the NOC. This work is ongoing and continual update of the classification is needed to keep it relevant for clinical practice. This is crucial to having standardized language for outcome measurement in nursing. Since the publication of the last edition, several outcomes have been submitted from students and practicing nurses. These submissions are very helpful to the development of the Classification. We recognize contributors to this work in the front of the book.

Additional efforts are needed to develop and validate family and community level outcomes. New family and community level outcomes, such as Community Violence Level and Family Resiliency, are included in this edition. Domains and classes for family and community outcomes were added to the NOC taxonomy for these areas in the second edition. The NOC focus groups persist in doing this work; however, graduate students also elect to develop some of the outcomes related to their clinical specialties as part of their graduate work. More family and community level outcomes need to be developed to make these areas complete. Input from specialty organizations is also helpful in these areas.

## SUMMARY

This chapter provides an overview of the current outcomes classification and changes made to this edition based on testing in practice. Common questions about NOC are posed and answered. Current and future work of the NOC team is reviewed, emphasizing clinical field testing of the reliability, validity, sensitivity, specificity, and usefulness of the outcome measures.

A classification of nursing-sensitive patient, family, and community outcomes will never be complete but will continue to expand and improve with further knowledge of the discipline and testing in practice. Readers and users of the classification are encouraged to provide feedback to the research team. Identification of problems, issues, and outcomes for future development is also encouraged. Appendix G contains a review form that can be completed and returned to the team.

Although there is increasing interest in outcomes management, quality assessment and improvement, and effectiveness research, nursing remains largely invisible in large data sets, and little nursing effectiveness research is being conducted. Those nursing studies completed are often done in a single health care system and most are not reported. The use of NOC provides data so that contributions made by the nursing profession to health care are documented and made visible. The health care organizations that adopt NOC will not only be able to demonstrate nursing's accountability and contributions to health care but will also be able to compare the achievement of outcomes of care across time and settings. Testing over the last 8 years has demonstrated that nurses can make dramatic improvements in outcomes in a short period. With shorter lengths of stay in acute care institutions, it is critical that we learn how to best use our time so that the interventions we choose are effective in improving outcomes. We also need to learn what interventions are not effective or poorly timed in our current practice strategies. We need to learn more about what outcomes are core to nursing practice and identify key outcomes for specialty practice. This will benefit both education and practice.

Classification work of this kind is essential to our future as a profession. We invite all nurses to join in the effort to include standardized nursing languages in all clinical information systems so that nursing data will be available in large local, national, and international data sets. We also invite our colleagues to assist with further testing of the psychometric integrity and clinical usefulness of the NOC outcomes. Of the outcomes, to date 161 have not been evaluated for reliability, validity, sensitivity, and clinical usefulness with clinical data; and a number of the 169 outcomes evaluated in the Phase III research need further testing. Research by nurse scientists, clinicians, and graduate students that is published and shared with the NOC research team will greatly advance this work that is so important for the nursing profession and the clients that nurses serve. Armed with data that demonstrate nursing effectiveness, nurses will influence health policy to optimally benefit the individuals, families, and communities to whom they provide care.

## References

1. American Nurses Association. (1986). *Standards of community health nursing practice.* Kansas City, MO: Author.
2. Bond, S., & Thomas, L. H. (1991). Issues in measuring outcomes on nursing. *Journal of Advanced Nursing, 16,* 1492-1502.
3. Erben, R., Franzkowiak, P., & Wenzel, E. (1992). Assessment of the outcomes of health intervention. *Social Science Medicine, 35,* 359-365.
4. Grobe, S. J. (1990). Nursing intervention lexicon and taxonomy study; language and classification methods. *Advances in Nursing Science, 13,* 22-33.
5. Hegyvary, S. T. (1991). Issues in outcomes research. *Journal of Nursing Quality Assurance, 5,* 1-6.
6. Iowa Intervention Project. (2000). *Nursing Interventions Classification (NIC)* (3rd ed.). St. Louis, MO: Mosby.
7. Kuss, T., Proulx-Girouard, L., Lovitt, S., Katz, C.B., & Kennelly, P. (1997). A public health nursing model. *Public Health Nursing, 14,* 81-91.
8. Lang, N. M., & Clinton, J. F. (1984). Assessment of quality of nursing care. In H. H. Werley & J. J. Fitzpatrick (Eds.), *Annual Review of Nursing Research* (Vol. 2, pp. 135-163). New York: Springer.
9. Lohr, K. (1988). Outcome measurement: Concepts and questions. *Inquiry, 25,* 37-50.
10. Marek, K. D. (1997). Measuring the effectiveness of nursing care. *Journal of Nursing Outcomes Management, 1,* 8-11.
11. Marek, K. D. (1989). Outcome measurement in nursing. *Journal of Nursing Quality Assurance, 4,* 1-9.
12. McCloskey, J. C., & Bulechek, G. M. (1994). Standardizing the language for nursing treatments: An overview of the issues. *Nursing Outlook, 42,* 56-63.
13. Nadzam, D. M. (1991). The agenda for change: Update on indicator development and possible implications for the nursing profession. *Journal of Nursing Quality Assurance, 5,* 18-22.
14. North American Nursing Diagnosis Association (NANDA International). (2003). *Nursing diagnoses: Definitions & classification, 2003-2004.* Philadelphia: Author.
15. Rantz, M. J., & LeMone, P. (Eds.). (1995). Classification of nursing diagnoses. *Proceedings of the Eleventh Conference of the North American Nursing Diagnosis Association.*
16. Saba, V. K. (1992). The classification of home health care nursing diagnoses and interventions. *Caring, 11,* 50-57.
17. Stanhope, M., & Lancaster, J. (1996). *Community health nursing: Promoting the health of aggregates, families, and individuals* (4th ed.). St. Louis, MO: Mosby.
18. Tarlov, A. R., Ware, J. E., Greenfield, S. Nelson, E. C., Perren, E., & Zubkoff, M. (1989). The Medical Outcomes Study: An application of methods for monitoring the results of medical care. *Journal of the American Medical Association, 262,* 925-930.
19. Werley, H. H., & Lang, N. M. (Eds.). (1988). *Identification of the Nursing Minimum Data Set.* New York: Springer.
20. Werley, H. H., & Devine, E. C. (1987). The Nursing Minimum Data Set: Status and implications (pp. 540-551). In Hanna, K.J., Reimer M., Mills, W.C., & LeTourneau S. (Eds.). *Clinical judgment and decision-making: The future of nursing diagnosis.* New York: John Wiley.

# CHAPTER THREE

# Testing the NOC Outcomes With Clinical Data

Nursing's concern about its accountability for patient outcomes has waxed and waned since the time of Florence Nightingale.[17] Most efforts to assess the quality of nursing care have examined process outcomes rather than patient outcomes. Although several typologies of patient outcomes sensitive to nursing interventions were developed, few had accompanying measures for clinical use,[8,13] and their use in studies of quality has been minimal. In recent years, concerns about the cost of health care and subsequent methods of cost control raised parallel concerns that quality might be sacrificed. This has renewed interest in patient outcomes and their linkage with interventions in studies of health care effectiveness.[10,11] The use of large clinical data sets to assess the effectiveness of health care is now of particular interest.

There is greater recognition of the need to define and measure outcomes that are sensitive to nursing interventions. However, nursing interventions and patient outcomes that are responsive to nursing interventions are largely absent from large clinical and national data sets. Without the ability to abstract uniform nursing data from local clinical documentation systems, the inclusion of a Nursing Minimum Data Set (NMDS)[4] in large national health care databases, such as the Hospital Discharge Data Set (HDDS), is impossible. This means that nursing is essentially not represented in national data sets that are routinely analyzed for health policy decisions. Moreover, for nursing to be a full interdisciplinary participant in health care, to demonstrate accountability to consumers, and to inform policy to optimally benefit patients and families, data must be included in national data sets that can be used to evaluate the effectiveness and cost-effectiveness of nursing interventions.[1] It is clear that the quality of health care cannot be adequately determined if the practice of the largest group of providers (nurses) is not evaluated. It is equally clear that the effectiveness of nursing interventions will largely not be evaluated unless nurse clinicians are confident of the usefulness, reliability, and validity of standardized nursing interventions and patient outcomes that are responsive to nursing, such as the Nursing Interventions Classification (NIC) and the Nursing Outcomes Classification (NOC). Without this confidence, standardized nursing languages are not likely to be widely implemented in electronic clinical documentation systems, and hence, will not be available for inclusion in large national data sets. This is why the research team undertook the testing of the NOC outcomes with actual clinical data.

Phase III research was enabled by 4 years of National Institute of Nursing funding (RO1-N03437). The research involved testing of the psychometric integrity and practicality of the 190 outcome measures and procedures with the exception of 16 outcomes that pertained to children, published in the first edition of the NOC book.[7] For evaluation of the NOC outcomes and measures, interrater reliability, construct or criterion-related validity, change in rating scores (sensitivity), and usefulness of the outcomes and measures were tested in 10 field sites representing the continuum of care. The field settings included two academic, tertiary hospitals; three private, community (intermediate) hospitals; one long-term care nursing home; one community-based parish nursing practice; one ambulatory, academic nursing center staffed by nurse practitioners; and two community health nursing agencies providing home care (Visiting Nurse Associations) in four Midwestern states.

## ASSIGNING THE OUTCOMES FOR TESTING

For the purpose of facilitating the distribution of outcomes among the field sites, procedures were developed to determine which outcomes could be tested in all sites and which ones should be assigned to specific sites. These procedures began with determining core outcomes that were expected to be used in all sites.

## Determining Core Outcomes

Core outcomes were defined as those outcomes used by nurses to assess the effectiveness of nursing interventions in all 10 field settings. For determination of the core outcomes, nurses in each of the settings were surveyed and asked to rate for what percent of their patients each of the 190 NOC outcomes was relevant on a scale from 0% to 100% of the time. Twenty-four outcomes were rated by the nurses as used at least 50% of the time for patients in each of the 10 settings and these were defined as core outcomes. Table 3-1 contains a list of the core outcomes. The outcomes that are italicized in Table 3-1 are some previously reported with the use of preliminary data.[15]

## Distribution of Outcomes Among the Data Collection Sites

Based on the ratings of the frequency of use by nurses in the field settings, all 174 NOC outcomes to be tested were distributed among the field settings for evaluation of interrater reliability, validity, sensitivity, and usefulness. Thus some outcomes were tested in all of the settings, some in three or more but fewer than 10 field settings, and some in only two of the settings. The 24 core outcomes were assigned to be tested in all 10 settings. The aim was to obtain data from at least 50 patients for each of the core outcomes. For the remainder, the aim was to obtain data from a minimum of 25 patients for each outcome.

| Table 3-1 | NOC Core Outcomes |
| --- | --- |

| NOC Core Outcomes |
| --- |
| Ambulation: Walking |
| Comfort Level |
| *Communication Ability* |
| Endurance |
| Energy Conservation |
| Health Promoting Behavior |
| *Infection Status* |
| Information Processing |
| Knowledge: Disease Process |
| Knowledge: Medication |
| *Mobility Level* |
| Nutritional Status: Nutrient Intake |
| Pain: Disruptive Effects |
| *Pain Level* |
| Participation: Health Care Decisions |
| Quality of Life |
| Rest |
| Safety Behavior: Fall Prevention |
| *Self Care: Activities of Daily Living (ADL)* |
| Self-Care: Hygiene |
| Sleep |
| Social Support |
| *Tissue Integrity: Skin & Mucous Membranes* |
| Vital Signs Status |

## DATA COLLECTION AND MANAGEMENT

A registered nurse research assistant (RNRA) was employed in each of the field settings to coordinate and oversee the data collection. The RNRAs were trained in the data collection procedures by the NOC investigators. Following their training, the RNRAs trained the nurses in each of the field sites in the process of data collection and documentation using study data collection forms.

Each day the RNRA, clinical nurses, or staff nurses identified those patients with outcomes that were to be tested. With the assistance of the RNRA, the clinical nurse assigned to the patient rated the outcomes for the patient as appropriate. The RNRA identified a second nurse and asked the second nurse to independently rate the same outcomes for the same patient to determine interrater reliability. In some cases these two ratings were completed between shifts by the two RN team raters, and in other cases by two nurses visiting the patient in the home. The patient's age, gender, race/ethnicity, medical diagnoses, medications, nursing diagnoses, nursing interventions, and NOC outcome ratings were extracted from documentation in the clinical record by the RNRA. These data were transferred to the University of Iowa College of Nursing, entered into an Access database, and analyzed by using the SPSS for Windows software (SPSS, Inc., Chicago, IL).

## Reliability

Interrater reliability ratings were done at a minimum each time a nurse completed an outcome that she or he had not previously rated. For interrater reliability, two registered nurses (RNs) who rated the patient independently were asked to do so within a prespecified period, depending on the nature of the outcome and the practice setting. For example, in acute care hospital settings, each outcome was rated by the two nurse raters for the same patient within the same ½- to 1-hour period. The paired ratings were done within the same 1-day period in the long-term care nursing home setting and at the same patient visit in home care settings and nursing ambulatory care centers. If the two raters' agreement was less that 80%, they discussed the reasons for the differences in the rating and each repeated the rating. Both ratings by the two nurses were reported, and discussion comments were captured for the researchers to analyze.

For assessment of the extent to which the outcome measures were stable and consistent across raters, two types of agreement were calculated for this study: near agreement and absolute agreement. Near agreement is defined as the numerical ratings that do not differ by more than 1 value on the five-point Likert-type scale for both the label and its indicators. For example, if Nurse A rated Pain Level as 1 and Nurse B rated the patient's Pain Level as 2, this is calculated as an agreement. Absolute agreement is the percentage of identical paired ratings for the same outcome label. Criteria of 0.80 for near agreement and 0.60 for absolute agreement were considered acceptable evidence of rater concordance among nurses in the field settings who, at the beginning of the study, were mostly not experienced in using the NOC outcomes. The criterion estimates of interrater agreement should be increased after the outcomes have been implemented and nurses have become experienced in using the outcomes as evaluative measures.

Originally the kappa statistic was proposed as the measure of interrater reliability. Kappa is a statistic that can be used to estimate the agreement of two individuals' attempts to measure the same thing. However, the kappa statistic was designed for use when rating categories are nominal rather than ordinal. Kramer and associates[12] assert emphatically that the kappa statistic should not be used when rating categories are ordered, as with our scales. Further, they also discourage the use of kappa as a measure of interrater reliability whenever there are more than two rating categories, such as the five options on our measurement scales. Intraclass correlations (ICCs), on the other hand, are designed for use with interval-level ratings and may appropriately be extended to use with ordinal-level ratings.[14] An ICC is an estimate of the concordance or agreement among multiple paired ratings of the same phenomenon among members of a group. Use of ICCs permits the explicit choice of a measure that reflects the fact that all ratings of an outcome were not done by the same pair of raters.[3] In a preliminary report of 15 NOC outcomes, the kappa statistic was used to assess the stability of concordance among pairs of ratings.[15] Because NOC measures are quantified with five-point Likert-type scales, ICC was chosen for the final analysis of interrater reliability.[14] An ICC of 0.70 or better is considered acceptable evidence of concordance stability or interrater reliability.

## Validity

For most of the outcomes, standardized tools that measure the same or a similar concept were identified and used to estimate the validity of the corresponding NOC outcome. A complete list of the NOC outcomes and the tools or patient data selected to assess the validity of each outcome can be found in Appendix C. In this edition, criterion tools for outcomes tested have a plus sign by the reference used for these tools. Measures that exactly matched the definition of each NOC outcome were often difficult to find in the literature. In many cases the concept in the established tool was broader than the NOC concept or contained multiple concepts. The tool that came closest to measuring the same concept as the NOC outcome was selected. Following data collection, the nurses who were part of the NOC team were asked to judge how closely the concept measured by a criterion tool corresponded to the concept measured by the NOC outcome to which it was matched. Outcomes and criterion tools were assigned to nurses according to their area of specialization. At this time 40 of the criterion tools have been rated in this way. Only about one third of the criterion tools were judged to be a close match with the outcome. An analysis of variance showed that the correlations of the NOC rating with the score on the criterion measure were significantly higher ($p < 0.001$) when the tool was judged to be a close match than when it was judged to be only moderately or less well related.

No standardized tools were located for 38 NOC outcomes, most of which describe discrete physiological status. For the purpose of estimating the validity of these physiological outcomes (e.g., Vital Signs Status), standardized measures that correspond to the NOC indicators were extracted from the patient's clinical record, and an overall rating was given as the criterion measure for these outcomes. Criterion tools matching the NOC outcomes were also not found for the knowledge outcomes. Patient ratings were obtained for each outcome with the NOC measure. Correlation of the two measures for the number of patients for whom data were obtained was used to assess the validity of each NOC knowledge outcome measure. Because many of the standardized tools used to assess the validity of the NOC outcome measures did not capture the exact meaning of the outcome concept, midrange correlation coefficients were expected and thought to be sufficient evidence that the intended patient state was being measured. Thus the criterion estimate for validity was set at $r = 0.50$ or higher, coupled with statistical significance $p < 0.05$, indicating that the result occurred by chance 5 or less times in 100 calculations.

## Sensitivity

Sensitivity to change is another important aspect of the adequacy of a measure, that is, the extent to which a measure captures change in a phenomenon.[8,19] Sensitivity also refers to the extent to which the measure distinguishes gradations of the phenomenon. In health outcomes research, this sensitivity to change is often called *responsiveness to change*.[5] Measures that are able to gauge small changes are more responsive and sensitive. This latter aspect of sensitivity was examined for the NOC outcomes by comparing two measurements of the same outcome. The measures could be applied at baseline and then at discharge or at some other time subsequent to baseline. It is also possible to obtain a series of measures over time.

## Usefulness

Clinical usefulness is a critical attribute of outcomes that will be used by nurses to monitor and evaluate the effects of interventions for patients. This means that the outcomes must describe salient patient states, behaviors, and perceptions that are responsive to nursing interventions. The outcomes must also be clear, with unambiguous definitions and measures that nurses can rate (score) with ease and confidence. For the purpose of assessing clinical usefulness, the field site nurses were asked to comment on data collection forms about any difficulties using the outcomes and measures and provide suggestions for revision. The narrative comments were read by the research team, entered into a database, evaluated, and used to make the revisions of the outcomes and measures that appear in this edition.

## RESULTS
## Demographics of Patients

Although demographic data for some patients were missing, the data collected provide an overall view of characteristics of the sample and distributions among the study sites. Two thousand three hundred thirty-three persons (2333) for whom the NOC outcomes were rated were distributed among the 10 field settings as shown in Table 3-2. Seven hundred forty-five were hospitalized in tertiary care settings in Iowa and Minnesota in heart transplant, medical, cardiac, orthopedic, surgical, and neurology patient care units; 710 were hospitalized in intermediate care hospitals in Iowa and Minnesota in mental health, obstetrical, medical-surgical, critical care, and women's health units; and 165 were in a nursing home in Iowa. Six hundred forty-six were cared for in their homes by visiting nurses in Michigan or were patients who visited a nursing primary care clinic in Detroit, Michigan; and 67 were clients of parish nurses in Illinois. Patients' ages ranged from 49 to 87 years. Nursing home patients, on average, were the oldest among those in the study, followed by persons cared for by parish nurses. Patients in the intermediate community hospitals were the youngest, on average, and those in home care and primary nursing care settings were next youngest. More female patients were rated in each setting except in the tertiary care hospitals where men outnumbered women. White patients outnumbered patients of other ethnic and minority groups by more that 4 to 1, although there were nearly equal numbers of African American and white patients rated in the home care and primary nursing clinic sites. More than three fourths of the total number of patients had a high school education or higher degree. More patients in the Michigan sites had less than a high school education than those in other sites, although the Michigan sites were exceeded only by the intermediate care hospitals in the proportion of patients who had education beyond a bachelor's degree, including eight patients with doctoral degrees.

### Medical Diagnoses

The most frequent medical diagnoses among patients in the sample were clearly a function of the type of setting, the specific patient care units where patients were located, and the number of patients sampled in each setting (see Table 3-2). For example, in tertiary care hospitals a cardiac care unit, a heart transplant unit, and an orthopedic unit were among the units from which patients were selected for outcome ratings. Thus it is not surprising that cardiovascular disease and repair of hip fractures were the most frequent medical diagnoses in these sites. Similarly, in intermediate care hospitals, depression and manual delivery were the most frequent medical diagnoses because many patients selected were located in psychiatric and obstetrical units. In the nursing home, two dementia diagnoses were most frequent, as might be expected. Parish nurses rated outcomes for patients whose most frequent medical diagnoses were diabetes and stress, whereas in the Michigan sites, the most frequent medical diagnoses were two types of hypertension. This is likely due to the larger number of African American patients who visited the Detroit nursing primary care clinic.

### Nursing Diagnoses, Interventions, Outcomes, and Linkages

As with the most frequent medical diagnoses, the most frequent nursing diagnoses in the study sites are somewhat predictable by the site and the patient care units from which patients were selected. In tertiary care hospitals the nursing diagnoses Pain and Altered Protection were most frequent and likely reflect the highly acute condition of patients and surgical intervention (Table 3-3). In intermediate care hospitals, Knowledge Deficit was the most frequent diagnosis,

| Table 3-2 | NUMBER RATED, DEMOGRAPHICS, MEDICAL DIAGNOSES, AND LOCATION OF PERSONS FOR WHOM OUTCOME RATINGS WERE OBTAINED BY FIELD SETTING* |
|---|---|

| | Tertiary Hospitals | Intermediate Hospitals | Nursing Home | Parish Nursing | VNA/ Primary Care | Total |
|---|---|---|---|---|---|---|
| Number rated | 745 | 710 | 165 | 67 | 646 | 2333 |
| *Average Age (yr)* | 64 | 49 | 87 | 71 | 55 | 58 |
| *Gender* | | | | | | |
| *Female* | 335 | 500 | 132 | 55 | 365 | 1387 |
| *Male* | 405 | 221 | 33 | 10 | 271 | 940 |
| *Race/ethnicity* | | | | | | |
| African American | 11 | 28 | — | — | 291 | 330 |
| Native American/ other | 30 | — | — | — | 4 | 34 |
| Latino | 3 | 10 | — | — | 11 | 25 |
| Asian American | 1 | 8 | — | — | 3 | 12 |
| White | 720 | 640 | 165 | 65 | 307 | 1897 |
| *Education†* | | | | | | |
| *Some high school or less* | 69 | 100 | 13 | 3 | 148 | 333 |
| *High school graduate* | 119 | 350 | 34 | 18 | 255 | 776 |
| *Technical degree/some college* | 68 | 81 | 25 | 21 | 124 | 319 |
| *College degree* | 20 | 102 | 24 | 15 | 54 | 215 |
| *Some master's work/degree* | 34 | 76 | 5 | 5 | 41 | 161 |
| *Doctoral degree* | — | — | — | — | 8 | 8 |
| *Medical diagnoses* | | | | | | |
| Most frequent | Cardio-vascular Disease | Depression | Alzheimer's | Diabetes | Malignant Essential Hypertension | Depression |
| Second most frequent | Repair of Hip | Manual Assisted Delivery | Senile Dementia | Stress | Unspecified Essential Hypertension | Cardio-vascular |

*VNA,* Visiting Nurse Association.
*All totals will not add to number rated because of missing data.
†One tertiary site did not report education of patients rated.

**Table 3-3**   MOST FREQUENT LINKAGES OF NIC INTERVENTIONS AND NOC OUTCOMES WITH MOST FREQUENT NURSING DIAGNOSES

| Linkages | Tertiary Hospitals | Intermediate Hospitals | Nursing Home | Parish Nursing | VNA/Primary Care |
|---|---|---|---|---|---|
| Nursing Diagnosis | Pain | Knowledge Deficit | Confusion | Potential for Enhanced Spiritual Well-Being | Altered Health Maintenance |
| **Outcomes** | | | | | |
| Most frequent | Pain Control | Knowledge: Medication | Cognitive Orientation | Spiritual Well-Being | Risk Detection |
| Second most frequent | Pain: Disruptive Effects | Knowledge: Health Behaviors | Cognitive Ability | Quality of Life | Risk Control |
| **Interventions** | | | | | |
| Most frequent | Pain Management | Discharge Planning | Cognitive Stimulation | Spiritual Support | Health Education |
| Second most frequent | Analgesic Administration | Teaching: Individual | Dementia Management | Emotional Support | Risk Identification |
| **Nursing Diagnosis** | Altered Protection | Pain | Risk for Injury | Knowledge Deficit | Knowledge Deficit |
| **Outcomes** | | | | | |
| Most frequent | Safety Behavior: Fall Prevention | Pain Level | Safety Behavior: Fall Prevention | Health Seeking Behavior | Knowledge: Diet |
| Second most frequent | Infection Status | Pain Control | Pain Level | Health Orientation | Knowledge: Medication |
| **Interventions** | | | | | |
| Most frequent | Surveillance: Safety | Analgesic Administration | Fall Prevention | Health Education | Active Listening |
| Second most frequent | Anxiety Reduction | Pain Management | | Support Group | Teaching: Prescribed Medication |

*VNA*, Visiting Nurse Association.

followed by Pain. Nursing home patients' most frequent nursing diagnosis was Confusion. Risk for Injury was the second most frequent nursing diagnosis in the nursing home. Potential for Enhanced Spiritual Well-Being and Knowledge Deficit, consistent with the nature of parish nursing, were the most frequent nursing diagnoses for patients treated by parish nurses. Altered Health Maintenance and Knowledge Deficit were the most frequent diagnoses in home care and primary care nursing settings.

The most frequent nursing interventions and nursing-sensitive outcomes linked with these nursing diagnoses are also among those that would be expected (Table 3-3). For example, in tertiary and intermediate care hospitals, the most frequent NOC outcomes linked with the nursing diagnosis Pain were Pain Control, Pain: Disruptive Effects, and Pain Level, respectively, with Pain Management and Analgesic Administration selected by nurses most often as interventions to achieve the outcomes. Likewise, nurses in more than one setting linked Knowledge outcomes with a Knowledge Deficit diagnosis and the interventions selected reflect the care emphasis of the setting. Discharge Planning was the intervention most frequently selected by nurses in intermediate care hospitals with a focus on increasing knowledge of medications and healthy behaviors. Parish nurses selected the intervention Health Education for the outcome Health Seeking Behaviors. Home care and primary care nurses chose the interventions Active Listening and Teaching: Prescribed Medication to reduce a deficit in patients' knowledge about diet and medication. Finally, in the nursing home, the most frequent outcomes and interventions focused on cognitive function, safety, and monitoring the level of pain. Overall, the linkages of nursing-sensitive outcomes and nursing interventions with the most frequent nursing diagnoses of the patients in the study sample were consistent with linkages proposed by Johnson and colleagues and provide them some clinical support.[9]

## Education of Clinical Nurse Raters

The majority of field site nurses who provided outcome ratings for the study were in tertiary and intermediate care hospitals, which is a function of the larger number of nurses employed in these settings (Table 3-4). Nearly one half of the nurses in tertiary care hospitals had a diploma or associate degree and slightly more in intermediate care hospitals reported having a diploma or an associate degree in nursing. Only the intermediate hospitals and nursing home had licensed practical nurses who provided patient ratings, although they comprised less than 3% of the nurses in both settings. All of the settings had a similar proportion of nurses with a bachelor's degree in nursing (BSN), although the parish nursing and Michigan sites had a greater proportion of nurses with BSNs than the other sites and there were also proportionately more nurses with master's degrees in these sites. Michigan sites had the highest percent of nurses with master's and doctoral degrees in nursing. The average number of years of experience for the nurses was fairly equal in the study sites. On average, the nurse raters in the nursing home had the fewest years of experience and the parish nurses had the most years of experience.

**Table 3-4** PERCENT OF HIGHEST DEGREE AND YEARS OF EXPERIENCE OF CLINICAL NURSE RATERS BY FIELD SETTING

| | Tertiary Hospital | Intermediate Hospital | Nursing Home | Parish Nursing | Michigan | |
|---|---|---|---|---|---|---|
| Percentage of Sample | 37.7 | 40.4 | 7.7 | 4.3 | 9.9 | |
| **Highest Degree** | | | | | | |
| Licensed Practical Nurse | — | 2.1 | 2.5 | — | — | |
| Diploma in Nursing | 18.3 | 19.3 | 15.5 | 18.2 | 5.9 | |
| Associate Degree in Nursing | 28.6 | 32.3 | 25.5 | — | 3.9 | |
| Bachelor's Degree in Nursing | 27.4 | 29.7 | 26.5 | 31.8 | 37.3 | |
| Bachelor's Degree in Other Field | 12.6 | 9.4 | 8.7 | 18.2 | | |
| Master's Degree in Nursing | 7.4 | 3.1 | 8.5 | 18.2 | 41.2 | |
| Master's Degree in Other Field | 2.9 | — | 1.7 | 9.1 | 2.0 | |
| PhD or Other Doctorate in Nursing | — | — | 0.3 | — | 3.9 | |
| Doctorate in Other Field | | | | | | |
| Other | 1.7 | 4.2 | 12 | — | 2.0 | |
| | | | | | | **Overall** |
| Average Years of Experience | 13.8 | 17.3 | 13.73 | 27.9 | 17.22 | 16.29 |

## ADEQUACY OF THE NOC OUTCOMES

We set out to collect a minimum of 50 patient ratings for each of the core outcomes and a minimum of 25 ratings for each of the remaining outcomes that were tested. We achieved this goal with all of the core outcomes except Information Processing (46 ratings) and Self-Care: Hygiene (33 ratings). Several core outcomes had more than 50 ratings. Some data were obtained for 168 of the 190 NOC outcomes in the first edition. No data were collected for the 16 outcomes in Table 3-5 because they described the health status of children and there were no children in our sample. When the data were examined, there were six additional outcomes without data. These are listed in Table 3-5 also. A number of these relate to outcomes more likely to be collected in an outpatient setting. Data were collected on one outcome, Maternal Status: Postpartum, that was not in the first edition, increasing the number of outcomes with data to 169. This outcome was completed when data collection began and was pertinent to some patients.

The number of ratings for interrater reliability ranged from 1 to 166 per outcome for near agreement, from 1 to 134 for absolute agreement, and from 5 to 147 for criterion validity. Four outcomes had insufficient data (0 or 1 rating) for calculating interrater reliability. Appendix D contains the NOC outcomes with ratings for 25 or more patients and the reliability and validity estimates that were obtained, followed by those obtained for fewer than 25 patients. Validity estimates were obtained for all but 17 of the 169 outcomes and for all but 2 of the outcomes that were rated for at least 25 patients. The patient N refers to the number of patients with at least 1 baseline rating for the outcome. The N for IRR can be greater than the patient N when more than one pair of ratings were done on a patient.

### Reliability

For the 109 outcomes with more than 25 ratings, near agreement (no more than one value difference on the five-point rating scale) ranged from 76% to 100%, and agreement was 88% or higher for the majority of these outcomes. Absolute agreement on the outcome labels ranged from 38% to 100%. Absolute agreement on the label was 60% or higher for 75 outcomes. Intraclass correlations ranged from 0.11 to 1.00 and were ≥0.70 for 63 of the 107 outcomes. Fifty-three outcomes with at least 25 patient ratings (49%) had near agreement ≥80%, absolute label agreement coefficients ≥60%, and intraclass correlation coefficients ≥0.70. Thirty-seven (37) of these 53 outcomes had ratings for 40 or more patients.

| Table 3-5 | FIRST EDITION OUTCOMES WITHOUT DATA |
|---|---|

| Outcomes Related to Children | Other Outcomes |
|---|---|
| Child Adaptation to Hospitalization | Abuse Cessation |
| Child Development: 2 Months | Abuse Protection |
| Child Development: 4 Months | Abuse Recovery: Financial |
| Child Development: 6 Months | Abusive Behavior Self-Control |
| Child Development: 12 Months | Breastfeeding Weaning |
| Child Development: 2 Years | Knowledge: Child Safety |
| Child Development: 3 Years | |
| Child Development: 4 Years | |
| Child Development: 5 Years | |
| Child Development: Middle Childhood (6-11 years) | |
| Child Development: Adolescence (12-17 years) | |
| Growth | |
| Physical Maturation: Female | |
| Physical Maturation: Male | |
| Play Participation | |
| Thermoregulation: Neonate | |

There were 60 outcomes with fewer than 25 patient ratings. Near-agreement scores ranged from 55% to 100%, with the majority 90% or higher (n=33) for these outcomes. Absolute agreement on the outcome labels ranged from 33% to 100%. As with the 109 outcomes with a minimum of 25 ratings, the majority of absolute agreements were 60% or higher (n=42). The range of ICC coefficients was 0.02 to 1.00 and was ≥0.70 for 29 of the 60 outcomes. Twenty-five of the outcomes with fewer than 25 ratings (42%) had near agreement ≥80%, absolute agreement ≥60%, and ICC ≥0.70. Twenty-five of the 52 ICCs computed for the NOC outcomes with fewer than 25 patient ratings were between 0.50 and 0.79 with 18 coefficients 0.80 or higher. A slightly lower proportion of these outcomes had ICC coefficients that were between 0.50 and 0.79 (42%) than those outcomes for which at least 25 patients were rated (49%), and a larger proportion of the outcomes with at least 25 patient ratings had ICCs that were 0.70 or higher (58% vs. 48%). For the 169 outcomes that had intraclass coefficients computed, 60% (N = 102) of the coefficients were 0.68 or higher. Overall, reliability estimates were better for outcomes that had at least 25 patient ratings.

All of the NOC core outcomes (see Table 3-1) achieved or exceeded 80% reliability for near agreement. All of the core outcomes except Endurance (49%), Nutritional Status: Nutrient Intake (59%), Participation: Health Care Decisions (53%), and Safety Behavior: Fall Prevention (58%) met or exceeded the reliability criterion of 60% for absolute agreement. However, only Endurance fell below 50% for absolute agreement. Six outcomes, Comfort Level (0.68), Endurance (0.60), Energy Conservation (0.56), Safety Behavior: Fall Prevention (0.44), Sleep (0.65), and Tissue Integrity:

## Table 3-6  INTERRATER AGREEMENT FOR CORE OUTCOMES

| NOC Outcome | Pt N | IRR Near Agreement | | IRR Absolute Agreement | | Intra-class Correlation | |
|---|---|---|---|---|---|---|---|
| | | N | % | N | % | N | ICC |
| Ambulation: Walking | 134 | 97 | 91 | 65 | 88 | 65 | 0.95 |
| Comfort Level | 156 | 124 | 91 | 49 | 65 | 49 | 0.68 |
| Communication Ability | 52 | 43 | 94 | 41 | 63 | 41 | 0.77 |
| Endurance | 72 | 47 | 91 | 43 | 49 | 43 | 0.60 |
| Energy Conservation | 105 | 76 | 90 | 57 | 63 | 57 | 0.56 |
| Health Promoting Behavior | 66 | 42 | 83 | 38 | 74 | 38 | 0.82 |
| Infection Status | 74 | 61 | 94 | 55 | 78 | 55 | 0.73 |
| Information Processing | 46 | 37 | 93 | 34 | 71 | 34 | 0.87 |
| Knowledge: Disease Process | 93 | 54 | 92 | 46 | 63 | 46 | 0.81 |
| Knowledge: Medication | 76 | 52 | 86 | 50 | 68 | 50 | 0.84 |
| Mobility Level | 140 | 87 | 95 | 72 | 92 | 72 | 0.97 |
| Nutritional Status: Nutrient Intake | 72 | 50 | 90 | 44 | 59 | 44 | 0.79 |
| Pain: Disruptive Effects | 67 | 52 | 89 | 43 | 70 | 43 | 0.82 |
| Pain Level | 166 | 130 | 92 | 82 | 70 | 82 | 0.78 |
| Participation: Health Care Decisions | 51 | 37 | 89 | 34 | 53 | 34 | 0.70 |
| Quality of Life | 61 | 49 | 89 | 42 | 64 | 42 | 0.80 |
| Rest | 54 | 42 | 94 | 38 | 63 | 38 | 0.72 |
| Safety Behavior: Fall Prevention | 72 | 58 | 87 | 53 | 58 | 53 | 0.44 |
| Self-Care: Activities of Daily Living (ADLs) | 186 | 166 | 94 | 134 | 84 | 134 | 0.84 |
| Self-Care: Hygiene | 33 | 27 | 93 | 25 | 88 | 25 | 0.95 |
| Sleep | 64 | 46 | 92 | 41 | 66 | 41 | 0.65 |
| Social Support | 53 | 43 | 92 | 40 | 73 | 40 | 0.75 |
| Tissue Integrity: Skin & Mucous Membranes | 82 | 60 | 94 | 55 | 62 | 55 | 0.59 |
| Vital Signs Status | 70 | 57 | 94 | 55 | 76 | 55 | 0.88 |

Skin & Mucous Membranes (0.59) did not meet the 0.70 criterion for ICC; however, the coefficients indicate a fair level of concordance between different pairs of nurse raters except for Safety Behavior: Fall Prevention. Endurance and Safety Behavior: Fall Prevention were the two outcomes that did not meet the criteria for absolute agreement and ICC. Sixteen (16) core outcomes meet the criteria for near agreement, absolute agreement, and ICC. Although intraclass correlation was used rather than the kappa statistic for the final analysis and cannot be directly compared, overall the estimates of reliability remain similar to those of the preliminary findings for 15 of the outcomes previously published using kappa.[15]

## Validity

For evidence of validity, 72 of the outcomes met or exceeded $r = 0.50$. All but four of these correlations were statistically significant. The proportions of outcomes that met this criterion were about equal for outcomes with 25 or more interrater reliability ratings, and those with fewer ratings were 43% and 42%, respectively. Eighteen additional outcomes had validity estimates between 0.40 and 0.49, and all but three were statistically significant. An additional 32 outcomes achieved estimates of validity between 0.25 and 0.39, and 19 of these correlations were not statistically significant; this may be partly due to the small number of patient ratings. The magnitude of the correlations for 30 outcomes was less than 0.25, and validity was not assessed for 17 of the outcomes.

Correlations between the outcome and the criterion measure were ≥0.50 for 10 of the 24 core outcomes. Eight additional core outcome measures were correlated 0.30 to 0.49 with a criterion measure. Thus only five outcomes were correlated less than 0.30 with a criterion—Mobility Level, Tissue Integrity: Skin & Mucous Membranes, Safety Behavior: Fall Prevention, Participation: Health Care Decisions, and Comfort Level. Only one of the outcomes, Self-Care: Hygiene, had no measure of validity because no tool was available.

## Sensitivity

A baseline and at least one follow-up rating were collected on 165 outcomes, and more than one follow-up rating was collected on 99 outcomes. There were 4215 ratings that included a baseline and at least one follow-up rating; 795 of these include at least two or more follow-up ratings. Information on the 165 outcomes with the baseline and second ratings appear in Appendix D. Change scores ranged from −3 to +4 with standard deviation (SD) scores ranging from 0.00 to 1.45. The majority of the outcomes had average change scores that were positive (N = 130) indicating that, on average, the patient state improved between ratings. Twenty (20) of the outcomes had average scores that were negative, indicating that the patient state, on average, deteriorated in relation to these outcomes between ratings. Fifteen of the outcomes had average change scores of 0.00, indicating that, on average, no change in patient state occurred between ratings.

Of the 15 ratings with an average change of zero, 3 had only one paired rating. Only one of the outcomes, Caregiving Endurance Potential with 6 ratings, showed no change in any of the scores. Transfer Performance had the widest range in change scores, −3 to +1 with an SD of 0.80. Blood Transfusion Reaction Control and Leisure Participation had a range in scores from −2 to +2 with SD of 1.22 and 1.03 respectively. Despite average change scores of 0.00, the only outcome that showed no change when more than one rating was done was Caregiving Endurance Potential. The outcomes with average change scores of 0.00 were not representative of any particular domain.

Fifty-nine (59), or approximately 36% of the ratings, showed a positive change ≥0.50 and 14 showed a change ≥1.00. The widest range in change scores for the 14 was for Distorted Thought Control, −3 to +4 with an SD of 1.33. Eight of the 14 outcomes are from the Psychosocial Domain, and a number of these were selected for patients on a psychiatric unit. The 20 change scores with average negative ratings showed a much smaller range, −0.03 to −0.73 with an SD of 0.35 and 1.17, respectively, than the change scores with positive ratings. Only three outcomes in this group had change scores ≥−0.50, and two of them had a small number of ratings.

There is a wide range in the average number of days between baseline and the second rating, 0 to 283 (Appendix D). Eleven outcomes had one fewer rating for days (Count) than the number of ratings (N) because times for the two ratings were not accurately recorded and therefore not counted in the average number of days between ratings. Sixty-two, or approximately 37% of the outcomes, had an average of ≥10 days between ratings compared to only 17 (10%) with ≥75 days between ratings. The difference in time between ratings was greatly influenced by the type of setting in which the outcome was measured. Outcomes with longer periods between ratings include a number that were collected in the nursing home setting; for example, outcomes that measured Cognitive Ability, Muscle Function, ADLs, and Urinary Continence. Others such as Health Beliefs were assessed in the nurse-managed clinics.

## Usefulness

Most clinical field nurses reported that the outcomes were clinically useful; however, the nurses also provided a great deal of feedback about how the outcomes, indicators, and scales might be revised to increase their usefulness and practicality. There were a number of suggestions for revisions of definitions of the outcomes, for changes in the indicators, and for changes in the scales. Some nurses also recommended new outcomes for development. The most frequent comments had to do with how to use the indicator rating to arrive at a rating of the outcome label and concerns about indicators that were stated awkwardly for the nurses to rate. For example, in an attempt to develop outcome labels that referred to a neutral or positive concept, a number of outcomes had indicators that were stated in the reverse of what would ordinarily be expected, such as "spasticity not present" and "seizure activity not present" for the outcome Neurological Status: Central Motor Control. The revisions that were made in response to the feedback from the clinical nurse raters and from the RNRAs in each site are discussed in Chapter 2.

## DISCUSSION

The results of the study indicate that nurses must be oriented to the NOC outcomes to use them effectively in their practice. Measurement of outcomes by nurses using a Likert-type scale, like those used with the NOC outcomes, is fairly rare. The tradition has been for nurses to use goals rather than outcomes and to simply document whether or not a goal was met. Thus the nurses in the field sites tended to be relatively inexperienced with use of the NOC outcomes at the beginning of the study, although they were all trained by the RNRA in each site. Many of the outcomes were also not familiar concepts to nurses as outcomes. As more ratings were performed on the same outcomes, the nurse raters became more accurate and more in agreement. The overall agreement was 67% at baseline, 77% for the second rating, and 80% at the third rating. This may be one reason that the outcomes that had a larger number of ratings tended to have higher interrater reliability coefficients. While this was not true for every outcome, it did occur for many. These results illustrate the importance of thorough training of nurses in the use of the outcomes before implementing their use in clinical documentation, as well as the importance of regular monitoring of nurse interrater reliability throughout the ongoing use of the outcomes.

In the field sites as a whole, the nurse raters had an average of 16 or more years of experience in nursing, which supports confidence in their ability to evaluate patient outcome status and rate the outcome measures. The proportion of nurse raters with a diploma and associate degree in nursing and the proportion with a bachelor's or higher degree were nearly equal in the tertiary care hospitals, intermediate care hospitals, and the nursing home. In contrast, 77.3% of parish nurses had a bachelor's or higher degree, and 84.4% of nurses in the Michigan settings had a bachelor's or higher degree. It was not possible to sort out in this study the separate effects on interrater reliability of the nurse raters' education level, how well the nurse raters knew the patient, the specific NOC outcomes rated, and the site, because all of these variables were highly correlated with one another for the outcome ratings done. To illustrate, the set of NOCs selected in the nursing home differed from those selected in other sites, and the nurse raters in the nursing home were much more likely to know the patient well than raters in other sites, especially the acute care sites. A study specifically designed to evaluate the effects of each of these variables would be highly desirable.

Further evaluation of the NOC field site data should include an assessment of the relationship of years of experience and education to reliability of outcome measurement. These results would better inform health care organizations about the training and experience needed for use of the NOC outcomes for clinical documentation and areas in which nurses need additional training. The results would also be helpful in hiring decisions and in determining the responsibilities that are assigned to nurses with specific amounts and types of nursing preparation.

Percent agreement estimates of interrater reliability of the core outcomes were all above the standard of 80% agreement that had been determined before data collection. Intraclass correlations were also mostly above or near the standard of 0.70. Safety Behavior: Fall Prevention and Energy Conservation had the lowest ICCs and should be a priority for further testing. This is especially important, since these are two outcomes most frequently used by nurses to monitor patient status following interventions for prevalent nursing diagnoses.

The higher near-agreement reliability coefficients may suggest that a three-point Likert-type scale would achieve more consistent interrater ratings of the outcomes. Raters often have difficulty discerning scores that are midway between the lowest score and the middle score and the middle score and the highest score, especially when there are no additional specific anchors. Three-point scales could be compared with five-point scales by using clinical data and nurses who are comfortable with the use of the NOC outcomes to determine whether they perform better psychometrically than the current five-point NOC scales. The value of a more precise interrater reliability must be weighed against the loss of discrimination and sensitivity to intervention effects with a five-point scale.

Although a higher percentage of outcomes with fewer than 25 patient ratings had validity coefficients that were not statistically significant, a number had quite good psychometric properties. Because a larger number of ratings might have resulted in statistical significance for the validity of many of these outcomes, the results support the reliability and validity of most of the 169 outcomes that were tested. For many outcomes, the standardized criterion measures did not match the outcome concept, and few ratings of the outcome and standardized measure were obtained for some. Yet many of the coefficients reached substantial magnitude, if not statistical significance. For these reasons and the expected midrange correlations of the NOC outcomes and standardized measures, the results support the validity of the majority of NOC outcomes and measures and support confidence in the integrity of the outcomes and measures.

Several of the measures of the NOC outcomes did not meet the correlation standard for criterion validity ($r \geq 0.50$), although most were in, or approaching, the moderately correlated range ($r = 0.40$ to $0.50$). As noted, moderate correlations are reasonable to expect, since many of the standardized measures that were located did not assess exactly the same concept as the NOC outcome. Although overall the study data provide support for the validity of most of the outcomes, further research to estimate validity is clearly needed. This is especially true for outcomes that had correlations below the correlation criterion of 0.50 and for those outcomes for which limited or no data were collected to assess their validity. The complete reliability and validity data for the 169 outcomes for which at least some data were collected can be found in Appendix D.

Careful evaluation of all of the data is needed to determine the adequacy and practicality of the NOC measures. Standardized measures that are currently used clinically, such as the commonly used 11-point Numeric Pain Intensity Scale[18] for Pain Level and the Mini-Mental State Examination (MMSE)[2,6] for Cognitive Ability, may perform better than the NOC measures. Because of the relatively low estimate of validity for Pain Level ($r = 0.28$) and the lower ICC ($r = 0.54$) for Cognitive Ability, these scales are not recommended as single outcome measures for clinical use until the NOC measures are tested more extensively. Clearly, the criterion tool that was used to test the validity of Tissue Integrity: Skin & Mucous Membranes was inappropriate, since the Braden Scale is a tool used to assess risk for skin breakdown rather than current status of skin integrity. Likewise, use of the MMSE is questionable for assessment of the cognitive ability of all persons. There is recent evidence that the MMSE is not the best tool for measuring the cognitive status of persons with dementia, a likely prevalent diagnosis among patients in most of the study settings.[16]

According to comments, the nurses found most of the outcomes and measures easy to use and were positive about the advantages of the outcomes, whether documented manually or electronically. Nurses who had electronic documentation systems, however, were more positive about use of outcomes because computerized documentation requires less time. Nonetheless, the field site nurses offered a number of suggestions to make the outcomes more useful. Some were easily accomplished, such as simple editorial changes. However, others are more difficult to resolve such as questions about whether or not to rate each indicator and how ratings of individual indicators should be used to rate the overall outcome. For example, should the indicator ratings only be used as a guide to decide the outcome rating, or should the indicator scores be averaged and that score used as the outcome score? In the study, the clinical field nurses used an average of 1.69 to 23 indicators in determining the score on the outcome scales. The average percentage of indicators used for the measurement of each outcome ranged from 16.9% to 100%.

A common concern among the clinical nurse raters was the difficulty of using indicators that were stated in the reverse of what would ordinarily be expected. A number of indicators were stated in this manner in an effort to not use negative outcome labels. An example is the outcome, Immune Status, with indicators "recurrent infections not present" and "chronic fatigue not present." Nurses found these indicators awkward and difficult to rate. As a result, the research team decided to split the indicators and scales, using two different scales for the same outcome. This enabled every indicator to be stated more simply and logically, such as "chronically fatigued" rather than "chronic fatigue not present." Outcomes that use two different scales to rate the indicators are included in this edition of the book. As mentioned previously, other revisions of the outcomes and indicators that were the result of feedback from the clinical field site nurses are discussed in more detail in Chapter 2.

## IMPLICATIONS AND FUTURE NEEDED RESEARCH

The research team is continuing to develop, validate, and classify outcomes and outcome measures for individuals, families, and communities. There is a list of outcomes to be developed and assessed for content validity that will require future clinical testing. Outcomes proposed for addition to the Classification are regularly received from clinicians throughout the United States. Proposed outcomes from international colleagues need to be received for inclusion as well. Cross-cultural studies of the reliability and validity of the NOC outcomes with clinical data are needed to evaluate their adequacy for use with ethnic and racial minorities and in international education, research, and practice.

There is a need to continue to examine the reliability and validity of the 169 NOC outcomes in a more comprehensive sample of settings and types of patient care units. Furthermore, 70 outcomes were added to the NOC in the second edition and 76 more, in this edition, for a total of 330 outcomes in the NOC. These additional outcomes should be tested with clinical data, along with those of the 190 published in the first edition of the NOC book, which were not tested in the phase III study (N=22). Nurses who choose to use these outcomes in their practice should remain aware that reliability and validity data are not available for the additional outcomes.

The NOC team encourages the use of the outcomes in education, research, and practice and hopes that nurse educators, researchers, and clinicians will assist in the evaluation of the integrity of the outcomes. Nurses who test any of the outcomes for reliability, validity, sensitivity, and/or usefulness are requested to contact the NOC investigators or the Center for Nursing Classification and Clinical Effectiveness, College of Nursing at The University of Iowa, to share the results of their research. Only through systematic testing by a large number of nurse users will the psychometric integrity of the outcomes be established and their clinical usefulness optimized. These goals are important to all nurses, the profession, and the clients whom nurses serve because of the importance of reliable and valid outcome data for the development of evidence-based nursing practice and the need for nursing to demonstrate its accountability for quality care.

Several issues emerged as a result of reliability and validity testing of the NOC outcomes and are being pursued. For example, the data indicate that the NOC scale (Extent of compromise) can be problematic. One of the adjustments used consistently in a number of sites was application of percentages to the scale. Examples of this can be found in Chapter 4 and a related appendix. Further evaluation of the scales by using percentages should be done. In an attempt to resolve the issue of whether or not the outcome indicators should be rated, and if so, how the final rating for the outcome should be determined, one site is rating the outcome and not the indicators. If these "outcome only" ratings are shown to be reliable and valid and a comparison with the reliability and validity estimates for the outcomes when indicators are rated is favorable, it may suggest that nurses need only rate the outcome labels. This is an important issue, given that most nurses are greatly concerned about the burden of documentation. The issue also has important implications for the development of electronic clinical nursing information systems. The NOC investigators will report the comparison of results when only the outcome label is rated versus rating the outcome label and indicators in a subsequent publication.

The issue of whether or not reliable and valid assessment of outcome status can be made without highly specific, descriptive anchors for scale values has existed for some time but was reinforced during the field testing of NOC outcomes. The RNRA coordinators reported that nurses were uncertain about how to decide the scale value for an outcome when they first used the NOC outcomes. The results of the field testing provide some data to help resolve this issue. Field site nurses' suggestions for the development of anchors will be used. Nurses who have had clinical experience with the outcomes will also be consulted to construct and test more specifically anchored scale values. The development of more specific anchors for some outcomes would likely improve interrater reliability, but the development of anchors is difficult and it remains to be seen whether they can be developed without making the outcomes too condition-specific. In regard to validity, some of the standardized tools that were questionable matches with the outcome concept may be the reason for lower correlation coefficients. Greater attention must be given to the development of theory to support the expected relationship between the NOC concept and the concept measured by the standardized tool to better assess criterion and construct validity.

Overall, the study findings provide support for the reliability and validity of a large number of the NOC outcomes. However, the findings indicate that revisions will be needed to enhance the reliability and validity of some outcomes and measures. Clearly, if reliability is compromised, validity will be affected.[10] Hence a priority for future research is to improve the consistency or stability with which some outcomes are rated. Revision of some outcomes and further testing are required. It is also necessary to systematically evaluate the "responsiveness" of the NOC outcomes to nursing interventions. Responsiveness has been assessed by using concept analyses but awaits empirical verification in effectiveness and efficacy studies. Only now are the data being used in a few studies to evaluate nursing interventions being implemented. Now that a comprehensive classification of patient outcomes has been developed with substantial evidence of the reliability and validity of a large number of the outcomes, nurse researchers can more easily examine the unique contribution of nursing interventions to changes in outcome status. This will provide empirical evidence of the responsiveness or nonresponsiveness of the outcomes to nursing interventions.

## CONCLUSION

Outcomes that are reliable, valid, and responsive to nursing interventions are needed for several reasons. Clinicians must have confidence in the integrity of outcome measures to monitor the progress, or lack of progress, of their patients. Administrators and clinician peers need dependable outcome data to evaluate competency and to hold individuals and groups of nurses accountable for a certain standard of practice. Clearly, standards of practice, quality and outcome management programs, and the selection of areas of needed knowledge development and dissemination among clinicians are dependent on reliable and valid measurement of patient outcomes that are responsive to nursing interventions. Finally, reliable and valid outcomes are needed for nursing efficacy and effectiveness research to further develop evidence-based practice and to influence health policy.

The study results indicate that many NOC outcomes are sufficiently reliable and valid for use in documenting the effectiveness of nursing interventions. Additional testing will be needed to refine some measures and to evaluate the outcomes and measures that continue to be developed. Although the findings are not conclusive for every one of the 169 outcomes that were tested, they are very encouraging. The findings indicate that nurses rate most outcomes with a high degree of agreement and that the development of valid measures of all patient outcomes is highly probable. The phase III results provide evidence that the majority of NOC standardized patient outcomes are adequate and useful for evaluating the effectiveness of nursing interventions and for comparisons among patient populations, care settings, and providers. The results should encourage and hasten the adoption of NOC outcomes in clinical settings and in computerized clinical information systems. As this occurs, the opportunities for nursing effectiveness research and effectiveness research on the interventions of other disciplines to inform patients, health care providers, and policy makers will multiply exponentially. It is difficult to overestimate the potential and importance of the contribution that this information will make to quality health care worldwide.

## References

1. American Nurses Association. (1997). *Nursing Informatics & Data Set Evaluation Center (NIDSEC) standards and scoring guidelines.* Washington, DC: Author.
2. Anthony, J. C., LeResche, L., Niaz, U., VonKorff, M. R., & Folstein, M. F. (1982). Limits of the "Mini-Mental State" as a screening test for dementia and delirium among hospital patients. *Psychological Medicine, 12,* 397-408.
3. Armstrong, G. (1981). The intraclass correlation as a measure of interrater reliability of subjective judgments. *Nursing Research, 30,* 14-15, 320A.
4. Brook, H. L. (1989). Practice guidelines and practicing: Are they compatible? *Journal of the American Medical Association, 262,* 3027-3030.
5. Epstein, R. S. (2000). Responsibilities in quality of life assessment: Nomenclature, determinants, and clinical applications. *Medical Care, 38*(Suppl. II), 91-94.
6. Folstein, M. F., Folstein, S. E., & McHugh, P. R. (1975). "Mini-Mental State": A practical method for grading the cognitive state of patients for the clinician. *Journal of Psychiatric Research, 12,* 189-195.
7. Iowa Outcomes Project. (1997). *Nursing Outcomes Classification (NOC)* (1st ed.). St. Louis, MO: Mosby.
8. Iowa Outcomes Project. (2000). *Nursing Outcomes Classification (NOC)* (2nd ed.). St. Louis, MO: Mosby.
9. Johnson, M., Bulechek, G., Dochterman, J., Maas, M., & Moorhead, S. (2001). *Nursing diagnoses, outcomes, and interventions: NANDA, NOC, NIC linkages.* St. Louis, MO: Mosby.
10. Johnson, M., & Maas, M. (1999). Nursing-sensitive patient outcomes: Development and importance for use in assessing health care effectiveness. In E. Cohen & V. DeBack. (Eds.), *Outcomes and collaboration in case management.* St. Louis, MO: Mosby.
11. Johnson, M., & Maas, M. (1995). Classification of nursing-sensitive patient outcomes. In ANA. *Nursing data systems: The emerging framework* (pp. 177-183). Washington, DC: The American Nurses Association.
12. Kramer, H. C., Periyakoil, V. S., & Noda, A. (2002). Kappa coefficients in medical research. *Statistics in Medicine, 21,* 2109-2129.
13. Lang, N. M., & Marek, K. D. (1990). The classification of patient outcomes. *Journal of Professional Nursing, 6,* 153-163.
14. Laschinger, H. K. (1992). Intraclass correlations as estimates of interrater reliability in nursing research. *Western Journal of Nursing Research, 14,* 241-247.
15. Maas, M., Reed, D., Reeder, K., Kerr, P., Specht, J., Johnson, M., et al. (2002). NOC outcomes: A preliminary report of field testing. *Journal of Nursing Outcomes Management, 6,* 112-119.
16. Pasqualetti, P., Moffa, F., Chiovenda, P., Carlesimo, G. A., Caltagirone, C., & Rossini, P. M. (2002). Mini-Mental State Examination and Mental Deterioration Battery: Analysis of the relationship and clinical implications. *Journal of the American Geriatric Society, 50,* 1577-1581.

17. Salive, M. E., Mayfield, J. A., & Weissman, N. W. (1990). Patient outcomes research teams and the Agency for Health Care Policy and Research. *Health Services Research, 25,* 697-708.
18. U. S. Department of Health and Human Services. (1992). *Acute pain management: Operative or medical procedures and trauma* (AHCPR Publication No. 92-0032). Rockville, MD: Public Health Service Agency for Health Care Policy and Research.
19. Ware, J. E., & Sherbourne, C. D. (1992). The MOS 36-item short-form health survey (SF-36), I. Conceptual framework and item selection. *Medical Care, 30,* 473-481.

# CHAPTER FOUR

# Using NOC in Clinical Settings

The Nursing Outcomes Classification (NOC) was developed to measure change in patient status for the purpose of evaluating the effects of nursing interventions. Although NOC was developed for nursing, other health professionals have found the outcomes useful for evaluating effects of their interventions. The authors encourage the use of the Classification by others and encourage other disciplines to contribute indicators specific to their practice. The outcomes measure patient status in a number of domains as identified in the taxonomy in Part Two. Measurement is not limited to functional and physiological status but includes measures of psychosocial, knowledge, and behavioral status. NOC also includes outcomes for an individual patient, a caregiver in the home setting, a family, and a community. This chapter discusses the selection and use of NOC outcomes in clinical practice. Although it is written from a nursing perspective, the process of selecting and using NOC outcomes can be applied to other disciplines.

## SELECTING THE OUTCOME

Selecting patient outcomes for a particular patient or a group of patients is one step in the nurse's clinical decision-making process. Variable outcomes, such as those in the NOC, will be selected in much the same manner as an outcome goal. The first judgment the nurse makes is to determine the pertinent health concerns and diagnoses associated with the patient's presenting condition. This judgment is generally based on a patient assessment that includes both data collection and data analysis. A variety of resources outline the steps and data sources used in the assessment process.[14,15] Once the health concerns and/or diagnoses have been identified, the nurse is ready to consider the selection of patient outcomes. A number of factors are considered in selection of an outcome including (1) the type of health concern, (2) the diagnosis or health problem with the defining characteristics and related factors or risk factors, (3) patient characteristics, (4) patient preferences, and (5) treatment options.[6,8]

### Type of Health Problem

Health concerns can be categorized as (1) problems for referral that are issues addressed primarily by other health providers, (2) interdisciplinary problems that are issues addressed collaboratively with other providers, and (3) nursing diagnoses that are issues for which the nurse has primary responsibility.[15] If the health concern falls into the first category, the primary responsibility for identifying the desired outcome will usually reside with the responsible health care provider. Examples of these concerns may be financial concerns referred to a social worker or spiritual concerns referred to a spiritual advisor. However, associated problems, such as anxiety or depression, may accompany these concerns and require the nurse to work collaboratively with the primary health care provider when outcomes are considered. If the health concern falls into the second category, the nurse and other responsible providers should work together to identify the outcome. This frequently occurs when the nurse and physical therapist or nurse and dietician collaborate about the outcomes that may be achieved in relation to a rehabilitation program or instructions about a new diet. If the health concern is a nursing diagnosis, the nurse should assume primary responsibility for identifying patient outcomes related to the diagnosis.

### Patient's Diagnosis or Health Problem

A diagnosis is a judgment based on an assessment and analysis of a patient's health status. It might be a nursing diagnosis, a medical diagnosis, or a diagnosis made by another health care practitioner. Although all health-related diagnoses are considered when the nurse selects an outcome, many of the outcomes of concern to nurses arise out of a nursing diagnosis. The nursing diagnosis might be related to another diagnosis, for example, a medical diagnosis, or may represent a patient health problem that is independent of other diagnoses. The common standardized language for nursing diagnoses is that of the North American Nursing Diagnosis Association (NANDA).[13] NANDA defines a nursing diagnosis as a "clinical judgment about individual, family, or community responses to actual or potential health problems/life processes" (p. 245)[13] that forms the basis for selecting nursing interventions to achieve patient outcomes. The diagnosis consists of a name, a definition, the defining characteristics, and risk factors if it is an actual diagnosis. If the diagnosis is a risk diagnosis, it includes the name, definition, and risk factors. Defining characteristics are the cues that cluster together and in essence characterize the diagnosis. Related factors are associated with the diagnosis as antecedent, contributing, or associated factors that increase vulnerability to the specific problem. Examples of an actual diagnosis and a risk diagnosis can be found in Boxes 4-1 and 4-2.

---

**Box 4-1**

## NANDA Activity Intolerance

**Activity Intolerance**

*Definition*

Insufficient physiological or psychological energy to endure or complete required or desired daily activities

*Defining Characteristics*

Verbal report of fatigue or weakness
Abnormal heart rate or blood pressure response to activity
Electrocardiographic changes reflecting arrhythmias or ischemia
Exertional discomfort or dyspnea

*Related Factors*

Bed rest or immobility
Generalized weakness
Imbalance between oxygen supply/demand
Sedentary lifestyle

---

**Box 4-2**

## NANDA Risk for Activity Intolerance

**Risk for Activity Intolerance**

*Definition*

At risk for experiencing insufficient physiological or psychological energy to endure or complete required or desired daily activities

*Risk Factors*

Inexperience with the activity
Presence of circulatory/respiratory problems
History of previous intolerance
Deconditioned status

When an outcome is selected for a patient, consideration should be given to the definition, defining characteristics, and related factors or the risk factors for a risk diagnosis. For example, based on the definition of Activity Intolerance, the nurse might select Activity Tolerance, Endurance, Psychomotor Energy, or Self-Care Status as an outcome pertinent to the definition. Activity Tolerance and Endurance are generally related to insufficient physiological energy, while Psychomotor Energy is related to insufficient psychological energy. The outcome Self-Care Status may be selected when the nurse is more interested in the patient's ability to carry out activities of daily living and other self-care activities. When the defining characteristics are considered, Vital Signs, Cardiac Pump Effectiveness, or Respiratory Status: Ventilation might be selected as intermediate outcomes that must improve if the patient is to increase his or her activity tolerance. Again, the related factors might indicate the selection of intermediate outcomes such as Mobility, Respiratory Status: Ventilation, or Respiratory Status: Gas Exchange, which address the immobility and oxygen imbalance. If the medical diagnosis is used as a basis for selecting an outcome, the signs and symptoms of the diagnosis, as well as the causative and other related factors, should be considered when an outcome is chosen. For example, pulmonary edema may be a symptom of the medical diagnosis Congestive Heart Failure and may suggest the selection of Fluid Overload Severity or Respiratory Status: Ventilation as an outcome.

Using the definition of the diagnosis Risk for Activity Intolerance, the nurse might select the same outcomes as those selected when the definition of the diagnosis Activity Intolerance is considered. Determination of the pertinent risk factors will suggest other possible outcomes such as Knowledge: Prescribed Activity, Knowledge: Body Mechanics, Cardiac Pump Effectiveness, Respiratory Status: Ventilation, Tissue Perfusion: Cardiac, Tissue Perfusion: Pulmonary, Personal Well-Being, and Physical Fitness. The fact that more than one outcome may be appropriate for a specific nursing diagnosis supports the clinical decision-making process. Each time the nurse selects an outcome for an individual patient, that nurse is making a clinical judgment based on the diagnosis and one or more of the factors described in the following sections.

## Outcomes Associated With a Diagnosis

Some medical and nursing diagnoses may have specific outcomes frequently associated with the specific diagnosis. For example, if the diagnosis is Diabetes Mellitus, blood glucose monitoring and control are specific medical and nursing outcomes for which the nurse may select the NOC outcome Blood Glucose Level. Two other outcomes specific to this medical diagnosis and associated with the nursing diagnoses of Deficient Knowledge and Ineffective or Effective Therapeutic Regimen Management are Knowledge: Diabetes Management and Diabetes Self-Management. Outcomes selected for standardized nursing care plans or critical paths are those that are pertinent to the medical diagnosis or to the nursing diagnoses commonly associated with the health problems accompanying the illness. Part Four contains a list of outcomes commonly associated with NANDA nursing diagnoses based primarily on expert opinion. Data collected during the evaluation of the outcomes in clinical sites were used if available. Examples of outcomes selected for two NANDA diagnoses by nurses in home care are shown in Table 4-1. Although this is a small sample taken from only one site, the variation in outcomes illustrates the multiple outcomes that can be considered for any diagnosis. Further data collection and analysis are needed to substantiate the associations presented in Part Four and to answer questions about the relationship between diagnoses and outcomes. Are some outcomes selected more frequently for a particular nursing diagnosis? Do the outcomes selected for a particular nursing diagnosis vary depending on the site of care, for example, in critical care, home care, or long-term care? Do the outcomes selected for a particular nursing diagnosis vary with patient age, sex, education, or social and economic status? This type of information will be invaluable in designing critical care paths, as well as in helping beginning practitioners to make judgments about the selection of appropriate patient outcomes.

| Table 4-1 | | NOC OUTCOMES SELECTED FOR NANDA DIAGNOSES FOR HOME CARE PATIENTS | | |
|---|---|---|---|---|
| Nanda Diagnoses | N | NOC Outcomes | N* | % |
| Knowledge Deficit | 73 | Knowledge: Health Resources | 15 | 20.5 |
| | | Knowledge: Diet | 11 | 15.1 |
| | | Knowledge: Treatment Procedures | 11 | 15.1 |
| | | Knowledge: Treatment Regimen | 11 | 15.1 |
| | | Knowledge: Disease Process | 10 | 13.7 |
| | | Knowledge: Medication | 8 | 11.0 |
| | | Knowledge: Prescribed Activity | 8 | 11.0 |
| | | Self-Care: Non-Parenteral Medication | 7 | 9.6 |
| | | Self-Care: Parenteral Medication | 7 | 9.6 |
| | | Knowledge: Energy Conservation | 6 | 8.2 |
| | | Knowledge: Infection Control | 4 | 5.5 |
| Caregiver Role Strain | 34 | Caregiver Performance: Direct Care | 13 | 38.2 |
| | | Caregiver Physical Health | 10 | 29.4 |
| | | Caregiver Performance: Indirect Care | 9 | 26.5 |
| | | Caregiver Lifestyle Disruption | 9 | 26.5 |
| | | Caregiver Home Care Readiness | 7 | 20.6 |
| | | Caregiver Well-Being | 7 | 20.6 |
| | | Caregiver-Patient Relationship | 7 | 20.6 |

*Fifteen outcomes were selected for each of the diagnoses; however, outcomes selected for fewer than four patients are not included. Nurses could select more than one outcome per patient.

## Patient Characteristics

Patient characteristics can affect the selection of an outcome and the degree to which an outcome can be achieved, and for this reason, patient characteristics may be referred to as *risk adjustment factors*. Broad areas to be considered include personal characteristics, illness or health-related characteristics, and resources available to the client.[16] Personal characteristics include demographic factors, psychological/cognitive processes, and personal and health beliefs or values. *Demographic factors* such as *age* and *gender* may play an important role in the selection of outcomes. Some NOC outcomes, such as the child development outcomes, are specific for certain ages, while others such as Cardiac Disease Self-Management are not appropriate for children. A number of outcomes, such as Maternal Status: Postpartum and Breastfeeding Establishment: Maternal, are obviously for females of childbearing age. *Race* and *ethnicity* can provide information important for consideration of predisposition to and response to illness and can indicate cultural beliefs that may affect the acceptance of outcomes by the patient or family. *Education level* is easy to collect and quantify and can act as a proxy for reading level, an important consideration in selecting outcomes related to knowledge and participation in health care.

*Psychological and cognitive* variables can include emotional states such as depression or anxiety and processes such as concentration, memory, information processing, and decision making. These factors influence the patient's response to illness, ability to learn, and motivation and therefore need to be considered when outcomes are selected for a particular patient. Knowledge outcomes will not be selected for the patient who has no short-term memory or cannot process information, while Anxiety Self-Control may be the most important outcome for the severely anxious patient. NOC has a number of outcomes that can be used to evaluate changes in psychological and cognitive function over time.

*Illness or health-related* variables such as *initial severity of illness* have a strong influence on outcome selection and outcome achievement. Nursing uses a number of patient acuity measures, as well as resource use measures, to capture severity of illness. Illness severity may dictate the elimination or inclusion of outcomes. For example, Mobility is generally not selected for a patient in a critical care unit, and Comfortable Death would be quite appropriate for a terminally ill patient. *Functional status* and ability to perform activities of daily living will also influence outcome selection. While ambulation is not an appropriate outcome for a patient with quadriplegia, Transfer Performance may be important, and Self-Direction of Care may be appropriate if the patient is mentally alert but unable to carry out physical self-care activities.

*Available resources* include all supportive resources that influence patient recovery and patient outcomes. These can include financial, social, family, and health resources that influence lifestyle, living conditions, and access to health care. They need to be considered in the selection of patient outcomes. Improvement in Compliance Behavior or Diabetes Self-Management is not likely to occur if the patient does not have the financial resources to purchase the medications or equipment required. *Social factors* include social support, social relationships, and the availability of someone to assist the patient as needed. Loneliness Severity or Caregiver Performance: Direct Care may become important outcomes if social support is absent or if a caregiver needs to learn multiple procedures and activities to provide care in the home.

## Patient Preferences

Including the patient and/or family in the decision-making process in selection of patient outcomes will ensure that patient preferences are considered. Preferences will be influenced by the patient's personal perceptions about health, desired health goals, preferences in relation to treatment, religious beliefs, and cultural beliefs and preferences. Each of these factors can affect which outcomes the patient or family finds acceptable. If the patient believes his or her health is satisfactory, he or she may be less inclined to accept outcomes aimed at measuring improvements in overall health such as Physical Fitness. If the patient is unable to accept emotional or psychological diagnoses because of religious or cultural beliefs, he or she is not likely to find outcomes such as Mood Equilibrium or Depression Level acceptable. In addition to collaborating in selection of the outcome, the patient should participate in determining where he or she wants to be on the outcome scale, that is, how much change he or she wants to accomplish. It may become important for the nurse to assist the patient in accepting a realistic outcome. An example would be a patient with pulmonary emphysema who wants to achieve a 5 (not compromised) on the outcome Respiratory Status: Ventilation when that is physiologically impossible.

## Treatment Potential

The availability of interventions and the potential for them to be delivered should be considered in the selection of an outcome. The Nursing Intervention Classification (NIC)[2] includes nursing interventions and recommendations for the level of nursing personnel required to provide the intervention. A first step is to determine whether an intervention is available to achieve an outcome for a particular patient. If the diagnosis for a patient is Chronic Confusion secondary to Alzheimer's disease, nursing interventions may be able to help the patient to maintain his or her current cognitive status for a period, but with current interventions, eventual decline in cognition can be expected. In such a case, the nurse would be unlikely to select Cognitive Orientation or Cognition as outcomes for which improvement is projected; and as cognition declines, other outcomes related to nutrition, safety, and hygiene may become more important. Likewise, if a patient has the diagnosis of Total Urinary Incontinence secondary to quadriplegia, treatments are not currently available to meet the outcome Urinary Continence, but maintaining a patient at a 5 rating on Infection Severity (none) or Tissue Integrity: Skin & Mucous Membranes (not compromised) may be the important outcome. A second factor to consider is whether the nursing personnel required to carry out an intervention are available. If teaching a patient or family and evaluating knowledge requires a professional nurse, then a nurse with the appropriate skills must be available to provide these services if a knowledge outcome is selected.

## Aids in Selection of Outcomes

There are a number of aids available that can assist in selecting outcomes for the individual patient, patient group, or standardized care plan or in teaching staff about the use of the Classification and outcomes. Publications that can be helpful can be found in Box 4-3. A number of these have been prepared by the authors of NIC and NOC or by users of the Classification and are available through the Center for Nursing Classification and Clinical Effectiveness (the Center) at the University of Iowa. These items can be ordered through the Center by e-mail (classification-center@uiowa.edu) or through the Center LISTSERV. The LISTSERV is maintained for users of NIC and/or NOC and anyone who has an interest in the languages. To subscribe to the LISTSERV, send the message "subscribe, end" to: classctr-request-@list.uiowa.edu. The words *subscribe* and *end* must appear on separate lines in the body of the message. Further information about the LISTSERV can be found on The University of Iowa, College of Nursing web site. Another aid is a list of NOC outcomes with behaviors corresponding to the knowledge outcomes in NOC. This list (see Table 5-1) can be helpful in assessing the effect of knowledge on the desired behavior. Chapter 5 and Appendix F also contain information related to teaching about the use of NOC in nursing programs. Although the discussions are in relation to educational programs, they provide insights that are helpful for educating staff in a practice setting. Another item that might prove helpful to the user is the list of core outcomes for nursing specialties found in Part Five.

---

**Box 4-3**

### Publications For Use When Implementing NOC

Burkhart, L., & Solari-Twadell, A. (2002). *Integration: A documentation system reporting whole person care.* St. Louis, MO: International Parish Nurse Resource Center, Deaconess Foundation. (www.parishnurses.org)

The Center for Nursing Classification. (2000). *NIC interventions & NOC outcomes linked to the OASIS information set.* Iowa City, IA: Author.

Cox, R.A. (2001). *Standardized nursing language in long-term care.* Iowa City, IA: Center for Nursing Classification.

Cox, R. (1998). Implementing nurse sensitive outcomes into care planning at a long-term care facility. *Journal of Nursing Care Quality, 12,* 41-51.

Denehy, J., & Poulton, S. (1999). The use of standardized language in individualized healthcare plans. *The Journal of School Nursing, 15,* 38-45.

Hayewski, C., Maupin, J., Rapp, D., Sitterding, M., & Pappas, J. (1998). Implementation of nursing intervention classification and nursing outcomes classification in a patient education plan. *Journal of Nursing Care Quality, 12*(5), 30-40.

Iowa Intervention Project. (1997). *NIC implementation manual.* Iowa City: The University of Iowa, Center for Nursing Classification.

Iowa Outcomes Project. (1997). *NOC use survey.* Iowa City: The University of Iowa, Center for Nursing Classification.

Johnson, M., Bulechek, G., Dochterman, J. M., Maas, M., & Moorhead, S. (2001). *Nursing diagnoses, outcomes, & interventions: NANDA, NOC, and NIC linkages.* St. Louis, MO: Mosby.

Moorhead, S., Clarke, M., Willits, M., & Tomsha, K. (1998). Nursing outcomes classification implementation projects across the care continuum. *Journal of Nursing Care Quality, 12,* 52-63.

Parris, K. M., Place, P. J., Orellana, E., Calder, J., Jackson, K., Karolys, A., et al. (1999). Integrating nursing diagnoses, interventions, and outcomes in public health nursing practice. *The Journal of Nursing Language and Classification, 10,* 49-56.

Scherb, C. A. (2002). Outcomes research: making a difference. *Outcomes Management, 6,* 22-26.

## COMPLETING THE OUTCOME

Once the outcomes for a patient or patient group are selected, information about the outcome is completed. The outcome Activity Tolerance is illustrated in Table 4-2. The outcome label, the outcome definition, and the measurement scale are standardized components of the outcome, meaning that the terminology for these elements should not change. Although minor changes can be made in the indicators, the indicator concept must remain the same if the indicators are rated and the information is kept for further analysis. Two items not included in previous outcomes are found in the upper right-hand corner of Table 4-2. These items are suggested because a number of users wanted to keep this data along with the outcome. The *Care Recipient* can be the patient, caregiver, parent (mother, father, both parents), family, or community. The *Data Source* can be the patient, a family member, a caregiver, direct observation by a health care provider, or the clinical record. Providers may wish to identify additional care recipients or data sources or make the list more specific by identifying the types of health care providers. The other pieces of information to be supplied include the patient rating on the outcome and the outcome target rating. The indicators may assist the nurse and the patient in making accurate judgments about these two items.

## Using the Outcome Indicators

Indicators can be considered more specific outcomes that are useful for determining the broader concept measured at the outcome level. The indicators are stated as briefly as possible to facilitate their use; however, a number of abbreviations previously used in the indicator statements have been spelled out so all users will be interpreting the indicators in the same way. The abbreviations IER (in expected range) and WNL (within normal limits), found in the second edition, have been deleted. As discussed in Chapter 2, the term *normal* is used in place of the other two terms; the norm for the term is what is expected of a healthy individual of approximately the same race, age, and sex. To shorten the indicator statement, abbreviations can be substituted if there is general agreement on the meaning of the abbreviations within the facility. Previous users will also note that terms such as *free of* or *absence of*, which users found difficult to use with the scales, have been eliminated. Scale terms were inverted and a second scale, in which these terms are used, was added for the negative conditions or symptoms that had included the terms *free of* and *absence of*. Examples of outcomes with two scales are Endurance and Mood Equilibrium (see Part Three). Although the language of the indicators should remain standardized as much as possible, practitioners may wish to add some indicators that are pertinent to a specialized area of practice or make the indicators more specific. For example, normal ranges for diagnostic test results or blood pressure can be substituted for test name or the term *blood pressure* in the outcome. Practitioners may also wish to delete indicators that aren't pertinent to an individual patient or patient group with a particular diagnosis.

After selecting the outcomes for an individual patient or for a standardized care plan, the nurse will want to select the indicators that will be used to determine patient status for an outcome, that is, the outcome rating the patient will receive on the measurement scale. In general, the staff should agree on the indicators to be used for the most frequently selected outcomes for their patient population. Some users have found they can limit the indicators for each outcome to four or five, while other users wish to select more indicators. Areas for further study are determining which indicators are most important for an outcome when selected for various patient populations and determining whether some of the indicators should carry more weight than others. This will eventually be accomplished if users share this information with others through the LISTSERV managed by the Center, through publications and conferences, or through contact with the authors so future editions can reflect how the indicators are being used in practice settings.

Rating the status of an individual patient on the selected indicators can help the nurse determine the patient's overall rating for the outcome. It will be noted that a column for not applicable (NA) has been added to the paper form. A computerized form could include both NA and not

## Table 4-2   Activity Tolerance Outcome

### Activity Tolerance (0005)

*Domain-Functional Health (I)*

*Class-Energy Maintenance (A)*

*Scale(s)—Severely compromised to Not compromised (a)*

*Care Recipient:*

*Data Source:*

**Definition:** Physiological response to energy-consuming movements with daily activities

OUTCOME TARGET RATING:     Maintain at_____ Increase to_____

| Activity Tolerance Overall Rating | Severely compromised 1 | Substantially compromised 2 | Moderately compromised 3 | Mildly compromised 4 | Not compromised 5 | |
|---|---|---|---|---|---|---|
| **INDICATORS:** | | | | | | |
| 000501 Oxygen saturation with activity | 1 | 2 | 3 | 4 | 5 | NA |
| 000502 Pulse rate with activity | 1 | 2 | 3 | 4 | 5 | NA |
| 000503 Respiratory rate with activity | 1 | 2 | 3 | 4 | 5 | NA |
| 000508 Ease of breathing with activity | 1 | 2 | 3 | 4 | 5 | NA |
| 000504 Systolic blood pressure with activity | 1 | 2 | 3 | 4 | 5 | NA |
| 000505 Diastolic blood pressure with activity | 1 | 2 | 3 | 4 | 5 | NA |
| 000506 Electrocardiogram findings | 1 | 2 | 3 | 4 | 5 | NA |
| 000507 Skin color | 1 | 2 | 3 | 4 | 5 | NA |
| 000509 Walking pace | 1 | 2 | 3 | 4 | 5 | NA |
| 000510 Walking distance | 1 | 2 | 3 | 4 | 5 | NA |
| 000511 Stair climbing tolerance | 1 | 2 | 3 | 4 | 5 | NA |
| 000516 Upper body strength | 1 | 2 | 3 | 4 | 5 | NA |
| 000517 Lower body strength | 1 | 2 | 3 | 4 | 5 | NA |
| 000518 Ease of performing activities of daily living (ADL) | 1 | 2 | 3 | 4 | 5 | NA |
| 000514 Ability to speak with physical activity | 1 | 2 | 3 | 4 | 5 | NA |

*Second edition 2000; Revised third edition.*

known (NK) if desired. Recording which indicators the nurse finds NA will provide data to determine whether some indicators are not pertinent and can be eliminated. As the nurse becomes familiar with the selected indicators, it may be unnecessary to rate patient status on each indicator, since the nurse will automatically consider the indicators when determining the patient's outcome rating. However, it must be recognized that data valuable for determining which indicators are most predictive of patient status will be lost when indicator ratings are not retained.

The source of data for the indicators and the outcome will vary. Data may be obtained from the patient record (e.g., biochemical measures or vital signs) or from direct observation or physical assessments (e.g., how well a patient can carry out treatments or whether certain signs and symptoms are present). Other indicators may require solicitation of information or perceptions from the patient or family (e.g., description of knowledge about the disease process or treatment, perceptions of health, and satisfaction with care). As noted earlier, the outcome form has a space in which to record the data source. If the outcomes are entered in a computerized database, the organization can provide codes for each of the sources likely to be used in that organization.

The indicators are less abstract than the outcome and may at times serve as intermediate outcomes in a standardized care plan. Indicators to be used in this way can be selected by members of the task force as they determine which outcomes are used frequently for the patient population served. If an indicator is considered an important measure of patient progress, nurses may choose to aggregate data on a particular indicator, as well as on the outcome. This may be particularly true for patients with short episodes of care in which progress in relation to the outcome may not be evident, but progress in relation to significant indicators may be achieved.

## Using the Measurement Scales

The current classification contains 13 measurement scales, which are illustrated in Chapter 2. Measurement scales are provided for both the outcome and the indicators, and in all instances the same scale is used, although it is inverted for indicators that represent negative conditions. Each scale is constructed so that the fifth point, or end point, reflects the most desirable patient condition relative to the outcome. The nurse can make a judgment about the outcome rating for a patient or patient group without using the indicators; however, most nurses find one or more of the indicators helpful for judging the patient rating on the outcome scale.

Although indicator ratings will assist in determining the patient's rating on the outcome scale, they currently are not weighted to provide a mean or summated rating. It is recommended that the practitioner use both the range and the frequency of patient ratings on the indicator scale as an aid in determining the outcome rating. In general, low ratings of 1 and 2 on important indicators will mean that the patient has a 1 or 2 rating on the outcome scale. For example, in the outcome illustrated in Table 4-2, equally distributed ratings of 1s and 2s on the indicators would suggest that Activity Tolerance should be rated as "severely compromised," since a number of the indicators are rated as severely compromised. However, if the indicator ratings range from "severely compromised" for ability to speak with physical activity to "mildly compromised" and "not compromised" for the remainder of the indicators, the nurse will want to determine how important the ability to speak with physical activity is for the patient situation when considering how it should affect the outcome rating. If the patient has always had difficult speaking with activity, the nurse may rate the patient as "mildly compromised" on the outcome. If this is a new symptom and particularly bothersome to the patient, the nurse may adjust the rating to "moderately compromised" or elect to monitor patient ratings for the indicator "ability to speak with physical activity," as well as for the outcome Activity Tolerance. If the user wishes to use intervening points on the scale and the database can handle these data, the nurse could rate the patient with ratings of 1 and 2 as 1.5.

After rating the patient on the selected outcome using the five-point measurement scale, the nurse can select the desired rating to be achieved following the care interventions. For example, a patient may enter the care situation with the outcome Endurance rated as "substantially compromised," and because the cause of the decreased endurance cannot be eliminated (e.g., myocardial myopathy), the desired goal for this patient may be to maintain a rating of "substantially compromised" for as long as possible. Another patient may have "extremely compromised" Endurance because of a condition that can be eliminated or partially controlled (e.g., congestive heart failure), and the desired outcome status following an episode of care may be "moderately compromised." As noted on the outcome Activity Tolerance, a space (Outcome Target Rating) has been provided to record the desired outcome rating. The nurse would indicate that the rating should be maintained at a 2 in the first instance and increased to a 3 in the second instance.

Outcomes stated as variable concepts and measured along a continuum allow goal statements to be individualized for each patient while maintaining standardized outcome language and measures. They also give recognition to what all nurses know: that not all patients will be able to achieve the most desirable outcome despite the most intensive care. Variable outcomes measured along a continuum allow the nurse to evaluate the amount of progress or lack of progress for individual patients. This information is not available when outcomes represent only the most desirable patient state and the evaluation at the conclusion of a care episode represents a goal met or not met.

## Using the Outcomes in Standardized Care Plans

The outcomes can also be used to identify goals in critical paths or in standardized care plans. In these situations, the outcome is stated with the desired or expected rating on the measurement scale to be achieved at a certain point in time (e.g., the first post-op day, the third home care visit). The desired goal at the end of an acute care episode for a patient who has had a stroke with "extremely compromised" Cognition at the time of admission might be "substantially compromised" with a goal of "moderately compromised" or "mildly compromised" following rehabilitation. If the acute care episode is extremely short, the goal may be to maintain the patient at the "extremely compromised" level with some improvement in specified indicators—the intermediate outcomes that indicate progress toward improvement in Cognition. The plan can project the expected outcome at the end of 6 months, and the patient's progress can be monitored at specified intervals if he or she is in a rehabilitation unit or a nursing home or can be checked at the next clinic visit. On the other hand, the desired goal for a patient with hepatic encephalopathy and "extremely compromised" Cognition at the time of admission may be to have the patient progress to "moderately compromised" or "mildly compromised" after an acute care episode.

## Concerns About Using the Scales

A concern frequently voiced by users is the *subjectivity of the scales*. The indicators have been provided to assist the nurse in determining the patient's status and consequent rating on the outcome scale, but they do not eliminate the need for a nursing judgment. Because the scale anchors are not specifically defined for each indicator and outcome, the nurse must make a nursing judgment about the patient status for the indicators, if used, and for the outcome. Although the accuracy of this judgment becomes more important when the nurse is quantifying outcomes, it requires the same judgment used when the nurse is determining whether the patient has met a goal, has improved in relation to a goal, has not met a goal, or has deteriorated in relation to the goal. Some organizations have elected to provide more specific anchors for the outcomes, as seen in the examples in Table 4-3. This approach is especially useful when the number of outcomes to be used with a particular population is limited, when the outcomes are used in a standard plan or when a limited number of outcomes are used in a research study. If nurses elect to do this, they need to provide this information in reports of their findings so other nurses can determine whether the rating has the same meaning and can be used to make comparisons across settings. As the outcomes are used in more settings, it is anticipated that more specificity of the scale anchors will be developed.

| Table 4-3 | EXAMPLES OF SPECIFIC ANCHORS FOR INDICATORS IN THE OUTCOME DIGNIFIED DYING AND THE KNOWLEDGE OUTCOMES* |
|---|---|

| Indicator Statement | Rating Scale | Operational Definition |
|---|---|---|
| Expresses symptom control | 1 = Not at all | 4 or more symptoms |
| | 2 = To a slight extent | 3 symptoms present |
| | 3 = To a moderate extent | 2 symptoms present |
| | 4 = To a great extent | 1 symptom present |
| | 5 = none | 0 symptoms present |
| Expresses pain relief | 1 = Not at all | Reports no change in pain; states level at 9-10 |
| | 2 = To a slight extent | Reports 1-2 points lower; states rate is 8 or lower |
| | 3 = To a moderate extent | Reports 3-4 points lower; states rate is 6 or lower |
| | 4 = To a great extent | Reports 5-6 points lower; states rate is 4 or lower |
| | 5 = None | Reports 7-10 points lower; states pain is 2 or lower |
| All knowledge outcomes | 1 = None | Dependent for all information |
| | 2 = Limited | Requires assistive person and resources |
| | 3 = Moderate | Requires assistive person |
| | 4 = Substantial | Independent with minimal cues |
| | 5 = Extensive | Independently verbalizes/ demonstrates information without cues |

*These examples are taken from Johnson, M., Maas, M., & Moorhead, S. (2000). *Nursing Outcomes Classification (NOC)*. St. Louis, MO: Mosby. The first two examples can be found in Appendix A in the hospice plan, and the knowledge example in the teaching plan from Columbus Regional Hospital. The outcome name for Dignified Dying has been changed to Dignified Life Closure in this edition, and the indicators have been moved to the outcome Comfortable Death. However, this illustrates how anchors can be made more specific and how measures from other tools can be used with a NOC outcome.

Another issue is *how to use published measurement scales* that appear in recognized patient assessment tools, for example, those used to assess pain, neurological status, pedal pulses, and edema or to grade pressure ulcers and burns. In general, these scales tend to measure a more specific or limited concept; in other words, the NOC outcome may be at a more abstract level. We recommend that users determine what they want to measure and whether the published measurement scale serves their need; they may elect to use that scale instead of a NOC outcome. For example, the 10-point pain scale that measures the patient report of pain can be used rather than the NOC outcome Pain Level if the patient report of pain is the only measure desired, or the scale grading pressure ulcers can be used in place of Wound Healing: Secondary Intention if it captures the dimensions of concern. The scales can also be used as assessment factors, and decisions can be made about how they correspond to the NOC outcome. For an example of how the 10-point pain scale has been used with a NOC outcome, see Table 4-3.

Another concern is the *patient rating on discharge* from a care episode. While it is recognized that the most desirable condition will not be achievable for all patients or patient groups, and therefore the expected outcome may be less than a "5" on the measurement scale, this is quite uncomfortable for many nurses who have been used to stating that goals are met when a patient is discharged. When NOC is introduced, staff education should include a discussion of how to use the measurement scales and what will be done when the patient does not achieve the desired outcome. The following example may be helpful in illustrating this. One of our test sites was an obstetrical unit that admitted a number of teen-age mothers. Two of the outcomes used were Knowledge: Infant Care and Knowledge: Postpartum Maternal Health. Initially, staff rated all mothers at a 4 or 5 on discharge from a 48-hour stay. When asked if all mothers met the criteria for that rating, staff acknowledged that many did not but they were concerned about the legal implications if they didn't rate the patient at a 4 or 5. This issue was discussed and staff decided to allow the mother with a 4 or 5 rating to go home without a referral for follow-up unless she chose to have one, to encourage follow-up for the mother with a 3 rating, and to require follow-up visits for the mother with a 1 or 2 rating. The staff believed the mother with a 3 rating or above was competent to care for herself and the baby until the scheduled follow-up visits with the physician or nurse, but that the mother with a 1 or 2 required additional teaching and assistance that would be provided by a follow-up nursing visit within the first 48 hours of returning home. It would be reasonable to assume that before the staff began using a rating scale, every patient left the hospital having met a goal that stated the patient had the necessary knowledge to care for her infant. The nursing care provided to these patients is now of a higher quality because it provides a rationale for the decisions based on patient status and provides a method for assisting the mother who needs additional help. The *legal implications* when a measurement scale is used are the same as those when a goal statement is used. If a goal is not met, a rationale for why the goal was not met (e.g., the patient's physiological status deteriorated, the patient was unable to comprehend the information) and the action taken should be provided. The same is true when a projected outcome rating is not achieved. For example, respiratory status is expected to continue to decline as a result of increased involvement of the lungs secondary to lung cancer; therefore the outcome Comfort Level is replacing the outcome Respiratory Status: Ventilation, indicating that the goal now is to keep the patient as comfortable as possible. Other examples of how these issues have been handled can be found in the case examples in Appendix E. As outcome data are collected and analyzed, patient and system characteristics that influence outcome achievement can be delineated, and the expected outcome ratings for various diagnoses or populations can be based on clinical evidence.

## Timing of Data Collection

The times at which outcomes should be evaluated are not specified, but the minimum requirement is that a rating should be obtained when the outcome is selected (i.e., the baseline measure) and when care is completed (i.e., the discharge measure). This may be sufficient in acute care settings if the patient has a short stay; however, staff in some acute care settings have chosen to evaluate patient status once a day or once a shift, depending on how rapidly changes in the outcome status are expected. Community agencies may elect to evaluate patient status at each visit, or at every other visit if the patient is seen frequently. Since measurement times are not standardized, reporting the date or patient care day when measures were obtained is important for making comparisons between populations and across units. Noting the times when outcomes are measured will provide information to recommend time intervals for the various outcomes and for varied patient populations.

At least two outcome (or indicator) ratings are necessary to determine whether change has occurred and the degree of change. This type of data will be some of the most valuable for evaluating how nursing interventions, other aspects of the patient's care, and the patient characteristics affect outcome achievement. If the desired change is not occurring in all patients, data will allow nursing to determine what, if any, differences exist between those who achieve the outcome target and those who do not. If it is the type of intervention or care program, these can be changed. If it is a patient characteristic that cannot be changed, such as age, race, or initial severity of illness, then the target outcome can be readjusted to be consistent with the findings. Examples of a few findings related to change in the completed outcome evaluation study are shown in Table 4-4.

| Table 4-4 | CHANGES IN OUTCOME RATINGS FROM BASELINE TO FOLLOW-UP MEASUREMENTS |
|---|---|

| Outcome* | N | Baseline[†] | Follow-up | Change | Setting/Unit |
|---|---|---|---|---|---|
| Ambulation: Walking | 4 | 2.25 | 2.50 | 0.25 | Nursing Home |
| (Ambulation) | 7 | 2.29 | 4.57 | 2.29 | Birth Center |
| | 6 | 3.83 | 4.50 | 0.67 | VNA |
| | 12 | 3.17 | 3.50 | 0.33 | Medical Unit |
| | 59 | 1.92 | 2.51 | 0.50 | Ortho Unit |
| Aggression Control | 5 | 3.60 | 4.60 | 1.00 | Stress Unit |
| | 13 | 2.23 | 3.62 | 1.38 | Behavioral Unit |
| Caregiver Emotional Health | 7 | 4.00 | 4.29 | 0.29 | Parish Nursing |
| | 5 | 4.00 | 4.00 | 0.00 | VNA |
| Breastfeeding Establishment: Maternal | 6 | 3.50 | 4.00 | 0.50 | VNA |
| | 40 | 3.00 | 3.78 | 0.78 | Birth Center |

*VNA,* Visiting Nurse Association.
*The outcome Ambulation: Walking has been changed to Ambulation in the current edition of NOC.
[†]The baseline and follow-up measures are averages of all ratings.

Although the process described for using the outcomes in practice is important, of equal importance are the processes associated with preparing to implement NOC in a clinical setting and in an electronic patient record. The next section provides a brief overview of these aspects of implementation, while the implementation examples in Appendix E illustrate aspects of the process in various settings.

## IMPLEMENTING THE CLASSIFICATION IN PRACTICE

There is increased recognition in clinical settings that standardized languages are a necessary component for the implementation of electronic medical records. Standardized outcomes are also important for evaluating the effectiveness of nursing interventions, facilitating the continuity of care in integrated health systems, and ensuring nursing accountability.[9] A recent Institute of Medicine report [3] on health care quality stresses the following six aims to be met by the health care system:

1. Safe: avoiding injury
2. Effective: avoiding overuse and underuse
3. Patient-centered: responding to patient preferences, needs, and values
4. Timely: reducing waits and delays
5. Efficient: avoiding waste
6. Equitable: providing care that does not vary in quality to all recipients

Evaluation of these aims requires measurement and tracking of patient outcomes, as well as measurement and tracking of other aspects of care. Given these factors, the opportunity for nursing to implement measures to assess nursing effectiveness is timely.

### Preparing for Clinical Implementation

Implementing NOC in the clinical setting requires organizational commitment and the development of an implementation plan. Advantages of using NOC must be identified and communicated to organizational leaders and nursing staff. Strengths of NOC that can be emphasized include[7]:

- Comprehensiveness: NOC includes outcomes for individuals, family caregivers, families, and communities that are applicable across clinical settings.

- Clinical usefulness: NOC can be used in a manual or electronic clinical information system. The outcomes can be used in critical paths and care plans and can be used to set expected patient goals for individual patients or groups of patients.
- Data measurement and analysis: Data can be collected from the patient record, quantified, and used in outcome analysis.
- Recognized nursing language: NOC is one of the nursing languages recognized by the American Nurses Association (ANA) Steering Committee on Databases to Support Clinical Nursing Practice; has been accepted by Healthcare 7 (HL7), an organization setting standards for the computerized record; and is scheduled to be incorporated into the reference language being developed by SNOMED CT.

Organizational leaders and staff may need to be educated about the importance of using standardized languages for nursing practice, although this may be less necessary as plans for the electronic medical record progress. A key person, one who is committed to the project and able to articulate the advantages of using standardized languages, needs to be responsible for the implementation process. The nurse in charge of nursing informatics or outcome management is often an ideal person to select as project leader for the implementation process.

Staff members who will use NOC need to be identified and educated about the Classification. In our research evaluating the use of NOC in clinical sites, we found that staff education is one of the most important factors for the successful implementation of NOC. All of the implementation examples address the need for education and discuss some of the methods used in their facility. The process for using NOC outcomes should be covered, as well as the issues and concerns that arise as nurses begin to use the outcomes. Staff should not have to become familiar with the use of NOC and a new computer system at the same time. If an organization is going to select a new computer system, the time used for evaluation and selection of the system should also be used to orient nurses to the NOC outcome system and to pilot written forms.

A task force of representatives from key areas and pilot sites should be established to assist the project leader with the implementation process.[4] The task force can assist with the development of the implementation plan and with staff education during the implementation process. The implementation plan should include the goals to be accomplished, steps for implementation with a list of the responsible individuals and a time line, the evaluation plan, and the costs associated with implementation. Planning should include the identification of other data that need to be collected in conjunction with the outcome data for clinical and administrative analyses. For example, patient characteristics, staff mix, nursing costs, and nursing diagnoses and interventions may need to be linked with outcome data to answer clinical and administrative questions. During this phase, the ability or inability of the electronic information system to link patient outcomes with other data should be evaluated, and if needed, plans to establish the necessary linkages to other databases should be developed. The ability to collect data on the links between nursing diagnoses, interventions, and outcomes should also be evaluated.

The initial planning should result in the development of a paper format that can be tested before implementation throughout the organization or placement in an electronic system. The format used for documenting with standardized languages should not be more time-consuming than that previously used in the organization; however, it must be recognized that documentation may take longer until the staff becomes familiar with the new system. A tri-fold paper form was created for initial use in medical critical care units at the University of Iowa Hospitals & Clinics. It includes information recorded on admission to the unit and provides a standardized format that can be used for nursing diagnoses related to the following nine areas of potential patient problems: (1) sensory, (2) pain, (3) neurological, (4) motor, (5) pulmonary, (6) cardiac, (7) integument and immune, (8) gastrointestinal and urinary, and (9) nutrition. Examples of how these are set up to include standardized languages are provided in Figs. 4-1 and 4-2. This format requires the nurse to make a judgment about the nursing diagnosis and the interventions and outcomes to be used with the diagnosis. Space is provided in the tri-fold form for additional

## CARDIAC PATIENT NURSING DIAGNOSIS (NANDA)

| Date/Time/Initial Initiated | Date/Time/Initial Resolved | |
|---|---|---|
| | | ☐ **Altered Tissue Perfusion Cardiopulmonary** |
| | | ☐ **Risk of Fluid Volume Imbalance (Excess/Deficit)** |
| | | ☐ **Decrease Cardiac Output** |

**Parameters:**

T  < _____ > _____
HR < _____ > _____
SBP< _____ > _____
DBP< _____ > _____
RR < _____ > _____
UO _____
SaO2 > _____
Other: _____

**Signs & Symptoms**

Edema
Oliguria or anuria
Weak or absent pulse
Altered mental status
Dyspnea/changes in respiratory pattern
Elevated pulmonary artery pressure

Arrhythmia
Jugular vein distention
Decrease Blood Pressure
Increase Pulse rate
Thirst
Changes in skin color/temp.

**Related Factors**

Excess fluid intake
Hypovolemia/Hypervolemia
Mechanical reduction of venous and/or arterial blood flow
Chest pain.  Cardiac ischemia/damage
Loss of fluid through abnormal routes (indwelling tubes, wounds/burns, diarrhea)
Impaired transport of the oxygen across alveolar and/or capillary membrane

## NURSING INTERVENTIONS (NIC) & ACTIVITIES

| Date/Time/Initial Initiated | |
|---|---|
| | **Blood Products Administration:** Administer per policy and protocol. |
| | **Cardiac Care: Acute:** R/O MI Protocol.  Monitor vital signs q 1-2 hrs or as needed.  CHAMPS MET level_____   Other: |
| | **Fluid/Electrolyte Management:** Monitor lab values relevant to fluid & electrolyte balance. |
| | **Invasive Hemodynamic Monitoring:** Cardiac Indices q_____   PCWP q_____ |
| | **Hemodynamic Regulation:**   Monitor Vital signs and pulses. Administer vasoactive or inotropic medications as ordered. |
| | **Shock Management:** Specify: |
| | **Teaching (Patient/Family):** Instruct the patient/family on cardiac monitor, I.V. lines, hemodynamic monitoring, and hemodynamic medications. Encourage realistic expectations for the patient and family.  Inform pt/family of any referral made.  Other: |

## PATIENT OUTCOME (NOC)

**Tissue Perfusion: Cardiac:** Extent to which blood flows through the coronary vasculature and maintains heart function

| Definition of Scale | 1 (0%) | 2 (25%) | 3 (50%) | 4 (75%) | 5 (100%) |
|---|---|---|---|---|---|
| Vital signs within normal limits | Extremely compromised | Substantially compromised | Moderately compromised | Mildly compromised | Not compromised |

**Day (level/initial)**

| 1 | 2 | 3 | 4 | 5 | 6 | 7 |
|---|---|---|---|---|---|---|
| 8 | 9 | 10 | 11 | 12 | 13 | 14 |

**Fig. 4-1** Cardiac patient diagnoses for a medical intensive care unit. (Greiner, J., Shelsky, C., Stenger, K., & Cram, E. (2002). *A-1b10 Nursing Diagnoses Standards Form Critical Care. University of Iowa Hospital & Clinics.*)

## PAIN PATIENT NURSING DIAGNOSIS (NANDA)

| Date/Time/Initial Initiated | Date/Time/Initial Resolved | | | | |
|---|---|---|---|---|---|
| | | ☐ **Pain** | ☐ **Chronic Pain** | **Acceptable pain level:** | |

| **Possible Signs & Symptoms** | **Related Factors** |
|---|---|
| states pain is present<br>states pain is present > 6 month<br>restless<br>diaphoresis<br>pressure | muscle guarding<br>facial expression of pain<br>moaning crying<br>autonomic responses | Injuring Agents (biological, chemical, physical, psychological)<br>Chronic physical/psychosocial disability<br>Surgery/ Invasive procedure<br>Cancer<br>Cardiac |

| Date/Time/Initial Initiated | |
|---|---|

### NURSING INTERVENTIONS (NIC) & ACTIVITIES

**Pain Management:** Assess for pain every two hrs & document on A-1c ICU Flowsheet.  Look for nonverbal clues.  Consider cultural influences.  Consider type & source of pain when selecting pain relief strategy.  Other:

**Analgesic Administration:** Administer analgesia per order.  Reassess 10-20 min for parenteral & 30 min to 1 hour for oral medications.  Titrate dosage based on intensity.  Other:

**Analgesic Administration: epidural:** NARCAN at bedside.  **DO NOT MANIPULATE, CHANGE DRESSING OR ADMINISTER ANYTHING VIA EPIDURAL CATHETER.**   For emergencies, if RR 8 or less or undue somnolence call anesthesiology (391) physician.  Other:

**Teaching (Patient/Family):** Instruct the patient/family about pain management & the effects of pain.  Review with patient/family medication taken in the past.  Provide comfort and reassurance.  Instruct to ask for PRN before pain is to severe.  Other:

### PATIENT OUTCOME

**Pain Level:** Amount of reported or demonstrated pain.

| Definition of Scale | 1 (0%) | 2 (25%) | 3 (50%) | 4 (75%) | 5 (100%) |
|---|---|---|---|---|---|
| Reported Pain (0-10) | Severe (8-10) | Substantial (6-7) | Moderate (5-4) | Slight (3-1) | None (0) |

| Day (level/initial) | | | | | | |
|---|---|---|---|---|---|---|
| 1 | 2 | 3 | 4 | 5 | 6 | 7 |
| 8 | 9 | 10 | 11 | 12 | 13 | 14 |

**Fig. 4-2** Pain patient diagnoses for a medical intensive care unit. (*Greiner, J., Shelsky, C., Stenger, K., & Cram, E. (2002). A-1b10 Nursing Diagnoses Standards Form Critical Care. University of Iowa Hospital & Clinics.*)

comments as necessary. Percentages have been applied to the five-point scale to make the scale more explicit; this technique was used by a number of sites in our evaluation study. Some used the percentage as noted in this example and some placed 100% with the 1 rating and 0% with the 5 rating. Since the rating is the number retained, the percentages can be presented in the manner that is most understandable for the staff.

It is recommended that the outcomes be implemented on one or more pilot units to assess and correct problems before house-wide implementation. The units selected should be ones in which a majority of the staff members are committed to the project. Once the pilot units are identified, the NOC outcomes used most frequently for the patient population in the unit need to be identified. This can be done by using the NOC Use Survey[5] or creating a task force of clinical staff to select the most frequently used outcomes. The survey tool is an efficient method for identifying outcomes for various patient populations and can be completed by all staff or by the task force. If the survey is not used and the unit has a list of the outcome goals used most frequently, the appropriate NOC outcomes can be substituted for the goals. If a needed outcome is not available, the task force can develop the outcome using the guidelines in Appendix G and submit the outcome to the NOC research team or inform the team of the need for a specific outcome.

## Preparing for Use in an Electronic Clinical Information System

One of the primary values of an electronic clinical information system is the ability to collect and analyze large amounts of data. Analyzing data requires that the system be developed in such a way that the information and linkages are available to answer the questions posed. Unfortunately, many current systems do not allow for the types of analyses that nurses need to do. Creation of systems that will provide the information nurses need for clinical and administrative decision making requires planning for the type of data sets that will be used and the linkages among the sets. One way to begin is by determining what such a system should do. It should provide a way to unify data from many information sources, provide a means of detecting trends and possible oversights in care, and provide a basis for outcomes management and a database for epidemiological studies.[11] An important step for nursing is to determine the data sets that are needed, the elements of the data sets, and the types of linkages they want between the data sets.

## Identifying Data Sets and Links

Data sets that are of interest to nursing include clinical data sets, provider data sets, fiscal data sets, and utilization data sets.[10] Nurses involved in the development of the electronic nursing system should know the data sets available in the organization and whether the sets can be linked with nursing data. One data set available in all hospital settings is the Uniform Hospital Discharge Data Set (UHDDS).[12] This set includes the 14 items found in Box 4-4, many of which are relevant for nursing. Clinical data sets generally represent the largest number of data sets, and in most cases, few of them are coded and organized in a similar fashion. They include data on patient medications, laboratory findings, surgical procedures, and radiology results, as well as diagnoses, treatments and interventions, and patient outcomes, to name a few. The electronic clinical nursing sets should contain information about the patient necessary for nursing practice and not contained elsewhere and the nursing diagnoses, interventions, and outcomes. In addition to the patient information contained in the UHDDS, nurses will want information discussed in the section on selecting an outcome. Nurses need to give careful consideration to the type of information they want retained about the diagnoses and outcomes. If NANDA diagnoses are used, retaining information about the defining characteristics and related factors or risk factors will increase the types of analyses that can be done. Likewise, obtaining as much information as possible about the outcomes, such as indicators selected and the data source, will serve this purpose. For the intervention, adequate information to capture important variance in the activities should be maintained.[16] The dose and frequency of the treatment will provide information about the strength of the treatment. The time of day the treatment is administered and the staff provid-

**Box 4-4**

---

### Elements in the Uniform Data Set

Personal identification
Date of birth
Gender
Race and ethnicity
Residence (zip code)
Hospital identification
Admission date
Discharge date
Physician identification – attending
Physician identification – operating
Diagnoses
Procedures and dates
Discharge disposition of patient
Expected principal source of payment

---

ing the treatment can be important information in analyzing the effectiveness of interventions. Perhaps one of the most important factors to consider in the nursing data sets is how linkages between the diagnoses, interventions, and outcomes will be provided. The linkage identifies the problem to be addressed by the intervention and the outcome expected as a result of the intervention.

Provider data sets include information about the nurse (such as age, education, and skill level) and information about the setting (such as unit size, staffing, and type of care delivery system) in addition to the type of organization. Fiscal data sets include information about costs and charges that are necessary to compute the cost of nursing and the income generated. The Nursing Management Minimum Data Set[1] includes methods for measuring many of these elements. Utilization data sets are available in most organizations that provide health care services; these sets are measures of the care provided[10] and will vary with the type of organization. In hospital settings, they will include patient days, hospital admissions, and discharges. In community settings, they will include number of visits, number of admissions, and discharges from the service. While many of the questions about patient care that clinical nurses will want answered will require links among clinical databases, many of the questions that nurse administrators want answered will require links among the clinical, provider, fiscal, and utilization databases. Nurses have a major opportunity to plan for data sets with the required links when new electronic systems are being put in place. Because electronic systems are costly, mistakes made with the introduction of new systems may be both difficult and costly to rectify at a later date.

## Implementing NOC Outcomes

In addition to questions about planning for implementation, a number of questions arise about the actual implementation of the NOC outcomes in an electronic system. One of the major problems that nurses encounter is the amount of space available in the software. There may not be adequate space to include both the outcome label and the definition, and often, space is not available for the inclusion of indicators. Eliminating the definition and using indicators as separate outcomes is one way in which nursing may address these problems. However, this eliminates the opportunity to analyze the indicators that might be most effective or useful for the outcome and may limit analyses that can be done with the data. Another method is to use a section of the system not intended for outcomes, for example, an assessment section with more space. A second space problem is related to the measurement scale; many of the software programs have traditionally provided space for two items, goal met and goal not met. Again, some nurses have addressed this problem by using parts of the program meant for other activities for the outcomes. The ideal solution is the development of software programs that will accommodate the information that nurses need to record and evaluate in conjunction with other data. Although there have been some initial efforts in this direction, much more needs to be accomplished. Software providers listen to users, and if nurses begin to demand what is needed for their data collection, changes will come about, especially as more emphasis is placed on designing systems for an electronic record.

## LICENSING THE OUTCOMES

A license is needed to use NOC if you put it on an electronic information system or if you use more than a few outcomes in a product for commercial gain. Mosby, now a part of Elsevier Science, holds the copyright for NOC. Requests for permission to use or license NOC should be sent to Mosby. The inside front cover contains information about whom to contact for permission to use NOC or to obtain a license. The research team elected to publish the Classification through a book publisher for a number of reasons. The team had no way to produce and market the product, to provide funding for continued development, or to protect the standardization of the language by protecting the copyright.

Copyright does not restrict fair use. The American Library Association recognizes fair use when the following guidelines are followed: (1) the portion copied is selective and not more than 10% of the work; (2) the materials are not used repeatedly; (3) no more than one copy is made for each person; (4) the source and copyright are included on each copy; and (5) persons are not assessed a fee for the copy beyond the cost of reproduction. Putting NOC on an electronic system requires a license because significant portions of the book will be available for use by multiple users. The use of significant portions of the Classification in a book or product that is being sold also requires a license. Fees for the use of NOC in an electronic system to be used in one organization depend on the number of users and average about $5.00 per user per year, an extremely reasonable fee when compared with fees for many other software products. If the user purchases a software product that uses NOC, the license fees will often be included as part of the product cost. Paying licensing fees for the use of nomenclatures or software is familiar to hospital administrators; often, it is nurses who are unaware that the organization is paying these fees for other information sets such as those for the pharmacy or laboratory.

Requests for permission to use the Classification, as well as for licenses, should be sent to Mosby. Many requests are consistent with fair use and therefore do not require fees. Fees are not required if the organization uses the outcomes in a paper format. However, the organization should purchase a sufficient number of books so they do not have to make multiple copies of the Classification. Fees are generally not required for schools of nursing that want to use NOC in educational products for their own students; however, if the school is using a significant portion of NOC, it is expected that students will purchase the books to use with the products produced by the schools. Fees are generally not required for research in which NOC is used. Fees for use in another publication will depend on the number of outcomes used; if only a few are provided as examples, no fee will be assessed for use.

A portion of the fees generated through license agreements and use are returned to the Center and help fund the upkeep of both NIC and NOC. To continue to evaluate NOC in clinical settings, to provide a means to update the language, and to keep the languages current with changes in federal requirements requires personnel and other resources. The American Nurses Association does not have the resources to fund the continued development of the languages they recognize, so development must be done by the authors. Thus the Center for Nursing Classification and Clinical Effectiveness was created at the University of Iowa for this purpose; however, long-term funding was not provided for the Center. The viability of the Center and its work is dependent on monies earned though publications, licenses, and other products and on donations made to an endowment fund whose purpose is to provide long-term funding for the continued support of the development of NIC and NOC.

## SUMMARY

Successful implementation of NOC in a practice setting requires strong leadership and administrative commitment during both the planning and implementation phases. An area of paramount importance that must receive adequate attention in both phases is staff education. Without adequate education and sufficient opportunity to practice the use of a scaled outcome rather than an outcome goal, the implementation process will be faced with unnecessary problems. Questions that staff frequently ask when they are using NOC have been discussed in the section on issues. In addition to planning for staff education, the plan must address the resources required to implement a new documentation method and the software requirements if an electronic system is used. The implementation examples provided in Appendix D illustrate how some organizations have proceeded with planning and implementation.

## References

1. Delaney, C., & Huber, D. (1996). *A Nursing Management Minimum Data Set (NMMDS): A report of an invitational conference*. Chicago: American Organization of Nurse Executives, 1996.
2. Dochterman, J. M., & Bulechek, G. M. (Eds.). (2004). *Nursing interventions classification (NIC)* (4th ed.). St. Louis, MO: Mosby.
3. Institute of Medicine. (2001). In J. M. Corrigan, M. S. Donaldson, & L. T. Kohn (Eds.), *Crossing the quality chasm: A new heath system for the 21st century*. Washington, DC: National Academy Press.
4. Iowa Intervention Project. (1997). *NIC implementation manual*. Iowa City: The University of Iowa.
5. Iowa Outcomes Project. (1997). *NOC use survey*. Iowa City: The University of Iowa.
6. Johnson, M. R. (2002). Variables for outcome analysis. *Outcomes Management, 6*, 95-98.
7. Johnson, M., & Maas, M. (1998). Implementing the nursing outcomes classification in a practice setting. *Outcomes Management for Nursing, 2*, 99-104.
8. Johnson, M., Bulechek, G., Dochterman, J. M., Maas, M., & Moorhead, S. (2001). *Nursing diagnoses, outcomes, and interventions: NANDA, NOC, NIC linkages*. St. Louis, MO: Mosby.
9. Keenan, G., & Aquilino, M. L. (1998). Standardized nomenclatures: Keys to continuity of care, nursing accountability and nursing effectiveness. *Outcomes Management for Nursing, 2*, 81-86.
10. Lagoe, R. J., Kurtzig, B. S., & Hohner, V. K. (1999). Health care data and their sources [Special issue]. *Journal of Nursing Care Quality, 1*, 7-24.
11. McDonald, C. J., Overhage, J. M., Dexter, P. R., Blevins, L., Meeks-Johnson, J., Suico, J. G., et al. (1998). Canopy computing: Using the Web in clinical practice. *Journal of the American Medical Association, 280*, 1325-1329.
12. National Center for Health Statistics. (1980). Uniform hospital discharge minimum data set (Department of Health Education and Welfare Publication No. PHS 80-1157). Washington, DC: Hyattsville, MO: Author.
13. NANDA International. (2003). *Nursing diagnoses: Definitions and classification 2003-2004*. Philadelphia: Author.
14. Pesut, D. J., & Herman, J. (1999). *Clinical reasoning: The art and science of critical & creative thinking*. Boston: Delmar.
15. Rubenfeld, M. G., & Scheffer, B. K. (1999). *Critical thinking in nursing: An interactive approach* (2nd ed.). Philadelphia: J. B. Lippincott.
16. Sidani, S., & Braden, C. J. (1998). *Evaluating nursing interventions A theory-driven approach*. Thousand Oaks, CA: Sage.

# CHAPTER FIVE
## Using NOC in Education and Research

For standardized, nursing languages such as the Nursing Outcomes Classification (NOC) to become consistently used in nursing, the incorporation of the languages in nursing education and research is required. The use of standardized languages in education is becoming more prevalent as new textbooks are beginning to use the languages and faculty are becoming more familiar with the languages. The use of standardized languages in nursing research is in its infancy, but the implementation of evidence-based practice and the electronic medical record will offer more opportunities to test the use of standardized languages in practice settings.

## IMPLEMENTING NOC IN EDUCATIONAL PROGRAMS

Implementation of standardized languages, including NOC, throughout a curriculum requires a high level of commitment on the part of faculty and academic administration. All facets of the curriculum—the philosophy, program goals, and individual course objectives—need to reflect this commitment. Frequently, one or more faculty members become interested in piloting a standardized language in a course, use the language in the course, and then encourage its adoption throughout the curriculum. They can act as the project leaders in educating other faculty and demonstrating how course content can be adapted to include NOC and other standardized languages.

### Selecting the Standardized Language(s)

Seldom is NOC the only standardized language introduced in a curriculum. Many programs have been using North American Nursing Diagnosis Association (NANDA) diagnoses and are moving toward the implementation of NOC and the Nursing Interventions Classification (NIC) to complete the process of identifying the diagnoses, outcomes, and interventions that students use as they learn the nursing process and plan care for their patients. The fact that the three languages have not been presented together has made implementation throughout the curriculum more difficult. However, recent movement toward bringing the languages closer together bodes well for expediting their use in curricula. One of the outcomes of the new cooperation has been the development of a taxonomy structure that can encompass all three languages.[3] The NOC outcomes have been placed in the taxonomy and are provided in Appendix B. This represents the first attempt to use the taxonomy for NOC outcomes, and changes will likely occur as all three languages are brought together within the taxonomy. Another development has been the publication of a book that links the three languages.[5] The linkages in the book use the terminology from the second edition of NOC[6] and are based on expert opinion rather than clinical data. In addition, studies of the linkages between the three languages are beginning to appear in the literature.[10]

Use of NANDA, NIC, and NOC as the standardized languages in a curriculum has a number of advantages. Many programs have been using NANDA diagnoses, thereby making it easier to incorporate NIC and NOC, two languages that can be used in conjunction with NANDA. The languages can be used in all clinical settings in which students have their learning experiences. The languages can be used throughout the curriculum and can serve as an organizing thread. The use of standardized languages will better prepare students for the future as electronic records become routine. Students and nurses who don't have to break other habits often find the languages easier to use than nurses who have not been exposed to standardized languages in their nursing programs.

## Implementation Strategies

A number of strategies can be used in planning how NOC will be implemented throughout the undergraduate curriculum. One strategy assumes the implementation of NANDA diagnoses, NIC, and NOC and includes the following steps.[1]

1. Determine which diagnoses are used in each course and clinical area. This can be done by individual faculty, by faculty in each course, or by the faculty as a whole.

2. Identify diagnoses used in more than one course and those not used in any of the courses. Determine how these will be handled—taught in more than one course, assigned to one course, not used in the curriculum. This task can be accomplished with a group representing all clinical courses or the faculty as a whole.

3. Select the NOC outcomes that are frequently used for each of the diagnoses. This can be done by using some of the linkage work or selecting the outcomes that can be used in place of previously used goal statements.

4. Identify the NIC interventions taught in each course. This can be done with a survey that lists all of the courses on the horizontal axis and the interventions on the vertical axis. It can also be accomplished by substituting the appropriate NIC intervention labels for the interventions currently taught in each course.

5. As a group, delete all interventions that will not be taught in the undergraduate curriculum.

6. Match all of the interventions that will be taught to one of the diagnoses and the associated outcomes. You may find some disparity, most likely some interventions that do not fit a diagnosis. Decide how these interventions will be handled—remain in the curriculum or be deleted.

The result should be a list of diagnoses matched to outcomes and interventions that will comprise the curriculum and reflect the goals of the program. The last step is to determine in which course each of the diagnoses and associated interventions and outcomes will be taught. Although time-consuming, this strategy preserves critical thinking and allows patient problems appropriate for the student level to drive the system.

Another strategy that can be used is to begin with the core interventions used by 39 clinical specialties[7] and determine which of these are appropriate for the undergraduate program. These interventions can be mapped to the interventions currently taught in the course, an exercise that can help faculty decide whether they want to eliminate some of the interventions previously taught or add to the interventions previously taught. Steps similar to those identified in the previous steps can than be used to link the selected interventions with the appropriate nursing diagnoses and patient outcomes.

## Aids for Curriculum Development and Teaching

Detailed suggestions for implementing the languages in a curriculum are in a manual by Finesilver and Metzler,[4] which can be obtained through the Center for Nursing Classification and Clinical Effectiveness. The manual describes courses in one undergraduate program and includes methods, forms, and teaching aids used in the classes. This and other aids that the educator might find helpful are listed in Box 5-1.

The linkages provided in this book, in the NIC book,[2] and in the NANDA, NOC, NIC (NNN) linkage book[5] can assist with the process. The linkage book also provides instructions for accessing a Web-based system that provides access to a customized care planning system based on the three languages. This system can be used as a teaching tool when students are first becoming familiar with the languages and beginning to plan care. An article by Yom and Yoo[10] provides a set of linkages developed for patients undergoing abdominal surgery in Korea. It can provide an opportunity to discuss similarities and differences in the outcomes for patients in Korea and the United States, as well as information to use in identifying the NNN linkages for use in the curriculum. (It should be noted that the column on page 85 of the article by Yim and Yoo is

---

**Box 5-1**

### Aids Useful for Educators

Denehy, J. (1998). Integrating nursing outcomes classification in nursing education. *Journal of Nursing Care Quality, 12,* 73-84.

Finesilver, C., & Metzler, D. (Eds.). (2002). *Curriculum guide for implementation of NANDA, NIC, and NOC into an undergraduate nursing curriculum.* Iowa City, IA: College of Nursing, Center for Nursing Classification and Clinical Effectiveness.

Maas, M. L., Buckwalter, K. C., Hardy, M. D., Tripp-Reimer, T., Titler, M., & Specht, J. P. (Eds.). (2001). *Nursing care of older adults: Diagnoses, outcomes, and interventions.* St. Louis, MO: Mosby. (An example of a text that uses NANDA, NOC, NIC)

The University of Iowa, Center for Nursing Classification and Clinical Effectiveness. NIC and NOC 101: The basics. Web course available at http://www.nursing.uiowa.edu/centers/cncce

---

mislabeled; the terms under the column "nursing intervention" are actually the nursing outcome terms.) Another resource is the LISTSERV available through the Center for Nursing Classification and Clinical Effectiveness at the University of Iowa. Directions for accessing the list can be found in Chapter 4 in the section on aids in selection of outcomes. The members comprise a diverse group that includes educators, as well as practitioners; and issues related to the use of NOC in education, as well as practice, are discussed.

We recognize that the knowledge outcomes, while important in their own right, are generally precursors to altering selected patient behaviors. For this reason, we have identified NOC outcomes that can be used to measure behaviors related to the NOC knowledge outcomes; these are provided in Table 5-1. The primary behavioral outcomes are those directly related to the knowledge outcome (e.g., Body Mechanics Performance for Knowledge: Body Mechanics). In general, the primary behavioral outcomes reflect both the knowledge definition and indicators found in the knowledge outcome. Secondary behavioral outcomes are those that are related less directly to the knowledge outcome; the relationship can be more directly tied to specific indicators than to the overall concept, for example, Transfer Performance for Knowledge: Body Mechanics. The secondary behavioral outcomes can also be more specific than the knowledge outcomes, for example, Asthma Self-Management for Knowledge: Disease Process, which is a more generic outcome.

### Examples of Implementation

Once decisions about the placement of the standardized languages in the curriculum are made, the next step is the implementation in course work. The description of the use of NOC in clinical practice in the previous chapter can provide a basis for the application of NOC in clinical courses. A major difference is the emphasis on teaching students clinical decision making. Appendix F contains a description of the processes and forms used in four educational programs.

### USING NOC IN RESEARCH

The Classification and individual outcomes can be used in evaluation research, effectiveness research, and traditional clinical or efficacy research. There is also a pressing need to continue research on the Classification itself, with particular attention to the reliability of the measures across populations and settings. These areas cannot be thoroughly addressed in this chapter; rather, this section discusses the need for further research on the Classification and touches on some of the other research areas and questions that need to be addressed.

| TABLE 5-1 | NOC PERFORMANCE OUTCOMES RELATED TO NOC KNOWLEDGE OUTCOMES | |
|---|---|---|
| **Knowledge Outcomes** | **Primary Behavioral Outcomes** | **Secondary Behavioral Outcomes** |
| All Knowledge: Outcomes | 1600 Adherence Behavior<br>1601 Compliance Behavior<br>1606 Participation in Health Care Decisions | 1705 Health Orientation<br>1209 Motivation<br>1614 Personal Autonomy |
| 1827 Knowledge: Body Mechanics | 1616 Body Mechanics Performance | 0200 Ambulation<br>0201 Ambulation: Wheelchair<br>0203 Body Positioning: Self-Initiated<br>0210 Transfer Performance |
| 1800 Knowledge: Breastfeeding | 1000 Breastfeeding Establishment: Infant<br>1001 Breastfeeding Establishment: Maternal<br>1002 Breastfeeding Maintenance<br>1003 Breastfeeding Weaning | 0110 Growth<br>1008 Nutritional Status: Food & Fluid Intake<br>1500 Parent-Infant Attachment |
| 1830 Knowledge: Cardiac Disease Management | 1617 Cardiac Disease Self-Management<br>1603 Health Seeking Behavior<br>1914 Risk Control: Cardiovascular Health<br>1608 Symptom Control | 1308 Adaptation to Physical Disability<br>0002 Energy Conservation<br>2605 Family Participation in Professional Care<br>2609 Family Support During Treatment<br>1008 Nutritional Status: Food & Fluid Intake<br>1305 Psychosocial Adjustment: Life Change<br>1902 Risk Control<br>1609 Treatment Behavior: Illness or Injury |
| 1801 Knowledge: Child Physical Safety | 2902 Parenting: Adolescent Physical Safety<br>2901 Parenting: Early/Middle Childhood Physical Safety<br>2900 Parenting: Infant/Toddler Physical Safety<br>2211 Parenting Performance | 2501 Abuse Protection<br>1901 Parenting: Psychosocial Safety<br>1910 Safe Home Environment |

*Continued*

| TABLE 5-1 | NOC PERFORMANCE OUTCOMES RELATED TO NOC KNOWLEDGE OUTCOMES—CONT'D | |
|---|---|---|
| **Knowledge Outcomes** | **Primary Behavioral Outcomes** | **Secondary Behavioral Outcomes** |
| 1821 Knowledge: Conception Prevention | 1907 Risk Control: Unintended Pregnancy | 1902 Risk Control<br>1905 Risk Control: Sexually Transmitted Diseases (STD) |
| 1820 Knowledge: Diabetes Management | 1619 Diabetes Self-Management<br>1603 Health Seeking Behavior<br>1608 Symptom Control<br>1612 Weight Control | 1008 Nutritional Status: Food & Fluid Intake<br>1902 Risk Control<br>1916 Risk Control: Visual Impairment<br>0119 Sexual Functioning<br>1609 Treatment Behavior: Illness or Injury<br>1611 Vision Compensation Behavior |
| 1802 Knowledge: Diet | 1603 Health Seeking Behavior<br>1008 Nutritional Status: Food & Fluid Intake<br>1612 Weight Control | 1607 Prenatal Health Behavior<br>1609 Treatment Behavior: Illness or Injury |
| 1803 Knowledge: Disease Process | 1603 Health Seeking Behavior<br>1608 Symptom Control<br>1609 Treatment Behavior: Illness or Injury | 1401 Aggression Self-Control<br>1402 Anxiety Self-Control<br>1918 Aspiration Prevention<br>0704 Asthma Self-Management<br>1616 Body Mechanics Performance<br>1617 Cardiac Disease Self-Management<br>1409 Depression Self-Control<br>1619 Diabetes Self-Management<br>1403 Distorted Thought Self-Control<br>1610 Hearing Compensation Behavior<br>1405 Impulse Self-Control<br>1618 Nausea & Vomiting Control |

| TABLE 5-1 | NOC PERFORMANCE OUTCOMES RELATED TO NOC KNOWLEDGE OUTCOMES | |
|---|---|---|
| **Knowledge Outcomes** | **Primary Behavioral Outcomes** | **Secondary Behavioral Outcomes** |
| | | 1615 Ostomy Self-Care<br>1605 Pain Control<br>1911 Personal Safety Behavior<br>1620 Seizure Control<br>1406 Self-Mutilation Restraint<br>1408 Suicide Self-Restraint<br>1611 Vision Compensation Behavior |
| 1804 Knowledge: Energy Conservation | 0002 Energy Conservation<br>1602 Health Promoting Behavior | 0200 Ambulation<br>1616 Body Mechanics Performance |
| 1828 Knowledge: Fall Prevention | 1909 Fall Prevention Behavior | 0200 Ambulation<br>0201 Ambulation: Wheelchair<br>1910 Safe Home Environment<br>0210 Transfer Performance |
| 1816 Knowledge: Fertility Promotion | 1607 Prenatal Health Behavior<br>0119 Sexual Functioning | 1905 Risk Control: Sexually Transmitted Diseases (STD)<br>1908 Risk Detection |
| 1805 Knowledge: Health Behavior | 1602 Health Promoting Behavior<br>1900 Immunization Behavior<br>1911 Personal Safety Behavior<br>1902 Risk Control<br>1903 Risk Control: Alcohol Use<br>1917 Risk Control: Cancer<br>1914 Risk Control: Cardiovascular Health<br>1904 Risk Control: Drug Use<br>1915 Risk Control: Hearing Impairment<br>1905 Risk Control: Sexually Transmitted Diseases (STD) | 1401 Aggression Self-Control<br>1402 Anxiety Self-Control<br>1616 Body Mechanics Performance<br>2801 Community Risk Control: Chronic Disease<br>2802 Community Risk Control: Communicable Disease<br>2803 Community Risk Control: Lead Exposure<br>2805 Community Risk Control: Violence<br>1302 Coping<br>0002 Energy Conservation |

*Continued*

| TABLE 5-1 | NOC Performance Outcomes Related to NOC Knowledge Outcomes—cont'd |
|---|---|

| Knowledge Outcomes | Primary Behavioral Outcomes | Secondary Behavioral Outcomes |
|---|---|---|
| | 1906 Risk Control: Tobacco Use<br>1907 Risk Control: Unintended Pregnancy<br>1916 Risk Control: Visual Impairment<br>1908 Risk Detection | 1909 Fall Prevention Behavior<br>1405 Impulse Self-Control<br>1604 Leisure Participation<br>1008 Nutritional Status: Food & Fluid Intake<br>1607 Prenatal Health Behavior<br>1612 Weight Control |
| 1823 Knowledge: Health Promotion | 1602 Health Promoting Behavior<br>1900 Immunization Behavior<br>1911 Personal Safety Behavior<br>1908 Risk Detection | 1903 Risk Control: Alcohol Use<br>1904 Risk Control: Drug Use<br>1905 Risk Control: Sexually Transmitted Diseases (STD)<br>1906 Risk Control: Tobacco Use<br>1612 Weight Control |
| 1806 Knowledge: Health Resources | 2206 Caregiver Performance: Indirect Care | 1308 Adaptation to Physical Disability<br>2700 Community Competence<br>2602 Family Functioning |
| 1824 Knowledge: Illness Care | 2205 Caregiver Performance: Direct Care<br>1603 Health Seeking Behavior<br>1618 Nausea & Vomiting Control<br>1605 Pain Control<br>1613 Self-Direction of Care<br>1608 Symptom Control<br>1609 Treatment Behavior: Illness or Injury | 1308 Adaptation to Physical Disability<br>1918 Aspiration Prevention<br>2206 Caregiver Performance: Indirect Care<br>1301 Child Adaptation to Hospitalization<br>0002 Energy Conservation<br>1909 Fall Prevention Behavior<br>2605 Family Participation in Professional Care<br>2609 Family Support During Treatment<br>1008 Nutritional Status: Food & Fluid Intake |

| TABLE 5-1 | NOC PERFORMANCE OUTCOMES RELATED TO NOC KNOWLEDGE OUTCOMES | |
|---|---|---|
| **Knowledge Outcomes** | **Primary Behavioral Outcomes** | **Secondary Behavioral Outcomes** |
| | | 1615 Ostomy Self-Care<br>1902 Risk Control<br>1612 Weight Control |
| 1819 Knowledge: Infant Care | 1500 Parent-Infant Attachment<br>2900 Parenting: Infant/ Toddler Physical Safety<br>2211 Parenting Performance<br>1901 Parenting: Psychosocial Safety | 2501 Abuse Protection<br>1400 Abusive Behavior Self-Restraint<br>1001 Breastfeeding Establishment: Maternal<br>2608 Family Resiliency<br>1900 Immunization Behavior |
| 1807 Knowledge: Infection Control | 1900 Immunization Behavior<br>2802 Community Risk Control: Communicable Disease<br>1905 Risk Control: Sexually Transmitted Diseases (STD) | 2800 Community Health Status: Immunity<br>1607 Prenatal Health Behavior<br>1902 Risk Control<br>1908 Risk Detection |
| 1817 Knowledge: Labor & Delivery | | 1302 Coping<br>0002 Energy Conservation<br>2605 Family Participation in Professional Care<br>1605 Pain Control |
| 1808 Knowledge: Medication | 2205 Caregiver Performance: Direct Care<br>0307 Self-Care: Non-Parenteral Medication<br>0309 Self-Care: Parenteral Medication | 1911 Personal Safety Behavior<br>1613 Self-Direction of Care |
| 1829 Knowledge: Ostomy Care | 1615 Ostomy Self-Care<br>1609 Treatment Behavior: Illness or Injury | 0305 Self-Care: Hygiene |
| 1826 Knowledge: Parenting | 2902 Parenting: Adolescent Physical Safety<br>2901 Parenting: Early/ Middle Childhood Physical Safety<br>2900 Parenting: Infant/ Toddler Physical Safety | 2501 Abuse Protection<br>2602 Family Functioning<br>2608 Family Resiliency<br>1500 Parent-Infant Attachment<br>0116 Play Participation<br>1501 Role Performance |

*Continued*

| TABLE 5-1 | NOC PERFORMANCE OUTCOMES RELATED TO NOC KNOWLEDGE OUTCOMES—CONT'D | |
|---|---|---|
| **Knowledge Outcomes** | **Primary Behavioral Outcomes** | **Secondary Behavioral Outcomes** |
| | 2211 Parenting Performance <br> 1901 Parenting: Psychosocial Safety | |
| 1809 Knowledge: Personal Safety | 1909 Fall Prevention Behavior <br> 1911 Personal Safety Behavior <br> 1910 Safe Home Environment | 1616 Body Mechanics Performance <br> 1405 Impulse Self-Control <br> 1902 Risk Control <br> 1903 Risk Control: Alcohol Use <br> 1904 Risk Control: Drug Use <br> 1908 Risk Detection <br> 0210 Transfer Performance |
| 1818 Knowledge: Postpartum Maternal Health | 1302 Coping <br> 1305 Psychosocial Adjustment: Life Change | 1001 Breastfeeding Establishment: Maternal <br> 0002 Energy Conservation <br> 2605 Family Participation in Professional Care <br> 1008 Nutritional Status: Food & Fluid Intake <br> 1907 Risk Control: Unintended Pregnancy |
| 1822 Knowledge: Preconception Maternal Health | 1602 Health Promoting Behavior <br> 1607 Prenatal Health Behavior | 1911 Personal Safety Behavior <br> 1905 Risk Control: Sexually Transmitted Diseases (STD) <br> 1908 Risk Detection <br> 1910 Safe Home Environment |
| 1810 Knowledge: Pregnancy | 1602 Health Promoting Behavior <br> 1607 Prenatal Health Behavior | 2501 Abuse Protection <br> 1616 Body Mechanics Performance <br> 0002 Energy Conservation <br> 1618 Nausea & Vomiting Control <br> 1008 Nutritional Status: Food & Fluid Intake |

| TABLE 5-1 | NOC PERFORMANCE OUTCOMES RELATED TO NOC KNOWLEDGE OUTCOMES | |
|---|---|---|
| **Knowledge Outcomes** | **Primary Behavioral Outcomes** | **Secondary Behavioral Outcomes** |
| | | 1902 Risk Control<br>1908 Risk Detection<br>1910 Safe Home Environment<br>1612 Weight Control |
| 1811 Knowledge: Prescribed Activity | 0200 Ambulation<br>1609 Treatment Behavior: Illness or Injury | 1308 Adaptation to Physical Disability<br>0201 Ambulation: Wheelchair<br>1616 Body Mechanics Performance<br>0203 Body Positioning: Self-Initiated<br>1607 Prenatal Health Behavior<br>0210 Transfer Performance |
| 1815 Knowledge: Sexual Functioning | 0119 Sexual Functioning | 1905 Risk Control: Sexually Transmitted Diseases (STD)<br>1907 Risk Control: Unintended Pregnancy |
| 1812 Knowledge: Substance Use Control | 1903 Risk Control: Alcohol Use<br>1904 Risk Control: Drug Use<br>1906 Risk Control: Tobacco Use | 1405 Impulse Self-Control<br>1911 Personal Safety Behavior |
| 1814 Knowledge: Treatment Procedure(s) | 2205 Caregiver Performance: Direct Care<br>1613 Self-Direction of Care<br>1609 Treatment Behavior: Illness or Injury | 1918 Aspiration Prevention<br>2609 Family Support During Treatment<br>1615 Ostomy Self-Care<br>0210 Transfer Performance |
| 1813 Knowledge: Treatment Regimen | 2205 Caregiver Performance: Direct Care<br>1613 Self-Direction of Care<br>1608 Symptom Control<br>1609 Treatment Behavior: Illness or Injury | 1308 Adaptation to Physical Disability<br>0704 Asthma Self-Management<br>1617 Cardiac Disease Self-Management<br>2206 Caregiver Performance: Indirect Care<br>1619 Diabetes Self-Management |

## Evaluating the Classification

The outcomes in the Classification require continued evaluation in clinical practice to ensure that they are reliable, valid measures of the concept being measured and that they remain current with practice. The use of outcomes in practice also requires study: How easy are they to use? How much time does it take to document with the outcomes? How useful is the information for nurses? and Does their use have an effect on the accuracy of clinical judgments made by nurses? These are just a few of the questions that might be addressed. A few articles addressing some of these issues by other investigators, as well as by the project team, are beginning to appear in the literature. Box 5-2 lists a few publications that others may find useful. The authors encourage further research on the outcomes and appreciate having the findings shared so changes can be made in the outcomes as new information becomes available.

## Evaluating Nursing Quality and Effectiveness

Outcomes are the trigger for the evaluation of quality and effectiveness, since they answer the question, "Did the patient benefit or not benefit from the care provided?"[9] For the purpose of facilitating improvement in care quality, information about patient outcomes should identify not only inadequate outcomes but also those that are marginal, adequate, and superior. The outcomes in NOC are concepts that reflect patient states, are generally neutral (e.g., mobility, hydration, coping), and can be measured on a continuum rather than as a goal that is met or not met. Because of these characteristics, they provide measures that can be aggregated in a number of ways—such as by nursing or medical diagnoses, by service unit, or by severity of illness—to study the effectiveness of nursing interventions. Questions about the combination of interventions that is most effective in achieving desired outcomes in a patient group or about the type of nursing care delivery system that produces the best outcomes can be addressed. They also allow for differences in outcome achievement to be analyzed by patient characteristics, such as age, gender, or functional status. Determining how patient characteristics affect outcome achievement is an important area for further research; results of this type of research will provide information about outcomes that can be realistically achieved with varied patient populations. "From a quality improvement perspective, it is important to be able to identify a realistic outcome to

---

**Box 5-2**

### Publications in which NOC Is Used in Research and Evaluation

Maas, M., Reed, D., Reeder, K. M., Kerr, P., Specht, J., Johnson, M., et al. (2002). Nursing outcomes classification: A preliminary report of field testing. *Outcomes Management, 6,* 112-119.

Morrison, R., Burroughs, C., Witt, M., Redden, J., & Leeper, J. D. (2000). Evaluation of NOC instruments with chronically ill patients. *Southern Online Journal of Nursing Research, 1,* 1-11. web site: http://www.snrs.org

Peters, R. M. (2000). Using NOC outcomes of risk control in prevention, early detection, and control of hypertension. *Outcomes Management for Nursing Practice, 4,* 39-45.

Scherb, C. (2001). Outcomes research: Making a difference in practice. *Outcomes Management 6,* 22-26.

Scherb, C. A., Rapp, C. G., Johnson, M., & Maas, M. (1998). The nursing outcomes classification (NOC): Validation by rehabilitation nurses. *Journal of Rehabilitation Nursing, 23,* 174-191.

Williams, J., Skirton, H., Reed, D., Johnson, M., Maas, M., & Daack-Hirsch, S. (2001). Genetic counseling outcomes validation by genetics nurses in the UK and US. *Journal of Nursing Scholarship, 33,* 369-374.

Yom, Y., & Yoo, H. S. (2002). Application of nursing diagnoses, interventions, and outcomes to patients undergoing abdominal surgery in Korea. *International Journal of Nursing Terminologies and Classifications, 13,* 77-87.

be achieved. Unrealistic outcome expectations are inefficient in that resources may be expended to no good effect" (p. 127).[8] The effect of patient characteristics on outcome achievement is also important when quality is being compared across organizations to ensure that the effects of structure and process on patient outcomes are being measured and not the effects of patient characteristics.

Effectiveness research requires the ability to quantify data, including patient outcomes. It generally relies on information obtained from large data sets to evaluate the effects of interventions provided by multiple providers in noncontrolled practice situations with patients receiving routine care. New techniques for data mining, data aggregation, and data analysis will foster the expansion of nursing effectiveness research if standardized nursing elements are coded and available in national data sets. At this time, a few investigators are beginning to use NOC outcomes to evaluate nursing effectiveness within an organization or patient group; some of their studies are listed in Box 5-2.

Clinical innovations are initially evaluated through controlled clinical studies with attention given to the measurement of desired or expected outcomes. Many clinical studies in nursing are conducted in one site and with relatively small samples. The ability to generalize findings can be increased by using meta-analysis if study variables are similar. The use of standardized patient outcomes as one of the study variables would increase the ease with which findings could be compared across studies. Because the current outcomes have not been tested as completely as instruments that are generally selected for controlled studies, we would encourage researchers to use the NOC outcomes that correspond to the instrument used in the study, compare results from the two measures, and report these findings when they report their research. The major concern that will need to be considered is whether the research instrument and the NOC outcome are measuring the same concept. If so, this type of testing would facilitate a more rapid evaluation of the outcomes.

## SUMMARY

The use of NOC in education is increasing as more textbooks and schools move toward the use of standardized languages. These are important steps for the nursing profession and will ensure that future nurses are better equipped to deal with the changes that will take place with the implementation of electronic records and electronic documentation. Although research studies in which NOC is used are just beginning to appear in the literature, it is hoped that critiques of the Classification and research making use of the Classification will increase. It is only through research in which patient outcomes are evaluated in relation to practice that nurses will have the data required to demonstrate the quality and effectiveness of our practice.

## REFERENCES

1. Delaney, C. (April 7, 1998). Personal communication via e-mail.
2. Dochterman, J., & Bulechek, G. (2004). *Nursing interventions classification (NIC)* (4th ed.). St. Louis, MO: Mosby.
3. Dochterman, J., & Jones, D. (2003). *Unifying nursing languages: The harmonization of NANDA, NIC and NOC.* Washington, DC: American Nurses Association.
4. Finesilver, C., & Metzler, D. (Eds.). (2002). *Curriculum guide for implementation of NANDA, NIC, and NOC into an undergraduate nursing curriculum.* Iowa City, IA: College of Nursing, Center for Nursing Classification and Clinical Effectiveness.
5. Johnson, M., Bulechek, G., Dochterman, J., Maas, M., & Moorhead, S. (2001). *Nursing diagnoses, outcomes, & interventions: NANDA, NOC, and NIC linkages.* St. Louis, MO: Mosby.
6. Johnson, M., Maas, M., & Moorhead, S. (2000). *Nursing outcomes classification (NOC).* St. Louis, MO: Mosby.
7. McCloskey, J., Bulechek, G., & Donahue, W. (1998). Nursing interventions core to specialty practice. *Nursing Outlook, 46,* 67-76.

8. Mills, W. C. (1994). Tacking through troubled waters: Toward desired outcomes. In R. M. Carroll-Johnson & M. Paquette (Eds.), *Classification of nursing diagnosis: Proceedings of the Tenth Conference* (pp. 126-130). Philadelphia: J. B. Lippincott.

9. Shaughnessy, P. W., & Crisler, K. S. (1995). *Outcome-based quality improvement: A manual for home care agencies on how to use outcomes.* Washington, DC: National Association for Home Care.

10. Yom, Y., & Yoo, H. S. (2002). Application of nursing diagnoses, interventions, and outcomes to patients undergoing abdominal surgery in Korea. *International Journal of Nursing Terminologies and Classifications, 13*, 77-87.

# PART TWO

# NOC Taxonomy

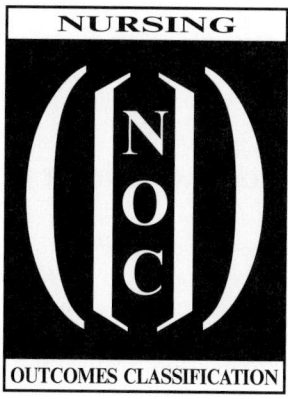

# Overview of the NOC Taxonomy

The following section contains the three-level taxonomy for the NOC. This taxonomic structure was developed during the second phase of the research and was first published in the second edition. The NOC taxonomy was created to: (1) provide a stable structure for outcome placement over time, (2) allow for the addition of new outcomes as they were developed, (3) allow for the identification of missing outcomes needed for future editions, and (4) assist nurses to identify and select outcomes for the diagnoses they treat for patients, families, and communities. Use of the taxonomy makes identification of possible outcomes for use in practice easier than an alphabetical list of the outcomes. The conceptual grouping of outcomes in the taxonomy has become even more important as the classification has grown over time. Each outcome is listed in only one place in the taxonomy.

## DEVELOPMENT OF THE TAXONOMY FOR NOC

The NOC taxonomic structure was developed using strategies refined by the Iowa Intervention Project.[1] The goal was to create a three-level taxonomic structure similar to the one developed for the Nursing Interventions Classification (NIC).[2] This required an inductive approach using qualitative similarity-dissimilarity analysis by many participants sorting outcomes into clusters. Participants assigned a concept label that they believedt captured the essence of the cluster. In the first sort 175 outcomes were grouped in this manner, and the participants were asked to create 15 to 25 clusters based on the sorting process. Hierarchical cluster analysis was then applied to combine the results of each participant's individual sort. This process created the class level of the NOC taxonomy, which when finalized created 24 classes. The classes created using this process are Energy Maintenance, Growth and Development, Mobility, Self-Care, Cardiopulmonary, Elimination, Fluid and Electrolytes, Immune Response, Metabolic Regulation, Neurocognitive, Nutrition, Tissue Integrity, Psychological Well-Being, Psychological Adaptation, Self-Control, Social Interaction, Health Behavior, Health Beliefs, Health Knowledge, Risk Control and Safety, Health and Life Quality, Symptom Status, Family Caregiver Status, and Maltreatment Resolution.

In the second phase of the development of the taxonomy, the 24 classes were sorted by participants to create the top level of the taxonomy. The results of this process identified six domains: Functional Health, Physiologic Health, Psychosocial Health, Health Knowledge and Behavior, Perceived Health, and Family Health. A more detailed description of the process used to create the taxonomy is available elsewhere.[3]

## REVISIONS MADE IN THE TAXONOMY SINCE ITS CREATION

The third edition has 7 Domains and 31 Classes in the taxonomic structure. The addition of 2 new classes resulted in some changes in the placement of outcomes within the taxonomy for this edition. Community Health was added as a domain to the taxonomy to allow for inclusion of outcomes focused on the community as the recipient of care. This domain contains outcomes that describe the health, well-being, and functioning of a community or population. Like the Family Domain, the focus of care is on a group rather than an individual. In this case the population might be an entire community, a neighborhood, or a population of patients with the same health concern.

In addition to the inclusion of two new classes, several other modifications were made in the class level of the taxonomy. The definition of the class Health Knowledge was modified for this edition. The performance aspect of this class was eliminated so the words "and skills" were removed from the definition. This was done to keep knowledge separate from behavior in the classification. The definition of Domain V, Perceived Health, was modified to describe an individual's health and health care. A new class was added to this domain to include the addition of the client satisfaction outcomes. This class, called Satisfaction with Care, includes outcomes that describe an individual's perceptions of the quality and adequacy of their health care. Due to this addition the definition of the class Health and Life Quality was modified. Several changes were made in Domain VI, Family Health. A new class was added called Parenting. This class contains outcomes that describe behaviors of parents that promote growth and development. The class Family Care Status was renamed Family Caregiver Performance to better reflect the outcomes in this class.

## CODING OF THE CLASSIFICATION

Once the taxonomic structure was created, coding of the NOC became a high priority for the second edition. Coding is important since it creates a way to: (1) represent each of the taxonomic elements, (2) facilitate use of NOC in computer systems, (3) create nursing data sets that can be linked with large regional and national health care databases, and (4) facilitate client outcome evaluation to improve the quality of patient care. The coding structure for NOC includes the domains, classes, outcomes, indicators of each outcome, measurement scales, and actual scores recorded by users.

Every effort has been made to retain codes used in the second edition in the third edition of this classification. With classification work it is important to keep coding of the outcomes consistent across editions. When changes were made in this edition, careful consideration of whether the outcome was a new outcome or a revision had to be made. Any outcome that was just updated and revised retained its original code. In a few cases the outcome revisions resulted in the creation of new outcomes from a previous outcome in the classification. In this case the old outcome was retired (along with its code), and the new outcome(s) were given new codes. Codes for any indicator eliminated from the outcome resulted in the retiring of the code assigned to that indicator. Each outcome had the code for the indicator "Other" retired for that outcome. This indicator was removed because testing in practice demonstrated that data from this indicator were not clinically useful. In many outcomes the indicators were organized in a new list, but the indicators retained their original code in spite of placement in the outcome.

The addition of a second scale to some outcomes has resulted in the need to modify the coding scheme for the scale data. Scales in the previous edition were coded with a letter of the alphabet. We continue to assign a letter to each scale, but the coding of the scales will need to account for the fact that two scales are in use for some outcomes. The coding will use a number to reflect what scale or scale combinations are used for that outcome, and, because there are more than nine scales, the codes for the scales will require two spaces in the structure (Table 1).

This coding structure allows for expansion of the NOC at every level of the taxonomy and creates a unique identification for each outcome, indicator, and measurement scale. For example, two additional domains can be added, and the classification can have up to 21 new classes, each containing up to 99 outcomes. This structure allows for substantial additions to the classifications without changing the coding structure. Since the first draft of the taxonomy was created, 155 new outcomes have been developed and placed in the taxonomy. Few changes in the structure have been needed to accomplish this. Changes in the outcomes for this edition are summarized in Appendix A.

| Table 1 | Coding Structure of NOC | | | | |
|---|---|---|---|---|---|
| Domain (1-9) | Class (A-Z) or (a-z) | Outcome (4 numbers) | Indicator (01-99) | Scale (01-99) | Scale Value (1-5) |
| # | A | #### | ## | ## | ### |

# References

1. Iowa Intervention Project. (1993). The NIC taxonomy structure. *Image: Journal of Nursing Scholarship, 25*(3), 187-192.
2. Iowa Intervention Project. J. C. McCloskey & G. M. Bulechek (Eds.). (1996). *Nursing interventions classification (NIC)* (2nd ed.). St. Louis: Mosby Year Book.
3. Moorhead, S., Head, B., Johnson, M. & Maas, M. (1998). The Nursing Outcomes Taxonomy: Development and coding. *Journal of Nursing Care Quality, 12*(6), 56-63.

| Level 1 Domains | (1) Domain I | (2) Domain II | |
|---|---|---|---|
| | **Functional Health**<br>Outcomes that describe capacity for and performance of basic tasks of life | **Physiologic Health**<br>Outcomes that describe organic functioning | |
| Level 2 Classes | **A-Energy Maintenance**<br>Outcomes that describe an individual's energy rejuvenation, conservation, and expenditure<br><br>**B-Growth & Development**<br>Outcomes that describe an individual's physical, emotional, and social maturation<br><br>**C-Mobility**<br>Outcomes that describe an individual's physical mobility and the sequelae of restricted movement<br><br>**D-Self-Care**<br>Outcomes that describe an individual's ability to accomplish basic and instrumental activities of daily living | **E-Cardiopulmonary**<br>Outcomes that describe an individual's cardiac, pulmonary, circulatory, or tissue perfusion status<br><br>**F-Elimination**<br>Outcomes that describe an individual's waste excretion, elimination patterns, and status<br><br>**G-Fluid & Electrolytes**<br>Outcomes that describe an individual's fluid and electrolyte status<br><br>**H-Immune Response**<br>Outcomes that describe an individual's physiological reaction to substances that are foreign or interpreted by the body as foreign<br><br>**I-Metabolic Regulation**<br>Outcomes that describe an individual's ability to regulate body metabolism<br><br>**J-Neurocognitive**<br>Outcomes that describe an individual's neurological and cognitive status<br><br>**K-Nutritional**<br>Outcomes that describe an individual's nutritional pattern | **a-Therapeutic Response**<br>Outcomes that describe an individual's systemic reaction to a remedial health treatment, agent, or method<br><br>**L-Tissue Integrity**<br>Outcomes that describe the condition and function of an individual's body tissues<br><br>**Y-Sensory Function**<br>Outcomes that describe an individual's perception and use of sensory information |

*Continued*

| *Level 1* *Domains* | **(3) Domain III** | **(4) Domain IV** | **(5) Domain V** |
|---|---|---|---|
| | **Psychosocial Health** Outcomes that describe psychological and social functioning | **Health Knowledge & Behavior** Outcomes that describe attitudes, comprehension, and actions with respect to health and illness | **Perceived Health** Outcomes that describe impressions of an individual's health and health care |
| *Level 2* *Classes* | **M-Psychological Well-Being** Outcomes that describe an individual's emotional health | **Q-Health Behavior** Outcomes that describe an individual's actions to promote, maintain, or restore health | **U-Health & Life Quality** Outcomes that describe an individual's perceived health status and related life circumstances |
| | **N-Psychosocial Adaptation** Outcomes that describe an individual's psychological and/or social adaptation to altered health or life circumstances | **R-Health Beliefs** Outcomes that describe an individual's ideas and perceptions that influence health behavior | **V-Symptom Status** Outcomes that describe an individual's indications of a disease, injury, or loss |
| | **O-Self-Control** Outcomes that describe an individual's ability to restrain behavior that may be emotionally or physically harmful to self or others | **S-Health Knowledge** Outcomes that describe an individual's understanding in applying information to promote, maintain, and restore health | **e-Satisfaction with Care** Outcomes that describe an individual's perceptions of the quality and adequacy of their health care |
| | **P-Social Interaction** Outcomes that describe an individual's relationships with others | **T-Risk Control & Safety** Outcomes that describe an individual's safety status and/or actions to avoid, limit, or control identifiable health threats | |

| Level 1 Domains | (6) Domain VI | (7) Domain VII |
|---|---|---|
| | **Family Health** Outcomes that describe health status, behavior, or functioning of the family as a whole or of an individual as a family member | **Community Health** Outcomes that describe the health, well-being, and functioning of a community or population |
| Level 2 Classes | **W-Family Caregiver Performance** Outcomes that describe the adaptation and performance of a family member caring for a dependent child or adult | **b-Community Well-Being** Outcomes that describe the overall health status and social competence of a population or community |
| | **Z-Family Member Health Status** Outcomes that describe the physical and emotional health of an individual family member | **c-Community Health Protection** Outcomes that describe the structures and programs of a community to eliminate or reduce health risks and increase community resistance to health threats |
| | **X-Family Well-Being** Outcomes that describe the family environment and the physical, emotional, and social health of a family as a unit | |
| | **d-Parenting** Outcomes that describe behaviors of parents that promote optimum growth and development | |

*Continued*

| Level 1 | **(1) Domain I–Functional Health**<br>Outcomes that describe capacity for and performance of basic tasks of life | |
|---|---|---|
| Level 2 | **A-Energy Maintenance**<br>Outcomes that describe an individual's energy rejuvenation, conservation, and expenditure | **B-Growth & Development**<br>Outcomes that describe an individual's physical, emotional, and social maturation |
| Level 3 | 0005-Activity Tolerance<br>0001-Endurance<br>0002-Energy Conservation<br>0006-Psychomotor Energy<br>0003-Rest<br>0004-Sleep | 0120-Child Development: 1 Month<br>0100-Child Development: 2 Months<br>0101-Child Development: 4 Months<br>0102-Child Development: 6 Months<br>0103-Child Development: 12 Months<br>0104-Child Development: 2 Years<br>0105-Child Development: 3 Years<br>0106-Child Development: 4 Years<br>0107-Child Development: Preschool<br>0108-Child Development:<br>    Middle Childhood<br>0109-Child Development: Adolescence<br>0111-Fetal Status: Antepartum<br>0112-Fetal Status: Intrapartum<br>0110-Growth<br>0118-Newborn Adaptation<br>0113-Physical Aging<br>0114-Physical Maturation: Female<br>0115-Physical Maturation: Male<br>0116-Play Participation<br>0117-Preterm Infant Organization<br>0119-Sexual Functioning |

**C-Mobility**

Outcomes that describe an individual's physical mobility and the sequelae of restricted movement

**D-Self-Care**

Outcomes that describe an individual's ability to accomplish basic and instrumental activities of daily living

0200-Ambulation
0201-Ambulation: Wheelchair
0202-Balance
0203-Body Positioning: Self-Initiated
0212-Coordinated Movement
0204-Immobility Consequences:
    Physiological
0205-Immobility Consequences:
    Psycho-Cognitive
0213-Joint Movement: Ankle
0214-Joint Movement: Elbow
0215-Joint Movement: Fingers
0216-Joint Movement: Hip
0217-Joint Movement: Knee
0218-Joint Movement: Neck
0219-Joint Movement: Shoulder
0220-Joint Movement: Spine
0221-Joint Movement: Wrist
0207-Joint Movement: Passive
0208-Mobility
0211-Skeletal Function
0210-Transfer Performance

0311-Discharge Readiness: Independent Living
0312-Discharge Readiness: Supported Living
0313-Self-Care Status
0300-Self-Care: Activities of Daily Living (ADL)
0301-Self-Care: Bathing
0302-Self-Care: Dressing
0303-Self-Care: Eating
0305-Self-Care: Hygiene
0306-Self-Care: Instrumental Activities of
    Daily Living (IADL)
0307-Self-Care: Non-Parenteral Medication
0308-Self-Care: Oral Hygiene
0309-Self-Care: Parenteral Medication
0310-Self-Care: Toileting

*Continued*

| Level 1 | (2) Domain II–Physiologic Health<br>Outcomes that describe organic functioning | | |
|---|---|---|---|
| Level 2 | **E-Cardiopulmonary**<br>Outcomes that describe an individual's cardiac, pulmonary, circulatory, or tissue perfusion status | | **F-Elimination**<br>Outcomes that describe an individual's waste excretion, elimination patterns, and status |
| Level 3 | 0409-Blood Coagulation<br>0413-Blood Loss<br>    Severity<br>0400-Cardiac Pump<br>    Effectiveness<br>0401-Circulation Status<br>0411-Mechanical<br>    Ventilation<br>    Response: Adult<br>0412-Mechanical<br>    Ventilation<br>    Weaning<br>    Response: Adult<br>0410-Respiratory Status:<br>    Airway Patency | 0402-Respiratory Status:<br>    Gas Exchange<br>0403-Respiratory Status:<br>    Ventilation<br>0404-Tissue Perfusion:<br>    Abdominal Organs<br>0405-Tissue Perfusion:<br>    Cardiac<br>0406-Tissue Perfusion:<br>    Cerebral<br>0407-Tissue Perfusion:<br>    Peripheral<br>0408-Tissue Perfusion:<br>    Pulmonary | 0500-Bowel Continence<br>0501-Bowel<br>    Elimination<br>0504-Kidney Function<br>0502-Urinary<br>    Continence<br>0503-Urinary<br>    Elimination |

| G-Fluid & Electrolytes | H-Immune Response | I-Metabolic Regulation |
|---|---|---|
| Outcomes that describe an individual's fluid and electrolyte status | Outcomes that describe an individual's physiological reaction to substances that are foreign or interpreted by the body as foreign | Outcomes that describe an individual's ability to regulate body metabolism |
| 0600-Electrolyte & Acid/ Base Balance<br>0601-Fluid Balance<br>0603-Fluid Overload Severity<br>0602-Hydration | 0705-Allergic Response: Localized<br>0706-Allergic Response: Systemic<br>0700-Blood Transfusion Reaction<br>0707-Immune Hypersensitivity Response<br>0702-Immune Status<br>0703-Infection Severity<br>0708-Infection Severity: Newborn | 0800-Thermoregulation<br>0801-Thermoregulation: Newborn<br>0802-Vital Signs<br>1006-Weight: Body Mass |

*Continued*

| Level 1 | (2) Domain II–Physiologic Health—cont'd<br>Outcomes that describe organic functioning | |
|---|---|---|
| **Level 2** | **J-Neurocognitive**<br>Outcomes that describe an individual's neurological and cognitive status | **K-Nutrition**<br>Outcomes that describe an individual's nutritional patterns |
| **Level 3** | 0900-Cognition<br>0901-Cognitive Orientation<br>0902-Communication<br>0903-Communication: Expressive<br>0904-Communication: Receptive<br>0905-Concentration<br>0906-Decision-Making<br>0915-Hyperactivity Level<br>0907-Information Processing<br>0908-Memory<br>0909-Neurological Status<br>0910-Neurological Status: Autonomic<br>0911-Neurological Status: Central Motor Control<br>0912-Neurological Status: Consciousness<br>0913-Neurological Status: Cranial Sensory/Motor Function<br>0914-Neurological Status: Spinal Sensory/Motor Function | 1014-Appetite<br>1000-Breastfeeding Establishment: Infant<br>1001-Breastfeeding Establishment: Maternal<br>1002-Breastfeeding Maintenance<br>1003 Breastfeeding Weaning<br>1004-Nutritional Status<br>1005-Nutritional Status: Biochemical Measures<br>1007-Nutritional Status: Energy<br>1008-Nutritional Status: Food & Fluid Intake<br>1009-Nutritional Status: Nutrient Intake<br>1010-Swallowing Status<br>1011-Swallowing Status: Esophageal Phase<br>1012-Swalloing Status: Oral Phase<br>1013-Swallowing Status: Pharyngeal Phase |

| a-Therapeutic Response | L-Tissue Integrity | Y-Sensory Function |
|---|---|---|
| Outcomes that describe an individual's systemic reaction to a remedial health treatment, agent, or method | Outcomes that describe the condition and function of an individual's body tissues | Outcomes that describe an individual's perception and use of sensory information |
| 2300-Blood Glucose Level<br>2301-Medication Response<br>2303-Post Procedure Recovery Status<br>2302-Systemic Toxin Clearance: Dialysis | 1104-Bone Healing<br>1105-Hemodialysis Access<br>1100-Oral Hygiene<br>1100-Tissue Integrity: Skin & Mucous Membranes<br>1102-Wound Healing: Primary Intention<br>1103-Wound Healing: Secondary Intention | 2405-Sensory Function Status<br>2400-Sensory Function: Cutaneous<br>2401-Sensory Function: Hearing<br>2402-Sensory Function: Proprioception<br>2403-Sensory Function: Taste & Smell<br>2404-Sensory Function: Vision |

*Continued*

| Level 1 | (3) Domain III–Psychosocial Health<br>Outcomes that describe psychological and social functioning | |
|---|---|---|
| Level 2 | **M-Psychological Well-Being**<br>Outcomes that describe<br>an individual's emotional health | **N-Psychosocial Adaptation**<br>Outcomes that describe an<br>individual's psychological and/or<br>social adaptation to altered health<br>or life circumstances |
| Level 3 | 1211-Anxiety Level<br>1200-Body Image<br>1208-Depression Level<br>1210-Fear Level<br>1213-Fear Level: Child<br>1201-Hope<br>1202-Identity<br>1203-Loneliness Severity<br>1204-Mood Equilibrium<br>1209-Motivation<br>1205-Self-Esteem<br>1207-Sexual Identity<br>1212-Stress Level<br>1206-Will to Live | 1300-Acceptance: Health Status<br>1308-Adaptation to Physical Disability<br>1301-Child Adaptation to<br>    Hospitalization<br>1302-Coping<br>1307-Dignified Life Closure<br>1304-Grief Resolution<br>1305-Psychosocial Adjustment:<br>    Life Change |

**O-Self-Control**
Outcomes that describe an individual's ability to restrain behavior that may be emotionally or physically harmful to self or others

1400-Abusive Behavior Self-Restraint
1401-Aggression Self-Control
1402-Anxiety Self-Control
1409-Depression Self-Control
1403-Distorted Thought Self-Control
1404-Fear Self-Control
1405-Impulse Self-Control
1406-Self-Mutilation Restraint
1407-Substance Addiction Consequences
1408-Suicide Self-Restraint

**P-Social Interaction**
Outcomes that describe an individual's relationships with others

1500-Parent-Infant Attachment
1501-Role Performance
1502-Social Interaction Skills
1503-Social Involvement
1504-Social Support

*Continued*

| | | |
|---|---|---|
| **Level 1** | **(4) Domain IV–Health Knowledge & Behavior**<br>Outcomes that describe attitudes, comprehension, and actions with respect to health and illness | |
| **Level 2** | **Q-Health Behavior**<br>Outcomes that describe an individual's actions to promote, maintain, or restore health | **R-Health Beliefs**<br>Outcomes that describe an individual's ideas and perceptions that influence health behavior |
| **Level 3** | 1600-Adherence Behavior<br>0704-Asthma Self-Management<br>1616-Body Mechanics Performance<br>1617-Cardiac Disease Self-Management<br>1601-Compliance Behavior<br>1619-Diabetes Self-Management<br>1602-Health Promoting Behavior<br>1603-Health Seeking Behavior<br>1610-Hearing Compensation Behavior<br>1604-Leisure Participation<br>1618-Nausea & Vomiting Control<br>1615-Ostomy Self-Care<br>1605-Pain Control<br>1606-Participation in Health Care Decisions<br>1614-Personal Autonomy<br>1607-Prenatal Health Behavior<br>1620-Seizure Control<br>1613-Self-Direction of Care<br>1608-Symptom Control<br>1609-Treatment Behavior: Illness or Injury<br>1611-Vision Compensation Behavior<br>1612-Weight Control | 1700-Health Beliefs<br>1701-Health Beliefs: Perceived Ability To Perform<br>1702-Health Beliefs: Perceived Control<br>1703-Health Beliefs: Perceived Resources<br>1704-Health Beliefs: Perceived Threat<br>1705-Health Orientation |

## S-Health Knowledge
Outcomes that describe an individual's understanding in applying information to promote, maintain, and restore health

1827-Knowledge: Body Mechanics
1800-Knowledge: Breastfeeding
1830-Knowledge: Cardiac Disease Management
1801-Knowledge: Child Physical Safety
1821-Knowledge: Conception Prevention
1820-Knowledge: Diabetes Management
1802-Knowledge: Diet
1803-Knowledge: Disease Process
1804-Knowledge: Energy Conservation
1828-Knowledge: Fall Prevention
1816-Knowledge: Fertility Promotion
1805-Knowledge: Health Behavior
1823-Knowledge: Health Promotion
1806-Knowledge: Health Resources
1824-Knowledge: Illness Care
1819-Knowledge: Infant Care
1807-Knowledge: Infection Control
1817-Knowledge: Labor & Delivery
1808-Knowledge: Medication
1829-Knowledge: Ostomy Care
1826-Knowledge: Parenting
1809-Knowledge: Personal Safety
1818-Knowledge: Postpartum Maternal Health
1822-Knowledge: Preconception Maternal Health
1810-Knowledge: Pregnancy
1811-Knowledge: Prescribed Activity
1815-Knowledge: Sexual Functioning
1812-Knowledge: Substance Use Control
1814-Knowledge: Treatment Procedure(s)
1813-Knowledge: Treatment Regimen

## T-Risk Control & Safety
Outcomes that describe an individual's safety status and/or actions to avoid, limit, or control identifiable health threats

1918-Aspiration Prevention
1909-Fall Prevention Behavior
1912-Falls Occurrence
1900-Immunization Behavior
1911-Personal Safety Behavior
1913-Physical Injury Severity
1902-Risk Control
1903-Risk Control: Alcohol Use
1917-Risk Control: Cancer
1914-Risk Control: Cardiovascular Health
1904-Risk Control: Drug Use
1915-Risk Control: Hearing Impairment
1905-Risk Control: Sexually Transmitted Diseases (STD)
1906-Risk Control: Tobacco Use
1907-Risk Control: Unintended Pregnancy
1916-Risk Control: Visual Impairment
1908-Risk Detection
1910-Safe Home Environment

*Continued*

| Level 1 | (5) Domain V—Perceived Health<br>Outcomes that describe impressions of an individual's health and health care | |
|---|---|---|
| Level 2 | U-Health & Life Quality<br>Outcomes that describe an individual's perceived health status and related life circumstances | V-Symptom Status<br>Outcomes that describe an individual's indications of a disease, injury, or loss |
| Level 3 | 2100-Comfort Level<br>2007-Comfortable Death<br>2006-Personal Health Status<br>2002-Personal Well-Being<br>2004-Physical Fitness<br>2000-Quality of Life<br>2001-Spiritual Health<br>2005-Student Health Status | 2106-Nausea & Vomiting: Disruptive Effects<br>2107-Nausea & Vomiting Severity<br>1306-Pain: Adverse Psychological Response<br>2101-Pain: Disruptive Effects<br>2102-Pain Level<br>2003-Suffering Severity<br>2103-Symptom Severity<br>2104-Symptom Severity: Perimenopause<br>2105-Symptom Severity: Premenstrual Syndrome (PMS) |

**e-Satisfaction with Care**
Outcomes that describe an individual's perceptions of the quality and adequacy of their health care

3000-Client Satisfaction: Access to Care Resources
3001-Client Satisfaction: Caring
3002-Client Satisfaction: Communication
3003-Client Satisfaction: Continuity of Care
3004-Client Satisfaction: Cultural Needs Fulfillment
3005-Client Satisfaction: Functional Assistance
3006-Client Satisfaction: Physical Care
3007-Client Satisfaction: Physical Environment
3008-Client Satisfaction: Protection of Rights
3009-Client Satisfaction: Psychological Care
3010-Client Satisfaction: Safety
3011-Client Satisfaction: Symptom Control
3012-Client Satisfaction: Teaching
3013-Client Satisfaction: Technical Aspects of Care

*Continued*

| Level 1 | (6) Domain VI—Family Health<br>Outcomes that describe health status, behavior, or functioning of the family as a whole or of an individual as a family member | |
|---------|---------------------------------------------------------------------------------------|---|
| Level 2 | **w-Family Caregiver Performance**<br>Outcomes that describe the adaptation and performance of a family member caring for a dependent child or adult | **z-Family Member Health Status**<br>Outcomes that describe the physical and emotional health of an individual family member |
| Level 3 | 2200-Caregiver Adaptation to Patient Institutionalization<br>2202-Caregiver Home Care Readiness<br>2203-Caregiver Lifestyle Disruption<br>2204-Caregiver-Patient Relationship<br>2205-Caregiver Performance: Direct Care<br>2206-Caregiver Performance: Indirect Care<br>2208-Caregiver Stressors<br>2210-Caregiving Endurance Potential | 2500-Abuse Cessation<br>2501-Abuse Protection<br>2514-Abuse Recovery Status<br>2502-Abuse Recovery: Emotional<br>2503-Abuse Recovery: Financial<br>2504-Abuse Recovery: Physical<br>2505-Abuse Recovery: Sexual<br>2506-Caregiver Emotional Health<br>2507-Caregiver Physical Health<br>2508-Caregiver Well-Being<br>2509-Maternal Status: Antepartum<br>2510-Maternal Status: Intrapartum<br>2511-Maternal Status: Postpartum<br>2513-Neglect Cessation<br>2512-Neglect Recovery |

| x-**Family Well-Being** | d-**Parenting** |
|---|---|
| Outcomes that describe the family environment and the physical, emotional, and social health of a family as a unit | Outcomes that describe behaviors of parents that promote optimum growth and development |
| 2600-Family Coping<br>2602-Family Functioning<br>2606-Family Health Status<br>2603-Family Integrity<br>2604-Family Normalization<br>2605-Family Participation in Professional Care<br>2607-Family Physical Environment<br>2608-Family Resiliency<br>2601-Family Social Climate<br>2609-Family Support During Treatment | 2902-Parenting: Adolescent Physical Safety<br>2901-Parenting: Early/Middle Childhood Physical Safety<br>2900-Parenting: Infant/Toddler Physical Safety<br>2211-Parenting Performance<br>1901-Parenting: Psychosocial Safety |

*Continued*

| Level 1 | **(7) Domain VII—Community Health**<br>Outcomes that describe the health, well-being, and functioning<br>of a community or population |
|---|---|
| Level 2 | **b-Community Well-Being**<br>Outcomes that describe the overall health status and social competence of<br>a population or community |
| Level 3 | 2700-Community Competence<br>2701-Community Health Status<br>2800-Community Health Status: Immunity<br>2702-Community Violence Level |

**c-Community Health Protection**

Actions that describe the structures and programs of a community to eliminate or reduce health risks and increase community resistance to health threats

2804-Community Disaster Readiness
2801-Community Risk Control: Chronic Disease
2802-Community Risk Control: Communicable Disease
2803-Community Risk Control: Lead Exposure
2805-Community Risk Control: Violence

# PART THREE

# Outcomes

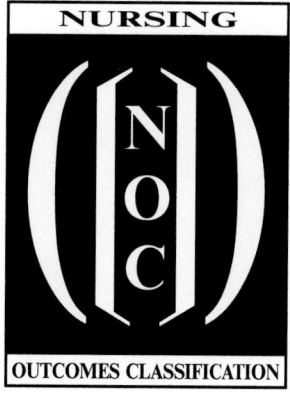

NURSING

N
O
C

OUTCOMES CLASSIFICATION

# *Abuse Cessation (2500)*

A

*Domain-Family Health (VI)*

*Class-Family Member Health Status (Z)*

*Scale(s)-None to Extensive (i)*

*Care Recipient:*

*Data Source:*

**Definition:** Evidence that the victim is no longer hurt or exploited

OUTCOME TARGET RATING:    Maintain at_____    Increase to_____

| Abuse Cessation Overall Rating | None 1 | Limited 2 | Moderate 3 | Substantial 4 | Extensive 5 | |
|---|---|---|---|---|---|---|
| **INDICATORS:** | | | | | | |
| 250002  Evidence that physical abuse has ceased | 1 | 2 | 3 | 4 | 5 | NA |
| 250003  Evidence that emotional abuse has ceased | 1 | 2 | 3 | 4 | 5 | NA |
| 250004  Evidence that sexual abuse has ceased | 1 | 2 | 3 | 4 | 5 | NA |
| 250006  Evidence that financial exploitation has ceased | 1 | 2 | 3 | 4 | 5 | NA |

*1st edition 1997; Revised 3rd edition*

Outcome Content References:

Amundson, M.J. (1989). Family crisis care: A home based intervention program for child abuse. *Issues in Mental Health Nursing, 10,* 285-296.

Cowen, P. (1991). *The Iowa Crisis Nursery Project as a factor in the prevention of abuse.* Unpublished doctoral dissertation, University of Iowa, Iowa City.

Marshall, E., Buckner, E., Perkins, J., Lowry, J., Hyatt, C., Campbell, C., & Helms, D. (1996). Effects of a child abuse prevention unit in health classes in four schools. *Journal of Community Health Nursing, 13*(2), 107-122.

Olds, D.L., Henderson, C.R., Chamberlin, R., & Tatelbaum, R. (1986). Preventing child abuse and neglect: A randomized trial of nurse home visitation. *Pediatrics, 78*(1), 65-78.

Pressel, D.M. (2000). Evaluation of physical abuse in children. *American Family Physician, 61*(10), 3057-3064.

Reuter, M.M. (1988). Parenting needs of abusing parents: Development of a tool for evaluation of parent education class. *Journal of Community Health Nursing, 5*(2), 129-140.

+Shepard, M., & Campbell, J.A. (1992). The abusive behavior inventory: A measure of psychological and physical abuse. *Journal of Interpersonal Violence, 7*(3), 291-305.

Silverman, J., & Hudson, M.F. (2000). Elder mistreatment: A guide for medical professionals. *North Carolina Medical Journal, 61*(5), 291-296.

**A**

# Abuse Protection (2501)

Domain-Family Health (VI)                                    Care Recipient:

Class-Family Member Health Status (Z)                        Data Source:

Scale(s)-Not adequate to Totally adequate (f)

**Definition:** Protection of self or dependent others from abuse

OUTCOME TARGET RATING:        Maintain at_____        Increase to_____

| Abuse Protection Overall Rating | Not adequate 1 | Slightly adequate 2 | Moderately adequate 3 | Substantially adequate 4 | Totally adequate 5 | |
|---|---|---|---|---|---|---|
| **INDICATORS:** | | | | | | |
| 250101 Plan for leaving situation | 1 | 2 | 3 | 4 | 5 | NA |
| 250102 Safety of residence | 1 | 2 | 3 | 4 | 5 | NA |
| 250103 Plan for avoiding abuse | 1 | 2 | 3 | 4 | 5 | NA |
| 250104 Implementation of plan to avoid abuse | 1 | 2 | 3 | 4 | 5 | NA |
| 250105 Safety of self | 1 | 2 | 3 | 4 | 5 | NA |
| 250106 Safety of children | 1 | 2 | 3 | 4 | 5 | NA |
| 250107 Limitation of contact with abuser by means of a restraining order | 1 | 2 | 3 | 4 | 5 | NA |
| 250108 Self-advocacy | 1 | 2 | 3 | 4 | 5 | NA |
| 250109 Facilitation of abuser obtaining counseling | 1 | 2 | 3 | 4 | 5 | NA |
| 250110 Withdrawal when relationship is unsafe | 1 | 2 | 3 | 4 | 5 | NA |
| 250111 Severance of relationship as needed | 1 | 2 | 3 | 4 | 5 | NA |

*1st edition 1997; Revised 3rd edition*

**Outcome Content References:**

Brendtro, M., & Bowker, L.H. (1989). Battered women: How can nurses help? *Issues in Mental Health Nursing, 10*(2), 169-180.

+Dutton, M.A. (1992). *Empowering and healing the battered women: A model for assessment and intervention.* New York: Springer.

Helton, A., McFarlane, J., & Anderson, E. (1987). Prevention of battering during pregnancy: Focus on nurse behavioral change. *Public Health Nursing, 4*(3), 166-174.

Hoff, L.A. (1992). Battered women: Understanding, identification, and assessment. A psychosocial perspective, Part 1. *Journal of the American Academy of Nurse Practitioners, 4*, 148-155.

Hoff, L.A. (1993). Battered women: Intervention and prevention. A psychosocial cultural perspective, Part 2. *Journal of the American Academy of Nurse Practitioners, 5*(1), 34-39.

Schiamberg, L.B., & Gans, D. (2000). Elder abuse by adult children: An applied ecological framework for understanding contextual risk factors and the intergenerational character of quality of life. *International Aging & Human Development, 50*(4), 329-359.

# *Abuse Recovery Status (2514)*

**A**

*Domain-Family Health (VI)*
*Class-Family Member Health Status (Z)*
*Scale(s)-None to Extensive (i)*

*Care Recipient:*
*Data Source:*

**Definition:** Extent of healing following physical or psychological abuse that may include sexual or financial exploitation

OUTCOME TARGET RATING: Maintain at_____ Increase to_____

| Abuse Recovery Status Overall Rating | None 1 | Limited 2 | Moderate 3 | Substantial 4 | Extensive 5 | |
|---|---|---|---|---|---|---|
| **INDICATORS:** | | | | | | |
| 251401 Recognition of abusive relationship(s) | 1 | 2 | 3 | 4 | 5 | NA |
| 251402 Healing of psychological injuries | 1 | 2 | 3 | 4 | 5 | NA |
| 251403 Healing of physical injuries | 1 | 2 | 3 | 4 | 5 | NA |
| 251404 Healing of physical injuries due to sexual abuse | 1 | 2 | 3 | 4 | 5 | NA |
| 251405 Healing of psychological injuries due to sexual abuse | 1 | 2 | 3 | 4 | 5 | NA |
| 251406 Control of personal finances following financial exploitation | 1 | 2 | 3 | 4 | 5 | NA |
| 251407 Control of legal matters following financial exploitation | 1 | 2 | 3 | 4 | 5 | NA |
| 251408 Demonstration of self-esteem | 1 | 2 | 3 | 4 | 5 | NA |
| 251409 Expressions of feeling empowered | 1 | 2 | 3 | 4 | 5 | NA |
| 251410 Demonstration of positive interpersonal relationships | 1 | 2 | 3 | 4 | 5 | NA |

*3rd edition*

**Outcome Content References:**

Bass, E., & Davis, L. (1994). *The courage to heal: A guide for women survivors of child sexual abuse* (3rd ed.). New York: Harper & Row.

Campbell J., McKenna, L.S., Torres, S., Sheridan, D., & Landenburger, K. (1993). Nursing care of abused women. In J. Campbell & J. Humphreys (Eds.), *Nursing care of survivors of family violence*. St. Louis: Mosby.

Hudson, M.F., & Johnson, T.F. (1986). Elder neglect and abuse: A review of the literature. *Annual Review of Nursing Research, 6*(3), 81-134.

Kaplan, S.J., Pelcovitz, D., & Labruna, V. (1999). Child and adolescent abuse and neglect research: A review of the past 10 years. Part I: Physical and emotional abuse and neglect. *Journal of the American Academy of Child & Adolescent Psychiatry, 38*(10), 1214-1222.

Smith, M.E., & Kelly, L.M. (2001). The journey of recovery after a rape experience. *Issues in Mental Health Nursing, 22*(4), 337-352.

Taylor, J.Y. (2000). Sisters of the Yam: African American women's healing and self-recovery from intimate male partner violence. *Issues in Mental Health Nursing, 21*(5), 515-531.

Walsh, K., & Bennett, G. (2000). Financial abuse of older people. *Journal of Adult Protection, 2*(1), 21-29.

**A**

# Abuse Recovery: Emotional (2502)

*Domain-Family Health (VI)*

*Class-Family Member Health Status (Z)*

*Scale(s)-None to Extensive (i) and Extensive to None (h)*

*Care Recipient:*

*Data Source:*

**Definition:** Extent of healing of psychological injuries due to abuse

OUTCOME TARGET RATING:      Maintain at_____      Increase to_____

| Abuse Recovery: Emotional Overall Rating | None 1 | Limited 2 | Moderate 3 | Substantial 4 | Extensive 5 | |
|---|---|---|---|---|---|---|

INDICATORS:

| | | None 1 | Limited 2 | Moderate 3 | Substantial 4 | Extensive 5 | |
|---|---|---|---|---|---|---|---|
| 250202 | Demonstration of confidence | 1 | 2 | 3 | 4 | 5 | NA |
| 250203 | Demonstration of self-esteem | 1 | 2 | 3 | 4 | 5 | NA |
| 250204 | Appropriate affect for situation | 1 | 2 | 3 | 4 | 5 | NA |
| 250212 | Demonstration of impulse control | 1 | 2 | 3 | 4 | 5 | NA |
| 250213 | Self-advocacy | 1 | 2 | 3 | 4 | 5 | NA |
| 250214 | Expressions of feeling empowered | 1 | 2 | 3 | 4 | 5 | NA |
| 250215 | Recognition of abusive relationship(s) | 1 | 2 | 3 | 4 | 5 | NA |
| 250217 | Demonstration of comfort with returning home | 1 | 2 | 3 | 4 | 5 | NA |
| 250218 | Demonstration of insight into abusive relationship | 1 | 2 | 3 | 4 | 5 | NA |
| 250219 | Demonstration of adequate social interactions | 1 | 2 | 3 | 4 | 5 | NA |
| 250220 | Demonstration of positive interpersonal relationships | 1 | 2 | 3 | 4 | 5 | NA |
| 250221 | Demonstration of positive adjustment to change in living arrangements | 1 | 2 | 3 | 4 | 5 | NA |

| | | Extensive | Substantial | Moderate | Limited | None | |
|---|---|---|---|---|---|---|---|
| 250201 | Depression | 1 | 2 | 3 | 4 | 5 | NA |
| 250205 | Suicide attempts | 1 | 2 | 3 | 4 | 5 | NA |
| 250206 | Trauma-induced psychoneurotic behaviors | 1 | 2 | 3 | 4 | 5 | NA |
| 250207 | Inappropriate attention seeking behaviors | 1 | 2 | 3 | 4 | 5 | NA |
| 250208 | Trauma-induced conduct disorders | 1 | 2 | 3 | 4 | 5 | NA |
| 250209 | Trauma-induced learning difficulties | 1 | 2 | 3 | 4 | 5 | NA |
| 250210 | Self-injurious behavior | 1 | 2 | 3 | 4 | 5 | NA |
| 250211 | Neurotic behaviors | 1 | 2 | 3 | 4 | 5 | NA |

*1st edition 1997; Revised 3rd edition*

Outcome Content References:

+Briere, J., & Runtz, M. (1989). The trauma symptom checklist (TSC-33): Early data on a new scale. *Journal of Interpersonal Violence, 4*(2) 151-163.

Campbell J., McKenna, L.S., Torres, S., Sheridan, D., & Landenburger, K. (1993). Nursing care of abused women. In J. Campbell & J. Humphreys (Eds.), *Nursing care of survivors of family violence*. St. Louis: Mosby.

Campbell, J., & Fishwick, N. (1993). Abuse of female partners. In J. Campbell & J. Humphreys (Eds.), *Nursing care of survivors of family violence*. St. Louis: Mosby.

Humphreys, J., Lee, K., Neylan, T., & Marmar, C. (2001). Psychological and physical distress of sheltered battered women. *Health Care for Women International, 22*(4), 401-414.

Kaplan, S.J., Pelcovitz, D., & Labruna, V. (1999). Child and adolescent abuse and neglect research: A review of the past 10 years. Part I: Physical and emotional abuse and neglect. *Journal of the American Academy of Child & Adolescent Psychiatry, 38*(10), 1214-1222.

Rosen, L.N., & Martin, L. (1998). Long-term effects of childhood maltreatment history on gender-related personality characteristics. *Child Abuse & Neglect, 22*(3), 197-211.

Taylor, J.Y. (2000). Sisters of the Yam: African American women's healing and self-recovery from intimate male partner violence. *Issues in Mental Health Nursing, 21*(5), 515-531.

**A**

# Abuse Recovery: Financial (2503)

*Domain-Family Health (VI)*

*Class-Family Member Health Status (Z)*

*Scale(s)-None to Extensive (i)*

*Care Recipient:*

*Data Source:*

**Definition:** Extent of control of monetary and legal matters following financial exploitation

OUTCOME TARGET RATING:    Maintain at_____    Increase to_____

| Abuse Recovery: Financial Overall Rating | None 1 | Limited 2 | Moderate 3 | Substantial 4 | Extensive 5 | |
|---|---|---|---|---|---|---|
| **INDICATORS:** | | | | | | |
| 250301 Control of personal possessions | 1 | 2 | 3 | 4 | 5 | NA |
| 250303 Control of personal finances | 1 | 2 | 3 | 4 | 5 | NA |
| 250306 Control of withdrawal of money from account(s) | 1 | 2 | 3 | 4 | 5 | NA |
| 250302 Control of social security and pension checks | 1 | 2 | 3 | 4 | 5 | NA |
| 250311 Control of earned income | 1 | 2 | 3 | 4 | 5 | NA |
| 250313 Control of court-ordered benefits | 1 | 2 | 3 | 4 | 5 | NA |
| 250304 Control of legal matters | 1 | 2 | 3 | 4 | 5 | NA |
| 250305 Exercise of legal rights | 1 | 2 | 3 | 4 | 5 | NA |
| 250307 Information about finances | 1 | 2 | 3 | 4 | 5 | NA |
| 250308 Information about legal matters | 1 | 2 | 3 | 4 | 5 | NA |
| 250309 Participation in financial planning | 1 | 2 | 3 | 4 | 5 | NA |
| 250310 Pursuit of vocation or occupation | 1 | 2 | 3 | 4 | 5 | NA |
| 250312 Protection of financial assets | 1 | 2 | 3 | 4 | 5 | NA |

*1st edition 1997; Revised 3rd edition*

Outcome Content References:

Anetzberger, G.J. (1987). *The etiology of elder abuse of adult offspring.* Springfield, IL: Charles C Thomas, Publisher.

Baumhover, L.A., Beall, S.C., & Pieroni, R.E. (1990). Elder abuse: An overview of social and medical indicators. *Journal of Health and Human Resources Administration, 12*(4), 414-443.

Hudson, M.F., & Johnson, T.F. (1986). Elder neglect and abuse: A review of the literature. *Annual Review of Nursing Research, 6*(3), 81-134.

Lavrisha, M. (1997). What can nurses do about financial exploitation of elders? *Journal of Gerontological Nursing, 23*(7), 49-50.

+Sullivan, C., Campbell, R., Angelique, H., Eby, K., & Davidson, W. (1994). An advocacy intervention program for women with abusive partners: Six-month follow-up. *American Journal of Community Psychology, 22*, 101-122.

Walsh, K., & Bennett, G. (2000). Financial abuse of older people. *Journal of Adult Protection, 2*(1), 21-29.

Weiler, K. (1989). Financial abuse of the elderly: Recognizing and acting on it. *Journal of Gerontological Nursing, 15*(8), 10-15.

# *Abuse Recovery: Physical (2504)*

A

Domain-Family Health (VI)

Class-Family Member Health Status (Z)

Scale(s)-None to Extensive (i)

Care Recipient:

Data Source:

**Definition:** Extent of healing of physical injuries due to abuse

OUTCOME TARGET RATING:    Maintain at_____    Increase to_____

| Abuse Recovery: Physical Overall Rating | None 1 | Limited 2 | Moderate 3 | Substantial 4 | Extensive 5 | |
|---|---|---|---|---|---|---|
| INDICATORS: | | | | | | |
| 250403  Timely treatment of injuries | 1 | 2 | 3 | 4 | 5 | NA |
| 250401  Healing of physical injuries | 1 | 2 | 3 | 4 | 5 | NA |
| 250407  Resolution of physical health problems | 1 | 2 | 3 | 4 | 5 | NA |
| 250404  Use of therapeutic health care when needed | 1 | 2 | 3 | 4 | 5 | NA |
| 250405  Use of preventive health care | 1 | 2 | 3 | 4 | 5 | NA |
| 250406  Demonstration of expected response to treatment | 1 | 2 | 3 | 4 | 5 | NA |
| 250408  Maintenance of nutritional requirements | 1 | 2 | 3 | 4 | 5 | NA |
| 250409  Urinary continence | 1 | 2 | 3 | 4 | 5 | NA |
| 250402  Regular bowel elimination | 1 | 2 | 3 | 4 | 5 | NA |

*1st edition 1997; Revised 3rd edition*

Outcome Content References:

+Briere, J., & Runtz, M. (1989). The trauma symptom checklist (TSC-33): Early data on a new scale. *Journal of Interpersonal Violence, 4*(2), 151-163.

Campbell, J., McKenna, L.S., Torres, S., Sheridan, D., & Landenburger, K. (1993). Nursing care of abused women. In J. Campbell & J. Humphreys (Eds.), *Nursing care of survivors of family violence.* St. Louis: Mosby.

Campbell, J., & Fishwick, N. (1993). Abuse of female partners. In J. Campbell & J. Humphreys (Eds.), *Nursing care of survivors of family violence.* St. Louis: Mosby.

Humphreys, J., Lee, K., Neylan, T., & Marmar, C. (2001). Psychological and physical distress of sheltered battered women. *Health Care for Women International, 22*(4), 401-414.

Kaplan, S.J., Pelcovitz, D., & Labruna, V. (1999). Child and adolescent abuse and neglect research: A review of the past 10 years. Part I: Physical and emotional abuse and neglect. *Journal of the American Academy of Child & Adolescent Psychiatry, 38*(10), 1214-1222.

Marshall, C.E., Benton, D., & Brazier, J.M. (2000). Elder abuse. Using clinical tools to identify clues of mistreatment. *Geriatrics, 55*(2), 42-44.

McFarlane, J., et al. (1996). Abuse during pregnancy: Associations with maternal health and infant birth weight. *Nursing Research, 45*(1), 37-42.

**A**

# Abuse Recovery: Sexual (2505)

*Domain-Family Health (VI)*

*Class-Family Member Health Status (Z)*

*Scale(s)-None to Extensive (i) and Extensive to None (h)*

*Care Recipient:*

*Data Source:*

**Definition:** Extent of healing of physical and psychological injuries due to sexual abuse or exploitation

OUTCOME TARGET RATING:     Maintain at_____     Increase to_____

| Abuse Recovery: Sexual Overall Rating | None 1 | Limited 2 | Moderate 3 | Substantial 4 | Extensive 5 | |
|---|---|---|---|---|---|---|
| INDICATORS: | | | | | | |
| 250502 Acknowledgment of right to disclose abusive situation | 1 | 2 | 3 | 4 | 5 | NA |
| 250505 Expressions of right to have been protected from abuse | 1 | 2 | 3 | 4 | 5 | NA |
| 250523 Healing of physical injuries | 1 | 2 | 3 | 4 | 5 | NA |
| 250509 Relief of anger in non-destructive ways | 1 | 2 | 3 | 4 | 5 | NA |
| 250510 Self-advocacy | 1 | 2 | 3 | 4 | 5 | NA |
| 250511 Expressions of feeling empowered | 1 | 2 | 3 | 4 | 5 | NA |
| 250512 Expressions of hope | 1 | 2 | 3 | 4 | 5 | NA |
| 250513 Consistency of behavior with social norms | 1 | 2 | 3 | 4 | 5 | NA |
| 250514 Evidence of appropriate same-sex relationships | 1 | 2 | 3 | 4 | 5 | NA |
| 250515 Evidence of appropriate opposite-sex relationships | 1 | 2 | 3 | 4 | 5 | NA |
| 250524 Expressions of comfort with gender identity | 1 | 2 | 3 | 4 | 5 | NA |
| 250525 Expressions of comfort with sexual orientation | 1 | 2 | 3 | 4 | 5 | NA |
| 250521 Verbalization of accurate information about sexual functioning | 1 | 2 | 3 | 4 | 5 | NA |

| | Extensive | Substantial | Moderate | Limited | None | |
|---|---|---|---|---|---|---|
| 250501 Verbalization of details of abuse | 1 | 2 | 3 | 4 | 5 | NA |
| 250503 Verbalization of feelings about the abuse | 1 | 2 | 3 | 4 | 5 | NA |
| 250504 Verbalization of feelings of guilt | 1 | 2 | 3 | 4 | 5 | NA |
| 250507 Sleep disturbances | 1 | 2 | 3 | 4 | 5 | NA |
| 250508 Depression | 1 | 2 | 3 | 4 | 5 | NA |
| 250518 Eating disorders | 1 | 2 | 3 | 4 | 5 | NA |
| 250519 Self-mutilation | 1 | 2 | 3 | 4 | 5 | NA |
| 250520 Suicide attempts | 1 | 2 | 3 | 4 | 5 | NA |

*1st edition 1997; Revised 3rd edition*

Outcome Content References:

Bass, E., & Davis, L. (1994). *The courage to heal: A guide for women survivors of child sexual abuse* (3rd ed.). New York: Harper & Row.

+Briere, J., & Runtz, M. (1989). The trauma symptom checklist (TSC-33): Early data on a new scale. *Journal of Interpersonal Violence, 4*(2), 151-163.

DePanfilis, D. (1986). *Literature review of sexual abuse* (DHHS Publication No. [OHDSA] 87-30530). Washington, DC: USDHHS, National Center on Child Abuse & Neglect.

Gries, L.T., Goh, D.S., Andrews, M.B., Gilbert, J., Praver, F., & Stelzer, D.N. (2000). Positive reaction to disclosure and recovery from child sexual abuse. *Journal of Child Sexual Abuse, 9*(1), 29-51.

Hill, E.L., Gold, S.N., & Bornstein, R.F. (2000). Interpersonal dependency among adult survivors of childhood sexual abuse in therapy. *Journal of Child Sexual Abuse, 9*(2), 71-86.

Sgroi, S.M. (1982). *Handbook of clinical intervention in child sexual abuse.* Lexington, MA: Lexington Books.

Sgroi, S.M. (Ed). (1988). *Vulnerable populations: Evaluation and treatment of sexually abused children and adult survivors* (Vol. 1). Lexington, MA: Lexington Books.

Sgroi, S.M. (Ed). (1988). *Vulnerable populations: Sexual abuse treatment for children, adult survivors, offenders, and persons with mental retardation* (Vol. 2). Lexington, MA: Lexington Books.

Smith, M.E., & Kelly, L.M. (2001). The journey of recovery after a rape experience. *Issues in Mental Health Nursing, 22*(4), 337-352.

Symes, L. (2000). Arriving at readiness to recover emotionally after sexual assault. *Archives of Psychiatric Nursing, 14*(1), 30-38.

Tremblay, C., Hebért, M., & Piché, C. (2000). Type I and type II posttraumatic stress disorder in sexually abused children. *Journal of Child Sexual Abuse, 9*(1), 65-90.

**A**

**A**

# *Abusive Behavior Self-Restraint (1400)*

*Domain-Psychosocial Health (III)*

*Class-Self-Control (O)*

*Scale(s)-Never demonstrated to Consistently demonstrated (m)*

Care Recipient:

Data Source:

**Definition:** Self-restraint of abusive and neglectful behaviors towards others

OUTCOME TARGET RATING:    Maintain at_____    Increase to_____

| Abusive Behavior Self-Restraint Overall Rating | | Never demonstrated 1 | Rarely demonstrated 2 | Sometimes demonstrated 3 | Often demonstrated 4 | Consistently demonstrated 5 | |
|---|---|---|---|---|---|---|---|
| INDICATORS: | | | | | | | |
| 140001 | Avoids physically abusive behavior | 1 | 2 | 3 | 4 | 5 | NA |
| 140002 | Avoids emotionally abusive behavior | 1 | 2 | 3 | 4 | 5 | NA |
| 140003 | Avoids sexually abusive behavior | 1 | 2 | 3 | 4 | 5 | NA |
| 140004 | Avoids neglect of dependent's basic needs | 1 | 2 | 3 | 4 | 5 | NA |
| 140005 | Uses alternative coping mechanisms for stress | 1 | 2 | 3 | 4 | 5 | NA |
| 140006 | Discusses the abusive behavior | 1 | 2 | 3 | 4 | 5 | NA |
| 140007 | Identifies factors contributing to abusive behavior | 1 | 2 | 3 | 4 | 5 | NA |
| 140008 | Expresses feelings about victim | 1 | 2 | 3 | 4 | 5 | NA |
| 140009 | Identifies available community resources for help | 1 | 2 | 3 | 4 | 5 | NA |
| 140010 | Expresses frustrations | 1 | 2 | 3 | 4 | 5 | NA |
| 140011 | Uses nurturing behavior toward victim | 1 | 2 | 3 | 4 | 5 | NA |
| 140012 | Demonstrates self-esteem | 1 | 2 | 3 | 4 | 5 | NA |
| 140013 | States expectations congruent with developmental level | 1 | 2 | 3 | 4 | 5 | NA |
| 140014 | Applies appropriate caregiving techniques | 1 | 2 | 3 | 4 | 5 | NA |
| 140015 | Uses support network | 1 | 2 | 3 | 4 | 5 | NA |
| 140016 | Expresses empathy for victim | 1 | 2 | 3 | 4 | 5 | NA |
| 140017 | Controls impulses | 1 | 2 | 3 | 4 | 5 | NA |
| 140018 | Uses correct role behaviors | 1 | 2 | 3 | 4 | 5 | NA |
| 140019 | Seeks treatment as needed | 1 | 2 | 3 | 4 | 5 | NA |
| 140020 | Participates in treatment as needed | 1 | 2 | 3 | 4 | 5 | NA |

*1st edition 1997; Revised 2nd edition 2000; Revised 3rd edition (formerly Abusive Behavior Self-Control)*

Outcome Content References:

Amundson, M.J. (1989). Family crisis care: A home based intervention program for child abuse. *Issues in Mental Health Nursing, 10*, 285-296.

Anderson, C.L. (1987). Assessing parenting potential for child abuse risk. *Pediatric Nursing, 13*(5), 323-327.

+Buss, A.H., & Perry, M. (1992). The Aggression Questionnaire. *Journal of Personality and Social Psychology, 63* (3), 452-459.

Cowen, P. (1991). *The Iowa Crisis Nursery Project as a factor in the prevention of child abuse.* Unpublished doctoral dissertation, University of Iowa, Iowa City.

Olds, D.L., Henderson, C.R., Chamberlin, R., & Tatelbaum, R. (1986). Preventing child abuse and neglect: A randomized trial of nurse home visitation. *Pediatrics, 78*(1), 65-78.

Marshall, E., Buckner, E., & Powell, K. (1991). Evaluation of a teen parent program designed to reduce child abuse and neglect and to strengthen families. *Journal of Child and Adolescent Psychiatric and Mental Health Nursing, 4*(3), 96-100.

Reuter, M.M. (1988). Parenting needs of abusing parents: Development of a tool for evaluation of parent education class. *Journal of Community Health Nursing, 5*(2), 129-140.

Taylor, D.K., & Beauchamp, C. (1988). Hospital-based primary prevention strategy in child abuse: A multi-level needs assessment. *Child Abuse and Neglect, 12*(3), 343-354.

Tolman, R.M., Edleson, J.L., & Fendrich, M. (1996). The applicability of the theory of planned behavior to abusive men's cessation of violent behavior. *Violence & Victims, 11*(4), 341-354.

A

**A**

# Acceptance: Health Status (1300)

*Domain-Psychosocial Health (III)*

*Class-Psychosocial Adaptation (N)*

*Scale(s)-Never demonstrated to Consistently demonstrated (m)*

Care Recipient:

Data Source:

**Definition:** Reconciliation to significant change in health circumstances

OUTCOME TARGET RATING:     Maintain at_____     Increase to_____

| Acceptance: Health Status Overall Rating | Never demonstrated 1 | Rarely demonstrated 2 | Sometimes demonstrated 3 | Often demonstrated 4 | Consistently demonstrated 5 | |
|---|---|---|---|---|---|---|
| **INDICATORS:** | | | | | | |
| 130002 Relinquishes previous concept of personal health | 1 | 2 | 3 | 4 | 5 | NA |
| 130008 Recognizes reality of health situation | 1 | 2 | 3 | 4 | 5 | NA |
| 130004 Demonstrates positive self-regard | 1 | 2 | 3 | 4 | 5 | NA |
| 130016 Maintains relationships | 1 | 2 | 3 | 4 | 5 | NA |
| 130007 Reports decreased need to verbalize feelings about health | 1 | 2 | 3 | 4 | 5 | NA |
| 130017 Adjusts to change in health status | 1 | 2 | 3 | 4 | 5 | NA |
| 130001 Appears peaceful | 1 | 2 | 3 | 4 | 5 | NA |
| 130003 Appears calm | 1 | 2 | 3 | 4 | 5 | NA |
| 130018 Demonstrates resilience | 1 | 2 | 3 | 4 | 5 | NA |
| 130009 Pursues information about health | 1 | 2 | 3 | 4 | 5 | NA |
| 130010 Copes with health situation | 1 | 2 | 3 | 4 | 5 | NA |
| 130011 Makes decisions about health | 1 | 2 | 3 | 4 | 5 | NA |
| 130012 Clarifies personal values | 1 | 2 | 3 | 4 | 5 | NA |
| 130019 Clarifies life priorities | 1 | 2 | 3 | 4 | 5 | NA |
| 130013 Reports sense of life being worth living | 1 | 2 | 3 | 4 | 5 | NA |
| 130014 Performs self-care tasks | 1 | 2 | 3 | 4 | 5 | NA |

*1st edition 1997; Revised 2nd edition 2000; Revised 3rd edition*

**Outcome Content References:**

Clayton, J.W. (1993). Paving the way to acceptance: Psychological adaptation to death and dying in cancer. *Professional Nurse, 8*(4), 206-211.

Kelley, M.P., & Henry, P. (1993). Open discussion can lead to acceptance: The psychosocial effects of stoma surgery. *Professional Nurse, 9*(2), 101-110.

Kubler-Ross, E. (1977). *On death and dying.* London: Tavistock Press.

Lazarus, R.S., & Folkman, S. (1984). *Stress, appraisal and coping.* New York: Springer.

Longo, M.B. (1993). Facilitating acceptance of a patient's decision to stop treatment. *Clinical Nurse Specialist, 7*(3), 233-243.

Melamed, S., Groswasser, Z., & Stern, M. (1992). Acceptance of disability, work involvement and subjective rehabilitation status of traumatic brain-injured (TBI) patients. *Brain Injury, 6*(3), 233-243.

Reynaud, S.N., & Meeker, B.J. (2002). Coping styles of older adults with ostomies. *Journal of Gerontological Nursing, 28*(5), 30-36.

+Wagnild, G.M., & Young, H. M. (1993). Development and psychometric evaluation of the resilience scale. *Journal of Nursing Measurement, 1*(2), 165-178.

# *Activity Tolerance (0005)*

Domain-Functional Health (I)

Class-Energy Maintenance (A)

Scale(s)-Severely compromised to Not compromised (a)

Care Recipient:

Data Source:

**Definition:** Physiologic response to energy-consuming movements with daily activities

OUTCOME TARGET RATING:　　Maintain at_____　　Increase to_____

| Activity Tolerance Overall Rating | Severely compromised 1 | Substantially compromised 2 | Moderately compromised 3 | Mildly compromised 4 | Not compromised 5 | |
|---|---|---|---|---|---|---|
| **INDICATORS:** | | | | | | |
| 000501 Oxygen saturation with activity | 1 | 2 | 3 | 4 | 5 | NA |
| 000502 Pulse rate with activity | 1 | 2 | 3 | 4 | 5 | NA |
| 000503 Respiratory rate with activity | 1 | 2 | 3 | 4 | 5 | NA |
| 000508 Ease of breathing with activity | 1 | 2 | 3 | 4 | 5 | NA |
| 000504 Systolic blood pressure with activity | 1 | 2 | 3 | 4 | 5 | NA |
| 000505 Diastolic blood pressure with activity | 1 | 2 | 3 | 4 | 5 | NA |
| 000506 Electrocardiogram findings | 1 | 2 | 3 | 4 | 5 | NA |
| 000507 Skin color | 1 | 2 | 3 | 4 | 5 | NA |
| 000509 Walking pace | 1 | 2 | 3 | 4 | 5 | NA |
| 000510 Walking distance | 1 | 2 | 3 | 4 | 5 | NA |
| 000511 Stair climbing tolerance | 1 | 2 | 3 | 4 | 5 | NA |
| 000516 Upper body strength | 1 | 2 | 3 | 4 | 5 | NA |
| 000517 Lower body strength | 1 | 2 | 3 | 4 | 5 | NA |
| 000518 Ease of performing activities of daily living (ADL) | 1 | 2 | 3 | 4 | 5 | NA |
| 000514 Ability to speak with physical activity | 1 | 2 | 3 | 4 | 5 | NA |

*2nd edition 2000; Revised 3rd edition*

## Outcome Content References:

Barnett-Damewood, M., & Carlson-Catalano, J. (2000). Physical activity deficit: A proposed nursing diagnosis. *Nursing Diagnosis, 11*(1), 24-31.

Buchner, D.M. (1995). Clinical assessments of physical activity in older adults. In L.Z. Rubenstein, D. Wieland, & R. Bernabei, *Geriatric Assessment Technology: The State of the Art* (pp. 147-159). New York: Springer Publishing.

Hosking, R., & Hiller, G. (1989). Using nursing diagnosis in a cardiovascular clinical nurse specialist practice. *Journal of Advanced Medical-Surgical Nursing, 1*(3), 33-41.

Larson, J.L., & Leidy, N.K. (1998). Chronic obstructive pulmonary disease: Strategies to improve functional status. *Annual Review of Nursing Research, 16,* 253-286.

Melillo, K.D., Houde, S.C., Williamson, E., & Futrell, M. (2000). Perceptions of nurse practitioners regarding their role in physical activity and exercise prescription for older adults. *Clinical Excellence for Nurse Practitioners, 4*(2), 108-116.

Mol, V.J., & Baker, C.A. (1991). Activity intolerance in the geriatric stroke patient. *Rehabilitation Nursing, 16*(6), 337-44.

Roberts, S.L., & White, B. (1992). Common nursing diagnoses for pulmonary alveolar edema patients. *Dimensions of Critical Care Nursing, 11*(1), 13-27.

Tack, B.B., & Gilliss, C.L. (1990). Nurse-monitored cardiac recovery: A description of the first 8 weeks. *Heart & Lung, 19*(5), 491-499.

Wieseke, A., Twibell, R., Bennett, S., Marine, M., & Schoger, J. (1994). A content validation study of five nursing diagnoses by critical care nurses. *Heart & Lung, 23*(4), 345-351.

**A**

# *Adaptation to Physical Disability (1308)*

*Domain-Psychosocial Health (III)*

*Class-Psychosocial Adaptation (N)*

*Scale(s)-Never demonstrated to Consistently demonstrated (m)*

Care Recipient:

Data Source:

**Definition:** Adaptive response to a significant functional challenge due to a physical disability

OUTCOME TARGET RATING:     Maintain at_____     Increase to_____

| Adaptation to Physical Disability Overall Rating | Never demonstrated 1 | Rarely demonstrated 2 | Sometimes demonstrated 3 | Often demonstrated 4 | Consistently demonstrated 5 | |
|---|---|---|---|---|---|---|
| **INDICATORS:** | | | | | | |
| 130801 Verbalizes ability to adjust to disability | 1 | 2 | 3 | 4 | 5 | NA |
| 130802 Verbalizes reconciliation to disability | 1 | 2 | 3 | 4 | 5 | NA |
| 130803 Adapts to functional limitations | 1 | 2 | 3 | 4 | 5 | NA |
| 130804 Modifies lifestyle to accommodate disability | 1 | 2 | 3 | 4 | 5 | NA |
| 130805 Modifies career goals to accommodate disability | 1 | 2 | 3 | 4 | 5 | NA |
| 130806 Uses strategies to reduce stress related to disability | 1 | 2 | 3 | 4 | 5 | NA |
| 130807 Identifies ways to increase sense of control | 1 | 2 | 3 | 4 | 5 | NA |
| 130808 Identifies ways to cope with life changes | 1 | 2 | 3 | 4 | 5 | NA |
| 130809 Identifies risk of complications associated with disability | 1 | 2 | 3 | 4 | 5 | NA |
| 130810 Identifies plan to meet activities of daily living | 1 | 2 | 3 | 4 | 5 | NA |
| 130811 Identifies plan to meet instrumental activities of daily living | 1 | 2 | 3 | 4 | 5 | NA |
| 130812 Accepts need for physical assistance | 1 | 2 | 3 | 4 | 5 | NA |
| 130813 Seeks information concerning disability | 1 | 2 | 3 | 4 | 5 | NA |
| 130814 Seeks community support group for disability | 1 | 2 | 3 | 4 | 5 | NA |
| 130815 Seeks professional help as appropriate | 1 | 2 | 3 | 4 | 5 | NA |
| 130816 Uses available social support | 1 | 2 | 3 | 4 | 5 | NA |
| 130817 Reports decrease in stress related to disability | 1 | 2 | 3 | 4 | 5 | NA |
| 130818 Reports decrease in negative feelings | 1 | 2 | 3 | 4 | 5 | NA |
| 130819 Reports decrease in negative body image | 1 | 2 | 3 | 4 | 5 | NA |
| 130820 Reports increase in psychological comfort | 1 | 2 | 3 | 4 | 5 | NA |

*3rd edition*

**Outcome Content References:**

Carlsson, E., Berglund, B., & Norgren, S. (2001). Living with an ostomy and short bowel syndrome: Practical aspects and impact on daily life. *Journal of Wocn, 28*(2), 96-105.

Gignac, M.A., Cott, C., & Badley, E.M. (2000). Adaptation to chronic illness and disability and its relationship to perceptions of independence and dependence. *Journal of Gerontology Series B-Psychological Sciences, 55*(6), P362-P372.

Livneh, H., Antonak, R.F., & Gerhardt, J. (1999). Psychosocial adaptation to amputation: The role of sociodemographic variables, disability-related factors and coping strategies. *International Journal of Rehabilitation Research, 22*(1), 21-31.

Wingate, S.J. (1986). Levels of pacemaker acceptance by patients. *Heart & Lung, 15*(1), 93-100.

**A**

# Adherence Behavior (1600)

Domain-Health Knowledge & Behavior (IV)

Class-Health Behavior (Q)

Scale(s)-Never demonstrated to Consistently demonstrated (m)

Care Recipient:

Data Source:

**Definition:** Self-initiated actions to promote wellness, recovery, and rehabilitation

OUTCOME TARGET RATING:     Maintain at_____     Increase to_____

| Adherence Behavior Overall Rating | Never demonstrated 1 | Rarely demonstrated 2 | Sometimes demonstrated 3 | Often demonstrated 4 | Consistently demonstrated 5 | |
|---|---|---|---|---|---|---|
| **INDICATORS:** | | | | | | |
| 160001 Asks health-related questions when indicated | 1 | 2 | 3 | 4 | 5 | NA |
| 160002 Seeks health-related information from a variety of sources | 1 | 2 | 3 | 4 | 5 | NA |
| 160003 Uses health-related information to develop health strategies | 1 | 2 | 3 | 4 | 5 | NA |
| 160004 Weighs risks/benefits of health behavior | 1 | 2 | 3 | 4 | 5 | NA |
| 160007 Provides rationale for adopting a health regimen | 1 | 2 | 3 | 4 | 5 | NA |
| 160008 Uses strategies to eliminate unhealthy behavior | 1 | 2 | 3 | 4 | 5 | NA |
| 160009 Uses strategies to maximize health | 1 | 2 | 3 | 4 | 5 | NA |
| 160010 Uses health services congruent with need | 1 | 2 | 3 | 4 | 5 | NA |
| 160011 Performs ADLs* consistent with energy and tolerance | 1 | 2 | 3 | 4 | 5 | NA |
| 160012 Performs self-screening | 1 | 2 | 3 | 4 | 5 | NA |
| 160013 Describes rationale for deviating from a recommended health regimen | 1 | 2 | 3 | 4 | 5 | NA |
| 160014 Performs self-monitoring of health status | 1 | 2 | 3 | 4 | 5 | NA |

*ADLs = Activities of daily living.

1st edition 1997; Revised 3rd edition

## Outcome Content References:

Burkhart, P.V., Dunbar-Jacob, J.M., & Rohay, J.M. (2001). Accuracy of children's self-reported adherence to treatment. *Journal of Nursing Scholarship, 33*(1), 27-32.

Epstein, L., & Cluss, P.A. (1982). A behavioral perspective on adherence to long-term medical regimens. *Journal of Consulting and Clinical Psychology, 50*, 950-971.

Folden, S.L. (1993). Definitions of health and health goals of participants in a community-based pulmonary rehabilitation program. *Public Health Nursing, 10*(1), 31-35

+Hettler, B. (1982). Wellness promotion and risk reduction on a university campus. In M. Faber & A. Reinhardt (Eds.), *Promoting health through risk reduction*. New York: Macmillan.

Jensen, L., & Allen, M. (1993). Wellness: The dialect of illness. *Image-the Journal of Nursing Scholarship, 25*(3), 220-224.

Konradi, D.B., & Lyon, B.L. (2000). Measuring adherence to a self-care fitness walking routine. *Journal of Community Health Nursing, 17*(3), 159-169.

Kravits, R., et al. (1993). Recall of recommendations and adherence to advice among patients with chronic medical conditions. *Archives of Internal Medicine, 153*(16), 1869-1878.

Miller, P., Wikoff, R., & Hiatt, A. (1972). Fishbein's Model of measured behavior of hypertensive patients. *Nursing Research, 41*(2), 104-109.

Pender, N.J. (1990). Expressing health through lifestyle patterns. *Nursing Science Quarterly, 3*(3), 115-122.

Pender, N.J., & Pender, A.R. (1986). Attitudes, subjective norms, and intentions of engagement in health behaviors. *Nursing Research, 35*(1), 15-18.

Shumaker, S.A., Schron, E.B., & Ockene, J.K. (1998). *The handbook of health behavior change* (2nd ed.). New York: Springer.

Toljamo, M., & Hentinen, M. (2001). Adherence to self-care and social support. *Journal of Clinical Nursing, 10*(5), 618-627.

Woods, N. (1989). Conceptualizations of self-care: Toward health-oriented models. *Advances in Nursing Science, 12*(1), 1-13.

A

# Aggression Self-Control (1401)

*Domain-Psychosocial Health (III)*

*Class-Self Control (O)*

*Scale(s)-Never demonstrated to Consistently demonstrated (m)*

*Care Recipient:*

*Data Source:*

**Definition:** Self-restraint of assaultive, combative, or destructive behaviors toward others

OUTCOME TARGET RATING:   Maintain at_____   Increase to_____

| Aggression Self-Control Overall Rating | Never demonstrated 1 | Rarely demonstrated 2 | Sometimes demonstrated 3 | Often demonstrated 4 | Consistently demonstrated 5 | |
|---|---|---|---|---|---|---|
| INDICATORS: | | | | | | |
| 140110 Identifies when angry | 1 | 2 | 3 | 4 | 5 | NA |
| 140111 Identifies when frustrated | 1 | 2 | 3 | 4 | 5 | NA |
| 140112 Identifies situations that precipitate hostility | 1 | 2 | 3 | 4 | 5 | NA |
| 140113 Identifies responsibility to maintain control | 1 | 2 | 3 | 4 | 5 | NA |
| 140114 Identifies when feeling aggressive | 1 | 2 | 3 | 4 | 5 | NA |
| 140115 Identifies alternatives to aggression | 1 | 2 | 3 | 4 | 5 | NA |
| 140116 Identifies alternatives to verbal outbursts | 1 | 2 | 3 | 4 | 5 | NA |
| 140107 Communicates needs appropriately | 1 | 2 | 3 | 4 | 5 | NA |
| 140108 Communicates feelings appropriately | 1 | 2 | 3 | 4 | 5 | NA |
| 140117 Vents negative feelings appropriately | 1 | 2 | 3 | 4 | 5 | NA |
| 140101 Refrains from verbal outbursts | 1 | 2 | 3 | 4 | 5 | NA |
| 140102 Refrains from violating others' personal space | 1 | 2 | 3 | 4 | 5 | NA |
| 140103 Refrains from striking others | 1 | 2 | 3 | 4 | 5 | NA |
| 140104 Refrains from harming others | 1 | 2 | 3 | 4 | 5 | NA |
| 140105 Refrains from harming animals | 1 | 2 | 3 | 4 | 5 | NA |
| 140106 Refrains from destroying property | 1 | 2 | 3 | 4 | 5 | NA |
| 140109 Controls impulses | 1 | 2 | 3 | 4 | 5 | NA |
| 140121 Uses physical outlets to reduce pent-up energy | 1 | 2 | 3 | 4 | 5 | NA |
| 140122 Uses specific techniques to control anger | 1 | 2 | 3 | 4 | 5 | NA |
| 140123 Uses specific techniques to control frustration | 1 | 2 | 3 | 4 | 5 | NA |
| 140118 Upholds contract to restrain aggressive behaviors | 1 | 2 | 3 | 4 | 5 | NA |
| 140119 Maintains self-control without supervision | 1 | 2 | 3 | 4 | 5 | NA |

*1st edition 1997; Revised 2nd edition 2000; Revised 3rd edition (formerly Aggression Control)*

*Continued*

Outcome Content References:

Berkowitz, L. (1993). *Aggression: Its causes, consequences, and control.* New York: McGraw-Hill.

+Buss, A.H., & Perry, M. (1992). The Aggression Questionnaire. *Journal of Personality and Social Psychology, 63* (3), 452-459.

Crowell, D.H., Evans, I.M., & O'Donnell, C.R. (Eds.). (1987). *Childhood aggression and violence.* New York: Plenum.

Grancola, P.R., & Zeichner, A. (1993). Aggressive behavior in the elderly: A critical review. *Clinical Gerontologist, 13*(2), 3-22.

Ingram, T.N. (2001). Risk for violence: Self-directed or directed at others. In M. Maas, K. Buckwalter, M. Hardy, T. Tripp-Reimer, M. Titler & J. Specht (Eds.), *Nursing care of older adults: Diagnoses, outcomes & interventions* (pp. 696-705). St. Louis: Mosby.

Mason, T., Chandley, M. (1999) *Managing violence and aggression: A manual for nurses and health care workers.* Edinburgh: Churchill Livingstone.

Maxfield, M.C., Lewis, R.E., & Connor, S. (1996). Training staff to prevent aggressive behavior of cognitively impaired elderly patients during bathing and grooming. *Journal of Gerontological Nursing, 22*(1), 37-43.

Pepler, D.J., & Rubin, K.H. (Eds.). (1991). *The development and treatment of childhood aggression.* Hillsdale, NJ: Erlbaum.

Rantz, M.J., & McShane, R.E. (1995). Nursing interventions for chronically confused nursing home residents. *Geriatric Nursing, 16*(1), 22-27.

Ryden, M.B. (1992). Aggressive behavior in persons with dementia who live in the community. *Alzheimer Disease and Associated Disorders, 2*(4), 342-355.

A

A

# *Allergic Response: Localized (0705)*

*Domain-Physiologic Health (II)*

*Class-Immune Response (H)*

*Scale(s)-Severe to None (n)*

Care Recipient:

Data Source:

**Definition:** Severity of localized hypersensitive immune response to a specific environmental (exogenous) antigen

OUTCOME TARGET RATING:     Maintain at_____     Increase to_____

| Allergic Response: Localized Overall Rating | Severe 1 | Substantial 2 | Moderate 3 | Mild 4 | None 5 | |
|---|---|---|---|---|---|---|
| **INDICATORS:** | | | | | | |
| 070501  Sinus pain | 1 | 2 | 3 | 4 | 5 | NA |
| 070502  Headache | 1 | 2 | 3 | 4 | 5 | NA |
| 070503  Conjunctivitis | 1 | 2 | 3 | 4 | 5 | NA |
| 070504  Lacrimation | 1 | 2 | 3 | 4 | 5 | NA |
| 070505  Rhinitis | 1 | 2 | 3 | 4 | 5 | NA |
| 070506  Sneezing | 1 | 2 | 3 | 4 | 5 | NA |
| 070507  Mucous secretions | 1 | 2 | 3 | 4 | 5 | NA |
| 070508  Circumoral edema | 1 | 2 | 3 | 4 | 5 | NA |
| 070509  Periorbital edema | 1 | 2 | 3 | 4 | 5 | NA |
| 070510  Dark circles under eyes | 1 | 2 | 3 | 4 | 5 | NA |
| 070511  Burning sensation of eyes | 1 | 2 | 3 | 4 | 5 | NA |
| 070512  Localized itching | 1 | 2 | 3 | 4 | 5 | NA |
| 070513  Localized rash | 1 | 2 | 3 | 4 | 5 | NA |
| 070514  Localized erythema | 1 | 2 | 3 | 4 | 5 | NA |
| 070515  Increased localized skin temperature | 1 | 2 | 3 | 4 | 5 | NA |
| 070516  Localized edema | 1 | 2 | 3 | 4 | 5 | NA |
| 070517  Localized pain | 1 | 2 | 3 | 4 | 5 | NA |
| 070518  Localized granuloma | 1 | 2 | 3 | 4 | 5 | NA |
| 070519  Localized necrotizing vasculitis | 1 | 2 | 3 | 4 | 5 | NA |

*3rd edition*

**Outcome Content References:**

Altman, G.B., Buchsel, P., & Coxon, V. (2000). *Delmar's fundamental & advanced nursing skills.* Albany, NY: Delmar/Thomson Learning.

Huether, S.E., & McCance, K.L. (2000). *Understanding pathophysiology* (2nd ed.). St. Louis: Mosby.

Lewis, S., Heitkemper, M., & Dirksen, S. (2000). *Medical-surgical nursing: Assessment and management of clinical problems* (5th ed.). St. Louis: Mosby.

McCance, K.L., & Huether, S.E., (2001). *Pathophysiology: The biological basis for disease in adults and children* (4th ed.). St. Louis: Mosby.

Mudge-Grout, C., (1992). *Immunologic disorders: Mosby's clinical nursing series.* St. Louis: Mosby.

Smeltzer, S.C., & Bare, B.G. (Eds.). (2003). *Brunner and Suddarth's textbook of medical-surgical nursing* (10th ed.). Philadelphia: Lippincott, Williams, & Wilkins.

Thelan, L., Urden, L., Lough, M., & Stacy, K., (1998). *Critical care nursing: Diagnosis and management* (3rd ed.). St. Louis: Mosby.

Tortora, G., & Grabowski, S. (1996). *Principles of anatomy and physiology* (8th ed.). New York, NY: Harper Collins Publishers.

# *Allergic Response: Systemic (0706)*

A

Domain-Physiologic Health (II)

Class-Immune Response (H)

Scale(s)-Severe to None (n)

Care Recipient:

Data Source:

Definition: Severity of systemic hypersensitive immune response to a specific environmental (exogenous) antigen

OUTCOME TARGET RATING:    Maintain at_____    Increase to_____

| Allergic Response: Systemic Overall Rating | Severe 1 | Substantial 2 | Moderate 3 | Mild 4 | None 5 | |
|---|---|---|---|---|---|---|
| **INDICATORS:** | | | | | | |
| 070601 Laryngeal edema | 1 | 2 | 3 | 4 | 5 | NA |
| 070602 Dyspnea at rest | 1 | 2 | 3 | 4 | 5 | NA |
| 070603 Wheezing | 1 | 2 | 3 | 4 | 5 | NA |
| 070604 Stridor | 1 | 2 | 3 | 4 | 5 | NA |
| 070605 Adventitious breath sounds | 1 | 2 | 3 | 4 | 5 | NA |
| 070606 Tachycardia | 1 | 2 | 3 | 4 | 5 | NA |
| 070607 Decreased blood pressure | 1 | 2 | 3 | 4 | 5 | NA |
| 070608 Dysrhythmia(s) | 1 | 2 | 3 | 4 | 5 | NA |
| 070609 Pulmonary edema | 1 | 2 | 3 | 4 | 5 | NA |
| 070610 Decreased level of consciousness | 1 | 2 | 3 | 4 | 5 | NA |
| 070611 Mucous secretions | 1 | 2 | 3 | 4 | 5 | NA |
| 070612 Facial edema | 1 | 2 | 3 | 4 | 5 | NA |
| 070613 Generalized itching | 1 | 2 | 3 | 4 | 5 | NA |
| 070614 Hives | 1 | 2 | 3 | 4 | 5 | NA |
| 070615 Body exfoliation | 1 | 2 | 3 | 4 | 5 | NA |
| 070616 Petechiae | 1 | 2 | 3 | 4 | 5 | NA |
| 070617 Erythema | 1 | 2 | 3 | 4 | 5 | NA |
| 070618 Increased skin temperature | 1 | 2 | 3 | 4 | 5 | NA |
| 070619 Fever | 1 | 2 | 3 | 4 | 5 | NA |
| 070620 Chills | 1 | 2 | 3 | 4 | 5 | NA |
| 070621 Nausea | 1 | 2 | 3 | 4 | 5 | NA |
| 070622 Vomiting | 1 | 2 | 3 | 4 | 5 | NA |
| 070623 Diarrhea | 1 | 2 | 3 | 4 | 5 | NA |
| 070624 Abdominal cramping | 1 | 2 | 3 | 4 | 5 | NA |
| 070625 Red blood cell hemolysis | 1 | 2 | 3 | 4 | 5 | NA |
| 070626 Increased bilirubin | 1 | 2 | 3 | 4 | 5 | NA |
| 070627 Enlarged spleen | 1 | 2 | 3 | 4 | 5 | NA |
| 070628 Enlarged lymph nodes | 1 | 2 | 3 | 4 | 5 | NA |
| 070629 Joint pain | 1 | 2 | 3 | 4 | 5 | NA |
| 070630 Muscle pain | 1 | 2 | 3 | 4 | 5 | NA |
| 070631 Anaphylactic shock | 1 | 2 | 3 | 4 | 5 | NA |

*3rd edition*

Outcome Content References:

Altman, G.B., Buchsel, P., & Coxon, V. (2000). *Delmar's fundamental & advanced nursing skills.* Albany, NY: Delmar/Thomson Learning.

Huether, S.E. & McCance, K.L. (2000). *Understanding pathophysiology* (2nd ed.). St. Louis: Mosby.

Lewis, S., Heitkemper, M., & Dirksen, S. (2000). *Medical-surgical nursing: Assessment and management of clinical problems* (5th ed.). St. Louis: Mosby.

McCance, K., & Huether, S., (2001). *Pathophysiology: The biological basis for disease in adults and children* (4th ed.). St. Louis: Mosby.

Mudge-Grout, C., (1992). *Immunologic disorders: Mosby's clinical nursing series.* St. Louis: Mosby.

Smeltzer, S.C., & Bare, B.G. (Eds.). (2003). *Brunner and Suddarth's textbook of medical-surgical nursing* (10th ed.). Philadelphia: Lippincott, Williams, & Wilkins.

Thelan, L., Urden, L., Lough, M., & Stacy, K., (1998). *Critical care nursing: Diagnosis and management* (3rd ed.). St. Louis: Mosby.

Tortora, G., & Grabowski, S. (1996). *Principles of anatomy and physiology* (8th ed.). New York, NY: Harper Collins Publishers.

**A**

# Ambulation (0200)

*Domain-Functional Health (I)*

*Class-Mobility (C)*

*Scale(s)-Severely compromised to Not compromised (a)*

*Care Recipient:*

*Data Source:*

**Definition:** Ability to walk from place to place independently with or without assistive device

OUTCOME TARGET RATING:     Maintain at_____     Increase to_____

| Ambulation Overall Rating | Severely compromised 1 | Substantially compromised 2 | Moderately compromised 3 | Mildly compromised 4 | Not compromised 5 | |
|---|---|---|---|---|---|---|
| **INDICATORS:** | | | | | | |
| 020001 Bears weight | 1 | 2 | 3 | 4 | 5 | NA |
| 020002 Walks with effective gait | 1 | 2 | 3 | 4 | 5 | NA |
| 020003 Walks at slow pace | 1 | 2 | 3 | 4 | 5 | NA |
| 020004 Walks at moderate pace | 1 | 2 | 3 | 4 | 5 | NA |
| 020005 Walks at fast pace | 1 | 2 | 3 | 4 | 5 | NA |
| 020006 Walks up steps | 1 | 2 | 3 | 4 | 5 | NA |
| 020007 Walks down steps | 1 | 2 | 3 | 4 | 5 | NA |
| 020008 Walks up inclines | 1 | 2 | 3 | 4 | 5 | NA |
| 020009 Walks down inclines | 1 | 2 | 3 | 4 | 5 | NA |
| 020010 Walks short distance (< 1 block) | 1 | 2 | 3 | 4 | 5 | NA |
| 020011 Walks moderate distance (> 1 block < 5 blocks) | 1 | 2 | 3 | 4 | 5 | NA |
| 020012 Walks long distance (5 blocks or >) | 1 | 2 | 3 | 4 | 5 | NA |
| 020014 Walks around room | 1 | 2 | 3 | 4 | 5 | NA |
| 020015 Walks around dwelling | 1 | 2 | 3 | 4 | 5 | NA |

*1st edition 1997; Revised 3rd edition (formerly Ambulation: Walking)*

**Outcome Content References:**

Green J., Forster A., & Young J. (2002). Reliability of gait speed measured by a timed walking test in patients one year after stroke. *Clinical Rehabilitation, 16*(3), 306-314.

+*Guide for the Uniform Data Set for Medical Rehabilitation* (including the FIM™ instrument), (version 5.1) (1997). Buffalo, NY: University at Buffalo.

Hoeman, S. (2002). *Rehabilitation nursing: Process, application, and outcomes* (3rd ed.). St. Louis: Mosby.

Jirovec, M.M. (1991). The impact of daily exercise on the mobility, balance, and urine control of cognitively impaired nursing home residents. *International Journal of Nursing Studies, 28*(2), 145-151.

Lord, S.R., & Menz, H.B. (2002). Physiologic, psychologic, and health predictors of 6-minute walk performance in older people. *Archives of Physical Medicine & Rehabilitation, 83*(7), 907-911.

Mikulic, M.A., Griffith, E.R., & Jebsen, R.H. (1976). Clinical application of a standardized mobility test. *Archives of Physical Medicine and Rehabilitation, 57*(3), 143-146.

Pomeroy, V. (1990). Development of an ADL-oriented assessment-of-mobility scale suitable for use for elderly people with dementia. *Physiotherapy, 76*(8), 446-448.

Tinetti, M.E. (1986). Performance-oriented assessment of mobility problems in elderly patients. *Journal of the American Geriatric Society, 34*(2), 119-126.

# *Ambulation: Wheelchair (0201)*

*Domain-Functional Health (I)*

*Class-Mobility (C)*

*Scale(s)-Severely compromised to Not compromised (a)*

*Care Recipient:*

*Data Source:*

**Definition:** Ability to move from place to place in a wheelchair

OUTCOME TARGET RATING:     Maintain at_____     Increase to_____

| Ambulation: Wheelchair Overall Rating | Severely compromised 1 | Substantially compromised 2 | Moderately compromised 3 | Mildly compromised 4 | Not compromised 5 | |
|---|---|---|---|---|---|---|
| **INDICATORS:** | | | | | | |
| 020101 Transfers to and from wheelchair | 1 | 2 | 3 | 4 | 5 | NA |
| 020102 Propels wheelchair safely | 1 | 2 | 3 | 4 | 5 | NA |
| 020103 Propels wheelchair short distance | 1 | 2 | 3 | 4 | 5 | NA |
| 020104 Propels wheelchair moderate distance | 1 | 2 | 3 | 4 | 5 | NA |
| 020105 Propels wheelchair long distance | 1 | 2 | 3 | 4 | 5 | NA |
| 020106 Maneuvers curbs | 1 | 2 | 3 | 4 | 5 | NA |
| 020107 Maneuvers doorways | 1 | 2 | 3 | 4 | 5 | NA |
| 020108 Maneuvers ramps | 1 | 2 | 3 | 4 | 5 | NA |

*1st edition 1997; Revised 3rd edition*

## Outcome Content References:

+*Guide for the Uniform Data Set for Medical Rehabilitation* (including the FIM™ instrument), (version 5.1) (1997). Buffalo, NY: University at Buffalo.

Hoeman, S. (2002). *Rehabilitation nursing: Process, application, and outcomes* (3rd ed.). St. Louis: Mosby.

Kane, R.L., & Kane, R.A. (2000). *Assessing older persons: Measures, meaning, and practical applications.* New York: Oxford University Press.

Lan, T.Y., Melzer, D., Tom, B.D., & Guralnik, J.M. (2002). Performance tests and disability: Developing an objective index of mobility-related limitation in older populations. *Journals of Gerontology Series A -Biological Sciences & Medical Sciences, 57*(5), M294-301.

Mikulic, M.A., Griffith, E.R., & Jebsen, R.H. (1976). Clinical application of a standardized mobility test. *Archives of Physical Medicine and Rehabilitation, 57*(3), 143-146.

**A**

# Anxiety Level (1211)

Domain-Psychosocial Health (III)

Class-Psychosocial Well-Being (M)

Scale(s)-Severe to None (n)

Care Recipient:

Data Source:

**Definition:** Severity of manifested apprehension, tension, or uneasiness arising from an unidentifiable source

OUTCOME TARGET RATING:   Maintain at_____   Increase to_____

| Anxiety Level Overall Rating | Severe 1 | Substantial 2 | Moderate 3 | Mild 4 | None 5 | |
|---|---|---|---|---|---|---|
| **INDICATORS:** | | | | | | |
| 121101 Restlessness | 1 | 2 | 3 | 4 | 5 | NA |
| 121102 Pacing | 1 | 2 | 3 | 4 | 5 | NA |
| 121103 Hand wringing | 1 | 2 | 3 | 4 | 5 | NA |
| 121104 Distress | 1 | 2 | 3 | 4 | 5 | NA |
| 121105 Uneasiness | 1 | 2 | 3 | 4 | 5 | NA |
| 121106 Muscle tension | 1 | 2 | 3 | 4 | 5 | NA |
| 121107 Facial tension | 1 | 2 | 3 | 4 | 5 | NA |
| 121108 Irritability | 1 | 2 | 3 | 4 | 5 | NA |
| 121109 Indecisiveness | 1 | 2 | 3 | 4 | 5 | NA |
| 121110 Outbursts of anger | 1 | 2 | 3 | 4 | 5 | NA |
| 121111 Problem behavior | 1 | 2 | 3 | 4 | 5 | NA |
| 121112 Difficulty concentrating | 1 | 2 | 3 | 4 | 5 | NA |
| 121113 Difficulty learning | 1 | 2 | 3 | 4 | 5 | NA |
| 121114 Difficulty problem solving | 1 | 2 | 3 | 4 | 5 | NA |
| 121115 Panic attack | 1 | 2 | 3 | 4 | 5 | NA |
| 121116 Verbalized apprehension | 1 | 2 | 3 | 4 | 5 | NA |
| 121117 Verbalized anxiety | 1 | 2 | 3 | 4 | 5 | NA |
| 121118 Exaggerated concern about life events | 1 | 2 | 3 | 4 | 5 | NA |
| 121119 Increased blood pressure | 1 | 2 | 3 | 4 | 5 | NA |
| 121120 Increased pulse rate | 1 | 2 | 3 | 4 | 5 | NA |
| 121121 Increased respiratory rate | 1 | 2 | 3 | 4 | 5 | NA |
| 121122 Dilated pupils | 1 | 2 | 3 | 4 | 5 | NA |
| 121123 Sweating | 1 | 2 | 3 | 4 | 5 | NA |
| 121124 Dizziness | 1 | 2 | 3 | 4 | 5 | NA |
| 121125 Fatigue | 1 | 2 | 3 | 4 | 5 | NA |
| 121126 Decreased productivity | 1 | 2 | 3 | 4 | 5 | NA |
| 121127 Decreased school achievement | 1 | 2 | 3 | 4 | 5 | NA |
| 121128 Withdrawal | 1 | 2 | 3 | 4 | 5 | NA |
| 121129 Sleep pattern disturbance | 1 | 2 | 3 | 4 | 5 | NA |
| 121130 Change in bowel pattern | 1 | 2 | 3 | 4 | 5 | NA |
| 121131 Change in eating pattern | 1 | 2 | 3 | 4 | 5 | NA |

3rd edition

A

Outcome Content References:

American Psychiatric Association. (2000). *Diagnostic and statistical manual of mental disorders* (4th ed. text revision). Washington DC: Author.

Byrne, B. (2000). Relationships between anxiety, fear, self-esteem, and coping strategies in adolescence. *Adolescence, 35*(137), 201-216.

Charron, H.S. (1998). Anxiety disorders. In E.M. Varcarolis (Ed.), *Foundations of Psychiatric Mental Health Nursing.* (3rd ed., pp. 443-477). Philadelphia: Saunders.

Kim, M., Sertella, R., Gulanick, M., Moyer, K., Parsons, E., Scherbel, J., Stafford, M., Suhayada, R., & Yocum, C. (1984). Clinical validation of cardiovascular nursing diagnoses. In M. Kim, G. McFarland, & A. McLane (Eds.), *Classification of nursing diagnoses: Proceedings of the fifth national conference* (pp. 128-137). St. Louis: Mosby.

Shuldham, C.M., Cunningham, G., Hiscock, M., & Luscombe, P. (1995). Assessment of anxiety in hospital patients. *Journal of Advanced Nursing 22(1),* 87-93.

Taylor-Loughran, A.E., O'Brien, M.E., LaChapelle, R., & Rangel, S. (1989). Defining characteristics of the nursing diagnoses fear and anxiety: A validation study. *Applied Nursing Research, 2*(4), 178-186.

Whitley, G.G., & Tousman, S.A. (1996). A multivariate approach for validation of anxiety and fear. *Nursing Diagnosis, 7*(3), 116-124.

**A**

# *Anxiety Self-Control (1402)*

*Domain-Psychosocial Health (III)*

*Class-Self Control (O)*

*Scale(s)-Never demonstrated to Consistently demonstrated (m)*

Care Recipient:

Data Source:

**Definition:** Personal actions to eliminate or reduce feelings of apprehension, tension, or uneasiness from an unidentifiable source

OUTCOME TARGET RATING:   Maintain at_____   Increase to_____

| Anxiety Self-Control Overall Rating | Never demonstrated 1 | Rarely demonstrated 2 | Sometimes demonstrated 3 | Often demonstrated 4 | Consistently demonstrated 5 | |
|---|---|---|---|---|---|---|
| INDICATORS: | | | | | | |
| 140201   Monitors intensity of anxiety | 1 | 2 | 3 | 4 | 5 | NA |
| 140202   Eliminates precursors of anxiety | 1 | 2 | 3 | 4 | 5 | NA |
| 140203   Decreases environ-mental stimuli when anxious | 1 | 2 | 3 | 4 | 5 | NA |
| 140204   Seeks information to reduce anxiety | 1 | 2 | 3 | 4 | 5 | NA |
| 140205   Plans coping strategies for stressful situations | 1 | 2 | 3 | 4 | 5 | NA |
| 140206   Uses effective coping strategies | 1 | 2 | 3 | 4 | 5 | NA |
| 140207   Uses relaxation techniques to reduce anxiety | 1 | 2 | 3 | 4 | 5 | NA |
| 140208   Monitors duration of episodes | 1 | 2 | 3 | 4 | 5 | NA |
| 140209   Monitors length of time between episodes | 1 | 2 | 3 | 4 | 5 | NA |
| 140210   Maintains role performance | 1 | 2 | 3 | 4 | 5 | NA |
| 140211   Maintains social relationships | 1 | 2 | 3 | 4 | 5 | NA |
| 140212   Maintains concentration | 1 | 2 | 3 | 4 | 5 | NA |
| 140213   Monitors sensory perceptual distortions | 1 | 2 | 3 | 4 | 5 | NA |
| 140214   Maintains adequate sleep | 1 | 2 | 3 | 4 | 5 | NA |
| 140215   Monitors physical manifestations of anxiety | 1 | 2 | 3 | 4 | 5 | NA |
| 140216   Monitors behavioral manifestations of anxiety | 1 | 2 | 3 | 4 | 5 | NA |
| 140217   Controls anxiety response | 1 | 2 | 3 | 4 | 5 | NA |

*1st edition 1997; Revised 2nd edition; Revised 3rd edition (formerly Anxiety Control)*

Outcome Content References:

+Hudson, W.W. (1992). *The WALMYR assessment scales scoring manual.* Tempe, AZ: WALMYR Publishing Co.

Laraia, M.T., Stuart, G.W., & Best, C.L. (1989). Behavioral treatment of panic-related disorders: A review. *Archives of Psychiatric Nursing, 3*(3), 125-133.

Moorhead, S.A., & Brighton, V.A. (2001). Anxiety and fear. In M. Maas, K. Buckwalter, M. Hardy, T. Tripp-Reimer, M. Titler & J. Specht (Eds.), *Nursing care of older adults: Diagnoses, outcomes & interventions* (pp. 571-592). St. Louis: Mosby.

Stuart, G.W., & Laraia, M.T. (2001). *Principles and practice of psychiatric nursing* (7th ed.). St. Louis: Mosby.

Tucker, S., Moore, W., & Luedtke, C. (2000). Outcomes of a brief inpatient treatment program for mood and anxiety disorders. *Outcomes Management for Nursing Practice, 4*(3), 117-123.

Waddell, K.L., & Demi, A.S. (1993). Effectiveness of an intensive partial hospitalization program for treatment of anxiety disorders. *Archives of Psychiatric Nursing, 7*(1), 2-10.

A

**A**

# *Appetite (1014)*

*Domain-Physiologic Health (II)*

*Class-Nutrition (K)*

*Scale-Severely compromised to Not compromised (a)*

*Care Recipient:*

*Data Source:*

**Definition:** Desire to eat when ill or receiving treatment

OUTCOME TARGET RATING:    Maintain at_____    Increase to_____

| Appetite Overall Rating | Severely compromised 1 | Substantially compromised 2 | Moderately compromised 3 | Mildly compromised 4 | Not compromised 5 | |
|---|---|---|---|---|---|---|
| **INDICATORS:** | | | | | | |
| 101401  Desire to eat | 1 | 2 | 3 | 4 | 5 | NA |
| 101402  Craving for food | 1 | 2 | 3 | 4 | 5 | NA |
| 101403  Enjoyment of food | 1 | 2 | 3 | 4 | 5 | NA |
| 101404  Pleasant taste of food | 1 | 2 | 3 | 4 | 5 | NA |
| 101405  Reports energy to eat | 1 | 2 | 3 | 4 | 5 | NA |
| 101406  Food intake | 1 | 2 | 3 | 4 | 5 | NA |
| 101407  Nutrient intake | 1 | 2 | 3 | 4 | 5 | NA |
| 101408  Fluid intake | 1 | 2 | 3 | 4 | 5 | NA |
| 101409  Stimulus to eat | 1 | 2 | 3 | 4 | 5 | NA |

*3rd edition*

**Outcome Content References:**

Anderson, K.N., Anderson, L.E., & Glanze, W.D. (2002). *Mosby's medical, nursing, & allied health dictionary* (6th ed). St. Louis: Mosby.

Dudek, S.G. (2001). *Nutrition essentials for nursing practice.* Philadelphia: Lippincott.

Lewis, S.M., Heitkemper, M.M., & Dirksen, S.R. (2000). *Medical surgical nursing: Assessment and management of clinical problems.* St. Louis: Mosby.

McCance, K.L., & Huether, S.E. (2002). *Pathophysiology: The biological basis for disease in adults and children* (4th ed.) St. Louis: Mosby.

Potter, P.A., & Perry, A.G. (2001). *Fundamentals of nursing* (5th ed). St. Louis: Mosby.

Thomas, C.L. (Ed.). (1993). *Taber's cylcopedic medical dictionary* (17th ed.). Philadelphia: F.A. Davis Company.

# *Aspiration Prevention (1918)*

*Domain-Health Knowledge & Behavior (IV)*

*Class-Risk Control & Safety (T)*

*Scale(s)-Never demonstrated to Consistently demonstrated (m)*

Care Recipient:

Data Source:

**Definition:** Personal actions to prevent the passage of fluid and solid particles into the lung

OUTCOME TARGET RATING:    Maintain at_____    Increase to_____

| Aspiration Prevention Overall Rating | Never demonstrated 1 | Rarely demonstrated 2 | Sometimes demonstrated 3 | Often demonstrated 4 | Consistently demonstrated 5 | |
|---|---|---|---|---|---|---|

INDICATORS:

| | | | | | | | |
|---|---|---|---|---|---|---|---|
| 191801 | Identifies risk factors | 1 | 2 | 3 | 4 | 5 | NA |
| 191802 | Avoids risk factors | 1 | 2 | 3 | 4 | 5 | NA |
| 191803 | Positions self upright for eating/ drinking | 1 | 2 | 3 | 4 | 5 | NA |
| 191804 | Selects foods according to swallowing ability | 1 | 2 | 3 | 4 | 5 | NA |
| 191805 | Positions self on side for eating and drinking as needed | 1 | 2 | 3 | 4 | 5 | NA |
| 191806 | Chooses liquids and foods of proper consistency | 1 | 2 | 3 | 4 | 5 | NA |
| 191808 | Uses liquid thickeners as needed | 1 | 2 | 3 | 4 | 5 | NA |

*2nd edition 2000; Revised 3rd edition (formerly Aspiration Control)*

Outcome Content References:

Clochesy, J.M., Brey, C., Cardin, S., Whittaker, A.A., & Rudy, E.B. (1996). *Critical Care Nursing* (2nd ed.). Philadelphia: W.B. Saunders.

Fellows, L.S., Miller, E.H., Frederickson, M., Bly, B., & Felt, P. (2000). Evidence-based practice for enteral feedings: Aspiration prevention strategies, bedside detection, and practice change. *Medsurg Nursing, 9*(1), 27-31.

The Joanna Briggs Institute for Evidence Based Nursing and Midwifery. (2000). Identification and nursing management of dysphagia in adults with neurological impairment. *Best Practice, 4*(2), Blackwell Science-Asia, Australia.

Lewis, S.M., Collier, I.C., Heitkermper, M.M., & Dirksen, S.R. (2000). *Medical-surgical nursing: Assessment & management of clinical problems* (5th ed.). St. Louis: Mosby.

McCance, K.L., & Huether, S.E. (2002). *Pathophysiology: The biologic basis for disease in adults and children* (4th ed.). St. Louis: Mosby

Smeltzer, S.C., & Bare, B.G. (Eds.). (2003). *Brunner and Suddarth's textbook of medical-surgical nursing* (10th ed.). Philadelphia: Lippincott, Williams, & Wilkins.

**A**

# *Asthma Self-Management (0704)*

Domain-Health Knowledge & Behavior (IV)   Care Recipient:

Class-Health Behavior (Q)   Data Source:

Scale(s)-Never demonstrated to Consistently demonstrated (m) and Consistently demonstrated to Never demonstrated (t)

**Definition:** Personal actions to reverse inflammatory condition resulting in bronchial constriction of the airways

OUTCOME TARGET RATING:   Maintain at_____   Increase to_____

| Asthma Self-Management Overall Rating | Never demonstrated 1 | Rarely demonstrated 2 | Sometimes demonstrated 3 | Often demonstrated 4 | Consistently demonstrated 5 | |
|---|---|---|---|---|---|---|
| INDICATORS: | | | | | | |
| 070418 Describes causal factors | 1 | 2 | 3 | 4 | 5 | NA |
| 070419 Recognizes onset of asthma | 1 | 2 | 3 | 4 | 5 | NA |
| 070401 Initiates action to avoid personal triggers | 1 | 2 | 3 | 4 | 5 | NA |
| 070402 Initiates action to manage personal triggers | 1 | 2 | 3 | 4 | 5 | NA |
| 070403 Makes appropriate environmental modifications | 1 | 2 | 3 | 4 | 5 | NA |
| 070420 Uses diary to monitor symptoms over time | 1 | 2 | 3 | 4 | 5 | NA |
| 070404 Seeks early treatment of infections | 1 | 2 | 3 | 4 | 5 | NA |
| 070405 Participates in age appropriate activities | 1 | 2 | 3 | 4 | 5 | NA |
| 070406 Sleeps through the night with no nocturnal cough or wheeze | 1 | 2 | 3 | 4 | 5 | NA |
| 070407 Wakes up rested | 1 | 2 | 3 | 4 | 5 | NA |
| 070408 Experiences no medication side effects | 1 | 2 | 3 | 4 | 5 | NA |
| 070409 Reports symptom-free state with minimal medication regimen | 1 | 2 | 3 | 4 | 5 | NA |
| 070410 Monitors peak flow routinely | 1 | 2 | 3 | 4 | 5 | NA |
| 070411 Monitors peak flow when symptoms occur | 1 | 2 | 3 | 4 | 5 | NA |
| 070412 Makes appropriate medication choices | 1 | 2 | 3 | 4 | 5 | NA |
| 070413 Demonstrates appropriate use of inhalers, spacers, and nebulizers | 1 | 2 | 3 | 4 | 5 | NA |

| Asthma Self-Management—cont'd | | Never demonstrated | Rarely demonstrated | Sometimes demonstrated | Often demonstrated | Consistently demonstrated | |
|---|---|---|---|---|---|---|---|
| 070414 | Self-manages exacerbations | 1 | 2 | 3 | 4 | 5 | NA |
| 070415 | Reports uncontrolled symptoms to health care professional | 1 | 2 | 3 | 4 | 5 | NA |
| 070416 | Accesses support and advocacy group | 1 | 2 | 3 | 4 | 5 | NA |
| 070421 | Reports asthma controlled | 1 | 2 | 3 | 4 | 5 | NA |

| | | Consistently demonstrated (4 + occurrences) | Often demonstrated (3 occurrences) | Sometimes demonstrated (2 occurrences) | Rarely demonstrated (1 occurrence) | Never demonstrated (no occurrence) | |
|---|---|---|---|---|---|---|---|
| 070422 | Emergency visits related to asthma within the last year | 1 | 2 | 3 | 4 | 5 | NA |
| 070423 | Hospitalizations related to asthma within the last year | 1 | 2 | 3 | 4 | 5 | NA |
| 070424 | School absences related to asthma within the school year | 1 | 2 | 3 | 4 | 5 | NA |
| 070425 | Work absences related to asthma within the last year | 1 | 2 | 3 | 4 | 5 | NA |

*2nd edition 2000; Revised 3rd edition (formerly Asthma Control)*

Outcome Content References:

Cross, S. (1997). Revised guidelines on asthma management. *Professional Nurse, 12*(6), 408-410.

Gallagher, C. (2002). Childhood asthma: Tools that help parents manage it. *American Journal of Nursing, 102*(8), 71-83.

Le, J.T., Pearlman, D.S., Nickals, R., Lowenthal, M., & Rosenthal, R. (1998). Algorithm for the diagnosis and management of asthma: A practice parameter update. *Annals of Allergy, Asthma and Immunology, 81*, 415-420.

National Heart, Lung, and Blood Institute. National Asthma Education Program. (1997). *Expert panel report 2: Guidelines for the diagnosis and management of asthma* (NIH Publication No. 97-4051). Bethesda, MD: U.S. Department of Health and Human Services.

Perry, C.S., & Toole, K.A. (2000). Impact of school nurse case management on asthma control in school-aged children. *Journal of School Health, 70*(7), 303-304.

Tettersell, M.J. (1993). Asthma patients' knowledge in relation to compliance with drug therapy. *Journal of Advanced Nursing, 18*(1), 103-113.

Yoos, H.L., & McMullen, A. (1999). Symptom perception and evaluation in childhood asthma. *Nursing Research, 48*(1) 2-8.

B

# *Balance (0202)*

*Domain-Functional Health (I)*

*Class-Mobility (C)*

*Scale(s)-Severely compromised to Not compromised (a) and Severe to None (n)*

*Care Recipient:*

*Data Source:*

**Definition:** Ability to maintain body equilibrium

OUTCOME TARGET RATING:    Maintain at_____    Increase to_____

| Balance Overall Rating | Severely compromised 1 | Substantially compromised 2 | Moderately compromised 3 | Mildly compromised 4 | Not compromised 5 | |
|---|---|---|---|---|---|---|
| **INDICATORS:** | | | | | | |
| 020201 Maintains balance while standing | 1 | 2 | 3 | 4 | 5 | NA |
| 020202 Maintains balance while sitting without back support | 1 | 2 | 3 | 4 | 5 | NA |
| 020203 Maintains balance while walking | 1 | 2 | 3 | 4 | 5 | NA |
| | **Severe** | **Substantial** | **Moderate** | **Mild** | **None** | |
| 020205 Weaving | 1 | 2 | 3 | 4 | 5 | NA |
| 020206 Dizziness | 1 | 2 | 3 | 4 | 5 | NA |
| 020207 Shakiness | 1 | 2 | 3 | 4 | 5 | NA |
| 020208 Stumbling | 1 | 2 | 3 | 4 | 5 | NA |

*1st edition 1997; Revised 3rd edition*

## Outcome Content References:

+Berg, K., Wood-Dauphinee, S., Williams, J.I., & Gayton, D. (1989). Measuring balance in the elderly: Preliminary development of an instrument. *Physiotherapy Canada, 41,* 304-311.

Dittmar, S. (1989). *Rehabilitation nursing: Process and application.* St. Louis: Mosby.

Gresham, G.E., Duncan, P.W., Stason, W.B., et al. (1995). *Post-stroke Rehabilitation. Clinical Practice Guideline,* No. 16. (AHCPR Publication No. 95-0062). Rockville, MD: U.S. Department of Health and Human Services. Public Health Services, Agency for Health Care Policy and Research.

Pettersson, A.F., Engardt, M., & Wahlund, L.O. (2002). Activity level and balance in subjects with mild Alzheimer's disease. *Dementia & Geriatric Cognitive Disorders, 13*(4), 213-216.

Pomeroy, V. (1990). Development of an ADL-oriented assessment-of-mobility scale suitable for use with elderly people with dementia. *Physiotherapy, 76*(8), 446-448.

Roberts, B.L. (1989). Effects of walking on balance among elders. *Nursing Research, 38*(3), 180-182.

Tinetti, M.E. (1986). Performance-oriented assessment of mobility problems in elderly patients. *Journal of the American Geriatric Society, 34*(2), 119-126.

# Blood Coagulation (0409)

*Domain-Physiologic Health (II)*

*Class-Cardiopulmonary (E)*

*Scale(s)-Severe deviation from normal range to No deviation from normal range (b) and Severe to None (n)*

*Care Recipient:*

*Data Source:*

**Definition:** Extent to which blood clots within normal period of time

OUTCOME TARGET RATING:    Maintain at_____    Increase to_____

| Blood Coagulation Overall Rating | Severe deviation from normal range 1 | Substantial deviation from normal range 2 | Moderate deviation from normal range 3 | Mild deviation from normal range 4 | No deviation from normal range 5 | |
|---|---|---|---|---|---|---|
| **INDICATORS:** | | | | | | |
| 040901 Clot formation | 1 | 2 | 3 | 4 | 5 | NA |
| 040912 Prothrombin time (PT) | 1 | 2 | 3 | 4 | 5 | NA |
| 040905 Prothrombin time - international normalized ratio (PT-INR) | 1 | 2 | 3 | 4 | 5 | NA |
| 040907 Partial thromboplastin time (PTT) | 1 | 2 | 3 | 4 | 5 | NA |
| 040913 Hemoglobin (Hgb) | 1 | 2 | 3 | 4 | 5 | NA |
| 040908 Platelet count | 1 | 2 | 3 | 4 | 5 | NA |
| 040909 Plasma fibrinogen | 1 | 2 | 3 | 4 | 5 | NA |
| 040914 Fibrin split products (FSP) | 1 | 2 | 3 | 4 | 5 | NA |
| 040910 Hematocrit (Hct) | 1 | 2 | 3 | 4 | 5 | NA |
| 040915 Activated clotting time (ACT) | 1 | 2 | 3 | 4 | 5 | NA |

| | Severe | Substantial | Moderate | Mild | None | |
|---|---|---|---|---|---|---|
| 040902 Bleeding | 1 | 2 | 3 | 4 | 5 | NA |
| 040903 Bruising | 1 | 2 | 3 | 4 | 5 | NA |
| 040904 Petechiae | 1 | 2 | 3 | 4 | 5 | NA |
| 040916 Ecchymosis | 1 | 2 | 3 | 4 | 5 | NA |
| 040917 Pupura | 1 | 2 | 3 | 4 | 5 | NA |
| 040918 Hematuria | 1 | 2 | 3 | 4 | 5 | NA |
| 040919 Blood in stool | 1 | 2 | 3 | 4 | 5 | NA |
| 040920 Hemoptysis | 1 | 2 | 3 | 4 | 5 | NA |
| 040921 Hematemesis | 1 | 2 | 3 | 4 | 5 | NA |
| 040922 Bleeding gums | 1 | 2 | 3 | 4 | 5 | NA |

*2nd edition 2000; Revised 3rd edition (formerly Coagulation Status)*

**Outcome Content References:**

Arnett, C. (1998). Thrombocytopenia in the newborn. *Neonatal Network – Journal of Neonatal Nursing, 17*(8), 27-37.

Beyth, R.J. (2001). Thromboembolic disease and anticoagulation in the elderly: Hemorrhagic complications of oral anticoagulant therapy (electronic version). *Clinics in Geriatric Medicine, 17*(1), 49-56.

Clochesy, J.M., Brey, C., Cardin, S., Whittaker, A.A., & Rudy, E.B. (1996). *Critical care nursing* (2nd ed.). Philadelphia: W.B. Saunders.

Fahey, V.A. (Ed.). (1999). *Vascular nursing.* (3rd ed.). Philadelphia: W.B. Saunders.

Fihn, S.D., Callahan, C.M., Martin, D., McDonell, M.B., Henikoff, J.G., & White, R.H. (1996). The risk for and severity of bleeding complications in elderly patients treated with warfarin. *Annals of Internal Medicine, 124*(11), 970-979.

Lewis, S.M., Collier, I.C., Heitkemper, M.M., & Dirksen, S.R. (2000). *Medical-surgical nursing: Assessment & management of clinical problems* (5th ed.). St. Louis: Mosby.

McCance, K.L., & Huether, S.E. (2002). *Pathophysiology: The biologic basis for disease in adults and children* (4th ed.). St. Louis: Mosby.

Smeltzer, S.C., & Bare, B.G. (Eds.). (2003). *Brunner and Suddarth's textbook of medical-surgical nursing* (10th ed.). Philadelphia: Lippincott, Williams, & Wilkins.

**B**

# *Blood Glucose Level (2300)*

*Domain Physiologic Health (II)*

*Class-Therapeutic Response (a)*

*Scale(s)-Severe deviation from normal range to No deviation from normal range (b)*

*Care Recipient:*

*Data Source:*

**Definition:** Extent to which glucose levels in plasma and urine are maintained in normal range

OUTCOME TARGET RATING:    Maintain at_____    Increase to_____

| Blood Glucose Level Overall Rating | Severe deviation from normal range 1 | Substantial deviation from normal range 2 | Moderate deviation from normal range 3 | Mild deviation from normal range 4 | No deviation from normal range 5 | |
|---|---|---|---|---|---|---|
| INDICATORS: | | | | | | |
| 230001  Blood glucose | 1 | 2 | 3 | 4 | 5 | NA |
| 230004  Glycosolated hemoglobin | 1 | 2 | 3 | 4 | 5 | NA |
| 230005  Fructosemine | 1 | 2 | 3 | 4 | 5 | NA |
| 230007  Urine glucose | 1 | 2 | 3 | 4 | 5 | NA |
| 230008  Urine ketones | 1 | 2 | 3 | 4 | 5 | NA |

*2nd edition 2000; Revised 3rd edition (formerly Blood Glucose Control)*

Outcome Content References:

American Diabetes Association. (1998). Standards of medical care for patients with diabetes mellitus. *Diabetes Care, 21* (Supp. 1), S23-S31.

American Diabetes Association. (1998). Testing of glycemia in diabetes. *Diabetes Care, 21*(Supp. 1), S69-S71.

Cryer, P.E. (2001). Hypoglycemia risk reduction in type 1 diabetes. *Experimental & Clinical Endocrinology & Diabetes, 109*(Suppl. 2), S412-S423.

Funnell, M.M., Hunt, C., Kulkarni, K., Rubin, R.R., & Yarborough, P.C. (Eds.) (1998). *A core curriculum for Association of Diabetes Educators.* Chicago: American Association of Diabetes Educators.

Kelley, D.B. (Ed.). (1998). *Intensive diabetes management.* (2nd ed.). Alexandria, VA: American Diabetes Association.

Lebovitz, H.E. (Ed.). (1998). *Therapy for diabetes mellitus and related disorders* (3rd ed.). Alexandria, VA: American Diabetes Association.

Lewis, S.M., Collier, I.C., Heitkermper, M.M., & Dirksen, S.R. (2000). *Medical-surgical nursing: Assessment & management of clinical problems* (5th ed.). St. Louis: Mosby.

McCance, K.L., & Huether, S.E. (2002). *Pathophysiology: The biologic basis for disease in adults and children* (4th ed.). St. Louis: Mosby.

**B**

# Blood Loss Severity (0413)

Domain-Physiologic Health (II)

Class-Cardiopulmonary (E)

Scale(s)-Severe to None (n)

Care Recipient:

Data Source:

**Definition:** Severity of internal or external bleeding/hemorrhage

OUTCOME TARGET RATING:  Maintain at_____  Increase to_____

| Blood Loss Severity Overall Rating | Severe 1 | Substantial 2 | Moderate 3 | Mild 4 | None 5 | |
|---|---|---|---|---|---|---|
| INDICATORS: | | | | | | |
| 041301 Visible blood loss | 1 | 2 | 3 | 4 | 5 | NA |
| 041302 Hematuria | 1 | 2 | 3 | 4 | 5 | NA |
| 041303 Frank blood from anus | 1 | 2 | 3 | 4 | 5 | NA |
| 041304 Hemoptysis | 1 | 2 | 3 | 4 | 5 | NA |
| 041305 Hematemesis | 1 | 2 | 3 | 4 | 5 | NA |
| 041306 Abdominal distention | 1 | 2 | 3 | 4 | 5 | NA |
| 041307 Vaginal bleeding | 1 | 2 | 3 | 4 | 5 | NA |
| 041308 Post surgical bleeding | 1 | 2 | 3 | 4 | 5 | NA |
| 041309 Decreased systolic blood pressure | 1 | 2 | 3 | 4 | 5 | NA |
| 041310 Decreased diastolic blood pressure | 1 | 2 | 3 | 4 | 5 | NA |
| 041311 Increased apical heart rate | 1 | 2 | 3 | 4 | 5 | NA |
| 041312 Loss of body heat | 1 | 2 | 3 | 4 | 5 | NA |
| 041313 Skin and mucous membrane pallor | 1 | 2 | 3 | 4 | 5 | NA |
| 041314 Anxiety | 1 | 2 | 3 | 4 | 5 | NA |
| 041315 Decreased cognition | 1 | 2 | 3 | 4 | 5 | NA |
| 041316 Decreased hemoglobin (Hgb) | 1 | 2 | 3 | 4 | 5 | NA |
| 041317 Decreased hematocrit (Hct) | 1 | 2 | 3 | 4 | 5 | NA |

Estimated blood loss_____(cc)

*3rd edition*

### Outcome Content References:

American College of Surgeons Committee on Trauma. (1997). *Advanced trauma life support for doctors.* Chicago: American College of Surgeons.

Blankenship, J.C. (1999). Bleeding complications of glycoprotein IIb-IIIa receptor inhibitors (electronic version). *American Heart Journal, 138,* 287-296.

deGuzman, E., Shankar, M.N., & Mattox, K.L. (1999). Limited volume resuscitation in penetrating thoracoabdominal trauma. *AACN Clinical Issues, 10,* 61-68.

Fihn, S.D., Callahan, C.M., Martin, D., McDonell, M.B., Henikoff, J.G., & White, R.H. (1996). The risk for and severity of bleeding complications in elderly patients treated with warfarin. *Annals of Internal Medicine, 124,* 970-979.

Maxson, J.H. (2000). Management of disseminated intravascular coagulation. *Critical Care Nursing Clinics of North America, 12,* 341-352.

Swearingin, P. L., & Keen, J. H. (2001). *Manual of critical care nursing: Nursing interventions and collaborative management* (4th ed.). St. Louis: Mosby.

B

# *Blood Transfusion Reaction (0700)*

*Domain-Physiologic Health (II)*

*Class-Immune Response (H)*

*Scale(s)-Severe to None (n)*

Care Recipient:

Data Source:

**Definition:** Severity of complications with blood transfusion reaction

OUTCOME TARGET RATING:     Maintain at_____     Increase to_____

| Blood Transfusion Reaction Overall Rating | Severe 1 | Substantial 2 | Moderate 3 | Mild 4 | None 5 | |
|---|---|---|---|---|---|---|

INDICATORS:

| | | | | | | |
|---|---|---|---|---|---|---|
| 070020 | Shortness of breath | 1 | 2 | 3 | 4 | 5 | NA |
| 070003 | Decreased urine output | 1 | 2 | 3 | 4 | 5 | NA |
| 070004 | Increased apical heart rate | 1 | 2 | 3 | 4 | 5 | NA |
| 070005 | Blood pressure change | 1 | 2 | 3 | 4 | 5 | NA |
| 070007 | Fever | 1 | 2 | 3 | 4 | 5 | NA |
| 070008 | Chills | 1 | 2 | 3 | 4 | 5 | NA |
| 070009 | Itching | 1 | 2 | 3 | 4 | 5 | NA |
| 070010 | Rash | 1 | 2 | 3 | 4 | 5 | NA |
| 070011 | Restlessness | 1 | 2 | 3 | 4 | 5 | NA |
| 070012 | Anxiety | 1 | 2 | 3 | 4 | 5 | NA |
| 070013 | Malaise | 1 | 2 | 3 | 4 | 5 | NA |
| 070021 | Nausea | 1 | 2 | 3 | 4 | 5 | NA |
| 070014 | Chest pain | 1 | 2 | 3 | 4 | 5 | NA |
| 070015 | Lumbar pain | 1 | 2 | 3 | 4 | 5 | NA |
| 070017 | Hemoglobinuria | 1 | 2 | 3 | 4 | 5 | NA |
| 070018 | Muscle spasms and twitching | 1 | 2 | 3 | 4 | 5 | NA |

*1st edition 1997; Revised 3rd edition (formerly Blood Transfusion Reaction Control)*

## Outcome Content References:

McCance, K.L., & Huether, S.E. (2002). *Pathophysiology: The biologic basis for disease in adults and children* (4th ed.). St. Louis: Mosby.

Raife, Thomas J. (1997). Adverse effects of transfusions caused by leukocytes. *Journal of Intravenous Nursing, 20*(5), 238-244.

Smeltzer, S.C., & Bare, B.G. (Eds.). (2003). *Brunner and Suddarth's textbook of medical-surgical nursing* (10th ed.). Philadelphia: Lippincott, Williams, & Wilkins.

B

# Body Image (1200)

Domain-Psychosocial Health (III)

Class-Psychological Well-Being (M)

Scale(s)-Never positive to Consistently positive (k)

Care Recipient:

Data Source:

**Definition:** Perception of own appearance and body functions

OUTCOME TARGET RATING:    Maintain at_____    Increase to_____

| Body Image Overall Rating | Never positive 1 | Rarely positive 2 | Sometimes positive 3 | Often positive 4 | Consistently positive 5 | |
|---|---|---|---|---|---|---|
| INDICATORS: | | | | | | |
| 120001 Internal picture of self | 1 | 2 | 3 | 4 | 5 | NA |
| 120002 Congruence between body reality, body ideal, and body presentation | 1 | 2 | 3 | 4 | 5 | NA |
| 120003 Description of affected body part | 1 | 2 | 3 | 4 | 5 | NA |
| 120004 Willingness to touch affected body part | 1 | 2 | 3 | 4 | 5 | NA |
| 120005 Satisfaction with body appearance | 1 | 2 | 3 | 4 | 5 | NA |
| 120006 Satisfaction with body function | 1 | 2 | 3 | 4 | 5 | NA |
| 120007 Adjustment to changes in physical appearance | 1 | 2 | 3 | 4 | 5 | NA |
| 120008 Adjustment to changes in body function | 1 | 2 | 3 | 4 | 5 | NA |
| 120009 Adjustment to changes in health status | 1 | 2 | 3 | 4 | 5 | NA |
| 120010 Willingness to use strategies to enhance appearance | 1 | 2 | 3 | 4 | 5 | NA |
| 120012 Willingness to use strategies to enhance function | 1 | 2 | 3 | 4 | 5 | NA |
| 120013 Adjustment to body changes due to injury | 1 | 2 | 3 | 4 | 5 | NA |
| 120014 Adjustment to body changes due to surgery | 1 | 2 | 3 | 4 | 5 | NA |
| 120015 Adjustment to body changes due to aging | 1 | 2 | 3 | 4 | 5 | NA |

*1st edition 1997; Revised 3rd edition*

Outcome Content References:

Comunale, D.L. (1992). Collaborative care planning with the arthritic client at home. *Journal of Home Health Care Practice, 4*(2), 8-15.

Dixon, J.B., Dixon, M.E., & O'Brien, P.E. (2002). Body image: Appearance orientation and evaluation in the severely obese. Changes with weight loss. *Obesity Surgery, 12*(1), 65-71.

Kater, K.J., Rohwer, J., & Londre, K. (2002). Evaluation of an upper elementary school program to prevent body image, eating, and weight concerns. *Journal of School Health, 72*(5), 199-204.

Key, A., George, C.L., Beattie, D., Stammers, K., Lacey, H., & Waller, G. (2002). Body image treatment within an inpatient program for anorexia nervosa: The role of mirror exposure in the desensitization process. *International Journal of Eating Disorders, 31*(2), 185-190.

LeMone, P. (1991). Analysis of human phenomenon: Self-concept. *Nursing Diagnosis, 2*(3), 129-130.

Low, M.B. (1993). Women's body image: The nurse's role in promotion of self-acceptance. *AWONN's Clinical Issues, 4*(2), 213-219.

MacGinley, K.J. (1993). Nursing care of the patient with altered body image. *British Journal of Nursing, 2*(22), 1098-1102.

Newell, R. (1991). Body-image disturbance: Cognitive behavioral formulation and intervention. *Journal of Advanced Nursing, 16*(12), 1400-1405.

*Continued*

**B**

Price, B. (1990). A model for body image care. *Journal of Advanced Nursing, 15*(5), 585-593.

Price, B. (1992). Living with altered body image: The cancer experience. *British Journal of Nursing, 1*(13), 641-645.

Price, B. (1993). Profiling the high-risk altered body image patient. *Senior Nurse, 13*(4), 17-21.

+Rosen, J.C., Srebnik, D., Saltzberg, E., & Wendt, S. (1991). Development of a body image avoidance questionnaire. *Psychological Assessment: A Journal of Consulting and Clinical Psychology, 3*(1), 32-37.

Van Deusen, J., Harlowe, D., & Baker, L. (1989). Body image perceptions of the community-based elderly. *The Occupational Therapy Journal of Research, 9*(4), 243-248.

Wasson, D., & Anderson, M.A. (1995). Chemical dependency and adolescent self-esteem. *Clinical Nursing Research, 4*(3), 274-289.

B

# Body Mechanics Performance (1616)

Domain-Health Knowledge & Behavior (IV)

Class-Health Behavior (Q)

Scale(s)-Never demonstrated to Consistently demonstrated (m)

Care Recipient:

Data Source:

**Definition:** Personal actions to maintain proper body alignment and to prevent muscular skeletal strain

OUTCOME TARGET RATING:    Maintain at_____    Increase to_____

| Body Mechanics Performance Overall Rating | Never demonstrated 1 | Rarely demonstrated 2 | Sometimes demonstrated 3 | Often demonstrated 4 | Consistently demonstrated 5 | |
|---|---|---|---|---|---|---|
| **INDICATORS:** | | | | | | |
| 161601 Uses correct standing posture | 1 | 2 | 3 | 4 | 5 | NA |
| 161602 Uses correct sitting posture | 1 | 2 | 3 | 4 | 5 | NA |
| 161603 Uses correct lying posture | 1 | 2 | 3 | 4 | 5 | NA |
| 161604 Uses correct lifting techniques | 1 | 2 | 3 | 4 | 5 | NA |
| 161605 Uses correct carrying techniques | 1 | 2 | 3 | 4 | 5 | NA |
| 161606 Uses correct technique for pushing heavy load | 1 | 2 | 3 | 4 | 5 | NA |
| 161607 Uses supportive devices correctly | 1 | 2 | 3 | 4 | 5 | NA |
| 161608 Obtains assistance with heavy load as needed | 1 | 2 | 3 | 4 | 5 | NA |
| 161609 Demonstrates muscle strength | 1 | 2 | 3 | 4 | 5 | NA |
| 161610 Demonstrates joint flexibility | 1 | 2 | 3 | 4 | 5 | NA |
| 161611 Uses prescribed exercises to prevent injury | 1 | 2 | 3 | 4 | 5 | NA |

*3rd edition*

## Outcome Content References:

Chan, D., Laporte, D.M., & Sveistrup, H. (1999). Rising from sitting in elderly people, Part 2: Strategies to facilitate rising. *British Journal of Occupational Therapy, 62*(2), 64-68.

Laporte, D.M., Chan, D., & Sveistrup, H. (1999). Rising from sitting in elderly people, Part 1: Implications of biomechanics and physiology. *British Journal of Occupational Therapy, 62*(1), 36-42.

Potter, P.A., & Perry, A.G. (2001). *Fundamentals of nursing* (5th ed.). St. Louis: Mosby.

**B**

# Body Positioning: Self-Initiated (0203)

Domain-Functional Health (I)

Class-Mobility (C)

Scale(s)-Severely compromised to Not compromised (a)

Care Recipient:

Data Source:

**Definition:** Ability to change own body position independently with or without assistive device

OUTCOME TARGET RATING:   Maintain at_____   Increase to_____

| Body Positioning: Self-Initiated Overall Rating | Severely compromised 1 | Substantially compromised 2 | Moderately compromised 3 | Mildly compromised 4 | Not compromised 5 | |
|---|---|---|---|---|---|---|
| INDICATORS: | | | | | | |
| 020302   Moves from lying to sitting | 1 | 2 | 3 | 4 | 5 | NA |
| 020303   Moves from sitting to lying | 1 | 2 | 3 | 4 | 5 | NA |
| 020304   Moves from sitting to standing | 1 | 2 | 3 | 4 | 5 | NA |
| 020305   Moves from standing to sitting | 1 | 2 | 3 | 4 | 5 | NA |
| 020306   Moves from standing to kneeling | 1 | 2 | 3 | 4 | 5 | NA |
| 020307   Moves from kneeling to standing | 1 | 2 | 3 | 4 | 5 | NA |
| 020308   Moves from standing to squatting | 1 | 2 | 3 | 4 | 5 | NA |
| 020309   Moves from squatting to standing | 1 | 2 | 3 | 4 | 5 | NA |
| 020310   Bends at waist while standing | 1 | 2 | 3 | 4 | 5 | NA |
| 020311   Moves from side to side while lying | 1 | 2 | 3 | 4 | 5 | NA |
| 020301   Moves from front to back while lying | 1 | 2 | 3 | 4 | 5 | NA |
| 020313   Moves from back to front while lying | 1 | 2 | 3 | 4 | 5 | NA |

*1st edition 1997; Revised 2nd edition 2000; Revised 3rd edition*

Outcome Content References:

+Berg, K., Wood-Dauphinee, S., Williams, J.I., & Gayton, D. (1989). Measuring balance in the elderly: Preliminary development of an instrument. *Physiotherapy Canada, 41*, 304-311.

Mikulic, M.A., Griffith, E.R., & Jebsen, R.H. (1976). Clinical application of a standardized mobility test. *Archives of Physical Medicine and Rehabilitation, 57*(3), 143-146.

# *Bone Healing (1104)*

*Domain-Physiologic Health (II)*

*Class-Tissue Integrity (L)*

*Scale(s)-None to Extensive (i) and Extensive to None (h)*

*Care Recipient:*

*Data Source:*

**B**

**Definition:** Extent of regeneration of cells and tissues following bone injury

OUTCOME TARGET RATING:    Maintain at_____    Increase to_____

| Bone Healing Overall Rating | None 1 | Limited 2 | Moderate 3 | Substantial 4 | Extensive 5 | |
|---|---|---|---|---|---|---|
| **INDICATORS:** | | | | | | |
| 110402  Cellular proliferation | 1 | 2 | 3 | 4 | 5 | NA |
| 110403  Callus formation | 1 | 2 | 3 | 4 | 5 | NA |
| 110404  Ossification, consolidation, and remodeling | 1 | 2 | 3 | 4 | 5 | NA |
| 110405  Intact peripheral circulation | 1 | 2 | 3 | 4 | 5 | NA |
| 110406  Return of skeletal function | 1 | 2 | 3 | 4 | 5 | NA |

| | Extensive | Substantial | Moderate | Limited | None | |
|---|---|---|---|---|---|---|
| 110401  Hematoma | 1 | 2 | 3 | 4 | 5 | NA |
| 110407  Pain | 1 | 2 | 3 | 4 | 5 | NA |
| 110408  Edema | 1 | 2 | 3 | 4 | 5 | NA |
| 110410  Infection in surrounding tissue | 1 | 2 | 3 | 4 | 5 | NA |
| 110411  Infection in bone | 1 | 2 | 3 | 4 | 5 | NA |

Site of fracture (# from skeleton) _____

*1st edition 1997; Revised 3rd edition*

## Outcome Content References:

Abdullah, D., Ford, T.R., Papaioannou, S., Nicholson, J., & McDonald, F. (2002). An evaluation of accelerated Portland cement as a restorative material. *Biomaterials, 23*(19), 4001-4010.

Mandracchia, V.J., Nelson, S.C., & Barp, E.A. (2001). Current concepts of bone healing. *Clinics in Podiatric Medicine & Surgery 18*(1), 55-77.

Porth, C.M. (2002). *Pathophysiology: Concepts of altered health states* (6th ed.). Philadelphia: Lippincott Williams & Wilkins.

Potter, P.A., & Perry, A.G. (2001). *Fundamentals of nursing* (5th ed.). St. Louis: Mosby.

Wade, R., & Richardson, J. (2001). Outcome in fracture healing: A review. *Injury, 32*(2), 109-14.

*Continued*

**B**

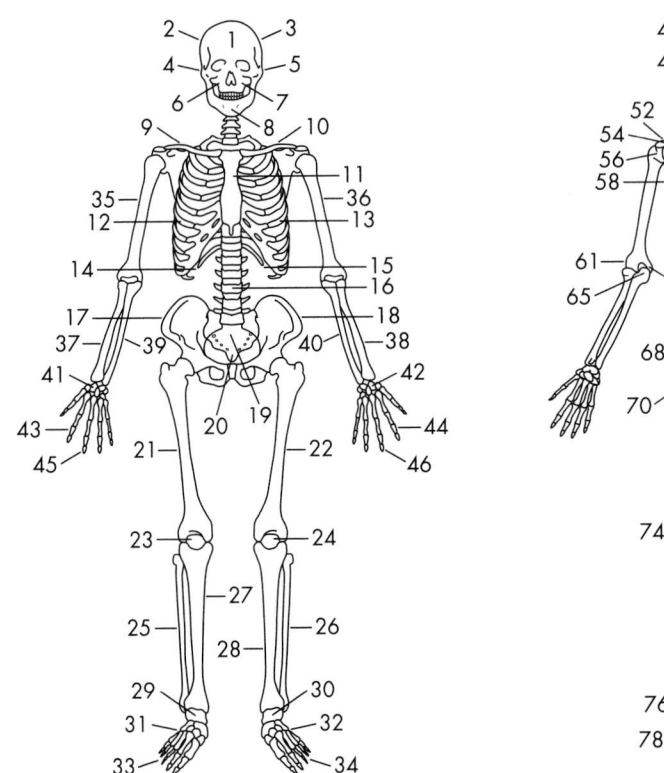

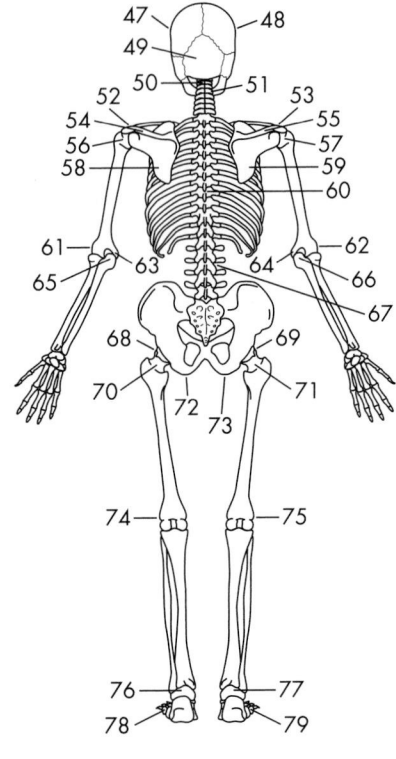

**Bones of the Head**
1. frontal
2. right temporal
3. left temporal
4. right zygomatic
5. left zygomatic
6. right maxilla
7. left maxilla
8. mandible
47. left parietal
48. right parietal
49. occipital

**Bones of the Neck and Chest**
9. right clavicle
10. left clavicle
11. sternum
12. right ribs
13. left ribs
14. right floating rib
15. left floating rib
16. vertebral column
50. atlas
51. cervical vertebra(e) specify ___
52. left acromion
53. right acromion
54. left spine of scapula
55. right spine of scapula
58. left scapula
59. right scapula
60. thoracic vertebra(e) specify___

**Bones of the Abdomen**
16. vertebral column
17. right ilium
18. left ilium
19. sacrum
20. coccyx
72. left ischium
73. right ischium
67. lumbar vertebra(e) specify___

**Bones of the Arm**
35. right humerus
36. left humerus
37. right radius
38. left radius
39. right ulna
40. left ulna
41. right carpals
42. left carpals
43. right metacarpals
44. left metacarpals
45. right phalanges
46. left phalanges
56. right head of humerus
57. left head of humerus
61. left epicondyle
62. right epicondyle
63. left epitrochlea
64. right epitrochlea
65. left olecranon
66. right olecranon

**Bones of the Leg**
21. right femur
22. left femur
23. right patella
24. left patella
25. right fibula
26. left fibula
27. right tibia
28. left tibia
29. right tarsals
30. left tarsals
31. right metatarsals
32. left metatarsals
33. right phalanges
34. left phalanges
68. left head of femur
69. right head of femur
70. left neck of femur
71. right neck of femur
74. left condyle of femur
75. right condyle of femur
76. left talus
77. right talus
78. left calcaneus
79. right calcaneus

# Bowel Continence (0500)

Domain-Physiologic Health (II)

Class-Elimination (F)

Scale(s)-Never demonstrated to Consistently demonstrated (m) and Consistently demonstrated to Never demonstrated (t)

Care Recipient:

Data Source:

**Definition:** Control of passage of stool from the bowel

OUTCOME TARGET RATING:    Maintain at_____    Increase to_____

| Bowel Continence Overall Rating | Never demonstrated 1 | Rarely demonstrated 2 | Sometimes demonstrated 3 | Often demonstrated 4 | Consistently demonstrated 5 | |
|---|---|---|---|---|---|---|
| **INDICATORS:** | | | | | | |
| 050008 Recognizes urge to defecate | 1 | 2 | 3 | 4 | 5 | NA |
| 050001 Maintains predictable pattern of stool evacuation | 1 | 2 | 3 | 4 | 5 | NA |
| 050002 Maintains control of stool passage | 1 | 2 | 3 | 4 | 5 | NA |
| 050003 Evacuates stool at least q 3 days | 1 | 2 | 3 | 4 | 5 | NA |
| 050006 Sphincter tone adequate to control defecation | 1 | 2 | 3 | 4 | 5 | NA |
| 050007 Sphincter innervation functional | 1 | 2 | 3 | 4 | 5 | NA |
| 050009 Responds to urge in timely manner | 1 | 2 | 3 | 4 | 5 | NA |
| 050010 Uses aids appropriately to achieve continence | 1 | 2 | 3 | 4 | 5 | NA |
| 050012 Gets to toilet between urge and evacuation of stool | 1 | 2 | 3 | 4 | 5 | NA |
| 050017 Maintains barrier-free environment for independent toileting | 1 | 2 | 3 | 4 | 5 | NA |
| 050013 Ingests adequate amount of fluid | 1 | 2 | 3 | 4 | 5 | NA |
| 050014 Ingests adequate amount of fiber | 1 | 2 | 3 | 4 | 5 | NA |
| 050015 Describes relationship of food intake to stool consistency | 1 | 2 | 3 | 4 | 5 | NA |
| 050018 Monitors amount and consistency of stool | 1 | 2 | 3 | 4 | 5 | NA |
| 050019 Toilets independently | 1 | 2 | 3 | 4 | 5 | NA |

*Continued*

**B**

| Bowel Continence—cont'd | Consistently demonstrated | Often demonstrated | Sometimes demonstrated | Rarely demonstrated | Never demonstrated | |
|---|---|---|---|---|---|---|
| 050004 Diarrhea | 1 | 2 | 3 | 4 | 5 | NA |
| 050005 Constipation | 1 | 2 | 3 | 4 | 5 | NA |
| 050020 Overuse of laxatives | 1 | 2 | 3 | 4 | 5 | NA |
| 050021 Overuse of enemas | 1 | 2 | 3 | 4 | 5 | NA |
| 050022 Soils under-clothing during day | 1 | 2 | 3 | 4 | 5 | NA |
| 050023 Soils underclothing or bedding during night | 1 | 2 | 3 | 4 | 5 | NA |

*1st edition 1997; Revised 3rd edition*

### Outcome Content References:

Hogstel, M.O., & Nelson, M. (1992). Anticipation and early detection can reduce bowel elimination complications. *Geriatric Nursing, 13*(1), 28-33.

Maas, M.L., & Specht, J.P. (2001). Bowel incontinence. In M. Maas, K. Buckwalter, M. Hardy, T. Tripp-Reimer, M. Titler & J. Specht (Eds.), *Nursing care of older adults: Diagnoses, outcomes & interventions* (pp. 238-251). St. Louis: Mosby.

McLane, A. (1987). *Classification of nursing diagnoses: Proceedings of the 7th conference*. St. Louis: Mosby.

+Morris, J.N., Hawes, C., et al. (1990). Designing the national resident assessment instrument for nursing homes. *Gerontologist 30*(3), 293-307.

# *Bowel Elimination (0501)*

Domain-Physiologic Health (II)

Class-Elimination (F)

Scale(s)-Severely compromised to Not compromised (a) and Severe to None (n)

Care Recipient:

Data Source:

**B**

---

**Definition:** Formation and evacuation of stool

OUTCOME TARGET RATING:    Maintain at_____    Increase to_____

| Bowel Elimination Overall Rating | Severely compromised 1 | Substantially compromised 2 | Moderately compromised 3 | Mildly compromised 4 | Not compromised 5 | |
|---|---|---|---|---|---|---|
| INDICATORS: | | | | | | |
| 050101 Elimination pattern | 1 | 2 | 3 | 4 | 5 | NA |
| 050102 Control of bowel movements | 1 | 2 | 3 | 4 | 5 | NA |
| 050103 Stool color | 1 | 2 | 3 | 4 | 5 | NA |
| 050104 Stool amount for diet | 1 | 2 | 3 | 4 | 5 | NA |
| 050105 Stool soft and formed | 1 | 2 | 3 | 4 | 5 | NA |
| 050112 Ease of stool passage | 1 | 2 | 3 | 4 | 5 | NA |
| 050113 Comfort of stool passage | 1 | 2 | 3 | 4 | 5 | NA |
| 050118 Sphincter tone | 1 | 2 | 3 | 4 | 5 | NA |
| 050119 Muscle tone to evacuate stool | 1 | 2 | 3 | 4 | 5 | NA |
| 050121 Passage of stool without aids | 1 | 2 | 3 | 4 | 5 | NA |

| | Severe | Substantial | Moderate | Mild | None | |
|---|---|---|---|---|---|---|
| 050107 Fat in stool | 1 | 2 | 3 | 4 | 5 | NA |
| 050108 Blood in stool | 1 | 2 | 3 | 4 | 5 | NA |
| 050109 Mucus in stool | 1 | 2 | 3 | 4 | 5 | NA |
| 050110 Constipation | 1 | 2 | 3 | 4 | 5 | NA |
| 050111 Diarrhea | 1 | 2 | 3 | 4 | 5 | NA |
| 050123 Abuse of elimination aids | 1 | 2 | 3 | 4 | 5 | NA |
| 050128 Pain with passage of stool | 1 | 2 | 3 | 4 | 5 | NA |

*1st edition 1997; Revised 3rd edition*

## Outcome Content References:

Heading, C. (1987). Factors affecting bowel functions. *Nursing, 3*(21), 773-783.

Hogstel, M.O., & Nelson, M. (1992). Anticipation and early detection can reduce bowel elimination complications. *Geriatric Nursing 13*(1), 28-33.

Lepshy, M.S., & Michael, A. (1993). Chronic diarrhea: Evaluation and treatment. *American Family Physician, 48*(8), 1461-1466.

Loening-Baucke, V. (1994). Management of chronic constipation in infants and toddlers. *American Family Physician, 46*(2), 397-406.

McKenna, S., Wallis, M., Brannelly, A., & Cawood, J. (2001). The nursing management of diarrhea and constipation before and after the implementation of a bowel management protocol. *Australian Critical Care, 14*(1), 10-6.

McLane, A.M., & McShane, R.E. (2001). Constipation. In M. Maas, K. Buckwalter, M. Hardy, T. Tripp-Reimer, M. Titler & J. Specht (Eds.), *Nursing care of older adults: Diagnoses, outcomes & interventions* (pp. 220-226). St. Louis: Mosby.

McShane, R.E., & McLane, A.M. (1988). Constipation: Impact of etiological factors. *Journal of Gerontological Nursing, 14*(4), 31-34.

Potter, P.A., & Perry, A.G. (2001). *Fundamentals of nursing* (5th ed.). St. Louis: Mosby.

Wadle, K.R. (2001). Diarrhea. In M. Maas, K. Buckwalter, M. Hardy, T. Tripp-Reimer, M. Titler & J. Specht (Eds.), *Nursing care of older adults: Diagnoses, outcomes & interventions* (pp. 227-237). St. Louis: Mosby.

**B**

# Breastfeeding Establishment: Infant (1000)

*Domain-Physiologic Health (II)*

*Class-Nutrition (K)*

*Scale(s)-Not adequate to Totally adequate (f)*

*Care Recipient:*

*Data Source:*

---

**Definition:** Infant attachment to and sucking from the mother's breast for nourishment during the first 3 weeks of breastfeeding

OUTCOME TARGET RATING:      Maintain at_____      Increase to_____

| Breastfeeding Establishment: Infant<br>Overall Rating | Not<br>adequate<br>1 | Slightly<br>adequate<br>2 | Moderately<br>adequate<br>3 | Substantially<br>adequate<br>4 | Totally<br>adequate<br>5 | |
|---|---|---|---|---|---|---|
| INDICATORS: | | | | | | |
| 100001   Proper alignment and latch on | 1 | 2 | 3 | 4 | 5 | NA |
| 100002   Proper areolar grasp | 1 | 2 | 3 | 4 | 5 | NA |
| 100003   Proper areolar compression | 1 | 2 | 3 | 4 | 5 | NA |
| 100004   Correct suck and tongue placement | 1 | 2 | 3 | 4 | 5 | NA |
| 100005   Audible swallow | 1 | 2 | 3 | 4 | 5 | NA |
| 100006   Swallowing a minimum of 5-10 minutes per breast | 1 | 2 | 3 | 4 | 5 | NA |
| 100007   Minimum 8 feedings per day | 1 | 2 | 3 | 4 | 5 | NA |
| 100008   Urinations per day appropriate for age | 1 | 2 | 3 | 4 | 5 | NA |
| 100009   Loose, yellow, seedy stools per day appropriate for age | 1 | 2 | 3 | 4 | 5 | NA |
| 100010   Weight gain appropriate for age | 1 | 2 | 3 | 4 | 5 | NA |
| 100011   Infant contentment after feeding | 1 | 2 | 3 | 4 | 5 | NA |

*1st edition 1997; Revised 3rd edition*

Outcome Content References:

Biancuzzo, M. (2003). *Breastfeeding the newborn* (2nd ed.). St. Louis: Mosby.

Henderson, A.M., Pincombe, J., & Stamp, G.E. (2000). Assisting women to establish breastfeeding: Exploring midwives' practices. *Breastfeeding Review, 8*(3), 11-17.

Lang, S. (2002). *Breastfeeding special care babies* (2nd ed.). London: Bailliere Tindall.

Lawrence, R.A., & Lawrence, R.M. (1999). *Breastfeeding: A guide for the medical profession* (5th ed.). St. Louis: Mosby.

Minchin, M.K. (1989). Positioning for breastfeeding. *Birth, 16*(2), 67-80.

+Muldford, C. (1992). The mother-baby assessment (MBA): An "Apgar Score" for breastfeeding. *Journal of Human Lactation 8*(2), 79-82.

Neifert, M.R., & Seacat, J.M. (1986). A guide to successful breastfeeding. *Contemporary Pediatrics, 3*, 1-14.

Page-Goertz, S. (1989). Discharge planning for the breastfeeding dyad. *Pediatric Nursing, 15*(5), 543-544.

Righard, L., & Alade, M.O. (1992). Sucking technique and its effect on success of breastfeeding. *Birth, 19*(4), 185-189.

Riordan, J., & Auerbach, K.G. (1999). *Breastfeeding and human lactation* (2nd ed.). Boston: Jones & Bartlett.

Shrago, L., & Bocar, D. (1990). The infant's contribution to breastfeeding. *Journal of Obstetric, Gynecologic, & Neonatal Nursing, 19*(3), 209-213.

Walker, M. (1989). Functional assessment of infant breastfeeding patterns. *Birth, 16*(3), 140-147.

## Breastfeeding Establishment: Maternal (1001)

Domain-Physiologic Health (II)                                        Care Recipient:

Class-Nutrition (K)                                                   Data Source:

Scale(s)-Not adequate to Totally adequate (f)

**Definition:** Maternal establishment of proper attachment of an infant to and sucking from the breast for nourishment during the first 3 weeks of breastfeeding

OUTCOME TARGET RATING:      Maintain at_____      Increase to_____

| Breastfeeding Establishment: Maternal Overall Rating | | Not adequate 1 | Slightly adequate 2 | Moderately adequate 3 | Substantially adequate 4 | Totally adequate 5 | |
|---|---|---|---|---|---|---|---|
| INDICATORS: | | | | | | | |
| 100101 | Comfort of position during nursing | 1 | 2 | 3 | 4 | 5 | NA |
| 100102 | Supports breast using "C" hold (cupping) | 1 | 2 | 3 | 4 | 5 | NA |
| 100103 | Breast fullness prior to feeding | 1 | 2 | 3 | 4 | 5 | NA |
| 100104 | Milk ejection (let-down) reflex | 1 | 2 | 3 | 4 | 5 | NA |
| 100106 | Recognition of infant swallowing | 1 | 2 | 3 | 4 | 5 | NA |
| 100107 | Breaking of suction before removing infant from breast | 1 | 2 | 3 | 4 | 5 | NA |
| 100108 | Freedom from nipple tenderness | 1 | 2 | 3 | 4 | 5 | NA |
| 100109 | Avoidance of artificial nipple use with infant | 1 | 2 | 3 | 4 | 5 | NA |
| 100110 | Avoidance of giving water to infant | 1 | 2 | 3 | 4 | 5 | NA |
| 100111 | Supplementation appropriate to infant's age and health status | 1 | 2 | 3 | 4 | 5 | NA |
| 100112 | Response to infant's temperament | 1 | 2 | 3 | 4 | 5 | NA |
| 100113 | Recognition of early hunger cues | 1 | 2 | 3 | 4 | 5 | NA |
| 100120 | Fluid intake of mother | 1 | 2 | 3 | 4 | 5 | NA |
| 100114 | Ability to hand express or use pump | 1 | 2 | 3 | 4 | 5 | NA |
| 100115 | Appropriate storage of milk | 1 | 2 | 3 | 4 | 5 | NA |
| 100117 | Use of community and family support as needed | 1 | 2 | 3 | 4 | 5 | NA |
| 100118 | Satisfaction with breastfeeding process | 1 | 2 | 3 | 4 | 5 | NA |

*1st edition 1997; Revised 3rd edition*

Outcome Content References:

Biancuzzo, M. (2003). *Breastfeeding the newborn* (2nd ed.). St. Louis: Mosby.

Henderson, A.M., Pincombe, J., & Stamp, G.E. (2000). Assisting women to establish breastfeeding: Exploring midwives' practices. *Breastfeeding Review, 8*(3), 11-17.

Hill, P., & Aldag, J. (1991). Potential indicators of insufficient milk supply syndrome. *Research in Nursing and Health, 14*(1), 11-19.

Lawrence, R.A., & Lawrence, R.M. (1999). *Breastfeeding: A guide for the medical profession* (5th ed.). St. Louis: Mosby.

Minchin, M.K. (1989). Positioning for breastfeeding. *Birth, 16*(2), 67-80.

+Muldford, C. (1992). The mother-baby assessment (MBA): An "Apgar Score" for breastfeeding. *Journal of Human Lactation 8*(2), 79-82.

Neifert, M.R., & Seacat, J.M. (1986). A guide to successful breastfeeding. *Contemporary Pediatrics, 3*, 1-14.

Page-Goertz, S. (1989). Discharge planning for the breastfeeding dyad. *Pediatric Nursing, 15*(5), 543-544.

Righard, L., & Alade, M.O. (1992). Sucking technique and its effect on success of breastfeeding. *Birth, 19*(4), 185-189.

Riordan, J., & Auerbach, K.G. (1999). *Breastfeeding and human lactation* (2nd ed.). Boston: Jones & Bartlett.

Shrago, L., & Bocar, D. (1990). The infant's contribution to breastfeeding. *Journal of Obstetric, Gynecologic, & Neonatal Nursing, 19*(3), 209-213.

Walker, M. (1989). Functional assessment of infant breastfeeding patterns. *Birth, 16*(3), 140-147.

B

# Breastfeeding Maintenance (1002)

*Domain-Physiologic Health (II)*

*Class-Nutrition (K)*

*Scale(s)-Not adequate to Totally adequate (f)*

Care Recipient:

Data Source:

**Definition:** Continuation of breastfeeding for nourishment of an infant/toddler

OUTCOME TARGET RATING:  Maintain at_____  Increase to_____

| Breastfeeding Maintenance Overall Rating | Not adequate 1 | Slightly adequate 2 | Moderately adequate 3 | Substantially adequate 4 | Totally adequate 5 | |
|---|---|---|---|---|---|---|
| **INDICATORS:** | | | | | | |
| 100201 Infant's growth in normal range | 1 | 2 | 3 | 4 | 5 | NA |
| 100202 Infant's development in normal range | 1 | 2 | 3 | 4 | 5 | NA |
| 100205 Mother's ability to safely collect and store breastmilk, if desired | 1 | 2 | 3 | 4 | 5 | NA |
| 100206 Child care provider's ability to safely thaw, warm and feed stored breastmilk | 1 | 2 | 3 | 4 | 5 | NA |
| 100207 Mother's freedom from breast tenderness | 1 | 2 | 3 | 4 | 5 | NA |
| 100208 Recognition of signs of decreased milk supply | 1 | 2 | 3 | 4 | 5 | NA |
| 100209 Recognition of signs of plugged ducts and mastitis | 1 | 2 | 3 | 4 | 5 | NA |
| 100210 Mother's avoidance of self-medication without checking with health care professional | 1 | 2 | 3 | 4 | 5 | NA |
| 100211 Support for continuation of lactation on return to work or school | 1 | 2 | 3 | 4 | 5 | NA |
| 100212 Written material reinforcing care instructions | 1 | 2 | 3 | 4 | 5 | NA |
| 100204 Family knowledge of benefits from continued breastfeeding | 1 | 2 | 3 | 4 | 5 | NA |
| 100213 Family recognition of community and health provider support | 1 | 2 | 3 | 4 | 5 | NA |
| 100214 Family expression of satisfaction with support available | 1 | 2 | 3 | 4 | 5 | NA |
| 100215 Family expression of satisfaction with breastfeeding process | 1 | 2 | 3 | 4 | 5 | NA |

*1st edition 1997; Revised 3rd edition*

Outcome Content References:

Bear, K., & Tigges, B.B. (1993). Management strategies for promoting successful breastfeeding. *Nurse Practitioner, 18*(6), 50, 53-54, 56-58, 60.

Coreil, J., & Murphy, J.E. (1988). Maternal commitment, lactation practices, and breastfeeding duration. *Journal of Obstetric, Gynecologic, & Neonatal Nursing, 17*(4), 273-278.

Dick, M.J., Evans, M.L., Arthurs, J.B., Barnes, J.K., Caldwell, R.S., Hutchins, S.S., & Johnson, L.K. (2002). Predicting early breastfeeding attrition. *Journal of Human Lactation, 18*(1), 21-28.

Hauck, Y., & Reinbold, J. (1996). Criteria for successful breastfeeding: Mothers' perceptions. *Journal – Australian College of Midwives, 9*(1), 21-7.

Lawrence, R.A. & Lawrence, R.M. (1999). *Breastfeeding: A guide for the medical profession* (5th ed.). St. Louis: Mosby.

Rentschler, D.D. (1991). Correlates of successful breastfeeding. *Image-the Journal of Nursing Scholarship, 23*(3), 151-154.

Riordan, J., & Auerbach, K.G. (1999). *Breastfeeding and human lactation* (2nd ed.). Boston: Jones & Bartlett.

# *Breastfeeding Weaning (1003)*

Domain-Physiologic Health (II)

Class-Nutrition (K)

Scale(s)-Not adequate to Totally adequate (f)

Care Recipient:

Data Source:

**Definition:** Progressive discontinuation of breastfeeding

OUTCOME TARGET RATING:      Maintain at_____      Increase to_____

| Breastfeeding Weaning Overall Rating | Not adequate 1 | Slightly adequate 2 | Moderately adequate 3 | Substantially adequate 4 | Totally adequate 5 | |
|---|---|---|---|---|---|---|
| INDICATORS: | | | | | | |
| 100301 Awareness that breastfeeding can continue beyond infancy | 1 | 2 | 3 | 4 | 5 | NA |
| 100302 Recognition of weaning readiness cues | 1 | 2 | 3 | 4 | 5 | NA |
| 100304 Knowledge of benefits of gradual weaning | 1 | 2 | 3 | 4 | 5 | NA |
| 100305 Knowledge of guidelines for rapid "emergency" weaning | 1 | 2 | 3 | 4 | 5 | NA |
| 100306 Mother's freedom from plugged ducts or mastitis | 1 | 2 | 3 | 4 | 5 | NA |
| 100307 Avoidance of solids before infant is 4 to 6 months old | 1 | 2 | 3 | 4 | 5 | NA |
| 100308 Replacement of one breastfeeding every few days | 1 | 2 | 3 | 4 | 5 | NA |
| 100309 Introduction of solid foods one at a time | 1 | 2 | 3 | 4 | 5 | NA |
| 100310 Introduction of solid foods using a spoon | 1 | 2 | 3 | 4 | 5 | NA |
| 100311 Additional touch and attention during time of weaning | 1 | 2 | 3 | 4 | 5 | NA |
| 100312 Written material reinforcing weaning information | 1 | 2 | 3 | 4 | 5 | NA |
| 100313 Recognition of resources available for support | 1 | 2 | 3 | 4 | 5 | NA |
| 100314 Use of available resources | 1 | 2 | 3 | 4 | 5 | NA |
| 100303 Family understanding of weaning options | 1 | 2 | 3 | 4 | 5 | NA |
| 100315 Family expression of satisfaction with support received | 1 | 2 | 3 | 4 | 5 | NA |
| 100316 Family expression of satisfaction with weaning process | 1 | 2 | 3 | 4 | 5 | NA |

*1st edition 1997; Revised 3rd edition*

Outcome Content References:

Castiglia, P.T. (1992). Weaning. *Journal of Pediatric Health Care, 6*(1), 38-39.

Hendricks, K.M., & Badruddin, S.H. (1992). Weaning recommendations: The scientific basis. *Nutrition Reviews, 50*(5), 125-133.

Hervada, A.R. (1992). Weaning: Historical perspectives, practical recommendations, and current controversies. *Current Problems in Pediatrics, 22*(5), 223-241.

Huggins, K., & Ziedrich, L. (1994). *The nursing mother's guide to weaning.* Boston: The Harvard Common Press.

Kleinman, R.E. (Ed.). (1998). *Pediatric nutrition handbook* (4th ed.). Elk Grove Village, IL: American Academy of Pediatrics.

Lawrence, R.A., & Lawrence, R.M. (1999). *Breastfeeding: A guide for the medical profession* (5th ed.). St. Louis: Mosby.

Riordan, J., & Auerbach, K.G. (1999). *Breastfeeding and human lactation* (2nd ed.). Boston: Jones & Bartlett.

Rogers, C.S., Morris, S., & Taper, L.J. (1987). Weaning from the breast: Influences on maternal decisions. *Pediatric Nursing, 13*(5), 341-345.

Spangler, A. (1992). *Amy Spangler's breastfeeding: A parent's guide.* Atlanta: Amy Spangler.

Walker, C. (1995). When to wean: Whose advice do mothers find helpful? *Health Visitor, 68*(3), 109-111.

C

# *Cardiac Disease Self-Management (1617)*

*Domain-Health Knowledge & Behavior (IV)*

*Class-Health Behavior (Q)*

*Scale(s)-Never demonstrated to Consistently demonstrated (m)*

Care Recipient:

Data Source:

**Definition:** Personal actions to manage heart disease and prevent disease progression

OUTCOME TARGET RATING:     Maintain at_____     Increase to_____

| Cardiac Disease Self-Management Overall Rating | Never demonstrated 1 | Rarely demonstrated 2 | Sometimes demonstrated 3 | Often demonstrated 4 | Consistently demonstrated 5 | |
|---|---|---|---|---|---|---|
| **INDICATORS:** | | | | | | |
| 161701 Accepts health care provider's diagnosis | 1 | 2 | 3 | 4 | 5 | NA |
| 161702 Seeks information about methods to maintain cardio-vascular health | 1 | 2 | 3 | 4 | 5 | NA |
| 161703 Participates in health care decision making process | 1 | 2 | 3 | 4 | 5 | NA |
| 161704 Participates in pre-scribed cardiac rehabilitation program | 1 | 2 | 3 | 4 | 5 | NA |
| 161705 Performs treatment regimen as prescribed | 1 | 2 | 3 | 4 | 5 | NA |
| 161706 Monitors symptom onset | 1 | 2 | 3 | 4 | 5 | NA |
| 161707 Monitors symptom persistence | 1 | 2 | 3 | 4 | 5 | NA |
| 161708 Monitors symptom severity | 1 | 2 | 3 | 4 | 5 | NA |
| 161709 Monitors symptom frequency | 1 | 2 | 3 | 4 | 5 | NA |
| 161710 Reports symptoms of worsening disease | 1 | 2 | 3 | 4 | 5 | NA |
| 161711 Reports signs and symptoms of depression | 1 | 2 | 3 | 4 | 5 | NA |
| 161712 Uses diary to monitor symptoms over time | 1 | 2 | 3 | 4 | 5 | NA |
| 161713 Uses preventive measures | 1 | 2 | 3 | 4 | 5 | NA |
| 161714 Uses relief measures | 1 | 2 | 3 | 4 | 5 | NA |
| 161715 Uses warning signs to seek health care | 1 | 2 | 3 | 4 | 5 | NA |
| 161716 Monitors pulse rate and rhythm | 1 | 2 | 3 | 4 | 5 | NA |
| 161717 Monitors blood pressure | 1 | 2 | 3 | 4 | 5 | NA |
| 161718 Limits sodium intake | 1 | 2 | 3 | 4 | 5 | NA |
| 161719 Limits fat and cholesterol intake | 1 | 2 | 3 | 4 | 5 | NA |

| Cardiac Disease Self-Management—cont'd | | Never demonstrated | Rarely demonstrated | Sometimes demonstrated | Often demonstrated | Consistently demonstrated | |
|---|---|---|---|---|---|---|---|
| 161720 | Follows recommended diet | 1 | 2 | 3 | 4 | 5 | NA |
| 161721 | Follows fluid restriction recommendations | 1 | 2 | 3 | 4 | 5 | NA |
| 161722 | Monitors effects of stimulants | 1 | 2 | 3 | 4 | 5 | NA |
| 161723 | Monitors body weight | 1 | 2 | 3 | 4 | 5 | NA |
| 161724 | Uses effective weight control strategies | 1 | 2 | 3 | 4 | 5 | NA |
| 161725 | Maintains optimum weight | 1 | 2 | 3 | 4 | 5 | NA |
| 161726 | Follows recommendations for alcohol use | 1 | 2 | 3 | 4 | 5 | NA |
| 161727 | Participates in smoking cessation regimen | 1 | 2 | 3 | 4 | 5 | NA |
| 161728 | Participates in recommended exercise program | 1 | 2 | 3 | 4 | 5 | NA |
| 161729 | Uses energy conserving techniques | 1 | 2 | 3 | 4 | 5 | NA |
| 161730 | Balances activity and rest | 1 | 2 | 3 | 4 | 5 | NA |
| 161731 | Performs usual life routine | 1 | 2 | 3 | 4 | 5 | NA |
| 161732 | Follows recommendations for sexual activity | 1 | 2 | 3 | 4 | 5 | NA |
| 161733 | Obtains needed medications | 1 | 2 | 3 | 4 | 5 | NA |
| 161734 | Uses medications as prescribed | 1 | 2 | 3 | 4 | 5 | NA |
| 161735 | Monitors prescribed medication effects | 1 | 2 | 3 | 4 | 5 | NA |
| 161736 | Uses only over-the-counter medications approved by health care professional | 1 | 2 | 3 | 4 | 5 | NA |
| 161737 | Uses stress management techniques | 1 | 2 | 3 | 4 | 5 | NA |
| 161738 | Obtains flu and pneumonia immunizations | 1 | 2 | 3 | 4 | 5 | NA |
| 161739 | Uses health care services congruent with needs | 1 | 2 | 3 | 4 | 5 | NA |
| 161740 | Participates in screening for cholesterol | 1 | 2 | 3 | 4 | 5 | NA |
| 161741 | Reports need for financial assistance to obtain supplies and medications | 1 | 2 | 3 | 4 | 5 | NA |

*Continued*

| Cardiac Disease Self-Management—cont'd | | Never demonstrated | Rarely demonstrated | Sometimes demonstrated | Often demonstrated | Consistently demonstrated | |
|---|---|---|---|---|---|---|---|
| 161742 | Keeps appointments with health care professional | 1 | 2 | 3 | 4 | 5 | NA |
| 161743 | Maintains plan for medical emergencies | 1 | 2 | 3 | 4 | 5 | NA |

*3rd edition*

Outcome Content References:

Cannon, C.P., Battler, A., Brindis, R.G., Cox, J.L., Ellis, S.G., Every, N.R., Flaherty, J.T., Harrington, R.A., Krumholz, H.M., Simoons, M.L., Van De Werf, F.J.J., & Weintraub, W.S. (2001). ACC key data elements and definitions for measuring the clinical management and outcomes of patients with acute coronary syndromes: A report of the American College of Cardiology task force on clinical data standards (acute coronary syndrome writing committee). *Journal of the American College of Cardiology, 38*, 2114-2130.

Dunbar, S.B., Jacobson, L.H., & Deaton, C. (1998). Heart failure: Strategies to enhance patient self-management. *AACN Clinical Issues: Advanced Practice in Acute & Critical Care, 9*, 244-256.

Dusseldorp, E., Van Elderan, T., Maes, S., Meulman, J., & Kraaij, V. (1999). A meta-analysis of psychoeducational programs for coronary heart disease patients. *Health Psychology, 18*, 506-519.

Hunt, S.A., Baker, D.W., Chin, M.H., Cinquegrani, M.P., Feldman, A.M., Grancis, G.S., Ganiats, T.G., Goldstein, S., Gregoratos, G., Jessup, M.L., Noble, R.J., Packer, M., Silver, M.A., & Steven, L.W. (2001). ACC/AHA guidelines for the evaluation and management of chronic heart failure in the adult: A report of the American College of Cardiology/American Heart Association Task Force on Practice Guidelines (Committee to revise the 1995 Guidelines for the Evaluation and Management of Heart Failure). *Journal of the American College of Cardiology, 38*, 2101-2113.

Johnson, J., & Pearson, V. (2000). The effects of a structured education course on stroke survivors living in the community...including commentary by Phipps, M. *Rehabilitation Nursing, 25*, 59-65.

Konstam, M., Dracup, K., Baker, D., et al. (1994). *Heart Failure: Management of Patients with Left-Ventricular Systolic Dysfunction. Clinical Practice Guideline No. 11.* AHCPR Publication No. 94-0612. Rockville, MD: Agency for Health Care Policy and Research, Public Health Service, U. S. Department of Health and Human Services.

Sheps, S.G., Black, H.R., Cohen, J.D., Kaplan, N. M., Ferdinand, K.C., Chobanian, A.V., Dustan, H.P., Gifford, R.W., Moser, M., et al. (1997). *The Sixth Report of the Joint National Committee on Prevention, Detection, Evaluation, & Treatment of High Blood Pressure.* NIH Publication No. 98-4080. Bethesda, MD: National Institutes of Health, National Heart, Lung, and Blood Institute (NHLBI), & National High Blood Pressure Education Program.

# Cardiac Pump Effectiveness (0400)

Domain-Physiologic Health (II)

Class-Cardiopulmonary (E)

Scale(s)-Severely compromised to Not compromised (a) and Severe to None (n)

Care Recipient:

Data Source:

C

**Definition:** Adequacy of blood volume ejected from the left ventricle to support systemic perfusion pressure

OUTCOME TARGET RATING:    Maintain at_____    Increase to_____

| Cardiac Pump Effectiveness Overall Rating | Severely compromised 1 | Substantially compromised 2 | Moderately compromised 3 | Mildly compromised 4 | Not compromised 5 | |
|---|---|---|---|---|---|---|
| INDICATORS: | | | | | | |
| 040001 Systolic blood pressure | 1 | 2 | 3 | 4 | 5 | NA |
| 040019 Diastolic blood pressure | 1 | 2 | 3 | 4 | 5 | NA |
| 040002 Apical heart rate | 1 | 2 | 3 | 4 | 5 | NA |
| 040003 Cardiac index | 1 | 2 | 3 | 4 | 5 | NA |
| 040004 Ejection fraction | 1 | 2 | 3 | 4 | 5 | NA |
| 040005 Activity tolerance | 1 | 2 | 3 | 4 | 5 | NA |
| 040006 Peripheral pulses | 1 | 2 | 3 | 4 | 5 | NA |
| 040007 Heart size | 1 | 2 | 3 | 4 | 5 | NA |
| 040008 Skin color | 1 | 2 | 3 | 4 | 5 | NA |
| 040020 Urinary output | 1 | 2 | 3 | 4 | 5 | NA |
| 040021 Cognitive status | 1 | 2 | 3 | 4 | 5 | NA |
| 040022 24-hour intake and output balance | 1 | 2 | 3 | 4 | 5 | NA |

| | Severe | Substantial | Moderate | Mild | None | |
|---|---|---|---|---|---|---|
| 040009 Neck vein distension | 1 | 2 | 3 | 4 | 5 | NA |
| 040010 Dysrhythmia | 1 | 2 | 3 | 4 | 5 | NA |
| 040011 Abnormal heart sounds | 1 | 2 | 3 | 4 | 5 | NA |
| 040012 Angina | 1 | 2 | 3 | 4 | 5 | NA |
| 040013 Peripheral edema | 1 | 2 | 3 | 4 | 5 | NA |
| 040014 Pulmonary edema | 1 | 2 | 3 | 4 | 5 | NA |
| 040015 Profuse diaphoresis | 1 | 2 | 3 | 4 | 5 | NA |
| 040016 Nausea | 1 | 2 | 3 | 4 | 5 | NA |
| 040017 Fatigue | 1 | 2 | 3 | 4 | 5 | NA |
| 040023 Dyspnea | 1 | 2 | 3 | 4 | 5 | NA |
| 040024 Weight gain | 1 | 2 | 3 | 4 | 5 | NA |

*1st edition 1997; Revised 3rd edition*

## Outcome Content References:

Bumann, R., & Speltz, M. (1989). Decreased cardiac output: A nursing diagnosis. *Dimensions of Critical Care Nursing, 8*(1), 6-15.

Dalton, J. (1985). A descriptive study: Defining characteristics of the nursing diagnosis cardiac output, alterations in: Decreased. *Image-the Journal of Nursing Scholarship, 17*(4), 113-117.

Dougherty, C. (1986). Decreased cardiac output: Validation of a nursing diagnosis. *Dimensions of Critical Care Nursing, 5*(3), 182-188.

Dougherty, C.M. (2001). Decreased cardiac output. In M. Maas, K. Buckwalter, M. Hardy, T. Tripp-Reimer, M. Titler & J. Specht (Eds.), *Nursing care of older adults: Diagnoses, outcomes & interventions* (pp. 285-297). St. Louis: Mosby.

Futrell, A. (1990). Decreased cardiac output: Case for a collaborative diagnosis. *Dimensions of Critical Care Nursing, 9*(4), 202-209.

U.S. Department of Health and Human Services. (1994). *Heart failure: Evaluation and care of patients with left-ventricular systolic dysfunction* (AHCPR Publication No. 94-0612). Rockville, MD: Public Health Service Agency for Health Care Policy and Research.

U.S. Department of Health and Human Services. (1994). *Unstable angina: Diagnosis and management* (AHCPR Publication No. 94-0602) Rockville, MD: Public Health Service Agency for Health Care Policy and Research.

C

# Caregiver Adaptation to Patient Institutionalization (2200)

*Domain-Family Health (VI)*

*Class-Family Caregiver Performance (W)*

*Scale(s)-Never demonstrated to Consistently demonstrated (m)*

*Care Recipient:*

*Data Source:*

> **Definition:** Adaptive response of family caregiver when the care recipient is moved to an institution

OUTCOME TARGET RATING:     Maintain at_____     Increase to_____

| Caregiver Adaptation to Patient Institutionalization Overall Rating | Never demonstrated 1 | Rarely demonstrated 2 | Sometimes demonstrated 3 | Often demonstrated 4 | Consistently demonstrated 5 | |
|---|---|---|---|---|---|---|
| INDICATORS: | | | | | | |
| 220001 Trusts non-family caregiver(s) | 1 | 2 | 3 | 4 | 5 | NA |
| 220002 Maintains desired control over care | 1 | 2 | 3 | 4 | 5 | NA |
| 220003 Participates in care as desired | 1 | 2 | 3 | 4 | 5 | NA |
| 220004 Maintains caregiver-care recipient relationship | 1 | 2 | 3 | 4 | 5 | NA |
| 220005 Communicates with health care provider(s) | 1 | 2 | 3 | 4 | 5 | NA |
| 220006 Reports decreased need to verbalize feelings about change | 1 | 2 | 3 | 4 | 5 | NA |
| 220007 Resolves feelings of guilt | 1 | 2 | 3 | 4 | 5 | NA |
| 220008 Resolves feelings of anger | 1 | 2 | 3 | 4 | 5 | NA |
| 220009 Uses conflict resolution methods | 1 | 2 | 3 | 4 | 5 | NA |
| 220010 Demonstrates comfort with role transition | 1 | 2 | 3 | 4 | 5 | NA |
| 220011 Provides consent for treatment(s) | 1 | 2 | 3 | 4 | 5 | NA |
| 220012 Provides information about patient's routine | 1 | 2 | 3 | 4 | 5 | NA |
| 220013 Provides patient's comfort items | 1 | 2 | 3 | 4 | 5 | NA |
| 220014 Communicates needs of nonverbal patient | 1 | 2 | 3 | 4 | 5 | NA |

*1st edition 1997; Revised 3rd edition*

Outcome Content References:

Gaugler, J.E., Pearlin, L.I., Leitsch, S.A., & Davey, A. (2001). Relinquishing in-home dementia care: Difficulties and perceived helpfulness during the nursing home transition. *American Journal of Alzheimer's Disease & Other Dementias, 16*(1), 32-42.

Kaus, K.J. (1990). Fostering family integrity. In Craft, M. & Denehy, J.A. (Eds.), *Nursing Interventions for infants and children* (pp.181-200). Philadelphia: W.B. Saunders Co.

Langford, M. (2001). A view from the front lines. Residential treatment: Have I done the right thing? *Premier Outlook, 2*(1), 16,18.

Lindgren, C.L. (1993). The caregiver career. *Image-the Journal of Nursing Scholarship, 25*(3), 214-219.

Lindsay, J. K., Roman, L., DeWys, M., Eager, M., Levick, J., & Quinn, M. (1993). Creative caring in the NICU: Parent to parent support. *Neonatal Network, 12*(4), 37-44.

Maas, M., Buckwalter, K, Swanson, E., Specht, J., Tripp-Reimer, T., & Hardy, M. (1994). The caring partnership: Staff and families of persons institutionalized with Alzheimer's disease. *The American Journal of Alzheimer's Care and Related Disorders & Research, 9*(6), 21-30.

+Montgomery, R.J.V., Gonyea, J.G., & Hooyman, N.R. (1985). Caregiving and the experience of subjective and objective burden. *Family Relations, 34*, 19-26.

Moyle, W., Edwards, H., & Clinton, M. (2002). Living with loss: Dementia and the family caregiver. *Australian Journal of Advanced Nursing, 19*(3), 25-31.

Olson, R. K., Heater, B. S., & Becker, A. M. (1990) A meta-analysis of the effects of nursing interventions on children and parents. *Maternal-Child Nursing, 15*(2), 104-108.

+Picot, S.J., Youngblut, J., & Zeller, R. (1997). Development and testing of a measure of perceived caregiver rewards in adults. *Journal of Nursing Measurement, 5* (1), 33-52.

Stevenson, J.E. (1990). Family stress related to home care of Alzheimer's disease patients and implications for support. *Journal of Neuroscience Nursing, 22*(3), 179-188.

Swanson, E., Jensen, D.P., Specht, J., Saylor, D., Johnson, M., & Maas, M. (1997). Caregiving: Concept analysis and outcomes, *Scholarly Inquiry for Nursing Practice, 11*(1), 65-79.

Wilson, H.S. (1989). Family caregiving for a relative with Alzheimer's dementia: Coping with negative choices. *Nursing Research, 38*(2), 94-98.

C

C

# Caregiver Emotional Health (2506)

*Domain-Family Health (VI)*

*Class-Family Member Health Status (Z)*

*Scale(s)-Severely compromised to Not compromised (a) and Severe to None (n)*

*Care Recipient:*

*Data Source:*

***Definition:*** Emotional well-being of a family care provider while caring for a family member

OUTCOME TARGET RATING:      Maintain at_____      Increase to_____

| Caregiver Emotional Health Overall Rating | Severely compromised 1 | Substantially compromised 2 | Moderately compromised 3 | Mildly compromised 4 | Not compromised 5 | |
|---|---|---|---|---|---|---|
| **INDICATORS:** | | | | | | |
| 250601  Satisfaction with life | 1 | 2 | 3 | 4 | 5 | NA |
| 250602  Sense of control | 1 | 2 | 3 | 4 | 5 | NA |
| 250603  Self-esteem | 1 | 2 | 3 | 4 | 5 | NA |
| 250610  Certainty about future | 1 | 2 | 3 | 4 | 5 | NA |
| 250611  Perceived social connectedness | 1 | 2 | 3 | 4 | 5 | NA |
| 250612  Perceived spiritual well-being | 1 | 2 | 3 | 4 | 5 | NA |
| 250614  Perceived adequacy of resources | 1 | 2 | 3 | 4 | 5 | NA |

| | Severe | Substantial | Moderate | Mild | None | |
|---|---|---|---|---|---|---|
| 250604  Anger | 1 | 2 | 3 | 4 | 5 | NA |
| 250605  Resentfulness | 1 | 2 | 3 | 4 | 5 | NA |
| 250606  Guilt | 1 | 2 | 3 | 4 | 5 | NA |
| 250607  Depression | 1 | 2 | 3 | 4 | 5 | NA |
| 250608  Frustration | 1 | 2 | 3 | 4 | 5 | NA |
| 250609  Ambivalence concerning situation | 1 | 2 | 3 | 4 | 5 | NA |
| 250613  Perceived burden | 1 | 2 | 3 | 4 | 5 | NA |
| 250615  Psychotropic drug(s) use | 1 | 2 | 3 | 4 | 5 | NA |

*1st edition 1997; Revised 3rd edition*

Outcome Content References:

Brown, M.A., & Powell-Cope, G.M. (1991). AIDS family caregiving: Transitions through uncertainty. *Nursing Research, 40*(6), 338-345.

Bull, M.J. (1990). Factors influencing family caregiver burden and health. *Western Journal of Nursing Research, 12*(6), 758-776.

Croog, S.H., Sudilovsky, A., Burleson, J.A., & Baume, R.M. (2001). Vulnerability of husband and wife caregivers of Alzheimer disease patients to caregiving stressors. *Alzheimer Disease & Associated Disorders, 15*(4), 201-210.

Ducharme, F., LeVesque, L., Gendron, M., & Legault, A. (2001). Development process and qualitative evaluation of a program to promote the mental health of family caregivers. *Clinical Nursing Research, 10*(2), 182-201.

Fruewirth, S.E. (1989). An application of Johnson's Behavioral Model: A case study. *Journal of Community Health Nursing, 6*(2), 61-71.

Given, B.A., Kozachik, S.L., Collins, C.E., DeVoss, D.N., & Given, C.W. (2001). Caregiver role strain. In M. Maas, K. Buckwalter, M. Hardy, T. Tripp-Reimer, M. Titler & J. Specht (Eds.), *Nursing care of older adults: Diagnoses, outcomes & interventions* (pp. 679-695). St. Louis: Mosby.

Grant, I., Adler, K.A., Patterson, T.L., Dimsdale, J.E., Ziegler, M.G., & Irwin, M.R. (2002). Health consequences of Alzheimer's caregiving transitions: Effects of placement and bereavement. *Psychosomatic Medicine, 64*(3), 477-486.

Haley, W.E., LaMonde, L.A., Han, B., Narramore, S., & Schonwetter, R. (2001). Family caregiving in hospice: Effects on psychological and health functioning among spousal caregivers of hospice patients with lung cancer or dementia. *Hospice Journal, 15*(4), 1-18.

Lindgren, C.L. (1990). Burnout and social support in family caregivers. *Western Journal of Nursing Research, 12*(4), 469-487.

Ptok, U., Papassotiropoulos, A., & Heun, R. (2001). Mental health in spouses of patients with gerontopsychiatric disorders. *International Journal of Geriatric Psychiatry, 16*(10), 1014-6.

Romeis, J.C. (1989). Caregiver strain. *Journal of Aging and Health, 1*(2), 188-208.

+Robinson, B.C. (1983). Validation of a caregiver strain index. *Journal of Gerontology, 38*(3), 344-348.

Thompson, E.H., Futterman, A.M., Gallagher-Thompson, D., Rose, J.M., & Lovett, S.B. (1993). Social support and caregiving burden in family caregivers of frail elders. *Journal of Gerontology, 48*(5), S245-S254.

# Caregiver Home Care Readiness (2202)

Domain-Family Health (VI)

Class-Family Caregiver Performance (W)

Scale(s)-Not adequate to Totally adequate (f)

Care Recipient:

Data Source:

**C**

**Definition:** Extent of preparedness of a caregiver to assume responsibility for the health care of a family member in the home

OUTCOME TARGET RATING:    Maintain at_____    Increase to_____

| Caregiver Home Care Readiness Overall Rating | Not adequate 1 | Slightly adequate 2 | Moderately adequate 3 | Substantially adequate 4 | Totally adequate 5 | |
|---|---|---|---|---|---|---|
| **INDICATORS:** | | | | | | |
| 220201 Willingness to assume caregiving role | 1 | 2 | 3 | 4 | 5 | NA |
| 220204 Participation in decisions about home care | 1 | 2 | 3 | 4 | 5 | NA |
| 220202 Knowledge about caregiving role | 1 | 2 | 3 | 4 | 5 | NA |
| 220203 Demonstration of positive regard for care recipient | 1 | 2 | 3 | 4 | 5 | NA |
| 220205 Knowledge of care recipient's disease process | 1 | 2 | 3 | 4 | 5 | NA |
| 220206 Knowledge of recommended treatment regimen | 1 | 2 | 3 | 4 | 5 | NA |
| 220207 Knowledge of recommended treatment procedures | 1 | 2 | 3 | 4 | 5 | NA |
| 220219 Knowledge of where to obtain needed equipment | 1 | 2 | 3 | 4 | 5 | NA |
| 220220 Knowledge of equipment operation | 1 | 2 | 3 | 4 | 5 | NA |
| 220208 Knowledge of prescribed activity | 1 | 2 | 3 | 4 | 5 | NA |
| 220209 Knowledge of follow-up care | 1 | 2 | 3 | 4 | 5 | NA |
| 220210 Knowledge of emergency care | 1 | 2 | 3 | 4 | 5 | NA |
| 220211 Knowledge of financial resources | 1 | 2 | 3 | 4 | 5 | NA |
| 220212 Financial resources | 1 | 2 | 3 | 4 | 5 | NA |
| 220213 Knowledge of when to contact health care professionals | 1 | 2 | 3 | 4 | 5 | NA |
| 220214 Social support for caregiving | 1 | 2 | 3 | 4 | 5 | NA |
| 220215 Confidence in ability to manage care at home | 1 | 2 | 3 | 4 | 5 | NA |
| 220217 Willingness to involve care recipient in planning care | 1 | 2 | 3 | 4 | 5 | NA |
| 220218 Evidence of plans for caregiver backup | 1 | 2 | 3 | 4 | 5 | NA |

*1st edition 1997; Revised 3rd edition*

## Outcome Content References:

Axelrod, J., Geismar, L., & Ross, R. (1994). Families of chronically mentally ill patients: Their structure, coping resources, and tolerance for deviant behavior. *Health & Social Work, 19*(4), 271-278.

Baginski, Y. (1994). Roadblocks to home care. *Continuing Care, 13*(8), 16-18, 24, 28-29.

Coppa, C., Hepburn, J., Strauss, D., & Yody, B.B. (1999). Return to home after acquired brain injury: Is the family ready? *Brain Injury Source, 3*(2), 18-20, 22.

Gennaro, S., & Bakewell-Sachs, S. (1992). Discharge planning and home care for low-birth weight infants. *NAACOGS Clinical Issues in Perinatal & Womens Health Nursing, 3*(1), 129-145.

Magilvy, J.K., & Lakomy, J.M. (1991). Transitions of older adults to home care. *Home Health Care Services Quarterly, 12*(4), 59-70.

+Picot, S.J., Youngblut, J., & Zeller, R. (1997). Development and testing of a measure of perceived caregiver rewards in adults. *Journal of Nursing Measurement, 5*(1), 33-52.

Titler, M.G., & Pettit, D.M. (1995). Discharge readiness assessment. *Journal of Cardiovascular Nursing, 9*(4), 64-74.

**C**

# Caregiver Lifestyle Disruption (2203)

*Domain-Family Health (VI)*

*Class-Family Caregiver Performance (W)*

*Scale(s)-Severe to None (n) and Severely compromised to Not compromised (a)*

Care Recipient:

Data Source:

**Definition:** Severity of disturbances in the lifestyle of a family member due to caregiving

OUTCOME TARGET RATING:     Maintain at_____     Increase to_____

| Caregiver Lifestyle Disruption Overall Rating | Severe 1 | Substantial 2 | Moderate 3 | Mild 4 | None 5 | |
|---|---|---|---|---|---|---|

INDICATORS:

| | | Severe 1 | Substantial 2 | Moderate 3 | Mild 4 | None 5 | |
|---|---|---|---|---|---|---|---|
| 220315 | Disruption of routine | 1 | 2 | 3 | 4 | 5 | NA |
| 220316 | Disruption of sleep | 1 | 2 | 3 | 4 | 5 | NA |
| 220317 | Disruption of family dynamics | 1 | 2 | 3 | 4 | 5 | NA |
| 220318 | Disruption of living environment | 1 | 2 | 3 | 4 | 5 | NA |
| 220319 | Financial burden to caregiver | 1 | 2 | 3 | 4 | 5 | NA |

| | | Severely compromised | Substantially compromised | Moderately compromised | Mildly compromised | Not compromised | |
|---|---|---|---|---|---|---|---|
| 220302 | Role performance | 1 | 2 | 3 | 4 | 5 | NA |
| 220303 | Role flexibility | 1 | 2 | 3 | 4 | 5 | NA |
| 220304 | Opportunities for privacy | 1 | 2 | 3 | 4 | 5 | NA |
| 220305 | Relationships with other family members | 1 | 2 | 3 | 4 | 5 | NA |
| 220306 | Social interactions | 1 | 2 | 3 | 4 | 5 | NA |
| 220307 | Social support | 1 | 2 | 3 | 4 | 5 | NA |
| 220308 | Diversional activities | 1 | 2 | 3 | 4 | 5 | NA |
| 220309 | Work productivity | 1 | 2 | 3 | 4 | 5 | NA |
| 220310 | Role responsibilities | 1 | 2 | 3 | 4 | 5 | NA |
| 220312 | Relationships with friends | 1 | 2 | 3 | 4 | 5 | NA |
| 220313 | Relationships with pets | 1 | 2 | 3 | 4 | 5 | NA |

*1st edition 1997; Revised 3rd edition*

Outcome Content References:

Baldwin, B.A., Kleeman, K.M., Stevens, G.L., & Rasin, J. (1989). Family caregiver stress: Clinical assessment and management. *International Psychogeriatrics, 1*(2), 183-193.

Gaynor, S.E. (1990). The long haul: The effects of home care on caregivers. *Image-the Journal of Nursing Scholarship, 22*(4), 208-212.

Given, B.A., & Given, C.W. (1991). Family caregiving for the elderly. *Annual Review of Nursing Research, 9*, 77-101.

Hinds, C. (1992). Suffering: A relatively unexplored phenomenon among family caregivers of non-institutionalized patients with cancer. *Journal of Advanced Nursing, 17*(8), 918-925.

Kuhlman, G.J., Wilson, H.S., Hutchison, S.A., & Wallhagen, M. (1991). Alzheimer's disease and family caregiving: Critical syntheses of the literature and research agenda. *Nursing Research, 40*(6), 331-337.

Lindgren, C.L. (1990). Burnout and social support in family caregivers. *Western Journal of Nursing Research, 12*(4), 469-487.

Lindgren, C.L. (1993). The caregiver career. *Image-the Journal of Nursing Scholarship, 25*(3), 214-219.

Oberst, M.T., Thomas, S.E., Gass, K.A., & Ward, S.E. (1989). Caregiving demands and appraisal of stress among family caregivers. *Cancer Nursing, 12*(4), 209-215.

+Robinson, B.C. (1983). Validation of a caregiver strain index. *Journal of Gerontology, 38*(3), 344-348.

Robinson, K. (1990). The relationships between social skills, social support, self-esteem and burden in adult caregivers. *Journal of Advanced Nursing, 15*(7), 788-795.

Robinson, K.M. (1989). Predictors of depression among wife caregivers. *Nursing Research, 38*(8), 359-363.

Stern, S., Doolan, M., Staples, E., Szmukler, G.L., & Eisler, I. (1999). Disruption and reconstruction: Narrative insights into the experience of family members caring for a relative diagnosed with serious mental illness. *Family Process, 38*(3), 353-369.

Stevenson, J.E. (1990). Family stress related to home care of Alzheimer's disease patients and implications for support. *Journal of Neuroscience Nursing, 22*(3), 179-188.

Thompson, E.H., Futterman, A.M., Gallagher-Thompson, D., Rose, J.M., & Lovette, S.B. (1993). Social support and caregiving burden in family caregivers of frail elders. *Journal of Gerontology, 48*(5), S245-S254.

C

# Caregiver-Patient Relationship (2204)

*Domain-Family Health (VI)*

*Class-Family Caregiver Performance (W)*

*Scale(s)-Severely compromised to Not compromised (a)*

*Care Recipient:*

*Data Source:*

**C**

**Definition:** Positive interactions and connections between the caregiver and care recipient

OUTCOME TARGET RATING:   Maintain at_____   Increase to_____

| Caregiver-Patient Relationship Overall Rating | Severely compromised 1 | Substantially compromised 2 | Moderately compromised 3 | Mildly compromised 4 | Not compromised 5 | |
|---|---|---|---|---|---|---|
| **INDICATORS:** | | | | | | |
| 220401 Effective communication | 1 | 2 | 3 | 4 | 5 | NA |
| 220402 Patience | 1 | 2 | 3 | 4 | 5 | NA |
| 220404 Calmness | 1 | 2 | 3 | 4 | 5 | NA |
| 220405 Nurturance and affirmation | 1 | 2 | 3 | 4 | 5 | NA |
| 220406 Companionship | 1 | 2 | 3 | 4 | 5 | NA |
| 220407 Caring | 1 | 2 | 3 | 4 | 5 | NA |
| 220408 Long-term commitment | 1 | 2 | 3 | 4 | 5 | NA |
| 220409 Mutual acceptance | 1 | 2 | 3 | 4 | 5 | NA |
| 220410 Mutual respect | 1 | 2 | 3 | 4 | 5 | NA |
| 220411 Collaborative problem solving | 1 | 2 | 3 | 4 | 5 | NA |
| 220412 Sense of responsibility | 1 | 2 | 3 | 4 | 5 | NA |
| 220413 Mutual sense of attachment | 1 | 2 | 3 | 4 | 5 | NA |

*1st edition 1997; Revised 3rd edition*

Outcome Content References:

Caldwell, S.M. (1993). Measuring family well-being: Conceptual model, reliability, validity and use. In C.F. Waltz & O.L. Strickland (Eds.), *Measuring client outcomes*. New York: Springer.

Clemen-Stone, S., McGuire, S., & Eigsti, D. (2002). *Comprehensive community health nursing: Family, aggregate and community practice* (6th ed.). St. Louis: Mosby.

Craft, M.J., & Willadsen, J.A. (1992). Interventions related to family. *Nursing Clinics of North America, 27*(20), 517-540.

+Picot, S.J., Youngblut, J., & Zeller, R. (1997). Development and testing of a measure of perceived caregiver rewards in adults. *Journal of Nursing Measurement, 5* (1), 33-52.

Gaynor, S.E. (1990). The long haul: The effects of home care on caregivers. *Image-the Journal of Nursing Scholarship, 22*(4), 208-212.

Hooyman, M., Gonyea, J., & Montgomery, R. (1985). Impact of in-home services termination on family caregivers. *The Gerontologist, 25*(2), 141-145.

O'Neill, C., & Sorenson, E.S. (1991). Home care of the elderly: A family perspective. *Advances in Nursing Science, 13*(4), 28-37.

Phillips, L.R. (1988). The fit of elder abuse with the family violence paradigm, and the implications of a paradigm shift for clinical practice. *Public Health Nursing, 5*(4), 222-229.

Printz-Feddersen, V. (1990). Group process effect on caregiver burden. *Journal of Neuroscience Nursing, 22*(3), 164-168.

+Vermooij-Dassen, M.J.F.J. (1993). *Dementia and home care: Determinants of the sense of competence of primary caregivers and the effect of professionally guided caregiver support* (in Dutch). Lisse, The Netherlands: Swets & Seitliger.

# Caregiver Performance: Direct Care (2205)

*Domain-Family Health (VI)*

*Class-Family Caregiver Performance (W)*

*Scale(s)-Not adequate to Totally adequate (f)*

Care Recipient:

Data Source:

**C**

**Definition:** Provision by family care provider of appropriate personal and health care for a family member

OUTCOME TARGET RATING:     Maintain at_____     Increase to_____

| Caregiver Performance: Direct Care Overall Rating | Not adequate 1 | Slightly adequate 2 | Moderately adequate 3 | Substantially adequate 4 | Totally adequate 5 | |
|---|---|---|---|---|---|---|
| **INDICATORS:** | | | | | | |
| 220503 Knowledge of disease process | 1 | 2 | 3 | 4 | 5 | NA |
| 220504 Knowledge of treatment plan | 1 | 2 | 3 | 4 | 5 | NA |
| 220505 Adherence to treatment plan | 1 | 2 | 3 | 4 | 5 | NA |
| 220507 Performance of treatments | 1 | 2 | 3 | 4 | 5 | NA |
| 220502 Assistance with care recipient's activities of daily living needs | 1 | 2 | 3 | 4 | 5 | NA |
| 220506 Assistance with care recipient's instrumental activities of daily living needs | 1 | 2 | 3 | 4 | 5 | NA |
| 220501 Provision of emotional support to care recipient | 1 | 2 | 3 | 4 | 5 | NA |
| 220508 Surveillance of health status of care recipient | 1 | 2 | 3 | 4 | 5 | NA |
| 220509 Surveillance of behavior of care recipient | 1 | 2 | 3 | 4 | 5 | NA |
| 220510 Anticipation of care recipient's needs | 1 | 2 | 3 | 4 | 5 | NA |
| 220511 Demonstration of unconditional positive regard for care recipient | 1 | 2 | 3 | 4 | 5 | NA |
| 220512 Demonstration of competence in monitoring own caregiving skill level | 1 | 2 | 3 | 4 | 5 | NA |
| 220513 Confidence in performing needed tasks | 1 | 2 | 3 | 4 | 5 | NA |
| 220515 Provision of safe, secure environment | 1 | 2 | 3 | 4 | 5 | NA |

*1st edition 1997; Revised 3rd edition*

Outcome Content References:

Given, B.A., Kozachik, S.L., Collins, C.E., DeVoss, D.N., & Given, C.W. (2001). Caregiver role strain. In M. Maas, K. Buckwalter, M. Hardy, T. Tripp-Reimer, M. Titler & J. Specht (Eds.), *Nursing care of older adults: Diagnoses, outcomes & interventions* (pp. 679-695). St. Louis: Mosby.

Given, B.A., & Given, C.W. (1991). Family caregiving for the elderly. *Annual Review of Nursing Research, 9,* 77-101.

Oberst, M.T., Thomas, S.E., Gass, K.A., & Ward, S.E. (1989). Caregiving demands and appraisal of stress among family caregivers. *Cancer Nursing, 12*(4), 209-215.

+Picot, S.J., Youngblut, J., & Zeller, R. (1997). Development and testing of a measure of perceived caregiver rewards in adults. *Journal of Nursing Measurement, 5*(1), 33-52.

Pierson, M.A., & Irons, K. (1992). Identification of a cluster of nursing diagnoses for a caregiver support group. *Nursing Diagnosis, 3*(1), 36-41.

Printz-Feddersen, V. (1990). Group process effect on caregiver burden. *Journal of Neuroscience Nursing, 22*(3), 164-168.

Thomas, V.M., Ellison, K., Howell, E.V., & Winters, K. (1992). Caring for the person receiving ventilatory support at home: Caregivers' needs and involvement. *Heart & Lung, 21*(2), 180-186.

+Vermooij-Dassen, M.J.F.J. (1993). *Dementia and home care: Determinants of the sense of competence of primary caregivers and the effect of professionally guided caregiver support* (in Dutch). Lisse, The Netherlands: Swets & Seitliger.

Wallhagen, M.I., & Kagan, S.H. (1993). Staying within bounds: Perceived control and the experience of elderly caregivers. *Journal of Aging Studies, 7*(2), 197-213.

# Caregiver Performance: Indirect Care (2206)

Domain-Family Health (VI)

Class-Family Caregiver Performance (W)

Scale(s)-Not adequate to Totally adequate (f)

Care Recipient:

Data Source:

**Definition:** Arrangement and oversight by family care provider of appropriate care for a family member

OUTCOME TARGET RATING:　　　Maintain at_____　　Increase to_____

| Caregiver Performance: Indirect Care Overall Rating | Not adequate 1 | Slightly adequate 2 | Moderately adequate 3 | Substantially adequate 4 | Totally adequate 5 | |
|---|---|---|---|---|---|---|
| **INDICATORS:** | | | | | | |
| 220601　Confidence in problem solving | 1 | 2 | 3 | 4 | 5 | NA |
| 220602　Recognition of changes in health status of care recipient | 1 | 2 | 3 | 4 | 5 | NA |
| 220603　Recognition of changes in behavior of care recipient | 1 | 2 | 3 | 4 | 5 | NA |
| 220604　Demonstration of ability to anticipate care recipient's needs | 1 | 2 | 3 | 4 | 5 | NA |
| 220605　Obtaining needed health care services for care recipient | 1 | 2 | 3 | 4 | 5 | NA |
| 220611　Obtaining needed transportation for care recipient | 1 | 2 | 3 | 4 | 5 | NA |
| 220612　Obtaining needed equipment and supplies for care recipient | 1 | 2 | 3 | 4 | 5 | NA |
| 220606　Skill in overseeing provision of care | 1 | 2 | 3 | 4 | 5 | NA |
| 220607　Demonstration of regard for care recipient's needs | 1 | 2 | 3 | 4 | 5 | NA |
| 220608　Skill in pursuing care problems with direct care providers | 1 | 2 | 3 | 4 | 5 | NA |
| 220609　Confidence in performing needed tasks | 1 | 2 | 3 | 4 | 5 | NA |
| 220613　Recognition of requirements for safety | 1 | 2 | 3 | 4 | 5 | NA |

1st edition 1997; Revised 3rd edition

Outcome Content References:

Bowers, B.J. (1987). Intergenerational caregiving: Adult caregivers and their aging parents. *Advances in Nursing Science, 9*(2), 20-31.

Given, B.A., Kozachik, S.L., Collins, C.E., DeVoss, D.N., & Given, C.W. (2001). Caregiver role strain. In M. Maas, K. Buckwalter, M. Hardy, T. Tripp-Reimer, M. Titler & J. Specht (Eds.), *Nursing care of older adults: Diagnoses, outcomes & interventions* (pp. 679-695). St. Louis: Mosby.

Given, B.A., & Given, C.W. (1991). Family caregiving for the elderly. *Annual Review of Nursing Research, 9*, 77-101.

Oberst, M.T., Thomas, S.E., Gass, K.A., & Ward, S.E. (1989). Caregiving demands and appraisal of stress among family caregivers. *Cancer Nursing, 12*(4), 209-215.

Pierson, M.A., & Irons, K. (1992). Identification of a cluster of nursing diagnoses for a caregiver support group. *Nursing Diagnosis, 3*(1), 36-41.

Printz-Feddersen, V. (1990). Group process effect on caregiver burden. *Journal of Neuroscience Nursing, 22*(3), 164-168.

Thomas, V.M., Ellison, K., Howell, E.V., & Winters, K. (1992). Caring for the person receiving ventilatory support at home: Caregivers' needs and involvement. *Heart & Lung, 21*(2), 180-186.

+Vermooij-Dassen, M.J.F.J. (1993). *Dementia and home care: Determinants of the sense of competence of primary caregivers and the effect of professionally guided caregiver support* (in Dutch). Lisse, The Netherlands: Swets & Seitliger.

Wallhagen, M.I., & Kagan, S.H. (1993). Staying within bounds: Perceived control and the experience of elderly caregivers. *Journal of Aging Studies, 7*(2), 197-213.

# Caregiver Physical Health (2507)

Domain-Family Health (VI)                                    Care Recipient:

Class-Family Member Health Status (Z)                        Data Source:

Scale(s)-Severely compromised to Not compromised (a)

**Definition:** Physical well-being of a family care provider while caring for a family member

OUTCOME TARGET RATING:        Maintain at_____        Increase to_____

| Caregiver Physical Health Overall Rating | Severely compromised 1 | Substantially compromised 2 | Moderately compromised 3 | Mildly compromised 4 | Not compromised 5 | |
|---|---|---|---|---|---|---|
| **INDICATORS:** | | | | | | |
| 250701 Physical health | 1 | 2 | 3 | 4 | 5 | NA |
| 250702 Sleep pattern | 1 | 2 | 3 | 4 | 5 | NA |
| 250703 Blood pressure | 1 | 2 | 3 | 4 | 5 | NA |
| 250704 Energy level | 1 | 2 | 3 | 4 | 5 | NA |
| 250705 Physical comfort | 1 | 2 | 3 | 4 | 5 | NA |
| 250706 Mobility level | 1 | 2 | 3 | 4 | 5 | NA |
| 250707 Resistance to infection | 1 | 2 | 3 | 4 | 5 | NA |
| 250708 Physical function | 1 | 2 | 3 | 4 | 5 | NA |
| 250709 Weight | 1 | 2 | 3 | 4 | 5 | NA |
| 250710 Gastrointestinal function | 1 | 2 | 3 | 4 | 5 | NA |
| 250711 Medication use | 1 | 2 | 3 | 4 | 5 | NA |
| 250712 Perceived general health | 1 | 2 | 3 | 4 | 5 | NA |

*1st edition 1997; Revised 3rd edition*

## Outcome Content References:

Collins, C.E., Given, B.A., & Given, C.W. (1994). Interventions with family caregivers of persons with Alzheimer's disease. *Nursing Clinics of North America, 29*(1), 127-131.

Given, B.A., Kozachik, S.L., Collins, C.E., DeVoss, D.N., & Given, C.W. (2001). Caregiver role strain. In M. Maas, K. Buckwalter, M. Hardy, T. Tripp-Reimer, M. Titler & J. Specht (Eds.), *Nursing care of older adults: Diagnoses, outcomes & interventions* (pp. 679-695). St. Louis: Mosby.

Given, B.A., & Given, C.W. (1991). Family caregiving for the elderly. *Annual Review of Nursing Research, 9*, 77-101.

Grant, I., Adler, K.A., Patterson, T.L., Dimsdale, J.E., Ziegler, M.G., & Irwin, M.R. (2002). Health consequences of Alzheimer's caregiving transitions: Effects of placement and bereavement. *Psychosomatic Medicine, 64*(3), 477-486.

Grasel E. (2002). When home care ends–changes in the physical health of informal caregivers caring for dementia patients: A longitudinal study. *Journal of American Geriatric Society, 50*(5), 843-849.

Haley, W.E., LaMonde, L.A., Han, B., Narramore, S., & Schonwetter, R. (2001). Family caregiving in hospice: Effects on psychological and health functioning among spousal caregivers of hospice patients with lung cancer or dementia. *Hospice Journal, 15*(4), 1-18.

Pepin, J.I. (1992). Family caring and caring in nursing: *Image-the Journal of Nursing Scholarship, 24*(2), 127-131.

+Robinson, B.C. (1983). Validation of a caregiver strain index. *Journal of Gerontology, 38*(3), 344-348.

Springer, D., & Brubaker, T.H. (1984). *Caregiving and the dependent elderly*. Newbury, CA: Sage.

Winslow, B., & O'Brien, R. (1992). Use of formal community resources by spouse caregivers of chronically ill adults. *Public Health Nursing, 9*(27), 128-132.

Zeisel, J., Hyde, J., & Levkoff, S. (1994). Best practices: An environment-behavior (E-B) model for Alzheimer special care units. *The American Journal of Alzheimer's Care and Related Disorders & Research, 9*(2), 4-21.

C

# Caregiver Stressors (2208)

Domain-Family Health (VI)

Class-Family Caregiver Performance (W)

Scale(s)-Severe to None (n)

Care Recipient:

Data Source:

**Definition:** Severity of biopsychosocial pressure on a family care provider caring for another over an extended period of time

OUTCOME TARGET RATING:     Maintain at_____     Increase to_____

| Caregiver Stressors Overall Rating | Severe 1 | Substantial 2 | Moderate 3 | Mild 4 | None 5 | |
|---|---|---|---|---|---|---|
| **INDICATORS:** | | | | | | |
| 220801 Reported stressors of caregiving | 1 | 2 | 3 | 4 | 5 | NA |
| 220802 Physical limitations for caregiving | 1 | 2 | 3 | 4 | 5 | NA |
| 220803 Psychological limitations for caregiving | 1 | 2 | 3 | 4 | 5 | NA |
| 220804 Cognitive limitations for caregiving | 1 | 2 | 3 | 4 | 5 | NA |
| 220805 Role conflict | 1 | 2 | 3 | 4 | 5 | NA |
| 220815 Sense of isolation | 1 | 2 | 3 | 4 | 5 | NA |
| 220807 Perceived lack of social support | 1 | 2 | 3 | 4 | 5 | NA |
| 220808 Perceived lack of health care system support | 1 | 2 | 3 | 4 | 5 | NA |
| 220816 Loss of personal time | 1 | 2 | 3 | 4 | 5 | NA |
| 220817 Balancing work with caregiving responsibilities | 1 | 2 | 3 | 4 | 5 | NA |
| 220811 Severity of care recipient illness | 1 | 2 | 3 | 4 | 5 | NA |
| 220812 Amount of care or oversight required | 1 | 2 | 3 | 4 | 5 | NA |
| 220813 Impairment of caregiver-patient relationship | 1 | 2 | 3 | 4 | 5 | NA |

*1st edition 1997; Revised 3rd edition*

Outcome Content References:

Andersson, A., Levin, L.A., Emtinger, B.G. (2002). The economic burden of informal care. *International Journal of Technology Assessment in Health Care, 18*(1), 46-54.

Brown, M.A., & Powell-Cope, G.M. (1991). AIDS family caregiving: Transitions through uncertainty. *Nursing Research, 40*(6), 338-345.

Davis, L.L. (2001). Altered family processes. In M. Maas, K. Buckwalter, M. Hardy, T. Tripp-Reimer, M. Titler & J. Specht (Eds.), *Nursing care of older adults: Diagnoses, outcomes & interventions* (pp. 719-727). St. Louis: Mosby.

Given, C.W., Given, B., Stommel, M., Collins, C., King, S., & Franklin, S. (1992). The Caregiver Reaction Assessment (CRA) for caregivers to persons with chronic physical and mental impairments. *Research in Nursing & Health, 15*(4), 271-283.

Glasscock, R. (2000). A phenomenological study of the experience of being a mother of a child with cerebral palsy. *Pediatric Nursing, 26*(4), 407-410.

Laidlaw, T.M., Coverdale, J.H., Falloon, I.R., & Kydd, R.R. (2002). Caregivers' stresses when living together or apart from patients with chronic schizophrenia. *Community Mental Health Journal, 38*(4), 303-310.

Levesque, L., Ducharme, F., & Lachance, L. (1999). Is there a difference between family caregiving of institutionalized elders with or without dementia? *Western Journal of Nursing Research, 21*(4), 472-497.

+Robinson, B.C. (1983). Validation of a caregiver strain index. *Journal of Gerontology, 38*(3), 344-348.

Stevenson, J.E. (1990). Family stress related to home care of Alzheimer's disease patients and implications for support. *Journal of Neuroscience Nursing, 22*(3), 179-188.

Thompson, E.H., Futterman, A.M., Gallagher-Thompson, D., Rose, J.M., & Lovett, S.B. (1993). Social support and caregiving burden in family caregivers of frail elders. *Journal of Gerontology, 48*(5), S245-S254.

Wallhagen, M.I. (1992). Caregiving demands: Their difficulty and effects on the well-being of elderly caregivers. *Scholarly Inquiry for Nursing Practice: An International Journal, 6*(2), 111-133.

# Caregiver Well-Being (2508)

*Domain-Family Health (VI)*
*Class-Family Member Health Status (Z)*
*Scale(s)-Not at all satisfied to Completely satisfied (s)*

*Care Recipient:*
*Data Source:*

**C**

**Definition:** Extent of positive perception of primary care provider's health status and life circumstances

OUTCOME TARGET RATING:    Maintain at_____    Increase to_____

| Caregiver Well-Being Overall Rating | Not at all satisfied 1 | Somewhat satisfied 2 | Moderately satisfied 3 | Very satisfied 4 | Completely satisfied 5 | |
|---|---|---|---|---|---|---|
| INDICATORS: | | | | | | |
| 250801 Physical health | 1 | 2 | 3 | 4 | 5 | NA |
| 250802 Psychological health | 1 | 2 | 3 | 4 | 5 | NA |
| 250803 Lifestyle | 1 | 2 | 3 | 4 | 5 | NA |
| 250804 Performance of usual roles | 1 | 2 | 3 | 4 | 5 | NA |
| 250805 Social support | 1 | 2 | 3 | 4 | 5 | NA |
| 250806 Support for instrumental activities of daily living | 1 | 2 | 3 | 4 | 5 | NA |
| 250807 Professional support | 1 | 2 | 3 | 4 | 5 | NA |
| 250808 Social relationships | 1 | 2 | 3 | 4 | 5 | NA |
| 250811 Family sharing of responsibilities for caregiving | 1 | 2 | 3 | 4 | 5 | NA |
| 250812 Availability for respite | 1 | 2 | 3 | 4 | 5 | NA |
| 250813 Ability to cope | 1 | 2 | 3 | 4 | 5 | NA |
| 250809 Caregiver role | 1 | 2 | 3 | 4 | 5 | NA |
| 250814 Financial resources for caregiving | 1 | 2 | 3 | 4 | 5 | NA |

*1st edition 1997; Revised 3rd edition*

## Outcome Content References:

Brown, M.A., & Powell-Cope, G.M. (1991). AIDS family caregiving: Transitions through uncertainty. *Nursing Research, 40*(6), 338-345.

Given, B.A., Kozachik, S.L., Collins, C.E., DeVoss, D.N., & Given, C.W. (2001). Caregiver role strain. In M. Maas, K. Buckwalter, M. Hardy, T. Tripp-Reimer, M. Titler & J. Specht (Eds.), *Nursing care of older adults: Diagnoses, outcomes & interventions* (pp. 679-695). St. Louis: Mosby.

Given, C.W., Given, B., Stommel, M., Collins, C., King, S., & Franklin, S. (1992). The Caregiver Reaction Assessment (CRA) for caregivers to persons with chronic physical and mental impairments. *Research in Nursing & Health, 15*(4), 271-283.

Jungbauer, J., & Angermeyer, M.C. (2002). Living with a schizophrenic patient: A comparative study of burden as it affects parents and spouses. Psychiatry, 65(2), 110-123.

Pender, N., Murdaugh, C., & Parsons, M.A. (2001). *Health promotion in nursing practice* (4th ed.). Upper Saddle River, New Jersey: Prentice Hall.

+Picot, S.J., Youngblut, J., & Zeller, R. (1997). Development and testing of a measure of perceived caregiver rewards in adults. *Journal of Nursing Measurement, 5* (1), 33-52.

Stevenson, J.E. (1990). Family stress related to home care of Alzheimer's disease patients and implications for support. *Journal of Neuroscience Nursing, 22*(3), 179-188.

Thompson, E.H., Futterman, A.M., Gallagher-Thompson, D., Rose, J.M., & Lovett, S.B. (1993). Social support and caregiving burden in family caregivers of frail elders. *Journal of Gerontology, 48*(5), S245-S254.

Wade, S.L., Taylor, H.G., Drotar, D., Stancin, T., Yeates, K.O., & Minich, N.M. (2002). A prospective study of long-term caregiver and family adaptation following brain injury in children. *Journal of Health Trauma Rehabilitation, 17*(2), 96-111.

Wallhagen, M.I. (1992). Caregiving demands: Their difficulty and effects on the well-being of elderly caregivers. *Scholarly Inquiry for Nursing Practice: An International Journal, 6*(2), 111-133.

Warfield, M.E. (2001). Employment, parenting, and well-being among mothers of children with disabilities. *Mental Retardation, 39*(4), 297-309.

C

# *Caregiving Endurance Potential (2210)*

*Domain-Family Health (VI)*

*Class-Family Caregiver Performance (W)*

*Scale(s)-Not adequate to Totally adequate (f)*

*Care Recipient:*

*Data Source:*

> **Definition:** Factors that promote family care provider continuance over an extended period of time

OUTCOME TARGET RATING:    Maintain at_____    Increase to_____

| Caregiving Endurance Potential Overall Rating | Not adequate 1 | Slightly adequate 2 | Moderately adequate 3 | Substantially adequate 4 | Totally adequate 5 | |
|---|---|---|---|---|---|---|
| **INDICATORS:** | | | | | | |
| 221001  Mutually satisfying care recipient caregiver relationship | 1 | 2 | 3 | 4 | 5 | NA |
| 221002  Mastery of direct care activities | 1 | 2 | 3 | 4 | 5 | NA |
| 221003  Mastery of indirect care activities | 1 | 2 | 3 | 4 | 5 | NA |
| 221004  Supplemental services to provide care | 1 | 2 | 3 | 4 | 5 | NA |
| 221006  Health care system support for caregiver | 1 | 2 | 3 | 4 | 5 | NA |
| 221007  Resources to provide care | 1 | 2 | 3 | 4 | 5 | NA |
| 221011  Financial resources | 1 | 2 | 3 | 4 | 5 | NA |
| 221005  Social support for caregiver | 1 | 2 | 3 | 4 | 5 | NA |
| 221008  Respite for caregiver | 1 | 2 | 3 | 4 | 5 | NA |
| 221009  Opportunities for caregiver leisure activities | 1 | 2 | 3 | 4 | 5 | NA |

*1st edition 1997; Revised 3rd edition*

## Outcome Content References:

Czaja, S.J., & Rubert, M.P. (2002). Telecommunications technology as an aid to family caregivers of persons with dementia. *Psychosomatic Medicine, 64*(3), 469-476.

Given, B.A., Stommel, M., Collins, C., King, S., & Given, C.W. (1990). Responses of elderly spouse caregivers. *Research in Nursing & Health, 13,* 77-85.

Oberst, M.T., Thomas, S.E., Gass, K.A., & Ward, S.E. (1989). Caregiving demands and appraisal of stress among family caregivers. *Cancer Nursing, 12*(4), 209-215.

+Picot, S.J., Youngblut, J., & Zeller, R. (1997). Development and testing of a measure of perceived caregiver rewards in adults. *Journal of Nursing Measurement, 5* (1), 33-52.

Rawlins, S.R. (1991). Using the connecting process to meet family caregiver needs. *Journal of Professional Nursing, 7*(4), 213-220.

Romeis, J.C. (1989). Caregiver strain. *Journal of Aging and Health, 1*(2), 188-208.

Stevenson, J.E. (1990). Family stress related to home care of Alzheimer's disease patients and implications for support. *Journal of Neuroscience Nursing, 22*(3), 179-188.

Thompson, E.H., Futterman, A.M., Gallagher-Thompson, D., Rose, J.M., & Lovett, S.B. (1993). Social support and caregiving burden in family caregivers of frail elders. *Journal of Gerontology, 48*(5), S245-S254.

Wallhagen, M.I. (1992). Caregiving demands: Their difficulty and effects on the well-being of elderly caregivers. *Scholarly Inquiry for Nursing Practice: An International Journal, 6*(2), 111-133.

Winslow, B., & O'Brien, R. (1992). Use of formal community resources by spouse caregivers of chronically ill adults. *Public Health Nursing, 9*(27), 128-132.

# Child Adaptation to Hospitalization (1301)

Domain-Psychosocial Health (III)

Class-Psychosocial Adaptation (N)

Care Recipient:

Data Source:

Scale(s)-Never demonstrated to Consistently demonstrated (m) and Consistently demonstrated to Never demonstrated (t)

**C**

**Definition:** Adaptive response of a child from 3 years through 17 years of age to hospitalization

OUTCOME TARGET RATING:     Maintain at_____     Increase to_____

| Child Adaptation to Hospitalization Overall Rating | Never demonstrated 1 | Rarely demonstrated 2 | Sometimes demonstrated 3 | Often demonstrated 4 | Consistently demonstrated 5 | |
|---|---|---|---|---|---|---|
| INDICATORS: | | | | | | |
| 130112 Interacts with parent(s) | 1 | 2 | 3 | 4 | 5 | NA |
| 130121 Maintains usual routine | 1 | 2 | 3 | 4 | 5 | NA |
| 130113 Recognizes need for hospitalization | 1 | 2 | 3 | 4 | 5 | NA |
| 130115 Participates in decision-making | 1 | 2 | 3 | 4 | 5 | NA |
| 130122 Asks about illness and treatment | 1 | 2 | 3 | 4 | 5 | NA |
| 130116 Describes illness and treatment | 1 | 2 | 3 | 4 | 5 | |
| 130108 Demonstrates sense of control | 1 | 2 | 3 | 4 | 5 | NA |
| 130118 Cooperates with procedures | 1 | 2 | 3 | 4 | 5 | NA |
| 130109 Responds to comfort measures | 1 | 2 | 3 | 4 | 5 | NA |
| 130110 Responds to diversional therapy | 1 | 2 | 3 | 4 | 5 | NA |
| 130111 Participates in social interaction | 1 | 2 | 3 | 4 | 5 | NA |
| 130119 Interacts with peers | 1 | 2 | 3 | 4 | 5 | NA |
| 130114 Demonstrates behavioral self-control | 1 | 2 | 3 | 4 | 5 | NA |
| 130117 Maintains pre-admission self-care behaviors | 1 | 2 | 3 | 4 | 5 | NA |

| | Consistently demonstrated | Often demonstrated | Sometimes demonstrated | Rarely demonstrated | Never demonstrated | |
|---|---|---|---|---|---|---|
| 130101 Agitation | 1 | 2 | 3 | 4 | 5 | NA |
| 130102 Separation anxiety | 1 | 2 | 3 | 4 | 5 | NA |
| 130103 Regressive behavior(s) | 1 | 2 | 3 | 4 | 5 | NA |
| 130104 Anxiety | 1 | 2 | 3 | 4 | 5 | NA |
| 130105 Fear | 1 | 2 | 3 | 4 | 5 | NA |
| 130106 Anger | 1 | 2 | 3 | 4 | 5 | NA |
| 130107 Behavioral disturbances | 1 | 2 | 3 | 4 | 5 | NA |

*1st edition 1997; Revised 3rd edition*

*Continued*

## Outcome Content References:

Coucouvanis, J.A. (1990). Behavior management. In M. Craft & J.A. Denehy (Eds.), *Nursing interventions for infants and children* (pp. 151-165). Philadelphia: W.B. Saunders.

Hockenberry, M.J., Wilson, D., Winkelstein, M.L., & Kline, N.E. (2003). *Wong's nursing care of infants and children* (7th ed.). St. Louis: Mosby.

Manion, J. (1990). Preparing children for hospitalization, procedures, or surgery. In M. Craft & J.A. Denehy (Eds.), *Nursing interventions for infants and children* (pp. 74-90). Philadelphia: W.B. Saunders.

Olson, R.K., Heater, B.S., & Becker, A.M. (1990). A meta-analysis of the effects of nursing interventions on children and parents. *Maternal-Child Nursing, 15*(2), 104-108.

Shields, L. (2001). A review of the literature from developed and developing countries relating to the effects of hospitalization on children and parents. *International Nursing Review, 48*(1), 29-37.

Wolfer, J.A., & Visintainer, M.A. (1975). Pediatric surgical patients' and parents' stress responses and adjustment as a function of psychologic preparation and stress-point nursing care. *Nursing Research, 24*(4), 244-255.

Ziegler, D.B., & Prior, M.M. (1994). Preparation for surgery and adjustment to hospitalization. *Nursing Clinics of North America, 29*(4), 655-669.

# Child Development: 1 Month (0120)

Domain-Functional Health (I)

Class-Growth & Development (B)

Scale(s)-Never demonstrated to Consistently demonstrated (m)

Care Recipient:

Data Source:

C

> **Definition**: Milestones of physical, cognitive, and psychosocial progression by 1 month of age

OUTCOME TARGET RATING:    Maintain at_____    Increase to_____

| Child Development: 1 Month Overall Rating | Never demonstrated 1 | Rarely demonstrated 2 | Sometimes demonstrated 3 | Often demonstrated 4 | Consistently demonstrated 5 | |
|---|---|---|---|---|---|---|
| **INDICATORS:** | | | | | | |
| 012001 Signals hunger | 1 | 2 | 3 | 4 | 5 | NA |
| 012002 Signals discomfort | 1 | 2 | 3 | 4 | 5 | NA |
| 012003 Responds to sounds | 1 | 2 | 3 | 4 | 5 | NA |
| 012004 Responds to voice | 1 | 2 | 3 | 4 | 5 | NA |
| 012005 Responds to face | 1 | 2 | 3 | 4 | 5 | NA |
| 012006 Coos | 1 | 2 | 3 | 4 | 5 | NA |
| 012007 Smiles spontaneously | 1 | 2 | 3 | 4 | 5 | NA |
| 012008 Eyes follow to mid-line | 1 | 2 | 3 | 4 | 5 | NA |
| 012009 Signals overstimulation | 1 | 2 | 3 | 4 | 5 | NA |
| 012010 Exhibits five sleep and alert states | 1 | 2 | 3 | 4 | 5 | NA |
| 012011 Flexes extremity | 1 | 2 | 3 | 4 | 5 | NA |
| 012012 Holds head erect momentarily | 1 | 2 | 3 | 4 | 5 | NA |
| 012013 Turns head side to side when prone | 1 | 2 | 3 | 4 | 5 | NA |
| 012014 Holds head in horizontal line with back when prone | 1 | 2 | 3 | 4 | 5 | NA |
| 012015 Moro reflex | 1 | 2 | 3 | 4 | 5 | NA |
| 012016 Tonic neck reflex | 1 | 2 | 3 | 4 | 5 | NA |
| 012017 Dance reflex | 1 | 2 | 3 | 4 | 5 | NA |
| 012018 Crawl reflex | 1 | 2 | 3 | 4 | 5 | NA |
| 012019 Babinski reflex | 1 | 2 | 3 | 4 | 5 | NA |
| 012020 Suck reflex | 1 | 2 | 3 | 4 | 5 | NA |
| 012021 Palmar reflex | 1 | 2 | 3 | 4 | 5 | NA |
| 012022 Plantar reflex | 1 | 2 | 3 | 4 | 5 | NA |
| 012023 Rooting reflex | 1 | 2 | 3 | 4 | 5 | NA |

*3rd edition*

## Outcome Content References:

Berger, K. S. (2001). *The developing person through the life span* (5th ed.). New York: Worth Publishers.

Broome, M.E., & Rollins, J.A. (Eds.). (1999). *Core curriculum for the nursing care of children and their families*. Pitman, New Jersey: Jannetti Publications.

Darrah, J., Redfern, L., Maguire, T.O., Beaulne, A.P., & Watt, J. (1998). Intra-individual stability of rate of gross motor development in full-term infants. *Early Human Development, 52*(2), 169-179.

Hockenberry, M.J., Wilson, D., Winkelstein, M.L., & Kline, N.E. (2003). *Wong's nursing care of infants and children* (7th ed.). St. Louis: Mosby.

Kimmel, S.R., Quinn, E.A., & Phelps, K.A. (1994). Assessing child development. *Primary Care 21*(4), 673-692.

Piper, M.C., Pinnell, L.E., Darrah, J., Maguire, T., & Byrne, P.J. (1992). Construction and validation of the Alberta Infant Motor Scale (AIMS). *Canadian Journal of Public Health, 83*(Suppl. 2), S46-S50.

Trachtenbarg, D.E., & Golemon, T.B. (1998). Care of the premature infant, Part 1: Monitoring growth and development. *American Family Physician 57*(9), 2123-2131.

## *Child Development: 2 Months (0100)*

Domain-Functional Health (I)

Class-Growth & Development (B)

Scale(s)-Never demonstrated to Consistently demonstrated (m)

Care Recipient:

Data Source:

**C**

*Definition:* Milestones of physical, cognitive, and psychosocial progression by 2 months of age

OUTCOME TARGET RATING:   Maintain at_____   Increase to_____

| Child Development: 2 Months Overall Rating | Never demonstrated 1 | Rarely demonstrated 2 | Sometimes demonstrated 3 | Often demonstrated 4 | Consistently demonstrated 5 | |
|---|---|---|---|---|---|---|
| **INDICATORS:** | | | | | | |
| 010002  Crawl reflex disappearance | 1 | 2 | 3 | 4 | 5 | NA |
| 010003  Lifts head, neck, and upper chest with support on fore-arms while in prone position | 1 | 2 | 3 | 4 | 5 | NA |
| 010004  Shows some head control in upright position | 1 | 2 | 3 | 4 | 5 | NA |
| 010005  Hands frequently open | 1 | 2 | 3 | 4 | 5 | NA |
| 010006  Grasp reflex fading | 1 | 2 | 3 | 4 | 5 | NA |
| 010007  Coos and vocalizes | 1 | 2 | 3 | 4 | 5 | NA |
| 010008  Shows interest in auditory stimuli | 1 | 2 | 3 | 4 | 5 | NA |
| 010009  Shows interest in visual stimuli | 1 | 2 | 3 | 4 | 5 | NA |
| 010010  Smiles | 1 | 2 | 3 | 4 | 5 | NA |
| 010011  Shows pleasure in interactions, espe-cially with primary caregivers | 1 | 2 | 3 | 4 | 5 | NA |

*1st edition 1997; Revised 3rd edition*

Outcome Content References:

Berger, K.S. (2001). *The developing person through the life span* (5th ed.). New York: Worth Publishers.

Bricker, D. (Ed.) (2002). *Assessment, Evaluation, and Programming System for infants and children* (2nd ed.). Baltimore: Paul H. Brookes Publishing.

Cowen, P., & Van Hoozer, H.L. (in press). *Building blocks for healthy tots.*

Darrah, J., Redfern, L., Maguire, T.O., Beaulne, A.P., & Watt, J. (1998). Intra-individual stability of rate of gross motor development in full-term infants. *Early Human Development, 52*(2), 169-179.

Green, M., & Palfrey, J.S. (Eds.). (2002). *Bright futures: Guidelines for health supervision of infants, children and adolescents.* Arlington, VA: National Center for Education in Maternal and Child Health.

Hockenberry, M.J., Wilson, D., Winkelstein, M.L., & Kline, N.E. (2003). *Wong's nursing care of infants and children* (7th ed.). St. Louis: Mosby.

# Child Development: 4 Months (0101)

Domain-Functional Health (I)                            Care Recipient:

Class-Growth & Development (B)                          Data Source:

Scale(s)-Never demonstrated to Consistently demonstrated (m)

**Definition:** Milestones of physical, cognitive, and psychosocial progression by 4 months of age

OUTCOME TARGET RATING:    Maintain at_____    Increase to_____

| Child Development: 4 Months Overall Rating | Never demonstrated 1 | Rarely demonstrated 2 | Sometimes demonstrated 3 | Often demonstrated 4 | Consistently demonstrated 5 | |
|---|---|---|---|---|---|---|
| INDICATORS: | | | | | | |
| 010101 Holds head erect and raises body on hands while in prone position | 1 | 2 | 3 | 4 | 5 | NA |
| 010102 Controls head well | 1 | 2 | 3 | 4 | 5 | NA |
| 010103 Rolls over from prone to supine | 1 | 2 | 3 | 4 | 5 | NA |
| 010104 Holds own hands | 1 | 2 | 3 | 4 | 5 | NA |
| 010105 Grasps rattle | 1 | 2 | 3 | 4 | 5 | NA |
| 010106 Reaches for objects | 1 | 2 | 3 | 4 | 5 | NA |
| 010107 Bats at objects | 1 | 2 | 3 | 4 | 5 | NA |
| 010108 Babbles and coos | 1 | 2 | 3 | 4 | 5 | NA |
| 010109 Recognizes parents' voices | 1 | 2 | 3 | 4 | 5 | NA |
| 010110 Recognizes parents' touch | 1 | 2 | 3 | 4 | 5 | NA |
| 010111 Looks at and becomes excited by mobile | 1 | 2 | 3 | 4 | 5 | NA |
| 010112 Smiles, laughs, and squeals | 1 | 2 | 3 | 4 | 5 | NA |
| 010113 Sleeps for at least 6 hours | 1 | 2 | 3 | 4 | 5 | NA |
| 010114 Comforts self (e.g., falls asleep by self without breast or bottle) | 1 | 2 | 3 | 4 | 5 | NA |

*1st edition 1997; Revised 3rd edition*

## Outcome Content References:

Berger, K.S. (2001). *The developing person through the life span* (5th ed.). New York: Worth Publishers.

Cowen, P., & Van Hoozer, H.L. (in press). *Building blocks for healthy tots.*

Green, M., & Palfrey, J.S. (Eds.). (2002). *Bright futures: Guidelines for health supervision of infants, children and adolescents.* Arlington, VA: National Center for Education in Maternal and Child Health.

Hockenberry, M.J., Wilson, D., Winkelstein, M.L., & Kline, N.E. (2003). *Wong's nursing care of infants and children* (7th ed.). St. Louis: Mosby.

C

# Child Development: 6 Months (0102)

*Domain-Functional Health (I)*

*Class-Growth & Development (B)*

*Scale(s)-Never demonstrated to Consistently demonstrated (m)*

*Care Recipient:*

*Data Source:*

**Definition:** Milestones of physical, cognitive, and psychosocial progression by 6 months of age

OUTCOME TARGET RATING:    Maintain at_____    Increase to_____

| Child Development: 6 Months Overall Rating | Never demonstrated 1 | Rarely demonstrated 2 | Sometimes demonstrated 3 | Often demonstrated 4 | Consistently demonstrated 5 | |
|---|---|---|---|---|---|---|
| **INDICATORS:** | | | | | | |
| 010201 Supports head when pulled to sit | 1 | 2 | 3 | 4 | 5 | NA |
| 010202 Rolls over | 1 | 2 | 3 | 4 | 5 | NA |
| 010203 Sits with support | 1 | 2 | 3 | 4 | 5 | NA |
| 010204 Stands when placed and bears weight | 1 | 2 | 3 | 4 | 5 | NA |
| 010205 Grasps and mouths objects | 1 | 2 | 3 | 4 | 5 | NA |
| 010206 Gestures (e.g., points, shakes head) | 1 | 2 | 3 | 4 | 5 | NA |
| 010207 Starts to self-feed | 1 | 2 | 3 | 4 | 5 | NA |
| 010208 Shows interest in toys | 1 | 2 | 3 | 4 | 5 | NA |
| 010209 Transfers small objects from hand to hand | 1 | 2 | 3 | 4 | 5 | NA |
| 010210 Vocalizes/sings syllables (dada, baba) | 1 | 2 | 3 | 4 | 5 | NA |
| 010211 Babbles reciprocally | 1 | 2 | 3 | 4 | 5 | NA |
| 010212 Smiles, laughs, squeals, imitates noise | 1 | 2 | 3 | 4 | 5 | NA |
| 010213 Turns to sounds | 1 | 2 | 3 | 4 | 5 | NA |
| 010214 Shows beginning signs of stranger anxiety | 1 | 2 | 3 | 4 | 5 | NA |
| 010215 Comforts self | 1 | 2 | 3 | 4 | 5 | NA |

*1st edition 1997; Revised 3rd edition*

Outcome Content References:

Berger, K. S. (2001). *The developing person through the life span* (5th ed.). New York: Worth Publishers.

Bricker, D. (Ed.). (2002). *Assessment, Evaluation, and Programming System for infants and children* (2nd ed.). Baltimore: Paul H. Brookes Publishing.

Cowen, P., & Van Hoozer, H.L. (in press). *Building blocks for healthy tots.*

Green, M., & Palfrey, J.S. (Eds.). (2002). *Bright futures: Guidelines for health supervision of infants, children and adolescents.* Arlington, VA: National Center for Education in Maternal and Child Health.

Hockenberry, M.J., Wilson, D., Winkelstein, M.L., & Kline, N.E. (2003). *Wong's nursing care of infants and children* (7th ed.). St. Louis: Mosby.

Rossetti, L.M. (1990). *Infant-toddler assessment: An interdisciplinary approach.* Boston: Little, Brown & Company.

# Child Development: 12 Months (0103)

*Domain-Functional Health (I)*

*Class-Growth & Development (B)*

*Scale(s)-Never demonstrated to Consistently demonstrated (m)*

Care Recipient:

Data Source:

**C**

**Definition:** Milestones of physical, cognitive, and psychosocial progression by 12 months of age

OUTCOME TARGET RATING:    Maintain at_____    Increase to_____

| Child Development: 12 Months Overall Rating | Never demonstrated 1 | Rarely demonstrated 2 | Sometimes demonstrated 3 | Often demonstrated 4 | Consistently demonstrated 5 | |
|---|---|---|---|---|---|---|
| **INDICATORS:** | | | | | | |
| 010301 Pulls to stand | 1 | 2 | 3 | 4 | 5 | NA |
| 010302 Cruises around furniture | 1 | 2 | 3 | 4 | 5 | NA |
| 010303 Attempts to take steps alone | 1 | 2 | 3 | 4 | 5 | NA |
| 010304 Precise pincer grasp | 1 | 2 | 3 | 4 | 5 | NA |
| 010305 Points with index fingers | 1 | 2 | 3 | 4 | 5 | NA |
| 010306 Bangs blocks together | 1 | 2 | 3 | 4 | 5 | NA |
| 010307 Drinks from cup | 1 | 2 | 3 | 4 | 5 | NA |
| 010308 Feeds self finger foods | 1 | 2 | 3 | 4 | 5 | NA |
| 010309 Feeds self with spoon | 1 | 2 | 3 | 4 | 5 | NA |
| 010310 Uses vocabulary of one to three words in addition to mama, dada | 1 | 2 | 3 | 4 | 5 | NA |
| 010311 Imitates vocalizations | 1 | 2 | 3 | 4 | 5 | NA |
| 010312 Looks for dropped or hidden object | 1 | 2 | 3 | 4 | 5 | NA |
| 010313 Plays social games | 1 | 2 | 3 | 4 | 5 | NA |
| 010314 Waves bye-bye | 1 | 2 | 3 | 4 | 5 | NA |

*1st edition 1997; Revised 3rd edition*

Outcome Content References:

Berger, K.S. (2001). *The developing person through the life span* (5th ed.). New York: Worth Publishers.

Bricker, D. (Ed.) (2002). *Assessment, Evaluation, and Programming System for infants and children* (2nd ed.). Baltimore: Paul H. Brookes Publishing.

Cowen, P., & Van Hoozer, H.L. (in press). *Building blocks for healthy tots.*

Green, M., & Palfrey, J.S. (Eds.). (2002). *Bright futures: Guidelines for health supervision of infants, children and adolescents.* Arlington, VA: National Center for Education in Maternal and Child Health.

Hockenberry, M.J., Wilson, D., Winkelstein, M.L., & Kline, N.E. (2003). *Wong's nursing care of infants and children* (7th ed.). St. Louis: Mosby.

Rossetti L.M. (1990). *Infant-toddler assessment: An interdisciplinary approach.* Boston: Little, Brown & Company.

Santos, D.C., Gabbard, C., & Goncalves, V.M. (2001). Motor development during the first year: A comparative study. *Journal of Genetic Psychology, 162*(2), 143-53.

Vaivre-Douret, L., & Burnod, Y. (2001). Development of a global motor rating scale for young children (0-4 years) including eye-hand grip coordination. *Child Care Health & Development, 27*(6), 515-534.

# Child Development: 2 Years (0104)

Domain-Functional Health (I)

Class-Growth & Development (B)

Scale(s)-Never demonstrated to Consistently demonstrated (m)

Care Recipient:

Data Source:

**Definition:** Milestones of physical, cognitive, and psychosocial progression by 2 years of age

OUTCOME TARGET RATING:    Maintain at_____    Increase to_____

| Child Development: 2 Years<br>Overall Rating | Never<br>demonstrated<br>1 | Rarely<br>demonstrated<br>2 | Sometimes<br>demonstrated<br>3 | Often<br>demonstrated<br>4 | Consistently<br>demonstrated<br>5 | |
|---|---|---|---|---|---|---|
| **INDICATORS:** | | | | | | |
| 010401  Walks quickly | 1 | 2 | 3 | 4 | 5 | NA |
| 010402  Stoops well | 1 | 2 | 3 | 4 | 5 | NA |
| 010403  Walks up and down stairs one step at a time | 1 | 2 | 3 | 4 | 5 | NA |
| 010404  Walks backwards | 1 | 2 | 3 | 4 | 5 | NA |
| 010405  Kicks a ball | 1 | 2 | 3 | 4 | 5 | NA |
| 010406  Throws a ball | 1 | 2 | 3 | 4 | 5 | NA |
| 010407  Makes circular and horizontal strokes with crayon | 1 | 2 | 3 | 4 | 5 | NA |
| 010408  Stacks five to six blocks | 1 | 2 | 3 | 4 | 5 | NA |
| 010409  Feeds self with spoon and fork | 1 | 2 | 3 | 4 | 5 | NA |
| 010410  Follows two-step commands | 1 | 2 | 3 | 4 | 5 | NA |
| 010411  Indicates wants verbally | 1 | 2 | 3 | 4 | 5 | NA |
| 010412  Uses phrases of two to three words | 1 | 2 | 3 | 4 | 5 | NA |
| 010413  Listens to story looking at pictures | 1 | 2 | 3 | 4 | 5 | NA |
| 010414  Points to some body parts | 1 | 2 | 3 | 4 | 5 | NA |
| 010415  Begins parallel play | 1 | 2 | 3 | 4 | 5 | NA |
| 010416  Imitates adults | 1 | 2 | 3 | 4 | 5 | NA |
| 010417  Interacts with adults in simple games | 1 | 2 | 3 | 4 | 5 | NA |

*1st edition 1997; Revised 3rd edition*

## Outcome Content References:

Berger, K. S. (2001). *The developing person through the life span* (5th ed.). New York: Worth Publishers.

Bricker, D. (Ed). (2002). *Assessment, Evaluation, and Programming System for infants and children* (2nd ed.). Baltimore: Paul H. Brookes Publishing.

Cowen, P., & Van Hoozer, H.L. (in press). *Building blocks for healthy tots.*

Green, M., & Palfrey, J.S. (Eds.). (2002). *Bright futures: Guidelines for health supervision of infants, children and adolescents.* Arlington, VA: National Center for Education in Maternal and Child Health.

Hockenberry, M.J., Wilson, D., Winkelstein, M.L., & Kline, N.E. (2003). *Wong's nursing care of infants and children* (7th ed.). St. Louis: Mosby.

Provost, B., Crowe, T.K., & McClain, C. (2000). Concurrent validity of the Bayley Scales of Infant Development II Motor Scale and the Peabody Developmental Motor Scales in two-year-old children. *Physical & Occupational Therapy in Pediatrics, 20*(1), 5-18.

Rossetti, L.M. (1990). *Infant-toddler assessment: An interdisciplinary approach.* Boston: Little, Brown & Company.

Vaivre-Douret, L., & Burnod, Y. (2001). Development of a global motor rating scale for young children (0-4 years) including eye-hand grip coordination. *Child Care Health & Development, 27*(6), 515-534.

# Child Development: 3 Years (0105)

Domain-Functional Health (I)                                    Care Recipient:

Class-Growth & Development (B)                              Data Source:

Scale(s)-Never demonstrated to Consistently demonstrated (m)

**Definition:** Milestones of physical, cognitive, and psychosocial progression by 3 years of age

OUTCOME TARGET RATING:     Maintain at_____     Increase to_____

| Child Development: 3 Years Overall Rating | Never demonstrated 1 | Rarely demonstrated 2 | Sometimes demonstrated 3 | Often demonstrated 4 | Consistently demonstrated 5 | |
|---|---|---|---|---|---|---|
| **INDICATORS:** | | | | | | |
| 010501  Balances on one foot | 1 | 2 | 3 | 4 | 5 | NA |
| 010502  Pedals a riding toy | 1 | 2 | 3 | 4 | 5 | NA |
| 010503  Dresses self | 1 | 2 | 3 | 4 | 5 | NA |
| 010504  Controls writing/ coloring instruments | 1 | 2 | 3 | 4 | 5 | NA |
| 010505  Copies a circle | 1 | 2 | 3 | 4 | 5 | NA |
| 010506  Copies a cross | 1 | 2 | 3 | 4 | 5 | NA |
| 010507  Controls bowel in daytime | 1 | 2 | 3 | 4 | 5 | NA |
| 010508  Controls bladder in daytime | 1 | 2 | 3 | 4 | 5 | NA |
| 010509  Distinguishes gender differences | 1 | 2 | 3 | 4 | 5 | NA |
| 010510  Gives own first name | 1 | 2 | 3 | 4 | 5 | NA |
| 010511  Gives own age | 1 | 2 | 3 | 4 | 5 | NA |
| 010512  Engages in magical thinking/fantasy | 1 | 2 | 3 | 4 | 5 | NA |
| 010513  Plays interactive games with peers | 1 | 2 | 3 | 4 | 5 | NA |
| 010514  Begins cooperative group play | 1 | 2 | 3 | 4 | 5 | NA |
| 010515  Uses sentences of three or four words | 1 | 2 | 3 | 4 | 5 | NA |
| 010516  Speech understood by strangers | 1 | 2 | 3 | 4 | 5 | NA |

*1st edition 1997; Revised 3rd edition*

**Outcome Content References:**

Berger, K. S. (2001). *The developing person through the life span* (5th ed.). New York: Worth Publishers.

Bricker, D. (Ed.). (2002). *Assessment, Evaluation, and Programming System for infants and children* (2nd ed.). Baltimore: Paul H. Brookes Publishing.

Cowen, P., & Van Hoozer, H.L. (in press). *Building blocks for healthy tots.*

Green, M., & Palfrey, J.S. (Eds.). (2002). *Bright futures: Guidelines for health supervision of infants, children and adolescents.* Arlington, VA: National Center for Education in Maternal and Child Health.

Hemgren, E., & Persson, K. (1999). A model for combined assessment of motor performance and behaviour in 3-year-old children. *Upsala Journal of Medical Sciences, 104*(1), 49-85.

Hockenberry, M.J., Wilson, D., Winkelstein, M.L., & Kline, N.E. (2003). *Wong's nursing care of infants and children* (7th ed.). St. Louis: Mosby.

Vaivre-Douret, L., & Burnod, Y. (2001). Development of a global motor rating scale for young children (0-4 years) including eye-hand grip coordination. *Child Care Health & Development, 27*(6), 515-534.

C

# *Child Development: 4 Years (0106)*

Domain-Functional Health (I)                                    Care Recipient:

Class-Growth & Development (B)                              Data Source:

Scale(s)-Never demonstrated to Consistently demonstrated (m)

**Definition:** Milestones of physical, cognitive, and psychosocial progression by 4 years of age

OUTCOME TARGET RATING:     Maintain at_____     Increase to_____

| Child Development: 4 Years Overall Rating | Never demonstrated 1 | Rarely demonstrated 2 | Sometimes demonstrated 3 | Often demonstrated 4 | Consistently demonstrated 5 | |
|---|---|---|---|---|---|---|

INDICATORS:

| | | | | | | | |
|---|---|---|---|---|---|---|---|
| 010601 | Walks, climbs, runs | 1 | 2 | 3 | 4 | 5 | NA |
| 010602 | Goes up and down stairs | 1 | 2 | 3 | 4 | 5 | NA |
| 010603 | Hops and jumps on one foot | 1 | 2 | 3 | 4 | 5 | NA |
| 010604 | Rides tricycle or bicycle with training wheels | 1 | 2 | 3 | 4 | 5 | NA |
| 010605 | Throws overhand ball | 1 | 2 | 3 | 4 | 5 | NA |
| 010606 | Builds tower of 10 blocks | 1 | 2 | 3 | 4 | 5 | NA |
| 010607 | Draws person with three parts | 1 | 2 | 3 | 4 | 5 | NA |
| 010608 | Gives first and last name | 1 | 2 | 3 | 4 | 5 | NA |
| 010609 | Uses sentences of four to five words, short paragraphs | 1 | 2 | 3 | 4 | 5 | NA |
| 010610 | Uses past tense in vocabulary | 1 | 2 | 3 | 4 | 5 | NA |
| 010611 | Describes a recent experience | 1 | 2 | 3 | 4 | 5 | NA |
| 010612 | Able to sing a song | 1 | 2 | 3 | 4 | 5 | NA |
| 010613 | Distinguishes fantasy from reality | 1 | 2 | 3 | 4 | 5 | NA |
| 010614 | Describes use of items used in the home (e.g., food and appliances) | 1 | 2 | 3 | 4 | 5 | NA |
| 010616 | Engages in creative play | 1 | 2 | 3 | 4 | 5 | NA |

*1st edition 1997; Revised 3rd edition*

Outcome Content References:

Berger, K. S. (2001). *The developing person through the life span* (5th ed.). New York: Worth Publishers.

Green, M., & Palfrey, J.S. (Eds.). (2002). *Bright futures: Guidelines for health supervision of infants, children and adolescents.* Arlington, VA: National Center for Education in Maternal and Child Health.

Hockenberry, M.J., Wilson, D., Winkelstein, M.L., & Kline, N.E. (2003). *Wong's nursing care of infants and children* (7th ed.). St. Louis: Mosby.

Vaivre-Douret, L., & Burnod, Y. (2001). Development of a global motor rating scale for young children (0-4 years) including eye-hand grip coordination. *Child Care Health & Development, 27*(6), 515-534.

# Child Development: Preschool (0107)

Domain-Functional Health (I)

Class-Growth & Development (B)

Scale(s)-Never demonstrated to Consistently demonstrated (m)

Care Recipient:

Data Source:

**C**

**Definition:** Milestones of physical, cognitive, and psychosocial progression from 3 years through 5 years of age

OUTCOME TARGET RATING:    Maintain at_____    Increase to_____

| Child Development: Preschool Overall Rating | Never demonstrated 1 | Rarely demonstrated 2 | Sometimes demonstrated 3 | Often demonstrated 4 | Consistently demonstrated 5 | |
|---|---|---|---|---|---|---|

INDICATORS:

| | | | | | | | |
|---|---|---|---|---|---|---|---|
| 010701 | Walks, climbs, runs with coordination | 1 | 2 | 3 | 4 | 5 | NA |
| 010702 | Able to skip | 1 | 2 | 3 | 4 | 5 | NA |
| 010703 | Dresses self without help | 1 | 2 | 3 | 4 | 5 | NA |
| 010704 | Draws a person with head, body, arms, and legs | 1 | 2 | 3 | 4 | 5 | NA |
| 010705 | Copies a triangle or square | 1 | 2 | 3 | 4 | 5 | NA |
| 010706 | Counts using fingers | 1 | 2 | 3 | 4 | 5 | NA |
| 010707 | Recognizes most letters of alphabet | 1 | 2 | 3 | 4 | 5 | NA |
| 010708 | Prints some letters | 1 | 2 | 3 | 4 | 5 | NA |
| 010709 | Uses complete sentence of five words | 1 | 2 | 3 | 4 | 5 | NA |
| 010710 | Uses future tense in vocabulary | 1 | 2 | 3 | 4 | 5 | NA |
| 010711 | Speaks short paragraphs | 1 | 2 | 3 | 4 | 5 | NA |
| 010712 | Gives own address | 1 | 2 | 3 | 4 | 5 | NA |
| 010713 | Gives own phone number | 1 | 2 | 3 | 4 | 5 | NA |
| 010714 | Follows simple rules of interactive games with peers | 1 | 2 | 3 | 4 | 5 | NA |
| 010716 | Engages in creative play | 1 | 2 | 3 | 4 | 5 | NA |

*1st edition 1997; Revised 3rd edition (formerly Child Development: 5 Years)*

Outcome Content References:

Berger, K. S. (2001). *The developing person through the life span* (5th ed.). New York: Worth Publishers.

Boucher, B.H., Doescher, S.M., & Sugawara, A.I. (1993). Preschool children's motor development and self-concept. *Perceptual & Motor Skills, 76*(1), 11-17.

Green, M., & Palfrey, J.S. (Eds.). (2002). *Bright futures: Guidelines for health supervision of infants, children and adolescents.* Arlington, VA: National Center for Education in Maternal and Child Health.

Hockenberry, M.J., Wilson, D., Winkelstein, M.L., & Kline, N.E. (2003). *Wong's nursing care of infants and children* (7th ed.). St. Louis: Mosby.

C

# Child Development: Middle Childhood (0108)

*Domain-Functional Health (I)*                                    *Care Recipient:*

*Class-Growth & Development (B)*                          *Data Source:*

*Scale(s)-Never demonstrated to Consistently demonstrated (m)*

**Definition:** Milestones of physical, cognitive, and psychosocial progression from 6 years through 11 years of age

OUTCOME TARGET RATING:      Maintain at_____      Increase to_____

| Child Development: Middle Childhood Overall Rating | Never demonstrated 1 | Rarely demonstrated 2 | Sometimes demonstrated 3 | Often demonstrated 4 | Consistently demonstrated 5 | |
|---|---|---|---|---|---|---|
| **INDICATORS:** | | | | | | |
| 010801 Practices good health habits | 1 | 2 | 3 | 4 | 5 | NA |
| 010802 Plays in groups | 1 | 2 | 3 | 4 | 5 | NA |
| 010803 Develops close friendships | 1 | 2 | 3 | 4 | 5 | NA |
| 010804 Identifies with same-sex peer group | 1 | 2 | 3 | 4 | 5 | NA |
| 010805 Assumes responsibility for selected household tasks | 1 | 2 | 3 | 4 | 5 | NA |
| 010806 Follows through with commitments to extracurricular activities | 1 | 2 | 3 | 4 | 5 | NA |
| 010807 Expresses feelings constructively | 1 | 2 | 3 | 4 | 5 | NA |
| 010808 Displays self-confidence | 1 | 2 | 3 | 4 | 5 | NA |
| 010809 Understands right and wrong | 1 | 2 | 3 | 4 | 5 | NA |
| 010810 Follows safety rules | 1 | 2 | 3 | 4 | 5 | NA |
| 010811 Expresses increasingly complex thoughts | 1 | 2 | 3 | 4 | 5 | NA |
| 010812 Shows creativity | 1 | 2 | 3 | 4 | 5 | NA |
| 010813 Comprehends increasingly complex ideas | 1 | 2 | 3 | 4 | 5 | NA |
| 010814 Assumes responsibility for homework | 1 | 2 | 3 | 4 | 5 | NA |
| 010815 Performs in school to level of ability | 1 | 2 | 3 | 4 | 5 | NA |

*1st edition 1997; Revised 3rd edition (formerly Child Development: Middle Childhood [6-11 Years])*

Outcome Content References:

Berger, K. S. (2001). *The developing person through the life span* (5th ed.). New York: Worth Publishers.

Green, M., & Palfrey, J.S. (Eds.). (2002). *Bright futures: Guidelines for health supervision of infants, children and adolescents.* Arlington, VA: National Center for Education in Maternal and Child Health.

Hockenberry, M.J., Wilson, D., Winkelstein, M.L., & Kline, N.E. (2003). *Wong's nursing care of infants and children* (7th ed.). St. Louis: Mosby.

# Child Development: Adolescence (0109)

Domain-Functional Health (I)

Class-Growth & Development (B)

Scale(s)-Never demonstrated to Consistently demonstrated (m)

Care Recipient:

Data Source:

**C**

**Definition:** Milestones of physical, cognitive, and psychosocial progression from 12 years through 17 years of age

OUTCOME TARGET RATING:      Maintain at_____      Increase to_____

| Child Development: Adolescence Overall Rating | Never demonstrated 1 | Rarely demonstrated 2 | Sometimes demonstrated 3 | Often demonstrated 4 | Consistently demonstrated 5 | |
|---|---|---|---|---|---|---|
| INDICATORS: | | | | | | |
| 010901 Practices good health habits | 1 | 2 | 3 | 4 | 5 | NA |
| 010902 Describes sexual development | 1 | 2 | 3 | 4 | 5 | NA |
| 010903 Expresses comfort with own sexual identity | 1 | 2 | 3 | 4 | 5 | NA |
| 010904 Uses effective social interaction skills | 1 | 2 | 3 | 4 | 5 | NA |
| 010905 Uses effective conflict resolution skills | 1 | 2 | 3 | 4 | 5 | NA |
| 010906 Maintains good peer relationships with same gender | 1 | 2 | 3 | 4 | 5 | NA |
| 010907 Maintains good peer relationships with opposite gender | 1 | 2 | 3 | 4 | 5 | NA |
| 010908 Shows capacity for intimacy | 1 | 2 | 3 | 4 | 5 | NA |
| 010909 Practices responsible sexual behaviors | 1 | 2 | 3 | 4 | 5 | NA |
| 010910 Avoids alcohol use | 1 | 2 | 3 | 4 | 5 | NA |
| 010918 Avoids tobacco use | 1 | 2 | 3 | 4 | 5 | NA |
| 010919 Avoids recreational drug use | 1 | 2 | 3 | 4 | 5 | NA |
| 010911 Uses effective coping behaviors | 1 | 2 | 3 | 4 | 5 | NA |
| 010912 Displays increasing levels of autonomy | 1 | 2 | 3 | 4 | 5 | NA |
| 010913 Describes personal value system | 1 | 2 | 3 | 4 | 5 | NA |
| 010914 Uses formal operational thinking | 1 | 2 | 3 | 4 | 5 | NA |
| 010915 Sets academic goals | 1 | 2 | 3 | 4 | 5 | NA |
| 010916 Performs in school to level of ability | 1 | 2 | 3 | 4 | 5 | NA |

*1st edition 1997; Revised 3rd edition (formerly Child Development: Adolescence [12-17 Years])*

Outcome Content References:

Berger, K. S. (2001). *The developing person through the life span* (5th ed.). New York: Worth Publishers.

Hockenberry, M.J., Wilson, D., Winkelstein, M.L., & Kline, N.E. (2003). *Wong's nursing care of infants and children* (7th ed.). St. Louis: Mosby.

Green, M., & Palfrey, J.S. (Eds.). (2002). *Bright futures: Guidelines for health supervision of infants, children and adolescents.* Arlington, VA: National Center for Education in Maternal and Child Health.

Krueger, D.W. (2001). Body self. Development, psychopathologies, and psychoanalytic significance. *Psychoanalytic Study of the Child, 56,* 238-259.

Mitchell, J.J. (1996). *Adolescent vulnerability: A sympathetic look at the frailties and limitations of youth.* Calgary, Alberta, Canada: Detselig Enterprises Ltd.

# Circulation Status (0401)

*Domain-Physiologic Health (II)*  
*Class-Cardiopulmonary (E)*  
*Scale(s)-Severely compromised to Not compromised (a) and Severe to None (n)*

*Care Recipient:*  
*Data Source:*

**Definition:** Unobstructed, unidirectional blood flow at an appropriate pressure through large vessels of the systemic and pulmonary circuits

OUTCOME TARGET RATING:  Maintain at_____  Increase to_____

| Circulation Status Overall Rating | Severely compromised 1 | Substantially compromised 2 | Moderately compromised 3 | Mildly compromised 4 | Not compromised 5 | |
|---|---|---|---|---|---|---|
| **INDICATORS:** | | | | | | |
| 040101 Systolic blood pressure | 1 | 2 | 3 | 4 | 5 | NA |
| 040102 Diastolic blood pressure | 1 | 2 | 3 | 4 | 5 | NA |
| 040103 Pulse pressure | 1 | 2 | 3 | 4 | 5 | NA |
| 040104 Mean blood pressure | 1 | 2 | 3 | 4 | 5 | NA |
| 040105 Central venous pressure | 1 | 2 | 3 | 4 | 5 | NA |
| 040106 Pulmonary wedge pressure | 1 | 2 | 3 | 4 | 5 | NA |
| 040125 Right carotid pulse rate | 1 | 2 | 3 | 4 | 5 | NA |
| 040126 Left carotid pulse rate | 1 | 2 | 3 | 4 | 5 | NA |
| 040127 Right brachial pulse rate | 1 | 2 | 3 | 4 | 5 | NA |
| 040128 Left brachial pulse rate | 1 | 2 | 3 | 4 | 5 | NA |
| 040129 Right radial pulse rate | 1 | 2 | 3 | 4 | 5 | NA |
| 040130 Left radial pulse rate | 1 | 2 | 3 | 4 | 5 | NA |
| 040131 Right femoral pulse rate | 1 | 2 | 3 | 4 | 5 | NA |
| 040132 Left femoral pulse rate | 1 | 2 | 3 | 4 | 5 | NA |
| 040133 Right pedal pulse rate | 1 | 2 | 3 | 4 | 5 | NA |
| 040134 Left pedal pulse rate | 1 | 2 | 3 | 4 | 5 | NA |
| 040135 $PaO_2$* | 1 | 2 | 3 | 4 | 5 | NA |
| 040136 $PaCO_2$* | 1 | 2 | 3 | 4 | 5 | NA |
| 040137 Oxygen saturation | 1 | 2 | 3 | 4 | 5 | NA |
| 040112 Arterial-venous oxygen difference | 1 | 2 | 3 | 4 | 5 | NA |
| 040122 Cognitive status | 1 | 2 | 3 | 4 | 5 | NA |
| 040138 Skin temperature | 1 | 2 | 3 | 4 | 5 | NA |
| 040139 Skin color | 1 | 2 | 3 | 4 | 5 | NA |
| 040140 Urinary output | 1 | 2 | 3 | 4 | 5 | NA |

| | Severe | Substantial | Moderate | Mild | None | |
|---|---|---|---|---|---|---|
| 040107 Orthostatic hypotension | 1 | 2 | 3 | 4 | 5 | NA |
| 040110 Angina | 1 | 2 | 3 | 4 | 5 | NA |
| 040113 Adventitious breath sounds | 1 | 2 | 3 | 4 | 5 | NA |

| Circulation Status—cont'd | | Severe | Substantial | Moderate | Mild | None | |
|---|---|---|---|---|---|---|---|
| 040118 | Large vessel bruits | 1 | 2 | 3 | 4 | 5 | NA |
| 040119 | Neck vein distention | 1 | 2 | 3 | 4 | 5 | NA |
| 040120 | Peripheral edema | 1 | 2 | 3 | 4 | 5 | NA |
| 040121 | Ascites | 1 | 2 | 3 | 4 | 5 | NA |
| 040123 | Extreme fatigue | 1 | 2 | 3 | 4 | 5 | NA |

*$PaO_2$ = partial pressure of oxygen in arterial blood; $PaCO_2$ = partial pressure of carbon dioxide in arterial blood.

*1st edition 1997; Revised 3rd edition*

## Outcome Content References:

Andreoli, K.G., Zipes, D.P., Wallace, A.G., Kinney, M.R., & Fowkes, V.K. (Eds.). (1996). *Comprehensive cardiac care* (8th ed.). St. Louis: Mosby.

Cullen, L. (1992). Interventions related to circulatory care. *Nursing Clinics of North America, 27*(2), 445-477.

Dougherty, C.M. (2001). Decreased cardiac output. In M. Maas, K. Buckwalter, M. Hardy, T. Tripp-Reimer, M. Titler & J. Specht (Eds.), *Nursing care of older adults: Diagnoses, outcomes & interventions* (pp. 285-297). St. Louis: Mosby.

Fahey, V.A. (Ed.). (1999). *Vascular nursing.* (3rd ed.) Philadelphia: W.B. Saunders.

Murphy, T.G., & Bennett, E.J. (1992). Low-tech, high-touch perfusion assessment. *American Journal of Nursing, 92*(5), 36-46.

Reischman, R.R. (2002). Critical care cardiovascular nurse expert and novice diagnostic cue utilization. *Journal of Advanced Nursing, 39*(1), 24-34.

Sheehy, S.B. (1999). *Manual of emergency care* (5th ed.). St. Louis: Mosby.

Smeltzer, S.C., & Bare, B.G. (Eds.). (2003). *Brunner and Suddarth's textbook of medical-surgical nursing* (10th ed.). Philadelphia: Lippincott Williams & Wilkins.

Smith, S.L. (1990). Postoperative perfusion deficits. *Critical Care Nursing Clinics of North America, 2*(4), 567-578.

C

C

# Client Satisfaction: Access to Care Resources (3000)

*Domain-Perceived Health (V)*

*Class-Satisfaction with Care (e)*

*Scale(s)-Not at all satisfied to Completely satisfied (s)*

*Care Recipient:*

*Data Source:*

**Definition:** Extent of positive perception of access to nursing staff, supplies, and equipment needed for care

OUTCOME TARGET RATING:     Maintain at_____     Increase to_____

| Client Satisfaction: Access to Care Resources Overall Rating | Not at all satisfied 1 | Somewhat satisfied 2 | Moderately satisfied 3 | Very satisfied 4 | Completely satisfied 5 | |
|---|---|---|---|---|---|---|
| **INDICATORS:** | | | | | | |
| 300001   Availability of registered nurses | 1 | 2 | 3 | 4 | 5 | NA |
| 300002   Availability of assistive staff | 1 | 2 | 3 | 4 | 5 | NA |
| 300003   Availability of supplies needed for care | 1 | 2 | 3 | 4 | 5 | NA |
| 300004   Availability of equipment needed for care | 1 | 2 | 3 | 4 | 5 | NA |
| 300005   Informed of registered nurse and assistive staff responsible for care | 1 | 2 | 3 | 4 | 5 | NA |
| 300006   Access to registered nurse responsible for care | 1 | 2 | 3 | 4 | 5 | NA |
| 300007   Assistance with gaining access to other health care providers | 1 | 2 | 3 | 4 | 5 | NA |
| 300008   Assistance with contacting physician | 1 | 2 | 3 | 4 | 5 | NA |
| 300009   Coordination of health care resources | 1 | 2 | 3 | 4 | 5 | NA |
| 300010   Coordination of health care providers | 1 | 2 | 3 | 4 | 5 | NA |
| 300011   Wait times for getting an appointment | 1 | 2 | 3 | 4 | 5 | NA |
| 300012   Wait times to be seen at appointment | 1 | 2 | 3 | 4 | 5 | NA |
| 300013   Access to support group(s) | 1 | 2 | 3 | 4 | 5 | NA |

*3rd edition*

## Outcome Content References:

Greeneich, D.S., Long, C.O., & Miller, B.K. (1992). Patient satisfaction update: Research applied to practice. *Applied Nursing Research, 5*(1), 43-48.

Linder-Pelz, S. (1982). Toward a theory of patient satisfaction. *Social Science & Medicine, 16*(5), 577-582.

Marsh, G.W. (1999). Measuring patient satisfaction outcomes across provider disciplines. *Journal of Nursing Measurement, 7*(1), 47-62.

Ware, J.E., Davies-Avery, A., & Stewart, A.I. (1978). The measurement and meaning of patient satisfaction. *Health & Medical Care Services Review, 1*(1), 1, 3-14.

# Client Satisfaction: Caring (3001)

Domain-Perceived Health (V)

Class-Satisfaction with Care (e)

Scale(s)-Not at all satisfied to Completely satisfied (s)

Care Recipient:

Data Source:

**C**

**Definition:** Extent of positive perception of nursing staff's concern for the client

OUTCOME TARGET RATING:    Maintain at_____    Increase to_____

| Client Satisfaction: Caring Overall Rating | Not at all satisfied 1 | Somewhat satisfied 2 | Moderately satisfied 3 | Very satisfied 4 | Completely satisfied 5 | |
|---|---|---|---|---|---|---|
| **INDICATORS:** | | | | | | |
| 300101 Courtesy shown by staff | 1 | 2 | 3 | 4 | 5 | NA |
| 300102 Compassion shown by staff | 1 | 2 | 3 | 4 | 5 | NA |
| 300103 Kindness shown by staff | 1 | 2 | 3 | 4 | 5 | NA |
| 300104 Respect shown by staff | 1 | 2 | 3 | 4 | 5 | NA |
| 300105 Consideration for feelings | 1 | 2 | 3 | 4 | 5 | NA |
| 300106 Consideration for opinions | 1 | 2 | 3 | 4 | 5 | NA |
| 300107 Concern shown for individual needs | 1 | 2 | 3 | 4 | 5 | NA |
| 300108 Relationship with nursing staff | 1 | 2 | 3 | 4 | 5 | NA |
| 300109 Frequency with which checked on by staff | 1 | 2 | 3 | 4 | 5 | NA |
| 300110 Promptness answering call light | 1 | 2 | 3 | 4 | 5 | NA |
| 300111 Promptness responding to inquires | 1 | 2 | 3 | 4 | 5 | NA |
| 300112 Emotional support provided | 1 | 2 | 3 | 4 | 5 | NA |
| 300113 Appropriate use of touch | 1 | 2 | 3 | 4 | 5 | NA |
| 300114 Orientation to room, equipment, and routines | 1 | 2 | 3 | 4 | 5 | NA |
| 300115 Visiting arrangements | 1 | 2 | 3 | 4 | 5 | NA |
| 300116 Family and friends made welcome | 1 | 2 | 3 | 4 | 5 | NA |
| 300117 Assistance with letter writing, as needed | 1 | 2 | 3 | 4 | 5 | NA |
| 300118 Leisure activities provided | 1 | 2 | 3 | 4 | 5 | NA |
| 300119 Information provided about options of care | 1 | 2 | 3 | 4 | 5 | NA |
| 300120 Consideration for cost of care | 1 | 2 | 3 | 4 | 5 | NA |
| 300121 Supplies and equipment not wasted | 1 | 2 | 3 | 4 | 5 | NA |
| 300122 Avoidance of unnecessary treatments and procedures | 1 | 2 | 3 | 4 | 5 | NA |

*3rd edition*

## Outcome Content References:

Abdellah, F.G., & Levine, E. (1957). Developing a measure of patient and personnel satisfaction with nursing care. *Nursing Research, 5*, 100-108.

Abramowitz, S., Cote, A.A., & Berry, E. (1987). *Quality Review Bulletin, 13*(4), 122-130.

Davis, B.A., & Bush, H.A. (1995). Developing effective measurement tools: A case study of the consumer emergency care satisfaction scale. *Journal of Nursing Care Quality, 9*(2), 26-35.

Davis, J., Davis, M., & Riggs, H. (1999). Taking the measure of patient satisfaction. *Nursing Times, 95*(24), 52-53.

*Continued*

C

Eriksen, L. (1988). Measuring patient satisfaction with nursing care: A magnitude estimation approach. In C. F. Waltz & O. W. Stickland (Eds.), *Measurement of nursing outcomes* (Vol. 1, pp. 523-527). New York: Springer.

Greeneich, D.S., Long, C.O., & Miller, B.K. (1992). Patient satisfaction update: Research applied to practice. *Applied Nursing Research, 5*(1), 43-48.

Hegedus, K.S. (1999). Providers' and consumers' perspective of nurses' caring behaviours. *Journal of Advanced Nursing, 30*(5), 1090-1096.

Hinshaw, A.S., & Atwood, J.R. (1982). A patient satisfaction instrument: Precision by replication. *Nursing Research, 31*(3), 170-175.

LaMonica, E.L., Oberst, M.T., Madea, A.R., & Wolf, R.M. (1986). Development of a patient satisfaction scale. *Research in Nursing and Health, 9*(1), 43-50.

Marsh, G.W. (1999). Measuring patient satisfaction outcomes across provider disciplines. *Journal of Nursing Measurement, 7*(1), 47-62.

Risser, N. L. (1975). Development of an instrument to measure patient satisfaction with nurses and nursing care in primary care settings. *Nursing Research, 24*(1), 45-52.

Ryden, M.B., Gross, C.R., Savik, K., Snyder, M., Oh, H.L., Jang, Y., Wang, J., & Krichbaum, K.E. (2000). Development of a measure of resident satisfaction with the nursing home. *Research in Nursing & Health, 23*(3), 237-245.

Walsh, M., & Walsh, A. (1999). Measuring patient satisfaction with nursing care: Experience of using the Newcastle Satisfaction with Nursing Scale. *Journal of Advanced Nursing, 29*(2), 307-315.

Ware, J.E., Davies-Avery, A., & Stewart, A.I. (1978). The measurement and meaning of patient satisfaction. *Health & Medical Care Services Review, 1*(1), 1, 3-14.

Wolf, L.R., Giardino, E.R., Osborne, P.A., & Ambrose, M.S. (1994). Dimensions of nurse caring. *Image -the Journal of Nursing Scholarship, 26*(2), 107-111.

# Client Satisfaction: Communication (3002)

Domain-Perceived Health (V)

Class-Satisfaction with Care (e)

Scale(s)-Not at all satisfied to Completely satisfied (s)

Care Recipient:

Data Source:

**C**

> **Definition:** Extent of positive perception of information exchanged between client and nursing staff

OUTCOME TARGET RATING:    Maintain at_____    Increase to_____

| Client Satisfaction: Communication Overall Rating | Not at all satisfied 1 | Somewhat satisfied 2 | Moderately satisfied 3 | Very satisfied 4 | Completely satisfied 5 | |
|---|---|---|---|---|---|---|
| **INDICATORS:** | | | | | | |
| 300201   Staff introduce self | 1 | 2 | 3 | 4 | 5 | NA |
| 300202   Use of client's preferred name | 1 | 2 | 3 | 4 | 5 | NA |
| 300203   Staff speak clearly | 1 | 2 | 3 | 4 | 5 | NA |
| 300204   Staff listen to client | 1 | 2 | 3 | 4 | 5 | NA |
| 300205   Staff encourage questions | 1 | 2 | 3 | 4 | 5 | NA |
| 300206   Staff repeat information as often as needed | 1 | 2 | 3 | 4 | 5 | NA |
| 300207   Staff take time when communicating | 1 | 2 | 3 | 4 | 5 | NA |
| 300208   Staff present information in understandable way | 1 | 2 | 3 | 4 | 5 | NA |
| 300209   Staff make sure information understood | 1 | 2 | 3 | 4 | 5 | NA |
| 300210   Staff use non-judgmental communication | 1 | 2 | 3 | 4 | 5 | NA |
| 300211   Questions answered clearly | 1 | 2 | 3 | 4 | 5 | NA |
| 300212   Questions answered completely | 1 | 2 | 3 | 4 | 5 | NA |
| 300213   Questions answered in a reasonable length of time | 1 | 2 | 3 | 4 | 5 | NA |
| 300214   Consistent information given by all nursing staff | 1 | 2 | 3 | 4 | 5 | NA |
| 300215   Personal values considered in communication | 1 | 2 | 3 | 4 | 5 | NA |
| 300216   Personal preferences considered | 1 | 2 | 3 | 4 | 5 | NA |
| 300217   Discrepancies in information are resolved in a timely manner | 1 | 2 | 3 | 4 | 5 | NA |
| 300218   Alternative communication methods used as needed | 1 | 2 | 3 | 4 | 5 | NA |

*3rd edition*

Outcome Content References:

Davis, J., Davis, M., & Riggs, H. (1999). Taking the measure of patient satisfaction. *Nursing Times, 95*(24), 52-53.

Greeneich, D.S., Long, C.O., & Miller, B.K. (1992). Patient satisfaction update: Research applied to practice. *Applied Nursing Research, 5*(1), 43-48.

Hegedus, K.S. (1999). Providers' and consumers' perspective of nurses' caring behaviours. *Journal of Advanced Nursing, 30*(5), 1090-1096.

Hinshaw, A.S., & Atwood, J.R. (1982). A patient satisfaction instrument: Precision by replication. *Nursing Research, 31*(3), 170-175.

LaMonica, E.L., Oberst, M.T., Madea, A.R., & Wolf, R.M. (1986). Development of a patient satisfaction scale. *Research in Nursing and Health, 9*(1), 43-50.

*Continued*

C

Lynn, M.R., & McMillen, B.J. (1999). Do nurses know what patients think is important in nursing care? *Journal of Nursing Care Quality, 13*(5), 65-74.

Risser, N. L. (1975). Development of an instrument to measure patient satisfaction with nurses and nursing care in primary care settings. *Nursing Research, 24*(1), 45-52.

Walsh, M., & Walsh, A. (1999). Measuring patient satisfaction with nursing care: Experience of using the Newcastle Satisfaction with Nursing Scale. *Journal of Advanced Nursing, 29*(2), 307-315.

Ware, J.E., Davies-Avery, A., & Stewart, A.I. (1978). The measurement and meaning of patient satisfaction. *Health & Medical Care Services Review, 1*(1), 1, 3-14.

Wolf, L.R., Giardino, E.R., Osborne, P.A., & Ambrose, M.S. (1994). Dimensions of nurse caring. *Image-the Journal of Nursing Scholarship, 26*(2), 107-111.

# Client Satisfaction: Continuity of Care (3003)

*Domain-Perceived Health (V)*

*Class-Satisfaction with Care (e)*

*Scale(s)-Not at all satisfied to Completely satisfied (s)*

*Care Recipient:*

*Data Source:*

**C**

> **Definition:** Extent of positive perception of coordination of care as the patient moves from one care setting to another

OUTCOME TARGET RATING:     Maintain at_____     Increase to_____

| Client Satisfaction: Continuity of Care Overall Rating | Not at all satisfied 1 | Somewhat satisfied 2 | Moderately satisfied 3 | Very satisfied 4 | Completely satisfied 5 | |
|---|---|---|---|---|---|---|
| **INDICATORS:** | | | | | | |
| 300301 Coordination of care | 1 | 2 | 3 | 4 | 5 | NA |
| 300302 Personal preferences included in care plan | 1 | 2 | 3 | 4 | 5 | NA |
| 300303 Patient/family included in planning care | 1 | 2 | 3 | 4 | 5 | NA |
| 300304 Client resources for providing care included in discharge plan | 1 | 2 | 3 | 4 | 5 | NA |
| 300305 Safety issues are addressed in care plan | 1 | 2 | 3 | 4 | 5 | NA |
| 300306 Time to prepare for transfer | 1 | 2 | 3 | 4 | 5 | NA |
| 300307 Information provided about what to expect when transferred | 1 | 2 | 3 | 4 | 5 | NA |
| 300308 Opportunity provided to express concerns about managing self-care | 1 | 2 | 3 | 4 | 5 | NA |
| 300309 Information provided to manage self-care | 1 | 2 | 3 | 4 | 5 | NA |
| 300310 Opportunity to demonstrate care activities | 1 | 2 | 3 | 4 | 5 | NA |
| 300311 Staff offer suggestions for solutions to concerns and questions | 1 | 2 | 3 | 4 | 5 | NA |
| 300312 Discussion of strategies to meet direct care needs the patient/ family cannot manage | 1 | 2 | 3 | 4 | 5 | NA |
| 300313 Discussion of strategies to meet household care needs the patient/family cannot manage | 1 | 2 | 3 | 4 | 5 | NA |
| 300314 Personal preparation to deal with potential health problems | 1 | 2 | 3 | 4 | 5 | NA |
| 300315 Discussion of guidelines for returning to sexual activities | 1 | 2 | 3 | 4 | 5 | NA |
| 300316 Discussion of strategies for returning to work | 1 | 2 | 3 | 4 | 5 | NA |
| 300317 Discussion of strategies for returning to homemaking activities | 1 | 2 | 3 | 4 | 5 | NA |
| 300318 Discussion of strategies for returning to community activities | 1 | 2 | 3 | 4 | 5 | NA |
| 300319 Assistance or referral regarding costs and finances | 1 | 2 | 3 | 4 | 5 | NA |
| 300320 Health care providers work as a team | 1 | 2 | 3 | 4 | 5 | NA |

*3rd edition*

*Continued*

Outcome Content References:

Eriksen, L. (1988). Measuring patient satisfaction with nursing care: A magnitude estimation approach. In C. F. Waltz & O. W. Stickland (Eds.), *Measurement of nursing outcomes* (Vol. 1, pp. 523-527). New York: Springer.

Greeneich, D.S., Long, C.O., & Miller, B.K. (1992). Patient satisfaction update: Research applied to practice. *Applied Nursing Research, 5*(1), 43-48.

Ware, J.E., Davies-Avery, A., & Stewart, A.I. (1978). The measurement and meaning of patient satisfaction. *Health & Medical Care Services Review, 1*(1), 1, 3-14.

C

# Client Satisfaction: Cultural Needs Fulfillment (3004)

Domain-Perceived Health (V)                      Care Recipient:

Class-Satisfaction with Care (e)                 Data Source:

Scale(s)-Not at all satisfied to Completely satisfied (s)

**C**

**Definition:** Extent of positive perception of integration of cultural beliefs, values, and social structures into nursing care

OUTCOME TARGET RATING:    Maintain at_____    Increase to_____

| Client Satisfaction: Cultural Needs Fulfillment Overall Rating | Not at all satisfied 1 | Somewhat satisfied 2 | Moderately satisfied 3 | Very satisfied 4 | Completely satisfied 5 | |
|---|---|---|---|---|---|---|
| **INDICATORS:** | | | | | | |
| 300401  Respect for cultural beliefs | 1 | 2 | 3 | 4 | 5 | NA |
| 300402  Respect for cultural health behaviors | 1 | 2 | 3 | 4 | 5 | NA |
| 300403  Respect for personal values | 1 | 2 | 3 | 4 | 5 | NA |
| 300404  Respect for personal perspectives | 1 | 2 | 3 | 4 | 5 | NA |
| 300405  Respect for background and traditions | 1 | 2 | 3 | 4 | 5 | NA |
| 300406  Respect for religious beliefs | 1 | 2 | 3 | 4 | 5 | NA |
| 300407  Respect for spiritual beliefs | 1 | 2 | 3 | 4 | 5 | NA |
| 300408  Incorporation of cultural beliefs in health teaching | 1 | 2 | 3 | 4 | 5 | NA |
| 300409  Care consistent with cultural beliefs | 1 | 2 | 3 | 4 | 5 | NA |
| 300410  Use of creative methods to establish communication due to language differences | 1 | 2 | 3 | 4 | 5 | NA |
| 300411  Consideration for cultural expectations | 1 | 2 | 3 | 4 | 5 | NA |
| 300412  Respect for family members' participation in care | 1 | 2 | 3 | 4 | 5 | NA |
| 300413  Respect for family members' participation in care | 1 | 2 | 3 | 4 | 5 | NA |

*3rd edition*

**Outcome Content References:**

Ali, N. S., & Khalil, H. Z. (1993). A comparison of American and Egyptian cancer patients' attitudes and unmet needs. *Cancer Nursing, 16*(3), 193-203.

Arruda, E. N., Larson, P. J., & Meleis, A. I. (1992). Comfort: Immigrant Hispanic cancer patient's views. *Cancer Nursing, 15*(6), 387-394.

Austin, W., Gallop, R., McCay, E., Peternelj-Taylor, C., & Bayer, M. (1999). Culturally competent care for psychiatric clients who have a history of sexual abuse. *Clinical Nursing Reasearch, 8*(1), 5-25.

Capers, C. F. (1994). Mental health issues and African-Americans. *Mental Health Nursing, 29*(1), 57-72.

Chmielarczyk, V. (1991). Transcultural nursing: Providing culturally congruent care to the Hausa of Northwest Africa. *Journal of Transcultural Nursing, 3*(1), 15-19.

Cravener, P. (1992). Establishing therapeutic alliance across cultural barriers. *Journal of Psychosocial Nursing, 30*(12), 10-14.

Denman-Vitale, S., & Murillo, E. K. (1999). Effective promotion of breastfeeding among Latin American women newly immigrated to the United States. *Holistic Nursing Practice, 13*(4), 51-60.

Granda-Cameron, C. (1999). The experience of having cancer in *Latin America. Cancer Nursing, 22*(1), 51-57.

Sommer, B. (1995). How we do it: Special considerations for Orthodox Jewish patients in the emergency department. *Journal of Emergency Nursing, 21*(6), 569-570.

Tripp-Reimer, T., Choi, E., Skemp Kelly, L., & Enslein, J. C. (2001). Cultural barriers to care: Inverting the problem. *Diabetes Spectrum, 14*(1), 13-22.

*Continued*

Weaver, H. N. (1999). Transcultural nursing with Native Americans: Critical knowledge, skills, and attitudes. *Journal of Transcultural Nursing, 10*(3), 197-202.

Willis, W. O. (1999). Culturally competent nursing care during the perinatal period. *Journal of Perinatal and Neonatal Nursing, 13*(3), 45-59.

Wilson, A. H., Pittman, K., & Wold, J. L. (2000). Listening to the quiet voices of Hispanic migrant children about health. *Journal of Pediatric Nursing, 15*(3), 137-147.

C

# Client Satisfaction: Functional Assistance (3005)

Domain-Perceived Health (V)

Class-Satisfaction with Care (e)

Scale(s)-Not at all satisfied to Completely satisfied (s)

Care Recipient:

Data Source:

**C**

**Definition:** Extent of positive perception of nursing assistance to achieve mobility and self-care as independently as health condition permits

OUTCOME TARGET RATING:    Maintain at_____    Increase to_____

| Client Satisfaction: Functional Assistance Overall Rating | Not at all satisfied 1 | Somewhat satisfied 2 | Moderately satisfied 3 | Very satisfied 4 | Completely satisfied 5 | |
|---|---|---|---|---|---|---|
| INDICATORS: | | | | | | |
| 300501 Included in planning for optimal mobility and self-care | 1 | 2 | 3 | 4 | 5 | NA |
| 300502 Included in planning time schedule for self-care | 1 | 2 | 3 | 4 | 5 | NA |
| 300503 Encouraged to be as active as possible | 1 | 2 | 3 | 4 | 5 | NA |
| 300504 Assistance with physical activity as needed | 1 | 2 | 3 | 4 | 5 | NA |
| 300505 Exercise routine provided to gain or maintain mobility | 1 | 2 | 3 | 4 | 5 | NA |
| 300506 Exercise routine provided to gain or maintain flexibility | 1 | 2 | 3 | 4 | 5 | NA |
| 300507 Equipment provided to enhance mobility | 1 | 2 | 3 | 4 | 5 | NA |
| 300508 Information provided to learn to use equipment or other adaptations | 1 | 2 | 3 | 4 | 5 | NA |
| 300509 Room space provided for equipment needed for functional independence | 1 | 2 | 3 | 4 | 5 | NA |
| 300510 Safety emphasized and taught in all activities | 1 | 2 | 3 | 4 | 5 | NA |
| 300511 Opportunity to do self-care unless assistance requested | 1 | 2 | 3 | 4 | 5 | NA |
| 300512 Assistance with care as needed | 1 | 2 | 3 | 4 | 5 | NA |
| 300513 Allowed to choose own clothing | 1 | 2 | 3 | 4 | 5 | NA |
| 300514 Allowed to choose food for meals | 1 | 2 | 3 | 4 | 5 | NA |
| 300515 Information provided to manage medication(s) | 1 | 2 | 3 | 4 | 5 | NA |

*3rd edition*

## Outcome Content References:

Greeneich, D.S., Long, C.O., & Miller, B.K. (1992). Patient satisfaction update: Research applied to practice. *Applied Nursing Research, 5*(1), 43-48.

Hinshaw, A.S., & Atwood, J.R. (1982). A patient satisfaction instrument: Precision by replication. *Nursing Research, 31*(3), 170-175.

LaMonica, E.L., Oberst, M.T., Madea, A.R., & Wolf, R.M. (1986). Development of a patient satisfaction scale. *Research in Nursing and Health, 9*(1), 43-50.

Risser, N. L. (1975). Development of an instrument to measure patient satisfaction with nurses and nursing care in primary care settings. *Nursing Research, 24*(1), 45-52.

Ware, J.E., Davies-Avery, A., & Stewart, A.I. (1978). The measurement and meaning of patient satisfaction. *Health & Medical Care Services Review, 1*(1), 1, 3-14.

C

# Client Satisfaction: Physical Care (3006)

*Domain-Perceived Health (V)*

*Class-Satisfaction with Care (e)*

*Scale(s)-Not at all satisfied to Completely satisfied (s)*

Care Recipient:

Data Source:

**Definition:** Extent of positive perception of nursing care to maintain body functions and cleanliness

OUTCOME TARGET RATING: Maintain at_____ Increase to_____

| Client Satisfaction: Physical Care Overall Rating | Not at all satisfied 1 | Somewhat satisfied 2 | Moderately satisfied 3 | Very satisfied 4 | Completely satisfied 5 | |
|---|---|---|---|---|---|---|
| **INDICATORS:** | | | | | | |
| 300601 Assistance with selecting foods and fluids | 1 | 2 | 3 | 4 | 5 | NA |
| 300602 Assistance with eating | 1 | 2 | 3 | 4 | 5 | NA |
| 300603 Time for uninterrupted meals | 1 | 2 | 3 | 4 | 5 | NA |
| 300604 Fluids available within restriction | 1 | 2 | 3 | 4 | 5 | NA |
| 300605 Assistance with mouth care | 1 | 2 | 3 | 4 | 5 | NA |
| 300606 Assistance with toileting | 1 | 2 | 3 | 4 | 5 | NA |
| 300607 Normal bowel habits maintained | 1 | 2 | 3 | 4 | 5 | NA |
| 300608 Normal bladder habits maintained | 1 | 2 | 3 | 4 | 5 | NA |
| 300609 Assistance with bath or shower | 1 | 2 | 3 | 4 | 5 | NA |
| 300610 Assistance with hair care | 1 | 2 | 3 | 4 | 5 | NA |
| 300611 Assistance with nail care | 1 | 2 | 3 | 4 | 5 | NA |
| 300612 Skin care routine maintained | 1 | 2 | 3 | 4 | 5 | NA |
| 300613 Special skin care needs followed | 1 | 2 | 3 | 4 | 5 | NA |
| 300614 Assistance with maintaining comfort | 1 | 2 | 3 | 4 | 5 | NA |
| 300615 Time for rest and sleep | 1 | 2 | 3 | 4 | 5 | NA |
| 300616 Sleep routine maintained | 1 | 2 | 3 | 4 | 5 | NA |
| 300617 Assistance with ambulation | 1 | 2 | 3 | 4 | 5 | NA |
| 300618 Opportunity for exercise | 1 | 2 | 3 | 4 | 5 | NA |
| 300619 Special exercises provided | 1 | 2 | 3 | 4 | 5 | NA |
| 300620 Assistance with turning or repositioning | 1 | 2 | 3 | 4 | 5 | NA |
| 300621 Assistance with transfer | 1 | 2 | 3 | 4 | 5 | NA |

*3rd edition*

Outcome Content References:

Davis, B.A., & Bush, H.A. (1995). Developing effective measurement tools: A case study of the consumer emergency care satisfaction scale. *Journal of Nursing Care Quality, 9*(2), 26-35.

Greeneich, D.S., Long, C.O., & Miller, B.K. (1992). Patient satisfaction update: Research applied to practice. *Applied Nursing Research, 5*(1), 43-48.

Hinshaw, A.S., & Atwood, J.R. (1982). A patient satisfaction instrument: Precision by replication. *Nursing Research, 31*(3), 170-175.

LaMonica, E.L., Oberst, M.T., Madea, A.R., & Wolf, R.M. (1986). Development of a patient satisfaction scale. *Research in Nursing and Health, 9*(1), 43-50.

Lynn, M.R., & McMillen, B.J. (1999). Do nurses know what patients think is important in nursing care? *Journal of Nursing Care Quality, 13*(5), 65-74.

Ryden, M.B., Gross, C.R., Savik, K., Snyder, M., Oh, H.L., Jang, Y., Wang, J., & Krichbaum, K.E. (2000). Development of a measure of resident satisfaction with the nursing home. *Research in Nursing & Health, 23*(3), 237-245.

Ware, J.E., Davies-Avery, A., & Stewart, A.I. (1978). The measurement and meaning of patient satisfaction. *Health & Medical Care Services Review, 1*(1), 1, 3-14.

Wolf, L.R., Giardino, E.R., Osborne, P.A., & Ambrose, M.S. (1994). Dimensions of nurse caring. *IMAGE—The Journal of Nursing Scholarship, 26*(2), 107-111.

# Client Satisfaction: Physical Environment (3007)

Domain-Perceived Health (V)                         Care Recipient:

Class-Satisfaction with Care (e)                     Data Source:

Scale(s)-Not at all satisfied to Completely satisfied (s)

C

**Definition:** Extent of positive perception of living environment, treatment environment, equipment and supplies in acute or long term care settings

OUTCOME TARGET RATING:        Maintain at_____        Increase to_____

| Client Satisfaction: Physical Environment Overall Rating | Not at all satisfied 1 | Somewhat satisfied 2 | Moderately satisfied 3 | Very satisfied 4 | Completely satisfied 5 | |
|---|---|---|---|---|---|---|
| **INDICATORS:** | | | | | | |
| 300701 Cleanliness of room | 1 | 2 | 3 | 4 | 5 | NA |
| 300702 Cleanliness of bathroom | 1 | 2 | 3 | 4 | 5 | NA |
| 300703 Cleanliness of equipment | 1 | 2 | 3 | 4 | 5 | NA |
| 300704 Control of room lighting | 1 | 2 | 3 | 4 | 5 | NA |
| 300705 Comfort of room temperature | 1 | 2 | 3 | 4 | 5 | NA |
| 300706 Comfort of bathroom temperature | 1 | 2 | 3 | 4 | 5 | NA |
| 300707 Comfort of treatment room temperature | 1 | 2 | 3 | 4 | 5 | NA |
| 300708 Comfort of room humidity | 1 | 2 | 3 | 4 | 5 | NA |
| 300709 Control of noise | 1 | 2 | 3 | 4 | 5 | NA |
| 300710 Control of number of people in room | 1 | 2 | 3 | 4 | 5 | NA |
| 300711 Supplies and equipment within reach | 1 | 2 | 3 | 4 | 5 | NA |
| 300712 Call light within reach | 1 | 2 | 3 | 4 | 5 | NA |
| 300713 Access to telephone | 1 | 2 | 3 | 4 | 5 | NA |
| 300714 Access to television | 1 | 2 | 3 | 4 | 5 | NA |
| 300715 Access to radio | 1 | 2 | 3 | 4 | 5 | NA |
| 300716 Attractiveness of room | 1 | 2 | 3 | 4 | 5 | NA |
| 300717 Availability of chairs for family and visitors | 1 | 2 | 3 | 4 | 5 | NA |
| 300718 Availability of space nearby for family and visitors | 1 | 2 | 3 | 4 | 5 | NA |
| 300719 Orientation of family and visitors to facilities | 1 | 2 | 3 | 4 | 5 | NA |
| 300720 Space in room for personal items | 1 | 2 | 3 | 4 | 5 | NA |

*3rd edition*

Outcome Content References:

Abdellah, F.G., & Levine, E. (1957). Developing a measure of patient and personnel satisfaction with nursing care. *Nursing Research, 5*, 100-108.

Eriksen, L. (1988). Measuring patient satisfaction with nursing care: A magnitude estimation approach. In C. F. Waltz & O. W. Stickland (Eds.), *Measurement of nursing outcomes* (Vol. 1, pp. 523-527). New York: Springer.

Greeneich, D.S., Long, C.O., & Miller, B.K. (1992). Patient satisfaction update: Research applied to practice. *Applied Nursing Research, 5*(1), 43-48.

Lynn, M.R., & McMillen, B.J. (1999). Do nurses know what patients think is important in nursing care? *Journal of Nursing Care Quality, 13*(5), 65-74.

Ryden, M.B., Gross, C.R., Savik, K., Snyder, M., Oh, H.L., Jang, Y., Wang, J., & Krichbaum, K.E. (2000). Development of a measure of resident satisfaction with the nursing home. *Research in Nursing & Health, 23*(3), 237-245.

Ware, J.E., Davies-Avery, A., & Stewart, A.I. (1978). The measurement and meaning of patient satisfaction. *Health & Medical Care Services Review, 1*(1), 1, 3-14.

C

# Client Satisfaction: Protection of Rights (3008)

Domain-Perceived Health (V)

Class-Satisfaction with Care (e)

Scale(s)-Not at all satisfied to Completely satisfied (s)

Care Recipient:

Data Source:

**Definition:** Extent of positive perception of protection of a client's legal and moral rights provided by nursing staff

OUTCOME TARGET RATING:      Maintain at_____      Increase to_____

| Client Satisfaction: Protection of Rights Overall Rating | Not at all satisfied 1 | Somewhat satisfied 2 | Moderately satisfied 3 | Very satisfied 4 | Completely satisfied 5 | |
|---|---|---|---|---|---|---|
| **INDICATORS:** | | | | | | |
| 300801 Maintenance of privacy | 1 | 2 | 3 | 4 | 5 | NA |
| 300802 Care consistent with religious and spiritual needs | 1 | 2 | 3 | 4 | 5 | NA |
| 300803 Confidentiality of client information maintained | 1 | 2 | 3 | 4 | 5 | NA |
| 300804 Requests respected | 1 | 2 | 3 | 4 | 5 | NA |
| 300805 Personal preferences for care considered | 1 | 2 | 3 | 4 | 5 | NA |
| 300806 Use of client's preferred name | 1 | 2 | 3 | 4 | 5 | NA |
| 300807 Introduced to staff | 1 | 2 | 3 | 4 | 5 | NA |
| 300808 Introduced to roommate(s) | 1 | 2 | 3 | 4 | 5 | NA |
| 300809 Information provided about available services of other disciplines | 1 | 2 | 3 | 4 | 5 | NA |
| 300810 Information provided about support groups and organizations | 1 | 2 | 3 | 4 | 5 | NA |
| 300811 Allowed to choose between care options | 1 | 2 | 3 | 4 | 5 | NA |
| 300812 Included in decisions about care | 1 | 2 | 3 | 4 | 5 | NA |
| 300813 Information provided about legal rights | 1 | 2 | 3 | 4 | 5 | NA |
| 300814 Information provided about advance directives | 1 | 2 | 3 | 4 | 5 | NA |
| 300815 Avoidance of repetitive questions by more than one provider | 1 | 2 | 3 | 4 | 5 | NA |

*3rd edition*

## Outcome Content References:

Eriksen, L. (1988). Measuring patient satisfaction with nursing care: A magnitude estimation approach. In C.F. Waltz & O.W. Stickland (Eds.), *Measurement of nursing outcomes* (Vol. 1, pp. 523-527). New York: Springer.

Greeneich, D.S., Long, C.O., & Miller, B.K. (1992). Patient satisfaction update: Research applied to practice. *Applied Nursing Research, 5*(1), 43-48.

Hegedus, K.S. (1999). Providers' and consumers' perspective of nurses' caring behaviours. *Journal of Advanced Nursing, 30*(5), 1090-1096.

LaMonica, E.L., Oberst, M.T., Madea, A.R., & Wolf, R.M. (1986). Development of a patient satisfaction scale. *Research in Nursing and Health, 9*(1), 43-50.

Ryden, M.B., Gross, C.R., Savik, K., Snyder, M., Oh, H.L., Jang, Y., Wang, J., & Krichbaum, K.E. (2000). Development of a measure of resident satisfaction with the nursing home. *Research in Nursing & Health, 23*(3), 237-245.

Ware, J.E., Davies-Avery, A., & Stewart, A.I. (1978). The measurement and meaning of patient satisfaction. *Health & Medical Care Services Review, 1*(1), 1, 3-14.

Wolf, L.R., Giardino, E.R., Osborne, P.A., & Ambrose, M.S. (1994). Dimensions of nurse caring. *IMAGE—The Journal of Nursing Scholarship, 26*(2), 107-111.

# Client Satisfaction: Psychological Care (3009)

Domain-Perceived Health (V)

Class-Satisfaction with Care (e)

Scale(s)-Not at all satisfied to Completely satisfied (s)

Care Recipient:

Data Source:

C

**Definition:** Extent of positive perception of nursing assistance to perform emotional and mental activities as independently as health condition permits

OUTCOME TARGET RATING:     Maintain at_____     Increase to_____

| Client Satisfaction: Psychological Care Overall Rating | Not at all satisfied 1 | Somewhat satisfied 2 | Moderately satisfied 3 | Very satisfied 4 | Completely satisfied 5 | |
|---|---|---|---|---|---|---|
| **INDICATORS:** | | | | | | |
| 300901 Information provided about course of illness | 1 | 2 | 3 | 4 | 5 | NA |
| 300902 Information provided about expected improvement | 1 | 2 | 3 | 4 | 5 | NA |
| 300903 Information provided about usual emotional responses to disease and treatment | 1 | 2 | 3 | 4 | 5 | NA |
| 300904 Assistance with identifying social support groups for client | 1 | 2 | 3 | 4 | 5 | NA |
| 300905 Assistance with identifying social support groups for family | 1 | 2 | 3 | 4 | 5 | NA |
| 300906 Discussion of strategies to cope with mental/ emotional impairments after discharge | 1 | 2 | 3 | 4 | 5 | NA |
| 300907 Emotional support provided when feeling sad, depressed, confused, anxious | 1 | 2 | 3 | 4 | 5 | NA |
| 300908 Counseling provided to improve mental functioning | 1 | 2 | 3 | 4 | 5 | NA |
| 300909 Counseling provided to improve emotional stability | 1 | 2 | 3 | 4 | 5 | NA |
| 300910 Counseling provided to improve social interactions | 1 | 2 | 3 | 4 | 5 | NA |
| 300911 Assistance with finding resources | 1 | 2 | 3 | 4 | 5 | NA |
| 300912 Support for finding own solutions to problems | 1 | 2 | 3 | 4 | 5 | NA |
| 300913 Support for expressing feelings | 1 | 2 | 3 | 4 | 5 | NA |
| 300914 Support for working through feelings of grief and loss | 1 | 2 | 3 | 4 | 5 | NA |
| 300915 Support for identifying ways to cope with stress | 1 | 2 | 3 | 4 | 5 | NA |
| 300916 Support for adjusting to body and/or functional changes | 1 | 2 | 3 | 4 | 5 | NA |

_3rd edition_

_Continued_

Outcome Content References:

Davis, B.A., & Bush, H.A. (1995). Developing effective measurement tools: A case study of the consumer emergency care satisfaction scale. *Journal of Nursing Care Quality, 9*(2), 26-35.

Greeneich, D.S., Long, C.O., & Miller, B.K. (1992). Patient satisfaction update: Research applied to practice. *Applied Nursing Research, 5*(1), 43-48.

Lynn, M.R., & McMillen, B.J. (1999). Do nurses know what patients think is important in nursing care? *Journal of Nursing Care Quality, 13*(5), 65-74.

Ryden, M.B., Gross, C.R., Savik, K., Snyder, M., Oh, H.L., Jang, Y., Wang, J., & Krichbaum, K.E. (2000). Development of a measure of resident satisfaction with the nursing home. *Research in Nursing & Health, 23*(3), 237-245.

Ware, J.E., Davies-Avery, A., & Stewart, A.I. (1978). The measurement and meaning of patient satisfaction. *Health & Medical Care Services Review, 1*(1), 1, 3-14.

# Client Satisfaction: Safety (3010)

Domain-Perceived Health (V)

Class-Satisfaction with Care (e)

Scale(s)-Not at all satisfied to Completely satisfied (s)

Care Recipient:

Data Source:

C

**Definition:** Extent of positive perception of procedures, information, and nursing care to prevent harm or injury

OUTCOME TARGET RATING:    Maintain at_____    Increase to_____

| Client Satisfaction: Safety Overall Rating | Not at all satisfied 1 | Somewhat satisfied 2 | Moderately satisfied 3 | Very satisfied 4 | Completely satisfied 5 | |
|---|---|---|---|---|---|---|
| INDICATORS: | | | | | | |
| 301001 Explanation of safety rules and procedures | 1 | 2 | 3 | 4 | 5 | NA |
| 301002 Prompt response to injury by staff | 1 | 2 | 3 | 4 | 5 | NA |
| 301003 Client identified before giving medication(s) | 1 | 2 | 3 | 4 | 5 | NA |
| 301004 Side rails and other protective devices used appropriately | 1 | 2 | 3 | 4 | 5 | NA |
| 301005 Assistance with transfer, as needed | 1 | 2 | 3 | 4 | 5 | NA |
| 301006 Assistance with ambulation, as needed | 1 | 2 | 3 | 4 | 5 | NA |
| 301007 Assistance with toileting, as needed | 1 | 2 | 3 | 4 | 5 | NA |
| 301008 Assistance with bath or shower, as needed | 1 | 2 | 3 | 4 | 5 | NA |
| 301009 Warning signs of high risk environment clearly displayed | 1 | 2 | 3 | 4 | 5 | NA |
| 301010 Floor kept free of clutter, obstructions, and slippery materials | 1 | 2 | 3 | 4 | 5 | NA |
| 301011 Information provided about treatment risks and complications | 1 | 2 | 3 | 4 | 5 | NA |
| 301012 Maintenance of safe environment when mental function is impaired | 1 | 2 | 3 | 4 | 5 | NA |
| 301013 Maintenance of protective environment when at risk for self-injury | 1 | 2 | 3 | 4 | 5 | NA |

*3rd edition*

## Outcome Content References:

Abdellah, F.G., & Levine, E. (1957). Developing a measure of patient and personnel satisfaction with nursing care. *Nursing Research, 5*, 100-108.

Eriksen, L. (1988). Measuring patient satisfaction with nursing care: A magnitude estimation approach. In C. F. Waltz & O. W. Stickland (Eds.), *Measurement of nursing outcomes* (Vol. 1, pp. 523-527). New York: Springer.

Greeneich, D.S., Long, C.O., & Miller, B.K. (1992). Patient satisfaction update: Research applied to practice. *Applied Nursing Research, 5*(1), 43-48.

Lynn, M.R., & McMillen, B.J. (1999). Do nurses know what patients think is important in nursing care? *Journal of Nursing Care Quality, 13*(5), 65-74.

Ryden, M.B., Gross, C.R., Savik, K., Snyder, M., Oh, H.L., Jang, Y., Wang, J., & Krichbaum, K.E. (2000). Development of a measure of resident satisfaction with the nursing home. *Research in Nursing & Health, 23*(3), 237-245.

Ware, J.E., Davies-Avery, A., & Stewart, A.I. (1978). The measurement and meaning of patient satisfaction. *Health & Medical Care Services Review, 1*(1), 1, 3-14.

C

# *Client Satisfaction: Symptom Control (3011)*

Domain-Perceived Health (V)

Class-Satisfaction with Care (e)

Scale(s)-Not at all satisfied to Completely satisfied (s)

Care Recipient:

Data Source:

**Definition:** Extent of positive perception of nursing care to relieve symptoms of illness

OUTCOME TARGET RATING:     Maintain at_____     Increase to_____

| Client Satisfaction: Symptom Control Overall Rating | Not at all satisfied 1 | Somewhat satisfied 2 | Moderately satisfied 3 | Very satisfied 4 | Completely satisfied 5 | |
|---|---|---|---|---|---|---|
| INDICATORS: | | | | | | |
| 301101 Patterns of symptoms identified | 1 | 2 | 3 | 4 | 5 | NA |
| 301102 Severity of symptoms identified | 1 | 2 | 3 | 4 | 5 | NA |
| 301103 Duration of symptoms identified | 1 | 2 | 3 | 4 | 5 | NA |
| 301104 Investigation of cause of symptoms | 1 | 2 | 3 | 4 | 5 | NA |
| 301105 Actions taken to prevent symptoms | 1 | 2 | 3 | 4 | 5 | NA |
| 301106 Symptoms responded to promptly | 1 | 2 | 3 | 4 | 5 | NA |
| 301107 Care to eliminate/reduce symptoms | 1 | 2 | 3 | 4 | 5 | NA |
| 301108 Care to eliminate/reduce pain | 1 | 2 | 3 | 4 | 5 | NA |
| 301109 Actions taken to provide comfort | 1 | 2 | 3 | 4 | 5 | NA |
| 301110 Symptoms regularly monitored | 1 | 2 | 3 | 4 | 5 | NA |
| 301111 Monitored for unusual symptoms | 1 | 2 | 3 | 4 | 5 | NA |
| 301112 Monitored for control of symptoms | 1 | 2 | 3 | 4 | 5 | NA |
| 301113 Monitored for comfort | 1 | 2 | 3 | 4 | 5 | NA |
| 301114 Referrals made to appropriate practitioners | 1 | 2 | 3 | 4 | 5 | NA |

*3rd edition*

**Outcome Content References:**

Greeneich, D.S., Long, C.O., & Miller, B.K. (1992). Patient satisfaction update: Research applied to practice. *Applied Nursing Research, 5*(1), 43-48.

Marsh, G.W. (1999). Measuring patient satisfaction outcomes across provider disciplines. *Journal of Nursing Measurement, 7*(1), 47-62.

Ryden, M.B., Gross, C.R., Savik, K., Snyder, M., Oh, H.L., Jang, Y., Wang, J., & Krichbaum, K.E. (2000). Development of a measure of resident satisfaction with the nursing home. *Research in Nursing & Health, 23*(3), 237-245.

Ware, J.E., Davies-Avery, A., & Stewart, A.I. (1978). The measurement and meaning of patient satisfaction. *Health & Medical Care Services Review, 1*(1), 1, 3-14.

# *Client Satisfaction: Teaching (3012)*

*Domain-Perceived Health (V)*

*Class-Satisfaction with Care (e)*

*Scale(s)-Not at all satisfied to Completely satisfied (s)*

*Care Recipient:*

*Data Source:*

**C**

**Definition:** Extent of positive perception of instruction provided by nursing staff to improve knowledge, understanding, and participation in care

OUTCOME TARGET RATING:      Maintain at_____   Increase to_____

| Client Satisfaction: Teaching Overall Rating | Not at all satisfied 1 | Somewhat satisfied 2 | Moderately satisfied 3 | Very satisfied 4 | Completely satisfied 5 | |
|---|---|---|---|---|---|---|
| INDICATORS: | | | | | | |
| 301201 Medical diagnosis explained in understandable terms | 1 | 2 | 3 | 4 | 5 | NA |
| 301202 Nursing care explained in understandable terms | 1 | 2 | 3 | 4 | 5 | NA |
| 301203 Explanation of diagnostic tests and preparation | 1 | 2 | 3 | 4 | 5 | NA |
| 301204 Explanation of results of diagnostic tests | 1 | 2 | 3 | 4 | 5 | NA |
| 301205 Explanation of effects of medication(s) | 1 | 2 | 3 | 4 | 5 | NA |
| 301206 Explanation of medication(s) side effects | 1 | 2 | 3 | 4 | 5 | NA |
| 301207 Explanation of reasons for treatment(s) | 1 | 2 | 3 | 4 | 5 | NA |
| 301208 Explanation of self-care responsibilities for treatment | 1 | 2 | 3 | 4 | 5 | NA |
| 301209 Explanation of self-care responsibilities for medication management | 1 | 2 | 3 | 4 | 5 | NA |
| 301210 Personal knowledge considered before teaching | 1 | 2 | 3 | 4 | 5 | NA |
| 301211 Information provided about signs of complications | 1 | 2 | 3 | 4 | 5 | NA |
| 301212 Explanation of activity restrictions | 1 | 2 | 3 | 4 | 5 | NA |
| 301213 Discussion of strategies to improve physical strength | 1 | 2 | 3 | 4 | 5 | NA |
| 301214 Discussion of strategies to improve physical endurance | 1 | 2 | 3 | 4 | 5 | NA |
| 301215 Discussion of strategies to improve health | 1 | 2 | 3 | 4 | 5 | NA |
| 301216 Explanation of available health resources | 1 | 2 | 3 | 4 | 5 | NA |
| 301217 Costs of care explained | 1 | 2 | 3 | 4 | 5 | NA |
| 301218 Time for patient learning | 1 | 2 | 3 | 4 | 5 | NA |
| 301219 Explanations provided in understandable terms | 1 | 2 | 3 | 4 | 5 | NA |
| 301220 Quality of instructional material provided | 1 | 2 | 3 | 4 | 5 | NA |
| 301221 Staff supportive of learning process | 1 | 2 | 3 | 4 | 5 | NA |

*3rd edition*

*Continued*

C

Outcome Content References:

Abramowitz, S., Cote, A.A., & Berry, E. (1987). *Quality Review Bulletin, 13*(4), 122-130.

Davis, B.A., & Bush, H.A. (1995). Developing effective measurement tools: A case study of the consumer emergency care satisfaction scale. *Journal of Nursing Care Quality, 9*(2), 26-35.

Greeneich, D.S., Long, C.O., & Miller, B.K. (1992). Patient satisfaction update: Research applied to practice. *Applied Nursing Research, 5*(1), 43-48.

Hinshaw, A.S., & Atwood, J.R. (1982). A patient satisfaction instrument: Precision by replication. *Nursing Research, 31*(3), 170-175.

Marsh, G.W. (1999). Measuring patient satisfaction outcomes across provider disciplines. *Journal of Nursing Measurement, 7*(1), 47-62.

Risser, N. L. (1975). Development of an instrument to measure patient satisfaction with nurses and nursing care in primary care settings. *Nursing Research, 24*(1), 45-52.

Ryden, M.B., Gross, C.R., Savik, K., Snyder, M., Oh, H.L., Jang, Y., Wang, J., & Krichbaum, K.E. (2000). Development of a measure of resident satisfaction with the nursing home. *Research in Nursing & Health, 23*(3), 237-245.

Ware, J.E., Davies-Avery, A., & Stewart, A.I. (1978). The measurement and meaning of patient satisfaction. *Health & Medical Care Services Review, 1*(1), 1, 3-14.

# Client Satisfaction: Technical Aspects of Care (3013)

Domain-Perceived Health (V)

Class-Satisfaction with Care (e)

Scale(s)-Not at all satisfied to Completely satisfied (s)

Care Recipient:

Data Source:

**C**

**Definition:** Extent of positive perception of nursing staff's knowledge and expertise used in providing care

OUTCOME TARGET RATING:      Maintain at_____      Increase to_____

| Client Satisfaction: Technical Aspects of Care Overall Rating | Not at all satisfied 1 | Somewhat satisfied 2 | Moderately satisfied 3 | Very satisfied 4 | Completely satisfied 5 | |
|---|---|---|---|---|---|---|
| **INDICATORS:** | | | | | | |
| 301301  Correct care provided | 1 | 2 | 3 | 4 | 5 | NA |
| 301302  Organization of care | 1 | 2 | 3 | 4 | 5 | NA |
| 301303  Thoroughness of care | 1 | 2 | 3 | 4 | 5 | NA |
| 301304  Capability of staff | 1 | 2 | 3 | 4 | 5 | NA |
| 301305  Registered nurse knowledge of disease process | 1 | 2 | 3 | 4 | 5 | NA |
| 301306  Registered nurse knowledge of treatments | 1 | 2 | 3 | 4 | 5 | NA |
| 301307  Registered nurse knowledge of medications | 1 | 2 | 3 | 4 | 5 | NA |
| 301308  Registered nurse knowledge of health history | 1 | 2 | 3 | 4 | 5 | NA |
| 301309  Consistency in performance of care | 1 | 2 | 3 | 4 | 5 | NA |
| 301310  Consistency of staff providing care | 1 | 2 | 3 | 4 | 5 | NA |
| 301311  Comfort attended to during treatments | 1 | 2 | 3 | 4 | 5 | NA |
| 301312  Gentleness of treatment providers | 1 | 2 | 3 | 4 | 5 | NA |
| 301313  Skillfulness of treatment providers | 1 | 2 | 3 | 4 | 5 | NA |
| 301314  Responsiveness of staff to emergencies | 1 | 2 | 3 | 4 | 5 | NA |
| 301315  Supplies and equipment not wasted | 1 | 2 | 3 | 4 | 5 | NA |

*3rd edition*

Outcome Content References:

Abdellah, F.G., & Levine, E. (1957). Developing a measure of patient and personnel satisfaction with nursing care. *Nursing Research, 5*, 100-108.

Eriksen, L. (1988). Measuring patient satisfaction with nursing care: A magnitude estimation approach. In C.F. Waltz & O.W. Stickland (Eds.), *Measurement of nursing outcomes* (Vol. 1, pp. 523-527). New York: Springer.

Greeneich, D.S., Long, C.O., & Miller, B.K. (1992). Patient satisfaction update: Research applied to practice. *Applied Nursing Research, 5*(1), 43-48.

Hinshaw, A.S., & Atwood, J.R. (1982). A patient satisfaction instrument: Precision by replication. *Nursing Research, 31*(3), 170-175.

LaMonica, E.L., Oberst, M.T., Madea, A.R., & Wolf, R.M. (1986). Development of a patient satisfaction scale. *Research in Nursing and Health, 9*(1), 43-50.

Marsh, G.W. (1999). Measuring patient satisfaction outcomes across provider disciplines. *Journal of Nursing Measurement, 7*(1), 47-62.

Risser, N. L. (1975). Development of an instrument to measure patient satisfaction with nurses and nursing care in primary care settings. *Nursing Research, 24*(1), 45-52.

Ware, J.E., Davies-Avery, A., & Stewart, A.I. (1978). The measurement and meaning of patient satisfaction. *Health & Medical Care Services Review, 1*(1), 1, 3-14.

Wolf, L.R., Giardino, E.R., Osborne, P.A., & Ambrose, M.S. (1994). Dimensions of nurse caring. *Image-the Journal of Nursing Scholarship, 26*(2), 107-111.

C

# Cognition (0900)

*Domain-Physiologic Health (II)*

*Class-Neurocognitive (J)*

*Scale(s)-Severely compromised to Not compromised (a)*

*Care Recipient:*

*Data Source:*

**Definition:** Ability to execute complex mental processes

OUTCOME TARGET RATING:      Maintain at_____      Increase to_____

| Cognition Overall Rating | Severely compromised 1 | Substantially compromised 2 | Moderately compromised 3 | Mildly compromised 4 | Not compromised 5 | |
|---|---|---|---|---|---|---|
| **INDICATORS:** | | | | | | |
| 090001 Communicates clearly and appropriately for age and ability | 1 | 2 | 3 | 4 | 5 | NA |
| 090013 Comprehends the meaning of events and situations | 1 | 2 | 3 | 4 | 5 | NA |
| 090003 Attentiveness | 1 | 2 | 3 | 4 | 5 | NA |
| 090004 Concentration | 1 | 2 | 3 | 4 | 5 | NA |
| 090005 Cognitive orientation | 1 | 2 | 3 | 4 | 5 | NA |
| 090006 Demonstrates immediate memory | 1 | 2 | 3 | 4 | 5 | NA |
| 090007 Demonstrates recent memory | 1 | 2 | 3 | 4 | 5 | NA |
| 090008 Demonstrates remote memory | 1 | 2 | 3 | 4 | 5 | NA |
| 090009 Processes information | 1 | 2 | 3 | 4 | 5 | NA |
| 090010 Weighs alternatives when making decisions | 1 | 2 | 3 | 4 | 5 | NA |
| 090011 Makes appropriate decisions | 1 | 2 | 3 | 4 | 5 | NA |

*1st edition 1997; Revised 3rd edition (formerly Cognitive Ability)*

## Outcome Content References:

Abraham, I., & Reel, S. (1993). Cognitive nursing interventions with long-term care residents: Effects on neurocognitive dimensions. *Archives of Psychiatric Nursing, 6*(6), 356-365.

Costa, P.T. Jr., Williams, T.F., Somerfield, M., et al. (1996). *Recognition and initial assessment of Alzheimer's disease and related dementias.* No. 19. (AHCPR Publication No. 97-0702). Rockville, MD: U.S. Department of Health and Human Services. Public Health Services, Agency for Health Care Policy and Research.

Dellasega, C. (1992). Home health nurses' assessments of cognition. *Applied Nursing Research, 5*(3), 127-133.

+Folstein, M.F., Folstein, S.E., & McHugh, P.R. (1975). "Mini-Mental State" A practical method for grading the cognitive state of patients for the clinician. *Journal of Psychiatric Research, 12*(3), 189-198.

Foreman, M., Gilles, D., & Wagner, D. (1989). Impaired cognition in the critically ill elderly patient: Clinical implications. *Critical Care Nursing Quarterly, 12*(1), 61-73.

Gerdner, L.A., & Hall, G.R. (2001). Chronic confusion. In M. Maas, K. Buckwalter, M. Hardy, T. Tripp-Reimer, M. Titler & J. Specht (Eds.), *Nursing care of older adults: Diagnoses, outcomes & interventions* (pp. 421-441). St. Louis: Mosby.

Inaba-Roland, K., & Maricle, R. (1992). Assessing delirium in the acute care setting. *Heart & Lung, 21*(1), 48-55.

Kupferer, S., Uebele, J., & Levin, D. (1988). Geriatric ambulatory surgery patients: Assessing cognitive functions. *AORN Journal, 47*(3), 752-766.

Mason, P. (1989). Cognitive assessment parameters and tools for the critically injured adult. *Critical Care Nursing Clinics of North America, 1*(1), 45-53.

Souder, E., & O'Sullivan, P.S. (2000). Nursing documentation versus standardized assessment of cognitive status in hospitalized medical patients. *Applied Nursing Research, 13*(1), 29-36.

Strub, R.L., & Black, F.W. (2000). *The mental status examination in neurology* (4th ed.). Philadelphia: F.A. Davis.

Wakefield, B., Mentes, J., Mobily, P., Tripp-Reimer, T., Culp, K.R., Rapp, C.G., Gaspar, P., Kundrat, M., Wadle, K.R., & Akins, J. (2001). Acute confusion. In M. Maas, K. Buckwalter, M. Hardy, T. Tripp-Reimer, M. Titler & J. Specht (Eds.), *Nursing care of older adults: Diagnoses, outcomes & interventions* (pp. 442-454). St. Louis: Mosby.

# *Cognitive Orientation (0901)*

Domain-Physiologic Health (II)

Class-Neurocognitive (J)

Scale(s)-Severely compromised to Not compromised (a)

Care Recipient:

Data Source:

**C**

**Definition:** Ability to identify person, place, and time accurately

OUTCOME TARGET RATING:    Maintain at_____    Increase to_____

| Cognitive Orientation Overall Rating | Severely compromised 1 | Substantially compromised 2 | Moderately compromised 3 | Mildly compromised 4 | Not compromised 5 | |
|---|---|---|---|---|---|---|
| **INDICATORS:** | | | | | | |
| 090101 Identifies self | 1 | 2 | 3 | 4 | 5 | NA |
| 090102 Identifies significant other | 1 | 2 | 3 | 4 | 5 | NA |
| 090103 Identifies current place | 1 | 2 | 3 | 4 | 5 | NA |
| 090104 Identifies correct day | 1 | 2 | 3 | 4 | 5 | NA |
| 090105 Identifies correct month | 1 | 2 | 3 | 4 | 5 | NA |
| 090106 Identifies correct year | 1 | 2 | 3 | 4 | 5 | NA |
| 090107 Identifies correct season | 1 | 2 | 3 | 4 | 5 | NA |
| 090109 Identifies significant current events | 1 | 2 | 3 | 4 | 5 | NA |

*1st edition 1997; Revised 3rd edition*

## Outcome Content References:

Abraham, I.L., & Reel, S.J. (1993). Cognitive nursing interventions and long-term care residents: Effects on neurocognitive dimensions. *Archives of Psychiatric Nursing, 6*(6), 356-365.

Agostinelli, B., Demers, K., Garrigan, D., & Waszynski, C. (1994). Targeted interventions: Use of the mini-mental state exam. *Journal of Gerontological Nursing, 20*(8), 15-23.

Dellasega, C. (1992). Home health nurses' assessments of cognition. *Applied Nursing Research, 5*(3), 127-133.

Foreman, M., Theis, S., & Anderson, M.A. (1993). Adverse events in the hospitalized elderly. *Clinical Nursing Research, 2*(3) 360-370.

Foreman, M., Gilles, D., & Wagner, D. (1989). Impaired cognition in the critically ill elderly patient: Clinical implications. *Critical Care Nursing Quarterly, 12*(1), 61-73.

Gerdner, L.A., & Hall, G.R. (2001). Chronic confusion. In M. Maas, K. Buckwalter, M. Hardy, T. Tripp-Reimer, M. Titler & J. Specht (Eds.), *Nursing care of older adults: Diagnoses, outcomes & interventions* (pp. 421-441). St. Louis: Mosby.

Inaba-Roland, K., & Maricle, R. (1992). Assessing delirium in the acute care setting. *Heart & Lung, 21*(1), 48-55.

Mason, P. (1989). Cognitive assessment parameters and tools for the critically injured adult. *Critical Care Nursing Clinics of North America, 1*(1), 45-53.

Meyer, J., Xu, G., Thornby, J., Chowdhury, M., & Quach, M. (2002). Longitudinal analysis of abnormal domains comprising mild cognitive impairment (MCI) during aging. *Journal of Neurological Sciences, 201*(1-2), 19-25.

+Pfeiffer, E. (1975). A short portable mental status questionnaire for the assessment of organic brain deficit in elderly patients. *American Geriatrics Society, 23*(10), 433-441.

Souder, E., & O'Sullivan, P.S. (2000). Nursing documentation versus standardized assessment of cognitive status in hospitalized medical patients. *Applied Nursing Research, 13*(1), 29-36.

Strub, R.L., & Black, F.W. (2000). *The mental status examination in neurology* (4th ed.). Philadelphia: F.A. Davis.

C

# *Comfort Level (2100)*

*Domain-Perceived Health (V)*

*Class-Health & Life Quality (U)*

*Scale(s)-Not at all satisfied to Completely satisfied (s)*

*Care Recipient:*

*Data Source:*

**Definition:** Extent of positive perception of physical and psychological ease

OUTCOME TARGET RATING:    Maintain at_____    Increase to_____

| Comfort Level Overall Rating | Not at all satisfied 1 | Somewhat satisfied 2 | Moderately satisfied 3 | Very satisfied 4 | Completely satisfied 5 | |
|---|---|---|---|---|---|---|
| **INDICATORS:** | | | | | | |
| 210001  Physical well-being | 1 | 2 | 3 | 4 | 5 | NA |
| 210002  Symptom control | 1 | 2 | 3 | 4 | 5 | NA |
| 210003  Psychological well-being | 1 | 2 | 3 | 4 | 5 | NA |
| 210004  Physical surroundings | 1 | 2 | 3 | 4 | 5 | NA |
| 210010  Room temperature | 1 | 2 | 3 | 4 | 5 | NA |
| 210005  Social relationships | 1 | 2 | 3 | 4 | 5 | NA |
| 210006  Spiritual life | 1 | 2 | 3 | 4 | 5 | NA |
| 210007  Level of independence | 1 | 2 | 3 | 4 | 5 | NA |
| 210008  Pain control | 1 | 2 | 3 | 4 | 5 | NA |

*1st edition 1997; Revised 2nd edition 2000; Revised 3rd edition*

## Outcome Content References:

Fleming, C., Scanlon, C., & D'Agostino, N.S. (1987). A study of the comfort needs of patients with advanced cancer. *Cancer Nursing, 10*(5), 237-243.

Gropper, E.I. (1992). Promoting health by promoting comfort. *Nursing Forum, 27*(2), 5-8.

Hamilton, J. (1989). Comfort and the hospitalized chronically ill. *Journal of Gerontological Nursing, 15*(4), 28-33.

Kennedy, G.T. (1991). *A nursing investigation of comfort and comforting care of the acutely ill patient.* Unpublished doctoral dissertation, The University of Texas, Austin.

+Kolcaba, K.Y. (1992). Holistic comfort: Operationalizing the construct as a nurse-sensitive outcome. *Advances in Nursing Science, 15*(1), 1-10.

Mobily, P., & Herr, K.A. (2001). Pain. In M. Maas, K. Buckwalter, M. Hardy, T. Tripp-Reimer, M. Titler & J. Specht (Eds.), *Nursing care of older adults: Diagnoses, outcomes & interventions* (pp. 455-475). St. Louis: Mosby.

Morse, J.M. (2000). On comfort and comforting. *American Journal of Nursing, 100*(9), 34-38.

Slater, K. (1985). *Human comfort.* Springfield, IL: Charles C Thomas.

# *Comfortable Death (2007)*

Domain-Perceived Health (V)

Class-Health & Life Quality (U)

Scale(s)-Severely compromised to Not compromised (a) and Severe to None (n)

Care Recipient:

Data Source:

**C**

---

**Definition:** Physical and psychological ease with the impending end of life

OUTCOME TARGET RATING:     Maintain at_____     Increase to_____

| Comfortable Death Overall Rating | Severely compromised 1 | Substantially compromised 2 | Moderately compromised 3 | Mildly compromised 4 | Not compromised 5 | |
|---|---|---|---|---|---|---|
| **INDICATORS:** | | | | | | |
| 200701 Calm and tranquil affect | 1 | 2 | 3 | 4 | 5 | NA |
| 200702 Comfort | 1 | 2 | 3 | 4 | 5 | NA |
| 200703 Airway patency | 1 | 2 | 3 | 4 | 5 | NA |
| 200704 Body temperature | 1 | 2 | 3 | 4 | 5 | NA |
| 200705 Comfortable position | 1 | 2 | 3 | 4 | 5 | NA |
| 200706 Muscles of neck, trunk, and extremities relaxed | 1 | 2 | 3 | 4 | 5 | NA |
| 200707 Support from friends and family | 1 | 2 | 3 | 4 | 5 | NA |
| 200708 Personal hygiene | 1 | 2 | 3 | 4 | 5 | NA |
| 200709 Oral hygiene | 1 | 2 | 3 | 4 | 5 | NA |
| 200710 Food and fluid intake as desired | 1 | 2 | 3 | 4 | 5 | NA |

| | Severe | Substantial | Moderate | Mild | None | |
|---|---|---|---|---|---|---|
| 200711 Moaning | 1 | 2 | 3 | 4 | 5 | NA |
| 200712 Suffering | 1 | 2 | 3 | 4 | 5 | NA |
| 200713 Thrashing | 1 | 2 | 3 | 4 | 5 | NA |
| 200714 Pain | 1 | 2 | 3 | 4 | 5 | NA |
| 200715 Itching | 1 | 2 | 3 | 4 | 5 | NA |
| 200716 Retching or vomiting | 1 | 2 | 3 | 4 | 5 | NA |
| 200717 Diarrhea | 1 | 2 | 3 | 4 | 5 | NA |
| 200718 Labored breathing | 1 | 2 | 3 | 4 | 5 | NA |
| 200719 Air hunger | 1 | 2 | 3 | 4 | 5 | NA |

*3rd edition*

---

Outcome Content References:

Byock, I. (1997). Dying well: *The prospect for growth at the end of life*. Riverhead Books: New York.

Callanan, M., & Kelley, P. (1992). *Final gifts: Understanding the special awareness, needs, and communications of the dying*. Poseidon Press: New York.

Ferrell, B.R. (1999). Caring at the end of life. *Reflections, 25*(4), 31-37.

Kozier, B., Erb, G., Glais, K., & Wilkinson, J.M. (Eds.). (1995). *Fundamentals of nursing* (5th ed.). Redwood City, CA: Addison Wesley.

Maliski, S.L. (1994). Coping with loss and grief. In V.B. Bolander (Ed.), *Sorensen and Luckmann's basic nursing: A psychophysiologic approach* (3rd ed., pp. 1533-1558). Philadelphia: W.B. Saunders.

Murphy, P.A., & Price, D.M. (1995). 'ACT' taking a positive approach to end-of-life care. *American Journal of Nursing, 95*(3), 42-43.

Potter, P.A., & Perry, A.G. (2001). *Fundamentals of nursing* (5th ed.). St. Louis: Mosby.

Rinear, E. (1976). Confronting expected death. In P.S. Chaney (Ed.), *Dealing with Death and Dying* (pp. 63-72). Jenkintown, PA: Intermead Communications.

Tarzian, A.J. (2000). Caring for dying patients who have air hunger. *Journal of Nursing Scholarship, 32*(2), 137-143.

C

# Communication (0902)

Domain-Physiologic Health (II)

Class-Neurocognitive (J)

Scale(s)-Severely compromised to Not compromised (a)

Care Recipient:

Data Source:

**Definition:** Reception, interpretation, and expression of spoken, written and non-verbal messages

OUTCOME TARGET RATING:    Maintain at_____    Increase to_____

| Communication Overall Rating | Severely compromised 1 | Substantially compromised 2 | Moderately compromised 3 | Mildly compromised 4 | Not compromised 5 | |
|---|---|---|---|---|---|---|
| INDICATORS: | | | | | | |
| 090201 Use of written language | 1 | 2 | 3 | 4 | 5 | NA |
| 090202 Use of spoken language | 1 | 2 | 3 | 4 | 5 | NA |
| 090203 Use of pictures and drawings | 1 | 2 | 3 | 4 | 5 | NA |
| 090204 Use of sign language | 1 | 2 | 3 | 4 | 5 | NA |
| 090205 Use of non-verbal language | 1 | 2 | 3 | 4 | 5 | NA |
| 090206 Acknowledgment of messages received | 1 | 2 | 3 | 4 | 5 | NA |
| 090210 Accurate interpretation of messages received | 1 | 2 | 3 | 4 | 5 | NA |
| 090207 Directs messages appropriately | 1 | 2 | 3 | 4 | 5 | NA |
| 090208 Exchanges messages accurately with others | 1 | 2 | 3 | 4 | 5 | NA |

1st edition 1997; Revised 3rd edition (formerly Communication Ability)

## Outcome Content References:

Arnold, E., & Boggs, K. (1999). Interpersonal relationships: Professional communications skills for nurses (3rd ed.). Philadelphia: W.B. Saunders.

Emick-Herring, B. (2001). Impaired communication. In M. Maas, K. Buckwalter, M. Hardy, T. Tripp-Reimer, M. Titler & J. Specht (Eds.), Nursing care of older adults: Diagnoses, outcomes & interventions (pp. 664-678). St. Louis: Mosby.

Gresham, G.E., Duncan, P.W., Stason, W.B., et al. (1995). Post-stroke Rehabilitation. Clinical Practice Guideline, No. 16. (AHCPR Publication No. 95-0062). Rockville, MD: U.S. Department of Health and Human Services. Public Health Services, Agency for Health Care Policy and Research.

+Harvey, R., & Jellinek, H. (1981). Functional performance assessment: A program approach. Archives Physical Medicine & Rehabilitation, 62(9), 456-460.

Potter, P.A., & Perry, A.G. (2001). Fundamentals of nursing (5th ed.). St. Louis: Mosby.

Strub, R.L., & Black, F.W. (2000). The mental status examination in neurology (4th ed.). Philadelphia: F.A. Davis.

# *Communication: Expressive (0903)*

*Domain-Physiologic Health (II)*

*Class-Neurocognitive (J)*

*Scale(s)-Severely compromised to Not compromised (a)*

Care Recipient:

Data Source:

**C**

**Definition:** Expression of meaningful verbal and/or non-verbal messages

OUTCOME TARGET RATING:    Maintain at_____    Increase to_____

| Communication: Expressive Overall Rating | Severely compromised 1 | Substantially compromised 2 | Moderately compromised 3 | Mildly compromised 4 | Not compromised 5 | |
|---|---|---|---|---|---|---|
| **INDICATORS:** | | | | | | |
| 090301 Use of written language | 1 | 2 | 3 | 4 | 5 | NA |
| 090302 Use of spoken language: vocal | 1 | 2 | 3 | 4 | 5 | NA |
| 090303 Use of spoken language: esophageal | 1 | 2 | 3 | 4 | 5 | NA |
| 090304 Clarity of speech | 1 | 2 | 3 | 4 | 5 | NA |
| 090305 Use of pictures and drawings to communicate | 1 | 2 | 3 | 4 | 5 | NA |
| 090306 Use of sign language | 1 | 2 | 3 | 4 | 5 | NA |
| 090307 Use of non-verbal language | 1 | 2 | 3 | 4 | 5 | NA |
| 090308 Directs messages appropriately | 1 | 2 | 3 | 4 | 5 | NA |

*1st edition 1997; Revised 3rd edition (formerly Communication: Expressive Ability)*

## Outcome Content References:

Arnold, E., & Boggs, K. (1999). *Interpersonal relationships: Professional communications skills for nurses* (3rd ed.). Philadelphia: W.B. Saunders.

Emick-Herring, B. (2001). Impaired communication. In M. Maas, K. Buckwalter, M. Hardy, T. Tripp-Reimer, M. Titler & J. Specht (Eds.), *Nursing care of older adults: Diagnoses, outcomes & interventions* (pp. 664-678). St. Louis: Mosby.

+Harvey, R., & Jellinek, H. (1981). Functional performance assessment: A program approach. *Archives Physical Medicine & Rehabilitation, 62*(9), 456-460.

Potter, P.A., & Perry, A.G. (2001). *Fundamentals of nursing* (5th ed.). St. Louis: Mosby.

Strub, R.L., & Black, F.W. (2000). *The mental status examination in neurology* (4th ed.). Philadelphia: F.A. Davis.

C

# Communication: Receptive (0904)

*Domain-Physiologic Health (II)*

*Class-Neurocognitive (J)*

*Scale(s)-Severely compromised to Not compromised (a)*

Care Recipient:

Data Source:

**Definition:** Reception and interpretation of verbal and/or non-verbal messages

OUTCOME TARGET RATING:    Maintain at_____    Increase to_____

| Communication: Receptive Overall Rating | Severely compromised 1 | Substantially compromised 2 | Moderately compromised 3 | Mildly compromised 4 | Not compromised 5 | |
|---|---|---|---|---|---|---|
| **INDICATORS:** | | | | | | |
| 090401 Interpretation of written language | 1 | 2 | 3 | 4 | 5 | NA |
| 090402 Interpretation of spoken language | 1 | 2 | 3 | 4 | 5 | NA |
| 090403 Interpretation of pictures and drawings | 1 | 2 | 3 | 4 | 5 | NA |
| 090404 Interpretation of sign language | 1 | 2 | 3 | 4 | 5 | NA |
| 090405 Interpretation of non-verbal language | 1 | 2 | 3 | 4 | 5 | NA |
| 090406 Acknowledgment of messages received | 1 | 2 | 3 | 4 | 5 | NA |

*1st edition 1997; Revised 2nd edition 2000; Revised 3rd edition (formerly Communication: Receptive Ability)*

## Outcome Content References:

Arnold, E., & Boggs, K. (1999). *Interpersonal relationships: Professional communications skills for nurses* (3rd ed.). Philadelphia: W.B. Saunders.

Emick-Herring, B. (2001). Impaired communication. In M. Maas, K. Buckwalter, M. Hardy, T. Tripp-Reimer, M. Titler & J. Specht (Eds.), *Nursing care of older adults: Diagnoses, outcomes & interventions* (pp. 664-678). St. Louis: Mosby.

+Harvey, R., & Jellinek, H. (1981). Functional performance assessment: A program approach. *Archives Physical Medicine & Rehabilitation, 62*(9), 456-460.

Potter, P.A., & Perry, A.G. (2001). *Fundamentals of nursing* (5th ed.). St. Louis: Mosby.

Strub, R.L., & Black, F.W. (2000). *The mental status examination in neurology* (4th ed.). Philadelphia: F.A. Davis.

# *Community Competence (2700)*

Domain-Community Health (VII)

Class-Community Well-Being (b)

Scale(s)-Poor to Excellent (r)

Care Recipient:

Data Source:

**Definition**: Capacity of a community to collectively problem solve to achieve community goals

OUTCOME TARGET RATING:    Maintain at_____    Increase to_____

| Community Competence Overall Rating | Poor 1 | Fair 2 | Good 3 | Very good 4 | Excellent 5 | |
|---|---|---|---|---|---|---|

INDICATORS:

| | | Poor 1 | Fair 2 | Good 3 | Very good 4 | Excellent 5 | |
|---|---|---|---|---|---|---|---|
| 270001 | Participation rates in community activities | 1 | 2 | 3 | 4 | 5 | NA |
| 270003 | Common and competing interests among groups are considered when solving community problems | 1 | 2 | 3 | 4 | 5 | NA |
| 270004 | Representation of all segments of the community in problem solving | 1 | 2 | 3 | 4 | 5 | NA |
| 270005 | Community issues articulated in media | 1 | 2 | 3 | 4 | 5 | NA |
| 270006 | Community issues articulated in community forums | 1 | 2 | 3 | 4 | 5 | NA |
| 270007 | Focus on community versus individual agendas | 1 | 2 | 3 | 4 | 5 | NA |
| 270008 | Collaboration among community groups to identify problems and needs | 1 | 2 | 3 | 4 | 5 | NA |
| 270009 | Consensus on goals and priorities | 1 | 2 | 3 | 4 | 5 | NA |
| 270010 | Consensus on actions to implement the goals | 1 | 2 | 3 | 4 | 5 | NA |
| 270011 | Communication among members and groups | 1 | 2 | 3 | 4 | 5 | NA |
| 270012 | Effective use of conflict management strategies | 1 | 2 | 3 | 4 | 5 | NA |
| 270013 | Obtains external resources | 1 | 2 | 3 | 4 | 5 | NA |
| 270014 | Uses external resources appropriately | 1 | 2 | 3 | 4 | 5 | NA |
| 270015 | Flexibility of structures and processes that guide interaction and decision-making at community forum | 1 | 2 | 3 | 4 | 5 | NA |
| 270016 | Participation rate in local government elections | 1 | 2 | 3 | 4 | 5 | NA |
| 270017 | Participation rate in school elections | 1 | 2 | 3 | 4 | 5 | NA |
| 270018 | Members attendance at community forums | 1 | 2 | 3 | 4 | 5 | NA |
| 270019 | Attainment of community goals | 1 | 2 | 3 | 4 | 5 | NA |

*2nd edition 2000; Revised 3rd edition*

Outcome Content References:

Denham, A., Quinn, S., & Gamble, D. (1998). Community organizing for health promotion in the rural south: An exploration of community competence. *Family and Community Health, 21*(1), 1-21

Eng, E., & Parker, E. (1994). Measuring community competence in the Mississippi Delta: The interface between program evaluation and empowerment. *Health Education Quarterly, 21*(2), 119-120.

Goeppinger, L., Lassiter, P., & Wilcox, B. (1982). Community health is community competence. *Nursing Outlook, 30*(8), 464-467.

Stanhope, M., & Lancaster, J. (2000). *Community health nursing* (5th ed.). St. Louis: Mosby.

**C**

# *Community Disaster Readiness (2804)*

*Domain-Community Health (VII)*

*Class-Community Health Protection (c)*

*Scale-Not adequate to Totally adequate (f)*

*Care Recipient:*

*Dara Source*

**Definition:** Community preparedness to respond to a natural or man-made calamitous event

OUTCOME TARGET RATING:     Maintain at_____     Increase to_____

| Community Disaster Readiness Overall Rating | Not adequate 1 | Slightly adequate 2 | Moderately adequate 3 | Substantially adequate 4 | Totally adequate 5 | |
|---|---|---|---|---|---|---|
| 280401 Identification of potential types of disasters | 1 | 2 | 3 | 4 | 5 | NA |
| 280402 Surveillance to protect water | 1 | 2 | 3 | 4 | 5 | NA |
| 280403 Surveillance to protect food supplies | 1 | 2 | 3 | 4 | 5 | NA |
| 280404 Policy designating temporary administrative authority (e.g., governor, public health director) to protect public's health | 1 | 2 | 3 | 4 | 5 | NA |
| 280405 Public health laboratory facilities | 1 | 2 | 3 | 4 | 5 | NA |
| 280406 Public health disease surveillance system | 1 | 2 | 3 | 4 | 5 | NA |
| 280407 Health information system | 1 | 2 | 3 | 4 | 5 | NA |
| 280408 Mass immunization plan | 1 | 2 | 3 | 4 | 5 | NA |
| 280409 "Surge capacity" of hospital resources | 1 | 2 | 3 | 4 | 5 | NA |
| 280410 Current written plan for mobilization of personnel, evacuation, triage, community and resource appropriation | 1 | 2 | 3 | 4 | 5 | NA |
| 280411 Essential agency involvement in planning, including response drills | 1 | 2 | 3 | 4 | 5 | NA |
| 280412 Assignment of agency responsibilities in the event of disaster | 1 | 2 | 3 | 4 | 5 | NA |
| 280413 Ongoing training for disaster response personnel | 1 | 2 | 3 | 4 | 5 | NA |
| 280414 Plan to protect health and safety of rescue and recovery personnel | 1 | 2 | 3 | 4 | 5 | NA |
| 280415 Notification network to alert response personnel | 1 | 2 | 3 | 4 | 5 | NA |
| 280416 Notification network to alert government and support agencies | 1 | 2 | 3 | 4 | 5 | NA |
| 280417 Operational communication equipment | 1 | 2 | 3 | 4 | 5 | NA |
| 280418 Plan for alternative communication among disaster personnel and agency networks at local, state and federal levels | 1 | 2 | 3 | 4 | 5 | NA |
| 280419 Functional warning mechanisms and equipment | 1 | 2 | 3 | 4 | 5 | NA |

| Community Disaster Readiness—cont'd | | Not adequate | Slightly adequate | Moderately adequate | Substantially adequate | Totally adequate | |
|---|---|---|---|---|---|---|---|
| 280420 | Operational alternative utility resources | 1 | 2 | 3 | 4 | 5 | NA |
| 280421 | Emergency power backup | 1 | 2 | 3 | 4 | 5 | NA |
| 280422 | Equipment and supply availability | 1 | 2 | 3 | 4 | 5 | NA |
| 280423 | Equipment and supply maintenance | 1 | 2 | 3 | 4 | 5 | NA |
| 280424 | Designated, equipped shelters | 1 | 2 | 3 | 4 | 5 | NA |
| 280425 | Emergency shelter capacity | 1 | 2 | 3 | 4 | 5 | NA |
| 280426 | Regular mock or mass casualty drills with evaluation | 1 | 2 | 3 | 4 | 5 | NA |
| 280427 | Public education on disaster warning and response | 1 | 2 | 3 | 4 | 5 | NA |
| 280428 | Media plan for public information updates | 1 | 2 | 3 | 4 | 5 | NA |
| 280429 | Plan for documentation and coordination of victim health care | 1 | 2 | 3 | 4 | 5 | NA |
| 280430 | Plan for availability of mental health services for victims, response and health care personnel | 1 | 2 | 3 | 4 | 5 | NA |
| 280431 | Post disaster plan including victim follow-up and referral mechanism, response personnel debriefing and evaluation of response | 1 | 2 | 3 | 4 | 5 | NA |

*3rd edition*

Outcome Content References:

American Public Health Association. (2002). *One year after the terrorist attacks: Is public health prepared?* Washington, DC: Author.

American Red Cross. (2001). *Disaster services.* http://www.redcross.org/services/disaster.

Federal Emergency Management Agency. (2001). *Preparedness, training, and exercises.* http://www.fema.gov/pte.prepare.htm.

Hassmiller, S. (2000). Disaster management. In M. Stanhope & J. Lancaster (Eds.), *Community and public health nursing* (5th ed.). St. Louis: Mosby.

Landesman, L.Y. (2001). *Public health management of disasters: The practice guide.* Washington, DC: American Public Health Association.

Santamaria, B. (1995). Nursing in a disaster. In C.M. Smith & F.A. Maurer (Eds.). *Community health nursing: Theory and practice.* Philadelphia: W.B. Saunders.

C

# Community Health Status (2701)

*Domain-Community Health (VII)*

*Class-Community Well-Being (b)*

*Scale(s)-Poor to Excellent (r)*

*Care Recipient:*

*Data Source:*

**C**

---

**Definition:** General state of well being of a community or population

---

OUTCOME TARGET RATING:    Maintain at_____    Increase to_____

| Community Health Status Overall Rating | Poor 1 | Fair 2 | Good 3 | Very good 4 | Excellent 5 | |
|---|---|---|---|---|---|---|

INDICATORS:

| | | Poor 1 | Fair 2 | Good 3 | Very good 4 | Excellent 5 | |
|---|---|---|---|---|---|---|---|
| 270111 | Health status of infants | 1 | 2 | 3 | 4 | 5 | NA |
| 270112 | Health status of children | 1 | 2 | 3 | 4 | 5 | NA |
| 270113 | Health status of adolescents | 1 | 2 | 3 | 4 | 5 | NA |
| 270114 | Health status of adults | 1 | 2 | 3 | 4 | 5 | NA |
| 270115 | Health status of elders | 1 | 2 | 3 | 4 | 5 | NA |
| 270132 | Health status of minority populations | 1 | 2 | 3 | 4 | 5 | NA |
| 270101 | Participation rates in preventive health services | 1 | 2 | 3 | 4 | 5 | NA |
| 270102 | Prevalence of health promotion programs | 1 | 2 | 3 | 4 | 5 | NA |
| 270103 | Prevalence of health protection programs | 1 | 2 | 3 | 4 | 5 | NA |
| 270104 | School enrollment rate | 1 | 2 | 3 | 4 | 5 | NA |
| 270105 | School attendance rate | 1 | 2 | 3 | 4 | 5 | NA |
| 270106 | Participation rates in worksite health programs | 1 | 2 | 3 | 4 | 5 | NA |
| 270107 | Participation rates in community health programs | 1 | 2 | 3 | 4 | 5 | NA |
| 270108 | Participation rates in school health programs | 1 | 2 | 3 | 4 | 5 | NA |
| 270109 | Evidence of health protection measures (e.g., immunizations, fluoridation, and sanitation) | 1 | 2 | 3 | 4 | 5 | NA |
| 270110 | Members with adequate health insurance coverage | 1 | 2 | 3 | 4 | 5 | NA |
| 270116 | Attendance at programs for healthy pregnancy | 1 | 2 | 3 | 4 | 5 | NA |
| 270117 | Compliance with environmental health standards | 1 | 2 | 3 | 4 | 5 | NA |
| 270118 | Rate of loss of two or more ADLs* | 1 | 2 | 3 | 4 | 5 | NA |
| 270124 | Mortality rates | 1 | 2 | 3 | 4 | 5 | NA |
| 270133 | Maternal mortality rates | 1 | 2 | 3 | 4 | 5 | NA |
| 270119 | Morbidity rates | 1 | 2 | 3 | 4 | 5 | NA |
| 270120 | Mental health illness rates | 1 | 2 | 3 | 4 | 5 | NA |
| 270125 | Chronic disease rates | 1 | 2 | 3 | 4 | 5 | NA |
| 270134 | Substance abuse rates adults | 1 | 2 | 3 | 4 | 5 | NA |
| 270135 | Substance abuse rates adolescents | 1 | 2 | 3 | 4 | 5 | NA |
| 270136 | Smoking rates | 1 | 2 | 3 | 4 | 5 | NA |
| 270126 | Sexually transmitted disease rates | 1 | 2 | 3 | 4 | 5 | NA |
| 270137 | Preterm birth rates | 1 | 2 | 3 | 4 | 5 | NA |
| 270138 | Low birth weights rates | 1 | 2 | 3 | 4 | 5 | NA |
| 270121 | Injury rates | 1 | 2 | 3 | 4 | 5 | NA |

| Community Health Status—cont'd | | Poor | Fair | Good | Very good | Excellent | |
|---|---|---|---|---|---|---|---|
| 270122 | Crime statistics | 1 | 2 | 3 | 4 | 5 | NA |
| 270139 | Homicide rates | 1 | 2 | 3 | 4 | 5 | NA |
| 270127 | Health surveillance data systems in place | 1 | 2 | 3 | 4 | 5 | NA |
| 270128 | Community health standards for health measurement and evaluation are defined | 1 | 2 | 3 | 4 | 5 | NA |
| 270129 | Monitoring of community health standards for health measurement and evaluation | 1 | 2 | 3 | 4 | 5 | NA |
| 270130 | Community demographics represented in health care planning and evaluation | 1 | 2 | 3 | 4 | 5 | NA |

*ADLs: Activities of daily living

*2nd edition 2000; Revised 3rd edition*

## Outcome Content References:

Deal, L. (1994). The effectiveness of community health nursing interventions: A literature review. *Public Health Nursing, 2*(5), 315-322.

Stanhope, M., & Lancaster, J. (2000). *Community health nursing* (5th ed.). St. Louis: Mosby.

Stoto, M. (1997). Sharing responsibility for the public's health: A new perspective from the Institute of Medicine. *Journal of Public Health Management and Practice, 3*(5), 22-34.

U.S. Department of Health and Human Services. (2000). *Healthy people 2010.* Washington, DC: Government Printing Office.

U.S. Department of Health and Human Services. (1998). *Clinician's handbook of preventive services: Put prevention into practice* (2nd ed.). Washington: DC: Government Printing Office.

U.S. Department of Health and Human Services. (1991). *Healthy people 2000: National health promotion and disease prevention objectives.* (DHHS Pub No (PHS) 91-50012). Washington DC: Government Printing Office.

U.S. Preventive Services Task Force. (1996). *Guide to clinical preventive services*, (2nd ed.). Baltimore: Williams & Wilkins.

C

C

# *Community Health Status: Immunity (2800)*

*Domain-Community Health (VII)*

*Class-Community Well-Being (b)*

*Scale(s)-Poor to Excellent (r)*

Care Recipient:

Data Source:

**Definition:** Resistance of community members to the invasion and spread of an infectious agent that could threaten public health

OUTCOME TARGET RATING:     Maintain at_____     Increase to_____

| Community Health Status: Immunity Overall Rating | Poor 1 | Fair 2 | Good 3 | Very good 4 | Excellent 5 | |
|---|---|---|---|---|---|---|

INDICATORS:

| | | Poor 1 | Fair 2 | Good 3 | Very good 4 | Excellent 5 | |
|---|---|---|---|---|---|---|---|
| 280001 | Immunization rates equal to or greater than current national standards | 1 | 2 | 3 | 4 | 5 | NA |
| 280002 | Incidence of vaccine preventable disease at or below recommended national rate | 1 | 2 | 3 | 4 | 5 | NA |
| 280003 | Prevalence of vaccine preventable disease at or below recommended national rate | 1 | 2 | 3 | 4 | 5 | NA |
| 280004 | Surveillance of immunization status in schools | 1 | 2 | 3 | 4 | 5 | NA |
| 280005 | Surveillance of immunization status in group living facilities (e.g., jails, group homes) | 1 | 2 | 3 | 4 | 5 | NA |
| 280006 | Surveillance of communicable disease | 1 | 2 | 3 | 4 | 5 | NA |
| 280007 | Screening of at-risk populations for infections | 1 | 2 | 3 | 4 | 5 | NA |
| 280008 | Compliance with immunization recommendations | 1 | 2 | 3 | 4 | 5 | NA |
| 280009 | Public education on the risks and benefits of immunization | 1 | 2 | 3 | 4 | 5 | NA |
| 280010 | Availability of low cost immunizations | 1 | 2 | 3 | 4 | 5 | NA |
| 280011 | Enforcement of preschool immunizations | 1 | 2 | 3 | 4 | 5 | NA |

*2nd edition 2000; Revised 3rd edition (formerly Community Health: Immunity)*

Outcome Content References:

Stanhope, M., & Lancaster, J. (2000). *Community health nursing* (5th ed.). St. Louis: Mosby.

U.S. Department of Health and Human Services. (2000). *Healthy people 2010*. Washington, DC: Government Printing Office.

U.S. Department of Health and Human Services. (1998). *Clinician's handbook of preventive services: Put prevention into practice* (2nd ed.). Washington: DC: Government Printing Office.

U.S. Department of Health and Human Services. (1991). *Healthy people 2000: National health promotion and disease prevention objectives*. DHHS Pub No (PHS) 91-50012. Washington DC: Government Printing Office.

U.S. Preventive Services Task Force. (1996). *Guide to clinical preventive services*, (2nd ed.) Baltimore: Williams & Wilkins.

# Community Risk Control: Chronic Disease (2801)

Domain-Community Health (VII)

Class-Community Health Protection (c)

Scale(s)-Poor to Excellent (r)

Care Recipient:

Data Source:

**C**

**Definition:** Community actions to reduce the risk of chronic diseases and related complications

OUTCOME TARGET RATING:      Maintain at_____      Increase to_____

| Community Risk Control: Chronic Disease Overall Rating | Poor 1 | Fair 2 | Good 3 | Very good 4 | Excellent 5 | |
|---|---|---|---|---|---|---|

INDICATORS:

| | | | | | | |
|---|---|---|---|---|---|---|
| 280101 | Provision of public education programs on chronic disease | 1 | 2 | 3 | 4 | 5 | NA |
| 280102 | Target population participation rates in risk reduction programs | 1 | 2 | 3 | 4 | 5 | NA |
| 280103 | Availability of preventive screening programs | 1 | 2 | 3 | 4 | 5 | NA |
| 280104 | Target population participation rates in preventive screening programs | 1 | 2 | 3 | 4 | 5 | NA |
| 280105 | Availability of chronic disease self-management education programs | 1 | 2 | 3 | 4 | 5 | NA |
| 280106 | Proportion of target population participation rates in chronic disease self-management education programs | 1 | 2 | 3 | 4 | 5 | NA |
| 280107 | Availability of chronic disease health care services | 1 | 2 | 3 | 4 | 5 | NA |
| 280108 | Target population obtaining chronic disease health care services | 1 | 2 | 3 | 4 | 5 | NA |
| 280109 | Monitoring of incidence and prevalence of chronic disease | 1 | 2 | 3 | 4 | 5 | NA |
| 280110 | Monitoring of chronic disease morbidity, mortality, and complications | 1 | 2 | 3 | 4 | 5 | NA |
| 280111 | Compliance with national standards for chronic disease prevention and management | 1 | 2 | 3 | 4 | 5 | NA |
| 280112 | Incidence of chronic disease at or below recommended state or national rates | 1 | 2 | 3 | 4 | 5 | NA |
| 280114 | Prevalence of chronic disease at or below recommended state or national rates | 1 | 2 | 3 | 4 | 5 | NA |
| 280115 | Public and private policies that promote health and prevent disease | 1 | 2 | 3 | 4 | 5 | NA |
| 280116 | Procurement and allocation of funding for chronic disease prevention programs | 1 | 2 | 3 | 4 | 5 | NA |
| 280117 | Evidence of advocacy efforts for prevention, treatment, and management of chronic illness | 1 | 2 | 3 | 4 | 5 | NA |

*2nd edition 2000; Revised 3rd edition*

Outcome Content References:

Clemen-Stone, S., McGuire, S.L., & Eigsti, D.G. (2002). *Comprehensive community health nursing: Family, aggregate, and community practice* (6th ed.). St. Louis: Mosby.

Stanhope, M., & Lancaster, J. (2000). *Community health nursing* (5th ed.). St. Louis: Mosby.

U.S. Department of Health and Human Services. (2000). *Healthy people 2010.* Washington, DC: Government Printing Office.

U.S. Department of Health and Human Services. (1991). *Healthy people 2000: National health promotion and disease prevention objectives.* DHHS Pub No (PHS) 91-50012. Washington DC: Government Printing Office.

U.S. Preventive Services Task Force. (1996). *Guide to clinical preventive services* (2nd ed.). Baltimore: Williams & Wilkins.

C

## Community Risk Control: Communicable Disease (2802)

*Domain-Community Health (VII)*

*Class-Community Health Protection (c)*

*Scale(s)-Poor to Excellent (r)*

Care Recipient:

Data Source:

**Definition:** Community actions to eliminate or reduce the spread of infectious agents that threaten public health

OUTCOME TARGET RATING: Maintain at_____ Increase to_____

| Community Risk Control: Communicable Disease Overall Rating | Poor 1 | Fair 2 | Good 3 | Very good 4 | Excellent 5 | |
|---|---|---|---|---|---|---|

INDICATORS:

| | | | | | | | |
|---|---|---|---|---|---|---|---|
| 280201 | Screening of all targeted high risk groups | 1 | 2 | 3 | 4 | 5 | NA |
| 280202 | Surveillance for infectious disease outbreaks including a system of data collection, reporting and follow-up | 1 | 2 | 3 | 4 | 5 | NA |
| 280203 | Investigation and notification of contacts concerning risk for infectious disease | 1 | 2 | 3 | 4 | 5 | NA |
| 280204 | Reporting disease occurrences as mandated by state laws and regulations | 1 | 2 | 3 | 4 | 5 | NA |
| 280205 | Availability of referral and treatment services for infected individuals | 1 | 2 | 3 | 4 | 5 | NA |
| 280206 | Provision of products to decrease disease spread | 1 | 2 | 3 | 4 | 5 | NA |
| 280207 | Established polices and programs for assuring safe food storage, handling, and preparation | 1 | 2 | 3 | 4 | 5 | NA |
| 280208 | Water testing consistent with local, state and federal regulations | 1 | 2 | 3 | 4 | 5 | NA |
| 280209 | Promotion of community-wide immunization | 1 | 2 | 3 | 4 | 5 | NA |
| 280210 | Enforcement of infection surveillance and control programs | 1 | 2 | 3 | 4 | 5 | NA |
| 280211 | Availability of chemoprophylaxis for travelers | 1 | 2 | 3 | 4 | 5 | NA |
| 280212 | Evidence of environmental controls | 1 | 2 | 3 | 4 | 5 | NA |
| 280213 | Enforcement of environmental monitoring policies | 1 | 2 | 3 | 4 | 5 | NA |
| 280214 | Enforcement of domestic animal vaccination | 1 | 2 | 3 | 4 | 5 | NA |
| 280215 | Availability of health services to treat communicable diseases | 1 | 2 | 3 | 4 | 5 | NA |
| 280216 | Access to health services | 1 | 2 | 3 | 4 | 5 | NA |
| 280217 | Public education about transmission and spread of infectious disease | 1 | 2 | 3 | 4 | 5 | NA |
| 280218 | Policies supporting control of infectious disease | 1 | 2 | 3 | 4 | 5 | NA |

*2nd edition 2000; Revised 3rd edition*

Outcome Content References:

Stanhope, M., & Lancaster, J. (2000). *Community health nursing* (5th ed.). St. Louis: Mosby.

U.S. Department of Health and Human Services. (2000). *Healthy people 2010.* Washington, DC: Government Printing Office.

U.S. Department of Health and Human Services. (1998). *Clinician's handbook of preventive services: Put prevention into practice* (2nd ed.). Washington: DC: Government Printing Office.

U.S. Department of Health and Human Services. (1991). *Healthy people 2000: National health promotion and disease prevention objectives.* (DHHS Pub No (PHS) 91-50012). Washington DC: Government Printing Office.

U.S. Preventive Services Task Force. (1996). *Guide to clinical preventive services* (2nd ed.). Baltimore: Williams & Wilkins.

# Community Risk Control: Lead Exposure (2803)

Domain-Community Health (VII)

Class-Community Health Protection (c)

Scale(s)-Poor to Excellent (r)

Care Recipient:

Data Source:

C

**Definition:** Community actions to reduce lead exposure and poisoning

OUTCOME TARGET RATING:    Maintain at_____    Increase to_____

| Community Risk Control: Lead Exposure Overall Rating | Poor 1 | Fair 2 | Good 3 | Very good 4 | Excellent 5 | |
|---|---|---|---|---|---|---|
| INDICATORS: | | | | | | |
| 280314  Problem assessment by community stake-holders and policy makers | 1 | 2 | 3 | 4 | 5 | NA |
| 280315  Planning and organization of lead screening programs that includes focus on preschools | 1 | 2 | 3 | 4 | 5 | NA |
| 280316  Culturally appropriate marketing of screening programs to high-risk groups | 1 | 2 | 3 | 4 | 5 | NA |
| 280301  Use of lead screening programs by tar-geted high-risk groups, especially children under age 5 | 1 | 2 | 3 | 4 | 5 | NA |
| 280317  Planning and organization of referral and treatment services for exposed individuals | 1 | 2 | 3 | 4 | 5 | NA |
| 280302  Referral of exposed individuals to treatment | 1 | 2 | 3 | 4 | 5 | NA |
| 280318  Treatment of individuals with exposure to lead | 1 | 2 | 3 | 4 | 5 | NA |
| 280303  Surveillance for sources of lead | 1 | 2 | 3 | 4 | 5 | NA |
| 280304  Abatement of known lead sources in the community | 1 | 2 | 3 | 4 | 5 | NA |
| 280305  Identification of programs to identify nutritional deficiencies in all targeted high-risk groups | 1 | 2 | 3 | 4 | 5 | NA |
| 280306  Adequacy of programs to correct nutri-tional deficiencies in all targeted high-risk groups | 1 | 2 | 3 | 4 | 5 | NA |
| 280307  Provision of culturally-appropriate public education about lead poisoning risks and exposure prevention | 1 | 2 | 3 | 4 | 5 | NA |
| 280319  Participation rates of high-risk groups in education programs | 1 | 2 | 3 | 4 | 5 | NA |
| 280308  Policies that require the removal of lead-based paint from all buildings | 1 | 2 | 3 | 4 | 5 | NA |
| 280309  Funds dedicated to screening and elimi-nation of lead hazards | 1 | 2 | 3 | 4 | 5 | NA |
| 280310  Incidence of elevated lead levels at or below recommended national standards | 1 | 2 | 3 | 4 | 5 | NA |
| 280311  Enforcement of home-buyer notification | 1 | 2 | 3 | 4 | 5 | NA |
| 280320  Advocacy on behalf of renters of pre-1950 homes | 1 | 2 | 3 | 4 | 5 | NA |
| 280312  Enforcement of emission standards | 1 | 2 | 3 | 4 | 5 | NA |

2nd edition 2000; Revised 3rd edition

Outcome Content References:

Morgan, L. (1996). Children and lead: A model of care for community health providers. Family and Community Health, 19(1), 42-48.

Needleman, H. (1998). Childhood lead poisoning: The promise and abandonment of primary prevention. American Journal of Public Health, 88(12), 1871-1876.

Needleman, H., Schell. A., Bellinger, D., Leviton, A., & Allred, E. (1990). The long-term effects of exposure to low doses of lead in childhood. The New England Journal of Medicine, 22(2), 83-90.

Schwartz, J. (1994). Societal benefits of reducing lead exposure. Environmental Research, 66(1), 105-124.

C

# Community Risk Control: Violence (2805)

Domain-Community Health (VII)

Class-Community Health Protection (c)

Scale(s)-Poor to Excellent (r)

Care Recipient:

Data Source:

**Definition:** Community actions to eliminate or reduce intentional violent acts resulting in serious physical or psychological harm

OUTCOME TARGET RATING:     Maintain at_____     Increase to_____

| Community Risk Control: Violence Overall Rating | Poor 1 | Fair 2 | Good 3 | Very good 4 | Excellent 5 | |
|---|---|---|---|---|---|---|
| **INDICATORS:** | | | | | | |
| 280501 Systematic assessment of at-risk groups | 1 | 2 | 3 | 4 | 5 | NA |
| 280502 Support programs for high-risk groups | 1 | 2 | 3 | 4 | 5 | NA |
| 280503 Intervention programs for high-risk groups | 1 | 2 | 3 | 4 | 5 | NA |
| 280504 Existence of weapon control policies | 1 | 2 | 3 | 4 | 5 | NA |
| 280505 Enforcement of weapon control policies | 1 | 2 | 3 | 4 | 5 | NA |
| 280506 Strategies to control violent content in the media | 1 | 2 | 3 | 4 | 5 | NA |
| 280507 Control of violent content in the media | 1 | 2 | 3 | 4 | 5 | NA |
| 280508 Educational programs on violence prevention | 1 | 2 | 3 | 4 | 5 | NA |
| 280509 Competence in recognizing violence by community leaders | 1 | 2 | 3 | 4 | 5 | NA |
| 280510 Competence in managing violence by community leaders | 1 | 2 | 3 | 4 | 5 | NA |
| 280511 Acceptance of population diversity | 1 | 2 | 3 | 4 | 5 | NA |
| 280512 Enforcement of laws against hate crimes by community leaders | 1 | 2 | 3 | 4 | 5 | NA |
| 280513 Systematic monitoring of community violence levels | 1 | 2 | 3 | 4 | 5 | NA |

*3rd edition*

## Outcome Content References:

Bell, C.C. (1997). Community violence: Causes, prevention, and intervention. *Journal of the National Medical Association, 89*(10), 657-662.

Campbell, J., & Landenburger, K. (2000). Violence and human abuse. In M. Stanhope & J. Lancaster (Eds.), *Community and public health nursing* (5th ed., pp. 747-778). St. Louis: Mosby.

Jones, F.C. (1997). Community violence, children and youth: Considerations for programs, policy and nursing roles. *Pediatric Nursing, 23*(2), 131-137.

Kroposki, M., & Alexander, J. (1998). Measuring community health nursing outcomes. South Carolina Nurse, 5(4), 17-18.

# Community Violence Level (2702)

*Domain-Community Health (VII)*

*Class-Community Well-Being (b)*

*Scale(s)-Poor to Excellent (r)*

*Care Recipient:*

*Data Source:*

**Definition**: Incidence of violent acts compared with local, state or national values

OUTCOME TARGET RATING:     Maintain at_____     Increase to_____

| Community Violence Level Overall Rating | Poor 1 | Fair 2 | Good 3 | Very good 4 | Excellent 5 | |
|---|---|---|---|---|---|---|

INDICATORS:

| | | Poor 1 | Fair 2 | Good 3 | Very good 4 | Excellent 5 | |
|---|---|---|---|---|---|---|---|
| 270201 | Homicide rate | 1 | 2 | 3 | 4 | 5 | NA |
| 270202 | Suicide rate | 1 | 2 | 3 | 4 | 5 | NA |
| 270203 | Sexual assault rate | 1 | 2 | 3 | 4 | 5 | NA |
| 270204 | Physical assault rate | 1 | 2 | 3 | 4 | 5 | NA |
| 270205 | Child abuse rate | 1 | 2 | 3 | 4 | 5 | NA |
| 270206 | Elder abuse rate | 1 | 2 | 3 | 4 | 5 | NA |
| 270207 | Partner abuse rate | 1 | 2 | 3 | 4 | 5 | NA |
| 270208 | Hate crime rate | 1 | 2 | 3 | 4 | 5 | NA |

*3rd edition*

Outcome Content References:

Bell, C.C. (1997). Community violence: Causes, prevention, and intervention. *Journal of the National Medical Association, 89*(10), 657-662.

Campbell, J., & Landenburger, K. (2000). Violence and human abuse. In M. Stanhope & J. Lancaster (Eds.), *Community and public health nursing* (5th ed., pp. 747-778). St. Louis: Mosby.

Jones, F.C. (1997). Community violence, children and youth: Considerations for programs, policy and nursing roles. *Pediatric Nursing, 23*(2), 131-137.

Lutenbacher, M., Cooper, W.O., & Faccia, K. (2002). Planning youth violence prevention efforts: Decision-making across community sectors. *Journal of Adolescent Health, 30*(5), 346-354.

U.S. Department of Health and Human Services. (2000). *Healthy People 2010*. Washington, DC: Government Printing Office.

C

# *Compliance Behavior (1601)*

Domain-Health Knowledge & Behavior (IV)

Class-Health Behavior (Q)

Scale(s)-Never demonstrated to Consistently demonstrated (m)

Care Recipient:

Data Source:

**Definition:** Personal actions to promote wellness, recovery, and rehabilitation based on professional advice

OUTCOME TARGET RATING:   Maintain at_____   Increase to_____

| Compliance Behavior Overall Rating | | Never demonstrated 1 | Rarely demonstrated 2 | Sometimes demonstrated 3 | Often demonstrated 4 | Consistently demonstrated 5 | |
|---|---|---|---|---|---|---|---|
| INDICATORS: | | | | | | | |
| 160104 | Accepts medical diagnosis | 1 | 2 | 3 | 4 | 5 | NA |
| 160101 | Seeks current information about illness and treatment | 1 | 2 | 3 | 4 | 5 | NA |
| 160102 | Discusses prescribed treatment regimen with health care professional | 1 | 2 | 3 | 4 | 5 | NA |
| 160103 | Performs treatment regimen as prescribed | 1 | 2 | 3 | 4 | 5 | NA |
| 160105 | Keeps appointments with health care professional | 1 | 2 | 3 | 4 | 5 | NA |
| 160111 | Reports changes in symptoms to health care professional | 1 | 2 | 3 | 4 | 5 | NA |
| 160106 | Modifies treatment regimen as directed by a health care professional | 1 | 2 | 3 | 4 | 5 | NA |
| 160112 | Monitors treatment response | 1 | 2 | 3 | 4 | 5 | NA |
| 160113 | Monitors medication response | 1 | 2 | 3 | 4 | 5 | NA |
| 160107 | Performs self-screening when directed | 1 | 2 | 3 | 4 | 5 | NA |
| 160108 | Performs ADLs* as prescribed | 1 | 2 | 3 | 4 | 5 | NA |
| 160109 | Seeks external reinforcement for performance of health behaviors | 1 | 2 | 3 | 4 | 5 | NA |

*ADLs = Activities of daily living.

*1st edition 1997; Revised 3rd edition*

## Outcome Content References:

Barotsky, I., Sergenbaker, P., & Mills, M. (1979). Compliance and quality of life assessment. In J. Cohen (Ed.), *New directions in patient compliance* (pp. 59-74). Lexington, MA: D.C. Health.

Burkhart, P.V., Dunbar-Jacob, J.M., & Rohay, J.M. (2001). Accuracy of children's self-reported adherence to treatment. *Journal of Nursing Scholarship, 33*(1), 27-32.

+DiMatteo, M.R., Hays, R.D., & Sherbourne, C.D. (1992). Adherence to cancer regimens: Implications for treating the older patient. *Oncology, 6*(2 Suppl.), 50-57.

Epstein, L., & Cluss, P.A. (1982). A behavioral perspective on adherence to long-term medical regimens. *Journal of Consulting and Clinical Psychology, 50*, 950-971.

Folden, S.L. (1993). Definitions of health and health goals of participants in a community-based pulmonary rehabilitation program. *Public Health Nursing, 10*(1), 31-35.

Heiby, E., & Carlson, J. (1986). The health compliance model. *The Journal of Compliance in Health Care, 1*(2), 135-152.

Jensen, L., & Allen, M. (1993). Wellness: The dialect of illness. *Image-the Journal of Nursing Scholarship, 25*(3), 220-224.

King, I.M. (1988). Measuring health goal attainment in patients. In C.F. Waltz & O.L. Strickland (Eds.), *Measurement of nursing outcomes* (Vol. I, pp. 108-127). New York: Springer.

Kravits, R., et al. (1993). Recall of recommendations and adherence to advice among patients with chronic medical conditions. *Archives of Internal Medicine, 153*(16), 1869-1878.

Oldridge, N. (1982). Compliance and exercise in primary and secondary prevention of coronary heart disease: A review. *Preventive Medicine, 11*(1), 56-70.

C

# Concentration (0905)

Domain-Physiologic Health (II)

Class-Neurocognitive (J)

Scale(s)-Severely compromised to Not compromised (a)

Care Recipient:

Data Source:

**C**

**Definition:** Ability to focus on a specific stimulus

OUTCOME TARGET RATING:     Maintain at_____     Increase to_____

| Concentration Overall Rating | Severely compromised 1 | Substantially compromised 2 | Moderately compromised 3 | Mildly compromised 4 | Not compromised 5 | |
|---|---|---|---|---|---|---|
| INDICATORS: | | | | | | |
| 090501 Maintains attention | 1 | 2 | 3 | 4 | 5 | NA |
| 090502 Maintains focus without being distracted | 1 | 2 | 3 | 4 | 5 | NA |
| 090503 Responds appropriately to visual cues | 1 | 2 | 3 | 4 | 5 | NA |
| 090504 Responds appropriately to auditory cues | 1 | 2 | 3 | 4 | 5 | NA |
| 090505 Responds appropriately to tactile cues | 1 | 2 | 3 | 4 | 5 | NA |
| 090506 Responds appropriately to olfactory cues | 1 | 2 | 3 | 4 | 5 | NA |
| 090507 Responds appropriately to language cues | 1 | 2 | 3 | 4 | 5 | NA |
| 090508 Spells 'world' backwards | 1 | 2 | 3 | 4 | 5 | NA |
| 090509 Counts backward from 20 by 3s, or from 100 by 7s | 1 | 2 | 3 | 4 | 5 | NA |
| 090510 Names the months of the year backward, starting with January | 1 | 2 | 3 | 4 | 5 | NA |
| 090511 Draws a circle | 1 | 2 | 3 | 4 | 5 | NA |
| 090514 Draws a triangle | 1 | 2 | 3 | 4 | 5 | NA |
| 090512 Draws a pentagon | 1 | 2 | 3 | 4 | 5 | NA |

*1st edition 1997; Revised 3rd edition*

Outcome Content References:

Abraham, I., & Reel, S. (1993). Cognitive nursing interventions with long-term care residents: Effects on neurocognitive dimensions. *Archives of Psychiatric Nursing, 6*(6), 356-365.

Agostinelli, B., Demers, K., Garrigan, D., & Waszynski, C. (1994). Targeted interventions: Use of the Mini-Mental State Exam. *Journal of Gerontological Nursing, 20*(8), 15-23.

Costa, P.T. Jr., Williams, T.F., Somerfield, M., et al. (1996). *Recognition and initial assessment of Alzheimer's disease and related dementias.* No. 19. (AHCPR Publication No. 97-0702). Rockville, MD: U.S. Department of Health and Human Services. Public Health Services, Agency for Health Care Policy and Research.

Dellasega, C. (1992). Home health nurses' assessments of cognition. *Applied Nursing Research, 5*(3), 127-133.

+Folstein, M.F., Folstein, S.E., & McHugh, P.R. (1975). "Mini-Mental State"-A practical method for grading the cognitive state of patients for the clinician. *Journal of Psychiatric Research, 12*(3), 189-198.

Foreman, M., Gilles, D., & Wagner, D. (1989). Impaired cognition in the critically ill elderly patient: Clinical implications. *Critical Care Nursing Quarterly, 12*(1), 61-73.

Kupferer, S., Uebele, J., & Levin, D. (1988). Geriatric ambulatory surgery patients: Assessing cognitive functions. *AORN Journal, 47*(3), 752-766.

Mason, P. (1989). Cognitive assessment parameters and tools for the critically injured adult. *Critical Care Nursing Clinics of North America, 1*(1), 45-53.

Norris, J. A., & Hoffman, P. R. (1996). Attaining, sustaining, and focusing attention: intervention for children with ADHD. *Seminars in Speech & Language, 17*(1), 59-71.

O'Keeffe, S.T., & Gosney, Margot A. (1997). Assessing attentiveness in older hospital patients: Global assessment versus tests of attention. *Journal of the American Geriatrics Society, 45*(4), 470-473.

Strub, R.L., & Black, F.W. (2000). *The mental status examination in neurology* (4th ed.). Philadelphia: F.A. Davis.

C

C

# *Coordinated Movement (0212)*

Domain-Functional Health (I)

Class-Mobility (C)

Scale(s)-Severely compromised to Not compromised (a)

Care Recipient:

Data Source:

**Definition:** Ability of muscles to work together voluntarily for purposeful movement

OUTCOME TARGET RATING:     Maintain at_____     Increase to_____

| Coordinated Movement Overall Rating | Severely compromised 1 | Substantially compromised 2 | Moderately compromised 3 | Mildly compromised 4 | Not compromised 5 | |
|---|---|---|---|---|---|---|
| **INDICATORS:** | | | | | | |
| 021201 Strength of muscle contraction | 1 | 2 | 3 | 4 | 5 | NA |
| 021202 Muscle tone | 1 | 2 | 3 | 4 | 5 | NA |
| 021203 Speed of movement | 1 | 2 | 3 | 4 | 5 | NA |
| 021204 Smooth movement | 1 | 2 | 3 | 4 | 5 | NA |
| 021205 Control of movement | 1 | 2 | 3 | 4 | 5 | NA |
| 021206 Steadiness of movement | 1 | 2 | 3 | 4 | 5 | NA |
| 021207 Balanced movement | 1 | 2 | 3 | 4 | 5 | NA |
| 021208 Muscle tension | 1 | 2 | 3 | 4 | 5 | NA |
| 021209 Movement in desired direction | 1 | 2 | 3 | 4 | 5 | NA |
| 021210 Movement with desired timing | 1 | 2 | 3 | 4 | 5 | NA |
| 021211 Movement at desired speed | 1 | 2 | 3 | 4 | 5 | NA |
| 021212 Movement with desired precision | 1 | 2 | 3 | 4 | 5 | NA |

*3rd edition*

Outcome Content References:

Buchner, D.M. (1995). Clinical assessments of physical activity in older adults. In L.Z. Rubenstein, D. Wieland, & R. Bernabei. *Geriatric Assessment Technology: The State of the Art* (pp. 147-159). New York: Springer Publishing.

Crawford, S.G., Wilson, B.N., & Dewey, D. (2001). Identifying developmental coordination disorder: Consistency between tests. *Physical & Occupational Therapy in Pediatrics, 20*(2/3), 29-50.

DiFabio, R.P., Paul, S., Emasithi, A., & Greany, J.F. (2001). Evaluating eye-body coordination during unrestrained functional activity in older persons. *Journals of Gerontology. Series A-Biological Sciences & Medical Sciences, 56*(9), M571-574.

Guyton, A.C. (1992). *Human physiology and mechanisms of disease* (5th ed.). Philadelphia: W.B. Saunders.

Harris, T. (1997). Muscle mass and strength: Relation to function in population studies. *Journal of Nutrition, 127*(Supp. 5), 1004S-1006S.

Junaid, K., Harris, S.R., Fulmer, K.A., & Carswell, A. (2000). Teachers' use of the MABC checklist to identify children with motor coordination difficulties. *Pediatric Physical Therapy, 12*(4), 158-163.

Matteson, M.A., McConnell, E.S., & Linton, A.D. (1997). *Gerontological nursing: Concepts and practice* (2nd ed.). Philadelphia: W.B. Saunders.

Novy, D.M., Simmonds, M.J., & Lee, C.E. (2002). Physical performance tasks: What are the underlying constructs? *Archives of Physical Medicine & Rehabilitation, 83*(1), 44-47.

Riggio, S., & Jagoda, A. (1999). The rapid neurologic examination, Part 2: Movement, reflexes, sensation, balance: Know the signs that lead to the site of the pathologic response. *Journal of Critical Illness, 14*(7), 368-372.

Schmitz, T.J. (2001). Coordination assessment. In S.B. O'Sullivan & T.J. Schmitz (Eds.), *Physical rehabilitation: Assessment and treatment* (4th ed., pp. 157-175). Philadelphia: F.A. Davis Company.

# Coping (1302)

*Domain-Psychosocial Health (III)*

*Class-Psychosocial Adaptation (N)*

*Scale(s)-Never demonstrated to Consistently demonstrated (m)*

*Care Recipient:*

*Data Source:*

C

**Definition:** Personal actions to manage stressors that tax an individual's resources

OUTCOME TARGET RATING:    Maintain at_____    Increase to_____

| Coping Overall Rating | | Never demonstrated 1 | Rarely demonstrated 2 | Sometimes demonstrated 3 | Often demonstrated 4 | Consistently demonstrated 5 | |
|---|---|---|---|---|---|---|---|
| INDICATORS: | | | | | | | |
| 130201 | Identifies effective coping patterns | 1 | 2 | 3 | 4 | 5 | NA |
| 130202 | Identifies ineffective coping patterns | 1 | 2 | 3 | 4 | 5 | NA |
| 130203 | Verbalizes sense of control | 1 | 2 | 3 | 4 | 5 | NA |
| 130204 | Reports decrease in stress | 1 | 2 | 3 | 4 | 5 | NA |
| 130205 | Verbalizes acceptance of situation | 1 | 2 | 3 | 4 | 5 | NA |
| 130206 | Seeks information concerning illness and treatment | 1 | 2 | 3 | 4 | 5 | NA |
| 130207 | Modifies lifestyle as needed | 1 | 2 | 3 | 4 | 5 | NA |
| 130208 | Adapts to life changes | 1 | 2 | 3 | 4 | 5 | NA |
| 130209 | Uses available social support | 1 | 2 | 3 | 4 | 5 | NA |
| 130210 | Uses behaviors to reduce stress | 1 | 2 | 3 | 4 | 5 | NA |
| 130211 | Identifies multiple coping strategies | 1 | 2 | 3 | 4 | 5 | NA |
| 130212 | Uses effective coping strategies | 1 | 2 | 3 | 4 | 5 | NA |
| 130213 | Avoids unduly stressful situations | 1 | 2 | 3 | 4 | 5 | NA |
| 130214 | Verbalizes need for assistance | 1 | 2 | 3 | 4 | 5 | NA |
| 130215 | Seeks help from a health care professional as appropriate | 1 | 2 | 3 | 4 | 5 | NA |
| 130216 | Reports decrease in physical symptoms of stress | 1 | 2 | 3 | 4 | 5 | NA |
| 130217 | Reports decrease in negative feelings | 1 | 2 | 3 | 4 | 5 | NA |
| 130218 | Reports increase in psychological comfort | 1 | 2 | 3 | 4 | 5 | NA |

*1st edition 1997; Revised 3rd edition*

## Outcome Content References:

Baldree, K., Murphy, S., & Powers, M. (1982). Stress identification and coping patterns in patients on hemodialysis. *Nursing Research, 31*(2), 107-112.

+Carver, C.S. (1997). You want to measure coping but your protocol's too long: Consider the Brief COPE. *International Journal of Behavioral Medicine,* 4, 92-100.

*Continued*

C

+Carver, C.S., Scheier, M.F., & Weintraub, J.K. (1989). Assessing coping strategies: A theoretically based approach. *Journal of Personality and Social Psychology, 56*(2), 267-283.

Folkman, S., Lazarus, R., Gruen, R., & Delongis, A. (1986). Appraisal, coping, health status, and psychological symptoms. *Journal of Personality and Social Psychology, 50*(3), 571-579.

McHaffie, H. (1992). The assessment of coping. *Clinical Nursing Research, 1*(1), 67-79.

Panzarine, S. (1985). Coping: Conceptual and methodological issues. *Advances in Nursing Science, 7*(4), 49-57.

Stolley, J.M. (2001). Ineffective individual coping. In M. Maas, K. Buckwalter, M. Hardy, T. Tripp-Reimer, M. Titler & J. Specht (Eds.), *Nursing care of older adults: Diagnoses, outcomes & interventions* (pp. 766-777). St. Louis: Mosby.

Whiting, G., & Buckwalter, K.C. (2001). Grieving. In M. Maas, K. Buckwalter, M. Hardy, T. Tripp-Reimer, M. Titler & J. Specht (Eds.), *Nursing care of older adults: Diagnoses, outcomes & interventions* (pp. 631-650). St. Louis: Mosby.

# *Decision-Making (0906)*

Domain-Physiologic Health (II)

Class-Neurocognitive (J)

Scale(s)-Severely compromised to Not compromised (a)

Care Recipient:

Data Source:

**D**

**Definition:** Ability to make judgments and choose between two or more alternatives

OUTCOME TARGET RATING:    Maintain at_____    Increase to_____

| Decision-Making<br>Overall Rating | Severely<br>compromised<br>1 | Substantially<br>compromised<br>2 | Moderately<br>compromised<br>3 | Mildly<br>compromised<br>4 | Not<br>compromised<br>5 | |
|---|---|---|---|---|---|---|
| **INDICATORS:** | | | | | | |
| 090601 Identifies relevant information | 1 | 2 | 3 | 4 | 5 | NA |
| 090602 Identifies alternatives | 1 | 2 | 3 | 4 | 5 | NA |
| 090603 Identifies potential consequences of each alternative | 1 | 2 | 3 | 4 | 5 | NA |
| 090604 Identifies resources necessary to support each alternative | 1 | 2 | 3 | 4 | 5 | NA |
| 090605 Recognizes contradiction with others' desires | 1 | 2 | 3 | 4 | 5 | NA |
| 090606 Acknowledges social context of the situation | 1 | 2 | 3 | 4 | 5 | NA |
| 090607 Acknowledges relevant legal implications | 1 | 2 | 3 | 4 | 5 | NA |
| 090608 Weighs alternatives | 1 | 2 | 3 | 4 | 5 | NA |
| 090609 Chooses among alternatives | 1 | 2 | 3 | 4 | 5 | NA |

*1st edition 1997; Revised 3rd edition*

**Outcome Content References:**

Abraham, I., & Reel, S. (1993). Cognitive nursing interventions with long-term care residents: Effects on neurocognitive dimensions. *Archives of Psychiatric Nursing, 6*(6), 356-365.

Agostinelli, B., Demers, K., Garrigan, D., & Waszynski, C. (1994). Targeted interventions: Use of the Mini-Mental State Exam. *Journal of Gerontological Nursing, 20*(8), 15-23.

Dellasega, C. (1992). Home health nurses' assessments of cognition. *Applied Nursing Research, 5*(3), 127-133.

Foreman, M., Gilles, D., & Wagner, D. (1989). Impaired cognition in the critically ill elderly patient: Clinical implications. *Critical Care Nursing Quarterly, 12*(1), 61-73.

+*Guide for the Uniform Data Set for Medical Rehabilitation* (including the FIM™ instrument), (version 5.1) (1997). Buffalo, NY: University at Buffalo.

Jubeck, M. (1992). Are you sensitive to the cognitive needs of the elderly? *Home Healthcare Nurse, 10*(5), 20-25.

Kendall, E., Shum, D., Halson, D., Bunning, S., & Teb, M. (1997). The assessment of social problem-solving ability following traumatic brain injury. *Journal of Head Trauma Rehabilitation, 12*(3), 68-78.

Kupferer, S., Uebele, J., & Levin, D. (1988). Geriatric ambulatory surgery patients: Assessing cognitive functions. *AORN Journal, 47*(3), 752-766.

Mason, P. (1989). Cognitive assessment parameters and tools for the critically injured adult. *Critical Care Nursing Clinics of North America, 1*(1), 45-53.

Strub, R.L., & Black, F.W. (2000). *The mental status examination in neurology* (4th ed.). Philadelphia: F.A. Davis.

# Depression Level (1208)

*Domain-Psychosocial Health (III)*

*Class-Psychological Well-Being (M)*

*Scale(s)-Severe to None (n)*

Care Recipient:

Data Source:

**Definition:** Severity of melancholic mood and loss of interest in life events

OUTCOME TARGET RATING:     Maintain at_____     Increase to_____

| Depression Level Overall Rating | Severe 1 | Substantial 2 | Moderate 3 | Mild 4 | None 5 | |
|---|---|---|---|---|---|---|

**INDICATORS:**

| | | Severe 1 | Substantial 2 | Moderate 3 | Mild 4 | None 5 | |
|---|---|---|---|---|---|---|---|
| 120801 | Depressed mood | 1 | 2 | 3 | 4 | 5 | NA |
| 120802 | Loss of interest in activities | 1 | 2 | 3 | 4 | 5 | NA |
| 120827 | Negative life events | 1 | 2 | 3 | 4 | 5 | NA |
| 120803 | Lack of pleasure in activities | 1 | 2 | 3 | 4 | 5 | NA |
| 120804 | Impaired concentration | 1 | 2 | 3 | 4 | 5 | NA |
| 120805 | Inappropriate guilt | 1 | 2 | 3 | 4 | 5 | NA |
| 120828 | Excessive guilt | 1 | 2 | 3 | 4 | 5 | NA |
| 120806 | Fatigue | 1 | 2 | 3 | 4 | 5 | NA |
| 120807 | Feelings of worthlessness | 1 | 2 | 3 | 4 | 5 | NA |
| 120808 | Psychomotor retardation | 1 | 2 | 3 | 4 | 5 | NA |
| 120829 | Psychomotor agitation | 1 | 2 | 3 | 4 | 5 | NA |
| 120809 | Insomnia | 1 | 2 | 3 | 4 | 5 | NA |
| 120830 | Hypersomnia | 1 | 2 | 3 | 4 | 5 | NA |
| 120810 | Weight gain | 1 | 2 | 3 | 4 | 5 | NA |
| 120831 | Weight loss | 1 | 2 | 3 | 4 | 5 | NA |
| 120811 | Increased appetite | 1 | 2 | 3 | 4 | 5 | NA |
| 120832 | Decreased appetite | 1 | 2 | 3 | 4 | 5 | NA |
| 120812 | Recurrent thoughts of death or suicide | 1 | 2 | 3 | 4 | 5 | NA |
| 120813 | Indecisiveness | 1 | 2 | 3 | 4 | 5 | NA |
| 120814 | Sadness | 1 | 2 | 3 | 4 | 5 | NA |
| 120815 | Crying spells | 1 | 2 | 3 | 4 | 5 | NA |
| 120816 | Anger | 1 | 2 | 3 | 4 | 5 | NA |
| 120817 | Hopelessness | 1 | 2 | 3 | 4 | 5 | NA |
| 120818 | Loneliness | 1 | 2 | 3 | 4 | 5 | NA |
| 120819 | Low self-esteem | 1 | 2 | 3 | 4 | 5 | NA |
| 120820 | Decreased libido | 1 | 2 | 3 | 4 | 5 | NA |
| 120821 | Decreased activity level | 1 | 2 | 3 | 4 | 5 | NA |
| 120822 | Lack of spontaneity | 1 | 2 | 3 | 4 | 5 | NA |
| 120823 | Irritability | 1 | 2 | 3 | 4 | 5 | NA |
| 120833 | Recreational drug use | 1 | 2 | 3 | 4 | 5 | NA |
| 120834 | Increased alcohol use | 1 | 2 | 3 | 4 | 5 | NA |
| 120825 | Poor personal hygiene/ grooming | 1 | 2 | 3 | 4 | 5 | NA |

*2nd edition 2000; Revised 3rd edition*

Outcome Content References:

American Psychiatric Association. (2000). *Diagnostic and statistical manual of mental disorders* (4th ed. text revision). Washington DC: Author.

Brink, T. L., Yesavage, J. A., Lum, O., Heersema, P.H., Adey, M., & Rose, T. L. (1982). Screening tests for geriatric depression. *Clinical Gerontologist 1*(1), 37-43.

Kendler, K.S., Karkowski, L.M., & Prescott, C.A. (1999). Causal relationship between stressful life events and the onset of major depression. *American Journal of Psychiatry, 156*(6), 837-841.

Kraaij, V., Arensman, E., & Spinhoven, P. (2002). Negative life events and depression in elderly persons: A meta-analysis. *Journal of Gerontology Series B-Psychological Sciences, 57*(1), P87-P94.

Lloyd-Williams, M., Friedman, T., & Rudd, N. (2001). An analysis of the validity of the Hospital Anxiety and Depression Scale as a screening tool in patients with advanced metastatic cancer. *Journal of Pain & Symptom Management, 22*(6), 990-996.

Oakley, L.D., & Kane, J. (1999). Personal and social illness demands related to depression. *Archives of Psychiatric Nursing, 13*(6), 294-302.

Raue, P.J., Brown, E.L., & Bruce, M.L. (2002). Assessing behavior health using OASIS: Part 1: Depression and suicidality. *Home Healthcare Nurse, 20*(3), 154-162.

U.S. Department of Health and Human Services. (1993). *Depression and primary care: Detection and diagnosis.* (Vol. 1) (AHCPR publication No. 93-0550). Rockville, MD: Government Printing Office.

U.S. Department of Health and Human Services. (1993). *Depression and primary care: Treatment of major depression.* (Vol. 2) (AHCPR publication No. 93-0551). Rockville, MD: Government Printing Office.

**D**

# Depression Self-Control (1409)

*Domain-Psychosocial Health (III)*

*Class-Self-Control (O)*

*Scale(s)-Never demonstrated to Consistently demonstrated (m)*

Care Recipient:

Data Source:

**D**

**Definition:** Personal actions to minimize melancholy and maintain interest in life events

OUTCOME TARGET RATING:     Maintain at_____     Increase to_____

| Depression Self-Control Overall Rating | Never demonstrated 1 | Rarely demonstrated 2 | Sometimes demonstrated 3 | Often demonstrated 4 | Consistently demonstrated 5 | |
|---|---|---|---|---|---|---|
| INDICATORS: | | | | | | |
| 140901 Monitors ability to concentrate | 1 | 2 | 3 | 4 | 5 | NA |
| 140902 Monitors intensity of depression | 1 | 2 | 3 | 4 | 5 | NA |
| 140903 Identifies precursors of depression | 1 | 2 | 3 | 4 | 5 | NA |
| 140904 Plans strategies to reduce effects of precursors | 1 | 2 | 3 | 4 | 5 | NA |
| 140905 Monitors behavioral manifestations of depression | 1 | 2 | 3 | 4 | 5 | NA |
| 140906 Reports adequate sleep | 1 | 2 | 3 | 4 | 5 | NA |
| 140907 Reports improved libido | 1 | 2 | 3 | 4 | 5 | NA |
| 140908 Monitors physical manifestations of depression | 1 | 2 | 3 | 4 | 5 | NA |
| 140909 Reports improved mood | 1 | 2 | 3 | 4 | 5 | NA |
| 140910 Maintains stable weight | 1 | 2 | 3 | 4 | 5 | NA |
| 140911 Follows treatment plan | 1 | 2 | 3 | 4 | 5 | NA |
| 140912 Takes medication as prescribed | 1 | 2 | 3 | 4 | 5 | NA |
| 140913 Follows exercise plan | 1 | 2 | 3 | 4 | 5 | NA |
| 140914 Adheres to therapy schedule | 1 | 2 | 3 | 4 | 5 | NA |
| 140915 Reports changes in symptoms to a health care provider | 1 | 2 | 3 | 4 | 5 | NA |
| 140920 Avoids alcohol misuse | 1 | 2 | 3 | 4 | 5 | NA |
| 140921 Avoids non-prescription drug misuse | 1 | 2 | 3 | 4 | 5 | NA |
| 140922 Avoids recreational drugs | 1 | 2 | 3 | 4 | 5 | NA |
| 140918 Maintains personal hygiene and grooming | 1 | 2 | 3 | 4 | 5 | NA |

*2nd edition 2000; Revised 3rd edition (formerly Depression Control)*

## Outcome Content References:

Adams, P. (2000). Insight: A mental health prevention intervention. *Nursing Clinics of North America, 35*(2), 329-338.

American Psychiatric Association. (2000). *Diagnostic and statistical manual of mental disorders* (4th ed. text revision). Washington DC: Author.

Cronin, J., Nash, V., Ray-Mihm, R., & Tucker, S. (2001). Relationship between psychiatric clinical assessment scores and patients' daily activities. *Journal of the American Psychiatric Nurses Association, 7*(5), 145-154.

Jaret, P. (1999). Fitness. Move the body, heal the mind. *Health, 13*(1), 50-51.

Johnson, C.D. (1999). Therapeutic recreation treats depression in the elderly. *Home Health Care Services Quarterly, 18*(2), 79-90.

Laliberte, R. (1999). How to manage your moods. *New Choices: Living Even Better After 50, 39*(6), 44-47.

Lantz, M.S. (2001). The psychiatric consultant. Suicide in late life: Identifying and managing at-risk older patients. *Geriatrics, 56*(7), 47-48.

Peden, A.R., Hall, L.A., Rayens, M.K., & Beebe, L.L. (2000). Reducing negative thinking and depressive symptoms in college women. *Journal of Nursing Scholarship, 32*(2), 145-151.

Tucker, S., & Darley, J. (2001). How to detect and manage depression in older people. *Nursing Times, 97*(45), 36-37.

U.S. Department of Health and Human Services. (1993). *Depression and primary care: Detection and diagnosis.* (Vol. 1) (AHCPR publication No. 93-0550). Rockville, MD: Government Printing Office.

U.S. Department of Health and Human Services. (1993). *Depression and primary care: Treatment of major depression.* (Vol. 2) (AHCPR publication No. 93-0551). Rockville, MD: Government Printing Office.

**D**

# Diabetes Self-Management (1619)

*Domain-Health Knowledge & Behavior (IV)*

*Class-Health Behavior (Q)*

*Scale(s)-Never demonstrated to Consistently demonstrated (m)*

*Care Recipient:*

*Data Source:*

**Definition:** Personal actions to manage diabetes mellitus and prevent disease progression

OUTCOME TARGET RATING:     Maintain at_____     Increase to_____

| Diabetes Self-Management Overall Rating | Never demonstrated 1 | Rarely demonstrated 2 | Sometimes demonstrated 3 | Often demonstrated 4 | Consistently demonstrated 5 | |
|---|---|---|---|---|---|---|
| INDICATORS: | | | | | | |
| 161901 Accepts health care provider's diagnosis | 1 | 2 | 3 | 4 | 5 | NA |
| 161902 Seeks information about methods to prevent complications | 1 | 2 | 3 | 4 | 5 | NA |
| 161903 Follows preventive foot care practices | 1 | 2 | 3 | 4 | 5 | NA |
| 161904 Obtains dilated vision examination as recommended | 1 | 2 | 3 | 4 | 5 | NA |
| 161905 Initiates changes in medication when acutely ill | 1 | 2 | 3 | 4 | 5 | NA |
| 161906 Reports non-healing breaks in skin to primary care provider | 1 | 2 | 3 | 4 | 5 | NA |
| 161907 Participates in health care decision making process | 1 | 2 | 3 | 4 | 5 | NA |
| 161908 Participates in prescribed educational program | 1 | 2 | 3 | 4 | 5 | NA |
| 161909 Performs treatment regimen as prescribed | 1 | 2 | 3 | 4 | 5 | NA |
| 161910 Demonstrates correct procedure for blood glucose testing | 1 | 2 | 3 | 4 | 5 | NA |
| 161911 Monitors blood glucose | 1 | 2 | 3 | 4 | 5 | NA |
| 161912 Treats symptoms of hyperglycemia | 1 | 2 | 3 | 4 | 5 | NA |
| 161913 Treats symptoms of hypoglycemia | 1 | 2 | 3 | 4 | 5 | NA |
| 161914 Monitors frequency of hypoglycemia episodes | 1 | 2 | 3 | 4 | 5 | NA |
| 161915 Reports symptoms of complications | 1 | 2 | 3 | 4 | 5 | NA |
| 161916 Uses diary to monitor blood glucose over time | 1 | 2 | 3 | 4 | 5 | NA |

D

| Diabetes Self-Management—cont'd | | Never demonstrated | Rarely demonstrated | Sometimes demonstrated | Often demonstrated | Consistently demonstrated | |
|---|---|---|---|---|---|---|---|
| 161917 | Uses measures to prevent complications | 1 | 2 | 3 | 4 | 5 | NA |
| 161918 | Seeks health care if blood glucose levels fluctuate outside of recommended parameters | 1 | 2 | 3 | 4 | 5 | NA |
| 161919 | Monitors urinary glucose and ketones | 1 | 2 | 3 | 4 | 5 | NA |
| 161920 | Follows recommended diet | 1 | 2 | 3 | 4 | 5 | NA |
| 161921 | Follows recommended activity level | 1 | 2 | 3 | 4 | 5 | NA |
| 161922 | Monitors body weight | 1 | 2 | 3 | 4 | 5 | NA |
| 161923 | Uses effective weight control strategies | 1 | 2 | 3 | 4 | 5 | NA |
| 161924 | Maintains optimum weight | 1 | 2 | 3 | 4 | 5 | NA |
| 161925 | Follows restrictions for alcohol use | 1 | 2 | 3 | 4 | 5 | NA |
| 161926 | Participates in smoking cessation regimen | 1 | 2 | 3 | 4 | 5 | NA |
| 161927 | Participates in recommended exercise program | 1 | 2 | 3 | 4 | 5 | NA |
| 161928 | Performs usual life routine | 1 | 2 | 3 | 4 | 5 | NA |
| 161929 | Demonstrates correct procedure for insulin administration | 1 | 2 | 3 | 4 | 5 | NA |
| 161930 | Stores insulin correctly | 1 | 2 | 3 | 4 | 5 | NA |
| 161931 | Obtains needed medications | 1 | 2 | 3 | 4 | 5 | NA |
| 161932 | Uses medications as prescribed | 1 | 2 | 3 | 4 | 5 | NA |
| 161933 | Monitors prescribed medication effects | 1 | 2 | 3 | 4 | 5 | NA |
| 161934 | Rotates injection sites | 1 | 2 | 3 | 4 | 5 | NA |
| 161935 | Uses only over-the-counter medications approved by health care professional | 1 | 2 | 3 | 4 | 5 | NA |
| 161936 | Obtains flu and pneumonia immunizations | 1 | 2 | 3 | 4 | 5 | NA |

D

*Continued*

| Diabetes Self-Management—cont'd | | Never demonstrated | Rarely demonstrated | Sometimes demonstrated | Often demonstrated | Consistently demonstrated | |
|---|---|---|---|---|---|---|---|
| 161937 | Uses health care services congruent with needs | 1 | 2 | 3 | 4 | 5 | NA |
| 161938 | Reports need for financial assistance to obtain supplies and medications | 1 | 2 | 3 | 4 | 5 | NA |
| 161939 | Keeps appointments with health care professional | 1 | 2 | 3 | 4 | 5 | NA |
| 161940 | Maintains plan for medical emergencies | 1 | 2 | 3 | 4 | 5 | NA |

*3rd edition*

**Outcome Content References:**

American Diabetes Association. (1998). Standards of medical care for patients with diabetes mellitus. *Diabetes Care, 21* (Supp. 1), S23-S31.

American Diabetes Association. (1998). Testing of glycemia in diabetes. *Diabetes Care, 21*(Supp. 1), S69-71.

Cryer, P.E. (2001). Hypoglycemia risk reduction in Type I Diabetes. *Experimental & Clinical Endocrinology & Diabetes, 109*(Suppl. 2), S412-S423.

Funnell, M.M., Hunt, C., Kulkarni, K., Rubin, R.R., & Yarborough, P.C. (Eds.). (1998). *A core curriculum for Association of Diabetes educators.* Chicago: American Association of Diabetes Educators.

Kelley, D.B. (Ed.). (1998). *Intensive diabetes management.* (2nd ed). Alexandria, VA: American Diabetes Association.

Lebovitz, H.E. (Ed.). (1998). *Therapy for diabetes mellitus and related disorders* (3rd ed.). Alexandria, VA: American Diabetes Association.

Lewis, S.M., Collier, I.C., Heitkemper, M.M., & Dirksen, S.R. (2000). *Medical-surgical nursing: Assessment & management of clinical problems* (5th ed.). St. Louis: Mosby.

McCance, K.L., & Huether, S.E. (2002). *Pathophysiology: The biologic basis for disease in adults and children* (4th ed.). St. Louis: Mosby.

# Dignified Life Closure (1307)

Domain-Psychosocial Health (III)

Class-Psychosocial Adaptation (N)

Scale(s)-Never demonstrated to Consistently demonstrated (m)

Care Recipient:

Data Source:

**D**

**Definition:** Personal actions to maintain control during approaching end of life

OUTCOME TARGET RATING:    Maintain at_____    Increase to_____

| Dignified Life Closure Overall Rating | Never demonstrated 1 | Rarely demonstrated 2 | Sometimes demonstrated 3 | Often demonstrated 4 | Consistently demonstrated 5 | |
|---|---|---|---|---|---|---|
| INDICATORS: | | | | | | |
| 130701 Puts affairs in order | 1 | 2 | 3 | 4 | 5 | NA |
| 130702 Expresses hopefulness | 1 | 2 | 3 | 4 | 5 | NA |
| 130703 Participates in decisions related to care | 1 | 2 | 3 | 4 | 5 | NA |
| 130704 Participates in decisions about hospitalization | 1 | 2 | 3 | 4 | 5 | NA |
| 130705 Participates in decisions about resuscitation status | 1 | 2 | 3 | 4 | 5 | NA |
| 130706 Controls decisions about organ donation | 1 | 2 | 3 | 4 | 5 | NA |
| 130707 Participates in planning funeral | 1 | 2 | 3 | 4 | 5 | NA |
| 130708 Maintains current will | 1 | 2 | 3 | 4 | 5 | NA |
| 130709 Maintains advance directives | 1 | 2 | 3 | 4 | 5 | NA |
| 130710 Resolves important issues and concerns | 1 | 2 | 3 | 4 | 5 | NA |
| 130711 Shares feelings about dying | 1 | 2 | 3 | 4 | 5 | NA |
| 130712 Reconciles relationships | 1 | 2 | 3 | 4 | 5 | NA |
| 130713 Completes meaningful goals | 1 | 2 | 3 | 4 | 5 | NA |
| 130714 Maintains sense of control of remaining time | 1 | 2 | 3 | 4 | 5 | NA |
| 130715 Exchanges affection with others | 1 | 2 | 3 | 4 | 5 | NA |
| 130716 Disengages gradually from significant others | 1 | 2 | 3 | 4 | 5 | NA |
| 130717 Recalls lifetime memories | 1 | 2 | 3 | 4 | 5 | NA |
| 130718 Reviews life's accomplishments | 1 | 2 | 3 | 4 | 5 | NA |
| 130719 Discusses spiritual experiences | 1 | 2 | 3 | 4 | 5 | NA |
| 130720 Discusses spiritual concerns | 1 | 2 | 3 | 4 | 5 | NA |
| 130721 Maintains physical independence | 1 | 2 | 3 | 4 | 5 | NA |
| 130722 Controls treatment choices | 1 | 2 | 3 | 4 | 5 | NA |
| 130723 Controls food/drink intake | 1 | 2 | 3 | 4 | 5 | NA |

*Continued*

| Dignified Life Closure—cont'd | | Never demonstrated | Rarely demonstrated | Sometimes demonstrated | Often demonstrated | Consistently demonstrated | |
|---|---|---|---|---|---|---|---|
| 130724 | Controls personal possessions | 1 | 2 | 3 | 4 | 5 | NA |
| 130725 | Expresses readiness for death | 1 | 2 | 3 | 4 | 5 | NA |

*3rd edition*

## Outcome Content References:

Callanan, M., & Kelley, P. (1992). *Final gifts*. New York: Poseidon Press.

Cicirelli, V.G. (1997). Elders' end-of-life decisions: implications for hospice care. *Hospice Journal Physical, Psychosocial, & Pastoral Care of the Dying.* 12(1), 57-72.

Ferrell, B.R. (1993). To know suffering. *Oncology Nursing Forum, 20*(10), 1471-1477.

McCanse, R.P. (1995). The McCanse Readiness for Death Instrument (MRDI): A reliable and valid measure for hospice care. *Hospice Journal, 10*(1), 15-26.

Potter, P.A., & Perry, A.G. (2001). *Fundamentals of nursing* (5th ed.). St. Louis: Mosby.

Quill, T.E. (1993). *Death and dignity: Making choices and taking charge.* New York: W. W. Norton & Co.

Schmele, J.A. (1995). Perceptions of a dying patient of the quality of care and caring: An interview with Ivan Hanson. *Journal of Nursing Care Quality, 9*(4), 31-42.

# Discharge Readiness: Independent Living (0311)

*Domain-Functional Health (I)*

*Class-Self-Care (D)*

*Scale-Never demonstrated to Consistently demonstrated (m) and Consistently demonstrated to Never demonstrated (t)*

*Care Recipient:*

*Data Source:*

**D**

**Definition:** Readiness of a patient to relocate from a health care institution to living independently

OUTCOME TARGET RATING:     Maintain at_____     Increase to_____

| Discharge Readiness: Independent Living Overall Rating | Never demonstrated 1 | Rarely demonstrated 2 | Sometimes demonstrated 3 | Often demonstrated 4 | Consistently demonstrated 5 | |
|---|---|---|---|---|---|---|
| **INDICATORS:** | | | | | | |
| 031104 Seeks assistance appropriately | 1 | 2 | 3 | 4 | 5 | NA |
| 031105 Uses available social support | 1 | 2 | 3 | 4 | 5 | NA |
| 031106 Describes signs & symptoms to health care professional | 1 | 2 | 3 | 4 | 5 | NA |
| 031107 Describes prescribed treatments | 1 | 2 | 3 | 4 | 5 | NA |
| 031108 Describes risks for complications | 1 | 2 | 3 | 4 | 5 | NA |
| 031109 Manages own medications | 1 | 2 | 3 | 4 | 5 | NA |
| 031110 Performs activities of daily living (ADLs) independently | 1 | 2 | 3 | 4 | 5 | NA |
| 031111 Performs instrumental activities of daily living (IADLs) independently | 1 | 2 | 3 | 4 | 5 | NA |
| 031112 Makes appropriate judgments | 1 | 2 | 3 | 4 | 5 | NA |

| | Consistently demonstrated | Often demonstrated | Sometimes demonstrated | Rarely demonstrated | Never demonstrated | |
|---|---|---|---|---|---|---|
| 031101 Fever | 1 | 2 | 3 | 4 | 5 | NA |
| 031102 Infection | 1 | 2 | 3 | 4 | 5 | NA |
| 031103 Confusion | 1 | 2 | 3 | 4 | 5 | NA |

*3rd edition*

## Outcome Content References:

Barnes, S. (2000). Ambulatory surgery. Are you watching the clock? Let criteria define discharge readiness. *Journal of Perianesthesia Nursing, 15*(3), 174-176.

Costa, M.J. (2001). The lived perioperative experience of ambulatory surgery patients. *AORN Journal, 74*(6), 874-876, 878-881.

Harris, M.D. (1999). Medicare & the nurse. 10 DRGs that can affect home care referrals. *Home Healthcare Nurse, 17*(2), 127-129.

Higson, J., & Bolland, R. (2001). Paediatric discharge criteria lead to improved outcomes. *Times, 97*(35), 30-31.

Kuc, J.A., & Pietro, J. (1999). Safe discharge from the PACU and ambulatory care setting. *Journal of Nursing Law, 6*(2), 7-14.

Walker, C.R., Watters, N., Nadon, C., Graham, K., & Niday, P. (1999). Discharge of mothers and babies from hospital after birth of a healthy full-term infant: Developing criteria through a community-wide consensus process. *Canadian Journal of Public Health, 90*(5), 313-315.

## Discharge Readiness: Supported Living (0312)

*Domain-Functional Health (I)*

*Class-Self-Care (D)*

*Scale-Never demonstrated to Consistently demonstrated (m)*

Care Recipient:

Data Source:

**D**

**Definition:** Readiness of a patient to relocate from a health care institution to a lower level of supported living

OUTCOME TARGET RATING:    Maintain at_____    Increase to_____

| Discharge Readiness: Supported Living Overall Rating | Never demonstrated 1 | Rarely demonstrated 2 | Sometimes demonstrated 3 | Often demonstrated 4 | Consistently demonstrated 5 | |
|---|---|---|---|---|---|---|
| INDICATORS: | | | | | | |
| 031201 Patient needs consistent with available staff support | 1 | 2 | 3 | 4 | 5 | NA |
| 031202 Patient needs consistent with available family support | 1 | 2 | 3 | 4 | 5 | NA |
| 031203 Oriented to care at new residence | 1 | 2 | 3 | 4 | 5 | NA |
| 031204 Accepts transfer to new residence | 1 | 2 | 3 | 4 | 5 | NA |
| 031205 Describes special needs | 1 | 2 | 3 | 4 | 5 | NA |
| 031206 Describes short term plan | 1 | 2 | 3 | 4 | 5 | NA |
| 031207 Describes long term plan | 1 | 2 | 3 | 4 | 5 | NA |
| 031208 Describes plan for continuity in care | 1 | 2 | 3 | 4 | 5 | NA |

*3rd edition*

Outcome Content References:

Bosek, M.S.D., Burton, L.A., & Savage, T.A. (1999). The patient who could not be discharged: How far should patient autonomy extend? *JONA's Healthcare Law, Ethics, & Regulation, 1*(4), 23-30.

Chan, L., & Ciol, M. (2000). Medicare's payment system: Its effect on discharges to skilled nursing facilities from rehabilitation hospitals. *Archives of Physical Medicine & Rehabilitation, 81*(6), 715-719.

# Distorted Thought Self-Control (1403)

Domain-Psychosocial Health (III)

Class-Self-Control (O)

Scale(s)-Never demonstrated to Consistently demonstrated (m)

Care Recipient:

Data Source:

**D**

**Definition:** Self-restraint of disruptions in perception, thought processes, and thought content

OUTCOME TARGET RATING:    Maintain at_____    Increase to_____

| Distorted Thought Self-Control Overall Rating | Never demonstrated 1 | Rarely demonstrated 2 | Sometimes demonstrated 3 | Often demonstrated 4 | Consistently demonstrated 5 | |
|---|---|---|---|---|---|---|
| **INDICATORS:** | | | | | | |
| 140301 Recognizes hallucinations or delusions are occurring | 1 | 2 | 3 | 4 | 5 | NA |
| 140302 Refrains from attending to hallucinations or delusions | 1 | 2 | 3 | 4 | 5 | NA |
| 140303 Refrains from responding to hallucinations or delusions | 1 | 2 | 3 | 4 | 5 | NA |
| 140304 Monitors frequency of hallucinations or delusions | 1 | 2 | 3 | 4 | 5 | NA |
| 140305 Describes content of hallucinations or delusions | 1 | 2 | 3 | 4 | 5 | NA |
| 140306 Reports decrease in hallucinations or delusions | 1 | 2 | 3 | 4 | 5 | NA |
| 140307 Asks for validation of reality | 1 | 2 | 3 | 4 | 5 | NA |
| 140308 Maintains affect consistent with mood | 1 | 2 | 3 | 4 | 5 | NA |
| 140309 Interacts with others appropriately | 1 | 2 | 3 | 4 | 5 | NA |
| 140310 Perceives environment accurately | 1 | 2 | 3 | 4 | 5 | NA |
| 140311 Exhibits logical thought flow patterns | 1 | 2 | 3 | 4 | 5 | NA |
| 140312 Exhibits reality-based thinking | 1 | 2 | 3 | 4 | 5 | NA |
| 140313 Exhibits appropriate thought content | 1 | 2 | 3 | 4 | 5 | NA |
| 140314 Exhibits ability to grasp ideas of others | 1 | 2 | 3 | 4 | 5 | NA |

*1st edition 1997; Revised 2nd edition 2000; Revised 3rd edition (formerly Distorted Thought Control)*

*Continued*

D

Outcome Content References:

Andreasen, N.C., & Black, D. (2001). *Introductory textbook of psychiatry* (3rd ed.). Washington DC: American Psychiatric Publishing.

Buccheri, R., Trygstad, L., Kanas, N., & Dowling, G. (1997). Symptom management of auditory hallucinations in schizophrenia: Results of 1-year follow up. *Journal of Psychosocial Nursing & Mental Health Services, 35*(12), 20-28, 37-38.

Buccheri, R., Trygstad, L., Kanas, N., Waldron, B., & Dowling, G. (1996). Auditory hallucinations in schizophrenia: Group experience in examining symptom management and behavioral strategies. *Journal of Psychosocial Nursing & Mental Health Services, 34*(2), 12-26, 44-45.

+Cummings, J.L., (1997). The Neuropsychiatric Inventory: Assessing psychopathology in dementia patients. *Neurology, 48* (Suppl. 6), S10-S16.

Frederick, J., & Cotanch, P. (1995). Self-help techniques for auditory hallucinations in schizophrenia. *Issues in Mental Health Nursing, 16*(3), 213-24.

Grimaldi, D., & Cousins, A. (1985). Paranoia. *Journal of Emergency Nursing, 11*(4), 201-204.

MacRae, A. (1997). The model of functional deficits associated with hallucinations. *American Journal of Occupational Therapy, 51*(1), 57-63.

Rosenthal, T.T., & McGuinness, T.M. (1986). Dealing with delusional patients: Discovering the distorted truth. *Issues in Mental Health Nursing, 8*(2), 143-154.

Stuart, G.W., & Laraia, M.T. (2001). *Principles and practice of psychiatric nursing* (7th ed.). St. Louis: Mosby.

# Electrolyte & Acid/Base Balance (0600)

Domain-Physiologic Health (II)

Class-Fluid & Electrolytes (G)

Scale(s)-Severely compromised to Not compromised (a)

Care Recipient:

Data Source:

**Definition:** Balance of electrolytes and non-electrolytes in the intracellular and extracellular compartments of the body

OUTCOME TARGET RATING:     Maintain at_____     Increase to_____

| Electrolyte & Acid/Base Balance Overall Rating | Severely compromised 1 | Substantially compromised 2 | Moderately compromised 3 | Mildly compromised 4 | Not compromised 5 | |
|---|---|---|---|---|---|---|
| INDICATORS: | | | | | | |
| 060001   Apical heart rate | 1 | 2 | 3 | 4 | 5 | NA |
| 060002   Apical heart rhythm | 1 | 2 | 3 | 4 | 5 | NA |
| 060003   Respiratory rate | 1 | 2 | 3 | 4 | 5 | NA |
| 060004   Respiratory rhythm | 1 | 2 | 3 | 4 | 5 | NA |
| 060005   Serum sodium | 1 | 2 | 3 | 4 | 5 | NA |
| 060006   Serum potassium | 1 | 2 | 3 | 4 | 5 | NA |
| 060007   Serum chloride | 1 | 2 | 3 | 4 | 5 | NA |
| 060008   Serum calcium | 1 | 2 | 3 | 4 | 5 | NA |
| 060009   Serum magnesium | 1 | 2 | 3 | 4 | 5 | NA |
| 060010   Serum pH | 1 | 2 | 3 | 4 | 5 | NA |
| 060011   Serum albumin | 1 | 2 | 3 | 4 | 5 | NA |
| 060012   Serum creatinine | 1 | 2 | 3 | 4 | 5 | NA |
| 060013   Serum bicarbonate | 1 | 2 | 3 | 4 | 5 | NA |
| 060014   Blood urea nitrogen | 1 | 2 | 3 | 4 | 5 | NA |
| 060015   Urine pH | 1 | 2 | 3 | 4 | 5 | NA |
| 060016   Mental alertness | 1 | 2 | 3 | 4 | 5 | NA |
| 060017   Cognitive orientation | 1 | 2 | 3 | 4 | 5 | NA |
| 060018   Muscle strength | 1 | 2 | 3 | 4 | 5 | NA |
| 060019   Neuromuscular non-irritability | 1 | 2 | 3 | 4 | 5 | NA |
| 060022   Urine specific gravity | 1 | 2 | 3 | 4 | 5 | NA |
| 060023   Sensation in extremities | 1 | 2 | 3 | 4 | 5 | NA |

*1st edition 1997; Revised 3rd edition*

Outcome Content References:

Cherry, R. (1992). Furosemide facts. *Emergency Medical Services, 21*(9), 79.

Cullen, L. (1992). Interventions related to fluid and electrolytes. *Nursing Clinics of North America, 27*(2), 60, 62, 79.

Innerarity, S.A. (1997). *Fluids and electrolytes* (3rd ed.). Springhouse, PA: Springhouse.

McCance, K.L., & Huether, S.E. (2002). *Pathophysiology: The biologic basis for disease in adults and children.* (4th ed.) St. Louis: Mosby.

Methany, N. (2000). *Fluid and electrolyte balance: Nursing considerations* (4th ed.). Philadelphia: Lippincott Williams & Wilkins.

Norris, C. (1982). *Concept clarification in nursing.* Rockville, MD: Aspen.

Schuller, D., Mitchell, J., Calendrino, F., & Schuster, D. (1991). Fluid balance during pulmonary edema: Is fluid gain a marker or a cause of post-operative outcome? *Chest, 100*(4), 1068-1075.

Vullo-Navich, K., Smith, S., Andrews, M., Levine, A.M., Tischer, J. F., & Veglia, J.M. (1998). Comfort and incidence of abnormal serum sodium, BUN, creatinine and osmolality in dehydration of terminal illness. *The American Journal of Hospice & Palliative Care, 15*(2) 77-84.

E

E

# *Endurance (0001)*

*Domain-Functional Health (I)*

*Class-Energy Maintenance (A)*

*Scale(s)-Severely compromised to Not compromised (a) and Severe to None (n)*

*Care Recipient:*

*Data Source:*

**Definition: Capacity to sustain activity**

OUTCOME TARGET RATING:     Maintain at_____     Increase to_____

| Endurance Overall Rating | Severely compromised 1 | Substantially compromised 2 | Moderately compromised 3 | Mildly compromised 4 | Not compromised 5 | |
|---|---|---|---|---|---|---|

INDICATORS:

| | | | | | | | |
|---|---|---|---|---|---|---|---|
| 000101 | Performance of usual routine | 1 | 2 | 3 | 4 | 5 | NA |
| 000102 | Activity | 1 | 2 | 3 | 4 | 5 | NA |
| 000103 | Rested appearance | 1 | 2 | 3 | 4 | 5 | NA |
| 000104 | Concentration | 1 | 2 | 3 | 4 | 5 | NA |
| 000105 | Interest in surroundings | 1 | 2 | 3 | 4 | 5 | NA |
| 000106 | Muscle endurance | 1 | 2 | 3 | 4 | 5 | NA |
| 000107 | Eating pattern | 1 | 2 | 3 | 4 | 5 | NA |
| 000108 | Libido | 1 | 2 | 3 | 4 | 5 | NA |
| 000109 | Energy restored after rest | 1 | 2 | 3 | 4 | 5 | NA |
| 000112 | Blood oxygen level | 1 | 2 | 3 | 4 | 5 | NA |
| 000113 | Hemoglobin | 1 | 2 | 3 | 4 | 5 | NA |
| 000114 | Hematocrit | 1 | 2 | 3 | 4 | 5 | NA |
| 000115 | Blood glucose | 1 | 2 | 3 | 4 | 5 | NA |
| 000116 | Serum electrolytes | 1 | 2 | 3 | 4 | 5 | NA |

| | | Severe | Substantial | Moderate | Mild | None | |
|---|---|---|---|---|---|---|---|
| 000110 | Exhaustion | 1 | 2 | 3 | 4 | 5 | NA |
| 000111 | Lethargy | 1 | 2 | 3 | 4 | 5 | NA |
| 000118 | Fatigue | 1 | 2 | 3 | 4 | 5 | NA |

*1st edition 1997; Revised 3rd edition*

Outcome Content References:

Ades, P.A., Ballor, D.L., Ashikaga, T., Utton, J.L., & Streekumaran Nair, K. (1996). Weight training improves walking endurance in healthy elderly persons, *Annals of Internal Medicine, 124*(6), 568-572.

+Dartmouth Primary Care Cooperative Information Project. (1987). *COOP Charts.* Hanover, NH: Department of Community and Family Medicine, Dartmouth Medical School.

Ellis, J.R., & Nowlis, E.A. (1994). *Providing nursing care within the nursing process* (5th ed.). Philadelphia: J.B. Lippincott.

Johns, M.E. (1991). Activity and exercise. In S. Wingate (Ed.), *Cardiac nursing: A clinical management and patient care resource* (pp. 141-145). Gaithersburg, MD: Aspen.

Lubkin, I.M. (2002). *Chronic illness: Impact and interventions* (5th ed.). Boston: Jones & Bartlett.

Potter, P.A., & Perry, A.G. (2001). *Fundamentals of nursing* (5th ed.). St. Louis: Mosby.

Pugh, L.C., & Milligan, R. (1993). A framework for the study of childbearing fatigue. *Advances in Nursing Science, 15*(4), 60-70.

Tiesinga, L.J., Dassen, T.W.N., & Halfens, R.J.G. (1996). Fatigue: A summary of the definitions, dimensions, and indicators. *Nursing Diagnosis, 7*(2), 51-62.

Titler, M.G. (2001). Activity intolerance. In M. Maas, K. Buckwalter, M. Hardy, T. Tripp-Reimer, M. Titler & J. Specht (Eds.), *Nursing care of older adults: Diagnoses, outcomes & interventions* (pp. 324-336). St. Louis: Mosby.

Topf, M. (1992). Effects of personal control over hospital noise on sleep. *Research in Nursing and Health, 15*(1), 19-28.

# *Energy Conservation (0002)*

Domain-Functional Health (I)                                Care Recipient:

Class-Energy Maintenance (A)                                Data Source:

Scale(s)-Never demonstrated to Consistently demonstrated (m)

**Definition:** Personal actions to manage energy for initiating and sustaining activity

OUTCOME TARGET RATING:     Maintain at_____     Increase to_____

| Energy Conservation Overall Rating | | Never demonstrated 1 | Rarely demonstrated 2 | Sometimes demonstrated 3 | Often demonstrated 4 | Consistently demonstrated 5 | |
|---|---|---|---|---|---|---|---|
| **INDICATORS:** | | | | | | | |
| 000201 | Balances activity and rest | 1 | 2 | 3 | 4 | 5 | NA |
| 000202 | Uses naps to restore energy | 1 | 2 | 3 | 4 | 5 | NA |
| 000203 | Recognizes energy limitations | 1 | 2 | 3 | 4 | 5 | NA |
| 000204 | Uses energy conservation techniques | 1 | 2 | 3 | 4 | 5 | NA |
| 000209 | Organizes activities to conserve energy | 1 | 2 | 3 | 4 | 5 | NA |
| 000205 | Adapts lifestyle to energy level | 1 | 2 | 3 | 4 | 5 | NA |
| 000206 | Maintains adequate nutrition | 1 | 2 | 3 | 4 | 5 | NA |
| 000207 | Reports adequate endurance for activity | 1 | 2 | 3 | 4 | 5 | NA |

*1st edition 1997; Revised 3rd edition*

Outcome Content References:

Dixon, J.K., Dixon, J.P., & Hickey, M. (1993). Energy as a central factor in the self assessment of health. *Advances in Nursing Science, 15*(4), 1-12.

+Lee, K.A., Hicks, G., & Nino-Murcia, G. (1991). Validity and reliability of a scale to assess fatigue. *Psychiatry Research, 36(3)*, 291-298.

Lubkin, I.M. (2002). *Chronic illness: Impact and interventions* (5th ed.). Boston: Jones & Bartlett.

McCance, K.L., & Huether, S.E. (2002). *Pathophysiology: The biologic basis for disease in adults and children.* (4th ed.). St. Louis: Mosby.

Potter, P.A., & Perry, A.G. (2001). *Fundamentals of nursing* (5th ed.). St. Louis: Mosby.

# Fall Prevention Behavior (1909)

*Domain-Health Knowledge & Behavior (IV)*

*Class-Risk Control & Safety (T)*

*Scale(s)-Never demonstrated to Consistently demonstrated (m)*

*Care Recipient:*

*Data Source:*

**F**

> **Definition:** Personal or family caregiver actions to minimize risk factors that might precipitate falls in the personal environment

OUTCOME TARGET RATING:    Maintain at_____    Increase to_____

| Fall Prevention Behavior Overall Rating | Never demonstrated 1 | Rarely demonstrated 2 | Sometimes demonstrated 3 | Often demonstrated 4 | Consistently demonstrated 5 | |
|---|---|---|---|---|---|---|
| **INDICATORS:** | | | | | | |
| 190903 Places barriers to prevent falls | 1 | 2 | 3 | 4 | 5 | NA |
| 190905 Uses handrails as needed | 1 | 2 | 3 | 4 | 5 | NA |
| 190915 Uses grab bars as needed | 1 | 2 | 3 | 4 | 5 | NA |
| 190914 Uses rubber mats in tub/shower | 1 | 2 | 3 | 4 | 5 | NA |
| 190910 Uses well-fitting tied shoes | 1 | 2 | 3 | 4 | 5 | NA |
| 190901 Uses assistive devices correctly | 1 | 2 | 3 | 4 | 5 | NA |
| 190918 Uses vision-correcting devices | 1 | 2 | 3 | 4 | 5 | NA |
| 190902 Provides assistance with mobility | 1 | 2 | 3 | 4 | 5 | NA |
| 190919 Uses safe transfer procedure | 1 | 2 | 3 | 4 | 5 | NA |
| 190922 Provides adequate lighting | 1 | 2 | 3 | 4 | 5 | NA |
| 190909 Uses stools/ladders appropriately | 1 | 2 | 3 | 4 | 5 | NA |
| 190906 Eliminates clutter, spills, glare from floors | 1 | 2 | 3 | 4 | 5 | NA |
| 190907 Removes rugs | 1 | 2 | 3 | 4 | 5 | NA |
| 190908 Arranges for removal of snow and ice from walking surfaces | 1 | 2 | 3 | 4 | 5 | NA |
| 190911 Adjusts toilet height as needed | 1 | 2 | 3 | 4 | 5 | NA |
| 190912 Adjusts chair height as needed | 1 | 2 | 3 | 4 | 5 | NA |
| 190913 Adjusts bed height as needed | 1 | 2 | 3 | 4 | 5 | NA |
| 190916 Controls agitation and restlessness | 1 | 2 | 3 | 4 | 5 | NA |
| 190917 Uses precautions when taking medications that increase risk for falls | 1 | 2 | 3 | 4 | 5 | NA |

*1st edition 1997; Revised 3rd edition (formerly Safety Behavior: Fall Prevention)*

## Outcome Content References:

Abreu, N., Hutchins, J., Matson, J., Polizzi, N., & Seymour, C.J. (1998). Effect of group versus home visit safety education and prevention strategies for falling in community-dwelling elderly persons. *Home Health Care Management & Practice, 10*(4), 57-65.

Kilpack, V., Boehm, J., Smith, N., & Mudge, B. (1991). Using research-based interventions to decrease patient falls. *Applied Nursing Research, 4*(2), 50-56.

Meller, J.L., & Shermeta, D.W. (1987). Falls in urban children. *American Journal of Diseases of Children, 14*(12), 1271-1275.

Moss, A.B. (1992). Are the elderly safe at home? *Journal of Community Health Nursing, 9*(1), 13-19.

O'Connor, M.S., Boyle, W.E., O'Connor, G.T., & Letellier, R. (1992). Self-reported safety practices in child care facilities. *American Journal of Preventative Medicine, 8*(1), 14-18.

Urton, M.M. (1991). A community home inspection approach to preventing falls among the elderly. *Public Health Reports, 106*(2), 192-196.

F

F

# *Falls Occurrence (1912)*

*Domain-Health Knowledge & Behavior (IV)*

*Class-Risk Control & Safety (T)*

*Scale(s)-10 and over to None (g)*

Care Recipient:

Data Source:

**Definition:** Number of falls in the past _____ (define period of time)

OUTCOME TARGET RATING:    Maintain at_____    Increase to_____

| Falls Occurrence Overall Rating | 10 and over 1 | 7-9 2 | 4-6 3 | 1-3 4 | None 5 | |
|---|---|---|---|---|---|---|
| INDICATORS: | | | | | | |
| 191201  Number of falls while standing still | 1 | 2 | 3 | 4 | 5 | NA |
| 191202  Number of falls while walking | 1 | 2 | 3 | 4 | 5 | NA |
| 191203  Number of falls while sitting | 1 | 2 | 3 | 4 | 5 | NA |
| 191204  Number of falls from bed | 1 | 2 | 3 | 4 | 5 | NA |
| 191205  Number of falls while transferring | 1 | 2 | 3 | 4 | 5 | NA |
| 191206  Number of falls climbing steps | 1 | 2 | 3 | 4 | 5 | NA |
| 191207  Number of falls descending steps | 1 | 2 | 3 | 4 | 5 | NA |

*1st edition 1997; Revised 3rd edition (formerly Safety Status: Falls Occurrence)*

**Outcome Content References:**

Baker, L. (1992). Developing a safety plan that works for patients and nurses. *Rehabilitation Nursing, 17*(5), 264-266.

Nelson, R.C., & Amin, M.A. (1990). Falls in the elderly. *Emergency Care of the Elderly, 8*(2), 309-323.

Schoenfelder, D.P., & Van Why, K. (1997). A fall prevention educational program for community dwelling seniors. *Public Health Nursing, 14*(6), 383-390.

Schroeder, P. (1995). Benchmarking patient falls. *Nursing Quality Connection, 4*(5), 5.

Sorock, G.S. (1988). Falls among the elderly: Epidemiology and prevention. *American Journal of Preventive Medicine, 4*(5), 282-288.

# Family Coping (2600)

Domain-Family Health (VI)

Class-Family Well-Being (X)

Scale(s)-Never demonstrated to Consistently demonstrated (m)

Care Recipient:

Data Source:

**Definition:** Family actions to manage stressors that tax family resources

OUTCOME TARGET RATING:     Maintain at_____     Increase to_____

**F**

| Family Coping Overall Rating | Never demonstrated 1 | Rarely demonstrated 2 | Sometimes demonstrated 3 | Often demonstrated 4 | Consistently demonstrated 5 | |
|---|---|---|---|---|---|---|
| INDICATORS: | | | | | | |
| 260001 Demonstrates role flexibility | 1 | 2 | 3 | 4 | 5 | NA |
| 260002 Enables member role flexibility | 1 | 2 | 3 | 4 | 5 | NA |
| 260003 Confronts family problems | 1 | 2 | 3 | 4 | 5 | NA |
| 260005 Manages family problems | 1 | 2 | 3 | 4 | 5 | NA |
| 260006 Involves family members in decision making | 1 | 2 | 3 | 4 | 5 | NA |
| 260007 Expresses feelings and emotions freely among members | 1 | 2 | 3 | 4 | 5 | NA |
| 260008 Uses strategies to manage anger among members | 1 | 2 | 3 | 4 | 5 | NA |
| 260009 Uses family-centered stress reduction activities | 1 | 2 | 3 | 4 | 5 | NA |
| 260010 Cares for needs of all family members | 1 | 2 | 3 | 4 | 5 | NA |
| 260011 Establishes family priorities | 1 | 2 | 3 | 4 | 5 | NA |
| 260012 Establishes schedule for family routines and activities | 1 | 2 | 3 | 4 | 5 | NA |
| 260019 Shares responsibility for family tasks | 1 | 2 | 3 | 4 | 5 | NA |
| 260013 Arranges for respite care | 1 | 2 | 3 | 4 | 5 | NA |
| 260014 Plans for emergencies | 1 | 2 | 3 | 4 | 5 | NA |
| 260015 Maintains financial stability | 1 | 2 | 3 | 4 | 5 | NA |
| 260016 Seeks family assistance when appropriate | 1 | 2 | 3 | 4 | 5 | NA |
| 260017 Uses available social support | 1 | 2 | 3 | 4 | 5 | NA |

*2nd edition 2000; Revised 3rd edition*

## Outcome Content References:

Friedman, M. (1991). An instrument to evaluate effectiveness in family functioning. *Western Journal of Nursing Research, 13*(2), 220-241.

Hymovich, D.P. (1983). The Chronicity Impact and Coping Instrument: Parent Questionnaire. *Nursing Research, 32*(5), 275-281.

Lohan, J.A., & Murphy, S.A. (2002). Family functioning and family typology after an adolescent or young adult's sudden violent death. *Journal of Family Nursing, 8*(1), 32-49.

McCubbin, H.I. (1987). Family Coping Inventory. In H.I. McCubbin, & A.I. Thomas (Eds.). *Family Assessment: Research and Practice.* Madison, WI: University of Wisconsin-Madison.

Ryan-Wenger, N.M. (1990). Development and psychometric properties of the Schoolagers' Coping Strategies Inventory. *Nursing Research, 39*(6), 344-349.

# Family Functioning (2602)

*Domain-Family Health (VI)*

*Class-Family Well-Being (X)*

*Scale(s)-Never demonstrated to Consistently demonstrated (m)*

*Care Recipient:*

*Data Source:*

F

**Definition:** Capacity of the family system to meet the needs of its members during developmental transitions

OUTCOME TARGET RATING:    Maintain at_____    Increase to_____

| Family Functioning Overall Rating | Never demonstrated 1 | Rarely demonstrated 2 | Sometimes demonstrated 3 | Often demonstrated 4 | Consistently demonstrated 5 | |
|---|---|---|---|---|---|---|

INDICATORS:

| | | | | | | | |
|---|---|---|---|---|---|---|---|
| 260201 | Socializes new family members | 1 | 2 | 3 | 4 | 5 | NA |
| 260202 | Cares for dependent members | 1 | 2 | 3 | 4 | 5 | NA |
| 260203 | Regulates behavior of members | 1 | 2 | 3 | 4 | 5 | NA |
| 260204 | Allocates responsibilities among members | 1 | 2 | 3 | 4 | 5 | NA |
| 260206 | Maintains stable core of traditions | 1 | 2 | 3 | 4 | 5 | NA |
| 260207 | Accepts change and new ideas | 1 | 2 | 3 | 4 | 5 | NA |
| 260208 | Adapts to developmental transitions | 1 | 2 | 3 | 4 | 5 | NA |
| 260209 | Adapts to unexpected crises | 1 | 2 | 3 | 4 | 5 | NA |
| 260210 | Obtains adequate resources to meet needs of members | 1 | 2 | 3 | 4 | 5 | NA |
| 260211 | Creates environment where members can freely express feelings | 1 | 2 | 3 | 4 | 5 | NA |
| 260212 | Accepts diversity among members | 1 | 2 | 3 | 4 | 5 | NA |
| 260213 | Involves members in problem solving | 1 | 2 | 3 | 4 | 5 | NA |
| 260214 | Involves members in conflict resolution | 1 | 2 | 3 | 4 | 5 | NA |
| 260205 | Members perform expected roles | 1 | 2 | 3 | 4 | 5 | NA |
| 260215 | Members support and help one another | 1 | 2 | 3 | 4 | 5 | NA |
| 260216 | Members spend time with one another | 1 | 2 | 3 | 4 | 5 | NA |
| 260217 | Members express commitment to family | 1 | 2 | 3 | 4 | 5 | NA |
| 260218 | Members express loyalty to family | 1 | 2 | 3 | 4 | 5 | NA |
| 260219 | Members participate in community activities | 1 | 2 | 3 | 4 | 5 | NA |

*2nd edition 2000; Revised 3rd edition*

Outcome Content References:

Friedman, M.M., Bowden V., & Jones, E. (2003). *Family nursing: Research theory, & practice* (5th ed.). New Jersey: Prentice Hall.

Friedman, M. (1991). An instrument to evaluate effectiveness in family functioning. *Western Journal of Nursing Research, 13*(2), 220-241.

Nishka, K.J. (2001). Mexican American family survival, continuity, and growth: The parental perspective. *Nursing Science Quarterly, 14*(4), 322-329.

Quayhagen, M.P., & Roth, P.A. (1989). From models to measures in assessment of mature families. *Journal of Professional Nursing, 5*(3), 144-151.

Roberts, C.S., & Feetham, S.A. (1982). Assessing family functioning across three areas of relationships. *Nursing Research, 31*(4), 231-235.

Swain, K.J., & Harrigan, M.P. (1995). *Measures of family functioning for research and practice.* New York: Springer Publishing.

Tamplin, A., & Goodyer, I.M. (2001). Family functioning in adolescents at high and low risk for major depressive disorder. *European Child & Adolescent Psychiatry, 10*(3), 170-190.

**F**

# *Family Health Status (2606)*

*Domain-Family Health (VI)*

*Class-Family Well-Being (X)*

*Scale(s)-Severely compromised to Not compromised (a) and Severe to None (n)*

*Care Recipient:*

*Data Source:*

**Definition:** Overall health and social competence of family unit

OUTCOME TARGET RATING:    Maintain at_____    Increase to_____

| Family Health Status Overall Rating | Severely compromised 1 | Substantially compromised 2 | Moderately compromised 3 | Mildly compromised 4 | Not compromised 5 | |
|---|---|---|---|---|---|---|
| INDICATORS: | | | | | | |
| 260605 Physical health of members | 1 | 2 | 3 | 4 | 5 | NA |
| 260606 Physical activity of members | 1 | 2 | 3 | 4 | 5 | NA |
| 260618 Mental health of members | 1 | 2 | 3 | 4 | 5 | NA |
| 260601 Immunization of members | 1 | 2 | 3 | 4 | 5 | NA |
| 260612 Physical development of members | 1 | 2 | 3 | 4 | 5 | NA |
| 260613 Psychosocial development of members | 1 | 2 | 3 | 4 | 5 | NA |
| 260617 Adjustment to disabilities | 1 | 2 | 3 | 4 | 5 | NA |
| 260602 Appropriate child care provisions | 1 | 2 | 3 | 4 | 5 | NA |
| 260603 Appropriate dependent adult care provisions | 1 | 2 | 3 | 4 | 5 | NA |
| 260604 Access to health care | 1 | 2 | 3 | 4 | 5 | NA |
| 260607 School attendance of members | 1 | 2 | 3 | 4 | 5 | NA |
| 260608 School achievement of members | 1 | 2 | 3 | 4 | 5 | NA |
| 260609 Parental employment | 1 | 2 | 3 | 4 | 5 | NA |
| 260610 Appropriate housing | 1 | 2 | 3 | 4 | 5 | NA |
| 260611 Nutritious food supply | 1 | 2 | 3 | 4 | 5 | NA |
| 260614 Access to financial resources | 1 | 2 | 3 | 4 | 5 | NA |
| 260615 Appropriate health care resources | 1 | 2 | 3 | 4 | 5 | NA |
| 260616 Appropriate social services resources | 1 | 2 | 3 | 4 | 5 | NA |

| | Severe | Substantial | Moderate | Mild | None | |
|---|---|---|---|---|---|---|
| 260620 Domestic violence | 1 | 2 | 3 | 4 | 5 | NA |
| 260621 Physical abuse of members | 1 | 2 | 3 | 4 | 5 | NA |
| 260624 Psychological abuse of members | 1 | 2 | 3 | 4 | 5 | NA |
| 260625 Alcohol abuse | 1 | 2 | 3 | 4 | 5 | NA |
| 260626 Tobacco use | 1 | 2 | 3 | 4 | 5 | NA |
| 260627 Recreational drug use | 1 | 2 | 3 | 4 | 5 | NA |

*2nd edition 2000; Revised 3rd edition*

## Outcome Content References:

Children's Defense Fund (1997). *The state of America's Children: Leave no child behind – Yearbook 1997.* Washington, DC: Author.

Cody, W.K. (1999). The view of family within the human becoming theory. In R.R. Parse (Ed.), *Illuminations: The human becoming theory in practice and research.* Sudbury, MA: Jones & Bartlett.

DeVoe, E.R., & Kantor, G.K. (2002). Measurement issues in child maltreatment and family violence prevention programs. *Trauma Violence & Abuse, 3*(1), 15-39.

Donnelly, E. (1993). Family health assessment. *Home Healthcare Nurse, 11*(2), 30-37.

Ford-Gilboe, M. (2002). Developing knowledge about family health promotion by testing the development model of health and nursing. *Journal of Family Nursing, 8*(2), 140-156.

Friedman, M. (1991). An instrument to evaluate effectiveness in family functioning. *Western Journal of Nursing Research, 13*(2), 220-241.

Garwick, A.W., Patterson, J.M., Meschke, L.L., Bennett, F.C., & Blum, R.W. (2002). The uncertainty of preadolescents' chronic health conditions and family distress. *Journal of Family Nursing, 8*(1), 11-31.

Graham, K.Y. (1995). Childbearing family health: A wake up call. *Public Health Nursing, 12*(3), 141.

Nishka, K.J. (2001). Mexican American family survival, continuity, and growth: The parental perspective. *Nursing Science Quarterly, 14*(4), 322-329.

Quayhagen, M.P., & Roth, P.A. (1989). From models to measures in assessment of mature families. *Journal of Professional Nursing, 5*(3), 144-151.

Reutter, L. (1984). Family health assessment–an integrated approach. *Journal of Advanced Nursing, 9*(4), 391-399.

**F**

# Family Integrity (2603)

*Domain-Family Health (VI)*

*Class-Family Well-Being (X)*

*Scale(s)-Never demonstrated to Consistently demonstrated (m)*

*Care Recipient:*

*Data Source:*

---

**Definition:** Family members' behaviors that collectively demonstrate cohesion, strength, and emotional bonding

OUTCOME TARGET RATING: Maintain at_____ Increase to_____

| Family Integrity Overall Rating | Never demonstrated 1 | Rarely demonstrated 2 | Sometimes demonstrated 3 | Often demonstrated 4 | Consistently demonstrated 5 | |
|---|---|---|---|---|---|---|

**INDICATORS:**

| | | Never 1 | Rarely 2 | Sometimes 3 | Often 4 | Consistently 5 | |
|---|---|---|---|---|---|---|---|
| 260305 | Interacts frequently with extended family | 1 | 2 | 3 | 4 | 5 | NA |
| 260308 | Involves members in conflict resolution | 1 | 2 | 3 | 4 | 5 | NA |
| 260309 | Involves members in problem solving | 1 | 2 | 3 | 4 | 5 | NA |
| 260310 | Encourages individual autonomy and independence | 1 | 2 | 3 | 4 | 5 | NA |
| 260311 | Prepares and eats meals together | 1 | 2 | 3 | 4 | 5 | NA |
| 260312 | Participates in leisure-time activities together | 1 | 2 | 3 | 4 | 5 | NA |
| 260313 | Participates in family rituals | 1 | 2 | 3 | 4 | 5 | NA |
| 260314 | Participates in family traditions | 1 | 2 | 3 | 4 | 5 | NA |
| 260315 | Provides support during times of crisis | 1 | 2 | 3 | 4 | 5 | NA |
| 260301 | Members express loyalty | 1 | 2 | 3 | 4 | 5 | NA |
| 260302 | Members express strong ties to family | 1 | 2 | 3 | 4 | 5 | NA |
| 260303 | Members express affection to one another | 1 | 2 | 3 | 4 | 5 | NA |
| 260304 | Members help one another in performing roles and daily tasks | 1 | 2 | 3 | 4 | 5 | NA |
| 260306 | Members share thoughts, feelings, interests, concerns | 1 | 2 | 3 | 4 | 5 | NA |
| 260307 | Members communicate openly and honestly with one another | 1 | 2 | 3 | 4 | 5 | NA |

*2nd edition 2000; Revised 3rd edition*

Outcome Content References:

Friedman, M.M., Bowden V., & Jones, E. (2003). *Family nursing: Research theory, & practice* (5th ed.). New Jersey: Prentice Hall.

Swain, K.J., & Harrigan, M.P. (1995). *Measures of family functioning for research and practice.* New York: Springer Publishing.

Thomasgard, M., & Metz, W.P. (1999). Parent-child relationship disorders: What do the Child Vulnerability Scale and the Parent Protection Scale measure? *Clinical Pediatrics, 38*(6), 347-356.

# *Family Normalization (2604)*

Domain-Family Health (VI)

Class-Family Well-Being (X)

Scale(s)-Never demonstrated to Consistently demonstrated (m)

Care Recipient:

Data Source:

**Definition:** Capacity of the family system to maintain routines and develop strategies for optimal functioning when a member has a chronic illness or disability

OUTCOME TARGET RATING:    Maintain at_____    Increase to_____

| Family Normalization Overall Rating | Never demonstrated 1 | Rarely demonstrated 2 | Sometimes demonstrated 3 | Often demonstrated 4 | Consistently demonstrated 5 | |
|---|---|---|---|---|---|---|
| INDICATORS: | | | | | | |
| 260401 Acknowledges existence of impairment and its potential to alter family routines | 1 | 2 | 3 | 4 | 5 | NA |
| 260402 Acknowledges family life as essentially normal | 1 | 2 | 3 | 4 | 5 | NA |
| 260403 Maintains usual family routines | 1 | 2 | 3 | 4 | 5 | NA |
| 260404 Adapts prescribed treatment regimen to fit family routines and values | 1 | 2 | 3 | 4 | 5 | NA |
| 260405 Adapts family routines to accommodate needs of affected individual | 1 | 2 | 3 | 4 | 5 | NA |
| 260406 Meets physical needs of non-affected members | 1 | 2 | 3 | 4 | 5 | NA |
| 260407 Meets psychosocial needs of non-affected members | 1 | 2 | 3 | 4 | 5 | NA |
| 260408 Meets developmental needs of non-affected members | 1 | 2 | 3 | 4 | 5 | NA |
| 260410 Communicates importance to maintain normal activities and routines as appropriate | 1 | 2 | 3 | 4 | 5 | NA |
| 260411 Maintains usual parenting expectations for affected child | 1 | 2 | 3 | 4 | 5 | NA |

F

*Continued*

| Family Normalization—cont'd | | Never demonstrated | Rarely demonstrated | Sometimes demonstrated | Often demonstrated | Consistently demonstrated | |
|---|---|---|---|---|---|---|---|
| 260412 | Provides age/ability appropriate activities for affected member | 1 | 2 | 3 | 4 | 5 | NA |
| 260413 | Structures activities to avoid attention to or embarrassment of affected member | 1 | 2 | 3 | 4 | 5 | NA |
| 260414 | Structures environment to avoid attention to or embarrassment of affected member | 1 | 2 | 3 | 4 | 5 | NA |
| 260415 | Uses resources, including support groups, as needed | 1 | 2 | 3 | 4 | 5 | NA |

*2nd edition 2000; Revised 3rd edition*

Outcome Content References:

Bossert, E., Holaday, B., Harkins. A., & Turner-Henson, A. (1990). Strategies of normalization used by parents of chronically ill school age children. *Journal of Child Psychiatric Nursing, 3*(2), 57-61.

Knafl, K., Brietmayer, B., Gallo, A., & Zoeller, L. (1996). Family response to childhood chronic illness: Description of management styles. *Journal of Pediatric Nursing, 11*(5), 315-316.

Knafl, K.A., & Deatrick, J.A. (1986). How families manage chronic conditions: An analysis of the concept of normalization. *Research in Nursing and Health, 9*(3), 215-222.

Knafl, K.A., & Gilliss, C.L. (2002). Families and chronic illness: A synthesis of current research. *Journal of Family Nursing, 8*(3), 178-198.

Wade, S.L., Taylor, H.G., Drotar, D., Stancin, T., Yeates, K.O., & Minich, N.M. (2002). A prospective study of long-term caregiver and family adaptation following brain injury in children. *Journal of Health Trauma Rehabilitation, 17*(2), 96-111.

# Family Participation in Professional Care (2605)

Domain-Family Health (VI)

Class-Family Well-Being (X)

Scale(s)-Never demonstrated to Consistently demonstrated (m)

Care Recipient:

Data Source:

> **Definition:** Family involvement in decision-making, delivery, and evaluation of care provided by health care personnel

OUTCOME TARGET RATING:      Maintain at_____      Increase to_____

| Family Participation in Professional Care Overall Rating | Never demonstrated 1 | Rarely demonstrated 2 | Sometimes demonstrated 3 | Often demonstrated 4 | Consistently demonstrated 5 | |
|---|---|---|---|---|---|---|
| **INDICATORS:** | | | | | | |
| 260501   Participates in planning care | 1 | 2 | 3 | 4 | 5 | NA |
| 260502   Participates in providing care | 1 | 2 | 3 | 4 | 5 | NA |
| 260503   Provides relevant information | 1 | 2 | 3 | 4 | 5 | NA |
| 260504   Obtains needed information | 1 | 2 | 3 | 4 | 5 | NA |
| 260505   Identifies factors that affect care | 1 | 2 | 3 | 4 | 5 | NA |
| 260506   Collaborates in determining treatment | 1 | 2 | 3 | 4 | 5 | NA |
| 260507   Defines needs and problems relevant to care | 1 | 2 | 3 | 4 | 5 | NA |
| 260508   Makes decisions when patient is unable to do so | 1 | 2 | 3 | 4 | 5 | NA |
| 260509   Participates in decisions with patient | 1 | 2 | 3 | 4 | 5 | NA |
| 260510   Participates in mutual goal setting for care | 1 | 2 | 3 | 4 | 5 | NA |
| 260511   Evaluates effectiveness of care | 1 | 2 | 3 | 4 | 5 | NA |

*2nd edition 2000*

## Outcome Content References:

Biley, F.C. (1992). Some determinants that effect patient participation in decision-making about nursing care. *Journal of Advanced Nursing, 17,* 414-421.

Brownlea, A. (1987). Participation: Myths, realities and prognosis. *Social Science and Medicine, 25*(6), 605-614.

Ende, J., Kazis, L., Ash, A., & Moskowitz, M.A. (1989). Measuring patients' desire for autonomy: Decision making and information-seeking preferences among medical patients. *Journal of General Internal Medicine, 4*(1), 23-30.

Janis, I.L., & Rodin, J. (1979). Attribution, control and decision making: Social psychology and health care. In G.D. Stone, F. Cohen & N.E. Adler (Eds.) *Health psychology.* San Francisco: Josey-Bass.

McEwen, J. (1985). Primary health care: The challenge of participation. In U. Laaser, R. Senault & H. Viefhues. (Eds.). *Primary health care in the making.* Hiedelberg: Springer-Verlag.

Richardson, A., & Bray, C. (1987). *Promoting health through participation.* London: Policy Studies Institute.

Stanhope, M., & Lancaster, J. (2000) *Community health nursing* (5th ed.). St Louis: Mosby.

# Family Physical Environment (2607)

*Domain-Family Health (VI)*

*Class-Family Well-Being (X)*

*Scale-Not adequate to Totally adequate (f)*

*Care Recipient:*

*Data Source:*

| **Definition:** Physical arrangements in the home that provide safety and stimulation to family members |
| --- |

OUTCOME TARGET RATING:    Maintain at_____    Increase to_____

| Family Physical Environment Overall Rating | Not adequate 1 | Slightly adequate 2 | Moderately adequate 3 | Substantially adequate 4 | Totally adequate 5 | |
| --- | --- | --- | --- | --- | --- | --- |
| **INDICATORS:** | | | | | | |
| 260701 Rooms have pictures or wall decorations appealing to members | 1 | 2 | 3 | 4 | 5 | NA |
| 260702 Interior of dwelling sufficiently lighted | 1 | 2 | 3 | 4 | 5 | NA |
| 260703 Sufficient, functional furniture | 1 | 2 | 3 | 4 | 5 | NA |
| 260704 Sufficient space to move safely in dwelling | 1 | 2 | 3 | 4 | 5 | NA |
| 260705 Dwelling reasonably clean and minimally cluttered | 1 | 2 | 3 | 4 | 5 | NA |
| 260706 At least 100 square feet (9x12 room) of living space available per person in the dwelling | 1 | 2 | 3 | 4 | 5 | NA |
| 260707 Noise level managed for family comfort and safety | 1 | 2 | 3 | 4 | 5 | NA |
| 260708 Building maintained to eliminate dangerous structural or health defects | 1 | 2 | 3 | 4 | 5 | NA |
| 260709 Outside environment safe and free of hazards | 1 | 2 | 3 | 4 | 5 | NA |
| 260710 Play equipment in the dwelling and outside of the dwelling safe and free of hazards | 1 | 2 | 3 | 4 | 5 | NA |
| 260711 Dwelling free of rodents and bugs | 1 | 2 | 3 | 4 | 5 | NA |
| 260712 Dwelling heated as needed | 1 | 2 | 3 | 4 | 5 | NA |
| 260713 Locks on windows and exterior doors | 1 | 2 | 3 | 4 | 5 | NA |
| 260714 Windows secured with safety guards and/or screens as needed | 1 | 2 | 3 | 4 | 5 | NA |
| 260715 Dwelling well ventilated | 1 | 2 | 3 | 4 | 5 | NA |
| 260716 Clean water available in the dwelling | 1 | 2 | 3 | 4 | 5 | NA |
| 260717 Cooking facilities present and working | 1 | 2 | 3 | 4 | 5 | NA |
| 260718 Light available for family activities | 1 | 2 | 3 | 4 | 5 | NA |
| 260719 Dwelling air conditioned as needed | 1 | 2 | 3 | 4 | 5 | NA |
| 260720 Dwelling free of tobacco smoke | 1 | 2 | 3 | 4 | 5 | NA |

*3rd edition*

F

Outcome Content References:

Caldwell, B., & Bradley, R. (1984). *Home observation for measurement of the environment.* Little Rock, Arkansas: University of Arkansas.

Bradley, R.H., Corwyn, R.F., & Whiteside-Mansell, L. (1996). Life at home: Same time, different places—An examination of the HOME Inventory in different cultures. *Early Development and Parenting, 5*(4), 251-269.

Smith, C.M., & Maurer, F.A. (1995). *Community Health Nursing* (pp. 645-651). Philadelphia, PA: W.B. Saunders.

F

# *Family Resiliency (2608)*

*Domain-Family Health (VI)*  
*Class-Family Well-Being (X)*  
*Scale-Never demonstrated to Consistently demonstrated (m)*

*Care Recipient:*  
*Data Source:*

---

**Definition:** Capacity of the family system to successfully adapt and function competently following significant adversity or crises

OUTCOME TARGET RATING:     Maintain at_____     Increase to_____

| Family Resiliency Overall Rating | Never demonstrated 1 | Rarely demonstrated 2 | Sometimes demonstrated 3 | Often demonstrated 4 | Consistently demonstrated 5 | |
|---|---|---|---|---|---|---|
| **INDICATORS:** | | | | | | |
| 260801 Mobilizes quickly following adversity | 1 | 2 | 3 | 4 | 5 | NA |
| 260802 Proposes practical, constructive solutions for disputes | 1 | 2 | 3 | 4 | 5 | NA |
| 260803 Adapts to adversities as challenges | 1 | 2 | 3 | 4 | 5 | NA |
| 260804 Tolerates separations when required | 1 | 2 | 3 | 4 | 5 | NA |
| 260805 Discusses meaning of crisis | 1 | 2 | 3 | 4 | 5 | NA |
| 260806 Expresses confidence in overcoming adversities | 1 | 2 | 3 | 4 | 5 | NA |
| 260807 Maintains values, goals, and dreams | 1 | 2 | 3 | 4 | 5 | NA |
| 260808 Exhibits warmth and low hostility | 1 | 2 | 3 | 4 | 5 | NA |
| 260809 Supports members | 1 | 2 | 3 | 4 | 5 | NA |
| 260810 Cooperates to meet challenges | 1 | 2 | 3 | 4 | 5 | NA |
| 260811 Nurtures members | 1 | 2 | 3 | 4 | 5 | NA |
| 260812 Protects members | 1 | 2 | 3 | 4 | 5 | NA |
| 260813 Communicates clearly among members | 1 | 2 | 3 | 4 | 5 | NA |
| 260814 Clarifies ambiguous communication | 1 | 2 | 3 | 4 | 5 | NA |
| 260815 Uses effective conflict management strategies | 1 | 2 | 3 | 4 | 5 | NA |
| 260816 Shares humor | 1 | 2 | 3 | 4 | 5 | NA |
| 260817 Reports learning and growth | 1 | 2 | 3 | 4 | 5 | NA |
| 260818 Maintains usual family routines | 1 | 2 | 3 | 4 | 5 | NA |
| 260819 Prepares for future challenges | 1 | 2 | 3 | 4 | 5 | NA |
| 260820 Supports individuality and independence among members | 1 | 2 | 3 | 4 | 5 | NA |
| 260821 Accepts respite from extended family | 1 | 2 | 3 | 4 | 5 | NA |

F

| Family Resiliency—cont'd | | Never demonstrated | Rarely demonstrated | Sometimes demonstrated | Often demonstrated | Consistently demonstrated | |
|---|---|---|---|---|---|---|---|
| 260822 | Accepts respite from friends | 1 | 2 | 3 | 4 | 5 | NA |
| 260823 | Accepts assistance with direct care from extended family | 1 | 2 | 3 | 4 | 5 | NA |
| 260824 | Accepts assistance with direct care from friends | 1 | 2 | 3 | 4 | 5 | NA |
| 260825 | Accepts assistance with IADLs from extended family | 1 | 2 | 3 | 4 | 5 | NA |
| 260826 | Accepts assistance with IADLs from friends | 1 | 2 | 3 | 4 | 5 | NA |
| 260827 | Seeks emotional support from extended family | 1 | 2 | 3 | 4 | 5 | NA |
| 260828 | Seeks emotional support from extended friends | 1 | 2 | 3 | 4 | 5 | NA |
| 260829 | Uses community resources for assistance when needed | 1 | 2 | 3 | 4 | 5 | NA |
| 260830 | Uses community groups for emotional support | 1 | 2 | 3 | 4 | 5 | NA |
| 260831 | Adjusts work and other schedules as able to support and assist members | 1 | 2 | 3 | 4 | 5 | NA |
| 260832 | Uses healthcare team for information and assistance | 1 | 2 | 3 | 4 | 5 | NA |

*IADLs= Instrumental activities of daily living.

*3rd edition*

Outcome Content References:

McCubbin, M., Balling, K., Possin, P., Frierdich, S., & Bryne, B. (2002). Family resiliency in childhood cancer. *Family Relations, 51*, 103-111.

Patterson, J.M. (2002). Integrating family resilience and family stress theory. *Journal of Marriage and Family, 64*, 349-360.

Walsh, F. (2002). A family resilience framework: Innovative practice applications. *Family Relations, 51*, 130-137.

F

# *Family Social Climate (2601)*

*Domain-Family Health (VI)*

*Class-Family Well-Being (X)*

*Scale(s)-Never demonstrated to Consistently demonstrated (m)*

Care Recipient:

Data Source:

> **Definition:** Supportive milieu as characterized by family member relationships and goals

OUTCOME TARGET RATING:     Maintain at_____     Increase to_____

**F**

| **Family Social Climate Overall Rating** | Never demonstrated 1 | Rarely demonstrated 2 | Sometimes demonstrated 3 | Often demonstrated 4 | Consistently demonstrated 5 | |
|---|---|---|---|---|---|---|
| INDICATORS: | | | | | | |
| 260101 Participates in activities together | 1 | 2 | 3 | 4 | 5 | NA |
| 260102 Participates in family traditions | 1 | 2 | 3 | 4 | 5 | NA |
| 260103 Attends religious services together | 1 | 2 | 3 | 4 | 5 | NA |
| 260104 Receives visits from friends and extended family members | 1 | 2 | 3 | 4 | 5 | NA |
| 260105 Participates in leisure activities | 1 | 2 | 3 | 4 | 5 | NA |
| 260119 Participates in community events | 1 | 2 | 3 | 4 | 5 | NA |
| 260106 Establishes family rules | 1 | 2 | 3 | 4 | 5 | NA |
| 260107 Follows schedule for family routines and activities | 1 | 2 | 3 | 4 | 5 | NA |
| 260108 Maintains clean/ neat home | 1 | 2 | 3 | 4 | 5 | NA |
| 260109 Supports one another | 1 | 2 | 3 | 4 | 5 | NA |
| 260110 Provides privacy for members | 1 | 2 | 3 | 4 | 5 | NA |
| 260111 Encourages individual autonomy and independence | 1 | 2 | 3 | 4 | 5 | NA |
| 260112 Shares the decision-making process | 1 | 2 | 3 | 4 | 5 | NA |
| 260113 Works together cooperatively to meet goals | 1 | 2 | 3 | 4 | 5 | NA |
| 260114 Shares feelings with one another | 1 | 2 | 3 | 4 | 5 | NA |
| 260120 Shares problems with one another | 1 | 2 | 3 | 4 | 5 | NA |
| 260115 Discusses issues relevant to family | 1 | 2 | 3 | 4 | 5 | NA |
| 260116 Solves problems together | 1 | 2 | 3 | 4 | 5 | NA |
| 260117 Promotes cohesion and family goals | 1 | 2 | 3 | 4 | 5 | NA |

*2nd edition 2000; Revised 3rd edition (formerly Family Environment: Internal)*

Outcome Content References:

Folden, S.L. (2001). The politics of the family. In P.L. Munhall (Ed.), *The emergence of family into the 21st century*. Sudbury, MA: Jones & Bartlett Publishers.

Moos, R.H. (1974). *Family Environment Scale – Form R*. Palo Alto, CA: Consulting Psychologists Press.

Swain, K.J., & Harrigan, M.P. (1995). *Measures of family functioning for research and practice*. New York: Springer Publishing.

F

# *Family Support During Treatment (2609)*

*Domain-Family Health (VI)*

*Class-Family Well-Being (X)*

*Scale(s)-Never demonstrated to Consistently demonstrated (m)*

*Care Recipient:*

*Data Source:*

**Definition:** Family presence and emotional support for an individual undergoing treatment

OUTCOME TARGET RATING:    Maintain at_____    Increase to_____

| Family Support During Treatment Overall Rating | Never demonstrated 1 | Rarely demonstrated 2 | Sometimes demonstrated 3 | Often demonstrated 4 | Consistently demonstrated 5 | |
|---|---|---|---|---|---|---|

**F**

INDICATORS:

| | | | | | | | |
|---|---|---|---|---|---|---|---|
| 260901 | Members express desire to support ill member | 1 | 2 | 3 | 4 | 5 | NA |
| 260902 | Members express feelings and emotions of concern for ill member | 1 | 2 | 3 | 4 | 5 | NA |
| 260903 | Members ask how they may assist | 1 | 2 | 3 | 4 | 5 | NA |
| 260904 | Requests information about process/procedure | 1 | 2 | 3 | 4 | 5 | NA |
| 260905 | Requests information about patient condition or status | 1 | 2 | 3 | 4 | 5 | NA |
| 260906 | Members maintain communication with ill member | 1 | 2 | 3 | 4 | 5 | NA |
| 260907 | Members encourage ill member | 1 | 2 | 3 | 4 | 5 | NA |
| 260908 | Members provide comforting touch to ill member | 1 | 2 | 3 | 4 | 5 | NA |
| 260909 | Seeks social and or spiritual support for ill member | 1 | 2 | 3 | 4 | 5 | NA |
| 260910 | Collaborates with ill member in determining care | 1 | 2 | 3 | 4 | 5 | NA |
| 260911 | Collaborates with health care providers in determining care | 1 | 2 | 3 | 4 | 5 | NA |
| 260912 | Members verbalize meaning of health crisis | 1 | 2 | 3 | 4 | 5 | NA |

| Family Support During Treatment—cont'd | | Never demonstrated | Rarely demonstrated | Sometimes demonstrated | Often demonstrated | Consistently demonstrated | |
|---|---|---|---|---|---|---|---|
| 260913 | Contacts other members as desired by ill member | 1 | 2 | 3 | 4 | 5 | NA |
| 260914 | Provides accurate information to other members | 1 | 2 | 3 | 4 | 5 | NA |

*3rd edition*

## Outcome Content References:

American Heart Association. (2000). Part 2: Ethical aspects of CPR and ECC. *Circulation, 102* (Suppl. 8), I12-I21.

Eichhorn, D.J., Meyers, T.A., Guzzetta, C.E., Clark, A.P., Klein, J.D., & Calvin, A.O. (2001). During invasive procedures and resuscitation: Hearing the voice of the patient. *American Journal of Nursing, 101*(5), 48-55.

Emergency Nurses Association. (1998). Emergency Nurses Association position statement: Family presence at the bedside during invasive procedures and/or resuscitation. *Journal of Emergency Nursing, 21*(2), 26A.

Emergency Nurses Association. (2000). *Presenting the option for family presence* (2nd ed.). Des Plaines, IL: Author.

Friedman, M. (1991). An instrument to evaluate effectiveness in family functioning. *Western Journal of Nursing Research, 13*(2), 220-241.

Hampe, S.O. (1975). Needs of a grieving spouse in a hospital setting. *Nursing Research, 24*(2), 113-120.

McPhee, A.T. (1983). Let the family in. *Nursing, 13*(1), 120.

Meyers, T.A., Eichhorn, D.J., & Guzzetta, C.E. (1998). Do families want to be present during CPR? A retrospective survey. *Journal of Emergency Nursing, 24*(5), 400-405.

Meyers, T.A., Eichhorn, D.J., Guzzetta, C.E., Clark, A.P., Klein, J.D., Taliaferro, E., & Calvin, A. (2000). Family presence during invasive procedures and resuscitation. *American Journal of Nursing, 100*(2), 32-42.

F

# Fear Level (1210)

Domain-Psychosocial Health (III)

Class-Psychological Well-Being (M)

Scale(s)-Severe to None (n)

Care Recipient:

Data Source:

**Definition:** Severity of manifested apprehension, tension, or uneasiness arising from an identifiable source

OUTCOME TARGET RATING:     Maintain at_____     Increase to_____

| Fear Level Overall Rating | Severe 1 | Substantial 2 | Moderate 3 | Mild 4 | None 5 | |
|---|---|---|---|---|---|---|

INDICATORS:

| | | Severe 1 | Substantial 2 | Moderate 3 | Mild 4 | None 5 | |
|---|---|---|---|---|---|---|---|
| 121001 | Distress | 1 | 2 | 3 | 4 | 5 | NA |
| 121002 | Tendency to blame others | 1 | 2 | 3 | 4 | 5 | NA |
| 121003 | Self absorption | 1 | 2 | 3 | 4 | 5 | NA |
| 121004 | Lack of self confidence | 1 | 2 | 3 | 4 | 5 | NA |
| 121005 | Restlessness | 1 | 2 | 3 | 4 | 5 | NA |
| 121006 | Irritability | 1 | 2 | 3 | 4 | 5 | NA |
| 121007 | Outbursts of anger | 1 | 2 | 3 | 4 | 5 | NA |
| 121008 | Difficulty concentrating | 1 | 2 | 3 | 4 | 5 | NA |
| 121009 | Difficulty learning | 1 | 2 | 3 | 4 | 5 | NA |
| 121010 | Difficulty problem solving | 1 | 2 | 3 | 4 | 5 | NA |
| 121011 | Decreased perceptual field | 1 | 2 | 3 | 4 | 5 | NA |
| 121012 | Perceived inadequacy in interpersonal relationships | 1 | 2 | 3 | 4 | 5 | NA |
| 121013 | Exaggerated concern about life events | 1 | 2 | 3 | 4 | 5 | NA |
| 121014 | Preoccupation with life events | 1 | 2 | 3 | 4 | 5 | NA |
| 121015 | Preoccupation with source of fear | 1 | 2 | 3 | 4 | 5 | NA |
| 121016 | Increased blood pressure | 1 | 2 | 3 | 4 | 5 | NA |
| 121017 | Increased radial pulse rate | 1 | 2 | 3 | 4 | 5 | NA |
| 121018 | Increased respiratory rate | 1 | 2 | 3 | 4 | 5 | NA |
| 121019 | Dilated pupils | 1 | 2 | 3 | 4 | 5 | NA |
| 121020 | Sweating | 1 | 2 | 3 | 4 | 5 | NA |
| 121021 | Feeling faint | 1 | 2 | 3 | 4 | 5 | NA |
| 121022 | Muscle tension | 1 | 2 | 3 | 4 | 5 | NA |
| 121023 | Facial tension | 1 | 2 | 3 | 4 | 5 | NA |
| 121024 | Frequent urination | 1 | 2 | 3 | 4 | 5 | NA |
| 121025 | Diarrhea | 1 | 2 | 3 | 4 | 5 | NA |
| 121026 | Inability to sleep | 1 | 2 | 3 | 4 | 5 | NA |
| 121027 | Skin pale | 1 | 2 | 3 | 4 | 5 | NA |
| 121028 | Fatigue | 1 | 2 | 3 | 4 | 5 | NA |
| 121029 | Withdrawal | 1 | 2 | 3 | 4 | 5 | NA |
| 121030 | Avoidance behavior | 1 | 2 | 3 | 4 | 5 | NA |
| 121031 | Verbalized fear | 1 | 2 | 3 | 4 | 5 | NA |
| 121032 | Crying | 1 | 2 | 3 | 4 | 5 | NA |

*3rd edition*

Outcome Content References:

American Psychiatric Association. (2000). *Diagnostic and statistical manual of mental disorders* (4th ed. text revision). Washington DC: Author.

Charron, H.S. (1998). Anxiety disorders. In E.M. Varcarolis (Ed.), *Foundations of psychiatric mental health nursing* (3rd ed., pp. 443-477). Philadelphia: Saunders.

Kim, M., Sertella, R., Gulanick, M., Moyer, K., Parsons, E., Scherbel, J., Stafford, M., Suhayada, R., & Yocum, C. (1984). Clinical validation of cardiovascular nursing diagnoses. In M. Kim, G. Mcfarland, & A. Mclane (Eds.), *Classification of nursing diagnoses: Proceedings of the fifth national conference* (pp. 128-137). St. Louis: Mosby.

Taylor-Loughran, A.E., O'Brien, M.E., Lachapelle, R., & Rangel, S. (1989). Defining characteristics of the nursing diagnoses fear and anxiety: A validation study. *Applied Nursing Research, 2*(4), 178-186.

Whitley, G.G., & Tousman, S.A. (1996). A multivariate approach for validation of anxiety and fear. *Nursing Diagnoses, 7*(3), 116-124.

# Fear Level: Child (1213)

Domain-Psychological Health (III)

Class-Psychological Well-Being (M)

Scale(s)-Severe to None (n)

Care Recipient:

Data Source:

**Definition:** Severity of manifested apprehension, tension, or uneasiness arising from an identifiable source in a child from 1 year through 17 years of age

OUTCOME TARGET RATING:     Maintain at_____     Increase to_____

| Fear Level: Child Overall Rating | Severe 1 | Substantial 2 | Moderate 3 | Mild 4 | None 5 | |
|---|---|---|---|---|---|---|
| **INDICATORS:** | | | | | | |
| 121301 Real or imagined illness | 1 | 2 | 3 | 4 | 5 | NA |
| 121302 Increased heart rate | 1 | 2 | 3 | 4 | 5 | NA |
| 121303 Headaches | 1 | 2 | 3 | 4 | 5 | NA |
| 121304 Stomachaches | 1 | 2 | 3 | 4 | 5 | NA |
| 121305 Frequent urination | 1 | 2 | 3 | 4 | 5 | NA |
| 121306 Frequent diarrhea | 1 | 2 | 3 | 4 | 5 | NA |
| 121307 Fatigue | 1 | 2 | 3 | 4 | 5 | NA |
| 121308 Weight loss | 1 | 2 | 3 | 4 | 5 | NA |
| 121309 Generalized aches and pains | 1 | 2 | 3 | 4 | 5 | NA |
| 121310 Sweating | 1 | 2 | 3 | 4 | 5 | NA |
| 121311 Crying | 1 | 2 | 3 | 4 | 5 | NA |
| 121312 Emotional lability | 1 | 2 | 3 | 4 | 5 | NA |
| 121313 Stammering | 1 | 2 | 3 | 4 | 5 | NA |
| 121314 Irritability | 1 | 2 | 3 | 4 | 5 | NA |
| 121315 Excessive giggling | 1 | 2 | 3 | 4 | 5 | NA |
| 121316 Avoidance behavior | 1 | 2 | 3 | 4 | 5 | NA |
| 121317 Withdrawal | 1 | 2 | 3 | 4 | 5 | NA |
| 121318 Increased school absence | 1 | 2 | 3 | 4 | 5 | NA |
| 121319 Cheating | 1 | 2 | 3 | 4 | 5 | NA |
| 121320 Difficulty staying on task | 1 | 2 | 3 | 4 | 5 | NA |
| 121321 Difficulty concentrating | 1 | 2 | 3 | 4 | 5 | NA |
| 121322 Tics | 1 | 2 | 3 | 4 | 5 | NA |
| 121323 Nail biting | 1 | 2 | 3 | 4 | 5 | NA |
| 121324 Finger sucking | 1 | 2 | 3 | 4 | 5 | NA |
| 121325 Hair chewing | 1 | 2 | 3 | 4 | 5 | NA |
| 121326 Chewing clothing | 1 | 2 | 3 | 4 | 5 | NA |
| 121327 Fidgeting | 1 | 2 | 3 | 4 | 5 | NA |
| 121328 Rocking motion | 1 | 2 | 3 | 4 | 5 | NA |
| 121329 Shaking | 1 | 2 | 3 | 4 | 5 | NA |
| 121330 Violent behavior | 1 | 2 | 3 | 4 | 5 | NA |
| 121331 Violence displayed in drawings | 1 | 2 | 3 | 4 | 5 | NA |
| 121332 Destructive behavior | 1 | 2 | 3 | 4 | 5 | NA |
| 121333 Stealing | 1 | 2 | 3 | 4 | 5 | NA |
| 121334 Regressive behavior | 1 | 2 | 3 | 4 | 5 | NA |
| 121335 Excessive approval seeking behavior | 1 | 2 | 3 | 4 | 5 | NA |
| 121336 Demanding behavior | 1 | 2 | 3 | 4 | 5 | NA |
| 121337 Fabrication of stories | 1 | 2 | 3 | 4 | 5 | NA |
| 121338 Continuous questioning | 1 | 2 | 3 | 4 | 5 | NA |
| 121339 Clinging behavior | 1 | 2 | 3 | 4 | 5 | NA |
| 121340 Injury faking behavior | 1 | 2 | 3 | 4 | 5 | NA |
| 121341 Self-destructive behavior | 1 | 2 | 3 | 4 | 5 | NA |
| 121342 Recreational drug use | 1 | 2 | 3 | 4 | 5 | NA |
| 121343 Alcohol use | 1 | 2 | 3 | 4 | 5 | NA |
| 121344 Excessive self-denigration | 1 | 2 | 3 | 4 | 5 | NA |

*3rd edition*

F

*Continued*

Outcome Content References:

Berliner, L., & Saunders, B.E. (1996). Treating fear and anxiety in sexually abused children. *Child Maltreatment, 1*(4), 294-310.

Byrne, B. (2000). Relationships between anxiety, fear, self-esteem and coping strategies in adolescence. *Adolescence, 35*(137), 201-216.

Carlson, K.L., Broome, M., & Vessey, J.A. (2000). Using distraction to reduce reported pain, fear and behavioral distress in children and adolescents: A multisite study. *Journal of the Society of Pediatric Nursing, 5*(2), 75-85.

Carr, T.D., Lemanek, K.L., & Armstrong, F.D. (1998). Pain and fear ratings: Clinical implications of age and gender differences. *Journal of Pain and Symptom Management, 15*(5), 305-313.

Carroll, M.K., & Ryan-Wenger, N.A. (1999). School-age children's fears, anxiety and human figure drawings. *Journal of Pediatric Health Care, 13*(1), 24-31.

Nicastro, E.A., & Whetsell, M.V. (1999). Children's fears. *Journal of Pediatric Nursing, 14*(6), 392-402.

Potter, P.A. & Perry, A.G. (2001). *Fundamentals of nursing* (5th ed.). St. Louis: Mosby.

Wilson, A.H., & Yorker, B. (1996). Fears of medical events among school-age children with emotional disorders, parents, and health care providers. *Issues in Mental Health Nursing, 18*(1), 57-71.

Wong, D.L., Hockenberry-Eaton, M., Wilson, D., Winkelstein, M.L., Ahmann, E., & DiVito-Thomas, P.A. (1999). *Whaley & Wong's nursing care of infants and children.* (6th ed.). St. Louis: Mosby.

**F**

# Fear Self-Control (1404)

*Domain-Psychosocial Health (III)*

*Class-Self Control (O)*

*Scale(s)-Never demonstrated to Consistently demonstrated (m)*

*Care Recipient:*

*Data Source:*

**Definition:** Personal actions to eliminate or reduce disabling feelings of apprehension, tension, or uneasiness from an identifiable source

OUTCOME TARGET RATING:    Maintain at_____    Increase to_____

| Fear Self-Control Overall Rating | Never demonstrated 1 | Rarely demonstrated 2 | Sometimes demonstrated 3 | Often demonstrated 4 | Consistently demonstrated 5 | |
|---|---|---|---|---|---|---|
| **INDICATORS:** | | | | | | |
| 140401 Monitors intensity of fear | 1 | 2 | 3 | 4 | 5 | NA |
| 140402 Eliminates precursors of fear | 1 | 2 | 3 | 4 | 5 | NA |
| 140403 Seeks information to reduce fear | 1 | 2 | 3 | 4 | 5 | NA |
| 140404 Avoids source of fear when possible | 1 | 2 | 3 | 4 | 5 | NA |
| 140405 Plans coping strategies for fearful situations | 1 | 2 | 3 | 4 | 5 | NA |
| 140406 Uses effective coping strategies | 1 | 2 | 3 | 4 | 5 | NA |
| 140407 Uses relaxation techniques to reduce fear | 1 | 2 | 3 | 4 | 5 | NA |
| 140408 Monitors duration of episodes | 1 | 2 | 3 | 4 | 5 | NA |
| 140409 Monitors length of time between episodes | 1 | 2 | 3 | 4 | 5 | NA |
| 140410 Maintains role performance | 1 | 2 | 3 | 4 | 5 | NA |
| 140411 Maintains social relationships | 1 | 2 | 3 | 4 | 5 | NA |
| 140412 Maintains concentration | 1 | 2 | 3 | 4 | 5 | NA |
| 140413 Maintains control over life | 1 | 2 | 3 | 4 | 5 | NA |
| 140414 Maintains physical functioning | 1 | 2 | 3 | 4 | 5 | NA |
| 140415 Maintains a sense of purpose despite fear | 1 | 2 | 3 | 4 | 5 | NA |
| 140416 Remains productive | 1 | 2 | 3 | 4 | 5 | NA |
| 140417 Controls fear response | 1 | 2 | 3 | 4 | 5 | NA |

*1st edition 1997; Revised 2nd edition 2000; Revised 3rd edition (formerly Fear Control)*

Outcome Content References:

+Marks, I. M., & Mathews, A. M. (1979). Brief standard self-rating for phobic patients. *Behavior Research and Therapy*, 17(3), 263-267.

McAuley, E., Mihalko, S.L., & Rosengren K. (1997). Self-efficacy and balance correlates of fear of falling in the elderly. *Journal of Aging and Physical Activity*, 5(4), 329-340.

McFarland, G.K., & McFarlane, E.A. (1997). *Nursing diagnosis & intervention: Planning for patient care* (3rd ed.). St. Louis: Mosby.

*Continued*

F

Moorhead, S.A., & Brighton, V.A. (2001). Anxiety and fear. In M. Maas, K. Buckwalter, M. Hardy, T. Tripp-Reimer, M. Titler & J. Specht (Eds.), *Nursing care of older adults: Diagnoses, outcomes & interventions* (pp. 571-592). St. Louis: Mosby.

Stuart, G.W., & Laraia, M.T. (2001). *Principles and practice of psychiatric nursing* (7th ed.). St. Louis: Mosby.

Whitley, G.G., & Tousman, S.A. (1996). A multivariate approach for validation of anxiety and fear. *Nursing Diagnosis, 7*(3), 116-124.

Wilson, A. H., & Yorker, B. (1997). Fears of medical events among school-age children with emotional disorders, parents, and health care providers. *Issues in Mental Health Nursing, 18*(1), 57-71.

F

# Fetal Status: Antepartum (0111)

*Domain-Functional Health (I)*

*Class-Growth & Development (B)*

*Scale(s)-Severe deviation from normal range to No deviation from normal range (b)*

*Care Recipient:*

*Data Source:*

> **Definition:** Extent to which fetal signs are within normal limits from conception to the onset of labor

OUTCOME TARGET RATING:    Maintain at_____    Increase to_____

| Fetal Status: Antepartum Overall Rating | Severe deviation from normal range 1 | Substantial deviation from normal range 2 | Moderate deviation from normal range 3 | Mild deviation from normal range 4 | No deviation from normal range 5 | |
|---|---|---|---|---|---|---|
| **INDICATORS:** | | | | | | |
| 011101 Fetal heart rate (120-160) | 1 | 2 | 3 | 4 | 5 | NA |
| 011102 Deceleration patterns in electronic fetal monitor findings | 1 | 2 | 3 | 4 | 5 | NA |
| 011103 Variability in electronic fetal monitor findings | 1 | 2 | 3 | 4 | 5 | NA |
| 011104 Fetal ultrasound growth measurements | 1 | 2 | 3 | 4 | 5 | NA |
| 011105 Fetal movement frequency | 1 | 2 | 3 | 4 | 5 | NA |
| 011106 Fetal movement pattern | 1 | 2 | 3 | 4 | 5 | NA |
| 011107 Nonstress test | 1 | 2 | 3 | 4 | 5 | NA |
| 011108 Contraction stress test | 1 | 2 | 3 | 4 | 5 | NA |
| 011109 Auscultated acceleration test | 1 | 2 | 3 | 4 | 5 | NA |
| 011110 Biophysical profile score | 1 | 2 | 3 | 4 | 5 | NA |
| 011111 Amniotic fluid sample findings | 1 | 2 | 3 | 4 | 5 | NA |
| 011112 Umbilical artery blood flow velocity | 1 | 2 | 3 | 4 | 5 | NA |

*2nd edition 2000; Revised 3rd edition*

## Outcome Content References:

Association of Women's Health, Obstetric and Neonatal Nurses. (1998). *Clinical competencies and education guide: Limited ultrasound examinations in obstetric and gynecologic/infertility settings.* Washington DC: Author.

Calhoun, S. (1990). "Ask the Experts": Daily fetal movement counts. *NAACOG Newsletter, 17*(8), p. 6.

Chez, B.F., Skurnick, J.H., Chez, R.A., Verklan, M.T., Biggs, S., & Hage, M.L. (1990). Interpretations of nonstress tests by obstetric nurses. *Journal of Obstetric, Gynecologic, and Neonatal Nursing, 19*(3), 227-232.

Gaffney, S., Solinger, L., & Vinzileos, A. (1990). The biophysical profile for fetal surveillance. *MCN: American Journal of Maternal Child Nursing, 15*(6), 356-360.

Gebauer, C., & Lowe, N. (1993). The biophysical profile: Antepartal assessment of fetal well-being. *Journal of Obstetric, Gynecologic, and Neonatal Nursing, 22*(2), 115-123.

Gegor C.L., & Paine, L.L. (1992). Antepartum fetal assessment techniques: An update for today's perinatal nurse. *Journal of Perinatal and Neonatal Nursing, 5*(4), 1-15.

Givens, S.R., & Moore, M.L. (1995). Status report on maternal and child health indicators. *Journal of Perinatal and Neonatal Nursing, 9*(1), 8-18.

Lowdermilk, D.L., & Perry, S.E. (2003). *Maternity Nursing* (6th ed.). St. Louis: Mosby.

Paine, L., et al. (1992). A comparison of the auscultated acceleration test and the nonstress test as predicators of perinatal outcomes. *Nursing Research, 41*(2), 87-91.

Petrikovsky, B.M. (1991). Antepartum fetal evaluation. A search for the ideal test. *Neonatal Intensive Care, 4*(5), 38-39.

Tucker, S.M. (2000). *Pocket guide to fetal monitoring and assessment* (4th ed.). St. Louis: Mosby.

F

# Fetal Status: Intrapartum (0112)

Domain-Functional Health (I)

Class-Growth & Development (B)

Scale(s)-Severe deviation from normal range to No deviation from normal range (b)

Care Recipient:

Data Source:

**Definition:** Extent to which fetal signs are within normal limits from onset of labor to delivery

OUTCOME TARGET RATING:     Maintain at_____     Increase to_____

| Fetal Status: Intrapartum Overall Rating | Severe deviation from normal range 1 | Substantial deviation from normal range 2 | Moderate deviation from normal range 3 | Mild deviation from normal range 4 | No deviation from normal range 5 | |
|---|---|---|---|---|---|---|
| **INDICATORS:** | | | | | | |
| 011201  Fetal heart rate (120-160) | 1 | 2 | 3 | 4 | 5 | NA |
| 011202  Deceleration patterns in electronic fetal monitor findings | 1 | 2 | 3 | 4 | 5 | NA |
| 011203  Variability in electronic fetal monitor findings | 1 | 2 | 3 | 4 | 5 | NA |
| 011204  Amniotic fluid color | 1 | 2 | 3 | 4 | 5 | NA |
| 011205  Amniotic fluid amount | 1 | 2 | 3 | 4 | 5 | NA |
| 011206  Fetal position | 1 | 2 | 3 | 4 | 5 | NA |
| 011207  Fetal presenting part | 1 | 2 | 3 | 4 | 5 | NA |
| 011209  Fetal scalp blood pH | 1 | 2 | 3 | 4 | 5 | NA |
| 011210  Fetal scalp stimulation response | 1 | 2 | 3 | 4 | 5 | NA |

*2nd edition 2000; Revised 3rd edition*

## Outcome Content References:

Dickason, E.J., Schultz, M.O., & Silverman, B.L. (1998). *Maternal-infant nursing care* (3rd ed.). St. Louis: Mosby.

Hodnett, E. (1996). Nursing support of the laboring woman. *Journal of Obstetric, and Neonatal Nursing, 25*(3), 257-263.

Lowe, N.K. (1996). The pain and discomfort of labor and birth. *Journal of Obstetric, and Neonatal Nursing, 25*(1), 82-92.

Mattson, S. (Ed.). (2000). *Core curriculum for maternal-newborn nursing* (2nd ed.). Philadelphia: W.B. Saunders.

Tucker, S.M. (2000). *Pocket guide to fetal monitoring and assessment* (4th ed.). St. Louis: Mosby.

# Fluid Balance (0601)

*Domain-Physiologic Health (II)*

*Care Recipient:*

*Class-Fluid & Electrolytes (G)*

*Data Source:*

*Scale(s)-Severely compromised to Not compromised (a) and Severe to None (n)*

**Definition:** Water balance in the intracellular and extracellular compartments of the body

OUTCOME TARGET RATING:   Maintain at_____   Increase to_____

| Fluid Balance Overall Rating | Severely compromised 1 | Substantially compromised 2 | Moderately compromised 3 | Mildly compromised 4 | Not compromised 5 | |
|---|---|---|---|---|---|---|
| **INDICATORS:** | | | | | | |
| 060101 Blood pressure | 1 | 2 | 3 | 4 | 5 | NA |
| 060122 Radial pulse rate | 1 | 2 | 3 | 4 | 5 | NA |
| 060102 Mean arterial pressure | 1 | 2 | 3 | 4 | 5 | NA |
| 060103 Central venous pressure | 1 | 2 | 3 | 4 | 5 | NA |
| 060104 Pulmonary wedge pressure | 1 | 2 | 3 | 4 | 5 | NA |
| 060105 Peripheral pulses | 1 | 2 | 3 | 4 | 5 | NA |
| 060107 24-hour intake and output balance | 1 | 2 | 3 | 4 | 5 | NA |
| 060109 Stable body weight | 1 | 2 | 3 | 4 | 5 | NA |
| 060116 Skin turgor | 1 | 2 | 3 | 4 | 5 | NA |
| 060117 Moist mucous membranes | 1 | 2 | 3 | 4 | 5 | NA |
| 060118 Serum electrolytes | 1 | 2 | 3 | 4 | 5 | NA |
| 060119 Hematocrit | 1 | 2 | 3 | 4 | 5 | NA |
| 060120 Urine specific gravity | 1 | 2 | 3 | 4 | 5 | NA |

| | Severe | Substantial | Moderate | Mild | None | |
|---|---|---|---|---|---|---|
| 060106 Orthostatic hypotension | 1 | 2 | 3 | 4 | 5 | NA |
| 060108 Adventitious breath sounds | 1 | 2 | 3 | 4 | 5 | NA |
| 060110 Ascites | 1 | 2 | 3 | 4 | 5 | NA |
| 060111 Neck vein distention | 1 | 2 | 3 | 4 | 5 | NA |
| 060112 Peripheral edema | 1 | 2 | 3 | 4 | 5 | NA |
| 060113 Soft, sunken eyeballs | 1 | 2 | 3 | 4 | 5 | NA |
| 060114 Confusion | 1 | 2 | 3 | 4 | 5 | NA |
| 060115 Thirst | 1 | 2 | 3 | 4 | 5 | NA |
| 060123 Muscle cramps | 1 | 2 | 3 | 4 | 5 | NA |
| 060124 Dizziness | 1 | 2 | 3 | 4 | 5 | NA |

*1st edition 1997; Revised 3rd edition*

## Outcome Content References:

Bosquet, G.L. (1990). Congestive heart failure: A review of nonpharmacologic therapies. *Journal of Cardiovascular Nursing, 4*(3), 35-46.

Coats, A.J.S., Adamopoulos, S., Meyer, T.E., Conway, J., & Sleight, P. (1990). Effects of physical training in chronic heart failure. *The Lancet, 335*(8681), 63-66.

Fukada, N. (1990). Outcome standards for the client with congestive heart failure. *Journal of Cardiovascular Nursing, 4*(3), 59-70.

Johanson, B.C., et al. (1988). *Standards for critical care* (3rd ed.). St. Louis: Mosby.

Kraft, P.A. (2000). The osmotic shift. *Journal of Intravenous Nursing, 23*(4), 220-224.

Medina, J. (2000). *Standards for acute and critical care nursing practice* (3rd ed.). Irvine, CA: American Association of Critical-Care Nurses.

*Continued*

Reese, J.L. (2001). Fluid volume deficit—dehydration: Isotonic, hypotonic, and hypertonic. In M. Maas, K. Buckwalter, M. Hardy, T. Tripp-Reimer, M. Titler & J. Specht (Eds.), *Nursing care of older adults: Diagnoses, outcomes & interventions* (pp. 183-200). St. Louis: Mosby.

Toto, K.H. (1998). Fluid balance assessment: The total perspective. *Critical Care Clinics of North America, 10*(4), 383-400.

Vullo-Navich, K., Smith, S., Andrews, M., Levine, A.M., Tischer, J. F., & Veglia, J.M. (1998). Comfort and incidence of abnormal serum sodium, BUN, creatinine and osmolality in dehydration of terminal illness. *The American Journal of Hospice & Palliative Care, 15*(2), 77-84.

F

# Fluid Overload Severity (0603)

Domain-Physiologic Health (II)

Class-Fluid & Electrolytes (G)

Scale(s)-Severe to None (n)

Care Recipient:

Data Source:

**Definition:** Severity of excess fluids in the intracellular and extracellular compartments of the body

OUTCOME TARGET RATING:      Maintain at_____      Increase to_____

| Fluid Overload Severity Overall Rating | | Severe 1 | Substantially 2 | Moderately 3 | Mild 4 | None 5 | |
|---|---|---|---|---|---|---|---|
| INDICATORS: | | | | | | | |
| 060301 | Periorbital edema | 1 | 2 | 3 | 4 | 5 | NA |
| 060302 | Hand edema | 1 | 2 | 3 | 4 | 5 | NA |
| 060303 | Sacral edema | 1 | 2 | 3 | 4 | 5 | NA |
| 060304 | Ankle edema | 1 | 2 | 3 | 4 | 5 | NA |
| 060305 | Leg edema | 1 | 2 | 3 | 4 | 5 | NA |
| 060306 | Ascites | 1 | 2 | 3 | 4 | 5 | NA |
| 060307 | Increased abdominal girth | 1 | 2 | 3 | 4 | 5 | NA |
| 060308 | Generalized edema | 1 | 2 | 3 | 4 | 5 | NA |
| 060309 | Venous congestion | 1 | 2 | 3 | 4 | 5 | NA |
| 060310 | Rales | 1 | 2 | 3 | 4 | 5 | NA |
| 060311 | Malaise | 1 | 2 | 3 | 4 | 5 | NA |
| 060312 | Lethargy | 1 | 2 | 3 | 4 | 5 | NA |
| 060313 | Headache | 1 | 2 | 3 | 4 | 5 | NA |
| 060314 | Confusion | 1 | 2 | 3 | 4 | 5 | NA |
| 060315 | Seizures | 1 | 2 | 3 | 4 | 5 | NA |
| 060316 | Coma | 1 | 2 | 3 | 4 | 5 | NA |
| 060317 | Increased blood pressure | 1 | 2 | 3 | 4 | 5 | NA |
| 060318 | Increased body weight | 1 | 2 | 3 | 4 | 5 | NA |
| 060319 | Decreased urinary output | 1 | 2 | 3 | 4 | 5 | NA |
| 060320 | Decreased specific urine gravity | 1 | 2 | 3 | 4 | 5 | NA |
| 060321 | Decreased urine color | 1 | 2 | 3 | 4 | 5 | NA |
| 060322 | Decreased serum sodium | 1 | 2 | 3 | 4 | 5 | NA |
| 060323 | Increased serum sodium | 1 | 2 | 3 | 4 | 5 | NA |

*3rd edition*

Outcome Content References:

Edwards, S.L. (2000). Fluid overload and monitoring indices. *Professional Nurse, 15*(9), 568-572.

Kelly, A.L. (1999). Left ventricular systolic heart failure resulting in acute pulmonary edema: Pathophysiology and nursing management in the emergency department. *Australian Emergency Nursing Journal, 2*(1), 5-9.

Smeltzer, S.C., & Bare, B.G. (Eds.). (2003). *Brunner and Suddarth's textbook of medical-surgical nursing* (10th ed.). Philadelphia: Lippincott, Williams, & Wilkins.

# Grief Resolution (1304)

*Domain-Psychosocial Health (III)*

*Class-Psychosocial Adaptation (N)*

*Scale(s)-Never demonstrated to Consistently demonstrated (m)*

*Care Recipient:*

*Data Source:*

| **Definition:** Adjustment to actual or impending loss |
|---|

OUTCOME TARGET RATING:    Maintain at_____    Increase to_____

| Grief Resolution Overall Rating | Never demonstrated 1 | Rarely demonstrated 2 | Sometimes demonstrated 3 | Often demonstrated 4 | Consistently demonstrated 5 | |
|---|---|---|---|---|---|---|
| **INDICATORS:** | | | | | | |
| 130401 Resolves feelings about loss | 1 | 2 | 3 | 4 | 5 | NA |
| 130402 Expresses spiritual beliefs about death | 1 | 2 | 3 | 4 | 5 | NA |
| 130403 Verbalizes reality of loss | 1 | 2 | 3 | 4 | 5 | NA |
| 130404 Verbalizes acceptance of loss | 1 | 2 | 3 | 4 | 5 | NA |
| 130405 Describes meaning of the loss or death | 1 | 2 | 3 | 4 | 5 | NA |
| 130406 Participates in planning funeral | 1 | 2 | 3 | 4 | 5 | NA |
| 130409 Discusses unresolved conflict(s) | 1 | 2 | 3 | 4 | 5 | NA |
| 130410 Reports absence of somatic distress | 1 | 2 | 3 | 4 | 5 | NA |
| 130411 Reports decreased preoccupation with loss | 1 | 2 | 3 | 4 | 5 | NA |
| 130412 Maintains living environment | 1 | 2 | 3 | 4 | 5 | NA |
| 130413 Maintains grooming and hygiene | 1 | 2 | 3 | 4 | 5 | NA |
| 130414 Reports absence of sleep disturbance | 1 | 2 | 3 | 4 | 5 | NA |
| 130415 Reports adequate nutritional intake | 1 | 2 | 3 | 4 | 5 | NA |
| 130416 Reports normal sexual desire | 1 | 2 | 3 | 4 | 5 | NA |
| 130417 Seeks social support | 1 | 2 | 3 | 4 | 5 | NA |
| 130418 Shares loss with significant others | 1 | 2 | 3 | 4 | 5 | NA |
| 130419 Reports involvement in social activities | 1 | 2 | 3 | 4 | 5 | NA |
| 130420 Progresses through stages of grief | 1 | 2 | 3 | 4 | 5 | NA |
| 130421 Expresses positive expectations about the future | 1 | 2 | 3 | 4 | 5 | NA |

*1st edition 1997; Revised 3rd edition*

**Outcome Content References:**

Batemen, A., Broderick, D., Gleason, L., Kardon, R., Flaherty, C., & Anderson, S. (1992). Dysfunctional grieving. *Journal of Psychosocial Nursing, 30*(12), 5-9.

Cooley, M.E. (1992). Bereavement care: A role for nurses. *Cancer Nursing, 15*(2), 125-129.

Freitag-Koontz, M.J. (1988). Parents' grief reaction to the diagnosis of their infants' severe neurologic impairment and static encephalopathy. *Journal of Perinatal and Neonatal Nursing, 2*(2), 45-57.

Gibbons, M.B. (1992). A child dies, a child survives: The impact of sibling loss. *Journal of Pediatric Health Care, 6*(2), 45-57.

Harrigan, R., Naber, M., Jensen, K., Tse, A., & Perez, D. (1993). Perinatal grief: Response to the loss of an infant. *Neonatal Network, 12*(5), 25-31.

Kallenberg, K., & Soderfeldt, B. (1992). Three years later: Grief, view of life, and personal crisis after the death of a family member. *Journal of Palliative Care, 8*(4), 13-19.

Kirschling, J.M., & McBride, A.B. (1989). Effects of age and sex on the experience of widowhood. *Western Journal of Nursing Research, 11*(2), 207-218.

Kuntz, B. (1991). Exploring the grief of adolescents after the death of a parent. *Journal of Child and Adolescent Psychiatric and Mental Health Nursing, 4*(3), 105-109.

+Prigerson, H.G., Maciejewski, P.K., Reynolds, C.F., Bierhals, A., Newsom, J.T., Fasiczka, A., Frank, E., Doman, J., & Miller, M. (1995). Inventory of complicated grief: A scale to measure maladaptive symptoms of loss. *Psychiatry Research, 59*(1-2), 65-79.

Whiting, G., & Buckwalter, K.C. (2001). Grieving. In M. Maas, K. Buckwalter, M. Hardy, T. Tripp-Reimer, M. Titler & J. Specht (Eds.), *Nursing care of older adults: Diagnoses, outcomes & interventions* (pp. 631-650). St. Louis: Mosby.

**G**

# Growth (0110)

Domain-Functional Health (I)

Class-Growth & Development (B)

Scale(s)-Severe deviation from normal range to No deviation from normal range (b)

Care Recipient:

Data Source:

**Definition:** Normal increase in bone size and body weight during growth years

OUTCOME TARGET RATING:     Maintain at_____     Increase to_____

| Growth Overall Rating | Severe deviation from normal range 1 | Substantial deviation from normal range 2 | Moderate deviation from normal range 3 | Mild deviation from normal range 4 | No deviation from normal range 5 | |
|---|---|---|---|---|---|---|
| **INDICATORS:** | | | | | | |
| 011001 Weight percentile for sex | 1 | 2 | 3 | 4 | 5 | NA |
| 011002 Weight percentile for age | 1 | 2 | 3 | 4 | 5 | NA |
| 011003 Weight percentile for height | 1 | 2 | 3 | 4 | 5 | NA |
| 011004 Rate of weight gain | 1 | 2 | 3 | 4 | 5 | NA |
| 011005 Rate of height gain | 1 | 2 | 3 | 4 | 5 | NA |
| 011006 Length/height percentile for age | 1 | 2 | 3 | 4 | 5 | NA |
| 011007 Length/height percentile for sex | 1 | 2 | 3 | 4 | 5 | NA |
| 011008 Head circumference percentile for age | 1 | 2 | 3 | 4 | 5 | NA |
| 011009 Bone mass index | 1 | 2 | 3 | 4 | 5 | NA |
| 011010 Mean body mass | 1 | 2 | 3 | 4 | 5 | NA |

*1st edition 1997; Revised 3rd edition*

### Outcome Content References:

Allen, K.D., Warzak, W.J., Greger, N.G., Bernotas, T.D., & Huseman, C.A. (1993). Psychosocial adjustment of children with isolated growth hormone deficiency. *Children's Health Care, 22*(1), 61-72.

Blinkin, N.J., Yip, R., Fleshood, L., & Trowbridge, F.L. (1988). Birth weight and childhood growth. *Pediatrics, 82*(6), 828-834.

Georgieff, M.K., Hoffman, J.S., Pereira, G.R., Bernbaum, J., & Hoffman-Williamson, M. (1985). Effect of neonatal caloric deprivation on head growth and 1-year developmental status in preterm infants. *Journal of Pediatrics, 107,* 581-587.

Hockenberry, M.J., Wilson, D., Winkelstein, M.L., & Kline, N.E. (2003). *Wong's nursing care of infants and children* (7th ed.). St. Louis: Mosby.

Jung, E., & Czajka-Narins, D.M. (1985). Birth weight doubling and tripling times: An updated look at the effects of birth weight, sex, race and type of feeding. *The American Journal of Clinical Nutrition, 42*(8), 182-189.

Sapala, S. (1994). Pediatric management problems. *Pediatric Nursing, 20*(1), 54-55.

Tanner, J.M., & Davies, P.S.W. (1985). Clinical longitudinal standards for height and height velocity for North American children. *The Journal of Pediatrics, 107*(3), 317-329.

G

# *Health Beliefs (1700)*

Domain-Health Knowledge & Behavior (IV)

Class-Health Beliefs (R)

Scale(s)-Very weak to Very strong (I)

Care Recipient:

Data Source:

**Definition:** Personal convictions that influence health behaviors

OUTCOME TARGET RATING:    Maintain at_____    Increase to_____

| Health Beliefs Overall Rating | Very weak 1 | Weak 2 | Moderate 3 | Strong 4 | Very strong 5 | |
|---|---|---|---|---|---|---|
| INDICATORS: | | | | | | |
| 170001 Perceived importance of taking action | 1 | 2 | 3 | 4 | 5 | NA |
| 170002 Perceived threat from inaction | 1 | 2 | 3 | 4 | 5 | NA |
| 170003 Perceived benefits of action | 1 | 2 | 3 | 4 | 5 | NA |
| 170004 Perceived internal control of action | 1 | 2 | 3 | 4 | 5 | NA |
| 170005 Perceived control of health outcome | 1 | 2 | 3 | 4 | 5 | NA |
| 170006 Perceived reduction of threat from action | 1 | 2 | 3 | 4 | 5 | NA |
| 170007 Perceived improvement in lifestyle from action | 1 | 2 | 3 | 4 | 5 | NA |
| 170008 Perceived ability to perform action | 1 | 2 | 3 | 4 | 5 | NA |
| 170009 Perceived resources to perform action | 1 | 2 | 3 | 4 | 5 | NA |
| 170010 Perceived absence of barriers to action | 1 | 2 | 3 | 4 | 5 | NA |

*1st edition 1997*

Outcome Content References:

+Champion, V.L. (1993). Instrument refinement for breast cancer screening behaviors. *Nursing Research, 42*(3), 139-143.

Gillis, A.J. (1993). Determinants of health promoting lifestyle: An integrative review. *Journal of Advanced Nursing, 18(3),* 345-353.

Glick, O. J., & Ressler, C. (2001). Altered health maintenance. In M. Maas, K. Buckwalter, M. Hardy, T. Tripp-Reimer, M. Titler, & J. Specht (Eds.), *Nursing care of older adults: Diagnoses, outcomes & interventions* (pp. 6-22). St. Louis: Mosby.

Hayes, D., & Ross, C. (1987). Concern with appearance, health beliefs, and eating habits. *Journal of Health and Social Behavior, 28*(6), 120-130.

+Kim, K.K., Horan, M.L., Gendler, P., & Patel, M.K. (1991). Development and evaluation of the osteoporosis health belief scale. *Research in Nursing and Health, 14*(2), 155-163.

Robertson, D., & Keller, C. (1992). Relationships among health beliefs, self-efficacy, and exercise adherence in patients with coronary artery disease. *Heart & Lung, 21*(1), 56-63.

Thompson, J., McFarland, G.K., & Hirsch, J.E. (2002). *Mosby's clinical nursing* (5th ed.). St. Louis: Mosby.

# Health Beliefs: Perceived Ability to Perform (1701)

Domain-Health Knowledge & Behavior (IV)

Class-Health Beliefs (R)

Scale(s)-Very weak to Very strong (l)

Care Recipient:

Data Source:

**Definition:** Personal conviction that one can carry out a given health behavior

OUTCOME TARGET RATING: Maintain at_____ Increase to_____

| Health Beliefs: Perceived Ability to Perform Overall Rating | Very weak 1 | Weak 2 | Moderate 3 | Strong 4 | Very strong 5 | |
|---|---|---|---|---|---|---|
| INDICATORS: | | | | | | |
| 170101 Perception that health behavior is not too complex | 1 | 2 | 3 | 4 | 5 | NA |
| 170102 Perception that health behavior requires reasonable effort | 1 | 2 | 3 | 4 | 5 | NA |
| 170103 Perception that the frequency of health behavior is not excessive | 1 | 2 | 3 | 4 | 5 | NA |
| 170104 Perception of likelihood of performing health behavior over time | 1 | 2 | 3 | 4 | 5 | NA |
| 170105 Confidence related to past experience with health behavior | 1 | 2 | 3 | 4 | 5 | NA |
| 170106 Confidence related to past experience with similar health behaviors | 1 | 2 | 3 | 4 | 5 | NA |
| 170107 Confidence related to observation of successful experiences of others | 1 | 2 | 3 | 4 | 5 | NA |
| 170108 Confidence in ability to perform health behavior | 1 | 2 | 3 | 4 | 5 | NA |

*1st edition 1997; Revised 3rd edition*

Outcome Content References:

+Champion, V.L. (1993). Instrument refinement for breast cancer screening behaviors. *Nursing Research, 42*(3), 139-143.

De Weerdt, I., Visser, A., & Van der Veen, E. (1989). Attitude behavior theories and diabetes education programs. *Patient Education and Counseling, 14*, 3-19.

Hayes, D., & Ross, C. (1987). Concern with appearance, health beliefs, and eating habits. *Journal of Health and Social Behavior, 28*(6), 120-130.

Jemmot, L., & Jemmot, J. (1992). Increasing condom-use intentions among sexually active black adolescent women. *Nursing Research, 41*(5), 273-278.

Jensen, K., Banwart, L., Venhaus, R., Popkess-Vawter, S., & Perkins, S.B. (1993). Advanced rehabilitation nursing care of coronary angioplasty patients using self-efficacy theory. *Journal of Advanced Nursing, 18(6)*, 926-931.

Kim, K.K., Horan, M.L., Gendler, P., & Patel, M.K. (1991). Development and evaluation of the Osteoporosis Health Belief Scale. *Research in Nursing and Health, 14*(2), 155-163.

Lowe, N.K. (1993). Maternal confidence for labor: Development of the Childbirth Self-Efficacy Inventory. *Research in Nursing and Health, 16*(2), 141-149.

Robertson, D., & Keller, C. (1992). Relationships among health beliefs, self-efficacy, and exercise adherence in patients with coronary artery disease. *Heart & Lung, 21*(1), 56-63.

+Smith, M.S., Wallston, K.A., & Smith, C.A. (1995). The development and validation of the Perceived Health Competence Scale. *Health Education Research, 10*(1), 51-64.

# Health Beliefs: Perceived Control (1702)

Domain-Health Knowledge & Behavior (IV)

Class-Health Beliefs (R)

Scale(s)-Very weak to Very strong (l)

Care Recipient:

Data Source:

**Definition:** Personal conviction that one can influence a health outcome

OUTCOME TARGET RATING:          Maintain at_____          Increase to_____

| Health Beliefs: Perceived Control Overall Rating | Very weak 1 | Weak 2 | Moderate 3 | Strong 4 | Very strong 5 | |
|---|---|---|---|---|---|---|
| **INDICATORS:** | | | | | | |
| 170201 Perceived responsibility for health decisions | 1 | 2 | 3 | 4 | 5 | NA |
| 170202 Requested involvement in health decisions | 1 | 2 | 3 | 4 | 5 | NA |
| 170203 Efforts at gathering information | 1 | 2 | 3 | 4 | 5 | NA |
| 170204 Belief that own decisions control health outcomes | 1 | 2 | 3 | 4 | 5 | NA |
| 170205 Belief that own actions control health outcomes | 1 | 2 | 3 | 4 | 5 | NA |
| 170206 Willingness to designate surrogate decision maker | 1 | 2 | 3 | 4 | 5 | NA |
| 170207 Willingness to have current living will | 1 | 2 | 3 | 4 | 5 | NA |

*1st edition 1997*

Outcome Content References:

Calnan, M., & Moss, S. (1984). The Health Belief Model and compliance with education given at a class in breast self-examination. *Journal of Health and Social Behavior, 25(2)*, 198-210.

+Champion, V.L. (1993). Instrument refinement for breast cancer screening behaviors. *Nursing Research, 42(3)*, 139-143.

Gillis, A.J. (1993). Determinants of health promoting lifestyle: An integrative review. *Journal of Advanced Nursing, 18(3)*, 345-353.

Hayes, D., & Ross, C. (1987). Concern with appearance, health beliefs, and eating habits. *Journal of Health and Social Behavior, 28(6)*, 120-130.

+Wallston, K.A., & Wallston, B.S. (1981). Health Locus of Control Scales. In H. Lefcourt (Ed.), *Research with the locus of control construct (Vol. 1*, pp. 189-243). New York: Academic Press.

+Wallston, K.A.., Wallston, B.S., DeVellis, R. (1978). Development of the Multidimensional Health Locus of Control (MHLC) Scales. *Health Education Monographs, 6*, 160-170.

**H**

# Health Beliefs: Perceived Resources (1703)

Domain-Health Knowledge & Behavior (IV)

Class-Health Beliefs (R)

Scale(s)-Very weak to Very strong (l)

Care Recipient:

Data Source:

**Definition:** Personal conviction that one has adequate means to carry out a health behavior

OUTCOME TARGET RATING:    Maintain at_____    Increase to_____

| Health Beliefs: Perceived Resources Overall Rating | Very weak 1 | Weak 2 | Moderate 3 | Strong 4 | Very strong 5 | |
|---|---|---|---|---|---|---|

INDICATORS:

| | | Very weak 1 | Weak 2 | Moderate 3 | Strong 4 | Very strong 5 | |
|---|---|---|---|---|---|---|---|
| 170301 | Perceived support of significant others | 1 | 2 | 3 | 4 | 5 | NA |
| 170302 | Perceived support of friends | 1 | 2 | 3 | 4 | 5 | NA |
| 170303 | Perceived support of neighbors | 1 | 2 | 3 | 4 | 5 | NA |
| 170304 | Perceived support of health care provider | 1 | 2 | 3 | 4 | 5 | NA |
| 170305 | Perceived support of self-help groups | 1 | 2 | 3 | 4 | 5 | NA |
| 170306 | Perceived functional ability | 1 | 2 | 3 | 4 | 5 | NA |
| 170307 | Perceived energy to act | 1 | 2 | 3 | 4 | 5 | NA |
| 170309 | Perceived adequacy of time | 1 | 2 | 3 | 4 | 5 | NA |
| 170310 | Perceived adequacy of personal finances | 1 | 2 | 3 | 4 | 5 | NA |
| 170311 | Perceived adequacy of health insurance | 1 | 2 | 3 | 4 | 5 | NA |
| 170318 | Perceived access to prescribed medications | 1 | 2 | 3 | 4 | 5 | NA |
| 170312 | Perceived access to equipment | 1 | 2 | 3 | 4 | 5 | NA |
| 170313 | Perceived access to supplies | 1 | 2 | 3 | 4 | 5 | NA |
| 170314 | Perceived access to services | 1 | 2 | 3 | 4 | 5 | NA |
| 170315 | Perceived access to transportation | 1 | 2 | 3 | 4 | 5 | NA |
| 170316 | Perceived access to physical assistance | 1 | 2 | 3 | 4 | 5 | NA |

*1st edition 1997; Revised 3rd edition*

## Outcome Content References:

+Becker, H., Stuifbergen, A.K., & Sands, D. (1991). Development of a scale to measure barriers to health promotion activities among persons with disabilities. *American Journal of Health Promotion, 5* (6), 449-454.

+Champion, V.L. (1993). Instrument refinement for breast cancer screening behaviors. *Nursing Research, 42*(3), 139-143.

Gillis, A.J. (1993). Determinants of health promoting lifestyle: An integrative review. *Journal of Advanced Nursing, 18(3),* 345-353.

Kim, K.K., Horan, M.L., Gendler, P., & Patel, M.K. (1991). Development and evaluation of the osteoporosis health belief scale. *Research in Nursing and Health, 14*(2), 155-163.

Robertson, D., & Keller, C. (1992). Relationships among health beliefs, self-efficacy, and exercise adherence in patients with coronary artery disease. *Heart & Lung, 21*(1), 56-63.

# Health Beliefs: Perceived Threat (1704)

Domain-Health Knowledge & Behavior (IV)

Class-Health Beliefs (R)

Scale(s)-Very weak to Very strong (I)

Care Recipient:

Data Source:

**Definition:** Personal conviction that a threatening health problem is serious and has potential negative consequences for lifestyle

OUTCOME TARGET RATING:      Maintain at_____      Increase to_____

| Health Beliefs: Perceived Threat Overall Rating | Very weak 1 | Weak 2 | Moderate 3 | Strong 4 | Very strong 5 | |
|---|---|---|---|---|---|---|
| **INDICATORS:** | | | | | | |
| 170401 Perceived threat to health | 1 | 2 | 3 | 4 | 5 | NA |
| 170403 Perceived vulnerability to progressive health problems | 1 | 2 | 3 | 4 | 5 | NA |
| 170404 Concern regarding illness or injury | 1 | 2 | 3 | 4 | 5 | NA |
| 170405 Concern regarding potential complications | 1 | 2 | 3 | 4 | 5 | NA |
| 170406 Perceived severity of illness or injury | 1 | 2 | 3 | 4 | 5 | NA |
| 170407 Perceived severity of complications | 1 | 2 | 3 | 4 | 5 | NA |
| 170408 Perceived threat of discomfort from illness or injury | 1 | 2 | 3 | 4 | 5 | NA |
| 170409 Perception that condition may be of long duration | 1 | 2 | 3 | 4 | 5 | NA |
| 170410 Perceived impact on current lifestyle | 1 | 2 | 3 | 4 | 5 | NA |
| 170411 Perceived impact on future lifestyle | 1 | 2 | 3 | 4 | 5 | NA |
| 170412 Perceived impact on functional status | 1 | 2 | 3 | 4 | 5 | NA |
| 170414 Perceived threat of death | 1 | 2 | 3 | 4 | 5 | NA |

*1st edition 1997; Revised 3rd edition*

## Outcome Content References:

+Champion, V.L. (1993). Instrument refinement for breast cancer screening behaviors. *Nursing Research, 42*(3), 139-143.

Calnan, M., & Moss, S. (1984). The health belief model and compliance with education given at a class in breast self-examination. *Journal of Health and Social Behavior, 25(2)*, 198-210.

De Weerdt, I., Visser, A., & Van Der Veen, E. (1989). Attitude behavior theories and diabetes education programs. *Patient Education and Counseling, 14*, 3-19.

Dunn, S., Beeney, L., Hoskins, P., & Turtle, J. (1990). Knowledge and attitude change as predictors of metabolic improvement in diabetes education. *Social Science Medicine, 31*(10), 1135-1141.

+Kim, K.K., Horan, M.L., Gendler, P., & Patel, M.K. (1991). Development and evaluation of the osteoporosis health belief scale. *Research in Nursing and Health, 14*(2), 155-163.

Robertson, D., & Keller, C. (1992). Relationships among health beliefs, self-efficacy, and exercise adherence in patients with coronary artery disease. *Heart & Lung, 21*(1), 56-63.

Thompson, J., McFarland, G., & Hirsch, J. (2002). *Mosby's clinical nursing* (5th ed.). St. Louis: Mosby.

H

# Health Orientation (1705)

Domain-Health Knowledge & Behavior (IV)

Class-Health Beliefs (R)

Scale(s)-Very weak to Very strong (l)

Care Recipient:

Data Source:

**Definition:** Personal commitment to health behaviors as lifestyle priorities

OUTCOME TARGET RATING:     Maintain at_____     Increase to_____

| Health Orientation Overall Rating | Very weak 1 | Weak 2 | Moderate 3 | Strong 4 | Very strong 5 | |
|---|---|---|---|---|---|---|

INDICATORS:

| | | Very weak 1 | Weak 2 | Moderate 3 | Strong 4 | Very strong 5 | |
|---|---|---|---|---|---|---|---|
| 170501 | Focus on wellness | 1 | 2 | 3 | 4 | 5 | NA |
| 170514 | Focus on maintaining health behaviors | 1 | 2 | 3 | 4 | 5 | NA |
| 170502 | Focus on disease prevention and management | 1 | 2 | 3 | 4 | 5 | NA |
| 170503 | Focus on maintaining role performance | 1 | 2 | 3 | 4 | 5 | NA |
| 170504 | Focus on maintaining functional abilities | 1 | 2 | 3 | 4 | 5 | NA |
| 170505 | Focus on adjustment to life situations | 1 | 2 | 3 | 4 | 5 | NA |
| 170506 | Focus on overall well-being | 1 | 2 | 3 | 4 | 5 | NA |
| 170507 | Expectation that individual is responsible for health-related choices | 1 | 2 | 3 | 4 | 5 | NA |
| 170508 | Perception that health behavior is relevant to ones health | 1 | 2 | 3 | 4 | 5 | NA |
| 170515 | Perceived importance of incorporating health behaviors with cultural beliefs | 1 | 2 | 3 | 4 | 5 | NA |
| 170512 | Perception that health is a high priority in making lifestyle choices | 1 | 2 | 3 | 4 | 5 | NA |

*1st edition 1997; Revised 3rd edition*

Outcome Content References:

Gillis, A.J. (1993). Determinants of health promoting lifestyle: An integrative review. *Journal of Advanced Nursing, 18,*(3), 345-353.

Glick, O.J., & Ressler, C. (2001). Altered health maintenance. In M. Maas, K. Buckwalter, M. Hardy, T. Tripp-Reimer, M. Titler, & J. Specht (Eds.), *Nursing care of older adults: Diagnoses, outcomes & interventions* (pp. 6-22). St. Louis: Mosby.

Kulbok, P., & Baldwin, J. (1992). From preventive health behavior to health promotion: Advancing a positive construct of health. *Advances in Nursing Science, 14*(4), 50-64.

Palank, C. (1991). Determinants of health promoting behavior. *Nursing Clinics of North America, 26*(4), 815-832.

Pender, N.J. (1990). Expressing health through lifestyle patterns. *Nursing Science Quarterly, 3*(3), 115-122.

+Walker, S.N., Sechrist, K.R., & Pender, N.J. (1995). *The Health-Promoting Lifestyle Profile II.* Omaha, NE: University of Nebraska at Omaha.

+Walker, S.N., Sechrist, K.R., & Pender, N.J. (1987). The Health-Promoting Lifestyle Profile: Development and psychometric characteristics. *Nursing Research, 36*(2), 76-81.

# Health Promoting Behavior (1602)

*Domain-Health Knowledge & Behavior (IV)*

*Class-Health Behavior (Q)*

*Scale(s)-Never demonstrated to Consistently demonstrated (m)*

Care Recipient:

Data Source:

**Definition:** Personal actions to sustain or increase wellness

OUTCOME TARGET RATING:     Maintain at_____     Increase to_____

| Health Promoting Behavior Overall Rating | Never demonstrated 1 | Rarely demonstrated 2 | Sometimes demonstrated 3 | Often demonstrated 4 | Consistently demonstrated 5 | |
|---|---|---|---|---|---|---|
| INDICATORS: | | | | | | |
| 160201 Uses risk avoidance behaviors | 1 | 2 | 3 | 4 | 5 | NA |
| 160202 Monitors environment for risks | 1 | 2 | 3 | 4 | 5 | NA |
| 160203 Monitors personal behavior for risks | 1 | 2 | 3 | 4 | 5 | NA |
| 160204 Seeks balance among exercise, work, leisure, rest and nutrition | 1 | 2 | 3 | 4 | 5 | NA |
| 160205 Uses effective stress reduction behaviors | 1 | 2 | 3 | 4 | 5 | NA |
| 160206 Maintains social relationships | 1 | 2 | 3 | 4 | 5 | NA |
| 160207 Performs healthy behaviors routinely | 1 | 2 | 3 | 4 | 5 | NA |
| 160208 Supports healthful public policy | 1 | 2 | 3 | 4 | 5 | NA |
| 160209 Uses financial and physical resources to promote health | 1 | 2 | 3 | 4 | 5 | NA |
| 160210 Uses social support to promote health | 1 | 2 | 3 | 4 | 5 | NA |
| 160212 Obtains recommended immunizations | 1 | 2 | 3 | 4 | 5 | NA |
| 160213 Obtains recommended health screenings | 1 | 2 | 3 | 4 | 5 | NA |
| 160214 Follows healthy diet | 1 | 2 | 3 | 4 | 5 | NA |
| 160215 Uses effective weight control methods | 1 | 2 | 3 | 4 | 5 | NA |
| 160216 Uses effective exercise program | 1 | 2 | 3 | 4 | 5 | NA |
| 160217 Avoids exposure to infections | 1 | 2 | 3 | 4 | 5 | NA |

*Continued*

| Health Promoting Behavior—cont'd | | Never demonstrated | Rarely demonstrated | Sometimes demonstrated | Often demonstrated | Consistently demonstrated | |
|---|---|---|---|---|---|---|---|
| 160218 | Avoids alcohol misuse | 1 | 2 | 3 | 4 | 5 | NA |
| 160219 | Avoids tobacco use | 1 | 2 | 3 | 4 | 5 | NA |
| 160220 | Avoids recreational drugs | 1 | 2 | 3 | 4 | 5 | NA |

*1st edition 1997; Revised 3rd edition*

Outcome Content References:

Green, L., & Raeburn, J. (1990). Contemporary development in health promotion. In N. Bracht, (Ed.), *Health promotion at the community level* (pp. 29-44). Newberry Park, CA: Sage.

Kulbok, P., & Baldwin, J. (1992). From preventive health behavior to health promotion: Advancing a positive construct of health. *Advances in Nursing Science, 14*(4), 50-64.

Leenerts, M.H., Teel, C.S., & Pendleton, M.K. (2002). Building a model of self-care for health promotion in aging. *Journal of Nursing Scholarship, 34*(4), 355-361.

Mechanic, D., & Cleary, P. (1980). Factors associated with maintenance of positive behavior. *Preventive Medicine, 9*(6), 805-814.

Resnick, B. (2000). Health promotion practices of the older adult. *Public Health Nursing, 17*(3), 160-168.

Seeman, T.E. (2000). Health promoting effects of friends and family on health outcomes in older adults. *American Journal of Health Promotion, 14*(6), 362-370.

Simons-Morton, D.G., Mullen, P.D., Mains, D.A., Tabak, E.R., & Green, L.W. (1992). Characteristics of controlled studies of patient education and counseling for preventive health behavior. *Patient Education and Counseling, 19*(2), 175-204.

Stevenson, J.S. (2001). Health seeking behaviors. In M. Maas, K. Buckwalter, M. Hardy, T. Tripp-Reimer, M. Titler, & J. Specht (Eds.), *Nursing care of older adults: Diagnoses, outcomes & interventions* (pp. 75-85). St. Louis: Mosby.

+Walker, S.N., Sechrist, K.R., & Pender, N.J. (1995). *The Health-Promoting Lifestyle Profile II*. Omaha, NE: University of Nebraska at Omaha.

+Walker, S.N., Sechrist, K.R., & Pender, N.J. (1987). The Health Promoting Lifestyle Profile: Development and psychometric characteristics. *Nursing Research, 36*(2), 76-81.

H

# Health Seeking Behavior (1603)

Domain-Health Knowledge & Behavior (IV)

Class-Health Behavior (Q)

Scale(s)-Never demonstrated to Consistently demonstrated (m)

Care Recipient:

Data Source:

**Definition:** Personal actions to promote optimal wellness, recovery, and rehabilitation

OUTCOME TARGET RATING:  Maintain at_____  Increase to_____

| Health Seeking Behavior Overall Rating | Never demonstrated 1 | Rarely demonstrated 2 | Sometimes demonstrated 3 | Often demonstrated 4 | Consistently demonstrated 5 | |
|---|---|---|---|---|---|---|
| **INDICATORS:** | | | | | | |
| 160301 Asks health-related questions when indicated | 1 | 2 | 3 | 4 | 5 | NA |
| 160302 Completes health-related tasks | 1 | 2 | 3 | 4 | 5 | NA |
| 160303 Performs self-screening when indicated | 1 | 2 | 3 | 4 | 5 | NA |
| 160304 Seeks assistance from health care professionals when indicated | 1 | 2 | 3 | 4 | 5 | NA |
| 160305 Performs ADLs* consistent with energy and tolerance | 1 | 2 | 3 | 4 | 5 | NA |
| 160306 Describes strategies to eliminate unhealthy behavior | 1 | 2 | 3 | 4 | 5 | NA |
| 160307 Adheres to self-developed strategies to eliminate unhealthy behavior | 1 | 2 | 3 | 4 | 5 | NA |
| 160308 Performs prescribed health behavior when indicated | 1 | 2 | 3 | 4 | 5 | NA |
| 160309 Seeks current health-related information | 1 | 2 | 3 | 4 | 5 | NA |
| 160310 Describes strategies to maximize health | 1 | 2 | 3 | 4 | 5 | NA |
| 160311 Adheres to self-developed strategies to maximize health | 1 | 2 | 3 | 4 | 5 | NA |

*ADLs = Activities of daily living.

*1st edition 1997; Revised 3rd edition*

H

*Continued*

Outcome Content References:

Folden, S.L. (1993). Definitions of health and health goals of participants in a community-based pulmonary rehabilitation program. *Public Health Nursing, 10*(1), 31-35.

Jensen, L., & Allen, M. (1993). Wellness: The dialect of illness. *Image - the Journal of Nursing Scholarship, 25*(3), 220-224.

Pender, N.J. (1990). Expressing health through lifestyle patterns. *Nursing Science Quarterly, 3*(3), 115-122.

Pender, N.J., & Pender, A.R. (1986). Attitudes, subjective norms, and intentions of engage in health behaviors. *Nursing Research, 35*(1), 15-18.

Stevenson, J.S. (2001). Health seeking behaviors. In M. Maas, K. Buckwalter, M. Hardy, T. Tripp-Reimer, M. Titler, & J. Specht (Eds.), *Nursing care of older adults: Diagnoses, outcomes & interventions* (pp. 75-85). St. Louis: Mosby.

+Walker, S.N., Sechrist, K.R., & Pender, N.J. (1995). *The Health-Promoting Lifestyle Profile II*. Omaha, NE: University of Nebraska at Omaha.

+Walker, S.N., Sechrist, K.R., & Pender, N.J. (1987). The Health Promoting Lifestyle Profile: Development and psychometric characteristics. *Nursing Research, 36*(2), 76-81.

Woods, N. (1989). Conceptualizations of self-care: Toward health-oriented models. *Advances in Nursing Science, 12*(1), 1-13.

**H**

# Hearing Compensation Behavior (1610)

Domain-Health Knowledge & Behavior (IV)

Class-Health Behavior (Q)

Scale(s)-Never demonstrated to Consistently demonstrated (m)

Care Recipient:

Data Source:

**Definition:** Personal actions to identify, monitor, and compensate for hearing loss

OUTCOME TARGET RATING:     Maintain at_____     Increase to_____

| Hearing Compensation Behavior Overall Rating | Never demonstrated 1 | Rarely demonstrated 2 | Sometimes demonstrated 3 | Often demonstrated 4 | Consistently demonstrated 5 | |
|---|---|---|---|---|---|---|
| INDICATORS: | | | | | | |
| 161001 Monitors symptoms of hearing deterioration | 1 | 2 | 3 | 4 | 5 | NA |
| 161002 Positions self to advantage hearing | 1 | 2 | 3 | 4 | 5 | NA |
| 161003 Reminds others to use techniques that advantage hearing | 1 | 2 | 3 | 4 | 5 | NA |
| 161004 Eliminates background noise | 1 | 2 | 3 | 4 | 5 | NA |
| 161005 Uses sign language | 1 | 2 | 3 | 4 | 5 | NA |
| 161006 Uses lip reading | 1 | 2 | 3 | 4 | 5 | NA |
| 161007 Uses closed captioning for television viewing | 1 | 2 | 3 | 4 | 5 | NA |
| 161009 Uses hearing supportive devices (e.g., light on telephone) | 1 | 2 | 3 | 4 | 5 | NA |
| 161008 Uses hearing assistive devices | 1 | 2 | 3 | 4 | 5 | NA |
| 161012 Uses hearing aid(s) correctly | 1 | 2 | 3 | 4 | 5 | NA |
| 161010 Cares for internal hearing assistive devices correctly | 1 | 2 | 3 | 4 | 5 | NA |
| 161011 Cares for external hearing assistive devices correctly | 1 | 2 | 3 | 4 | 5 | NA |
| 161013 Uses support services for hearing impaired | 1 | 2 | 3 | 4 | 5 | NA |

*2nd edition 2000; Revised 3rd edition*

**Outcome Content References:**

Burrell, L.O. (Ed). (1992). *Adult nursing in hospital and community settings*. Norwalk, CT: Appleton & Lange.

Phipps, W.J., Monahan, F.D., Sands J.K., Marek, J., & Neighbors, M. (Eds.). (2003). *Medical-surgical nursing: Concepts and clinical practice* (7th ed). St. Louis: Mosby.

Smeltzer, S.C., & Bare, B.G. (Eds.). (2003). *Brunner and Suddarth's textbook of medical-surgical nursing* (10th ed.). Philadelphia: Lippincott, Williams, & Wilkins.

# Hemodialysis Access (1105)

*Domain-Physiologic Health (II)*

*Class-Tissue Integrity (L)*

*Care Recipient:*

*Data Source:*

*Scale(s)-Severely compromised to Not compromised (a) and Severe to None (n)*

**Definition:** Functionality of a dialysis access site

OUTCOME TARGET RATING:    Maintain at_____     Increase to_____

| Hemodialysis Access Overall Rating | Severely compromised 1 | Substantially compromised 2 | Moderately compromised 3 | Mildly compromised 4 | Not compromised 5 | |
|---|---|---|---|---|---|---|
| **INDICATORS:** | | | | | | |
| 110501 Blood volume flow through fistula/shunt | 1 | 2 | 3 | 4 | 5 | NA |
| 110502 Site skin color | 1 | 2 | 3 | 4 | 5 | NA |
| 110517 Access site skin temperature | 1 | 2 | 3 | 4 | 5 | NA |
| 110505 Bruit | 1 | 2 | 3 | 4 | 5 | NA |
| 110506 Thrill | 1 | 2 | 3 | 4 | 5 | NA |
| 110509 Distal peripheral pulses | 1 | 2 | 3 | 4 | 5 | NA |
| 110510 Distal peripheral skin temperature | 1 | 2 | 3 | 4 | 5 | NA |
| 110511 Distal peripheral skin color | 1 | 2 | 3 | 4 | 5 | NA |
| 110514 Clotting time | 1 | 2 | 3 | 4 | 5 | NA |

| | Severe | Substantial | Moderate | Mild | None | |
|---|---|---|---|---|---|---|
| 110503 Drainage at site | 1 | 2 | 3 | 4 | 5 | NA |
| 110507 Hematoma at site | 1 | 2 | 3 | 4 | 5 | NA |
| 110508 Bleeding at site | 1 | 2 | 3 | 4 | 5 | NA |
| 110512 Distal peripheral edema | 1 | 2 | 3 | 4 | 5 | NA |
| 110515 Tenderness at site | 1 | 2 | 3 | 4 | 5 | NA |
| 110513 Cannula displacement | 1 | 2 | 3 | 4 | 5 | NA |

*2nd edition 2000; Revised 3rd edition (formerly Dialysis Access Integrity)*

**Outcome Content References:**

Eisenbud, M.D. (1996). *The handbook of dialysis access*. Columbus, OH: Anadem Publishing.

Lancaster, L.E. (Ed.). (1995). *ANNA's core curriculum for nephrology nurses* (3rd ed.) (Section X). Pitman, NJ: Janetti.

Levine, D.Z. (1997). *Caring for the renal patient* (3rd ed.). Philadelphia: W.B. Saunders.

Gutch, C.F., Stoner, M.H., & Corea, A.L. (1999). *Review of hemodialysis for nurses and dialysis personnel* (6th ed.). St. Louis: Mosby.

# *Hope (1201)*

Domain-Psychosocial Health (III)

Class-Psychological Well-Being (M)

Scale(s)-Never demonstrated to Consistently demonstrated (m)

Care Recipient:

Data Source:

**Definition:** Optimism that is personally satisfying and life-supporting

OUTCOME TARGET RATING:     Maintain at_____     Increase to_____

| Hope Overall Rating | Never demonstrated 1 | Rarely demonstrated 2 | Sometimes demonstrated 3 | Often demonstrated 4 | Consistently demonstrated 5 | |
|---|---|---|---|---|---|---|
| INDICATORS: | | | | | | |
| 120101 Expresses expectation of a positive future | 1 | 2 | 3 | 4 | 5 | NA |
| 120102 Expresses faith | 1 | 2 | 3 | 4 | 5 | NA |
| 120103 Expresses will to live | 1 | 2 | 3 | 4 | 5 | NA |
| 120104 Expresses reasons to live | 1 | 2 | 3 | 4 | 5 | NA |
| 120105 Expresses meaning in life | 1 | 2 | 3 | 4 | 5 | NA |
| 120106 Expresses optimism | 1 | 2 | 3 | 4 | 5 | NA |
| 120107 Expresses belief in self | 1 | 2 | 3 | 4 | 5 | NA |
| 120108 Expresses belief in others | 1 | 2 | 3 | 4 | 5 | NA |
| 120109 Expresses inner peace | 1 | 2 | 3 | 4 | 5 | NA |
| 120110 Expresses sense of self-control | 1 | 2 | 3 | 4 | 5 | NA |
| 120111 Exhibits a zest for life | 1 | 2 | 3 | 4 | 5 | NA |
| 120112 Sets goals | 1 | 2 | 3 | 4 | 5 | NA |

*1st edition 1997; Revised 3rd edition*

Outcome Content References:

+Beckman, E.E., Leber, W.R., Watkins, J.T., Boyer, J.L., & Cook, J.B. (1986). Development of an instrument to measure Beck's cognitive triad: The Cognitive Triad Inventory. *Journal of Consulting and Clinical Psychology, 54*(4), 566-567.

Farran, C.J. (2001). Hopelessness. In M. Maas, K. Buckwalter, M. Hardy, T. Tripp-Reimer, M. Titler, & J. Specht (Eds.), *Nursing care of older adults: Diagnoses, outcomes & interventions* (pp. 601-612). St. Louis: Mosby.

Hall, B. (1990). The struggle of the diagnosed terminally ill person to maintain hope. *Nursing Science Quarterly, 3*(4), 177-184.

Herth, K. (1993). Hope in the family caregiver of terminally ill people. *Journal of Advanced Nursing, 18*(4), 538-548.

Hunt-Raleigh, E. (1992). Sources of hope in chronic illness. *Oncology Nursing Forum, 3*(19), 443-448.

Owen, D. (1989). Nurses perspectives on the meaning of hope in patients with cancer: A qualitative study. *Oncology Nursing Forum, 1*(16), 75-79.

Stephenson, C. (1991). The concept of hope revisited for nursing. *Journal of Advanced Nursing, 16*(12), 1456-1461.

H

# Hydration (0602)

*Domain-Physiologic Health (II)*

*Class-Fluid & Electrolytes (G)*

*Scale(s)-Severely compromised to Not compromised (a) and Severe to None (n)*

*Care Recipient:*

*Data Source:*

---

**Definition:** Adequate water in the intracellular and extracellular compartments of the body

OUTCOME TARGET RATING:   Maintain at_____   Increase to_____

| Hydration Overall Rating | Severely compromised 1 | Substantially compromised 2 | Moderately compromised 3 | Mildly compromised 4 | Not compromised 5 | |
|---|---|---|---|---|---|---|
| **INDICATORS:** | | | | | | |
| 060201 Skin turgor | 1 | 2 | 3 | 4 | 5 | NA |
| 060202 Moist mucous membranes | 1 | 2 | 3 | 4 | 5 | NA |
| 060215 Adequate fluid intake | 1 | 2 | 3 | 4 | 5 | NA |
| 060211 Urine output | 1 | 2 | 3 | 4 | 5 | NA |
| 060216 Serum sodium | 1 | 2 | 3 | 4 | 5 | NA |
| 060217 Tissue perfusion | 1 | 2 | 3 | 4 | 5 | NA |
| 060218 Cognitive function | 1 | 2 | 3 | 4 | 5 | NA |

| | Severe | Substantial | Moderate | Mild | None | |
|---|---|---|---|---|---|---|
| 060205 Thirst | 1 | 2 | 3 | 4 | 5 | NA |
| 060219 Dark urine | 1 | 2 | 3 | 4 | 5 | NA |
| 060208 Soft, sunken eyeballs | 1 | 2 | 3 | 4 | 5 | NA |
| 060220 Sunken fontanel | 1 | 2 | 3 | 4 | 5 | NA |
| 060212 Decreased blood pressure | 1 | 2 | 3 | 4 | 5 | NA |
| 060221 Rapid thready pulse | 1 | 2 | 3 | 4 | 5 | NA |
| 060213 Increased hematocrit | 1 | 2 | 3 | 4 | 5 | NA |
| 060222 Increased blood urea nitrogen | 1 | 2 | 3 | 4 | 5 | NA |
| 060223 Weight loss | 1 | 2 | 3 | 4 | 5 | NA |
| 060224 Muscle cramps | 1 | 2 | 3 | 4 | 5 | NA |
| 060225 Muscle twitching | 1 | 2 | 3 | 4 | 5 | NA |
| 060226 Diarrhea | 1 | 2 | 3 | 4 | 5 | NA |

*1st edition 1997; Revised 3rd edition*

## Outcome Content References:

Arieff, A. (1986). Hyponatremia, convulsions, respiratory arrest, and permanent brain damage after elective surgery in healthy women. *The New England Journal of Medicine, 314*(24), 1529-1534.

Carcillo, J.A., Davis, A.L., & Zaritsky, A. (1991). Role of early fluid resuscitation in pediatric septic shock. *Journal of the American Medical Association, 266*(9), 1242-1245.

Gilski, D. (1993). Controversies in patient management after cardiac surgery. *Journal of Cardiovascular Nursing, 7*(4), 1-13.

Hill, P., & Aldag, J. (1991). Potential indicators of insufficient milk supply syndrome. *Research in Nursing and Health, 14(1)*, 11-19.

Innerarity, S.A. (1997). *Fluids and electrolytes* (3rd ed.). Springhouse, PA: Springhouse.

The Joanna Briggs Institute for Evidence Based Nursing and Midwifery. (2000). Identification and nursing management of dysphagia in adults with neurological impairment. *Best Practice, 4*(2), Blackwell Science-Asia, Australia.

Mentes, J., Culp, K., Wakefield, B., Gaspar, P., Rapp, C., Mobily, P., & Tripp-Reimer, T. (1998). Dehydration as a precipitating factor in the development of acute confusion in the frail elderly. In B. Vellas, J. Albarde, & P. Garry (Eds.), *Facts, research, and intervention in geriatrics: Hydration and aging.* Paris: Serdi Publisher.

Reese, J.L. (2001). Fluid volume deficit—dehydration: Isotonic, hypotonic, and hypertonic. In M. Maas, K. Buckwalter, M. Hardy, T. Tripp-Reimer, M. Titler, & J. Specht (Eds.), *Nursing care of older adults: Diagnoses, outcomes & interventions* (pp. 183-200). St. Louis: Mosby.

Wakefield, B., Mentes, J., Digglemann, L., & Culp, K. (2002). Monitoring hydration status in elderly veterans. *Western Journal of Nursing Research, 24*(2), 132-142.

# *Hyperactivity Level (0915)*

Domain-Physiologic Health (II)                                    Care Recipient:

Class-Neurocognitive (J)                                          Data Source:

Scale-Severe to None (n)

**Definition:** Severity of patterns of inattention or impulsivity in a child from 1 year through 17 years of age

OUTCOME TARGET RATING:        Maintain at_____    Increase to_____

| Hyperactivity Level Overall Rating | Severe 1 | Substantial 2 | Moderate 3 | Mild 4 | None 5 | |
|---|---|---|---|---|---|---|

INDICATORS:

| | | Severe 1 | Substantial 2 | Moderate 3 | Mild 4 | None 5 | |
|---|---|---|---|---|---|---|---|
| 091501 | Inattention | 1 | 2 | 3 | 4 | 5 | NA |
| 091502 | Lack of active listening | 1 | 2 | 3 | 4 | 5 | NA |
| 091503 | Difficulty organizing tasks | 1 | 2 | 3 | 4 | 5 | NA |
| 091504 | Inability to stay "on task" | 1 | 2 | 3 | 4 | 5 | NA |
| 091505 | Lack of follow-through or completion of activities | 1 | 2 | 3 | 4 | 5 | NA |
| 091506 | Difficulty with tasks that require sustained mental effort | 1 | 2 | 3 | 4 | 5 | NA |
| 091507 | Careless mistakes | 1 | 2 | 3 | 4 | 5 | NA |
| 091508 | Frequency of losing things | 1 | 2 | 3 | 4 | 5 | NA |
| 091509 | Excessive distractibility | 1 | 2 | 3 | 4 | 5 | NA |
| 091510 | Excessive forgetfulness | 1 | 2 | 3 | 4 | 5 | NA |
| 091511 | Impulsivity | 1 | 2 | 3 | 4 | 5 | NA |
| 091512 | Excessive fidgeting | 1 | 2 | 3 | 4 | 5 | NA |
| 091513 | Inability to remain seated | 1 | 2 | 3 | 4 | 5 | NA |
| 091514 | Excessive running and/or climbing | 1 | 2 | 3 | 4 | 5 | NA |
| 091515 | Excessive motor behavior | 1 | 2 | 3 | 4 | 5 | NA |
| 091516 | Difficulty playing quietly | 1 | 2 | 3 | 4 | 5 | NA |
| 091517 | Excessive talking | 1 | 2 | 3 | 4 | 5 | NA |
| 091518 | Blurts out answers before the question is completed | 1 | 2 | 3 | 4 | 5 | NA |
| 091519 | Difficulty "waiting turn" | 1 | 2 | 3 | 4 | 5 | NA |
| 091520 | Excessive interrupting of others | 1 | 2 | 3 | 4 | 5 | NA |
| 091521 | Intrusive, abrasive, loud, interpersonal interactions | 1 | 2 | 3 | 4 | 5 | NA |
| 091522 | Inappropriate aggressive behavior | 1 | 2 | 3 | 4 | 5 | NA |
| 091523 | Difficulty keeping hands to self | 1 | 2 | 3 | 4 | 5 | NA |

*3rd edition*

Outcome Content References:

American Psychiatric Association. (2000). *Diagnostic and statistical manual of mental disorders* (4th ed. text revision). Washington DC: Author.

Novak, L.L. (1999). Attention deficit hyperactivity disorder. In M.R. Dambro (Ed.), *Griffith's 5-minute clinical consult.* Philadelphia: Lippincott.

Sharma, V., Newcorn, J.H., Matier-Sharma, K., & Halperin, J. M. (1997). Attention-deficient and disruptive behavior disorders. In A. Tasman (Ed.). *Psychiatriy.* Philadelphia: Saunders.

Hechtman, L. (2000). Assessment and diagnosis of attention deficit/hyperactive disorder. *Child and Adolescent Psychiatric Clinics of North America 9*(3), 481-498.

H

# Identity (1202)

*Domain-Psychosocial Health (III)*

*Class-Psychological Well-Being (M)*

*Scale(s)-Never demonstrated to Consistently demonstrated (m)*

*Care Recipient:*

*Data Source:*

**Definition**: Distinguishes between self and non-self and characterizes one's essence

OUTCOME TARGET RATING:     Maintain at_____     Increase to_____

| Identity Overall Rating | Never demonstrated 1 | Rarely demonstrated 2 | Sometimes demonstrated 3 | Often demonstrated 4 | Consistently demonstrated 5 | |
|---|---|---|---|---|---|---|
| **INDICATORS:** | | | | | | |
| 120201 Verbalizes affirmations of personal identity | 1 | 2 | 3 | 4 | 5 | NA |
| 120202 Exhibits congruent verbal and non-verbal behavior about self | 1 | 2 | 3 | 4 | 5 | NA |
| 120203 Verbalizes clear sense of personal identity | 1 | 2 | 3 | 4 | 5 | NA |
| 120204 Differentiates self from environment | 1 | 2 | 3 | 4 | 5 | NA |
| 120205 Differentiates self from other human beings | 1 | 2 | 3 | 4 | 5 | NA |
| 120206 Perceives environment accurately | 1 | 2 | 3 | 4 | 5 | NA |
| 120207 Performs social roles | 1 | 2 | 3 | 4 | 5 | NA |
| 120208 Verbalizes own value system | 1 | 2 | 3 | 4 | 5 | NA |
| 120209 Challenges faulty beliefs about self | 1 | 2 | 3 | 4 | 5 | NA |
| 120210 Challenges negative images of self | 1 | 2 | 3 | 4 | 5 | NA |
| 120211 Recognizes interpersonal versus intra-personal conflict | 1 | 2 | 3 | 4 | 5 | NA |
| 120212 Establishes personal boundaries | 1 | 2 | 3 | 4 | 5 | NA |
| 120213 Verbalizes trust in self | 1 | 2 | 3 | 4 | 5 | NA |

*1st edition 1997; Revised 3rd edition*

## Outcome Content References:

Barnard, D. (1990). Healing the damaged self: Identity, intimacy, and meaning in the lives of the chronically ill. *Perspectives in Biology & Medicine, 33*(4), 535-546.

Erickson, E. (1968). *Identity, youth and crisis.* New York: W.W. Norton & Co.

Gara, M.A., Rosenberg, S., & Cohen, B. (1987). Personal identity and the schizophrenic process: An integration. *Psychiatry, 50(3),* 267-278.

Grotevant, H.D., & Adams, G.R. (1984). Development of an objective measure to assess ego identity in adolescence: Validation and replication. *Journal of Youth and Adolescence, 13*(5), 419-437.

Hernandez, J.T., & Diclemente, R.J. (1992). Self-control and ego identity development as predictors of unprotected sex in late adolescent males. *Journal of Adolescence, 15(4),* 437-447.

Marcia, J.E. (1966). Development and validations of ego identity status. *Journal of Personality and Social Psychology, 3,* 551-558.

Marcia, J.E. (1967). Ego identity status: Relationships to change in self-esteem, general adjustment, and authoritarianism. *Journal of Personality, 35,* 118-133.

Oldaker, S. (1985). Identity confusion: Nursing diagnoses for adolescents. *Nursing Clinics of North America, 20(4),* 763-773.

Streitmatter, J. (1993). Gender differences in identity development: An examination of longitudinal data. *Adolescence, 28(109),* 55-66.

Streitmatter, J. (1993). Identity status and identity style: A replication study. *Journal of Adolescence, 16(2),* 211-215.

Stuart, G.W., & Laraia, M.T. (2001). *Principles and practice of psychiatric nursing* (7th ed.). St. Louis: Mosby.

+Tan, A. L., Kendis, R.J., Fine, J.T., & Porac, J. (1977). A short measure of Ericksonian ego identity. *Journal of Personality Assessment, 41,* 279-284.

I

# *Immobility Consequences: Physiological (0204)*

*Domain-Functional Health (I)*

*Class-Mobility (C)*

*Scale(s)-Severe to None (n) and Severely compromised to Not compromised (a)*

*Care Recipient:*

*Data Source:*

| **Definition:** Severity of compromise in physiological functioning due to impaired physical mobility |
|---|

OUTCOME TARGET RATING:    Maintain at_____    Increase to_____

| Immobility Consequences: Physiological Overall Rating | Severe 1 | Substantial 2 | Moderate 3 | Mild 4 | None 5 | |
|---|---|---|---|---|---|---|

INDICATORS:

| | | Severe 1 | Substantial 2 | Moderate 3 | Mild 4 | None 5 | |
|---|---|---|---|---|---|---|---|
| 020401 | Pressure sore(s) | 1 | 2 | 3 | 4 | 5 | NA |
| 020402 | Constipation | 1 | 2 | 3 | 4 | 5 | NA |
| 020403 | Stool impaction | 1 | 2 | 3 | 4 | 5 | NA |
| 020405 | Hypoactive bowel | 1 | 2 | 3 | 4 | 5 | NA |
| 020406 | Paralytic ileus | 1 | 2 | 3 | 4 | 5 | NA |
| 020407 | Urinary calculi | 1 | 2 | 3 | 4 | 5 | NA |
| 020408 | Urinary retention | 1 | 2 | 3 | 4 | 5 | NA |
| 020409 | Fever | 1 | 2 | 3 | 4 | 5 | NA |
| 020410 | Urinary tract infection | 1 | 2 | 3 | 4 | 5 | NA |
| 020413 | Bone fracture | 1 | 2 | 3 | 4 | 5 | NA |
| 020415 | Contracted joints | 1 | 2 | 3 | 4 | 5 | NA |
| 020416 | Ankylosed joints | 1 | 2 | 3 | 4 | 5 | NA |
| 020417 | Orthostatic hypotension | 1 | 2 | 3 | 4 | 5 | NA |
| 020418 | Venous thrombosis | 1 | 2 | 3 | 4 | 5 | NA |
| 020419 | Lung congestion | 1 | 2 | 3 | 4 | 5 | NA |
| 020422 | Pneumonia | 1 | 2 | 3 | 4 | 5 | NA |

| | | Severely compromised | Substantially compromised | Moderately compromised | Mildly compromised | Not compromised | |
|---|---|---|---|---|---|---|---|
| 020404 | Nutritional status | 1 | 2 | 3 | 4 | 5 | NA |
| 020411 | Muscle strength | 1 | 2 | 3 | 4 | 5 | NA |
| 020412 | Muscle tone | 1 | 2 | 3 | 4 | 5 | NA |
| 020414 | Joint movement | 1 | 2 | 3 | 4 | 5 | NA |
| 020420 | Cough effectiveness | 1 | 2 | 3 | 4 | 5 | NA |
| 020421 | Vital capacity | 1 | 2 | 3 | 4 | 5 | NA |

*1st edition 1997; Revised 2nd edition 2000; Revised 3rd edition*

**Outcome Content References:**

Bloomfield, S.A. (1997). Changes in musculoskeletal structure and function with prolonged bed rest. *Medicine & Science in Sports & Exercise, 29*(2), 197-206.

Greenleaf, J.E. (1997). Intensive exercise training during bed rest attenuates deconditioning. *Medicine & Science in Sports & Exercise, 29* (2), 207-215.

Kottke, F.J., & Lehmann, J.F. (1990). *Krusen's handbook of physical medicine and rehabilitation* (4th ed.). Philadelphia: W.B. Saunders.

Maas, M., & Specht, J.P. (2001). Impaired physical mobility. In M. Maas, K. Buckwalter, M. Hardy, T. Tripp-Reimer, M. Titler, & J. Specht (Eds.), *Nursing care of older adults: Diagnoses, outcomes & interventions* (pp. 337-365). St. Louis: Mosby.

Milde, F.K. (1981). Physiological immobilization. In L. Hart, J. Reese & M. Fearing (Eds.), *Concepts common to acute illness: Identification and management* (pp. 67-109). St. Louis: Mosby.

Olson, E.V., Johnson, B.J., Thompson, L.F., McCarthy, J.S., Edmonds, R.E., Schroeder, L.M., & Wade, M. (1967). The hazards of immobility. *American Journal of Nursing, 67*(4), 780-797.

Potter, P.A., & Perry, A.G. (1997). Mobility and immobility. In P.A. Potter & A.G. Perry (Eds.), *Fundamentals of nursing: Concepts, process, and practice* (4th ed., pp. 1460-1520). St. Louis: Mosby.

Rubin, M. (1988). The physiology of bedrest. *American Journal of Nursing, 88*(1), 50-55.

# *Immobility Consequences: Psycho-Cognitive (0205)*

*Domain-Functional Health (I)*

*Class-Mobility (C)*

*Scale(s)-Severe to None (n) and Severely compromised to Not compromised (a)*

*Care Recipient:*

*Data Source:*

**Definition:** Severity of compromise in psycho-cognitive functioning due to impaired physical mobility

OUTCOME TARGET RATING:     Maintain at_____     Increase to_____

| Immobility Consequences: Psycho-Cognitive Overall Rating | | Severe 1 | Substantial 2 | Moderate 3 | Mild 4 | None 5 | |
|---|---|---|---|---|---|---|---|
| INDICATORS: | | | | | | | |
| 020504 | Perceptual distortions | 1 | 2 | 3 | 4 | 5 | NA |
| 020507 | Exaggerated emotions | 1 | 2 | 3 | 4 | 5 | NA |
| 020508 | Sleep disturbances | 1 | 2 | 3 | 4 | 5 | NA |
| 020510 | Negative body image | 1 | 2 | 3 | 4 | 5 | NA |
| 020513 | Depression | 1 | 2 | 3 | 4 | 5 | NA |
| 020514 | Apathy | 1 | 2 | 3 | 4 | 5 | NA |
| | | Severely compromised | Substantially compromised | Moderately compromised | Mildly compromised | Not compromised | |
| 020501 | Alertness | 1 | 2 | 3 | 4 | 5 | NA |
| 020502 | Cognitive orientation | 1 | 2 | 3 | 4 | 5 | NA |
| 020503 | Attentiveness | 1 | 2 | 3 | 4 | 5 | NA |
| 020505 | Kinesthetic sense | 1 | 2 | 3 | 4 | 5 | NA |
| 020509 | Self-esteem | 1 | 2 | 3 | 4 | 5 | NA |
| 020511 | Ability to act | 1 | 2 | 3 | 4 | 5 | NA |

*1st edition 1997; Revised 3rd edition*

Outcome Content References:

Friedrich, R.M., & Lively, S.I. (1981). Psychological immobilization. In L. Hart, J. Reese, & M. Fearing (Eds.), *Concepts common to acute illness: Identification and management* (pp. 51-66). St. Louis: Mosby.

Greenleaf, J.E. (1997). Intensive exercise training during bed rest attenuates deconditioning. *Medicine & Science in Sports & Exercise, 29*(2), 207-215.

Maas, M., & Specht, J.P. (2001). Impaired physical mobility. In M. Maas, K. Buckwalter, M. Hardy, T. Tripp-Reimer, M. Titler, & J. Specht (Eds.), *Nursing care of older adults: Diagnoses, outcomes & interventions* (pp. 337-365). St. Louis: Mosby.

Rubin, M. (1988). How bedrest changes perception. *American Journal of Nursing, 88*(1), 55-56.

# Immune Hypersensitivity Response (0707)

*Domain-Physiologic Health (II)*

*Class-Immune Response (H)*

*Scale(s)-Severe to None (n) and Severely compromised to Not compromised (a)*

*Care Recipient:*

*Data Source:*

**Definition:** Severity of inappropriate immune responses

OUTCOME TARGET RATING:   Maintain at_____   Increase to_____

| Immune Hypersensitivity Response Overall Rating | Severe 1 | Substantial 2 | Moderate 3 | Mild 4 | None 5 | |
|---|---|---|---|---|---|---|
| INDICATORS: | | | | | | |
| 070701 Alterations in skin | 1 | 2 | 3 | 4 | 5 | NA |
| 070702 Alterations in mucosa | 1 | 2 | 3 | 4 | 5 | NA |
| 070703 Allergic reactions | 1 | 2 | 3 | 4 | 5 | NA |
| 070704 Localized inflammatory responses | 1 | 2 | 3 | 4 | 5 | NA |
| 070705 Autoimmune events | 1 | 2 | 3 | 4 | 5 | NA |
| 070706 Vasculitis | 1 | 2 | 3 | 4 | 5 | NA |
| 070707 Transplant rejection | 1 | 2 | 3 | 4 | 5 | NA |
| 070708 Graft versus host response | 1 | 2 | 3 | 4 | 5 | NA |
| 070709 Itching | 1 | 2 | 3 | 4 | 5 | NA |
| 070710 Jaundice | 1 | 2 | 3 | 4 | 5 | NA |
| 070711 Level of auto-antibodies or auto-antigens | 1 | 2 | 3 | 4 | 5 | NA |
| 070712 Increased bilirubin | 1 | 2 | 3 | 4 | 5 | NA |
| 070713 Alterations in complete blood count | 1 | 2 | 3 | 4 | 5 | NA |
| 070714 Alterations in differential white blood count | 1 | 2 | 3 | 4 | 5 | NA |
| 070715 Alterations in complement levels | 1 | 2 | 3 | 4 | 5 | NA |
| 070716 Alterations in T4-cell level | 1 | 2 | 3 | 4 | 5 | NA |
| 070717 Alterations in T8-cell level | 1 | 2 | 3 | 4 | 5 | NA |

| | Severely compromised | Substantially compromised | Moderately compromised | Mildly compromised | Not compromised | |
|---|---|---|---|---|---|---|
| 070718 Respiratory function | 1 | 2 | 3 | 4 | 5 | NA |
| 070719 Cardiac function | 1 | 2 | 3 | 4 | 5 | NA |
| 070720 Gastrointestinal function | 1 | 2 | 3 | 4 | 5 | NA |
| 070721 Renal function | 1 | 2 | 3 | 4 | 5 | NA |
| 070722 Neurological function | 1 | 2 | 3 | 4 | 5 | NA |
| 070723 Joint mobility | 1 | 2 | 3 | 4 | 5 | NA |

*3rd edition*

## Outcome Content References:

Birney, M.H. (1991). Psychoneuroimmunology: A holistic framework for the study of stress and illness. *Holistic Nursing Practice, 5*(4), 32-38.

Brandt, B. (1990). Nursing protocol for the patient with neutropenia. *Oncology Nursing Forum, 17*(Suppl. 1), 9-15.

McCance, K.L., & Huether, S.E. (2002). *Pathophysiology: The biologic basis for disease in adults and children* (4th ed.). St. Louis: Mosby.

Phillips, M.C., & Olson, L.R. (1993). The immunologic role of the gastrointestinal tract. *Critical Care Nursing Clinics of North America, 5*(1), 107-118.

Van Wynsberghe, D., Noback, C.R., & Carola, R. (1995). *Human anatomy and physiology* (3rd ed.). New York: McGraw-Hill.

Workman, M.L. (1993). The immune system: Your defensive partner and offensive foe. *AACN, 4*(3), 453-470.

I

# *Immune Status (0702)*

Domain-Physiologic Health (II)

Class-Immune Response (H)

Scale-Severely compromised to Not compromised (a) and Severe to None (n)

Care Recipient:

Data Source:

**Definition:** Natural and acquired appropriately targeted resistance to internal and external antigens

OUTCOME TARGET RATING:    Maintain at_____    Increase to_____

| Immune Status Overall Rating | Severely compromised 1 | Substantially compromised 2 | Moderately compromised 3 | Mildly compromised 4 | Not compromised 5 | |
|---|---|---|---|---|---|---|
| **INDICATORS:** | | | | | | |
| 070203 Gastrointestinal function | 1 | 2 | 3 | 4 | 5 | NA |
| 070204 Respiratory function | 1 | 2 | 3 | 4 | 5 | NA |
| 070205 Genitourinary function | 1 | 2 | 3 | 4 | 5 | NA |
| 070207 Body temperature | 1 | 2 | 3 | 4 | 5 | NA |
| 070208 Skin integrity | 1 | 2 | 3 | 4 | 5 | NA |
| 070209 Mucosa integrity | 1 | 2 | 3 | 4 | 5 | NA |
| 070211 Immunizations current | 1 | 2 | 3 | 4 | 5 | NA |
| 070212 Antibody titers | 1 | 2 | 3 | 4 | 5 | NA |
| 070213 Appropriate skin test reaction with exposure | 1 | 2 | 3 | 4 | 5 | NA |
| 070214 Absolute white blood count | 1 | 2 | 3 | 4 | 5 | NA |
| 070215 Differential white blood count | 1 | 2 | 3 | 4 | 5 | NA |
| 070216 T4-cell level | 1 | 2 | 3 | 4 | 5 | NA |
| 070217 T8-cell level | 1 | 2 | 3 | 4 | 5 | NA |
| 070218 Complement levels | 1 | 2 | 3 | 4 | 5 | NA |
| 070219 Thymus x-ray findings | 1 | 2 | 3 | 4 | 5 | NA |
| | **Severe** | **Substantial** | **Moderate** | **Mild** | **None** | |
| 070201 Recurrent infections | 1 | 2 | 3 | 4 | 5 | NA |
| 070202 Tumors | 1 | 2 | 3 | 4 | 5 | NA |
| 070206 Weight loss | 1 | 2 | 3 | 4 | 5 | NA |
| 070210 Chronic fatigue | 1 | 2 | 3 | 4 | 5 | NA |

*1st edition 1997; Revised 3rd edition*

### Outcome Content References:

Birney, M.H. (1991). Psychoneuroimmunology: A holistic framework for the study of stress and illness. *Holistic Nursing Practice, 5*(4), 32-38.

Brandt, B. (1990). Nursing protocol for the patient with neutropenia. *Oncology Nursing Forum, 17*(Suppl. 1), 9-15.

Hymes, D.J. (1985). Primary immunodeficiency disorders in the neonate. *Neonatal Network-The Journal of Neonatal Nursing, 3*(4), 40-48.

McCance, K.L., & Huether, S.E. (2002). *Pathophysiology: The biologic basis for disease in adults and children* (4th ed.). St. Louis: Mosby.

Phillips, M.C., & Olson, L.R. (1993). The immunologic role of the gastrointestinal tract. *Critical Care Nursing Clinics of North America, 5*(1), 107-118.

Ungvarski, P.J., & Flaskerud, J.H. (1999). *HIV/AIDS: A guide to primary care management* (4th ed.). Philadelphia: W.B. Saunders.

Van Wynsberghe, D., Noback, C.R., & Carola, R. (1995). *Human anatomy and physiology* (3rd ed.). New York: McGraw-Hill.

Workman, M.L. (1993). The immune system: Your defensive partner and offensive foe. *AACN, 4*(3), 453-470.

# *Immunization Behavior (1900)*

Domain-Health Knowledge & Behavior (IV)

Class-Risk Control & Safety (T)

Scale(s)-Never demonstrated to Consistently demonstrated (m)

Care Recipient:

Data Source:

**Definition:** Personal actions to obtain immunization to prevent a communicable disease

OUTCOME TARGET RATING:     Maintain at_____     Increase to_____

| Immunization Behavior Overall Rating | Never demonstrated 1 | Rarely demonstrated 2 | Sometimes demonstrated 3 | Often demonstrated 4 | Consistently demonstrated 5 | |
|---|---|---|---|---|---|---|
| INDICATORS: | | | | | | |
| 190001  Acknowledges disease risk without immunization | 1 | 2 | 3 | 4 | 5 | NA |
| 190002  Describes risks associated with specific immunization | 1 | 2 | 3 | 4 | 5 | NA |
| 190003  Describes contra-indications to specific immunization | 1 | 2 | 3 | 4 | 5 | NA |
| 190004  Brings updated vaccination card to each visit | 1 | 2 | 3 | 4 | 5 | NA |
| 190005  Obtains immunizations recommended for age by the AAP* or USPHS* | 1 | 2 | 3 | 4 | 5 | NA |
| 190006  Describes relief measures for vaccine side effects | 1 | 2 | 3 | 4 | 5 | NA |
| 190007  Reports any adverse reactions | 1 | 2 | 3 | 4 | 5 | NA |
| 190009  Confirms date of next immunization | 1 | 2 | 3 | 4 | 5 | NA |
| 190010  Obtains immunizations recommended with chronic illness by the AAP or USPHS | 1 | 2 | 3 | 4 | 5 | NA |
| 190011  Obtains immunizations recommended for occupational risk by the AAP or USPHS | 1 | 2 | 3 | 4 | 5 | NA |
| 190012  Obtains immunizations recommended for travel by the AAP or USPHS | 1 | 2 | 3 | 4 | 5 | NA |
| 190013  Identifies community resources for immunization | 1 | 2 | 3 | 4 | 5 | NA |

*AAP = American Academy of Pediatrics; USPHS = United States Public Health Service.

1st edition 1997; Revised 2nd edition 2000; Revised 3rd edition

*Continued*

Outcome Content References:

Forshner, L., & Garza, A. (1999). Childhood vaccines: An update. *RN, 62*(4), 32-37.

Notice to readers: Recommended childhood immunization schedule–United States, 2002. (2002). *Morbidity and Mortality Weekly Report, 51*(2), 31-33.

Paulson, P.R., & Hammer, A.L. (2002). Updates & kidbits. Pediatric immunization update 2002. *Pediatric Nursing, 28*(2), 173-181.

Preboth, M. (2000). Practice guidelines. ACIP recommendations for the prevention of hepatitis A through immunization. *American Family Physician, 61*(7), 2246-2248.

Selekman, J. (1994). The guidelines for immunizations have changed again! *Pediatric Nursing, 20*(4), 376-378.

Sharts-Hopko, N.C. (1994). Current immunization guidelines. *MCN: American Journal of Maternal Child Nursing, 19*(2), 82-84.

Smith, C., & Maurer, F. (1995). *Community health nursing: Theory and practice*. Philadelphia: W.B. Saunders.

U.S. Department of Health and Human Services. (1994). *Clinician's handbook of preventive service: Put prevention into practice*. Washington, DC: Government Printing Office.

Zimmerman, R.K., & Ball, J.A. (2001). Adult vaccinations. *Primary Care: Clinics in Office Practice, 28*(4), 763-790.

I

# Impulse Self-Control (1405)

Domain-Psychosocial Health (III)

Class-Self-Control (O)

Scale(s)-Never demonstrated to Consistently demonstrated (m)

Care Recipient:

Data Source:

---

**Definition:** Self-restraint of compulsive or impulsive behaviors

OUTCOME TARGET RATING:    Maintain at_____    Increase to_____

| Impulse Self-Control Overall Rating | Never demonstrated 1 | Rarely demonstrated 2 | Sometimes demonstrated 3 | Often demonstrated 4 | Consistently demonstrated 5 | |
|---|---|---|---|---|---|---|
| **INDICATORS:** | | | | | | |
| 140501 Identifies harmful impulsive behaviors | 1 | 2 | 3 | 4 | 5 | NA |
| 140502 Identifies feelings that lead to impulsive actions | 1 | 2 | 3 | 4 | 5 | NA |
| 140503 Identifies behaviors that lead to impulsive actions | 1 | 2 | 3 | 4 | 5 | NA |
| 140504 Identifies consequences of impulsive actions to self or others | 1 | 2 | 3 | 4 | 5 | NA |
| 140505 Recognizes risks in environment | 1 | 2 | 3 | 4 | 5 | NA |
| 140506 Avoids high-risk environments and situations | 1 | 2 | 3 | 4 | 5 | NA |
| 140507 Controls impulses | 1 | 2 | 3 | 4 | 5 | NA |
| 140508 Seeks help when experiencing impulses | 1 | 2 | 3 | 4 | 5 | NA |
| 140509 Uses available social support | 1 | 2 | 3 | 4 | 5 | NA |
| 140510 Accepts referrals for treatment | 1 | 2 | 3 | 4 | 5 | NA |
| 140511 Upholds contract to control behavior | 1 | 2 | 3 | 4 | 5 | NA |
| 140512 Maintains self-control without supervision | 1 | 2 | 3 | 4 | 5 | NA |

*1st edition 1997; Revised 2nd edition 2000; Revised 3rd edition (formerly Impulse Control)*

## Outcome Content References:

American Psychiatric Association Practice Guidelines. (1993). *American Journal of Psychiatry, 150*(2), 207-228.

Dyckoff, D., Goldstein, L., & Levine-Schacht, L. (1996). The investigation of behavioral contracting in patients with borderline personality disorder. *Journal of the American Psychiatric Nurses Association, 2*(3), 71-76.

Gallop, R. (1992). Self-destructive and impulsive behavior in the patient with borderline personality disorder: Rethinking hospital treatment and management. *Archives of Psychiatric Nursing, 6*(6), 366-373.

Gallop, R., McCay, E., & Esplen, M.T. (1992). The conceptualization of impulsivity for psychiatric nursing practice. *Archives of Psychiatric Nursing, 6*(6), 366-373.

Ingram, T.N. (2001). Risk for violence: Self-Directed or directed at others. In M. Maas, K. Buckwalter, M. Hardy, T. Tripp-Reimer, M. Titler, & J. Specht (Eds.), *Nursing care of older adults: Diagnoses, outcomes & interventions* (pp. 696-705). St. Louis: Mosby.

*Continued*

+Lazzaro, T.A., Beggs, D.L., & McNeil, K.A. (1969). The development and validation of the Self-Report Test of Impulse Control. *Journal of Clinical Psychology, 25(4)*, 434-438.

Miller, L.J. (1990). The formal treatment contract in the inpatient management of borderline personality disorder. *Hospital and Community Psychiatry, 41*(9) 985-987.

Staples, N.R., & Schwartz, M. (1990). Anorexia nervosa support group: Providing transitional support. *Journal of Psychosocial Nursing and Mental Health Services, 28*(2), 6-10.

Stuart, G.W., & Laraia, M.T. (2001). *Principles and practice of psychiatric nursing* (7th ed.). St. Louis: Mosby.

**I**

# *Infection Severity (0703)*

Domain-Physiologic Health (II)

Class-Immune Response (H)

Scale(s)-Severe to None (n)

Care Recipient:

Data Source:

**Definition:** Severity of infection and associated symptoms

OUTCOME TARGET RATING:    Maintain at_____    Increase to_____

| Infection Severity Overall Rating | Severe 1 | Substantial 2 | Moderate 3 | Mild 4 | None 5 | |
|---|---|---|---|---|---|---|
| INDICATORS: | | | | | | |
| 070301  Rash | 1 | 2 | 3 | 4 | 5 | NA |
| 070302  Uncrusted vesicles | 1 | 2 | 3 | 4 | 5 | NA |
| 070303  Foul-smelling discharge | 1 | 2 | 3 | 4 | 5 | NA |
| 070304  Purulent sputum | 1 | 2 | 3 | 4 | 5 | NA |
| 070305  Purulent drainage | 1 | 2 | 3 | 4 | 5 | NA |
| 070306  Pyuria | 1 | 2 | 3 | 4 | 5 | NA |
| 070307  Fever | 1 | 2 | 3 | 4 | 5 | NA |
| 070329  Hypothermia | 1 | 2 | 3 | 4 | 5 | NA |
| 070330  Temperature instability | 1 | 2 | 3 | 4 | 5 | NA |
| 070308  Pain/tenderness | 1 | 2 | 3 | 4 | 5 | NA |
| 070309  Gastrointestinal symptoms | 1 | 2 | 3 | 4 | 5 | NA |
| 070310  Lymphadenopathy | 1 | 2 | 3 | 4 | 5 | NA |
| 070311  Malaise | 1 | 2 | 3 | 4 | 5 | NA |
| 070312  Chilling | 1 | 2 | 3 | 4 | 5 | NA |
| 070313  Unexplained cognitive impairment | 1 | 2 | 3 | 4 | 5 | NA |
| 070331  Lethargy | 1 | 2 | 3 | 4 | 5 | NA |
| 070332  Loss of appetite | 1 | 2 | 3 | 4 | 5 | NA |
| 070319  Chest x-ray infiltration | 1 | 2 | 3 | 4 | 5 | NA |
| 070320  Blood culture colonization | 1 | 2 | 3 | 4 | 5 | NA |
| 070321  Sputum culture colonization | 1 | 2 | 3 | 4 | 5 | NA |
| 070322  Cerebrospinal fluid culture colonization | 1 | 2 | 3 | 4 | 5 | NA |
| 070323  Wound site culture colonization | 1 | 2 | 3 | 4 | 5 | NA |
| 070324  Urine culture colonization | 1 | 2 | 3 | 4 | 5 | NA |
| 070325  Stool culture colonization | 1 | 2 | 3 | 4 | 5 | NA |
| 070326  White blood count elevation | 1 | 2 | 3 | 4 | 5 | NA |
| 070327  White blood count depression | 1 | 2 | 3 | 4 | 5 | NA |

Site of infection_____

*1st edition 1997; Revised 3rd edition (formerly Infection Status)*

## Outcome Content References:

Albrutyn, E., & Talbot, G.H. (1987). Surveillance strategies: A primer. *Infection Control, 8*(11), 459-464.

Birnbaum, D. (1987). Nosocomial infection surveillance programs. *Infection Control, 8*(11), 474-479.

Burns, M.V. (1998). Pathophysiology: A self-instructional program (pp. 151-207). Stamford, CT: Appleton & Lange.

Carter, C., & Pottinger, J.M. (2001). Risk for infection. In M. Maas, K. Buckwalter, M. Hardy, T. Tripp-Reimer, M. Titler, & J. Specht (Eds.), *Nursing care of older adults: Diagnoses, outcomes & interventions* (pp. 47-62). St. Louis: Mosby.

Haley, R.W., Aber, R.C., & Bennett, J.V. (1986). Surveillance of nosocomial infections. In J.V. Bennett & D. S. Brachman (Eds.), *Hospital infections* (2nd ed., pp. 51-71). Boston: Little, Brown.

# Infection Severity: Newborn (0708)

Domain-Physiologic Health (II)

Class-Immune Response (H)

Scale(s)-Severe to None (n)

Care Recipient:

Data Source:

**Definition:** Severity of infection and associated symptoms during the first 28 days of life

OUTCOME TARGET RATING:   Maintain at_____   Increase to_____

| Infection Severity: Newborn Overall Rating | Severe 1 | Substantial 2 | Moderate 3 | Mild 4 | None 5 | |
|---|---|---|---|---|---|---|
| **INDICATORS:** | | | | | | |
| 070801 Temperature instability | 1 | 2 | 3 | 4 | 5 | NA |
| 070802 Hypothermia | 1 | 2 | 3 | 4 | 5 | NA |
| 070803 Tachypnea | 1 | 2 | 3 | 4 | 5 | NA |
| 070804 Tachycardia | 1 | 2 | 3 | 4 | 5 | NA |
| 070805 Bradycardia | 1 | 2 | 3 | 4 | 5 | NA |
| 070806 Arrhythmias | 1 | 2 | 3 | 4 | 5 | NA |
| 070807 Hypotension | 1 | 2 | 3 | 4 | 5 | NA |
| 070808 Hypertension | 1 | 2 | 3 | 4 | 5 | NA |
| 070809 Pale | 1 | 2 | 3 | 4 | 5 | NA |
| 070810 Mottled skin | 1 | 2 | 3 | 4 | 5 | NA |
| 070811 Cyanosis | 1 | 2 | 3 | 4 | 5 | NA |
| 070812 Cold, clammy skin | 1 | 2 | 3 | 4 | 5 | NA |
| 070813 Vomiting | 1 | 2 | 3 | 4 | 5 | NA |
| 070814 Diarrhea | 1 | 2 | 3 | 4 | 5 | NA |
| 070815 Abdominal distension | 1 | 2 | 3 | 4 | 5 | NA |
| 070816 Feeding intolerance | 1 | 2 | 3 | 4 | 5 | NA |
| 070817 Lethargy | 1 | 2 | 3 | 4 | 5 | NA |
| 070818 Irritability | 1 | 2 | 3 | 4 | 5 | NA |
| 070819 Seizures | 1 | 2 | 3 | 4 | 5 | NA |
| 070820 Jitteriness | 1 | 2 | 3 | 4 | 5 | NA |
| 070821 High-pitched cry | 1 | 2 | 3 | 4 | 5 | NA |
| 070822 Rash | 1 | 2 | 3 | 4 | 5 | NA |
| 070823 Uncrusted vesicles | 1 | 2 | 3 | 4 | 5 | NA |
| 070824 Foul-smelling discharge | 1 | 2 | 3 | 4 | 5 | NA |
| 070825 Purulent drainage | 1 | 2 | 3 | 4 | 5 | NA |
| 070826 Conjunctivitis | 1 | 2 | 3 | 4 | 5 | NA |
| 070827 Infected umbilicus | 1 | 2 | 3 | 4 | 5 | NA |
| 070828 Blood culture colonization | 1 | 2 | 3 | 4 | 5 | NA |
| 070829 Wound site culture colonization | 1 | 2 | 3 | 4 | 5 | NA |
| 070830 Urine culture colonization | 1 | 2 | 3 | 4 | 5 | NA |
| 070831 Stool culture colonization | 1 | 2 | 3 | 4 | 5 | NA |
| 070832 Chest x-ray infiltration | 1 | 2 | 3 | 4 | 5 | NA |
| 070833 Cerebrospinal fluid culture colonization | 1 | 2 | 3 | 4 | 5 | NA |
| 070834 White blood count elevation | 1 | 2 | 3 | 4 | 5 | NA |
| 070835 White blood count depression | 1 | 2 | 3 | 4 | 5 | NA |

Site of infection_____

*3rd edition*

**Outcome Content References:**

Albrutyn, E., & Talbot, G.H. (1987). Surveillance strategies: A primer. *Infection Control, 8*(11), 459-464.

Deacon, J., & O'Neill, P. (Eds.). (1999). *Core curriculum for neonatal intensive care nursing* (2nd ed.). Philadelphia: W.B. Saunders.

Mattson, S., & Smith, J.E. (Eds.). (2000). *Core curriculum for maternal-newborn nursing* (2nd ed.). Philadelphia: W.B. Saunders.

# *Information Processing (0907)*

Domain-Physiologic Health (II)

Class-Neurocognitive (J)

Scale(s)-Severely compromised to Not compromised (a)

Care Recipient:

Data Source:

**Definition:** Ability to acquire, organize, and use information

OUTCOME TARGET RATING:     Maintain at_____     Increase to_____

| Information Processing Overall Rating | Severely compromised 1 | Substantially compromised 2 | Moderately compromised 3 | Mildly compromised 4 | Not compromised 5 | |
|---|---|---|---|---|---|---|
| INDICATORS: | | | | | | |
| 090701  Identifies common objects correctly | 1 | 2 | 3 | 4 | 5 | NA |
| 090702  Reads and understands a short sentence or paragraph | 1 | 2 | 3 | 4 | 5 | NA |
| 090703  Verbalizes a coherent message | 1 | 2 | 3 | 4 | 5 | NA |
| 090704  Exhibits organized thought processes | 1 | 2 | 3 | 4 | 5 | NA |
| 090705  Exhibits logical thought processes | 1 | 2 | 3 | 4 | 5 | NA |
| 090706  Explains similarity or dissimilarity between two items | 1 | 2 | 3 | 4 | 5 | NA |
| 090707  Adds or subtracts several numbers | 1 | 2 | 3 | 4 | 5 | NA |

*1st edition 1997; Revised 3rd edition*

Outcome Content References:

Abraham, I., & Reel, S. (1993). Cognitive nursing interventions with long-term care residents: Effects on neurocognitive dimensions. *Archives of Psychiatric Nursing, 6*(6), 356-365.

Agostinelli, B., Demers, K., Garrigan, D., & Waszynski, C. (1994). Targeted interventions: Use of the mini-mental state exam. *Journal of Gerontological Nursing, 20*(8), 15-23.

Costa, P.T. Jr., Williams, T.F., Somerfield, M., et al. (1996). *Recognition and Initial Assessment of Alzheimer's Disease and Related Dementias.* No. 19. (AHCPR Publication No. 97-0702). Rockville, MD: U.S. Department of Health and Human Services. Public Health Services, Agency for Health Care Policy and Research.

Dellasega, C. (1992). Home health nurses' assessments of cognition. *Applied Nursing Research, 5*(3), 127-133.

+Folstein, M.F., Folstein, S.E., & McHugh, P.R. (1975). "Mini-Mental State"—A practical method for grading the cognitive state of patients for the clinician. *Journal of Psychiatric Research, 12,* 189-198.

Foreman, M., Theis, S., & Anderson, M.A. (1993). Adverse events in the hospitalized elderly. *Clinical Nursing Research, 2*(3) 360-370.

Gerdner, L.A., & Hall, G.R. (2001). Chronic confusion. In M. Maas, K. Buckwalter, M. Hardy, T. Tripp-Reimer, M. Titler, & J. Specht (Eds.), *Nursing care of older adults: Diagnoses, outcomes & interventions* (pp. 421-441). St. Louis: Mosby.

Inaba-Roland, K., & Maricle, R. (1992). Assessing delirium in the acute care setting. *Heart & Lung, 21*(1), 48-55.

Mason, P. (1989). Cognitive assessment parameters and tools for the critically injured adult. *Critical Care Nursing Clinics of North America, 1*(1), 45-53.

Strub, R.L., & Black, F.W. (2000). *The mental status examination in neurology* (4th ed.). Philadelphia: F.A. Davis.

# *Joint Movement: Ankle (0213)*

*Domain-Functional Health (I)*

*Class-Mobility (C)*

*Scale(s)-Severe deviation from normal range to No deviation from normal range (b)*

*Care Recipient:*

*Data Source:*

**Definition:** Active range of motion of the ankle with self-initiated movement

OUTCOME TARGET RATING:   Maintain at_____   Increase to_____

| Joint Movement: Ankle Overall Rating | Severe deviation from normal range 1 | Substantial deviation from normal range 2 | Moderate deviation from normal range 3 | Mild deviation from normal range 4 | No deviation from normal range 5 | |
|---|---|---|---|---|---|---|
| **INDICATORS:** | | | | | | |
| 021301 Dorsal flexion 20 degrees (R) | 1 | 2 | 3 | 4 | 5 | NA |
| 021302 Plantar flexion 45 degrees (R) | 1 | 2 | 3 | 4 | 5 | NA |
| 021303 Inversion 30 degrees (R) | 1 | 2 | 3 | 4 | 5 | NA |
| 021304 Eversion 20 degrees (R) | 1 | 2 | 3 | 4 | 5 | NA |
| 021305 Rotation (R) | 1 | 2 | 3 | 4 | 5 | NA |
| 021306 Dorsal flexion 20 degrees (L) | 1 | 2 | 3 | 4 | 5 | NA |
| 021307 Plantar flexion 45 degrees (L) | 1 | 2 | 3 | 4 | 5 | NA |
| 021308 Inversion 30 degrees (L) | 1 | 2 | 3 | 4 | 5 | NA |
| 021309 Eversion 20 degrees (L) | 1 | 2 | 3 | 4 | 5 | NA |
| 021310 Rotation (L) | 1 | 2 | 3 | 4 | 5 | NA |

Specify: Right (R)____ Left (L)____ Both____

*3rd edition*

**Outcome Content References:**

Bickley, L. (2002). *Bates' guide to physical examination and history taking* (8th ed.). Philadelphia: Lippincott, Williams, & Wilkins.

Hoeman, S. (2002). *Rehabilitation nursing: Process, application, and outcomes* (3rd ed.). St. Louis: Mosby.

Seidel, H.M., Ball, J.W., Dains, J.E., & Benedict, G.W. (2003). *Mosby's guide to physical examination* (5th ed.). St. Louis: Mosby.

J

# Joint Movement: Elbow (0214)

Domain-Functional Health (I)

Class-Mobility (C)

Scale(s)-Severe deviation from normal range to No deviation from normal range (b)

Care Recipient:

Data Source:

**Definition:** Active range of motion of the elbow with self-initiated movement

OUTCOME TARGET RATING:    Maintain at_____    Increase to_____

| Joint Movement: Elbow Overall Rating | Severe deviation from normal range 1 | Substantial deviation from normal range 2 | Moderate deviation from normal range 3 | Mild deviation from normal range 4 | No deviation from normal range 5 | |
|---|---|---|---|---|---|---|

INDICATORS:

| | | | | | | | |
|---|---|---|---|---|---|---|---|
| 021401 | Extension 0 degrees (R) | 1 | 2 | 3 | 4 | 5 | NA |
| 021402 | Flexion 160 degrees (R) | 1 | 2 | 3 | 4 | 5 | NA |
| 021403 | Supination 90 degrees (R) | 1 | 2 | 3 | 4 | 5 | NA |
| 021404 | Pronation 90 degrees (R) | 1 | 2 | 3 | 4 | 5 | NA |
| 021405 | Extension 0 degrees (L) | 1 | 2 | 3 | 4 | 5 | NA |
| 021406 | Flexion 160 degrees (L) | 1 | 2 | 3 | 4 | 5 | NA |
| 021407 | Supination 90 degrees (L) | 1 | 2 | 3 | 4 | 5 | NA |
| 021408 | Pronation 90 degrees (L) | 1 | 2 | 3 | 4 | 5 | NA |

Specify: Right (R)____ Left (L)____ Both____

*3rd edition*

Outcome Content References:

Bickley, L. (2002). *Bates' guide to physical examination and history taking* (8th ed.). Philadelphia: Lippincott, Williams, & Wilkins.

Hoeman, S. (2002). *Rehabilitation nursing: Process, application, and outcomes* (3rd ed.). St. Louis: Mosby.

Seidel, H.M., Ball, J.W., Dains, J.E., & Benedict, G.W. (2003). *Mosby's guide to physical examination* (5th ed.). St. Louis: Mosby.

J

# Joint Movement: Fingers (0215)

*Domain-Functional Health (I)*

*Class-Mobility (C)*

*Scale(s)-Severe deviation from normal range to No deviation from normal range (b)*

*Care Recipient:*

*Data Source:*

**Definition:** Active range of motion of the fingers with self-initiated movement

OUTCOME TARGET RATING:   Maintain at_____   Increase to_____

| Joint Movement: Fingers Overall Rating | | Severe deviation from normal range 1 | Substantial deviation from normal range 2 | Moderate deviation from normal range 3 | Mild deviation from normal range 4 | No deviation from normal range 5 | |
|---|---|---|---|---|---|---|---|
| INDICATORS: | | | | | | | |
| 021501 | Metacarpophalangeal extension 0 degrees (R) | 1 | 2 | 3 | 4 | 5 | NA |
| 021502 | Metacarpophalangeal flexion 90 degrees (R) | 1 | 2 | 3 | 4 | 5 | NA |
| 021503 | Metacarpophalangeal hyperflexion 30 degrees (R) | 1 | 2 | 3 | 4 | 5 | NA |
| 021504 | Proximal interphalangeal extension 0 degrees (R) | 1 | 2 | 3 | 4 | 5 | NA |
| 021505 | Proximal interphalangeal flexion 100-120 degrees (R) | 1 | 2 | 3 | 4 | 5 | NA |
| 021506 | Distal interphalangeal extension 0 degrees (R) | 1 | 2 | 3 | 4 | 5 | NA |
| 021507 | Distal interphalangeal flexion 45-80 degrees (R) | 1 | 2 | 3 | 4 | 5 | NA |
| 021508 | Metacarpophalangeal extension 0 degrees (L) | 1 | 2 | 3 | 4 | 5 | NA |
| 021509 | Metacarpophalangeal flexion 90 degrees (L) | 1 | 2 | 3 | 4 | 5 | NA |
| 021510 | Metacarpophalangeal hyperflexion 30 degrees (L) | 1 | 2 | 3 | 4 | 5 | NA |
| 021511 | Proximal interphalangeal extension 0 degrees (L) | 1 | 2 | 3 | 4 | 5 | NA |
| 021512 | Proximal interphalangeal flexion 100-120 degrees (L) | 1 | 2 | 3 | 4 | 5 | NA |
| 021513 | Distal interphalangeal extension 0 degrees (L) | 1 | 2 | 3 | 4 | 5 | NA |
| 021514 | Distal interphalangeal flexion 45-80 degrees (L) | 1 | 2 | 3 | 4 | 5 | NA |

Specify: Right (R)____ Left (L)____ Both____

*3rd edition*

Outcome Content References:

Bickley, L. (2002). *Bates' guide to physical examination and history taking* (8th ed.). Philadelphia: Lippincott, Williams, & Wilkins.
Hoeman, S. (2002). *Rehabilitation nursing: Process, application, and outcomes* (3rd ed.). St. Louis: Mosby.
Seidel, H.M., Ball, J.W., Dains, J.E., & Benedict, G.W. (2003). *Mosby's guide to physical examination* (5th ed.). St. Louis: Mosby.

J

# *Joint Movement: Hip (0216)*

Domain-Functional Health (I)                                   Care Recipient:

Class-Mobility (C)                                             Data Source:

Scale(s)-Severe deviation from normal range to No deviation from normal range (b)

**Definition:** Active range of motion of the hip with self-initiated movement

OUTCOME TARGET RATING:      Maintain at_____      Increase to_____

| Joint Movement: Hip Overall Rating | Severe deviation from normal range 1 | Substantial deviation from normal range 2 | Moderate deviation from normal range 3 | Mild deviation from normal range 4 | No deviation from normal range 5 | |
|---|---|---|---|---|---|---|
| **INDICATORS:** | | | | | | |
| 021601 Flexion knee straight 90 degrees (R) | 1 | 2 | 3 | 4 | 5 | NA |
| 021602 Extension knee straight 0 degrees (R) | 1 | 2 | 3 | 4 | 5 | NA |
| 021603 Hyperextension knee straight 15 degrees (R) | 1 | 2 | 3 | 4 | 5 | NA |
| 021604 Flexion knee bent 120 degrees (R) | 1 | 2 | 3 | 4 | 5 | NA |
| 021605 Abduction 45 degrees (R) | 1 | 2 | 3 | 4 | 5 | NA |
| 021606 Adduction 30 degrees (R) | 1 | 2 | 3 | 4 | 5 | NA |
| 021607 Internal rotation 40 degrees (R) | 1 | 2 | 3 | 4 | 5 | NA |
| 021608 External rotation 45 degrees (R) | 1 | 2 | 3 | 4 | 5 | NA |
| 021609 Flexion knee straight 90 degrees (L) | 1 | 2 | 3 | 4 | 5 | NA |
| 021610 Extension knee straight 0 degrees (L) | 1 | 2 | 3 | 4 | 5 | NA |
| 021611 Hyperextension knee straight 15 degrees (L) | 1 | 2 | 3 | 4 | 5 | NA |
| 021612 Flexion knee bent 120 degrees (L) | 1 | 2 | 3 | 4 | 5 | NA |
| 021613 Abduction 45 degrees (L) | 1 | 2 | 3 | 4 | 5 | NA |
| 021614 Adduction 30 degrees (L) | 1 | 2 | 3 | 4 | 5 | NA |
| 021615 Internal rotation 40 degrees (L) | 1 | 2 | 3 | 4 | 5 | NA |
| 021616 External rotation 45 degrees (L) | 1 | 2 | 3 | 4 | 5 | NA |

Specify: Right (R)_____  Left (L)_____  Both_____

*3rd edition*

**Outcome Content References:**

Bickley, L. (2002). *Bates' guide to physical examination and history taking* (8th ed.). Philadelphia: Lippincott, Williams, & Wilkins.
Hoeman, S. (2002). *Rehabilitation nursing: Process, application, and outcomes* (3rd ed.). St. Louis: Mosby.
Seidel, H.M., Ball, J.W., Dains, J.E., & Benedict, G.W. (2003). *Mosby's guide to physical examination* (5th ed.). St. Louis: Mosby.

# *Joint Movement: Knee (0217)*

Domain-Functional Health (I)

Class-Mobility (C)

Scale(s)-Severe deviation from normal range to No deviation from normal range (b)

Care Recipient:

Data Source:

## Definition: Active range of motion of the knee with self-initiated movement

OUTCOME TARGET RATING:     Maintain at_____     Increase to_____

| Joint Movement: Knee<br>Overall Rating | Severe<br>deviation<br>from normal<br>range<br>1 | Substantial<br>deviation<br>from normal<br>range<br>2 | Moderate<br>deviation<br>from normal<br>range<br>3 | Mild<br>deviation<br>from normal<br>range<br>4 | No<br>deviation<br>from normal<br>range<br>5 | |
|---|---|---|---|---|---|---|
| **INDICATORS:** | | | | | | |
| 021701  Extension 0 degrees (R) | 1 | 2 | 3 | 4 | 5 | NA |
| 021702  Flexion 130 degrees (R) | 1 | 2 | 3 | 4 | 5 | NA |
| 021703  Hyperextension<br>15 degrees (R) | 1 | 2 | 3 | 4 | 5 | NA |
| 021704  Extension 0 degrees (L) | 1 | 2 | 3 | 4 | 5 | NA |
| 021705  Flexion 130 degrees (L) | 1 | 2 | 3 | 4 | 5 | NA |
| 021706  Hyperextension<br>15 degrees (L) | 1 | 2 | 3 | 4 | 5 | NA |

Specify: Right (R)____ Left (L)____ Both____

*3rd edition*

### Outcome Content References:

Bickley, L. (2002). *Bates' guide to physical examination and history taking* (8th ed.). Philadelphia: Lippincott, Williams, & Wilkins.

Hoeman, S. (2002). *Rehabilitation nursing: Process, application, and outcomes* (3rd ed.). St. Louis: Mosby.

Seidel, H.M., Ball, J.W., Dains, J.E., & Benedict, G.W. (2003). *Mosby's guide to physical examination* (5th ed.). St. Louis: Mosby.

J

# Joint Movement: Neck (0218)

*Domain-Functional Health (I)*

*Class-Mobility (C)*

*Scale(s)-Severe deviation from normal range to No deviation from normal range (b)*

Care Recipient:

Data Source:

**Definition:** Active range of motion of the neck with self-initiated movement

OUTCOME TARGET RATING:    Maintain at_____    Increase to_____

| Joint Movement: Neck Overall Rating | Severe deviation from normal range 1 | Substantial deviation from normal range 2 | Moderate deviation from normal range 3 | Mild deviation from normal range 4 | No deviation from normal range 5 | |
|---|---|---|---|---|---|---|
| **INDICATORS:** | | | | | | |
| 021801   Flexion 45 degrees | 1 | 2 | 3 | 4 | 5 | NA |
| 021802   Extension 55 degrees | 1 | 2 | 3 | 4 | 5 | NA |
| 021803   Lateral bending 40 degrees (R) | 1 | 2 | 3 | 4 | 5 | NA |
| 021804   Lateral bending 40 degrees (L) | 1 | 2 | 3 | 4 | 5 | NA |
| 021805   Rotation | 1 | 2 | 3 | 4 | 5 | NA |

*3rd edition*

**Outcome Content References:**

Bickley, L. (2002). *Bates' guide to physical examination and history taking* (8th ed.). Philadelphia: Lippincott, Williams, & Wilkins.
Hoeman, S. (2002). *Rehabilitation nursing: Process, application, and outcomes* (3rd ed.). St. Louis: Mosby.
Seidel, H.M., Ball, J.W., Dains, J.E., & Benedict, G.W. (2003). *Mosby's guide to physical examination* (5th ed.). St. Louis: Mosby.

# *Joint Movement: Passive (0207)*

Domain-Functional Health (I)                                   Care Recipient:

Class-Mobility (C)                                             Data Source:

Scale-Severe deviation from normal range to No deviation from normal range (b)

***Definition:*** Joint movement with assistance

OUTCOME TARGET RATING:    Maintain at_____    Increase to_____

| Joint Movement: Passive Overall Rating | Severe deviation from normal range 1 | Substantial deviation from normal range 2 | Moderate deviation from normal range 3 | Mild deviation from normal range 4 | No deviation from normal range 5 | |
|---|---|---|---|---|---|---|
| **INDICATORS:** | | | | | | |
| 020702    Neck | 1 | 2 | 3 | 4 | 5 | NA |
| 020703    Fingers (right) | 1 | 2 | 3 | 4 | 5 | NA |
| 020705    Thumb (right) | 1 | 2 | 3 | 4 | 5 | NA |
| 020707    Wrist (right) | 1 | 2 | 3 | 4 | 5 | NA |
| 020709    Elbow (right) | 1 | 2 | 3 | 4 | 5 | NA |
| 020711    Shoulder (right) | 1 | 2 | 3 | 4 | 5 | NA |
| 020713    Ankle (right) | 1 | 2 | 3 | 4 | 5 | NA |
| 020715    Knee (right) | 1 | 2 | 3 | 4 | 5 | NA |
| 020717    Hip (right) | 1 | 2 | 3 | 4 | 5 | NA |
| 020704    Fingers (left) | 1 | 2 | 3 | 4 | 5 | NA |
| 020706    Thumb (left) | 1 | 2 | 3 | 4 | 5 | NA |
| 020708    Wrist (left) | 1 | 2 | 3 | 4 | 5 | NA |
| 020710    Elbow (left) | 1 | 2 | 3 | 4 | 5 | NA |
| 020712    Shoulder (left) | 1 | 2 | 3 | 4 | 5 | NA |
| 020714    Ankle (left) | 1 | 2 | 3 | 4 | 5 | NA |
| 020716    Knee (left) | 1 | 2 | 3 | 4 | 5 | NA |
| 020718    Hip (left) | 1 | 2 | 3 | 4 | 5 | NA |

*1st edition 1997; Revised 3rd edition*

## Outcome Content References:

Bickley, L. (2002). *Bates' guide to physical examination and history taking* (8th ed.). Philadelphia: Lippincott, Williams, & Wilkins.

Hoeman, S. (2002). *Rehabilitation nursing: Process, application, and outcomes* (3rd ed.). St. Louis: Mosby.

Seidel, H.M., Ball, J.W., Dains, J.E., & Benedict, G.W. (2003). *Mosby's guide to physical examination* (5th ed.). St. Louis: Mosby.

J

# Joint Movement: Shoulder (0219)

*Domain-Functional Health (I)*

*Class-Mobility (C)*

*Scale(s)-Severe deviation from normal range to No deviation from normal range (b)*

*Care Recipient:*

*Data Source:*

**Definition:** Active range of motion of the shoulder with self-initiated movement

OUTCOME TARGET RATING:      Maintain at_____      Increase to_____

| Joint Movement: Shoulder Overall Rating | Severe deviation from normal range 1 | Substantial deviation from normal range 2 | Moderate deviation from normal range 3 | Mild deviation from normal range 4 | No deviation from normal range 5 | |
|---|---|---|---|---|---|---|
| INDICATORS: | | | | | | |
| 021901  Forward flexion 180 degrees (R) | 1 | 2 | 3 | 4 | 5 | NA |
| 021902  Extension 50 degrees (R) | 1 | 2 | 3 | 4 | 5 | NA |
| 021903  External rotation 90 degrees (R) | 1 | 2 | 3 | 4 | 5 | NA |
| 021904  Internal rotation 90 degrees (R) | 1 | 2 | 3 | 4 | 5 | NA |
| 021905  Abduction 180 degrees (R) | 1 | 2 | 3 | 4 | 5 | NA |
| 021906  Adduction 50 degrees (R) | 1 | 2 | 3 | 4 | 5 | NA |
| 021907  Forward flexion 180 degrees (L) | 1 | 2 | 3 | 4 | 5 | NA |
| 021908  Extension 50 degrees (L) | 1 | 2 | 3 | 4 | 5 | NA |
| 021909  External rotation 90 degrees (L) | 1 | 2 | 3 | 4 | 5 | NA |
| 021910  Internal rotation 90 degrees (L) | 1 | 2 | 3 | 4 | 5 | NA |
| 021911  Abduction 180 degrees (L) | 1 | 2 | 3 | 4 | 5 | NA |
| 021912  Adduction 50 degrees (L) | 1 | 2 | 3 | 4 | 5 | NA |

Specify: Right (R)____ Left (L)____ Both____

*3rd edition*

Outcome Content References:

Bickley, L. (2002). *Bates' guide to physical examination and history taking* (8th ed.). Philadelphia: Lippincott, Williams, & Wilkins.
Hoeman, S. (2002). *Rehabilitation nursing: Process, application, and outcomes* (3rd ed.). St. Louis: Mosby.
Seidel, H.M., Ball, J.W., Dains, J.E., & Benedict, G.W. (2003). *Mosby's guide to physical examination* (5th ed.). St. Louis: Mosby.

# *Joint Movement: Spine (0220)*

Domain-Functional Health (I)                                Care Recipient:

Class-Mobility (C)                                          Data Source:

Scale(s)-Severe deviation from normal range to No deviation from normal range (b)

**Definition:** Active range of motion of the spine with self-initiated movement

OUTCOME TARGET RATING:     Maintain at_____     Increase to_____

| Joint Movement: Spine Overall Rating | Severe deviation from normal range 1 | Substantial deviation from normal range 2 | Moderate deviation from normal range 3 | Mild deviation from normal range 4 | No deviation from normal range 5 | |
|---|---|---|---|---|---|---|
| INDICATORS: | | | | | | |
| 022001  Extension 30 degrees | 1 | 2 | 3 | 4 | 5 | NA |
| 022002  Flexion 90 degrees | 1 | 2 | 3 | 4 | 5 | NA |
| 022003  Lateral bending 35 degrees (R) | 1 | 2 | 3 | 4 | 5 | NA |
| 022004  Rotation (R) | 1 | 2 | 3 | 4 | 5 | NA |
| 022005  Lateral bending 35 degrees (L) | 1 | 2 | 3 | 4 | 5 | NA |
| 022006  Rotation (L) | 1 | 2 | 3 | 4 | 5 | NA |

*3rd edition*

Outcome Content References:

Bickley, L. (2002). *Bates' guide to physical examination and history taking* (8th ed.). Philadelphia: Lippincott, Williams, & Wilkins.

Hoeman, S. (2002). *Rehabilitation nursing: Process, application, and outcomes* (3rd ed.). St. Louis: Mosby.

Seidel, H.M., Ball, J.W., Dains, J.E., & Benedict, G.W. (2003). *Mosby's guide to physical examination* (5th ed.). St. Louis: Mosby.

J

# Joint Movement: Wrist (0221)

*Domain-Functional Health (I)*

*Class-Mobility (C)*

*Scale(s)-Severe deviation from normal range to No deviation from normal range (b)*

Care Recipient:

Data Source:

**Definition:** Active range of motion of the wrist with self-initiated movement

OUTCOME TARGET RATING:     Maintain at_____     Increase to_____

| Joint Movement: Wrist Overall Rating | | Severe deviation from normal range 1 | Substantial deviation from normal range 2 | Moderate deviation from normal range 3 | Mild deviation from normal range 4 | No deviation from normal range 5 | |
|---|---|---|---|---|---|---|---|
| INDICATORS: | | | | | | | |
| 022101 | Radial deviation 20 degrees (R) | 1 | 2 | 3 | 4 | 5 | NA |
| 022102 | Ulnar deviation 55 degrees (R) | 1 | 2 | 3 | 4 | 5 | NA |
| 022103 | Flexion 90 degrees (R) | 1 | 2 | 3 | 4 | 5 | NA |
| 022104 | Extension 70 degrees (R) | 1 | 2 | 3 | 4 | 5 | NA |
| 022105 | Radial deviation 20 degrees (L) | 1 | 2 | 3 | 4 | 5 | NA |
| 022106 | Ulnar deviation 55 degrees (L) | 1 | 2 | 3 | 4 | 5 | NA |
| 022107 | Flexion 90 degrees (L) | 1 | 2 | 3 | 4 | 5 | NA |
| 022108 | Extension 70 degrees (L) | 1 | 2 | 3 | 4 | 5 | NA |

Specify: Right (R)____ Left (L)____ Both____

*3rd edition*

Outcome Content References:

Bickley, L. (2002). *Bates' guide to physical examination and history taking* (8th ed.). Philadelphia: Lippincott, Williams, & Wilkins.
Hoeman, S. (2002). *Rehabilitation nursing: Process, application, and outcomes* (3rd ed.). St. Louis: Mosby.
Seidel, H.M., Ball, J.W., Dains, J.E., & Benedict, G.W. (2003). *Mosby's guide to physical examination* (5th ed.). St. Louis: Mosby.

# *Kidney Function (0504)*

Domain-Physiologic Health (II)

Class-Elimination (F)

Scale(s)-Severely compromised to Not compromised (a) and Severe to None (n)

Care Recipient:

Data Source:

**Definition:** Filtration of blood and elimination of metabolic waste products through the formation of urine

OUTCOME TARGET RATING:     Maintain at_____     Increase to_____

| Kidney Function Overall Rating | Severely compromised 1 | Substantially compromised 2 | Moderately compromised 3 | Mildly compromised 4 | Not compromised 5 | |
|---|---|---|---|---|---|---|
| INDICATORS: | | | | | | |
| 050401 Intake of adequate fluid | 1 | 2 | 3 | 4 | 5 | NA |
| 050402 24-hour intake and output balance | 1 | 2 | 3 | 4 | 5 | NA |
| 050403 Blood urea nitrogen | 1 | 2 | 3 | 4 | 5 | NA |
| 050404 Serum creatinine | 1 | 2 | 3 | 4 | 5 | NA |
| 050405 Urine specific gravity | 1 | 2 | 3 | 4 | 5 | NA |
| 050406 Urine color | 1 | 2 | 3 | 4 | 5 | NA |
| 050407 Urine proteins | 1 | 2 | 3 | 4 | 5 | NA |
| 050408 Urine pH | 1 | 2 | 3 | 4 | 5 | NA |
| 050409 Urine electrolytes | 1 | 2 | 3 | 4 | 5 | NA |
| 050410 Arterial bicarbonate ($HCO_3$) | 1 | 2 | 3 | 4 | 5 | NA |
| 050411 Arterial pH | 1 | 2 | 3 | 4 | 5 | NA |
| 050412 Serum electrolytes | 1 | 2 | 3 | 4 | 5 | NA |

| | Severe | Substantial | Moderate | Mild | None | |
|---|---|---|---|---|---|---|
| 050413 Urine glucose | 1 | 2 | 3 | 4 | 5 | NA |
| 050414 Hematuria | 1 | 2 | 3 | 4 | 5 | NA |
| 050415 Urine ketones | 1 | 2 | 3 | 4 | 5 | NA |
| 050416 Urine abnormal microscopic findings | 1 | 2 | 3 | 4 | 5 | NA |
| 050417 Kidney stone formation | 1 | 2 | 3 | 4 | 5 | NA |
| 050418 Weight gain | 1 | 2 | 3 | 4 | 5 | NA |
| 050419 Hypertension | 1 | 2 | 3 | 4 | 5 | NA |
| 050420 Nausea | 1 | 2 | 3 | 4 | 5 | NA |
| 050421 Fatigue | 1 | 2 | 3 | 4 | 5 | NA |
| 050422 Malaise | 1 | 2 | 3 | 4 | 5 | NA |
| 050423 Anemia | 1 | 2 | 3 | 4 | 5 | NA |

*3rd edition*

Outcome Content References:

Brundage, D.J., & Linton, A.D. (1997). Age related changes in the genitourinary system. In M.A. Matteson, E.S. McConnell, & A.D. Linton (Eds.), *Gerontological nursing: Concepts in practice* (2nd ed.). Philadelphia, W.B. Saunders.

Culp, K., Flanigan, M., Dudley, J., Taylor, L., Bissen, T., & Garrison, S. (1998). Using the Quetelet Body Mass Index as a prognostic indicator for patients starting renal replacement therapy. *American Nephrology Nurses Association Journal, 25*(3), 321-332.

Culp, K., Flanigan, M., & Hayajneh, Y. (1999). Body weight and hemodialysis adequacy: An analysis of urea reduction ratios. *American Nephrology Nurses Association Journal, 26*(4), 391-402.

Culp, K., Flanigan, M., Lowie, E., Lew, N., & Zimmerman, B. (1996). Modeling mortality risk in hemodialysis patients using laboratory values as time-dependent covariates. *American Journal of Kidney Diseases, 28*(5), 741-746.

Guyton, A.C., Hall, J.E., & Schmitt, W. (1997). *Human physiology and mechanisms of disease* (6th ed.). New York: Harcourt Brace & Company.

Morton, P.G. (1989). *Health assessment in nursing.* Springhouse, PA: Springhouse.

Potter, P.A., & Perry, A.G. (2001). *Fundamentals of nursing* (5th ed.). St. Louis: Mosby.

Roth, C., & Culp, K. (2001). Renal osteodystrophy in elderly patients with end-stage renal disease. *Journal of Gerontological Nursing, 27*(7), 46-51.

# *Knowledge: Body Mechanics (1827)*

*Domain-Health Knowledge & Behavior (IV)*

*Class-Health Knowledge (S)*

*Scale(s)-None to Extensive (i)*

Care Recipient:

Data Source:

**Definition:** Extent of understanding conveyed about proper body alignment, balance and coordinated movement

OUTCOME TARGET RATING:    Maintain at_____    Increase to_____

| Knowledge: Body Mechanics Overall Rating | None 1 | Limited 2 | Moderate 3 | Substantial 4 | Extensive 5 | |
|---|---|---|---|---|---|---|
| **INDICATORS:** | | | | | | |
| 182701 Description of the 3 natural spinal curves | 1 | 2 | 3 | 4 | 5 | NA |
| 182702 Description of proper standing posture | 1 | 2 | 3 | 4 | 5 | NA |
| 182703 Description of proper sitting posture | 1 | 2 | 3 | 4 | 5 | NA |
| 182704 Description of proper lying posture | 1 | 2 | 3 | 4 | 5 | NA |
| 182705 Description of proper lifting techniques | 1 | 2 | 3 | 4 | 5 | NA |
| 182706 Description of exercises to improve posture | 1 | 2 | 3 | 4 | 5 | NA |
| 182707 Description of exercises to improve muscle flexibility | 1 | 2 | 3 | 4 | 5 | NA |
| 182708 Description of exercises to increase joint mobility | 1 | 2 | 3 | 4 | 5 | NA |
| 182709 Description of exercises to increase muscle strength | 1 | 2 | 3 | 4 | 5 | NA |
| 182710 Description of exercises to strengthen lower abdominal muscles | 1 | 2 | 3 | 4 | 5 | NA |
| 182711 Description of possible positional causes of muscle or joint pain from sitting | 1 | 2 | 3 | 4 | 5 | NA |
| 182712 Description of possible positional causes of muscle or joint pain from lying | 1 | 2 | 3 | 4 | 5 | NA |
| 182713 Description of possible positional causes of muscle or joint pain from lifting | 1 | 2 | 3 | 4 | 5 | NA |
| 182714 Description of symptoms of potential back injury | 1 | 2 | 3 | 4 | 5 | NA |
| 182715 Description of personal risk activities | 1 | 2 | 3 | 4 | 5 | NA |

*3rd edition*

Outcome Content References:

American Physical Therapy Association. (1996). *Taking care of your back: A physical therapist's perspective*. Washington, DC: Author.

American Physical Therapy Association. (2000). *The secret of good posture: A physical therapist's perspective*. Washington, DC: Author.

Lieber, S.J., Rudy, T.E., & Boston, R. (1999). Effects of body mechanics training on performance of repetitive lifting. *The American Journal of Occupational Therapy, 54*(2), 166-175.

Perry, A.G., & Potter, P.A. (1998). *Clinical nursing skills and techniques*. (4th ed., pp. 877-884). St. Louis: Mosby.

Porteau-Cassard L. Zabraniecki L. Dromer C. Fournie B. (1999). A back school program at the Toulouse-Purpan teaching hospital. Evaluation of 144 patients. *Revue Du Rhumatisme, English Edition, 66*(10), 477-483.

Sorrentino, S.A. (2000). *Mosby's textbook for nursing assistants*. (5th ed., pp. 242–247). St. Louis: Mosby.

K

# Knowledge: Breastfeeding (1800)

*Domain-Health Knowledge & Behavior (IV)*  
*Class-Health Knowledge (S)*  
*Scale(s)-None to Extensive (i)*

*Care Recipient:*  
*Data Source:*

**Definition:** Extent of understanding conveyed about lactation and nourishment of infant through breastfeeding

OUTCOME TARGET RATING:     Maintain at_____     Increase to_____

| Knowledge: Breastfeeding Overall Rating | None 1 | Limited 2 | Moderate 3 | Substantial 4 | Extensive 5 | |
|---|---|---|---|---|---|---|
| **INDICATORS:** | | | | | | |
| 180001 Description of benefits of breastfeeding | 1 | 2 | 3 | 4 | 5 | NA |
| 180002 Description of physiology of lactation | 1 | 2 | 3 | 4 | 5 | NA |
| 180020 Description of adequate fluid intake for mother | 1 | 2 | 3 | 4 | 5 | NA |
| 180003 Description of breastmilk composition, letdown process, foremilk versus hindmilk | 1 | 2 | 3 | 4 | 5 | NA |
| 180004 Description of early infant hunger cues | 1 | 2 | 3 | 4 | 5 | NA |
| 180005 Description of proper technique for attaching infant to the breast | 1 | 2 | 3 | 4 | 5 | NA |
| 180006 Description of proper infant positioning while nursing | 1 | 2 | 3 | 4 | 5 | NA |
| 180007 Description of nutritive versus nonnutritive suck | 1 | 2 | 3 | 4 | 5 | NA |
| 180008 Description of evaluation of infant swallowing | 1 | 2 | 3 | 4 | 5 | NA |
| 180009 Description of proper technique to break infant suction | 1 | 2 | 3 | 4 | 5 | NA |
| 180010 Description of signs of adequate milk supply | 1 | 2 | 3 | 4 | 5 | NA |
| 180011 Description of signs of adequately nourished infant | 1 | 2 | 3 | 4 | 5 | NA |
| 180012 Description of nipple evaluation | 1 | 2 | 3 | 4 | 5 | NA |
| 180013 Description of signs of mastitis, blocked ducts, nipple trauma | 1 | 2 | 3 | 4 | 5 | NA |
| 180014 Description of reasons for early avoidance of artificial nipples | 1 | 2 | 3 | 4 | 5 | NA |
| 180021 Description of reasons for early avoidance of water and supplements | 1 | 2 | 3 | 4 | 5 | NA |
| 180015 Description of proper breastmilk expression and storage techniques | 1 | 2 | 3 | 4 | 5 | NA |
| 180016 Description of substances that transfer from mother to infant though breastmilk | 1 | 2 | 3 | 4 | 5 | NA |
| 180022 Description of relationship between breastfeeding and infant immunity | 1 | 2 | 3 | 4 | 5 | NA |
| 180017 Description of weaning readiness | 1 | 2 | 3 | 4 | 5 | NA |
| 180018 Description of how to access health care system | 1 | 2 | 3 | 4 | 5 | NA |

*1st edition 1997; Revised 3rd edition*

*Continued*

Outcome Content References:

Lawrence, R.A., & Lawrence, R.M. (1999). *Breastfeeding: A guide for the medical profession* (5th ed.). St. Louis: Mosby.

Minchin, M.K. (1989). Positioning for breastfeeding. *Birth: Issues in Perinatal Care and Education, 16*(2), 67-80.

Righard, L., & Alade, M. (1992). Sucking technique and its effect on success of breastfeeding. *Birth: Issues in Perinatal Care and Education, 19(4)*, 185-189.

Riordan, J., & Auerbach, K.G. (1999). *Breastfeeding and human lactation* (2nd ed.). Boston: Jones & Bartlett.

Shrago, L., & Bocar, D. (1990). The infant's contribution to breastfeeding. *Journal of Obstetric, Gynecologic, and Neonatal Nursing, 19(3)*, 209-213.

Spangler, A. (1992). *Amy Spangler's breastfeeding: A parent's guide*. Atlanta: A. Spangler Publications.

Walker, M. (1989). Functional assessment of infant breastfeeding patterns. *Birth: Issues in Perinatal Care and Education, 16*(3), 140-147.

**K**

# Knowledge: Cardiac Disease Management (1830)

Domain-Health Knowledge & Behavior (IV)

Class–Health Knowledge (S)

Scale(s)-None to Extensive (i)

Care Recipient:

Data Source

**Definition:** Extent of understanding conveyed about heart disease and the prevention of complications

OUTCOME TARGET RATING:       Maintain at_____       Increase to_____

| Knowledge: Cardiac Disease Management Overall Rating | None 1 | Limited 2 | Moderate 3 | Substantial 4 | Extensive 5 | |
|---|---|---|---|---|---|---|
| INDICATORS: | | | | | | |
| 183001 Description of usual course of disease process | 1 | 2 | 3 | 4 | 5 | NA |
| 183002 Description of symptoms of early disease | 1 | 2 | 3 | 4 | 5 | NA |
| 183003 Description of symptoms of worsening disease | 1 | 2 | 3 | 4 | 5 | NA |
| 183004 Description of benefits of disease management | 1 | 2 | 3 | 4 | 5 | NA |
| 183005 Description of ways to manage controllable risk factors | 1 | 2 | 3 | 4 | 5 | NA |
| 183006 Description of importance of completing recommended cardiac rehabilitation program | 1 | 2 | 3 | 4 | 5 | NA |
| 183007 Description of family caregivers role in treatment plan | 1 | 2 | 3 | 4 | 5 | NA |
| 183008 Description of methods to obtain blood pressure and pulse rate | 1 | 2 | 3 | 4 | 5 | NA |
| 183009 Identification of ways to limit sodium intake | 1 | 2 | 3 | 4 | 5 | NA |
| 183010 Explanation of rationale for following a low-fat, low cholesterol diet | 1 | 2 | 3 | 4 | 5 | NA |
| 183011 Description of strategies for diet adherence | 1 | 2 | 3 | 4 | 5 | NA |
| 183012 Description of ways to limit fluid intake | 1 | 2 | 3 | 4 | 5 | NA |
| 183013 Explanation of rationale for monitoring weight | 1 | 2 | 3 | 4 | 5 | NA |
| 183014 Description of need for alcohol restriction | 1 | 2 | 3 | 4 | 5 | NA |
| 183015 Description of importance of tobacco abstinence | 1 | 2 | 3 | 4 | 5 | NA |
| 183016 Description of recreation, leisure, and work activity recommendations | 1 | 2 | 3 | 4 | 5 | NA |
| 183017 Explanation of rationale for regular exercise | 1 | 2 | 3 | 4 | 5 | NA |
| 183018 Description of energy conservation techniques | 1 | 2 | 3 | 4 | 5 | NA |
| 183019 Description of guidelines for sexual activity after cardiovascular event | 1 | 2 | 3 | 4 | 5 | NA |

K

*Continued*

| Knowledge: Cardiac Disease Management—cont'd | | None | Limited | Moderate | Substantial | Extensive | |
|---|---|---|---|---|---|---|---|
| 183020 | Discussion of potential sexual difficulties and coping strategies | 1 | 2 | 3 | 4 | 5 | NA |
| 183021 | Description of effects of medications | 1 | 2 | 3 | 4 | 5 | NA |
| 183022 | Description of strategies for managing stress | 1 | 2 | 3 | 4 | 5 | NA |
| 183023 | Description of importance of obtaining flu and pneumonia vaccines | 1 | 2 | 3 | 4 | 5 | NA |
| 183024 | Description of when to seek help from health care provider | 1 | 2 | 3 | 4 | 5 | NA |
| 183025 | Description of options in assistance with medical emergencies | 1 | 2 | 3 | 4 | 5 | NA |
| 183026 | Identification of importance of family learning cardiopulmonary resuscitation | 1 | 2 | 3 | 4 | 5 | NA |
| 183027 | Discussion of cultural beliefs that affect adherence to treatment plan | 1 | 2 | 3 | 4 | 5 | NA |

*3rd edition*

**Outcome Content References:**

Cannon, C.P., Battler, A., Brindis, R.G., Cox, J.L., Ellis, S.G., Every, N.R., Flaherty, J.T., Harrington, R.A., Krumholz, H.M., Simoons, M.L., Van De Werf, F.J.J., & Weintraub, W.S. (2001). ACC key data elements and definitions for measuring the clinical management and outcomes of patients with acute coronary syndromes: A report of the American College of Cardiology task force on clinical data standards (acute coronary syndrome writing committee). *Journal of the American College of Cardiology, 38,* 2114-2130.

Dunbar, S.B., Jacobson, L.H., & Deaton, C. (1998). Heart failure: Strategies to enhance patient self-management. *AACN Clinical Issues: Advanced Practice in Acute & Critical Care, 9,* 244-256.

Dusseldorp, E., Van Elderan, T., Maes, S., Meulman, J, & Kraaij, V. (1999). A meta-analysis of psychoeducational programs for coronary heart disease patients. *Health Psychology, 18,* 506-519.

Hunt, S.A., Baker, D.W., Chin, M.H., Cinquegrani, M.P., Feldman, A.M., Grancis, G.S., Ganiats, T.G., Goldstein, S., Gregoratos, G., Jessup, M.L., Noble, R.J., Packer, M., Silver, M.A., & Steven, L. W. (2001). ACC/AHA guidelines for the evaluation and management of chronic heart failure in the adult: A report of the American College of Cardiology/American Heart Association Task Force on Practice Guidelines (Committee to revise the 1995 Guidelines for the Evaluation and Management of Heart Failure). *Journal of the American College of Cardiology, 38,* 2101-2113.

Johnson, J., & Pearson, V. (2000). The effects of a structured education course on stroke survivors living in the community...including commentary by Phipps, M. *Rehabilitation Nursing, 25,* 59-65.

Konstam, M., Dracup, K., Baker, D., et al. (1994). *Heart Failure: Management of Patients with Left-Ventricular Systolic Dysfunction. Clinical Practice Guideline No. 11.* (AHCPR Publication No. 94-0612). Rockville, MD: Agency for Health Care Policy and Research, Public Health Service, U. S. Department of Health and Human Services.

Sheps, S.G., Black, H.R., Cohen, J.D., Kaplan, N.M., Ferdinand, K.C., Chobanian, A.V., Dustan, H.P., Gifford, R.W., Moser, M., et al. (1997). *The Sixth Report of the Joint National Committee on Prevention, Detection, Evaluation, & Treatment of High Blood Pressure.* NIH Publication No. 98-4080. Bethesda, MD: National Institutes of Health, National Heart, Lung, and Blood Institute (NHLBI), & National High Blood Pressure Education Program.

K

# *Knowledge: Child Physical Safety (1801)*

Domain-Health Knowledge & Behavior (IV)

Class-Health Knowledge (S)

Scale(s)-None to Extensive (i)

Care Recipient:

Data Source:

---

**Definition:** Extent of understanding conveyed about safely caring for a child from 1 year through 17 years of age

---

OUTCOME TARGET RATING:        Maintain at_____    Increase to_____

| Knowledge: Child Physical Safety Overall Rating | None 1 | Limited 2 | Moderate 3 | Substantial 4 | Extensive 5 | |
|---|---|---|---|---|---|---|
| **INDICATORS:** | | | | | | |
| 180101  Description of appropriate activities for child's developmental level | 1 | 2 | 3 | 4 | 5 | NA |
| 180119  Description of diving hazards | 1 | 2 | 3 | 4 | 5 | NA |
| 180103  Description of methods to prevent drowning | 1 | 2 | 3 | 4 | 5 | NA |
| 180104  Description of methods to prevent electrical shock | 1 | 2 | 3 | 4 | 5 | NA |
| 180105  Description of benefits of protective helmets | 1 | 2 | 3 | 4 | 5 | NA |
| 180106  Description of methods to prevent choking on objects | 1 | 2 | 3 | 4 | 5 | NA |
| 180120  Description of first aid techniques | 1 | 2 | 3 | 4 | 5 | NA |
| 180108  Description of correct use of safety seats and seat belts | 1 | 2 | 3 | 4 | 5 | NA |
| 180121  Description of age appropriate cardiopulmonary resuscitation techniques | 1 | 2 | 3 | 4 | 5 | NA |
| 180122  Description of Heimlich maneuver | 1 | 2 | 3 | 4 | 5 | NA |
| 180111  Description of methods to prevent farm accidents | 1 | 2 | 3 | 4 | 5 | NA |
| 180123  Description of methods to prevent vehicle accidents | 1 | 2 | 3 | 4 | 5 | NA |
| 180112  Description of methods to prevent falls | 1 | 2 | 3 | 4 | 5 | NA |
| 180113  Description of methods to prevent playground accidents | 1 | 2 | 3 | 4 | 5 | NA |
| 180114  Description of methods to prevent burns | 1 | 2 | 3 | 4 | 5 | NA |
| 180115  Description of use of functioning smoke detectors | 1 | 2 | 3 | 4 | 5 | NA |
| 180116  Description of proper surveillance of outdoor play | 1 | 2 | 3 | 4 | 5 | NA |
| 180117  Description of teaching stranger awareness | 1 | 2 | 3 | 4 | 5 | NA |

*1st edition 1997; Revised 3rd edition (formerly Knowledge: Child Safety)*

Outcome Content References:

Eichelberger, M.R., Gotschall, C.S., Feely, H.B., Harstad, P., & Bowman, L.M. (1990). Parental attitudes and knowledge of child safety. *American Journal of Diseases of Children, 144*(6), 714-720.

Gilk, D., Kronenfeld, J., & Jackson, K. (1993). Safety behaviors among parents of preschoolers. *Health Values, 17*(1), 18-25.

Grossman, D.C., & Rivera, F. P. (1992). Injury control in childhood. *Pediatric Clinics of North America, 39*(3), 471-484.

Rivera, F.P., & Howard, D. (1982). Parental knowledge of child development and injury risks. *Developmental and Behavioral Pediatrics, 3*(2), 103-105.

Wortel E., Geus, G.H., Kok, G., & van Woerkum, C. (1994). Injury control in pre-school children: A review of parental safety measures and the behavioral determinants. *Health Education Research, 9*(2), 201-213.

K

# Knowledge: Conception Prevention (1821)

*Domain-Health Knowledge & Behavior (IV)*

*Class-Health Knowledge (S)*

*Scale(s)-None to Extensive (i)*

*Care Recipient:*

*Data Source:*

**Definition:** Extent of understanding conveyed about prevention of unintended pregnancy

OUTCOME TARGET RATING:   Maintain at_____   Increase to_____

| Knowledge: Conception Prevention Overall Rating | None 1 | Limited 2 | Moderate 3 | Substantial 4 | Extensive 5 | |
|---|---|---|---|---|---|---|

INDICATORS:

| | | | | | | | |
|---|---|---|---|---|---|---|---|
| 182101 | Description of how chosen contraceptive method works | 1 | 2 | 3 | 4 | 5 | NA |
| 182102 | Description of correct use of chosen contraceptive method | 1 | 2 | 3 | 4 | 5 | NA |
| 182103 | Description of effectiveness of chosen contraceptive method(s) | 1 | 2 | 3 | 4 | 5 | NA |
| 182104 | Description of effect of chosen contraceptive method on STD* transmission | 1 | 2 | 3 | 4 | 5 | NA |
| 182105 | Description of how conception occurs | 1 | 2 | 3 | 4 | 5 | NA |
| 182106 | Description of advantages and disadvantages of having a child | 1 | 2 | 3 | 4 | 5 | NA |
| 182107 | Description of influence of personal and religious values on contraception | 1 | 2 | 3 | 4 | 5 | NA |
| 182108 | Description of periodic rhythm method | 1 | 2 | 3 | 4 | 5 | NA |
| 182109 | Description of chemical barrier methods | 1 | 2 | 3 | 4 | 5 | NA |
| 182110 | Description of hormonal therapy methods | 1 | 2 | 3 | 4 | 5 | NA |
| 182111 | Description of mechanical barrier methods | 1 | 2 | 3 | 4 | 5 | NA |
| 182112 | Description of surgical intervention methods | 1 | 2 | 3 | 4 | 5 | NA |
| 182113 | Description of patterns of contraceptive use | 1 | 2 | 3 | 4 | 5 | NA |

*STD = Sexually transmitted disease.

*2nd edition 2000; Revised 3rd edition*

Outcome Content References:

Hatcher, R.A., et al. (1998). *Contraceptive Technology*, (17th ed.). New York: Irvington Publishers.

Howard, M. (1991). *How to help your teenager postpone sexual involvement.* Lexington, NY: Continuum Publishing Co.

Miller, B., Card, J., Paikoff, R.J., & Peterson, J. (1992). *Preventing adolescent pregnancy.* Newbury Park, CA: Sage Publications.

# Knowledge: Diabetes Management (1820)

*Domain-Health Knowledge & Behavior (IV)*

*Class-Health Knowledge (S)*

*Scale(s)-None to Extensive (i)*

*Care Recipient:*

*Data Source:*

**Definition:** Extent of understanding conveyed about diabetes mellitus and the prevention of complications

OUTCOME TARGET RATING:        Maintain at_____    Increase to_____

| Knowledge: Diabetes Management Overall Rating | None 1 | Limited 2 | Moderate 3 | Substantial 4 | Extensive 5 | |
|---|---|---|---|---|---|---|
| **INDICATORS:** | | | | | | |
| 182001 Description of insulin function | 1 | 2 | 3 | 4 | 5 | NA |
| 182002 Description of role of diet in controlling blood glucose level | 1 | 2 | 3 | 4 | 5 | NA |
| 182003 Description of prescribed meal plan | 1 | 2 | 3 | 4 | 5 | NA |
| 182004 Description of strategies for diet adherence | 1 | 2 | 3 | 4 | 5 | NA |
| 182005 Description of role of exercise in controlling blood glucose level | 1 | 2 | 3 | 4 | 5 | NA |
| 182006 Description of hyperglycemia and related symptoms | 1 | 2 | 3 | 4 | 5 | NA |
| 182007 Description of hyperglycemia prevention | 1 | 2 | 3 | 4 | 5 | NA |
| 182008 Description of procedures to be followed in treating hyperglycemia | 1 | 2 | 3 | 4 | 5 | NA |
| 182009 Description of hypoglycemia and related symptoms | 1 | 2 | 3 | 4 | 5 | NA |
| 182010 Description of hypoglycemia prevention | 1 | 2 | 3 | 4 | 5 | NA |
| 182011 Description of procedures to be followed in treating hypoglycemia | 1 | 2 | 3 | 4 | 5 | NA |
| 182012 Description of importance of maintaining blood glucose in target range | 1 | 2 | 3 | 4 | 5 | NA |
| 182013 Description of impact of acute illness on blood glucose level | 1 | 2 | 3 | 4 | 5 | NA |
| 182026 Description of the correct procedure for blood glucose testing | 1 | 2 | 3 | 4 | 5 | NA |
| 182015 Description of actions to be taken in relation to blood glucose levels | 1 | 2 | 3 | 4 | 5 | NA |
| 182016 Description of prescribed insulin regimen | 1 | 2 | 3 | 4 | 5 | NA |
| 182027 Description of proper technique to draw up and administer insulin | 1 | 2 | 3 | 4 | 5 | NA |
| 182018 Description of plan for rotation of injection sites | 1 | 2 | 3 | 4 | 5 | NA |
| 182019 Description of onset, peak, and duration of prescribed insulin(s) | 1 | 2 | 3 | 4 | 5 | NA |
| 182020 Description of prescribed regimen for oral agents | 1 | 2 | 3 | 4 | 5 | NA |
| 182021 Description of when to seek help from health care professional | 1 | 2 | 3 | 4 | 5 | NA |
| 182028 Description of correct procedure for urine ketone testing | 1 | 2 | 3 | 4 | 5 | NA |

K

*Continued*

| Knowledge: Diabetes Management—cont'd | | None | Limited | Moderate | Substantial | Extensive | |
|---|---|---|---|---|---|---|---|
| 182029 | Description of importance for dilated eye exam and vision testing by an ophthalmologist | 1 | 2 | 3 | 4 | 5 | NA |
| 182023 | Description of preventive foot care practices | 1 | 2 | 3 | 4 | 5 | NA |
| 182024 | Description of benefits of disease management | 1 | 2 | 3 | 4 | 5 | NA |

*2nd edition 2000; Revised 3rd edition*

### Outcome Content References:

Anderson, S. (1994). 7 Caretips for managing patients with diabetes. *American Journal of Nursing, 94*(9), 36-38.

Brody, G. (1992). Diabetic ketoacidosis and hyperosmolar hyperglycemic nonketotic coma. *Topics of Emergency Medicine, 14*(1), 12-22.

Cameron, B.L. (2002). Making diabetes management routine: How often do you and your patients screen for complications? *American Journal of Nursing, 102*(2), 26-33.

Carlson, M. (1994). Diabetic emergencies: A clinical review. *Journal of the American Academy of Physician Assistants, 7*(2), 79-86.

Clark, A. (1994). Complications and management of diabetes. *Critical Care Nursing of North America, 6*(4), 723-733.

Franz, M.J. (Ed.) (2000). *A core curriculum for diabetes education* (4th ed.). Chicago, IL: American Association of Diabetes Educators.

Jones, T. (1994). From diabetic ketoacidosis to hyperglycemic hyperosmolar nonketotic syndrome. *Critical Care Nursing Clinics of North America, 6*(4), 703-721.

Loewen, S., & Haas, L. (1991). Complications of diabetes: Acute and chronic. *Nurse Practitioner Forum, 2*(3), 181-187.

Norton, R. (1995). The right mix of diet and exercise, *RN, 58*(4), 20-24.

Peragallo-Dittko, V. (1995). Diabetes 2000: Acute complications. *RN, 58*(8), 36-41.

Reising, D.L. (1995). Acute hypoglycemia: Keeping the bottom from falling out. *Nursing, 25*(2), 41-48.

**K**

# *Knowledge: Diet (1802)*

Domain-Health Knowledge & Behavior (IV)

Class-Health Knowledge (S)

Scale(s)-None to Extensive (i)

Care Recipient:

Data Source:

**Definition:** Extent of understanding conveyed about recommended diet

OUTCOME TARGET RATING:    Maintain at_____    Increase to_____

| Knowledge: Diet<br>Overall Rating | None<br>1 | Limited<br>2 | Moderate<br>3 | Substantial<br>4 | Extensive<br>5 | |
|---|---|---|---|---|---|---|

INDICATORS:

| | | | | | | |
|---|---|---|---|---|---|---|
| 180201 | Description of diet | 1 | 2 | 3 | 4 | 5 | NA |
| 180202 | Description of rationale for diet | 1 | 2 | 3 | 4 | 5 | NA |
| 180203 | Description of advantages of diet | 1 | 2 | 3 | 4 | 5 | NA |
| 180204 | Description of dietary goals | 1 | 2 | 3 | 4 | 5 | NA |
| 180205 | Description of relationships among<br>diet, exercise, and body weight | 1 | 2 | 3 | 4 | 5 | NA |
| 180206 | Description of foods allowed in diet | 1 | 2 | 3 | 4 | 5 | NA |
| 180207 | Description of foods to be avoided | 1 | 2 | 3 | 4 | 5 | NA |
| 180208 | Description of how to interpret food<br>labels | 1 | 2 | 3 | 4 | 5 | NA |
| 180209 | Description of guidelines for food<br>preparation | 1 | 2 | 3 | 4 | 5 | NA |
| 180210 | Description of how to select foods | 1 | 2 | 3 | 4 | 5 | NA |
| 180211 | Description of menu planning using<br>dietary guidelines | 1 | 2 | 3 | 4 | 5 | NA |
| 180212 | Description of strategies to change<br>dietary habits | 1 | 2 | 3 | 4 | 5 | NA |
| 180213 | Description of diet plans for social<br>situations | 1 | 2 | 3 | 4 | 5 | NA |
| 180217 | Description of self-monitoring<br>activities | 1 | 2 | 3 | 4 | 5 | NA |
| 180215 | Description of potential for food and<br>medication interaction | 1 | 2 | 3 | 4 | 5 | NA |

Specify diet_____

*1st edition 1997; Revised 3rd edition*

Outcome Content References:

Bloomgarden, Z.T., Karmally, W., Metzger, J., Brothers, M., Nechemias, C., Bookman, J., Faierman, D., Ginsberg-Fellner, F., Rayfield, E., & Brown, W.V. (1987). Randomized controlled trial of diabetic patient education: Improved knowledge without improved metabolic status. *Diabetes Care, 10*(3), 263-272.

Bushnell, F. (1992). Self-care teaching for congestive heart failure patients. *Journal of Gerontological Nursing, 18*(10), 27-32.

Conn, V.S., Armer, J.M., & Hayes, K.S. (2001). Knowledge deficit. In M. Maas, K. Buckwalter, M. Hardy, T. Tripp-Reimer, M. Titler, & J. Specht (Eds.), *Nursing care of older adults: Diagnoses, outcomes & interventions* (pp. 503-515). St. Louis: Mosby.

Devins, G.M., Binik, Y.M., Mandin, H., Litourneau, P.K., Hollomby, D.J., Barre, P.E., & Prichard, S. (1990). The Kidney Disease Questionnaire: A test for measuring patient knowledge about end-stage renal disease. *Journal of Clinical Epidemiology, 43*(3), 297-307.

Garrard, J., Joynes, J.O., Mullen, L., McNeil, L., Mensing, C., Feste, C., & Etzwiler, D.D. (1987). Psychometric study of patient knowledge test. *Diabetes Care, 10*(4), 500-509.

Gilden, J.L., Hendryx, M., Casia, C., & Singh, S.P. (1989). The effectiveness of diabetes education programs for older patients and their spouses. *Journal of American Geriatrics Society, 37*(11), 1023-1030.

Mazzuca, S.A., Moorman, N.H., Wheeler, M.L., Norton, J.A., Fineberg, N.S., Vinicor, F., Cohen, S.J., & Clark, C.M. (1986). The diabetes education study: A controlled trial of the effects of diabetes patient education. *Diabetes Care, 9*(1), 1-10.

Redman, B. (1993). Knowledge deficit (specify). In J.M. Thompson, G.K. McFarland, J.E. Hirsch, & S.M. Tucker (Eds.), *Mosby's clinical nursing* (3rd ed., pp. 1548-1552). St. Louis: Mosby.

Scherer, Y.K., Janelli, L.M., & Schmieder, L.E. (1992). A time-series perspective of effectiveness of a health teaching program on chronic obstructive pulmonary disease. *Journal of Healthcare Education and Training, 6*(3), 7-13.

Smith, M.M., Hicks, V.L., & Heyward, V.H. (1991). Coronary disease knowledge test: Developing a valid and reliable tool. *Nurse Practitioner, 16*(4), 28, 31, 35-38.

# Knowledge: Disease Process (1803)

*Domain-Health Knowledge & Behavior (IV)*

*Class-Health Knowledge (S)*

*Scale(s)-None to Extensive (i)*

*Care Recipient:*

*Data Source:*

**Definition**: Extent of understanding conveyed about a specific disease process

OUTCOME TARGET RATING:    Maintain at_____    Increase to_____

| Knowledge: Disease Process<br>Overall Rating | None<br>1 | Limited<br>2 | Moderate<br>3 | Substantial<br>4 | Extensive<br>5 | |
|---|---|---|---|---|---|---|

INDICATORS:

| | | None<br>1 | Limited<br>2 | Moderate<br>3 | Substantial<br>4 | Extensive<br>5 | |
|---|---|---|---|---|---|---|---|
| 180302 | Description of specific disease process | 1 | 2 | 3 | 4 | 5 | NA |
| 180303 | Description of cause or contributing factors | 1 | 2 | 3 | 4 | 5 | NA |
| 180304 | Description of risk factors | 1 | 2 | 3 | 4 | 5 | NA |
| 180305 | Description of effects of disease | 1 | 2 | 3 | 4 | 5 | NA |
| 180306 | Description of signs and symptoms | 1 | 2 | 3 | 4 | 5 | NA |
| 180307 | Description of usual disease course | 1 | 2 | 3 | 4 | 5 | NA |
| 180308 | Description of measures to minimize disease progression | 1 | 2 | 3 | 4 | 5 | NA |
| 180309 | Description of complications | 1 | 2 | 3 | 4 | 5 | NA |
| 180310 | Description of signs and symptoms of complications | 1 | 2 | 3 | 4 | 5 | NA |
| 180311 | Description of precautions to prevent complications | 1 | 2 | 3 | 4 | 5 | NA |

Specify disease_____

*1st edition 1997; Revised 3rd edition*

Outcome Content References:

Bushnell, F. (1992). Self-care teaching for congestive heart failure patients. *Journal of Gerontological Nursing, 18*(10), 27-32.

Conn, V.S., Armer, J.M., & Hayes, K.S. (2001). Knowledge deficit. In M. Maas, K. Buckwalter, M. Hardy, T. Tripp-Reimer, M. Titler, & J. Specht (Eds.), *Nursing care of older adults: Diagnoses, outcomes & interventions* (pp. 503-515). St. Louis: Mosby.

Devins, G.M., Binik, Y.M., Mandin, H., Litourneau, P.K., Hollomby, D.J., Barre, P.E., & Prichard, S. (1990). The Kidney Disease Questionnaire: A test for measuring patient knowledge about end-stage renal disease. *Journal of Clinical Epidemiology, 43*(3), 297-307.

Garrard, J., Joynes, J.O., Mullen, L., McNeil, L., Mensing, C., Feste, C., & Etzwiler, D.D. (1987). Psychometric study of patient knowledge test. *Diabetes Care, 10*(4), 500-509.

Gilden, J.L., Hendryx, M., Casia, C., & Singh, S.P. (1989). The effectiveness of diabetes education programs for older patients and their spouses. *Journal of American Geriatrics Society, 37*(11), 1023-1030.

Mazzuca, S.A., Moorman, N.H., Wheeler, M.L., Norton, J.A., Fineberg, N.S., Vinicor, F., Cohen, S.J., & Clark, C.M. (1986). The diabetes education study: A controlled trial of the effects of diabetes patient education. *Diabetes Care, 9*(1), 1-10.

Redman, B. (1993). Knowledge deficit (specify). In J.M. Thompson, G.K. McFarland, J.E. Hirsch, & S.M. Tucker (Eds.), *Mosby's clinical nursing* (3rd ed., pp. 1548-1552). St. Louis: Mosby.

Scherer, Y.K., Janelli, L.M., & Schmieder, L.E. (1992). A time-series perspective of effectiveness of a health teaching program on chronic obstructive pulmonary disease. *Journal of Healthcare Education and Training, 6*(3), 7-13.

Smith, M.M., Hicks, V.L., & Heyward, V.H. (1991). Coronary Disease Knowledge Test: Developing a valid and reliable tool. *Nurse Practitioner, 16*(4), 28, 31, 35-38.

Wright, L.K. (2001). Sexual dysfunction. In M. Maas, K. Buckwalter, M. Hardy, T. Tripp-Reimer, M. Titler, & J. Specht (Eds.), *Nursing care of older adults: Diagnoses, outcomes & interventions* (pp. 733-749). St. Louis: Mosby.

# Knowledge: Energy Conservation (1804)

Domain-Health Knowledge & Behavior (IV)

Class-Health Knowledge (S)

Scale(s)-None to Extensive (i)

Care Recipient:

Data Source:

**Definition:** Extent of understanding conveyed about energy conservation techniques

OUTCOME TARGET RATING:        Maintain at_____        Increase to_____

| Knowledge: Energy Conservation Overall Rating | None 1 | Limited 2 | Moderate 3 | Substantial 4 | Extensive 5 | |
|---|---|---|---|---|---|---|
| INDICATORS: | | | | | | |
| 180401 Description of recommended activity level | 1 | 2 | 3 | 4 | 5 | NA |
| 180402 Description of activity restrictions | 1 | 2 | 3 | 4 | 5 | NA |
| 180403 Description of appropriate activities | 1 | 2 | 3 | 4 | 5 | NA |
| 180404 Description of factors that increase energy expenditure | 1 | 2 | 3 | 4 | 5 | NA |
| 180405 Description of factors that decrease energy expenditure | 1 | 2 | 3 | 4 | 5 | NA |
| 180406 Description of energy limitations | 1 | 2 | 3 | 4 | 5 | NA |
| 180407 Description of how to balance rest and activity | 1 | 2 | 3 | 4 | 5 | NA |
| 180416 Description of methods to conserve energy | 1 | 2 | 3 | 4 | 5 | NA |
| 180417 Description of pulse taking technique | 1 | 2 | 3 | 4 | 5 | NA |
| 180418 Description of controlled breathing | 1 | 2 | 3 | 4 | 5 | NA |
| 180419 Description of proper body mechanics | 1 | 2 | 3 | 4 | 5 | NA |
| 180420 Description of work simplification techniques | 1 | 2 | 3 | 4 | 5 | NA |
| 180421 Description of how to use assistive devices | 1 | 2 | 3 | 4 | 5 | NA |

*1st edition 1997; Revised 3rd edition*

## Outcome Content References:

Conn, V.S., Armer, J.M., & Hayes, K.S. (2001). Knowledge deficit. In M. Maas, K. Buckwalter, M. Hardy, T. Tripp-Reimer, M. Titler, & J. Specht (Eds.), *Nursing care of older adults: Diagnoses, outcomes & interventions* (pp. 503-515). St. Louis: Mosby.

Hart, L.K., & Freel, M.I. (1982). Fatigue. In C.M. Norris (Ed.), *Concept clarification in nursing* (pp. 251-261). Rockville, MD: Aspen.

Lubkin, I.M. (2002). *Chronic illness: Impact and interventions* (5th ed.). Boston: Jones & Bartlett.

McFarlane, E.A. (1993). Activity intolerance. In J.M. Thompson, G.K. McFarland, J.E. Hirsch, & S.M. Tucker (Eds.), *Clinical nursing* (3rd ed., pp. 1498-1500). St. Louis: Mosby.

McFarlane, E.A. (1993). High risk for activity intolerance. In J.M. Thompson, G.K. McFarland, J.E. Hirsch, & S.M. Tucker (Eds.), *Clinical nursing* (3rd ed., pp. 1497-1498). St. Louis: Mosby.

Mock, V.L. (1993). Fatigue. In J.M. Thompson, G.K. McFarland, J.E. Hirsch, & S.M. Tucker (Eds.), *Clinical nursing* (3rd ed., pp. 1504-1506). St. Louis: Mosby.

Morris, M.L. (1982). Tiredness and fatigue. In C.M. Norris (Ed.), *Concept clarification in nursing* (pp. 263-275). Rockville, MD: Aspen.

K

# Knowledge: Fall Prevention (1828)

*Domain-Health Knowledge & Behavior (IV)*

*Class-Health Knowledge (S)*

*Scale(s)-None to Extensive (i)*

*Care Recipient:*

*Data Source:*

**Definition:** Extent of understanding conveyed about prevention of falls

OUTCOME TARGET RATING:      Maintain at_____   Increase to_____

| Knowledge: Fall Prevention Overall Rating | None 1 | Limited 2 | Moderate 3 | Substantial 4 | Extensive 5 | |
|---|---|---|---|---|---|---|
| **INDICATORS:** | | | | | | |
| 182801  Description of correct use of assistive devices | 1 | 2 | 3 | 4 | 5 | NA |
| 182802  Description of use and purpose of safety devices | 1 | 2 | 3 | 4 | 5 | NA |
| 182803  Description of appropriate footwear | 1 | 2 | 3 | 4 | 5 | NA |
| 182804  Description of use of grab bars | 1 | 2 | 3 | 4 | 5 | NA |
| 182805  Description of correct use of child gates | | | | | | |
| 182806  Description of correct use of window guards | 1 | 2 | 3 | 4 | 5 | NA |
| 182807  Description of correct use of environmental lighting | 1 | 2 | 3 | 4 | 5 | NA |
| 182808  Description of when to ask for personal assistance | 1 | 2 | 3 | 4 | 5 | NA |
| 182809  Description of use of safe transfer procedure | 1 | 2 | 3 | 4 | 5 | NA |
| 182810  Description of reason for restraints | 1 | 2 | 3 | 4 | 5 | NA |
| 182811  Description of exercises to reduce risk of falling | 1 | 2 | 3 | 4 | 5 | NA |
| 182812  Description of medications that increase risk of falling | 1 | 2 | 3 | 4 | 5 | NA |
| 182813  Description of chronic condition that increase risk of falling | 1 | 2 | 3 | 4 | 5 | NA |
| 182814  Description of acute illnesses that increase risk of falling | 1 | 2 | 3 | 4 | 5 | NA |
| 182815  Description of blood pressure changes that increase risk of falling | 1 | 2 | 3 | 4 | 5 | NA |
| 182816  Description of non-prescription drugs that increase risk of falling | 1 | 2 | 3 | 4 | 5 | NA |
| 182817  Description of how to safely ambulate | 1 | 2 | 3 | 4 | 5 | NA |
| 182818  Description of need to maintain clear walkway | 1 | 2 | 3 | 4 | 5 | NA |
| 182819  Description of appropriate use of stools/ladders | 1 | 2 | 3 | 4 | 5 | NA |
| 182820  Description of use of tub/ shower mats | 1 | 2 | 3 | 4 | 5 | NA |
| 182821  Description of how to keep floor surfaces safe | 1 | 2 | 3 | 4 | 5 | NA |

*3rd edition*

Outcome Content References:

Bexon, J., Echevarria, K.H., & Smith, G.B. (1999). Nursing outcome indicator: Preventing falls for elderly people. *Outcomes Management for Nursing Practice, 3*(3), 112-116.

Edwards, B.J., & Lee, S. (1998). Gait disorders and falls in a retirement home: A pilot study. *Annals of Long-Term Care, 6*(4), 140-143.

Fleck, M.M., & Forrester, D.A. (2001). The efficacy of an educational program to improve direct caregiver knowledge regarding fall prevention. *Journal for Nurses in Staff Development, 17*(1), 27-33.

Hendrich, A.L. (1996). *Falls, immobility, and restraints: A resource manual.* St. Louis: Mosby.

Malmivaara, A., Heliovaara, M., Knekt, P., Reunanen, A., & Aromaa, A. (1993). Risk factors for injurious falls leading to hospitalization or death in a cohort of 19,500 adults. *American Journal of Epidemiology, 138*(6), 384-394.

Patient information. Decreasing your risks of falls. *American Family Physician, 56*(7), 1823.

Schoenfelder, D.P., Crowell, C.M., & The Nursing Diagnosis Extension and Classification Research Team (1999). From risk for trauma to unintentional injury risk: Falls—a concept analysis. *Nursing Diagnoses, 10*(4), 149-157.

Stevens, J.A., & Olson, S. (2000). Reducing falls and resulting hip fractures among older women. *Morbidity & Mortality Weekly Report, 49*(RR-2), 1-12.

Wortel, E., & de Geus, G.H. (1993). Prevention of home related injuries of pre-school children: Safety measures taken by mothers. *Health Education Research, 8*(2), 217-231.

K

# Knowledge: Fertility Promotion (1816)

*Domain-Health Knowledge & Behavior (IV)*

*Class-Health Knowledge (S)*

*Scale(s)-None to Extensive (i)*

*Care Recipient:*

*Data Source:*

---

**Definition**: Extent of understanding conveyed about fertility testing and the conditions that affect conception

---

OUTCOME TARGET RATING:     Maintain at_____     Increase to_____

| Knowledge: Fertility Promotion Overall Rating | None 1 | Limited 2 | Moderate 3 | Substantial 4 | Extensive 5 | |
|---|---|---|---|---|---|---|
| **INDICATORS:** | | | | | | |
| 181601  Description of effect of age | 1 | 2 | 3 | 4 | 5 | NA |
| 181602  Description of effect of coital frequency | 1 | 2 | 3 | 4 | 5 | NA |
| 181603  Description of effect of nutrition | 1 | 2 | 3 | 4 | 5 | NA |
| 181604  Description of hazards of weight loss | 1 | 2 | 3 | 4 | 5 | NA |
| 181606  Description of effect of heat on sperm count | 1 | 2 | 3 | 4 | 5 | NA |
| 181607  Description of effect of tight clothes on sperm count | 1 | 2 | 3 | 4 | 5 | NA |
| 181608  Description of effect of physical anomalies | 1 | 2 | 3 | 4 | 5 | NA |
| 181609  Description of effect of pelvic surgery | 1 | 2 | 3 | 4 | 5 | NA |
| 181610  Description of effect of pelvic infections | 1 | 2 | 3 | 4 | 5 | NA |
| 181611  Description of influence of vaginal/ uterine environment | 1 | 2 | 3 | 4 | 5 | NA |
| 181612  Description of the effect of hormone levels | 1 | 2 | 3 | 4 | 5 | NA |
| 181613  Description of the effect of thyroid function | 1 | 2 | 3 | 4 | 5 | NA |
| 181614  Description of use of basal body temperature to predict ovulation | 1 | 2 | 3 | 4 | 5 | NA |
| 181615  Description of symptothermal method | 1 | 2 | 3 | 4 | 5 | NA |
| 181616  Description of ultrasonography | 1 | 2 | 3 | 4 | 5 | NA |
| 181617  Description of influence of semen characteristics | 1 | 2 | 3 | 4 | 5 | NA |
| 181618  Description of influence of sperm count | 1 | 2 | 3 | 4 | 5 | NA |
| 181619  Description of postcoital test | 1 | 2 | 3 | 4 | 5 | NA |
| 181620  Description of fertility monitoring devices | 1 | 2 | 3 | 4 | 5 | NA |
| 181621  Description of options to reverse sterilization | 1 | 2 | 3 | 4 | 5 | NA |
| 181622  Description of methods for sample collection | 1 | 2 | 3 | 4 | 5 | NA |

*2nd edition 2000; Revised 3rd edition*

---

Outcome Content References:

Fehring, R.J. (1991). New technology in natural family planning. *Journal of Obstetric, Gynecologic, and Neonatal Nursing, 20*(3), 199-205.

Grodstein, F., Goldman, M.B., & Cramer, D.W. (1994). Infertility in women and moderate alcohol use. *American Journal of Public Health, 84*(9), 1429-1432.

Halman, L.J., Abbey, A., & Andrews, F.M. (1992). Attitudes about infertility interventions among fertile and infertile couples. *American Journal of Public Health, 82*(2), 191-194.

Rudy, E.B., & Estok, P. (1992). Professional and lay interrater reliability of urinary luteinizing hormone surges measured by OvuQuick test. *Journal of Obstetric, Gynecologic, and Neonatal Nursing, 21*(5), 407-410.

Shane, J.M. (1993). Evaluation and treatment of infertility. *Clinical Symposia, 45*(2), 2-32.

Toner, J.P., & Flood, J.T. (1993). Fertility after the age of 40. *Obstetrics and Gynecology Clinics of North America, 20*(2), 261-272.

**K**

# Knowledge: Health Behavior (1805)

*Domain-Health Knowledge & Behavior (IV)*

*Class-Health Knowledge (S)*

*Scale(s)-None to Extensive (i)*

*Care Recipient:*

*Data Source:*

**Definition:** Extent of understanding conveyed about the promotion and protection of health

OUTCOME TARGET RATING:     Maintain at_____     Increase to_____

| Knowledge: Health Behavior Overall Rating | None 1 | Limited 2 | Moderate 3 | Substantial 4 | Extensive 5 | |
|---|---|---|---|---|---|---|
| **INDICATORS:** | | | | | | |
| 180501 Description of healthy nutritional practices | 1 | 2 | 3 | 4 | 5 | NA |
| 180502 Description of benefits of activity and exercise | 1 | 2 | 3 | 4 | 5 | NA |
| 180503 Description of effective stress management techniques | 1 | 2 | 3 | 4 | 5 | NA |
| 180504 Description of effective sleep-wake patterns | 1 | 2 | 3 | 4 | 5 | NA |
| 180505 Description of methods of family planning | 1 | 2 | 3 | 4 | 5 | NA |
| 180506 Description of adverse health effects of tobacco use | 1 | 2 | 3 | 4 | 5 | NA |
| 180507 Description of adverse health effects of alcohol misuse | 1 | 2 | 3 | 4 | 5 | NA |
| 180508 Description of adverse health effects of recreational drug use | 1 | 2 | 3 | 4 | 5 | NA |
| 180509 Description of safe use of prescription drugs | 1 | 2 | 3 | 4 | 5 | NA |
| 180510 Description of safe use of non-prescription drugs | 1 | 2 | 3 | 4 | 5 | NA |
| 180511 Description of effect of caffeine use | 1 | 2 | 3 | 4 | 5 | NA |
| 180512 Description of measures to reduce the risk of accidental injury | 1 | 2 | 3 | 4 | 5 | NA |
| 180513 Description of measures to avoid exposure to environmental hazards | 1 | 2 | 3 | 4 | 5 | NA |
| 180514 Description of measures to prevent transmission of infectious disease | 1 | 2 | 3 | 4 | 5 | NA |
| 180515 Description of health promotion and protection services | 1 | 2 | 3 | 4 | 5 | NA |
| 180516 Description of appropriate use of self-screening | 1 | 2 | 3 | 4 | 5 | NA |

*1st edition 1997; Revised 3rd edition (formerly Knowledge: Health Behaviors)*

Outcome Content References:

Conn, V.S., Armer, J.M., & Hayes, K.S. (2001). Knowledge deficit. In M. Maas, K. Buckwalter, M. Hardy, T. Tripp-Reimer, M. Titler, & J. Specht (Eds.), *Nursing care of older adults: Diagnoses, outcomes & interventions* (pp. 503-515). St. Louis: Mosby.

Simons-Morton, D.G., Mullen, P.D., Mains, D.A., Tabak, E.R., & Green, L.W. (1992). Characteristics of controlled studies of patient education and counseling for preventive health behaviors. *Patient Education and Counseling, 19*(2), 174-204.

Spellbring, A.M. (1991). Nursing's role in health promotion. *Nursing Clinics of North America, 16*(4), 805-814.

Tanner, E.K.W. (1991). Assessment of a health-promotive lifestyle. *Nursing Clinics of North America, 26*(4), 845-854.

U.S. Department of Health and Human Services. (1990). *Healthy people 2000. National health promotion and disease prevention objectives.* Washington, DC: Government Printing Office.

U.S. Department of Health and Human Services. (1998). *Clinician's handbook of preventive services: Put prevention into practice.* (2nd ed.) Washington, DC: Government Printing Office.

# Knowledge: Health Promotion (1823)

*Domain-Health Knowledge & Behavior (IV)*

*Class-Health Knowledge (S)*

*Scale(s)-None to Extensive (i)*

*Care Recipient:*

*Data Source:*

**Definition:** Extent of understanding conveyed about information needed to obtain and maintain optimal health

OUTCOME TARGET RATING:    Maintain at_____    Increase to_____

| Knowledge: Health Promotion Overall Rating | None 1 | Limited 2 | Moderate 3 | Substantial 4 | Extensive 5 | |
|---|---|---|---|---|---|---|
| INDICATORS: | | | | | | |
| 182308  Description of behaviors that promote health | 1 | 2 | 3 | 4 | 5 | NA |
| 182309  Description of effective coping strategies for stress | 1 | 2 | 3 | 4 | 5 | NA |
| 182310  Description of recommended health screening | 1 | 2 | 3 | 4 | 5 | NA |
| 182311  Description of recommended immunizations | 1 | 2 | 3 | 4 | 5 | NA |
| 182312  Description of relevant health care resources | 1 | 2 | 3 | 4 | 5 | NA |
| 182313  Description of prevention and control of infection | 1 | 2 | 3 | 4 | 5 | NA |
| 182314  Description of behaviors to prevent unintentional injuries | 1 | 2 | 3 | 4 | 5 | NA |
| 182315  Description of behaviors to protect skin from sun exposure | 1 | 2 | 3 | 4 | 5 | NA |
| 182316  Description of managing medication use safely | 1 | 2 | 3 | 4 | 5 | NA |
| 182317  Description of adverse effects of alcohol, tobacco, and drug use | 1 | 2 | 3 | 4 | 5 | NA |
| 182318  Description of a healthy diet | 1 | 2 | 3 | 4 | 5 | NA |
| 182319  Description of effective weight control measures | 1 | 2 | 3 | 4 | 5 | |
| 182320  Description of effective exercise program | 1 | 2 | 3 | 4 | 5 | NA |

*2nd edition 2000; Revised 3rd edition*

Outcome Content References:

This is a general outcome that combines the following: Knowledge: Health Behaviors, Knowledge: Health Resources, Knowledge: Infection Control, Knowledge: Personal Safety, Knowledge: Substance Use Control, Knowledge: Diet.

K

# Knowledge: Health Resources (1806)

*Domain-Health Knowledge & Behavior (IV)*

*Class-Health Knowledge (S)*

*Scale(s)-None to Extensive (i)*

*Care Recipient:*

*Data Source:*

---

**Definition:** Extent of understanding conveyed about relevant health care resources

OUTCOME TARGET RATING:   Maintain at_____   Increase to_____

| Knowledge: Health Resources Overall Rating | None 1 | Limited 2 | Moderate 3 | Substantial 4 | Extensive 5 | |
|---|---|---|---|---|---|---|
| **INDICATORS:** | | | | | | |
| 180601 Description of resources that enhance health | 1 | 2 | 3 | 4 | 5 | NA |
| 180602 Description of when to contact a health care professional | 1 | 2 | 3 | 4 | 5 | NA |
| 180603 Description of emergency measures | 1 | 2 | 3 | 4 | 5 | NA |
| 180604 Description of resources for emergency care | 1 | 2 | 3 | 4 | 5 | NA |
| 180605 Description of need for follow-up care | 1 | 2 | 3 | 4 | 5 | NA |
| 180606 Description of plan for follow-up care | 1 | 2 | 3 | 4 | 5 | NA |
| 180607 Description of community resources available for assistance | 1 | 2 | 3 | 4 | 5 | NA |
| 180608 Description of how to connect with needed services | 1 | 2 | 3 | 4 | 5 | NA |

*1st edition 1997; Revised 3rd edition*

Outcome Content References:

Bull, M.J. (1994). Patients' and professionals' perceptions of quality in discharge planning. *Journal of Nursing Care Quality, 8*(2), 47-61.

Conn, V.S., Armer, J.M., & Hayes, K.S. (2001). Knowledge deficit. In M. Maas, K. Buckwalter, M. Hardy, T. Tripp-Reimer, M. Titler, & J. Specht (Eds.), *Nursing care of older adults: Diagnoses, outcomes & interventions* (pp. 503-515). St. Louis: Mosby.

Redman, B. (1993). Knowledge deficit (specify). In J.M. Thompson, G.K. McFarland, J.E. Hirsch, & S.M. Tucker (Eds.), *Mosby's clinical nursing* (3rd ed., pp. 1548-1552). St. Louis: Mosby.

Wyness, M.A. (1990). Evaluation of an educational program for patients taking warfarin. *Journal of Advanced Nursing, 15*(9), 1052-1063.

# Knowledge: Illness Care (1824)

Domain-Health Knowledge & Behavior (IV)

Class-Health Knowledge (S)

Scale(s)-None to Extensive (i)

Care Recipient:

Data Source:

**Definition:** Extent of understanding conveyed about illness-related information needed to achieve and maintain optimal health

OUTCOME TARGET RATING:　　Maintain at_____　　Increase to_____

| Knowledge: Illness Care Overall Rating | None 1 | Limited 2 | Moderate 3 | Substantial 4 | Extensive 5 | |
|---|---|---|---|---|---|---|
| **INDICATORS:** | | | | | | |
| 182401　Description of recommended diet | 1 | 2 | 3 | 4 | 5 | NA |
| 182402　Description of specific disease process | 1 | 2 | 3 | 4 | 5 | NA |
| 182403　Description of energy conservation techniques | 1 | 2 | 3 | 4 | 5 | NA |
| 182404　Description of prevention and control of infection | 1 | 2 | 3 | 4 | 5 | NA |
| 182405　Description of safe use of medication | 1 | 2 | 3 | 4 | 5 | NA |
| 182406　Description of prescribed activity and exercise | 1 | 2 | 3 | 4 | 5 | NA |
| 182407　Description of treatment procedure(s) | 1 | 2 | 3 | 4 | 5 | NA |
| 182408　Description of treatment regimen | 1 | 2 | 3 | 4 | 5 | NA |
| 182409　Description of relevant healthcare resources | 1 | 2 | 3 | 4 | 5 | NA |

*2nd edition 2000; Revised 3rd edition*

## Outcome Content References:

This is a general outcome that combines the following: Knowledge: Diet, Knowledge: Disease Process, Knowledge: Energy Conservation, Knowledge: Infection Control, Knowledge: Medication, Knowledge: Prescribed Activity, Knowledge: Treatment Procedure(s), Knowledge: Treatment Regimen, Knowledge: Health Resources.

K

# Knowledge: Infant Care (1819)

*Domain-Health Knowledge & Behavior (IV)*

*Class-Health Knowledge (S)*

*Scale(s)-None to Extensive (i)*

*Care Recipient:*

*Data Source:*

---

**Definition:** Extent of understanding conveyed about caring for a baby from birth to 1st birthday

---

OUTCOME TARGET RATING:     Maintain at_____     Increase to_____

| Knowledge: Infant Care Overall Rating | None 1 | Limited 2 | Moderate 3 | Substantial 4 | Extensive 5 | |
|---|---|---|---|---|---|---|
| INDICATORS: | | | | | | |
| 181901  Description of normal infant characteristics | 1 | 2 | 3 | 4 | 5 | NA |
| 181902  Description of normal infant development | 1 | 2 | 3 | 4 | 5 | NA |
| 181903  Description of proper holding of the infant | 1 | 2 | 3 | 4 | 5 | NA |
| 181904  Description of proper positioning of the infant | 1 | 2 | 3 | 4 | 5 | NA |
| 181905  Description of infant safety practices | 1 | 2 | 3 | 4 | 5 | NA |
| 181906  Description of swaddling | 1 | 2 | 3 | 4 | 5 | NA |
| 181928  Description of infant cardiopulmonary resuscitation techniques | 1 | 2 | 3 | 4 | 5 | NA |
| 181908  Description of nutritive versus nonnutritive suck | 1 | 2 | 3 | 4 | 5 | NA |
| 181909  Description of pros and cons of infant feeding choices | 1 | 2 | 3 | 4 | 5 | NA |
| 181910  Description of infant feeding technique | 1 | 2 | 3 | 4 | 5 | NA |
| 181911  Description of signs of dehydration | 1 | 2 | 3 | 4 | 5 | NA |
| 181912  Description of signs of jaundice | 1 | 2 | 3 | 4 | 5 | NA |
| 181913  Description of bathing the infant | 1 | 2 | 3 | 4 | 5 | NA |
| 181914  Description of umbilical cord care | 1 | 2 | 3 | 4 | 5 | NA |
| 181915  Description of infant diapering | 1 | 2 | 3 | 4 | 5 | NA |
| 181916  Description of proper clothing | 1 | 2 | 3 | 4 | 5 | NA |
| 181917  Description of body temperature taking techniques | 1 | 2 | 3 | 4 | 5 | NA |
| 181918  Description of infant sleep-wake patterns | 1 | 2 | 3 | 4 | 5 | NA |
| 181919  Description of infant communication | 1 | 2 | 3 | 4 | 5 | NA |
| 181920  Description of infant stimulation methods | 1 | 2 | 3 | 4 | 5 | NA |
| 181921  Description of infant relaxation techniques | 1 | 2 | 3 | 4 | 5 | NA |
| 181922  Description of family adjustments to addition of an infant | 1 | 2 | 3 | 4 | 5 | NA |
| 181923  Description of special care needs | 1 | 2 | 3 | 4 | 5 | NA |
| 181924  Description of considerations when choosing a childcare provider | 1 | 2 | 3 | 4 | 5 | NA |
| 181925  Description of community resources for infant care | 1 | 2 | 3 | 4 | 5 | NA |
| 181926  Description of precautions when pets are in the household | 1 | 2 | 3 | 4 | 5 | NA |

---

*2nd edition 2000; Revised 3rd edition*

Outcome Content References:

Association of Women's Health, Obstetricians and Neonatal Nurses. (1998). *Standards & guidelines for the professional nursing practice in the care of women and newborns* (5th ed.). Washington, DC: Author

Nichols, F., & Humenick, S. (2000). *Childbirth education: Practice, research and theory* (2nd ed.). Philadelphia: W.B. Saunders.

Reeder, S.J., Martin, L.L., & Koniak-Griffin, D. (1997). *Maternity nursing: Family, newborn, and women's health care* (18th ed.). Philadelphia: Lippincott.

K

# *Knowledge: Infection Control (1807)*

*Domain-Health Knowledge & Behavior (IV)*          Care Recipient:

*Class-Health Knowledge (S)*          Data Source:

*Scale(s)-None to Extensive (i)*

---

**Definition:** Extent of understanding conveyed about prevention and control of infection

OUTCOME TARGET RATING:     Maintain at_____     Increase to_____

| Knowledge: Infection Control Overall Rating | None 1 | Limited 2 | Moderate 3 | Substantial 4 | Extensive 5 | |
|---|---|---|---|---|---|---|
| **INDICATORS:** | | | | | | |
| 180701   Description of mode of transmission | 1 | 2 | 3 | 4 | 5 | NA |
| 180702   Description of factors contributing to transmission | 1 | 2 | 3 | 4 | 5 | NA |
| 180703   Description of practices that reduce transmission | 1 | 2 | 3 | 4 | 5 | NA |
| 180704   Description of signs and symptoms | 1 | 2 | 3 | 4 | 5 | NA |
| 180705   Description of screening procedures | 1 | 2 | 3 | 4 | 5 | NA |
| 180706   Description of monitoring procedures | 1 | 2 | 3 | 4 | 5 | NA |
| 180707   Description of activities to increase resistance to infection | 1 | 2 | 3 | 4 | 5 | NA |
| 180708   Description of treatment for diagnosed infection | 1 | 2 | 3 | 4 | 5 | NA |
| 180709   Description of follow-up for diagnosed infection | 1 | 2 | 3 | 4 | 5 | NA |

*1st edition 1997*

Outcome Content References:

Centers for Disease Control and Prevention, National Center for HIV, STD, and TB Prevention & Division of Tuberculosis Elimination. (2000). *Core curriculum on tuberculosis* (4th ed.). Atlanta, GA: U.S. Department of Health and Human Services.

Conn, V.S., Armer, J.M., & Hayes, K.S. (2001). Knowledge deficit. In M. Maas, K. Buckwalter, M. Hardy, T. Tripp-Reimer, M. Titler, & J. Specht (Eds.), *Nursing care of older adults: Diagnoses, outcomes & interventions* (pp. 503-515). St. Louis: Mosby.

National Center for Nursing Research. (1990). *HIV infection: Prevention and care*. Bethesda, MD: U.S. Department of Health and Human Services.

Rotheram-Borus, M.J., Reid, M.A., & Rosario, M. (1994). Factors mediating changes in sexual HIV risk behaviors among gay and bisexual male adolescents. *American Journal of Public Health, 84*(12), 1938-1946.

Simons-Morton, D.G., Mullen, P.D., Mains, D.A., Tabak, E.R., & Green, L.W. (1992). Characteristics of controlled studies of patient education and counseling for preventive health behaviors. *Patient Education and Counseling, 19*(2), 174-204.

Statton, P., & Alexander, N.J. (1993). Prevention of sexually transmitted infections: Physical and chemical barrier methods. *Infectious Disease Clinics of North America, 7*(4), 841-859.

Ungvarski, P.J., & Flaskerud, J.H. (1999). *HIV/AIDS: A guide to primary care management* (4th ed.). Philadelphia: W.B. Saunders.

# Knowledge: Labor & Delivery (1817)

Domain-Health Knowledge & Behavior (IV)

Class-Health Knowledge (S)

Scale(s)-None to Extensive (i)

Care Recipient:

Data Source:

**Definition:** Extent of understanding conveyed about labor and vaginal delivery

OUTCOME TARGET RATING:        Maintain at_____    Increase to_____

| Knowledge: Labor & Delivery Overall Rating | None 1 | Limited 2 | Moderate 3 | Substantial 4 | Extensive 5 | |
|---|---|---|---|---|---|---|
| **INDICATORS:** | | | | | | |
| 181701  Description of birthing options | 1 | 2 | 3 | 4 | 5 | NA |
| 181702  Description of role of the support person/coach | 1 | 2 | 3 | 4 | 5 | NA |
| 181703  Description of signs and symptoms of labor | 1 | 2 | 3 | 4 | 5 | NA |
| 181704  Description of stages and phases of labor and delivery | 1 | 2 | 3 | 4 | 5 | NA |
| 181705  Description of pain control methods | 1 | 2 | 3 | 4 | 5 | NA |
| 181706  Description of effective breathing techniques | 1 | 2 | 3 | 4 | 5 | NA |
| 181707  Description of effective relaxation techniques | 1 | 2 | 3 | 4 | 5 | NA |
| 181708  Description of effective positioning | 1 | 2 | 3 | 4 | 5 | NA |
| 181709  Description of potential medical procedures | 1 | 2 | 3 | 4 | 5 | NA |
| 181710  Description of potential complications | 1 | 2 | 3 | 4 | 5 | NA |
| 181711  Description of effective pushing techniques during delivery | 1 | 2 | 3 | 4 | 5 | NA |
| 181712  Description of delivery of the placenta | 1 | 2 | 3 | 4 | 5 | NA |

*2nd edition 2000; Revised 3rd edition*

Outcome Content References:

Association of Women's Health, Obstetricians and Neonatal Nurses. (1998). *Standards & guidelines for the professional nursing practice in the care of women and newborns* (5th ed.). Washington, DC: Author

Nichols, F., & Humenick, S. (2000). *Childbirth education: Practice, research and theory* (2nd ed.). Philadelphia: W.B. Saunders.

Reeder, S.J., Martin, L.L., & Koniak-Griffin, D. (1997). *Maternity nursing: Family, newborn, and women's health care* (18th ed.). Philadelphia: Lippincott.

K

# *Knowledge: Medication (1808)*

Domain-Health Knowledge & Behavior (IV)

Class-Health Knowledge (S)

Scale(s)-None to Extensive (i)

Care Recipient:

Data Source:

**Definition:** Extent of understanding conveyed about the safe use of medication

OUTCOME TARGET RATING:    Maintain at_____    Increase to_____

| Knowledge: Medication Overall Rating | None 1 | Limited 2 | Moderate 3 | Substantial 4 | Extensive 5 | |
|---|---|---|---|---|---|---|
| **INDICATORS:** | | | | | | |
| 180801 Recognition of need to inform health professional of all medications being taken | 1 | 2 | 3 | 4 | 5 | NA |
| 180802 Identification of correct name of medication(s) | 1 | 2 | 3 | 4 | 5 | NA |
| 180803 Description of appearance of medication(s) | 1 | 2 | 3 | 4 | 5 | NA |
| 180804 Description of actions of medication(s) | 1 | 2 | 3 | 4 | 5 | NA |
| 180805 Description of side effects of medication(s) | 1 | 2 | 3 | 4 | 5 | NA |
| 180806 Description of precautions for medication(s) | 1 | 2 | 3 | 4 | 5 | NA |
| 180807 Description of use of memory aids | 1 | 2 | 3 | 4 | 5 | NA |
| 180808 Description of potential adverse reactions when taking multiple medications | 1 | 2 | 3 | 4 | 5 | NA |
| 180809 Description of potential for interaction with other agents other then prescribed medications | 1 | 2 | 3 | 4 | 5 | NA |
| 180810 Description of correct administration of medication(s) | 1 | 2 | 3 | 4 | 5 | NA |
| 180811 Description of self-monitoring techniques | 1 | 2 | 3 | 4 | 5 | NA |
| 180812 Description of proper storage of medication(s) | 1 | 2 | 3 | 4 | 5 | NA |
| 180813 Description of proper care of administration devices | 1 | 2 | 3 | 4 | 5 | NA |
| 180814 Description of how to obtain required medication(s) and supplies | 1 | 2 | 3 | 4 | 5 | NA |
| 180815 Description of proper disposal of unused medications | 1 | 2 | 3 | 4 | 5 | NA |
| 180816 Description of needed laboratory tests | 1 | 2 | 3 | 4 | 5 | NA |
| 180817 Description of proper use of medication alert identification | 1 | 2 | 3 | 4 | 5 | NA |

Specify medication(s)_____

*1st edition 1997; Revised 3rd edition*

Outcome Content References:

Barry, K. (1993). Patient self-medication: An innovative approach to medication teaching. *Journal of Nursing Care Quality, 8*(1), 75-82.

Colley, C.A., & Lucas, L.M. (1993). Polypharmacy: The cure becomes the disease. *Journal of General Internal Medicine, 8*(5), 278-283.

Conn, V.S., Armer, J.M., & Hayes, K.S. (2001). Knowledge deficit. In M. Maas, K. Buckwalter, M. Hardy, T. Tripp-Reimer, M. Titler, & J. Specht (Eds.), *Nursing care of older adults: Diagnoses, outcomes & interventions* (pp. 503-515). St. Louis: Mosby.

Everitt, D.E., & Avorn, J. (1986). Drug prescribing for the elderly. *Archives of Internal Medicine, 146*(12), 2393-2396.

Kleoppel, J.W., & Henry, D.W. (1987). Teaching patients, families, and communities about their medications. In C.E. Smith (Ed.), *Patient education: Nurses in partnership with other health professionals,* (pp. 271-296). Philadelphia: W.B. Saunders.

Proos, M., Reiley, P., Eagan, J., Stengrevics, S., Castile, J., & Arian, D. (1992). A study of the effects of self-medication on patients' knowledge of and compliance with their medication regimen. *Journal of Nursing Care Quality,* (Special Report), 18-26.

Simons-Morton, D.G., Mullen, P.D., Mains, D.A., Tabak, E.R., & Green, L.W. (1992). Characteristics of controlled studies of patient education and counseling for preventive health behaviors. *Patient Education and Counseling, 19*(2), 174-204.

Togger, D.A., & Brenner, P.S. (2001). Metered dose inhalers. *American Journal of Nursing, 101*(10), 26-32, 38-39.

U.S. Department of Health and Human Services. (1990). *Healthy people 2000: National health promotion and disease prevention objectives.* Washington, DC: Government Printing Office.

U.S. Department of Health and Human Services. (1998). *Clinician's handbook of prevention services: Put prevention into practice.* (2nd ed.) Washington, DC: Government Printing Office.

Waddell, D.L., Hummel, M.E., & Sumners, A.D. (2001). Three herbs you should get to know. *American Journal of Nursing, 101*(4), 48-54.

Weitzel, E.A. (2001). Risk for poisoning: Drug toxicity. In M. Maas, K. Buckwalter, M. Hardy, T. Tripp-Reimer, M. Titler, & J. Specht (Eds.), *Nursing care of older adults: Diagnoses, outcomes & interventions* (pp. 34-46). St. Louis: Mosby.

K

# Knowledge: Ostomy Care (1829)

Domain-Health Knowledge & Behavior (IV)

Class-Health Knowledge (S)

Scale(s)-None to Extensive (i)

Care Recipient:

Data Source:

**Definition:** Extent of understanding conveyed about maintenance of an ostomy for elimination

OUTCOME TARGET RATING:    Maintain at_____    Increase to_____

| Knowledge: Ostomy Care Overall Rating | None 1 | Limited 2 | Moderate 3 | Substantial 4 | Extensive 5 | |
|---|---|---|---|---|---|---|
| 182901 | Description of functioning of ostomy | 1 | 2 | 3 | 4 | 5 | NA |
| 182902 | Description of purpose of ostomy | 1 | 2 | 3 | 4 | 5 | NA |
| 182903 | Description of skin care around ostomy | 1 | 2 | 3 | 4 | 5 | NA |
| 182904 | Description of irrigation technique | 1 | 2 | 3 | 4 | 5 | NA |
| 182905 | Description of how to measure stoma | 1 | 2 | 3 | 4 | 5 | NA |
| 182906 | Description of procedure to change/empty ostomy pouch | 1 | 2 | 3 | 4 | 5 | NA |
| 182907 | Description of complications related to stoma/skin | 1 | 2 | 3 | 4 | 5 | NA |
| 182908 | Description of schedule for changing ostomy pouch | 1 | 2 | 3 | 4 | 5 | NA |
| 182909 | Description of supplies needed to care for ostomy | 1 | 2 | 3 | 4 | 5 | NA |
| 182910 | Identification of flatus-producing foods | 1 | 2 | 3 | 4 | 5 | NA |
| 182911 | Description of diet modifications | 1 | 2 | 3 | 4 | 5 | NA |
| 182912 | Description of need for adequate fluid intake | 1 | 2 | 3 | 4 | 5 | NA |
| 182913 | Description of odor control mechanisms | 1 | 2 | 3 | 4 | 5 | NA |
| 182914 | Description of modifications on daily activities | 1 | 2 | 3 | 4 | 5 | NA |

*3rd edition*

Outcome Content References:

Bryant, D., & Fleischer, I. (2000). Changing an ostomy appliance. *Nursing, 30*(11), 51-53.

O'Shea, H.S. (2001). Teaching the adult ostomy patient. *Journal of Wound, Ostomy, and Continence Nursing, 28*(1), 47-54.

Thompson, J. (2000). A practical ostomy guide. *RN, 63*(11), 61-68.

# Knowledge: Parenting (1826)

Domain-Health Knowledge & Behavior (IV)

Class-Health Knowledge (S)

Scale(s)-None to Extensive (i)

Care Recipient:

Data Source:

**Definition:** Extent of understanding conveyed about provision of a nurturing and constructive environment for a child from 1 year through 17 years of age

OUTCOME TARGET RATING:        Maintain at_____    Increase to_____

| Knowledge: Parenting Overall Rating | None 1 | Limited 2 | Moderate 3 | Substantial 4 | Extensive 5 | |
|---|---|---|---|---|---|---|
| INDICATORS: | | | | | | |
| 182601  Description of normal growth and development | 1 | 2 | 3 | 4 | 5 | NA |
| 182602  Description of normal child behavior | 1 | 2 | 3 | 4 | 5 | NA |
| 182603  Description of safety needs | 1 | 2 | 3 | 4 | 5 | NA |
| 182604  Description of injury prevention | 1 | 2 | 3 | 4 | 5 | NA |
| 182605  Description of nutritional needs | 1 | 2 | 3 | 4 | 5 | NA |
| 182606  Description of physical care needs | 1 | 2 | 3 | 4 | 5 | NA |
| 182607  Description of psychological needs | 1 | 2 | 3 | 4 | 5 | NA |
| 182608  Description of emotional needs | 1 | 2 | 3 | 4 | 5 | NA |
| 182609  Description of stimulation needs | 1 | 2 | 3 | 4 | 5 | NA |
| 182610  Description of socialization needs | 1 | 2 | 3 | 4 | 5 | NA |
| 182611  Description of spiritual needs | 1 | 2 | 3 | 4 | 5 | NA |
| 182612  Description of moral guidance needs | 1 | 2 | 3 | 4 | 5 | NA |
| 182613  Description of health supervision needs | 1 | 2 | 3 | 4 | 5 | NA |
| 182614  Description of illness prevention | 1 | 2 | 3 | 4 | 5 | NA |
| 182615  Description of management of common health problems | 1 | 2 | 3 | 4 | 5 | NA |
| 182616  Description of age-appropriate expectations | 1 | 2 | 3 | 4 | 5 | NA |
| 182617  Description of discipline appropriate to age, development and situation | 1 | 2 | 3 | 4 | 5 | NA |
| 182618  Description of meeting basic care needs | 1 | 2 | 3 | 4 | 5 | NA |
| 182619  Description of effective communication | 1 | 2 | 3 | 4 | 5 | NA |

*3rd edition*

## Outcome Content References:

Craft-Rosenberg, M., & Denehy, J. (Eds.) (2001). *Nursing interventions for infants, children, and families.* Thousand Oaks, CA: Sage Publications.

Friedman, M. (1998). *Family nursing: Research, theory and practice* (4th ed.). Stamford, CT: Appleton & Lange.

Green, M., Palfrey, J.S. (Eds.). (2002). *Bright futures: Guidelines for health supervision of infants, children, and adolescents.* Arlington, VA: National Center for Education in Maternal and Child Health.

Murray, R., & Zenter, J. (1997). *Health assessment & promotion strategies through the life span* (6th ed.). Stamford, CT: Appleton & Lange.

K

# Knowledge: Personal Safety (1809)

Domain-Health Knowledge & Behavior (IV)

Class-Health Knowledge (S)

Scale(s)-None to Extensive (i)

Care Recipient:

Data Source:

**Definition:** Extent of understanding conveyed about prevention of unintentional injuries

OUTCOME TARGET RATING:    Maintain at_____    Increase to_____

| Knowledge: Personal Safety Overall Rating | None 1 | Limited 2 | Moderate 3 | Substantial 4 | Extensive 5 | |
|---|---|---|---|---|---|---|
| INDICATORS: | | | | | | |
| 180901 Description of suffocation prevention measures | 1 | 2 | 3 | 4 | 5 | NA |
| 180902 Description of fall prevention measures | 1 | 2 | 3 | 4 | 5 | NA |
| 180903 Description of risk reduction measures | 1 | 2 | 3 | 4 | 5 | NA |
| 180904 Description of home safety measures | 1 | 2 | 3 | 4 | 5 | NA |
| 180905 Description of water safety precautions | 1 | 2 | 3 | 4 | 5 | NA |
| 180906 Description of fire safety measures | 1 | 2 | 3 | 4 | 5 | NA |
| 180907 Description of burn prevention | 1 | 2 | 3 | 4 | 5 | NA |
| 180908 Description of electrocution prevention | 1 | 2 | 3 | 4 | 5 | NA |
| 180909 Description of poison prevention | 1 | 2 | 3 | 4 | 5 | NA |
| 180910 Description of bicycle safety guidelines | 1 | 2 | 3 | 4 | 5 | NA |
| 180911 Description of pedestrian safety measures | 1 | 2 | 3 | 4 | 5 | NA |
| 180912 Description of benefits of protective helmets | 1 | 2 | 3 | 4 | 5 | NA |
| 180913 Description of firearm safety measures | 1 | 2 | 3 | 4 | 5 | NA |
| 180915 Description of motor vehicle safety measures | 1 | 2 | 3 | 4 | 5 | NA |
| 180916 Description of emergency procedures | 1 | 2 | 3 | 4 | 5 | NA |
| 180917 Description of age-specific safety risks | 1 | 2 | 3 | 4 | 5 | NA |
| 180918 Description of personal high-risk behaviors | 1 | 2 | 3 | 4 | 5 | NA |
| 180919 Description of work safety risks | 1 | 2 | 3 | 4 | 5 | NA |
| 180920 Description of community safety risks | 1 | 2 | 3 | 4 | 5 | NA |

*1st edition 1997; Revised 3rd edition*

Outcome Content References:

Conn, V.S., Armer, J.M., & Hayes, K.S. (2001). Knowledge deficit. In M. Maas, K. Buckwalter, M. Hardy, T. Tripp-Reimer, M. Titler, & J. Specht (Eds.), *Nursing care of older adults: Diagnoses, outcomes & interventions* (pp. 503-515). St. Louis: Mosby.

Simons-Morton, D.G., Mullen, P.D., Mains, D.A., Tabak, E.R., & Green, L.W. (1992). Characteristics of controlled studies of patient education and counseling for preventive health behaviors. *Patient Education and Counseling, 19*(2), 174-204.

U.S. Department of Health and Human Services. (1990). *Healthy people 2000. National health promotion and disease prevention objectives.* Washington, DC: Government Printing Office.

U.S. Department of Health and Human Services. (1998). *Clinician's handbook of prevention services: Put prevention into practice.* (2nd ed.) Washington, DC: Government Printing Office.

K

# Knowledge: Postpartum Maternal Health (1818)

Domain-Health Knowledge & Behavior (IV)

Class-Health Knowledge (S)

Scale(s)-None to Extensive (i)

Care Recipient:

Data Source:

**Definition:** Extent of understanding conveyed about maternal health following delivery

OUTCOME TARGET RATING:    Maintain at_____    Increase to_____

| Knowledge: Postpartum Maternal Health Overall Rating | None 1 | Limited 2 | Moderate 3 | Substantial 4 | Extensive 5 | |
|---|---|---|---|---|---|---|
| **INDICATORS:** | | | | | | |
| 181801 Description of normal physical sensations following delivery | 1 | 2 | 3 | 4 | 5 | NA |
| 181802 Description of routine monitoring | 1 | 2 | 3 | 4 | 5 | NA |
| 181803 Description of vaginal discharge | 1 | 2 | 3 | 4 | 5 | NA |
| 181804 Description of breast changes | 1 | 2 | 3 | 4 | 5 | NA |
| 181805 Description of uterine involution patterns | 1 | 2 | 3 | 4 | 5 | NA |
| 181806 Description of fundal massage | 1 | 2 | 3 | 4 | 5 | NA |
| 181807 Description of perineal care | 1 | 2 | 3 | 4 | 5 | NA |
| 181808 Description of episiotomy care | 1 | 2 | 3 | 4 | 5 | NA |
| 181809 Description of cesarean section care | 1 | 2 | 3 | 4 | 5 | NA |
| 181810 Description of coughing techniques following surgery | 1 | 2 | 3 | 4 | 5 | NA |
| 181811 Description of appropriate fluid and nutrient intake | 1 | 2 | 3 | 4 | 5 | NA |
| 181812 Description of appropriate rest and activity | 1 | 2 | 3 | 4 | 5 | NA |
| 181813 Description of appropriate exercise | 1 | 2 | 3 | 4 | 5 | NA |
| 181814 Description of time frame for resumption of sexual activity | 1 | 2 | 3 | 4 | 5 | NA |
| 181815 Description of contraceptive options | 1 | 2 | 3 | 4 | 5 | NA |
| 181816 Description of psychological changes | 1 | 2 | 3 | 4 | 5 | NA |
| 181817 Description of effective coping mechanisms | 1 | 2 | 3 | 4 | 5 | NA |
| 181818 Description of plan for social support | 1 | 2 | 3 | 4 | 5 | NA |

*2nd edition 2000; Revised 3rd edition (formerly Knowledge: Postpartum)*

**Outcome Content References:**

Association of Women's Health, Obstetricians and Neonatal Nurses. (1998). *Standards & guidelines for the professional nursing practice in the care of women and newborns* (5th ed.). Washington, DC: Author

Crowell, D.T. (1995). Weight change in the postpartum period. A review of the literature. *Journal of Nurse Midwifery, 40*(5), 418-423.

Nichols, F., & Humenick, S. (2000). *Childbirth education: Practice, research and theory* (2nd ed.). Philadelphia: W.B. Saunders.

Reeder, S.J., Martin, L.L., & Koniak-Griffin, D. (1997). *Maternity nursing: Family, newborn, and women's health care* (18th ed.). Philadelphia: Lippincott.

**K**

# Knowledge: Preconception Maternal Health (1822)

Domain-Health Knowledge & Behavior (IV)

Class-Health Knowledge (S)

Scale(s)-None to Extensive (i)

Care Recipient:

Data Source:

**Definition:** Extent of understanding conveyed about maternal health prior to conception to insure a healthy pregnancy

OUTCOME TARGET RATING:     Maintain at_____     Increase to_____

| Knowledge: Preconception Maternal Health Overall Rating | None 1 | Limited 2 | Moderate 3 | Substantial 4 | Extensive 5 | |
|---|---|---|---|---|---|---|
| **INDICATORS:** | | | | | | |
| 182201 Description of factors to consider when deciding to become a parent | 1 | 2 | 3 | 4 | 5 | NA |
| 182202 Description of a healthy pregnancy | 1 | 2 | 3 | 4 | 5 | NA |
| 182203 Description of a healthy diet | 1 | 2 | 3 | 4 | 5 | NA |
| 182204 Description of appropriate rest and exercise | 1 | 2 | 3 | 4 | 5 | NA |
| 182205 Description of adverse effects of alcohol, tobacco, and drug use | 1 | 2 | 3 | 4 | 5 | NA |
| 182206 Description of maternal risk factors | 1 | 2 | 3 | 4 | 5 | NA |
| 182207 Description of environmental hazards at home that could affect fetal development | 1 | 2 | 3 | 4 | 5 | NA |
| 182211 Description of environmental hazards at work that could affect fetal development | 1 | 2 | 3 | 4 | 5 | NA |
| 182208 Description of risk for hereditary disease | 1 | 2 | 3 | 4 | 5 | NA |
| 182209 Description of potential adjustments to pregnancy | 1 | 2 | 3 | 4 | 5 | NA |
| 182212 Description of potential adjustments to addition of new family member | 1 | 2 | 3 | 4 | 5 | NA |

*2nd edition 2000; Revised 3rd edition (formerly Knowledge: Preconception)*

Outcome Content References:

Aneshensel, C.S., Becerra, R.M., Fielder, E.P., & Schuler, R.H. (1990). Onset of fertility-related events during adolescence: A prospective comparison of Mexican American and non-Hispanic White females. *American Journal of Public Health, 80*(8), 959-963.

Fehring, R.J. (1991). New technology in natural family planning. *Journal of Obstetric, Gynecologic, & Neonatal Nursing, 20*(3), 199-205.

Grodstein, F., Goldman, M.B., & Cramer, D.W. (1994). Infertility in women and moderate alcohol use. *American Journal of Public Health, 84*(9), 1429-1432.

Halman, L.J., Abbey, A., & Andrews, F.M. (1992). Attitudes about infertility interventions among fertile and infertile couples. *American Journal of Public Health, 82*(2), 191-194.

Rudy, E.B., & Estok, P. (1992). Professional and lay interrater reliability of urinary luteinizing hormone surges measured by OvuQuik test. *Journal of Obstetric, Gynecologic, & Neonatal Nursing, 21*(5), 407-411.

Shane, JM (1993). Evaluation and treatment of infertility. *Clinical Symposia, 45*(2), 2-32.

Summers, L. (1993). Preconception care: An opportunity to maximize health in pregnancy. *Journal of Nurse Midwifery, 38*(4), 188-198.

Toner, J.P., & Flood, J.T. (1993). Fertility after the age of 40. *Obstetrics & Gynecology Clinics of North America, 20*(2), 261-272.

# Knowledge: Pregnancy (1810)

Domain-Health Knowledge & Behavior (IV)

Class-Health Knowledge (S)

Scale(s)-None to Extensive (i)

Care Recipient:

Data Source:

**Definition:** Extent of understanding conveyed about promotion of a healthy pregnancy and prevention of complications

OUTCOME TARGET RATING:      Maintain at_____      Increase to_____

| Knowledge: Pregnancy Overall Rating | None 1 | Limited 2 | Moderate 3 | Substantial 4 | Extensive 5 | |
|---|---|---|---|---|---|---|

INDICATORS:

| | | None 1 | Limited 2 | Moderate 3 | Substantial 4 | Extensive 5 | |
|---|---|---|---|---|---|---|---|
| 181026 | Description of importance of prenatal care | 1 | 2 | 3 | 4 | 5 | NA |
| 181027 | Description of importance of prenatal education | 1 | 2 | 3 | 4 | 5 | NA |
| 181003 | Description of warning signs of pregnancy complications | 1 | 2 | 3 | 4 | 5 | NA |
| 181004 | Description of major fetal developmental milestones | 1 | 2 | 3 | 4 | 5 | NA |
| 181005 | Description of physical and physiological changes of pregnancy | 1 | 2 | 3 | 4 | 5 | NA |
| 181006 | Description of psychological changes of pregnancy | 1 | 2 | 3 | 4 | 5 | NA |
| 181007 | Description of appropriate rest and sleep | 1 | 2 | 3 | 4 | 5 | NA |
| 181008 | Description of proper body mechanics | 1 | 2 | 3 | 4 | 5 | NA |
| 181009 | Description of appropriate exercise | 1 | 2 | 3 | 4 | 5 | NA |
| 181010 | Description of healthy nutrition | 1 | 2 | 3 | 4 | 5 | NA |
| 181011 | Description of healthy weight gain pattern | 1 | 2 | 3 | 4 | 5 | NA |
| 181012 | Description of correct use of nutritional supplements and medications | 1 | 2 | 3 | 4 | 5 | NA |
| 181013 | Description of importance of dental care | 1 | 2 | 3 | 4 | 5 | NA |
| 181014 | Description of appropriate self-care for discomforts of pregnancy | 1 | 2 | 3 | 4 | 5 | NA |
| 181015 | Description of safe sexual activity | 1 | 2 | 3 | 4 | 5 | NA |
| 181016 | Description of proper use of auto safety devices | 1 | 2 | 3 | 4 | 5 | NA |
| 181017 | Description of types of health care professionals available for prenatal care and childbirth | 1 | 2 | 3 | 4 | 5 | NA |
| 181018 | Description of signs of labor | 1 | 2 | 3 | 4 | 5 | NA |
| 181019 | Description of techniques to facilitate effective labor | 1 | 2 | 3 | 4 | 5 | NA |
| 181020 | Description of methods to prevent infection | 1 | 2 | 3 | 4 | 5 | NA |
| 181021 | Description of methods to escape domestic violence | 1 | 2 | 3 | 4 | 5 | NA |
| 181022 | Description of ways to prepare family members | 1 | 2 | 3 | 4 | 5 | NA |
| 181023 | Description of environmental hazards | 1 | 2 | 3 | 4 | 5 | NA |
| 181024 | Description of teratogenic agents | 1 | 2 | 3 | 4 | 5 | NA |

*2nd edition 2000; Revised 3rd edition*

*Continued*

Outcome Content References:

Bell, R., & O'Neill M. (1994). Exercise and pregnancy: A review. *Birth, 21*(2), 85-95.

Freda, M.C., et al. (1993). What pregnant women want to know: A comparison of client and provider perceptions. *Journal of Obstetric, Gynecologic, and Neonatal Nursing, 22*(3), 237.

Kearney, M.H., Murphy, S., Irwin, K., & Rosenbaum, M. (1995). Salvaging self: A grounded theory of pregnancy on crack cocaine. *Nursing Research, 44*(4), 208-213.

Lowdermilk, D.L., & Perry, S.E. (2003). *Maternity Nursing* (6th ed.). St. Louis: Mosby.

McFarlane, J., et al. (1996). Abuse during pregnancy: Associations with maternal health and infant birth weight. *Nursing Research, 45*(1), 37-42.

Olds, S.B., London, M.L., & Ladewig, P.W. (1996). *Maternal-newborn nursing: A family-centered approach* (5th ed.). Menlo Park, CA: Addison-Wesley.

Shapiro, H.R. (1993). Prenatal education in the work place. *AWHONNS Clinical Issues in Perinatal & Women's Health Nursing, 4*(1), 113-121.

**K**

# *Knowledge: Prescribed Activity (1811)*

Domain-Health Knowledge & Behavior (IV)

Class-Health Knowledge (S)

Scale(s)-None to Extensive (i)

Care Recipient:

Data Source:

**Definition:** Extent of understanding conveyed about prescribed activity and exercise

OUTCOME TARGET RATING:     Maintain at_____     Increase to_____

| Knowledge: Prescribed Activity Overall Rating | None 1 | Limited 2 | Moderate 3 | Substantial 4 | Extensive 5 | |
|---|---|---|---|---|---|---|
| INDICATORS: | | | | | | |
| 181101 Description of prescribed activity | 1 | 2 | 3 | 4 | 5 | NA |
| 181102 Description of purpose of activity | 1 | 2 | 3 | 4 | 5 | NA |
| 181103 Description of expected effects of activity | 1 | 2 | 3 | 4 | 5 | NA |
| 181104 Description of activity restrictions | 1 | 2 | 3 | 4 | 5 | NA |
| 181105 Description of activity precautions | 1 | 2 | 3 | 4 | 5 | NA |
| 181106 Description of factors that decrease the ability to perform activity | 1 | 2 | 3 | 4 | 5 | NA |
| 181107 Description of strategies for gradual activity increase | 1 | 2 | 3 | 4 | 5 | NA |
| 181108 Description of how to monitor activity | 1 | 2 | 3 | 4 | 5 | NA |
| 181115 Description of self-monitoring techniques | 1 | 2 | 3 | 4 | 5 | NA |
| 181110 Description of obstacles to implementing exercise routine | 1 | 2 | 3 | 4 | 5 | NA |
| 181111 Description of realistic exercise plan | 1 | 2 | 3 | 4 | 5 | NA |
| 181112 Description of proper performance of exercise | 1 | 2 | 3 | 4 | 5 | NA |

*1st edition 1997; Revised 3rd edition*

Outcome Content References:

Bushnell, F. (1992). Self-care teaching for congestive heart failure patients. *Journal of Gerontological Nursing,* 18(10), 27-32.

Conn, V.S., Armer, J.M., & Hayes, K.S. (2001). Knowledge deficit. In M. Maas, K. Buckwalter, M. Hardy, T. Tripp-Reimer, M. Titler, & J. Specht (Eds.), *Nursing care of older adults: Diagnoses, outcomes & interventions* (pp. 503-515). St. Louis: Mosby.

Devins, G.M., Binik, Y.M., Mandin, H., Litourneau, P.K., Hollomby, D.J., Barre, P.E., & Prichard, S. (1990). The Kidney Disease Questionnaire: A test for measuring patient knowledge about end-stage renal disease. *Journal of Clinical Epidemiology,* 43(3), 297-307.

Garrard, J., Joynes, J.O., Mullen, L., McNeil, L., Mensing, C., Feste, C., & Etzwiler, D.D. (1987). Psychometric study of patient knowledge test. *Diabetes Care,* 10(4), 500-509.

Gilden, J.L., Hendryx, M., Casia, C., & Singh, S.P. (1989). The effectiveness of diabetes education programs for older patients and their spouses. *Journal of American Geriatrics Society,* 37(11), 1023-1030.

Mazzuca S.A., Moorman, N.H., Wheeler, M.L., Norton, J.A., Fineberg, N.S., Vinicor, F., Cohen, S.J., & Clark, C.M. (1986). The diabetes education study: A controlled trial of the effects of diabetes patient education. *Diabetes Care,* 9(1), 1-10.

Redman, B. (1993). Knowledge deficit (specify). In J.M. Thompson, G.K. McFarland, J.E. Hirsch, & S.M. Tucker (Eds.), *Mosby's clinical nursing* (3rd ed., pp. 1548-1552). St. Louis: Mosby.

Scherer, Y.K., Janelli, L.M., & Schmieder, L.E. (1992). A time-series perspective of effectiveness of a health teaching program on chronic obstructive pulmonary disease. *Journal of Healthcare Education and Training,* 6(3), 7-13.

Smith, M.M., Hicks, V.L., & Heyward, V.H. (1991). Coronary Disease Knowledge Test: Developing a valid and reliable tool. *Nurse Practitioner,* 16(4), 28, 31, 35-38.

K

# *Knowledge: Sexual Functioning (1815)*

*Domain-Health Knowledge & Behavior (IV)*

*Class-Health Knowledge (S)*

*Scale(s)-None to Extensive (i)*

Care Recipient:

Data Source:

**Definition:** Extent of understanding conveyed about sexual development and responsible sexual practices

OUTCOME TARGET RATING:     Maintain at_____     Increase to_____

| Knowledge: Sexual Functioning Overall Rating | None 1 | Limited 2 | Moderate 3 | Substantial 4 | Extensive 5 | |
|---|---|---|---|---|---|---|
| **INDICATORS:** | | | | | | |
| 181501 Description of sexual anatomy | 1 | 2 | 3 | 4 | 5 | NA |
| 181502 Description of function of sexual anatomy | 1 | 2 | 3 | 4 | 5 | NA |
| 181503 Description of physical changes with puberty | 1 | 2 | 3 | 4 | 5 | NA |
| 181504 Description of emotional changes with puberty | 1 | 2 | 3 | 4 | 5 | NA |
| 181505 Description of reproduction | 1 | 2 | 3 | 4 | 5 | NA |
| 181506 Description of physical changes with aging | 1 | 2 | 3 | 4 | 5 | NA |
| 181507 Description of emotional changes with aging | 1 | 2 | 3 | 4 | 5 | NA |
| 181508 Description of societal influences on sexual behavior | 1 | 2 | 3 | 4 | 5 | NA |
| 181509 Description of safe sexual practices | 1 | 2 | 3 | 4 | 5 | NA |
| 181510 Description of effective contraception | 1 | 2 | 3 | 4 | 5 | NA |
| 181511 Description of techniques to prevent STDs* | 1 | 2 | 3 | 4 | 5 | NA |

*STDs = Sexually transmitted diseases.

*2nd edition 2000; Revised 3rd edition*

**Outcome Content References:**

Howard, M. (1991). *How to help your teenager postpone sexual involvement.* Lexington, NY: Continuum Publishing Co.

Nass, G., Libby, R., & Fischer, M.P. (1989). *Sexual choices: An introduction to human sexuality* (2nd ed.). Monterey, CA: Wadsworth Health Sciences.

Neinstein, L.S. (2002). *Adolescent health care: A practical guide.* Philadelphia: Lippincott Williams & Wilkins.

Tuttle, B. (1984). Adult sexual response. In L.P. Higgins, & J.W. Hawkins (Eds.), *Human sexuality across the life span: Implications for nursing practice* (p.p. 39-76). Monterey, CA: Wadsworth Health Sciences Division.

Wright, L.K. (2001). Altered sexuality patterns. In M. Maas, K. Buckwalter, M. Hardy, T. Tripp-Reimer, M. Titler, & J. Specht (Eds.), *Nursing care of older adults: Diagnoses, outcomes & interventions* (pp. 750-761). St. Louis: Mosby.

# Knowledge: Substance Use Control (1812)

Domain-Health Knowledge & Behavior (IV)

Class-Health Knowledge (S)

Scale(s)-None to Extensive (i)

Care Recipient:

Data Source:

**Definition:** Extent of understanding conveyed about controlling the use of drugs, tobacco, or alcohol

OUTCOME TARGET RATING:    Maintain at_____    Increase to_____

| Knowledge: Substance Use Control Overall Rating | None 1 | Limited 2 | Moderate 3 | Substantial 4 | Extensive 5 | |
|---|---|---|---|---|---|---|
| **INDICATORS:** | | | | | | |
| 181201 Description of own risk for substance misuse | 1 | 2 | 3 | 4 | 5 | NA |
| 181202 Description of adverse health effects of substance use | 1 | 2 | 3 | 4 | 5 | NA |
| 181203 Description of benefits of eliminating substance use | 1 | 2 | 3 | 4 | 5 | NA |
| 181204 Description of dangers of substance use | 1 | 2 | 3 | 4 | 5 | NA |
| 181205 Description of social consequences of substance use | 1 | 2 | 3 | 4 | 5 | NA |
| 181206 Description of personal responsibility in managing substance use | 1 | 2 | 3 | 4 | 5 | NA |
| 181207 Description of threats to substance use control | 1 | 2 | 3 | 4 | 5 | NA |
| 181208 Description of support for substance use control | 1 | 2 | 3 | 4 | 5 | NA |
| 181209 Description of actions to prevent substance use | 1 | 2 | 3 | 4 | 5 | NA |
| 181210 Description of actions to manage substance use | 1 | 2 | 3 | 4 | 5 | NA |
| 181211 Description of benefits of ongoing self monitoring | 1 | 2 | 3 | 4 | 5 | NA |
| 181212 Description of potential for relapse in efforts to control substance use | 1 | 2 | 3 | 4 | 5 | NA |
| 181213 Description of actions to prevent and manage relapses in substance use | 1 | 2 | 3 | 4 | 5 | NA |
| 181214 Description of signs of dependence during substance withdrawal | 1 | 2 | 3 | 4 | 5 | NA |

Specify substance_____

*1st edition 1997; Revised 3rd edition*

Outcome Content References:

Eells, M.A.W. (1991). Strategies for promotion of avoiding harmful substances. *Nursing Clinics of North America, 26*(40), 915-927.

Simons-Morton, D.G., Mullen, P.D., Mains, D.A., Tabak, E.R., & Green, L.W. (1992). Characteristics of controlled studies of patient education and counseling for preventive health behaviors. *Patient Education and Counseling, 19*(2), 174-204.

Tanner, E.K. (1991). Assessment of a health-promotive lifestyle. *Nursing Clinics of North America, 26*(4), 845-854.

U.S. Department of Health and Human Services. (1990). *Healthy people 2000, National health promotion and disease prevention objectives.* Washington, DC: Government Printing Office.

U.S. Department of Health and Human Services. (1998). *Clinician's handbook of prevention services: Put prevention into practice.* (2nd ed.) Washington, DC: Government Printing Office.

K

# *Knowledge: Treatment Procedure(s) (1814)*

*Domain-Health Knowledge & Behavior (IV)*

*Class-Health Knowledge (S)*

*Scale(s)-None to Extensive (i)*

Care Recipient:

Data Source:

**Definition:** Extent of understanding conveyed about procedure(s) required as part of a treatment regimen

OUTCOME TARGET RATING:     Maintain at_____     Increase to_____

| Knowledge: Treatment Procedure(s) Overall Rating | None 1 | Limited 2 | Moderate 3 | Substantial 4 | Extensive 5 | |
|---|---|---|---|---|---|---|
| **INDICATORS:** | | | | | | |
| 181401 Description of treatment procedure(s) | 1 | 2 | 3 | 4 | 5 | NA |
| 181402 Explanation of purpose of procedure(s) | 1 | 2 | 3 | 4 | 5 | NA |
| 181403 Description of steps in procedure(s) | 1 | 2 | 3 | 4 | 5 | NA |
| 181405 Description of precautions related to procedure(s) | 1 | 2 | 3 | 4 | 5 | NA |
| 181406 Description of restrictions related to procedure(s) | 1 | 2 | 3 | 4 | 5 | NA |
| 181404 Description of use of equipment | 1 | 2 | 3 | 4 | 5 | NA |
| 181407 Describes proper care of equipment | 1 | 2 | 3 | 4 | 5 | NA |
| 181409 Description of appropriate action for complications | 1 | 2 | 3 | 4 | 5 | NA |
| 181410 Description of potential side effects | 1 | 2 | 3 | 4 | 5 | NA |
| 181412 Description of contraindication for procedure(s) | 1 | 2 | 3 | 4 | 5 | NA |

Specify procedure _____

*1st edition 1997; Revised 3rd edition*

**Outcome Content References:**

Conn, V.S., Armer, J.M., & Hayes, K.S. (2001). Knowledge deficit. In M. Maas, K. Buckwalter, M. Hardy, T. Tripp-Reimer, M. Titler, & J. Specht (Eds.), *Nursing care of older adults: Diagnoses, outcomes & interventions* (pp. 503-515). St. Louis: Mosby.

Redman, B.K. (2001). *The practice of patient education.* (9th ed.). St. Louis: Mosby.

Roe, B.H. (1990). Study of the effects of education on the management of urine drainage systems by patients and carers. *Journal of Advanced Nursing, 15*(5), 517-524.

Sarisley, C. (1987). Designing a teaching program for outpatient antibiotic therapy. *Journal of Nursing Staff Development, 3*(3), 128-135.

Smith, C.E. (1987). *Patient education: Nurses in partnership with other health professionals.* Orlando, FL: Gruen & Stratton.

Togger, D.A., & Brenner, P.S. (2001). Metered dose inhalers. *American Journal of Nursing, 101*(10), 26-32, 38-39.

# Knowledge: Treatment Regimen (1813)

*Domain-Health Knowledge & Behavior (IV)*

*Class-Health Knowledge (S)*

*Scale(s)-None to Extensive (i)*

*Care Recipient:*

*Data Source:*

**Definition:** Extent of understanding conveyed about a specific treatment regimen

OUTCOME TARGET RATING:      Maintain at_____      Increase to_____

| Knowledge: Treatment Regimen Overall Rating | None 1 | Limited 2 | Moderate 3 | Substantial 4 | Extensive 5 | |
|---|---|---|---|---|---|---|
| INDICATORS: | | | | | | |
| 181310 Description of specific disease process | 1 | 2 | 3 | 4 | 5 | NA |
| 181301 Description of rationale for treatment regimen | 1 | 2 | 3 | 4 | 5 | NA |
| 181302 Description of self-care responsibilities for ongoing treatment | 1 | 2 | 3 | 4 | 5 | NA |
| 181303 Description of self-care responsibilities for emergency situations | 1 | 2 | 3 | 4 | 5 | NA |
| 181315 Description of self-monitoring techniques | 1 | 2 | 3 | 4 | 5 | NA |
| 181304 Description of expected effects of treatment | 1 | 2 | 3 | 4 | 5 | NA |
| 181305 Description of prescribed diet | 1 | 2 | 3 | 4 | 5 | NA |
| 181306 Description of prescribed medication(s) | 1 | 2 | 3 | 4 | 5 | NA |
| 181307 Description of prescribed activity | 1 | 2 | 3 | 4 | 5 | NA |
| 181308 Description of prescribed exercise | 1 | 2 | 3 | 4 | 5 | NA |
| 181309 Description of prescribed procedure(s) | 1 | 2 | 3 | 4 | 5 | NA |
| 181316 Description of benefits of disease management | 1 | 2 | 3 | 4 | 5 | NA |

*1st edition 1997; Revised 2nd edition 2000; Revised 3rd edition*

Outcome Content References:

Bushnell, F. (1992). Self-care teaching for congestive heart failure patients. *Journal of Gerontological Nursing,* 18(10), 27-32.

Conn, V.S., Armer, J.M., & Hayes, K.S. (2001). Knowledge deficit. In M. Maas, K. Buckwalter, M. Hardy, T. Tripp-Reimer, M. Titler, & J. Specht (Eds.), *Nursing care of older adults: Diagnoses, outcomes & interventions* (pp. 503-515). St. Louis: Mosby.

Devins, G.M., Binik, Y.M., Mandin, H., Litourneau, P.K., Hollomby, D.J., Barre, P.E., & Prichard, S. (1990). The Kidney Disease Questionnaire: A test for measuring patient knowledge about end-stage renal disease. *Journal of Clinical Epidemiology,* 43(3), 297-307.

Garrard, J., Joynes, J.O., Mullen, L., McNeil, L., Mensing, C., Feste, C., & Etzwiler, D.D. (1987). Psychometric study of patient knowledge test. *Diabetes Care,* 10(4), 500-509.

Gilden, J.L., Hendryx, M., Casia, C., & Singh, S.P. (1989). The effectiveness of diabetes education programs for older patients and their spouses. *Journal of American Geriatrics Society,* 37(11), 1023-1030.

Mazzuca, S.A., Moorman, N.H., Wheeler, M.L., Norton, J.A., Fineberg, N.S., Vinicor, F., Cohen, S.J., & Clark, C.M. (1986). The diabetes education study: A controlled trial of the effects of diabetes patient education. *Diabetes Care,* 9(1), 1-10.

Redman, B. (1993). Knowledge deficit (specify). In J.M. Thompson, G.K. McFarland, J.E. Hirsch, & S.M. Tucker (Eds.), *Mosby's clinical nursing* (3rd ed., pp. 1548-1552). St. Louis: Mosby.

Scherer, Y.K., Janelli, L.M., & Schmieder, L.E. (1992). A time-series perspective of effectiveness of a health teaching program on chronic obstructive pulmonary disease. *Journal of Healthcare Education & Training,* 6(3), 7-13.

Smith, M.M., Hicks, V.L., & Heyward, V.H. (1991). Coronary Disease Knowledge Test: Developing a valid and reliable tool. *Nurse Practitioner,* 16(4), 28, 31, 35-38.

Zwygart-Stauffacher, M. (2001). Ineffective management of therapeutic regimen. In M. Maas, K. Buckwalter, M. Hardy, T. Tripp-Reimer, M. Titler, & J. Specht (Eds.), *Nursing care of older adults: Diagnoses, outcomes & interventions* (pp. 86-92). St. Louis: Mosby.

K

# Leisure Participation (1604)

*Domain-Health Knowledge & Behavior (IV)*

*Class-Health Behavior (Q)*

*Scale(s)-Never demonstrated to Consistently demonstrated (m)*

Care Recipient:

Data Source:

**Definition:** Use of relaxing, interesting, and enjoyable activities to promote well-being

OUTCOME TARGET RATING:    Maintain at_____    Increase to_____

| Leisure Participation Overall Rating | Never demonstrated 1 | Rarely demonstrated 2 | Sometimes demonstrated 3 | Often demonstrated 4 | Consistently demonstrated 5 | |
|---|---|---|---|---|---|---|

**INDICATORS:**

| | | Never demonstrated 1 | Rarely demonstrated 2 | Sometimes demonstrated 3 | Often demonstrated 4 | Consistently demonstrated 5 | |
|---|---|---|---|---|---|---|---|
| 160401 | Participates in activities other than regular work | 1 | 2 | 3 | 4 | 5 | NA |
| 160410 | Participates in high physical demand leisure activities | 1 | 2 | 3 | 4 | 5 | NA |
| 160411 | Participates in low physical demand leisure activities | 1 | 2 | 3 | 4 | 5 | NA |
| 160412 | Selects leisure activities of interest | 1 | 2 | 3 | 4 | 5 | NA |
| 160402 | Expresses satisfaction with leisure activities | 1 | 2 | 3 | 4 | 5 | NA |
| 160403 | Uses appropriate social and interactional skills | 1 | 2 | 3 | 4 | 5 | NA |
| 160404 | Feels relaxed from leisure activities | 1 | 2 | 3 | 4 | 5 | NA |
| 160413 | Enjoys leisure activities | 1 | 2 | 3 | 4 | 5 | NA |
| 160405 | Exhibits creativity through leisure activities | 1 | 2 | 3 | 4 | 5 | NA |
| 160406 | Chooses own leisure activities | 1 | 2 | 3 | 4 | 5 | NA |
| 160407 | Identifies recreational options | 1 | 2 | 3 | 4 | 5 | NA |

*1st edition 1997; Revised 3rd edition*

**Outcome Content References:**

Ansello, E.F. (1985). *The activity coordinator as environmental press.* New York: The Haworth Press.

+Drummond, A.E.R., & Walker, M.F. (1994). The Nottingham Leisure Questionnaire for stroke patients. *British Journal of Occupational Therapy, 57*(11), 414-418.

Everard, K.M., Lach, H.W., Fisher, E.B., & Baum, M.C. (2000). Relationship of activity and social support to the functional health of older adults. *Journal of Gerontology Series B-Social Sciences, 55*(4), P208-P212.

Godin, G., Jobin, J., & Bouillon, J. (1986). Assessment of leisure time exercise behavior by self-report: A concurrent validity study. *Canadian Journal of Public Health, 77*(5), 359-362.

Gordon, M.D. (1987). Pediatric recreational therapy after thermal injury. *Journal of Burn Rehabilitation, 8*(4), 336-340.

Johnson, S.W., McSweeney, M., & Webster, R.E. (1989). Leisure: How to promote inpatient motivation after discharge. *Journal of Psychosocial Nursing, 27*(9), 29-31.

Jongbloed, L., & Morgan, D. (1991). An investigation of involvement in leisure activities after a stroke. *The American Journal of Occupational Therapy, 45*(5), 420-427.

Klein, M.M. (1985). The therapeutics of recreation. *Physical Occupational Therapy Pediatrics, 4*(3): 9-11.

Peterson, C.A., & Stumbo, N.J. (1999). *Therapeutic recreation program design: Principles and procedures.* (3rd ed.). San Francisco: Benjamin Cummings.

Rantz, M.J., & Popejoy, L. (2001). Diversional activity deficit. In M. Maas, K. Buckwalter, M. Hardy, T. Tripp-Reimer, M. Titler, & J. Specht (Eds.), *Nursing care of older adults: Diagnoses, outcomes & interventions* (pp. 385-396). St. Louis: Mosby.

# Loneliness Severity (1203)

*Domain-Psychosocial Health (III)*

*Class-Psychological Well-Being (M)*

*Scale(s)-Severe to None (n)*

*Care Recipient:*

*Data Source:*

**Definition:** Severity of emotional, social, or existential isolation response

OUTCOME TARGET RATING:     Maintain at_____     Increase to_____

| Loneliness Severity Overall Rating | Severe 1 | Substantial 2 | Moderate 3 | Mild 4 | None 5 | |
|---|---|---|---|---|---|---|
| INDICATORS: | | | | | | |
| 120301 Sense of unfounded dread | 1 | 2 | 3 | 4 | 5 | NA |
| 120302 Sense of desperation | 1 | 2 | 3 | 4 | 5 | NA |
| 120303 Sense of extreme restlessness | 1 | 2 | 3 | 4 | 5 | NA |
| 120304 Sense of hopelessness | 1 | 2 | 3 | 4 | 5 | NA |
| 120305 Sense of not belonging | 1 | 2 | 3 | 4 | 5 | NA |
| 120306 Sense of loss due to separation from another | 1 | 2 | 3 | 4 | 5 | NA |
| 120307 Sense of social isolation | 1 | 2 | 3 | 4 | 5 | NA |
| 120308 Sense of not being understood | 1 | 2 | 3 | 4 | 5 | NA |
| 120309 Sense of being excluded | 1 | 2 | 3 | 4 | 5 | NA |
| 120310 Sense that time seems endless | 1 | 2 | 3 | 4 | 5 | NA |
| 120311 Difficulty in planning | 1 | 2 | 3 | 4 | 5 | NA |
| 120312 Difficulty in establishing contact with other people | 1 | 2 | 3 | 4 | 5 | NA |
| 120313 Difficulty overcoming separateness | 1 | 2 | 3 | 4 | 5 | NA |
| 120314 Difficulty in effecting a mutual relationship | 1 | 2 | 3 | 4 | 5 | NA |
| 120315 Demonstration of mood fluctuations | 1 | 2 | 3 | 4 | 5 | NA |
| 120316 Impaired concentration | 1 | 2 | 3 | 4 | 5 | NA |
| 120317 Demonstration of non-assertiveness | 1 | 2 | 3 | 4 | 5 | NA |
| 120318 Difficulty making decisions | 1 | 2 | 3 | 4 | 5 | NA |
| 120319 Eating disturbances | 1 | 2 | 3 | 4 | 5 | NA |
| 120320 Sleep disturbances | 1 | 2 | 3 | 4 | 5 | NA |
| 120321 Headaches | 1 | 2 | 3 | 4 | 5 | NA |
| 120322 Nausea | 1 | 2 | 3 | 4 | 5 | NA |
| 120323 Decreased activity level | 1 | 2 | 3 | 4 | 5 | NA |
| 120324 Pain | 1 | 2 | 3 | 4 | 5 | NA |
| 120325 Spiritual discomfort | 1 | 2 | 3 | 4 | 5 | NA |
| 120327 Depression | 1 | 2 | 3 | 4 | 5 | NA |

*1st edition 1997; Revised 3rd edition (formerly Loneliness)*

L

Outcome Content References:

Copel, L.C. (1988). Loneliness: A conceptual model. *Journal of Psychosocial Nursing, 26*(1), 14-19.

Ellison, C.W. (1978). Loneliness: A social-developmental analysis. *Journal of Psychology and Theology, 6*(1), 3-17.

Peplau, H.E. (1955). Loneliness. *American Journal of Nursing, 55*(12), 1476-1481.

Peplau, L.A., & Pearlman, D. (Eds.). (1982). *Loneliness: A sourcebook of current theory, research, and therapy.* New York: John Wiley.

+Russell, D., Peplau, L.A., & Cutrona, C.E. (1980). The revised UCLA Loneliness Scale: Concurrent and discriminant validity evidence. *Journal of Personality and Social Psychology, 39*(3), 472-480.

+Russell, D., Peplau, L.A., & Ferguson, M. (1978). Developing a measure of loneliness. *Journal of Personality Assessment, 42*(3), 290-294.

Weiss, R.S. (Ed.). (1973). *Loneliness: The experience of emotional and social isolation.* Cambridge, MA: The MIT Press.

West, D.A., Kellner, R., & Moore-West, M. (1986). The effects of loneliness: A review of the literature. *Comparative Psychiatry, 27*(4), 351-363.

# Maternal Status: Antepartum (2509)

*Domain-Family Health (VI)*

*Class-Family Member Health Status (Z)*

*Scale(s)-Severe deviation from normal range to No deviation from normal range (b) and Severe to None (n)*

*Care Recipient:*

*Data Source:*

> **Definition:** Extent to which maternal well-being is within normal limits from conception to the onset of labor

OUTCOME TARGET RATING:     Maintain at_____     Increase to_____

| Maternal Status: Antepartum Overall Rating | Severe deviation from normal range 1 | Substantial deviation from normal range 2 | Moderate deviation from normal range 3 | Mild deviation from normal range 4 | No deviation from normal range 5 | |
|---|---|---|---|---|---|---|
| **INDICATORS:** | | | | | | |
| 250901 Emotional attachment to fetus | 1 | 2 | 3 | 4 | 5 | NA |
| 250902 Coping with discomforts of pregnancy | 1 | 2 | 3 | 4 | 5 | NA |
| 250903 Mood lability | 1 | 2 | 3 | 4 | 5 | NA |
| 250904 Weight change | 1 | 2 | 3 | 4 | 5 | NA |
| 250907 Cognitive orientation | 1 | 2 | 3 | 4 | 5 | NA |
| 250908 Visual acuity | 1 | 2 | 3 | 4 | 5 | NA |
| 250910 Neurological reflexes | 1 | 2 | 3 | 4 | 5 | NA |
| 250916 Blood pressure | 1 | 2 | 3 | 4 | 5 | NA |
| 250917 Radial pulse rate | 1 | 2 | 3 | 4 | 5 | NA |
| 250926 Apical heart rate | 1 | 2 | 3 | 4 | 5 | NA |
| 250918 Body temperature | 1 | 2 | 3 | 4 | 5 | NA |
| 250919 Urine protein | 1 | 2 | 3 | 4 | 5 | NA |
| 250920 Urine glucose | 1 | 2 | 3 | 4 | 5 | NA |
| 250921 Blood glucose | 1 | 2 | 3 | 4 | 5 | NA |
| 250922 Hemoglobin | 1 | 2 | 3 | 4 | 5 | NA |
| 250923 Liver enzymes | 1 | 2 | 3 | 4 | 5 | NA |
| 250924 Blood count | 1 | 2 | 3 | 4 | 5 | NA |

| | Severe | Substantial | Moderate | Mild | None | |
|---|---|---|---|---|---|---|
| 250905 Edema | 1 | 2 | 3 | 4 | 5 | NA |
| 250906 Headache | 1 | 2 | 3 | 4 | 5 | NA |
| 250909 Seizure activity | 1 | 2 | 3 | 4 | 5 | NA |
| 250911 Nausea | 1 | 2 | 3 | 4 | 5 | NA |
| 250928 Vomiting | 1 | 2 | 3 | 4 | 5 | NA |
| 250912 Abdominal pain | 1 | 2 | 3 | 4 | 5 | NA |
| 250913 Epigastric pain | 1 | 2 | 3 | 4 | 5 | NA |
| 250914 Vaginal bleeding | 1 | 2 | 3 | 4 | 5 | NA |
| 250915 Vaginal discharge | 1 | 2 | 3 | 4 | 5 | NA |
| 250927 Heart burn | 1 | 2 | 3 | 4 | 5 | NA |

*2nd edition 2000; Revised 3rd edition*

M

Outcome Content References:

Association of Women's Health, Obstetricians and Neonatal Nurses. (1998). *Standards & guidelines for the professional nursing practice in the care of women and newborns* (5th ed.). Washington, DC: Author.

Association of Women's Health, Obstetric and Neonatal Nurses. (1998). *Clinical competencies and educational guide: Limited ultrasound examinations in obstetric and gynecologic/infertility settings.* Washington DC: Author.

Chez, B.F., Skurnick, J.H., Chez, R.A., Verklan, M.T., Biggs, S., & Hage, M.L. (1990). Interpretations of nonstress tests by obstetric nurses. *Journal of Obstetric, Gynecologic, and Neonatal Nursing, 19*(3), 227-232.

Givens, S.R. & Moore, M.L. (1995). Status report on maternal and child health indicators. *Journal of Perinatal and Neonatal Nursing, 9*(1), 8-18.

Lowdermilk, D.L., & Perry, S.E. (2003) *Maternity Nursing* (6th ed.). St. Louis: Mosby.

Nichols, F., & Humenick, S. (2000). *Childbirth education: Practice, research and theory* (2nd ed.). Philadelphia: W.B. Saunders.

Nurses Association of the American College of Obstetricians and Gynecologists. (1991). *NAACOBG standards for the nursing care of women and newborns* (4th ed.). Washington, DC: Author.

Reeder, S.J., Martin, L.L., & Koniak-Griffin, D. (1997). *Maternity nursing: Family, newborn, and women's health care* (18th ed.). Philadelphia: Lippincott.

**M**

# *Maternal Status: Intrapartum (2510)*

*Domain-Family Health (VI)*

*Class-Family Member Health Status (Z)*

*Scale(s)-Severe deviation from normal range to No deviation from normal range (b) and Severe to None (n)*

*Care Recipient:*

*Data Source:*

*Definition:* Extent to which maternal well-being is within normal limits from onset of labor to delivery

OUTCOME TARGET RATING: Maintain at_____ Increase to_____

| Maternal Status: Intrapartum Overall Rating | Severe deviation from normal range 1 | Substantial deviation from normal range 2 | Moderate deviation from normal range 3 | Mild deviation from normal range 4 | No deviation from normal range 5 | |
|---|---|---|---|---|---|---|
| **INDICATORS:** | | | | | | |
| 251001 Coping with discomforts of labor | 1 | 2 | 3 | 4 | 5 | NA |
| 251003 Use of techniques to facilitate labor | 1 | 2 | 3 | 4 | 5 | NA |
| 251004 Uterine contraction frequency | 1 | 2 | 3 | 4 | 5 | NA |
| 251005 Uterine contraction duration | 1 | 2 | 3 | 4 | 5 | NA |
| 251006 Uterine contraction intensity | 1 | 2 | 3 | 4 | 5 | NA |
| 251007 Progression of cervical dilation | 1 | 2 | 3 | 4 | 5 | NA |
| 251009 Blood pressure | 1 | 2 | 3 | 4 | 5 | NA |
| 251010 Radial pulse rate | 1 | 2 | 3 | 4 | 5 | NA |
| 251021 Apical heart rate | 1 | 2 | 3 | 4 | 5 | NA |
| 251011 Blood glucose | 1 | 2 | 3 | 4 | 5 | NA |
| 251012 Body temperature | 1 | 2 | 3 | 4 | 5 | NA |
| 251013 Urine output | 1 | 2 | 3 | 4 | 5 | NA |
| 251014 Visual acuity | 1 | 2 | 3 | 4 | 5 | NA |
| 251015 Cognitive orientation | 1 | 2 | 3 | 4 | 5 | NA |
| 251016 Neurological reflexes | 1 | 2 | 3 | 4 | 5 | NA |

| | Severe | Substantial | Moderate | Mild | None | |
|---|---|---|---|---|---|---|
| 251008 Vaginal bleeding | 1 | 2 | 3 | 4 | 5 | NA |
| 251017 Seizure activity | 1 | 2 | 3 | 4 | 5 | NA |
| 251018 Headache | 1 | 2 | 3 | 4 | 5 | NA |
| 251019 Epigastric pain | 1 | 2 | 3 | 4 | 5 | NA |
| 251022 Pain with contractions | 1 | 2 | 3 | 4 | 5 | NA |
| 251023 Back pain | 1 | 2 | 3 | 4 | 5 | NA |
| 251024 Nausea | 1 | 2 | 3 | 4 | 5 | NA |
| 251025 Vomiting | 1 | 2 | 3 | 4 | 5 | NA |

*2nd edition 2000; Revised 3rd edition*

Outcome Content References:

Dickason, E.J., Schultz, M.O., & Silverman, B.L. (1994). *Maternal-infant nursing care* (3rd ed.). St. Louis: Mosby.
Hodnett, E. (1996). Nursing support of the laboring woman. *Journal of Obstetric, and Neonatal Nursing, 25*(3), 257-263.
Lowe, N.K. (1996). The pain and discomfort of labor and birth. *Journal of Obstetric, and Neonatal Nursing, 25*(1), 82-92.
Mattson, S. (Ed.). (2000). *Core curriculum for maternal-newborn nursing* (2nd ed.). Philadelphia: W.B. Saunders.

# Maternal Status: Postpartum (2511)

Domain-Family Health (VI)

Class-Family Member Health Status (Z)

Scale(s)-Severe deviation from normal range to No deviation from normal range (b) and Severe to None (n)

Care Recipient:

Data Source:

**Definition:** Extent to which maternal well-being is within normal limits from delivery of placenta to completion of involution

OUTCOME TARGET RATING:  Maintain at_____  Increase to_____

| Maternal Status: Postpartum Overall Rating | Severe deviation from normal range 1 | Substantial deviation from normal range 2 | Moderate deviation from normal range 3 | Mild deviation from normal range 4 | No deviation from normal range 5 | |
|---|---|---|---|---|---|---|
| **INDICATORS:** | | | | | | |
| 251101 Mood equilibrium | 1 | 2 | 3 | 4 | 5 | NA |
| 251102 Comfort | 1 | 2 | 3 | 4 | 5 | NA |
| 251103 Blood pressure | 1 | 2 | 3 | 4 | 5 | NA |
| 251104 Apical heart rate | 1 | 2 | 3 | 4 | 5 | NA |
| 251123 Radial pulse rate | 1 | 2 | 3 | 4 | 5 | NA |
| 251105 Peripheral circulation | 1 | 2 | 3 | 4 | 5 | NA |
| 251106 Uterine fundal height | 1 | 2 | 3 | 4 | 5 | NA |
| 251107 Lochia amount | 1 | 2 | 3 | 4 | 5 | NA |
| 251124 Lochia color | 1 | 2 | 3 | 4 | 5 | NA |
| 251108 Breast fullness | 1 | 2 | 3 | 4 | 5 | NA |
| 251109 Breast comfort | 1 | 2 | 3 | 4 | 5 | NA |
| 251110 Perineal healing | 1 | 2 | 3 | 4 | 5 | NA |
| 251111 Incisional healing | 1 | 2 | 3 | 4 | 5 | NA |
| 251112 Body temperature | 1 | 2 | 3 | 4 | 5 | NA |
| 251114 Urinary elimination | 1 | 2 | 3 | 4 | 5 | NA |
| 251115 Bowel elimination | 1 | 2 | 3 | 4 | 5 | NA |
| 251116 Food and fluid intake | 1 | 2 | 3 | 4 | 5 | NA |
| 251117 Physical activity | 1 | 2 | 3 | 4 | 5 | NA |
| 251118 Endurance | 1 | 2 | 3 | 4 | 5 | NA |
| 251119 Liver enzymes | 1 | 2 | 3 | 4 | 5 | NA |
| 251120 Hemoglobin | 1 | 2 | 3 | 4 | 5 | NA |
| 251121 White blood count | 1 | 2 | 3 | 4 | 5 | NA |

| | Severe | Substantial | Moderate | Mild | None | |
|---|---|---|---|---|---|---|
| 251113 Infection | 1 | 2 | 3 | 4 | 5 | NA |
| 251125 Incisional pain | 1 | 2 | 3 | 4 | 5 | NA |
| 251126 Fatigue | 1 | 2 | 3 | 4 | 5 | NA |
| 251127 Vaginal bleeding | 1 | 2 | 3 | 4 | 5 | NA |
| 251128 Depression | 1 | 2 | 3 | 4 | 5 | NA |

*2nd edition 2000; Revised 3rd edition*

Outcome Content References:

Association of Women's Health, Obstetricians and Neonatal Nurses. (1998). *Standards & guidelines for the professional nursing practice in the care of women and newborns* (5th ed.). Washington, DC: Author.

Beck, C.T. (1992). The lived experience of postpartum depression: A phenomenological study. *Nursing Research, 41*(3), 166-170.

Bond, L. (1993). Physiological changes. In S. Mattson & J.E. Smith (Eds.), *AWHONN: Core Curriculum for maternal newborn nursing*. Philadelphia: W.B. Saunders.

Nichols, F., & Humenick, S. (2000). *Childbirth education: Practice, research and theory* (2nd ed.). Philadelphia: W.B. Saunders.

Reeder, S.J., Martin, L.L., & Koniak-Griffin, D. (1997). *Maternity nursing: Family, newborn, and women's health care* (18th ed.). Philadelphia: Lippincott.

M

## Mechanical Ventilation Response: Adult (0411)

*Domain-Physiologic Health (II)*

*Class-Cardiopulmonary (E)*

*Scale(s)-Severely compromised to Not compromised (a) and Severe to None (n)*

*Care Recipient:*

*Data Source:*

**Definition:** Alveolar exchange and tissue perfusion are supported by mechanical ventilation

OUTCOME TARGET RATING:   Maintain at_____   Increase to_____

| Mechanical Ventilation Response: Adult Overall Rating | Severely compromised 1 | Substantially compromised 2 | Moderately compromised 3 | Mildly compromised 4 | Not compromised 5 | |
|---|---|---|---|---|---|---|
| INDICATORS: | | | | | | |
| 041101  Auscultated breath sounds | 1 | 2 | 3 | 4 | 5 | NA |
| 041102  Respiratory rate | 1 | 2 | 3 | 4 | 5 | NA |
| 041103  Respiratory rhythm | 1 | 2 | 3 | 4 | 5 | NA |
| 041104  Depth of inspiration | 1 | 2 | 3 | 4 | 5 | NA |
| 041105  Lung compliance | 1 | 2 | 3 | 4 | 5 | NA |
| 041106  Tidal volume | 1 | 2 | 3 | 4 | 5 | NA |
| 041107  Vital capacity | 1 | 2 | 3 | 4 | 5 | NA |
| 041108  $FiO_2$* meets oxygen demand | 1 | 2 | 3 | 4 | 5 | NA |
| 041109  $PaO_2$* | 1 | 2 | 3 | 4 | 5 | NA |
| 041110  $PaCO_2$* | 1 | 2 | 3 | 4 | 5 | NA |
| 041111  Arterial pH | 1 | 2 | 3 | 4 | 5 | NA |
| 041112  Oxygen saturation | 1 | 2 | 3 | 4 | 5 | NA |
| 041113  Peripheral tissue perfusion | 1 | 2 | 3 | 4 | 5 | NA |
| 041114  End tidal carbon dioxide | 1 | 2 | 3 | 4 | 5 | NA |
| 041115  Pulmonary function tests | 1 | 2 | 3 | 4 | 5 | NA |
| 041116  Chest x-ray findings | 1 | 2 | 3 | 4 | 5 | NA |
| 041117  Ventilation perfusion balance | 1 | 2 | 3 | 4 | 5 | NA |
| 041118  Integrity of lips and oral mucosa | 1 | 2 | 3 | 4 | 5 | NA |
| 041119  Integrity of nasal pharyngeal structures | 1 | 2 | 3 | 4 | 5 | NA |
| 041120  Integrity of tracheostomy site | 1 | 2 | 3 | 4 | 5 | NA |
| 041121  Able to communicate needs | 1 | 2 | 3 | 4 | 5 | NA |

| | Severe | Substantial | Moderate | Mild | None | |
|---|---|---|---|---|---|---|
| 041122  Asymmetrical chest wall movement | 1 | 2 | 3 | 4 | 5 | NA |
| 041123  Asymmetrical chest wall expansion | 1 | 2 | 3 | 4 | 5 | NA |
| 041124  Difficulty breathing with ventilator | 1 | 2 | 3 | 4 | 5 | NA |
| 041125  Anxiety | 1 | 2 | 3 | 4 | 5 | NA |

Type and mode of ventilation_____

*$FiO_2$ = fraction of inspired oxygen; $PaO_2$ = partial pressure of oxygen in arterial blood; $PaCO_2$ = partial pressure of carbon dioxide in arterial blood.

*3rd edition*

*Continued*

## Outcome Content References:

Abel, M., (2001). Fast track protocol for patients undergoing cardiopulmonary bypass. Fast track protocol – Anesthesiology Department Website, Mayo Medical Center; http://anesthesia.mayo.edu/DIVISIONS/cvt/Procedures/FastTrackProtoco.htm.

Bickley, L.S., & Hoekelman, R.A. (1998). *Bates' guide to physical examination and history taking* (7th ed.). Philadelphia: Lippincott.

Chlan, L., (2000). Music therapy as a nursing intervention for patients supported by mechanical ventilation. *AACN Clinical Issues, 11*(1), 128-138.

Coates, L., (2000). Care of the ventilated patient. *Nursing Standard, 14*(28), 60.

Hanneman, S., (1999). Protocols for practice, applying research at the bedside. *Critical Care Nurse, 9*(5), 86-89.

Henderson, N. (1999). Mechanical ventilation. *Nursing Standard, 13*(44), 49-54.

Kelly-Heidenthal, P., & O'Connor, M. (1994). Nursing assessment of portable AP chest x-rays. *Dimensions of Critical Care Nursing, 13*(3), 127-132.

**M**

## Mechanical Ventilation Weaning Response: Adult (0412)

Domain-Physiologic Health (II)

Class-Cardiopulmonary (E)

Scale(s)-Severely compromised to Not compromised (a) and Severe to None (n)

Care Recipient:

Data Source:

**Definition:** Respiratory and psychological adjustment to progressive removal of mechanical ventilation

OUTCOME TARGET RATING:  Maintain at_____  Increase to_____

| Mechanical Ventilation Weaning Response: Adult Overall Rating | Severely compromised 1 | Substantially compromised 2 | Moderately compromised 3 | Mildly compromised 4 | Not compromised 5 | |
|---|---|---|---|---|---|---|
| INDICATORS: | | | | | | |
| 041201 Drive to breathe | 1 | 2 | 3 | 4 | 5 | NA |
| 041202 Spontaneous respiratory rate | 1 | 2 | 3 | 4 | 5 | NA |
| 041203 Spontaneous respiratory rhythm | 1 | 2 | 3 | 4 | 5 | NA |
| 041204 Spontaneous respiratory depth | 1 | 2 | 3 | 4 | 5 | NA |
| 041205 Apical heart rate | 1 | 2 | 3 | 4 | 5 | NA |
| 041206 Intact gag reflex | 1 | 2 | 3 | 4 | 5 | NA |
| 041207 Intact cough reflex | 1 | 2 | 3 | 4 | 5 | NA |
| 041208 $PaO_2$* | 1 | 2 | 3 | 4 | 5 | NA |
| 041209 $PaCO_2$* | 1 | 2 | 3 | 4 | 5 | NA |
| 041210 Arterial pH | 1 | 2 | 3 | 4 | 5 | NA |
| 041211 Oxygen saturation | 1 | 2 | 3 | 4 | 5 | NA |
| 041212 Vital capacity | 1 | 2 | 3 | 4 | 5 | NA |
| 041213 Tidal volume | 1 | 2 | 3 | 4 | 5 | NA |
| 041214 Minute ventilation <10 L/minute | 1 | 2 | 3 | 4 | 5 | NA |
| 041215 Positive end expiratory pressure | 1 | 2 | 3 | 4 | 5 | NA |
| 041216 Response to setting changes in mechanical ventilation | 1 | 2 | 3 | 4 | 5 | NA |
| 041217 Chest abdominal synchrony | 1 | 2 | 3 | 4 | 5 | NA |
| 041218 Auscultated breath sounds | 1 | 2 | 3 | 4 | 5 | NA |
| 041219 Chest x-ray findings | 1 | 2 | 3 | 4 | 5 | NA |
| 041220 Ventilation perfusion balance | 1 | 2 | 3 | 4 | 5 | NA |
| 041221 Comfort | 1 | 2 | 3 | 4 | 5 | NA |
| 041222 Able to communicate needs | 1 | 2 | 3 | 4 | 5 | NA |

M

| Mechanical Ventilation Weaning Response: Adult—cont'd | | Severe | Substantial | Moderate | Mild | None | |
|---|---|---|---|---|---|---|---|
| 041223 | Difficulty breathing on own | 1 | 2 | 3 | 4 | 5 | NA |
| 041224 | Respiratory secretions | 1 | 2 | 3 | 4 | 5 | NA |
| 041225 | Anxiety | 1 | 2 | 3 | 4 | 5 | NA |
| 041226 | Fear | 1 | 2 | 3 | 4 | 5 | NA |

*$PaO_2$ = partial pressure of oxygen in arterial blood; $PaCO_2$ = partial pressure of carbon dioxide in arterial blood.

*3rd edition*

Outcome Content References:

Abel, M., (2001). Fast track protocol for patients undergoing cardiopulmonary bypass. Fast track protocol – Anesthesiology Department Website, Mayo Medical Center;
   http://anesthesia.mayo.edu/DIVISIONS/cvt/Procedures/ FastTrackProtoco.htm.

Burns, S.M., et al. (1991). Weaning from mechanical ventilation: A method for assessment and intervention. *AACN Clinical Issues for Critical Care Nurses, 2*(3), 372-387.

Chlan, L., (2000). Music therapy as a nursing intervention for patients supported by mechanical ventilation. *AACN Clinical Issues, 11*(1), 128-138.

Coates, L., (2000). Care of the ventilated patient. *Nursing Standard, 14*(28), 60.

Hanneman, S., (1999). Protocols for practice, applying research at the bedside. *Critical Care Nurse, 9*(5), 86-89.

Henderson, N., (1999). Mechanical ventilation. *Nursing Standard, 13*(44), 49-54.

Kelly-Heidenthal, P., & O'Connor, M., (1994). Nursing assessment of portable AP chest x-rays. *Dimensions of Critical Care Nursing, 13*(3), 127-132.

Morganroth, M.L., et al. (1984). Criteria for weaning from prolonged mechanical ventilation. *Archives Internal Medicine, 144*(5), 1012-1016.

Urban, N., Greenlee, K., Krumberger, J., & Winkelman, C. (1995). *Guidelines for Critical Care Nursing.* Mosby: St. Louis.

Yang, K.L., & Tobin, M.J. (1991). A prospective study of indexes predicting the outcome trials of weaning a patient from mechanical ventilation. *New England Journal of Medicine, 324*(21), 1445-1450.

**M**

# *Medication Response (2301)*

*Domain-Physiologic Health (II)*
*Class-Therapeutic Response (a)*
*Scale(s)-Severely compromised to Not compromised (a) and Severe to None (n)*

*Care Recipient:*
*Data Source:*

**Definition:** Therapeutic and adverse effects of prescribed medication

OUTCOME TARGET RATING:    Maintain at_____    Increase to_____

| Medication Response Overall Rating | Severely compromised 1 | Substantially compromised 2 | Moderately compromised 3 | Mildly compromised 4 | Not compromised 5 | |
|---|---|---|---|---|---|---|
| **INDICATORS:** | | | | | | |
| 230101 Expected thera-peutic effects | 1 | 2 | 3 | 4 | 5 | NA |
| 230102 Expected change in blood chemistries | 1 | 2 | 3 | 4 | 5 | NA |
| 230103 Expected change in symptoms | 1 | 2 | 3 | 4 | 5 | NA |
| 230104 Maintenance of therapeutic blood levels of medication | 1 | 2 | 3 | 4 | 5 | NA |
| | **Severe** | **Substantial** | **Moderate** | **Mild** | **None** | |
| 230105 Allergic reaction | 1 | 2 | 3 | 4 | 5 | NA |
| 230106 Adverse effects | 1 | 2 | 3 | 4 | 5 | NA |
| 230107 Drug interaction | 1 | 2 | 3 | 4 | 5 | NA |
| 230108 Drug intolerance | 1 | 2 | 3 | 4 | 5 | NA |

*2nd edition 2000; Revised 3rd edition*

## Outcome Content References:

Arnold, G.J. (1998). Clinical recognition of adverse drug reactions: Obstacles and opportunities for the nursing profession. *Journal of Nursing Care Quality, 13*(2), 45-55.

Hodgson, B.B., & Kizior, R.J. (2003). *Saunders nursing drug book 2003* (3rd ed.). Philadelphia: W.B. Saunders.

Katzung, B.G. (Ed.). (2000). *Basic and clinical pharmacology* (8th ed.). Norwalk, CT: Appleton & Lange.

Shannon, M.T., Wilson, B.A., & Stang, C.L. (1995). *Drugs and nursing implications* (8th ed.). Norwalk, CT: Appleton & Lange.

Springhouse. (1998). *Nurse practitioner's drug handbook* (2nd ed.). Springhouse, PA: Author.

# Memory (0908)

Domain-Physiologic Health (II)                                  Care Recipient:

Class-Neurocognitive (J)                                        Data Source:

Scale(s)-Severely compromised to Not compromised (a)

**Definition:** Ability to cognitively retrieve and report previously stored information

OUTCOME TARGET RATING:     Maintain at_____     Increase to_____

| Memory Overall Rating | Severely compromised 1 | Substantially compromised 2 | Moderately compromised 3 | Mildly compromised 4 | Not compromised 5 | |
|---|---|---|---|---|---|---|
| **INDICATORS:** | | | | | | |
| 090801 Recalls immediate information accurately | 1 | 2 | 3 | 4 | 5 | NA |
| 090802 Recalls recent information accurately | 1 | 2 | 3 | 4 | 5 | NA |
| 090803 Recalls remote information accurately | 1 | 2 | 3 | 4 | 5 | NA |

*1st edition 1997; Revised 3rd edition*

Outcome Content References:

Abraham, I., & Reel, S. (1993). Cognitive nursing interventions with long-term residents: Effects on neurocognitive dimensions. *Archives of Psychiatric Nursing, 6*(6), 356-365.

Agostinelli, B., Demers, K., Garrigan, D., & Waszynski, C. (1994). Targeted interventions: Use of the Mini-Mental State Exam. *Journal of Gerontological Nursing, 20*(8), 15-23.

Costa, P.T. Jr., Williams, T.F., Somerfield, M., et al. (1996). *Recognition and initial assessment of Alzheimer's disease and related dementias.* No. 19. (AHCPR Publication No. 97-0702). Rockville, MD: U.S. Department of Health and Human Services. Public Health Services, Agency for Health Care Policy and Research.

Dellasega, C. (1992). Home health nurses' assessments of cognition. *Applied Nursing Research, 5*(3), 127-133.

Foreman, M., Theis, S., & Anderson, M.A. (1993). Adverse events in the hospitalized elderly. *Clinical Nursing Research, 2*(3), 360-370.

Gerdner, L.A., & Hall, G.R. (2001). Chronic confusion. In M. Maas, K. Buckwalter, M. Hardy, T. Tripp-Reimer, M. Titler, & J. Specht (Eds.), *Nursing care of older adults: Diagnoses, outcomes & interventions* (pp. 421-441). St. Louis: Mosby.

Mason, P. (1989). Cognitive assessment parameters and tools for the critically injured adult. *Critical Care Nursing Clinics of North America, 1*(1), 45-53.

+Pfeiffer, E. (1975). A short portable mental status questionnaire for the assessment of organic brain deficit in elderly patients. *American Geriatrics Society, 23*(10), 433-441.

Strub, R.L., & Black, F.W. (2000). *The mental status examination in neurology* (4th ed.). Philadelphia: F.A. Davis.

**M**

# *Mobility (0208)*

Domain-Functional Health (I)                                    Care Recipient:

Class-Mobility (C)                                              Data Source:

Scale(s)-Severely compromised to Not compromised (a)

**Definition:** Ability to move purposefully in own environment independently with or without assistive device

OUTCOME TARGET RATING:      Maintain at_____      Increase to_____

| Mobility Overall Rating | Severely compromised 1 | Substantially compromised 2 | Moderately compromised 3 | Mildly compromised 4 | Not compromised 5 | |
|---|---|---|---|---|---|---|

INDICATORS:

| | | | | | | |
|---|---|---|---|---|---|---|
| 020801 | Balance | 1 | 2 | 3 | 4 | 5 | NA |
| 020809 | Coordination | 1 | 2 | 3 | 4 | 5 | NA |
| 020810 | Gait | 1 | 2 | 3 | 4 | 5 | NA |
| 020803 | Muscle movement | 1 | 2 | 3 | 4 | 5 | NA |
| 020804 | Joint movement | 1 | 2 | 3 | 4 | 5 | NA |
| 020802 | Body positioning performance | 1 | 2 | 3 | 4 | 5 | NA |
| 020805 | Transfer performance | 1 | 2 | 3 | 4 | 5 | NA |
| 020811 | Running | 1 | 2 | 3 | 4 | 5 | NA |
| 020812 | Jumping | 1 | 2 | 3 | 4 | 5 | NA |
| 020813 | Crawling | | | | | | |
| 020806 | Walking | 1 | 2 | 3 | 4 | 5 | NA |
| 020814 | Moves with ease | 1 | 2 | 3 | 4 | 5 | NA |

*1st edition 1997; Revised 3rd edition (formerly Mobility Level)*

Outcome Content References:

Gresham, G.E., Duncan, P.W., Stason, W.B., et al. (1995). *Post-stroke Rehabilitation. Clinical practice guideline*, No. 16. (AHCPR Publication No. 95-0062). Rockville, MD: U.S. Department of Health and Human Services. Public Health Services, Agency for Health Care Policy and Research.

Maas, M.L., & Specht, J.P. (2001). Impaired physical mobility. In M. Maas, K. Buckwalter, M. Hardy, T. Tripp-Reimer, M. Titler, & J. Specht (Eds.), *Nursing care of older adults: Diagnoses, outcomes & interventions* (pp. 337-365). St. Louis: Mosby.

+Podsiadlo, D. & Richardson, S. (1991). The timed "Up & Go": A test of basic functional mobility for frail elderly persons. *Journal of American Geriatrics Society, 39*(2), 142-148.

Rukenstein, L.Z., Wieland, D., & Bernakei, R. (Eds.). (1995). *Geriatric assessment technology: The state of the art.* New York: Springer.

# Mood Equilibrium (1204)

*Domain-Psychosocial Health (III)*

*Class-Psychological Well-Being (M)*

*Care Recipient:*

*Data Source:*

*Scale(s)-Never demonstrated to Consistently demonstrated (m) and Consistently demonstrated to Never demonstrated (t)*

**Definition:** Appropriate adjustment of prevailing emotional tone in response to circumstances

OUTCOME TARGET RATING:    Maintain at_____    Increase to_____

| Mood Equilibrium Overall Rating | Never demonstrated 1 | Rarely demonstrated 2 | Sometimes demonstrated 3 | Often demonstrated 4 | Consistently demonstrated 5 | |
|---|---|---|---|---|---|---|
| INDICATORS: | | | | | | |
| 120401 Exhibits appropriate affect | 1 | 2 | 3 | 4 | 5 | NA |
| 120402 Exhibits non-labile mood | 1 | 2 | 3 | 4 | 5 | NA |
| 120403 Exhibits impulse control | 1 | 2 | 3 | 4 | 5 | NA |
| 120404 Reports adequate sleep (at least 5 hr/24 hr) | 1 | 2 | 3 | 4 | 5 | NA |
| 120405 Exhibits concentration | 1 | 2 | 3 | 4 | 5 | NA |
| 120406 Speaks at moderate pace | 1 | 2 | 3 | 4 | 5 | NA |
| 120410 Exhibits appropriate grooming and hygiene | 1 | 2 | 3 | 4 | 5 | NA |
| 120411 Wears appropriate clothing for situation and weather | 1 | 2 | 3 | 4 | 5 | NA |
| 120412 Maintains stable weight | 1 | 2 | 3 | 4 | 5 | NA |
| 120413 Exhibits normal appetite | 1 | 2 | 3 | 4 | 5 | NA |
| 120414 Reports compliance with medication and therapeutic regimen | 1 | 2 | 3 | 4 | 5 | NA |
| 120415 Shows interest in surroundings | 1 | 2 | 3 | 4 | 5 | NA |
| 120417 Exhibits appropriate energy level | 1 | 2 | 3 | 4 | 5 | NA |
| 120418 Accomplishes daily tasks | 1 | 2 | 3 | 4 | 5 | NA |

| | Consistently demonstrated | Often demonstrated | Sometimes demonstrated | Rarely demonstrated | Never demonstrated | |
|---|---|---|---|---|---|---|
| 120407 Flight of ideas | 1 | 2 | 3 | 4 | 5 | NA |
| 120408 Grandiosity | 1 | 2 | 3 | 4 | 5 | NA |
| 120409 Euphoria | 1 | 2 | 3 | 4 | 5 | NA |
| 120416 Suicide ideation | 1 | 2 | 3 | 4 | 5 | NA |
| 120420 Depression | 1 | 2 | 3 | 4 | 5 | NA |
| 120421 Lethargy | 1 | 2 | 3 | 4 | 5 | NA |
| 120422 Hyperactivity | 1 | 2 | 3 | 4 | 5 | NA |

*1st edition 1997; Revised 3rd edition*

M

*Continued*

Outcome Content References:

George, L.K., Blazer, D.B., Hughes, D.C., & Fowler N. (1989). Social support and the outcome of major depression. *British Journal of Psychiatry, 154,* 478-485.

Keitner, G.I., & Miller, I.W. (1990). Family functioning and major depression: An overview. *American Journal of Psychiatry, 147*(9), 1128-1137.

Maynard, C.K. (1993). Comparison of effectiveness of group interventions for depression in women. *Archives of Psychiatric Nursing, 7*(5), 277-283.

Maynard, C. (1993). Psychoeducational approach to depression in women. *Journal of Psychosocial Nursing and Mental Health Services, 31*(12), 9-14.

Piven, M.L., & Buckwalter, K.C. (2001). Depression. In M. Maas, K. Buckwalter, M. Hardy, T. Tripp-Reimer, M. Titler, & J. Specht (Eds.), *Nursing care of older adults: Diagnoses, outcomes & interventions* (pp. 521-542). St. Louis: Mosby.

Porth, C.M. (2002). *Pathophysiology: Concepts of altered health states* (6th ed.). Philadelphia: Lippincott Williams & Wilkins.

Stuart, G.W., & Laraia, M.T. (2001). *Principles and practice of psychiatric nursing* (7th ed.). St. Louis: Mosby.

+Underwood, B., & Froming, W.J. (1980). The Mood Survey: A personality measure of happy and sad moods. *Journal of Personality Assessment, 44*(4), 404-413.

U.S. Department of Health and Human Services. (1993). *Depression in primary care: Detection and diagnosis (Vol. 1)* (AHCPR Publication No. 93-0550). Rockville, MD: Public Health Service Agency for Health Care Policy and Research.

U.S. Department of Health and Human Services. (1993). *Depression in primary care: Treatment of major depression (Vol. 2)* (AHCPR Publication No. 93-0551). Rockville, MD: Public Health Service Agency for Health Care Policy and Research.

**M**

# Motivation (1209)

Domain-Psychosocial Health (III)

Class-Psychological Well-Being (M)

Scale(s)-Never demonstrated to Consistently demonstrated (m)

Care Recipient:

Data Source:

**Definition:** Inner urge that moves or prompts an individual to positive action(s)

OUTCOME TARGET RATING:    Maintain at_____    Increase to_____

| Motivation Overall Rating | Never demonstrated 1 | Rarely demonstrated 2 | Sometimes demonstrated 3 | Often demonstrated 4 | Consistently demonstrated 5 | |
|---|---|---|---|---|---|---|

INDICATORS:

| | | | | | | | |
|---|---|---|---|---|---|---|---|
| 120901 | Plans for the future | 1 | 2 | 3 | 4 | 5 | NA |
| 120902 | Develops an action plan | 1 | 2 | 3 | 4 | 5 | NA |
| 120903 | Obtains needed resources | 1 | 2 | 3 | 4 | 5 | NA |
| 120904 | Obtains needed support | 1 | 2 | 3 | 4 | 5 | NA |
| 120905 | Self-initiates goal directed behavior | 1 | 2 | 3 | 4 | 5 | NA |
| 120906 | Seeks new experiences | 1 | 2 | 3 | 4 | 5 | NA |
| 120907 | Maintains positive self-esteem | 1 | 2 | 3 | 4 | 5 | NA |
| 120908 | Welcomes opportunity to make contributions | 1 | 2 | 3 | 4 | 5 | NA |
| 120909 | Demonstrates flexibility | 1 | 2 | 3 | 4 | 5 | NA |
| 120910 | Expresses belief in ability to perform action | 1 | 2 | 3 | 4 | 5 | NA |
| 120911 | Expresses that performance will lead to desired outcome | 1 | 2 | 3 | 4 | 5 | NA |
| 120912 | Completes tasks or activities | 1 | 2 | 3 | 4 | 5 | NA |
| 120913 | Accepts responsibility for actions | 1 | 2 | 3 | 4 | 5 | NA |
| 120914 | Anticipates intrinsic and extrinsic reward | 1 | 2 | 3 | 4 | 5 | NA |
| 120915 | Expresses intent to act | 1 | 2 | 3 | 4 | 5 | NA |

M

*3rd edition*

Outcome Content References:

Ellis, J. R., & Hartley, C. L. (1999). *Managing and coordinating nursing care* (3rd ed.). Philadelphia: Lippincott.

Glickstein, J. (1990). Motivation in geriatric rehabilitation. *Focus on Geriatric Care and Rehabilitation, 3*(8), 1-3.

Mali, P. (1978). *Improving total productivity: MBO strategies for business, government, and not-for-profit organizations.* New York: Wiley.

Marriner-Tomey, A. (1996). *Guide to Nursing Management and Leadership* (5th ed.). St. Louis: Mosby.

Resnick, B. (1998). Motivating older adults to perform functional activities. *Journal of Gerontological Nursing, 24*(11), 23-20.

Resnick, B., Zimmerman, S. I., Magaziner, J., & Adelman, A. (1998). Use of the apathy evaluation scale as a measure of motivation in elderly people. *Rehabilitation Nursing, 23*(3), 141-147.

Vroom, V. (1964). *Work and motivation.* New York: Wiley.

# *Nausea & Vomiting Control (1618)*

*Domain-Health Knowledge & Behavior (IV)*

*Class-Health Behavior (Q)*

*Scale-Never demonstrated to Consistently demonstrated (m)*

Care Recipient:

Data Source:

**Definition:** Personal actions to control nausea, retching, and vomiting symptoms

OUTCOME TARGET RATING:   Maintain at_____   Increase to_____

| Nausea & Vomiting Control Overall Rating | | Never demonstrated 1 | Rarely demonstrated 2 | Sometimes demonstrated 3 | Often demonstrated 4 | Consistently demonstrated 5 | |
|---|---|---|---|---|---|---|---|
| **INDICATORS:** | | | | | | | |
| 161801 | Recognizes onset of nausea | 1 | 2 | 3 | 4 | 5 | NA |
| 161802 | Describes causal factors | 1 | 2 | 3 | 4 | 5 | NA |
| 161803 | Recognizes precipitating stimuli | 1 | 2 | 3 | 4 | 5 | NA |
| 161804 | Uses diary to monitor symptoms over time | 1 | 2 | 3 | 4 | 5 | NA |
| 161805 | Uses preventive measures | 1 | 2 | 3 | 4 | 5 | NA |
| 161806 | Avoids causal factors when possible | 1 | 2 | 3 | 4 | 5 | NA |
| 161807 | Avoids disagreeable odors | 1 | 2 | 3 | 4 | 5 | NA |
| 161808 | Uses antiemetic medications appropriately | 1 | 2 | 3 | 4 | 5 | NA |
| 161809 | Reports failure of antiemetic regimen | 1 | 2 | 3 | 4 | 5 | NA |
| 161810 | Reports bothersome side effects from antiemetics | 1 | 2 | 3 | 4 | 5 | NA |
| 161811 | Reports uncontrolled symptoms to health care professional | 1 | 2 | 3 | 4 | 5 | NA |
| 161812 | Reports nausea, retching, and vomiting controlled | 1 | 2 | 3 | 4 | 5 | NA |

*3rd edition*

Outcome Content References:

Brown, J.K., & Hogan, C.M. (1990). Chemotherapy. In S.L. Groenwald, M.H. Frogge, M. Goodman, & C.H. Yarbro (Eds.), *Cancer nursing: Principles and practice* (pp. 230-283). Boston: Jones & Bartlett.

Engstrom, C., Hernandez, I., Haywood, J., & Lilenbaum, R. (1999). The efficacy and cost effectiveness of new antiemetic guidelines. *Oncology Nursing Forum, 26*(9), 1453-1458.

Houston, D. (1997). Supportive therapies for cancer chemotherapy patients and the role of the oncology nurse. *Cancer Nursing, 20*(6), 409-413.

Nolte, J.J., Berkery, R., Pizzo, B., Baltzer, L., Grossano, D., Lucarelli, C.D., & Kris, M.G. (1998). Assuring the optimal use of serotonin antagonist antiemetics: The process for development and implementation of institutional antiemetic guidelines at Memorial Sloan-Kettering Cancer Center. *Journal of Clinical Oncology, 16*(2), 771-778.

Rhodes, V.A., McDaniel, R.W., Simms, S.G., & Johnson, M. (1995). Nurses' perceptions of antiemetic effectiveness. *Oncology Nursing Forum, 22*(8), 1243-1252.

Wickham, R. (1999). Nausea and vomiting. In C.H. Yarbro, M.H. Frogge, & M. Goodman (Eds.), *Cancer symptom management* (pp. 228-263). Boston: Jones & Bartlett.

## *Nausea & Vomiting: Disruptive Effects (2106)*

Domain-Perceived Health (V)                                        Care Recipient:

Class-Symptom Status (V)                                           Data Source:

Scale(s)-Severe to None (n)

**Definition:** Severity of observed or reported disruptive effects of nausea, retching, and vomiting on daily functioning

OUTCOME TARGET RATING:        Maintain at_____    Increase to_____

| Nausea & Vomiting: Disruptive Effects<br>Overall Rating | Severe<br>1 | Substantial<br>2 | Moderate<br>3 | Mild<br>4 | None<br>5 | |
|---|---|---|---|---|---|---|
| **INDICATORS:** | | | | | | |
| 210601 Decreased fluid intake | 1 | 2 | 3 | 4 | 5 | NA |
| 210602 Decreased food intake | 1 | 2 | 3 | 4 | 5 | NA |
| 210603 Decreased urinary output | 1 | 2 | 3 | 4 | 5 | NA |
| 210604 Altered fluid balance | 1 | 2 | 3 | 4 | 5 | NA |
| 210605 Altered serum electrolytes | 1 | 2 | 3 | 4 | 5 | NA |
| 210606 Altered acid/base balance | 1 | 2 | 3 | 4 | 5 | NA |
| 210607 Altered nutritional status | 1 | 2 | 3 | 4 | 5 | NA |
| 210608 Weight loss | 1 | 2 | 3 | 4 | 5 | NA |
| 210609 Malaise | 1 | 2 | 3 | 4 | 5 | NA |
| 210610 Lethargy | 1 | 2 | 3 | 4 | 5 | NA |
| 210611 Intolerance of movement | 1 | 2 | 3 | 4 | 5 | NA |
| 210612 Impaired physical activity | 1 | 2 | 3 | 4 | 5 | NA |
| 210613 Disrupted sleep | 1 | 2 | 3 | 4 | 5 | NA |
| 210614 Withdrawal from interpersonal relationships | 1 | 2 | 3 | 4 | 5 | NA |
| 210615 Impaired role performance | 1 | 2 | 3 | 4 | 5 | NA |
| 210616 Impaired work performance | 1 | 2 | 3 | 4 | 5 | NA |
| 210617 Interference with leisure, recreation, or social activities | 1 | 2 | 3 | 4 | 5 | NA |
| 210618 Interference with activities of daily living (ADLs) | 1 | 2 | 3 | 4 | 5 | NA |
| 210619 Anxiety | 1 | 2 | 3 | 4 | 5 | NA |
| 210620 Depression | 1 | 2 | 3 | 4 | 5 | NA |
| 210621 Emotional stress | 1 | 2 | 3 | 4 | 5 | NA |
| 210622 Helplessness | 1 | 2 | 3 | 4 | 5 | NA |
| 210623 Side effects from antiemetic medications | 1 | 2 | 3 | 4 | 5 | NA |
| 210624 Treatment delays due to symptom severity | 1 | 2 | 3 | 4 | 5 | NA |

*3rd edition*

### Outcome Content References:

Cotanch, P.H. (1988). Measuring nausea and vomiting. In M. Frank-Stromborg (Ed.), *Instruments for clinical nursing research* (pp. 313-321). Norwalk, CT: Appleton & Lange.

Engelking, C., Wickham, R., & Iwamoto, R. (1996). Cancer-related gastrointestinal symptoms: Dilemmas in assessment and management. *Developments in Supportive Cancer Care, 1*(1), 3-10.

Ezzone, S., Baker, C., Rosselet, R., & Terepka, E. (1998). Music as an adjunct to antiemetic therapy. *Oncology Nursing Forum, 25*(9), 1551-1556.

Low, K.G. (1996). Nausea and vomiting in pregnancy: A review of the research. *Journal of Gender, Culture, and Health, 1*(3), 151-172.

Rhodes, V.A., & McDaniel, R.W. (1997). Measuring nausea, vomiting, and retching. In M. Frank-Stromborg & S. J. Olsen (Eds.), *Instruments for Clinical Health-Care Research* (2nd ed., pp. 509-517). Boston: Jones & Bartlett.

Wickham, R. (1999). Nausea and vomiting. In C.H. Yarbro, M.H. Frogge, & M. Goodman (Eds.), *Cancer symptom management* (pp. 228-263). Boston: Jones & Bartlett.

# Nausea & Vomiting Severity (2107)

Domain-Perceived Health (V)

Class-Symptom Status (V)

Scale(s)-Severe to None (n)

Care Recipient:

Data Source:

**Definition:** Severity of nausea, retching, and vomiting symptoms

OUTCOME TARGET RATING:    Maintain at_____    Increase to_____

| Nausea & Vomiting Severity Overall Rating | Severe 1 | Substantial 2 | Moderate 3 | Mild 4 | None 5 | |
|---|---|---|---|---|---|---|
| INDICATORS: | | | | | | |
| 210701    Frequency of nausea | 1 | 2 | 3 | 4 | 5 | NA |
| 210702    Intensity of nausea | 1 | 2 | 3 | 4 | 5 | NA |
| 210703    Distress of nausea | 1 | 2 | 3 | 4 | 5 | NA |
| 210704    Frequency of retching | 1 | 2 | 3 | 4 | 5 | NA |
| 210705    Intensity of retching | 1 | 2 | 3 | 4 | 5 | NA |
| 210706    Distress of retching | 1 | 2 | 3 | 4 | 5 | NA |
| 210707    Frequency of vomiting | 1 | 2 | 3 | 4 | 5 | NA |
| 210708    Intensity of vomiting | 1 | 2 | 3 | 4 | 5 | NA |
| 210709    Distress of vomiting | 1 | 2 | 3 | 4 | 5 | NA |
| 210710    Excessive secretion of saliva | 1 | 2 | 3 | 4 | 5 | NA |
| 210711    Alteration in taste | 1 | 2 | 3 | 4 | 5 | NA |
| 210712    Intolerance of odors | 1 | 2 | 3 | 4 | 5 | NA |
| 210713    Weight loss | 1 | 2 | 3 | 4 | 5 | NA |
| 210714    Heartburn | 1 | 2 | 3 | 4 | 5 | NA |
| 210715    Gastric pain | 1 | 2 | 3 | 4 | 5 | NA |
| 210716    Projectile vomiting | 1 | 2 | 3 | 4 | 5 | NA |
| 210717    Blood in emesis | 1 | 2 | 3 | 4 | 5 | NA |
| 210718    Coffee ground emesis | 1 | 2 | 3 | 4 | 5 | NA |
| 210719    Fecal odor of emesis | 1 | 2 | 3 | 4 | 5 | NA |

Duration of nausea: ____(hours) ____(days) ____(months)

Amount of emesis _____(cc)

*3rd edition*

Outcome Content References:

Cotanch, P.H. (1988). Measuring nausea and vomiting. In M. Frank-Stromborg (Ed.), *Instruments for clinical nursing research* (pp. 313-321). Norwalk, CT: Appleton & Lange.

Engstrom, C., Hernandez, I., Haywood, J., & Lilenbaum, R. (1999). The efficacy and cost effectiveness of new antiemetic guidelines. *Oncology Nursing Forum, 26*(9), 1453-1458.

Rhodes, V.A., & McDaniel, R.W. (1997). Measuring nausea, vomiting, and retching. In M. Frank-Stromborg & S.J. Olsen (Eds.), *Instruments for clinical health-care research* (2nd ed., pp. 509-517). Boston: Jones & Bartlett.

Rhodes, V.A., & McDaniel, R.W. (1999). The index of nausea, vomiting, and retching: A new format of the index of nausea and vomiting. *Oncology Nursing Forum, 26*(5), 889-894.

Wickham, R. (1999). Nausea and vomiting. In C. H. Yarbro, M.H. Frogge, & M. Goodman (Eds.), *Cancer symptom management* (pp. 228-263). Boston: Jones & Bartlett.

N

# Neglect Cessation (2513)

Domain-Family Health (VI)

Class-Family Member Health Status (Z)

Scale(s)-None to Extensive (i)

Care Recipient:

Data Source:

**Definition:** Evidence that the victim is no longer receiving substandard care

OUTCOME TARGET RATING:    Maintain at_____    Increase to_____

| Neglect Cessation Overall Rating | None 1 | Limited 2 | Moderate 3 | Substantial 4 | Extensive 5 | |
|---|---|---|---|---|---|---|

INDICATORS:

| | | None 1 | Limited 2 | Moderate 3 | Substantial 4 | Extensive 5 | |
|---|---|---|---|---|---|---|---|
| 251301 | Evidence that physical neglect has ceased | 1 | 2 | 3 | 4 | 5 | NA |
| 251302 | Evidence that emotional neglect has ceased | 1 | 2 | 3 | 4 | 5 | NA |
| 251303 | Evidence that financial neglect has ceased | 1 | 2 | 3 | 4 | 5 | NA |
| 251304 | Evidence that spiritual neglect has ceased | 1 | 2 | 3 | 4 | 5 | NA |
| 251305 | Evidence that healthcare neglect has ceased | 1 | 2 | 3 | 4 | 5 | NA |

*3rd edition*

Outcome Content References:

Aber, J.L., Allen, J.P., Carlson, V., & Cicchetti, D. (1990). The effects of maltreatment on development during early childhood: Recent studies and their theoretical, clinical, and policy implications. In D. Cicchetti & V. Carlson (Eds.), *Child maltreatment: Theory and research on the causes and consequences of child abuse and neglect* (pp. 579-619). New York: Cambridge University Press.

Cicchetti, D., & Carlson, V. (Eds.). (1989). *Child maltreatment: Theory and research on the causes and consequences of child abuse and neglect.* New York: Cambridge University Press.

Cowen, P.S. (2001). Elder mistreatment. In M. Maas, K. Buckwalter, M. Hardy, T. Tripp-Reimer, M. Titler, & J. Specht (Eds.), *Nursing care of older adults: Diagnoses, outcomes & interventions* (pp. 93-114). St. Louis: Mosby.

Fulmer, T., & Ashley, J. (1989). Clinical indicators of elder neglect. *Applied Nursing Research, 2*(4), 161-167.

Hudson, M.F., & Johnson, T.F. (1986). Elder neglect and abuse: A review of the literature [Monograph]. *Annual Review of Nursing Research, 6,* 81-134.

Lobo, M.L., Barnard, K.E., & Coombs, J.B. (1992). Failure to thrive: A parent-infant interaction perspective. *Journal of Pediatric Nursing, 7*(4), 251-261.

Olds, D.L., Henderson, C.R., Chamberlin, R., & Tatelbaum R. (1986). Preventing child abuse and neglect: A randomized trial of nurse home visitation. *Pediatrics, 78*(1), 65-78.

Silverman, J., & Hudson, M.F. (2000). Elder mistreatment: A guide for medical professionals. *North Carolina Medical Journal, 61*(5), 291-296.

Weinman, M.L., Schreiber, N.B., & Robinson, M. (1992). Adolescent mothers: Were there any gains in a parent education program? *Family and Community Health, 15*(3), 1-10.

Young, L. (1981). *Physical child neglect.* Chicago: The National Committee for Prevention of Child Abuse.

N

# Neglect Recovery (2512)

*Domain-Family Health (VI)*

*Class-Family Member Health Status (Z)*

*Scale(s)-None to Extensive (i) and Extensive to None (h)*

*Care Recipient:*

*Data Source:*

---

**Definition:** Extent of healing following the cessation of substandard care

OUTCOME TARGET RATING:    Maintain at_____    Increase to_____

| Neglect Recovery Overall Rating | None 1 | Limited 2 | Moderate 3 | Substantial 4 | Extensive 5 | |
|---|---|---|---|---|---|---|
| **INDICATORS:** | | | | | | |
| 251201 Maintenance of personal hygiene | 1 | 2 | 3 | 4 | 5 | NA |
| 251205 Appropriate clothing for weather | 1 | 2 | 3 | 4 | 5 | NA |
| 251206 Cleanliness of living environment | 1 | 2 | 3 | 4 | 5 | NA |
| 251207 Safety of living environment | 1 | 2 | 3 | 4 | 5 | NA |
| 251209 Provision of supervision required | 1 | 2 | 3 | 4 | 5 | NA |
| 251210 Demonstration of interest in life | 1 | 2 | 3 | 4 | 5 | NA |
| 251211 Expressions of pride in self | 1 | 2 | 3 | 4 | 5 | NA |
| 251212 Expressions of hope | 1 | 2 | 3 | 4 | 5 | NA |
| 251213 Timely meeting of emotional needs | 1 | 2 | 3 | 4 | 5 | NA |
| 251214 Provision of appropriate health care | 1 | 2 | 3 | 4 | 5 | NA |
| 251215 Provision of recommended diet | 1 | 2 | 3 | 4 | 5 | NA |
| 251216 Provision of recommended medication regimen | 1 | 2 | 3 | 4 | 5 | NA |
| 251217 Use of appropriate equipment or appliance | 1 | 2 | 3 | 4 | 5 | NA |
| 251220 Normal development | 1 | 2 | 3 | 4 | 5 | NA |
| 251218 Normal growth | 1 | 2 | 3 | 4 | 5 | NA |
| 251219 Provision of cognitive stimulation | 1 | 2 | 3 | 4 | 5 | NA |
| 251221 Expectations of responsibilities reasonable for age | 1 | 2 | 3 | 4 | 5 | NA |
| 251224 Consistency of behavior with social norms | 1 | 2 | 3 | 4 | 5 | NA |

| | Extensive | Substantial | Moderate | Limited | None | |
|---|---|---|---|---|---|---|
| 251202 Hunger | 1 | 2 | 3 | 4 | 5 | NA |
| 251208 Skin breakdown | 1 | 2 | 3 | 4 | 5 | NA |
| 251223 Substance abuse | 1 | 2 | 3 | 4 | 5 | NA |
| 251226 Inappropriate attention seeking behavior | 1 | 2 | 3 | 4 | 5 | NA |
| 251227 Fatigue | 1 | 2 | 3 | 4 | 5 | NA |
| 251228 Malnutrition | 1 | 2 | 3 | 4 | 5 | NA |
| 251229 Dehydration | 1 | 2 | 3 | 4 | 5 | NA |

*1st edition 1997, Revised 3rd edition*

## Outcome Content References:

Aber, J.L., Allen, J.P., Carlson, V., & Cicchetti, D. (1990). The effects of maltreatment on development during early childhood: Recent studies and their theoretical, clinical, and policy implications. In D. Cicchetti & V. Carlson (Eds.), *Child maltreatment: Theory and research on the causes and consequences of child abuse and neglect* (pp. 579-619). New York: Cambridge University Press.

Cicchetti, D., & Carlson, V. (Eds.). (1989). *Child maltreatment: Theory and research on the causes and consequences of child abuse and neglect*. New York: Cambridge University Press.

Cowen, P.S. (2001). Elder mistreatment. In M. Maas, K. Buckwalter, M. Hardy, T. Tripp-Reimer, M. Titler, & J. Specht (Eds.), *Nursing care of older adults: Diagnoses, outcomes & interventions* (pp. 93-114). St. Louis: Mosby.

Fulmer, T., & Ashley, J. (1989). Clinical indicators of elder neglect. *Applied Nursing Research, 2*(4), 161-167.

Fulmer, T., & Paveza, G. (1998). Neglect in the elderly patient. *Nursing Clinics of North America, 33*(3), 457-466.

Hudson, M.F., & Johnson, T.F. (1986). Elder neglect and abuse: A review of the literature [Monograph]. *Annual Review of Nursing Research, 6*, 81-134.

Lobo, M.L., Barnard, K.E., & Coombs, J.B. (1992). Failure to thrive: A parent-infant interaction perspective. *Journal of Pediatric Nursing, 7*(4), 251-261.

Olds, D.L., Henderson, C.R., Chamberlin, R., & Tatelbaum R. (1986). Preventing child abuse and neglect: A randomized trial of nurse home visitation. *Pediatrics, 78*(1), 65-78.

Polansky, N.A., Halley, C., & Polansky, N.F. (1977). *Profile of neglect: A survey of the state of knowledge*. Washington, DC: U.S. Department of Health, Education, and Welfare.

Weinman, M.L., Schreiber, N.B., & Robinson, M. (1992). Adolescent mothers: Were there any gains in a parent education program? *Family and Community Health, 15*(3), 1-10.

Young, L. (1981). *Physical child neglect*. Chicago: The National Committee for Prevention of Child Abuse.

N

# *Neurological Status (0909)*

*Domain-Physiologic Health (II)*

*Class-Neurocognitive (J)*

*Scale(s)-Severely compromised to Not compromised (a) and Severe to None (n)*

Care Recipient:

Data Source:

**Definition:** Ability of the peripheral and central nervous system to receive, process, and respond to internal and external stimuli

OUTCOME TARGET RATING:   Maintain at_____   Increase to_____

| Neurological Status Overall Rating | Severely compromised 1 | Substantially compromised 2 | Moderately compromised 3 | Mildly compromised 4 | Not compromised 5 | |
|---|---|---|---|---|---|---|
| **INDICATORS:** | | | | | | |
| 090901 Consciousness | 1 | 2 | 3 | 4 | 5 | NA |
| 090902 Central motor control | 1 | 2 | 3 | 4 | 5 | NA |
| 090903 Cranial sensory/ motor function | 1 | 2 | 3 | 4 | 5 | NA |
| 090904 Spinal sensory/ motor function | 1 | 2 | 3 | 4 | 5 | NA |
| 090905 Autonomic function | 1 | 2 | 3 | 4 | 5 | NA |
| 090906 Intracranial pressure | 1 | 2 | 3 | 4 | 5 | NA |
| 090907 Communication appropriate to situation | 1 | 2 | 3 | 4 | 5 | NA |
| 090908 Pupil size | 1 | 2 | 3 | 4 | 5 | NA |
| 090909 Pupil reactivity | 1 | 2 | 3 | 4 | 5 | NA |
| 090910 Eye movement pattern | 1 | 2 | 3 | 4 | 5 | NA |
| 090911 Breathing pattern | 1 | 2 | 3 | 4 | 5 | NA |
| 090913 Rest-sleep pattern | 1 | 2 | 3 | 4 | 5 | NA |
| 090917 Blood pressure | 1 | 2 | 3 | 4 | 5 | NA |
| 090918 Pulse pressure | 1 | 2 | 3 | 4 | 5 | NA |
| 090919 Respiratory rate | 1 | 2 | 3 | 4 | 5 | NA |
| 090920 Hyperthermia | 1 | 2 | 3 | 4 | 5 | NA |
| 090921 Apical heart rate | 1 | 2 | 3 | 4 | 5 | NA |
| 090922 Radial pulse rate | 1 | 2 | 3 | 4 | 5 | NA |
| 090923 Cognitive orientation | 1 | 2 | 3 | 4 | 5 | NA |
| 090924 Cognitive ability | 1 | 2 | 3 | 4 | 5 | NA |
| | Severe | Substantial | Moderate | Mild | None | |
| 090914 Seizure activity | 1 | 2 | 3 | 4 | 5 | NA |
| 090915 Headaches | 1 | 2 | 3 | 4 | 5 | NA |

*1st edition 1997; Revised 3rd edition*

Outcome Content References:

American Nurses' Association Council on Medical-Surgical Nursing Practice and American Association of Neuroscience Nurses. (1986). *Neuroscience nursing practice: process and outcome criteria for selected diagnoses.* Washington, DC: Government Printing Office.

Gresham, G.E., Duncan, P.W., Stason, W.B., et al. (1995). *Post-stroke Rehabilitation. Clinical practice guideline*, No. 16. (AHCPR Publication No. 95-0062). Rockville, MD: U.S. Department of Health and Human Services. Public Health Services, Agency for Health Care Policy and Research.

Hickey, J.V. (2002). *The clinical practice of neurological and neurosurgical nursing* (5th ed.). Philadelphia: J.B. Lippincott.

Mitchell, P.H., Hodges, L.C., Muwaswes, M., & Walleck, C.A. (Eds.). (1988). *AANN's neuroscience nursing: phenomena and practice.* Norwalk, CT: Appleton & Lange.

Riess, P.C. (1995). *Validity and reliability of the Riess Intracranial Aneurysm Assessment Tool and the Glasgow Coma Scale in the aneurysm population.* Master's thesis, The University of Iowa, Iowa City.

Smeltzer, S.C., & Bare, B.G. (Eds.). (2003). *Brunner and Suddarth's textbook of medical-surgical nursing* (10th ed.). Philadelphia: Lippincott, Williams, & Wilkins.

+Teasdale, G., & Jennett, B. (1974). Assessment of coma and impaired consciousness: A practical scale. *Lancet, 2,* 81-84.

**N**

# *Neurological Status: Autonomic (0910)*

Domain-Physiologic Health (II)

Class-Neurocognitive (J)

Scale(s)-Severely compromised to Not compromised (a) and Severe to None (n)

Care Recipient:

Data Source:

**Definition:** Ability of the autonomic nervous system to coordinate visceral and homeostatic function

OUTCOME TARGET RATING:    Maintain at_____    Increase to_____

| Neurological Status: Autonomic Overall Rating | Severely compromised 1 | Substantially compromised 2 | Moderately compromised 3 | Mildly compromised 4 | Not compromised 5 | |
|---|---|---|---|---|---|---|
| INDICATORS: | | | | | | |
| 091001 Apical heart rate | 1 | 2 | 3 | 4 | 5 | NA |
| 091020 Radial pulse rate | 1 | 2 | 3 | 4 | 5 | NA |
| 091002 Systolic blood pressure | 1 | 2 | 3 | 4 | 5 | NA |
| 091003 Diastolic blood pressure | 1 | 2 | 3 | 4 | 5 | NA |
| 091004 Cardiac pump effectiveness | 1 | 2 | 3 | 4 | 5 | NA |
| 091005 Vasodilatation response | 1 | 2 | 3 | 4 | 5 | NA |
| 091006 Vasoconstriction response | 1 | 2 | 3 | 4 | 5 | NA |
| 091007 Perspiration response pattern | 1 | 2 | 3 | 4 | 5 | NA |
| 091008 Goose bumps response pattern | 1 | 2 | 3 | 4 | 5 | NA |
| 091009 Bowel elimination pattern | 1 | 2 | 3 | 4 | 5 | NA |
| 091010 Intestinal motility | 1 | 2 | 3 | 4 | 5 | NA |
| 091011 Urinary elimination pattern | 1 | 2 | 3 | 4 | 5 | NA |
| 091021 Pupil reactivity | 1 | 2 | 3 | 4 | 5 | NA |
| 091013 Thermoregulation | 1 | 2 | 3 | 4 | 5 | NA |
| 091014 Peripheral tissue perfusion | 1 | 2 | 3 | 4 | 5 | NA |
| 091015 Sexual organ response | 1 | 2 | 3 | 4 | 5 | NA |

| | Severe | Substantial | Moderate | Mild | None | |
|---|---|---|---|---|---|---|
| 091016 Bronchospasms | 1 | 2 | 3 | 4 | 5 | NA |
| 091017 Intestinal spasms | 1 | 2 | 3 | 4 | 5 | NA |
| 091018 Bladder spasms | 1 | 2 | 3 | 4 | 5 | NA |
| 091022 Headaches | 1 | 2 | 3 | 4 | 5 | NA |
| 091023 Dilated pupils | 1 | 2 | 3 | 4 | 5 | NA |
| 091024 Constricted pupils | 1 | 2 | 3 | 4 | 5 | NA |
| 091025 Hyperthermia | 1 | 2 | 3 | 4 | 5 | NA |
| 091026 Dysreflexia | 1 | 2 | 3 | 4 | 5 | NA |

*1st edition 1997; Revised 3rd edition*

Outcome Content References:

McCance, K.L., & Huether, S.E. (2002). *Pathophysiology: The biologic basis for disease in adults and children* (4th ed.). St. Louis: Mosby.

Smeltzer, S.C., & Bare, B.G. (Eds.). (2003). *Brunner and Suddarth's textbook of medical-surgical nursing* (10th ed.). Philadelphia: Lippincott, Williams, & Wilkins.

# *Neurological Status: Central Motor Control (0911)*

Domain-Physiologic Health (II)

Class-Neurocognitive (J)

Scale(s)-Severely compromised to Not compromised (a) and Severe to None (n)

Care Recipient:

Data Source:

**Definition:** Ability of the central nervous system to coordinate skeletal muscle activity for body movement

OUTCOME TARGET RATING:    Maintain at_____    Increase to_____

| Neurological Status: Central Motor Control Overall Rating | Severely compromised 1 | Substantially compromised 2 | Moderately compromised 3 | Mildly compromised 4 | Not compromised 5 | |
|---|---|---|---|---|---|---|
| **INDICATORS:** | | | | | | |
| 091101 Balance | 1 | 2 | 3 | 4 | 5 | NA |
| 091103 Maintenance of posture | 1 | 2 | 3 | 4 | 5 | NA |
| 091104 Infantile reflexes (automatisms) | 1 | 2 | 3 | 4 | 5 | NA |
| 091105 Babinski's reflex | 1 | 2 | 3 | 4 | 5 | NA |
| 091106 Deep tendon reflexes | 1 | 2 | 3 | 4 | 5 | NA |
| 091112 Purposeful movement on command | 1 | 2 | 3 | 4 | 5 | NA |
| | **Severe** | **Substantial** | **Moderate** | **Mild** | **None** | |
| 091113 Gait abnormalities | 1 | 2 | 3 | 4 | 5 | NA |
| 091107 Spasticity | 1 | 2 | 3 | 4 | 5 | NA |
| 091108 Involuntary movements | 1 | 2 | 3 | 4 | 5 | NA |
| 091109 Nystagmus | 1 | 2 | 3 | 4 | 5 | NA |
| 091110 Seizure activity | 1 | 2 | 3 | 4 | 5 | NA |

*1st edition 1997; Revised 3rd edition*

Outcome Content References:

American Nurses' Association Council on Medical-Surgical Nursing Practice and American Association of Neuroscience Nurses. (1986). *Neuroscience nursing practice: Process and outcome criteria for selected diagnoses.* Washington, DC: Government Printing Office.

Bickley, L. (2002). *Bates' guide to physical examination and history taking* (8th ed.). Philadelphia: Lippincott, Williams, & Wilkins.

Hickey, J.V. (2002). *The clinical practice of neurological and neurosurgical nursing* (5th ed.). Philadelphia: J.B. Lippincott.

Mitchell, P.H., Hodges, L.C., Muwaswes, M., & Walleck, C.A. (Eds.). (1988). *AANN's neuroscience nursing: Phenomena and practice.* Norwalk, CT: Appleton & Lange.

Smeltzer, S.C., & Bare, B.G. (Eds.). (2003). *Brunner and Suddarth's textbook of medical-surgical nursing* (10th ed.). Philadelphia: Lippincott, Williams, & Wilkins.

N

# Neurological Status: Consciousness (0912)

Domain-Physiologic Health (II)

Class-Neurocognitive (J)

Scale(s)-Severely compromised to Not compromised (a) and Severe to None (n)

Care Recipient:

Data Source:

**Definition:** Arousal, orientation, and attention to the environment

OUTCOME TARGET RATING:    Maintain at_____    Increase to_____

| Neurological Status: Consciousness Overall Rating | Severely compromised 1 | Substantially compromised 2 | Moderately compromised 3 | Mildly compromised 4 | Not compromised 5 | |
|---|---|---|---|---|---|---|
| **INDICATORS:** | | | | | | |
| 091201 Opens eyes to external stimuli | 1 | 2 | 3 | 4 | 5 | NA |
| 091202 Cognitive orientation | 1 | 2 | 3 | 4 | 5 | NA |
| 091203 Communication appropriate to situation | 1 | 2 | 3 | 4 | 5 | NA |
| 091204 Obeys commands | 1 | 2 | 3 | 4 | 5 | NA |
| 091205 Motor responses to noxious stimuli | 1 | 2 | 3 | 4 | 5 | NA |
| 091206 Attends to environmental stimuli | 1 | 2 | 3 | 4 | 5 | NA |
| | Severe | Substantial | Moderate | Mild | None | |
| 091207 Seizure activity | 1 | 2 | 3 | 4 | 5 | NA |
| 091209 Abnormal flexion | 1 | 2 | 3 | 4 | 5 | NA |
| 091210 Abnormal extension | 1 | 2 | 3 | 4 | 5 | NA |

Glasgow Coma Scale score_____

*1st edition 1997; Revised 3rd edition*

## Outcome Content References:

American Nurses' Association Council on Medical-Surgical Nursing Practice and American Association of Neuroscience Nurses. (1986). *Neuroscience nursing practice: Process and outcome criteria for selected diagnoses.* Washington, DC: Government Printing Office.

Hickey, J.V. (2002). *The clinical practice of neurological and neurosurgical nursing* (5th ed.). Philadelphia: J.B. Lippincott.

Mitchell, P.H., Hodges, L.C., Muwaswes, M., & Walleck, C.A. (Eds.). (1988). *AANN's neuroscience nursing: Phenomena and practice.* Norwalk, CT: Appleton & Lange.

Riess, P.C. (1995). *Validity and reliability of the Riess Intracranial Aneurysm Assessment Tool and the Glasgow Coma Scale in the aneurysm population.* Master's thesis, The University of Iowa: Iowa City.

Smeltzer, S.C., & Bare, B.G. (Eds.). (2003). *Brunner and Suddarth's textbook of medical-surgical nursing* (10th ed.). Philadelphia: Lippincott, Williams, & Wilkins.

# Neurological Status: Cranial Sensory/Motor Function (0913)

Domain-Physiologic Health (II)

Class-Neurocognitive (J)

Scale(s)-Severely compromised to Not compromised (a) and Severe to None (n)

Care Recipient:

Data Source

**Definition:** Ability of the cranial nerves to convey sensory and motor impulses

OUTCOME TARGET RATING:    Maintain at_____    Increase to_____

| Neurological Status: Cranial Sensory/Motor Function Overall Rating | Severely compromised 1 | Substantially compromised 2 | Moderately compromised 3 | Mildly compromised 4 | Not compromised 5 | |
|---|---|---|---|---|---|---|
| INDICATORS: | | | | | | |
| 091301 Olfaction | 1 | 2 | 3 | 4 | 5 | NA |
| 091302 Vision | 1 | 2 | 3 | 4 | 5 | NA |
| 091303 Corneal reflex | 1 | 2 | 3 | 4 | 5 | NA |
| 091304 Taste | 1 | 2 | 3 | 4 | 5 | NA |
| 091305 Hearing | 1 | 2 | 3 | 4 | 5 | NA |
| 091317 Speech | 1 | 2 | 3 | 4 | 5 | NA |
| 091306 Facial sensation | 1 | 2 | 3 | 4 | 5 | NA |
| 091307 Facial muscle movement | 1 | 2 | 3 | 4 | 5 | NA |
| 091318 Facial symmetry | 1 | 2 | 3 | 4 | 5 | NA |
| 091319 Bilateral muscle strength | 1 | 2 | 3 | 4 | 5 | NA |
| 091308 Swallowing | 1 | 2 | 3 | 4 | 5 | NA |
| 091309 Gag reflex | 1 | 2 | 3 | 4 | 5 | NA |
| 091310 Tongue movement | 1 | 2 | 3 | 4 | 5 | NA |
| 091312 Purposeful head movement | 1 | 2 | 3 | 4 | 5 | NA |
| 091320 Purposeful shoulder movement | 1 | 2 | 3 | 4 | 5 | NA |

| | Severe | Substantial | Moderate | Mild | None | |
|---|---|---|---|---|---|---|
| 091314 Dizziness | 1 | 2 | 3 | 4 | 5 | NA |
| 091315 Pronator drift | 1 | 2 | 3 | 4 | 5 | NA |
| 091321 Involuntary head movement | 1 | 2 | 3 | 4 | 5 | NA |
| 091322 Involuntary facial movement | 1 | 2 | 3 | 4 | 5 | NA |
| 091323 Tics | 1 | 2 | 3 | 4 | 5 | NA |
| 091324 Hoarseness | 1 | 2 | 3 | 4 | 5 | NA |
| 091325 Nasal tone to voice | 1 | 2 | 3 | 4 | 5 | NA |
| 091326 Unilateral facial paralysis | 1 | 2 | 3 | 4 | 5 | NA |

1st edition 1997; Revised 3rd edition

Outcome Content References:

Bickley, L. (2002). *Bates' guide to physical examination and history taking* (8th ed.). Philadelphia: Lippincott, Williams, & Wilkins.

McCance, K.L., & Huether, S.E. (2002). *Pathophysiology: The biologic basis for disease in adults and children* (4th ed.). St. Louis: Mosby.

Riess, P.C. (1995). *Validity and reliability of the Riess Intracranial Aneurysm Assessment Tool and the Glasgow Coma Scale in the aneurysm population.* Master's thesis, The University of Iowa: Iowa City.

Smeltzer, S.C., & Bare, B.G. (Eds.). (2003). *Brunner and Suddarth's textbook of medical-surgical nursing* (10th ed.). Philadelphia: Lippincott, Williams, & Wilkins.

N

# Neurological Status: Spinal Sensory/Motor Function (0914)

*Domain-Physiologic Health (II)*

*Class-Neurocognitive (J)*

*Scale(s)-Severely compromised to Not compromised (a) and Severe to None (n)*

*Care Recipient:*

*Data Source:*

**Definition:** Ability of the spinal nerves to convey sensory and motor impulses

OUTCOME TARGET RATING: Maintain at_____ Increase to_____

| Neurological Status: Spinal Sensory Motor/Function Overall Rating | Severely compromised 1 | Substantially compromised 2 | Moderately compromised 3 | Mildly compromised 4 | Not compromised 5 | |
|---|---|---|---|---|---|---|
| **INDICATORS:** | | | | | | |
| 091401 Head and shoulder movement | 1 | 2 | 3 | 4 | 5 | NA |
| 091402 Autonomic function | 1 | 2 | 3 | 4 | 5 | NA |
| 091403 Deep tendon reflexes | 1 | 2 | 3 | 4 | 5 | NA |
| 091404 Upper body skin sensation | 1 | 2 | 3 | 4 | 5 | NA |
| 091409 Lower body skin sensation | 1 | 2 | 3 | 4 | 5 | NA |
| 091405 Upper body strength | 1 | 2 | 3 | 4 | 5 | NA |
| 091410 Lower body strength | 1 | 2 | 3 | 4 | 5 | NA |
| | **Severe** | **Substantial** | **Moderate** | **Mild** | **None** | |
| 091406 Flaccidity | 1 | 2 | 3 | 4 | 5 | NA |
| 091407 Pronator drift | 1 | 2 | 3 | 4 | 5 | NA |
| 091411 Involuntary movement | 1 | 2 | 3 | 4 | 5 | NA |
| 091412 Fasciculation | 1 | 2 | 3 | 4 | 5 | NA |

*1st edition 1997; Revised 3rd edition*

**Outcome Content References:**

Bickley, L. (2002). *Bates' guide to physical examination and history taking* (8th ed.). Philadelphia: Lippincott, Williams, & Wilkins.

Riess, P.C. (1995). *Validity and reliability of the Riess Intracranial Aneurysm Assessment Tool and the Glasgow Coma Scale in the aneurysm population.* Master's thesis, The University of Iowa: Iowa City.

Smeltzer, S.C., & Bare, B.G. (Eds.). (2003). *Brunner and Suddarth's textbook of medical-surgical nursing* (10th ed.). Philadelphia: Lippincott, Williams, & Wilkins.

**N**

# Newborn Adaptation (0118)

*Domain-Functional Health (I)*

*Class-Growth & Development (B)*

*Scale(s)-Severe deviation from normal range to No deviation from normal range (b)*

*Care Recipient:*

*Data Source:*

**Definition:** Adaptive response to the extrauterine environment by a physiologically mature newborn during the first 28 days

OUTCOME TARGET RATING:   Maintain at_____   Increase to_____

| Newborn Adaptation Overall Rating | Severe deviation from normal range 1 | Substantial deviation from normal range 2 | Moderate deviation from normal range 3 | Mild deviation from normal range 4 | No deviation from normal range 5 | |
|---|---|---|---|---|---|---|
| **INDICATORS:** | | | | | | |
| 011801 Apgar score | 1 | 2 | 3 | 4 | 5 | NA |
| 011802 Gestational age index | 1 | 2 | 3 | 4 | 5 | NA |
| 011803 Apical heart rate (100-160) | 1 | 2 | 3 | 4 | 5 | NA |
| 011804 Respiratory rate (30-60) | 1 | 2 | 3 | 4 | 5 | NA |
| 011805 Blood pressure ratio of arm to leg | 1 | 2 | 3 | 4 | 5 | NA |
| 011806 Oxygen saturation >90% | 1 | 2 | 3 | 4 | 5 | NA |
| 011807 Thermoregulation | 1 | 2 | 3 | 4 | 5 | NA |
| 011808 Skin color | 1 | 2 | 3 | 4 | 5 | NA |
| 011809 Eyes clear | 1 | 2 | 3 | 4 | 5 | NA |
| 011810 Cord drying | 1 | 2 | 3 | 4 | 5 | NA |
| 011811 Weight | 1 | 2 | 3 | 4 | 5 | NA |
| 011812 Feeding tolerance | 1 | 2 | 3 | 4 | 5 | NA |
| 011813 Suck reflex | 1 | 2 | 3 | 4 | 5 | NA |
| 011814 Muscle tone | 1 | 2 | 3 | 4 | 5 | NA |
| 011815 Smooth, synchronous movement | 1 | 2 | 3 | 4 | 5 | NA |
| 011816 Attentiveness to stimuli | 1 | 2 | 3 | 4 | 5 | NA |
| 011817 Response to stimuli | 1 | 2 | 3 | 4 | 5 | NA |
| 011818 Sustained alertness during interaction | 1 | 2 | 3 | 4 | 5 | NA |
| 011819 Interaction with caregiver | 1 | 2 | 3 | 4 | 5 | NA |
| 011820 Self-consolability | 1 | 2 | 3 | 4 | 5 | NA |
| 011821 Blood glucose | 1 | 2 | 3 | 4 | 5 | NA |
| 011822 Coombs test | 1 | 2 | 3 | 4 | 5 | NA |
| 011823 Bilirubin level | 1 | 2 | 3 | 4 | 5 | NA |
| 011824 Bowel elimination | 1 | 2 | 3 | 4 | 5 | NA |
| 011825 Urinary elimination | 1 | 2 | 3 | 4 | 5 | NA |

*2nd edition 2000; Revised 3rd edition*

Outcome Content References:

American Academy of Pediatrics & The American College of Obstetricians and Gynecologists. (1997). *Guidelines for perinatal care* (4th ed.). Washington, DC: American College of Obstetricians and Gynecologists.

Association of Women's Health, Obstetricians and Neonatal Nurses. (1998). *Standards & guidelines for the professional nursing practice in the care of women and newborns* (5th ed.). Washington, DC: Author

AWHONN Voice. (1996). Clinical commentary: Physiologic assessment of the healthy newborn. *Journal of Obstetric, Gynecologic, and Neonatal Nursing 4*(6), 5-6.

Committee on Fetus and Newborn (1993). Routine evaluation of blood pressure, hematocrit, and glucose in newborns. *Pediatrics, 92*(3), 474-476.

Murray, S.S., McKinney, E.S., & Gorrie, T.M. (2002). *Foundations of maternal-newborn nursing* (3rd ed.). Philadelphia: W.B. Saunders.

Simpson, K.R., et al. (2001). *AWHONN's perinatal nursing* (2nd ed.). Philadelphia: Lippincott.

# *Nutritional Status (1004)*

*Domain-Physiologic Health (II)*

*Care Recipient:*

*Class-Nutrition (K)*

*Data Source:*

*Scale(s)-Severe deviation from normal range to No deviation from normal range (b)*

---

**Definition:** Extent to which nutrients are available to meet metabolic needs

OUTCOME TARGET RATING:      Maintain at_____      Increase to_____

| Nutritional Status Overall Rating | Severe deviation from normal range 1 | Substantial deviation from normal range 2 | Moderate deviation from normal range 3 | Mild deviation from normal range 4 | No deviation from normal range 5 | |
|---|---|---|---|---|---|---|
| **INDICATORS:** | | | | | | |
| 100401   Nutrient intake | 1 | 2 | 3 | 4 | 5 | NA |
| 100402   Food intake | 1 | 2 | 3 | 4 | 5 | NA |
| 100408   Fluid intake | 1 | 2 | 3 | 4 | 5 | NA |
| 100403   Energy | 1 | 2 | 3 | 4 | 5 | NA |
| 100405   Weight/height ratio | 1 | 2 | 3 | 4 | 5 | NA |
| 100409   Hematocrit | 1 | 2 | 3 | 4 | 5 | NA |
| 100410   Muscle tone | 1 | 2 | 3 | 4 | 5 | NA |
| 100411   Hydration | 1 | 2 | 3 | 4 | 5 | NA |

*1st edition 1997; Revised 3rd edition*

---

**Outcome Content References:**

Chang, B.L., Uman, G.C., Linn, L.S., Ware, J.E., & Kane, R.L. (1985). Adherence to healthcare regimens among elderly women. *Nursing Research, 34*(1), 27-31.

Collinsworth, R., & Boyle, K. (1989). Nutritional assessment of the elderly. *Journal of Gerontological Nursing, 15*(12), 17-21.

Curtas, S., Chapman, G., & Meguid, M. (1989). Evaluation of nutritional status. *Nursing Clinics of North America, 24*(2), 301-313.

Folsom, A.R., Kaye, S.A., Sellers, T.A., Hang, C.P., Cerhan, J.R., Potter, J.D., & Prineas, R.J. (1993). Body fat distribution and five year risk of death in older women. *Journal of the American Medical Association, 269*(4), 483-487.

Gianino, S., & St. John, R.E. (1993). Nutritional assessment of the patient in the intensive care unit. *Critical Care Nursing Clinics of North America, 5*(1), 1-16.

+Guigoz, Y., Vallas, B., & Garry, P.J. (1996). Mini Nutritional Assessment: A practical assessment tool for grading the nutritional state of elderly patients. *Facts and Research in Gerontology, 4*(Suppl. 2), 15-59.

Tandy, L., & Malan, S. (2001). Impaired swallowing. In M. Maas, K. Buckwalter, M. Hardy, T. Tripp-Reimer, M. Titler, & J. Specht (Eds.), *Nursing care of older adults: Diagnoses, outcomes & interventions* (pp. 158-171). St. Louis: Mosby.

Wakefield, B. (2001). Altered nutrition: Less than body requirements. In M. Maas, K. Buckwalter, M. Hardy, T. Tripp-Reimer, M. Titler, & J. Specht (Eds.), *Nursing care of older adults: Diagnoses, outcomes & interventions* (pp. 145-157). St. Louis: Mosby.

N

# Nutritional Status: Biochemical Measures (1005)

*Domain-Physiologic Health (II)*                                    *Care Recipient:*

*Class-Nutrition (K)*                                               *Data Source:*

*Scale(s)-Severe deviation from normal range to No deviation from normal range (b)*

**Definition**: Body fluid components and chemical indices of nutritional status

OUTCOME TARGET RATING:    Maintain at_____    Increase to_____

| Nutritional Status: Biochemical Measures Overall Rating | Severe deviation from normal range 1 | Substantial deviation from normal range 2 | Moderate deviation from normal range 3 | Mild deviation from normal range 4 | No deviation from normal range 5 | |
|---|---|---|---|---|---|---|
| **INDICATORS:** | | | | | | |
| 100501 Serum albumin | 1 | 2 | 3 | 4 | 5 | NA |
| 100502 Serum prealbumin | 1 | 2 | 3 | 4 | 5 | NA |
| 100514 Serum creatinine | 1 | 2 | 3 | 4 | 5 | NA |
| 100503 Hematocrit | 1 | 2 | 3 | 4 | 5 | NA |
| 100504 Hemoglobin | 1 | 2 | 3 | 4 | 5 | NA |
| 100510 Serum transferrin | 1 | 2 | 3 | 4 | 5 | NA |
| 100505 Total iron binding capacity | 1 | 2 | 3 | 4 | 5 | NA |
| 100506 Lymphocyte count | 1 | 2 | 3 | 4 | 5 | NA |
| 100507 Blood glucose | 1 | 2 | 3 | 4 | 5 | NA |
| 100508 Blood cholesterol | 1 | 2 | 3 | 4 | 5 | NA |
| 100509 Blood triglycerides | 1 | 2 | 3 | 4 | 5 | NA |
| 100511 24-hour urinary creatinine | 1 | 2 | 3 | 4 | 5 | NA |
| 100512 Urinary urea nitrogen | 1 | 2 | 3 | 4 | 5 | NA |

*1st edition 1997; Revised 3rd edition*

**N**

Outcome Content References:

Chang, B.L., Uman, G.C., Linn, L.S., Ware, J.E., & Kane, R.L. (1985). Adherence to healthcare regimens among elderly women. *Nursing Research, 34*(1), 27-31.

Collinsworth, R., & Boyle, K. (1989). Nutritional assessment of the elderly. *Journal of Gerontological Nursing, 15*(12), 17-21.

Curtas, S., Chapman, G., & Meguid, M. (1989). Evaluation of nutritional status. *Nursing Clinics of North America, 24*(2), 301-313.

Folsom, A.R., Kaye, S.A., Sellers, T.A., Hang, C.P., Cerhan, J.R., Potter, J.D., & Prineas, R.J. (1993). Body fat distribution and five year risk of death in older women. *Journal of the American Medical Association, 269*(4), 483-487.

Gianino, S., & St. John, R.E. (1993). Nutritional assessment of the patient in the intensive care unit. *Critical Care Nursing Clinics of North America, 5*(1), 1-16.

# Nutritional Status: Energy (1007)

*Domain-Physiologic Health (II)*

*Class-Nutrition (K)*

*Scale(s)-Severe deviation from normal range to No deviation from normal range (b)*

Care Recipient:

Data Source:

**Definition:** Extent to which nutrients and oxygen provide cellular energy

OUTCOME TARGET RATING:    Maintain at_____    Increase to_____

| Nutritional Status: Energy Overall Rating | Severe deviation from normal range 1 | Substantial deviation from normal range 2 | Moderate deviation from normal range 3 | Mild deviation from normal range 4 | No deviation from normal range 5 | |
|---|---|---|---|---|---|---|
| **INDICATORS:** | | | | | | |
| 100701  Stamina | 1 | 2 | 3 | 4 | 5 | NA |
| 100702  Endurance | 1 | 2 | 3 | 4 | 5 | NA |
| 100703  Hand grip strength | 1 | 2 | 3 | 4 | 5 | NA |
| 100708  Muscle tone | 1 | 2 | 3 | 4 | 5 | NA |
| 100704  Tissue healing | 1 | 2 | 3 | 4 | 5 | NA |
| 100705  Infection resistance | 1 | 2 | 3 | 4 | 5 | NA |
| 100706  Growth (children) | 1 | 2 | 3 | 4 | 5 | NA |

*1st edition 1997; Revised 3rd edition*

Outcome Content References:

Chang, B.L., Uman, G.C., Linn, L.S., Ware, J.E., & Kane, R.L. (1985). Adherence to healthcare regimens among elderly women. *Nursing Research, 34*(1), 27-31.

Collinsworth, R., & Boyle, K. (1989). Nutritional assessment of the elderly. *Journal of Gerontological Nursing, 15*(12), 17-21.

Curtas, S., Chapman, G., & Meguid, M. (1989). Evaluation of nutritional status. *Nursing Clinics of North America, 24*(2), 301-313.

+Dartmouth Primary Care Cooperative Information Project (1987). *COOP Charts.* Hanover, NH: Department of Community and Family Medicine, Dartmouth Medical School.

Folsom, A.R., Kaye, S.A., Sellers, T.A., Hang, C.P., Cerhan, J.R., Potter, J.D., Prineas, R.J. (1993). Body fat distribution and 5 year risk of death in older women. *Journal of the American Medical Association, 269*(4), 483-487.

Gianino, S., & St. John, R.E. (1993). Nutritional assessment of the patient in the intensive care unit. *Critical Care Nursing Clinics of North America, 5*(1), 1-16.

N

# Nutritional Status: Food & Fluid Intake (1008)

Domain-Physiologic Health (II)

Class-Nutrition (K)

Scale(s)-Not adequate to Totally adequate (f)

Care Recipient:

Data Source:

**Definition:** Amount of food and fluid taken into the body over a 24-hour period

OUTCOME TARGET RATING:    Maintain at_____    Increase to_____

| Nutritional Status: Food & Fluid Intake Overall Rating | Not adequate 1 | Slightly adequate 2 | Moderately adequate 3 | Substantially adequate 4 | Totally adequate 5 | |
|---|---|---|---|---|---|---|
| **INDICATORS:** | | | | | | |
| 100801  Oral food intake | 1 | 2 | 3 | 4 | 5 | NA |
| 100802  Tube feeding intake | 1 | 2 | 3 | 4 | 5 | NA |
| 100803  Oral fluid intake | 1 | 2 | 3 | 4 | 5 | NA |
| 100804  Intravenous fluid intake | 1 | 2 | 3 | 4 | 5 | NA |
| 100805  Parenteral nutrition intake | 1 | 2 | 3 | 4 | 5 | NA |

*1st edition 1997; Revised 3rd edition*

## Outcome Content References:

Champagne, M.T., & Ashley, M.L. (1989). Nutritional support in the critically ill elderly patient. *Critical Care Nursing Quarterly, 12*(1), 15-25.

Duggal, A., & Lawrence, R.M. (2001). Aspects of food refusal in the elderly: The "hunger strike." *International Journal of Eating Disorders, 30*(2), 213-216.

Gianino, S., & St. John, R.E. (1993). Nutritional assessment of the patient in the intensive care unit. *Critical Care Nursing Clinics of North America, 5*(1), 1-16.

Keithley, J.K., & Kohn, C.L. (1990). Managing nutritional problems in people with AIDS. *Oncology Nursing Forum, 17*(1), 23-27.

N

# *Nutritional Status: Nutrient Intake (1009)*

*Domain-Physiologic Health (II)*

*Class-Nutrition (K)*

*Scale(s)-Not adequate to Totally adequate (f)*

*Care Recipient:*

*Data Source:*

**Definition:** Adequacy of usual pattern of nutrient intake

OUTCOME TARGET RATING:     Maintain at_____     Increase to_____

| Nutritional Status: Nutrient Intake Overall Rating | Not adequate 1 | Slightly adequate 2 | Moderately adequate 3 | Substantially adequate 4 | Totally adequate 5 | |
|---|---|---|---|---|---|---|
| **INDICATORS:** | | | | | | |
| 100901   Caloric intake | 1 | 2 | 3 | 4 | 5 | NA |
| 100902   Protein intake | 1 | 2 | 3 | 4 | 5 | NA |
| 100903   Fat intake | 1 | 2 | 3 | 4 | 5 | NA |
| 100904   Carbohydrate intake | 1 | 2 | 3 | 4 | 5 | NA |
| 100910   Fiber intake | 1 | 2 | 3 | 4 | 5 | NA |
| 100905   Vitamin intake | 1 | 2 | 3 | 4 | 5 | NA |
| 100906   Mineral intake | 1 | 2 | 3 | 4 | 5 | NA |
| 100907   Iron intake | 1 | 2 | 3 | 4 | 5 | NA |
| 100908   Calcium intake | 1 | 2 | 3 | 4 | 5 | NA |
| 100911   Sodium intake | 1 | 2 | 3 | 4 | 5 | NA |

*1st edition 1997; Revised 3rd edition*

Outcome Content References:

Champagne, M.T., & Ashley, M.L. (1989). Nutritional support in the critically ill elderly patient. *Critical Care Nursing Quarterly, 12*(1), 15-25.

Gianino, S., & St. John, R.E. (1993). Nutritional assessment of the patient in the intensive care unit. *Critical Care Nursing Clinics of North America, 5*(1), 1-16.

Keithley, J.K., & Kohn, C.L. (1990). Managing nutritional problems in people with AIDS. *Oncology Nursing Forum, 17*(1), 23-27.

N

# *Oral Hygiene (1100)*

Domain-Physiologic Health (II)                                    Care Recipient:

Class-Tissue Integrity (L)                                        Data Source:

Scale(s)-Severely compromised to Not compromised (a) and Severe to None (n)

**Definition:** Condition of the mouth, teeth, gums, and tongue

OUTCOME TARGET RATING:      Maintain at_____      Increase to_____

| Oral Hygiene Overall Rating | Severely compromised 1 | Substantially compromised 2 | Moderately compromised 3 | Mildly compromised 4 | Not compromised 5 | |
|---|---|---|---|---|---|---|
| INDICATORS: | | | | | | |
| 110001 Cleanliness of mouth | 1 | 2 | 3 | 4 | 5 | NA |
| 110002 Cleanliness of teeth | 1 | 2 | 3 | 4 | 5 | NA |
| 110003 Cleanliness of gums | 1 | 2 | 3 | 4 | 5 | NA |
| 110004 Cleanliness of tongue | 1 | 2 | 3 | 4 | 5 | NA |
| 110005 Cleanliness of dentures | 1 | 2 | 3 | 4 | 5 | NA |
| 110006 Cleanliness of dental appliances | 1 | 2 | 3 | 4 | 5 | NA |
| 110007 Fit of dentures | 1 | 2 | 3 | 4 | 5 | NA |
| 110008 Fit of dental appliances | 1 | 2 | 3 | 4 | 5 | NA |
| 110009 Moistness of lips | 1 | 2 | 3 | 4 | 5 | NA |
| 110010 Moisture of oral mucosa and tongue | 1 | 2 | 3 | 4 | 5 | NA |
| 110011 Color of mucosa membranes | 1 | 2 | 3 | 4 | 5 | NA |
| 110012 Oral mucosa integrity | 1 | 2 | 3 | 4 | 5 | NA |
| 110013 Tongue integrity | 1 | 2 | 3 | 4 | 5 | NA |
| 110014 Gum integrity | 1 | 2 | 3 | 4 | 5 | NA |
| 110020 Adequate teeth for chewing | 1 | 2 | 3 | 4 | 5 | NA |

| | Severe | Substantial | Moderate | Mild | None | |
|---|---|---|---|---|---|---|
| 110017 Halitosis | 1 | 2 | 3 | 4 | 5 | NA |
| 110018 Bleeding | 1 | 2 | 3 | 4 | 5 | NA |
| 110021 Pain | 1 | 2 | 3 | 4 | 5 | NA |
| 110022 Oral mucosa lesions | 1 | 2 | 3 | 4 | 5 | NA |
| 110023 Dental caries | 1 | 2 | 3 | 4 | 5 | NA |
| 110024 Gingivitis | 1 | 2 | 3 | 4 | 5 | NA |
| 110025 Periodontal disease | 1 | 2 | 3 | 4 | 5 | NA |

Dental Prosthesis YES / NO

*1st edition 1997; Revised 3rd edition (formerly Oral Health)*

**Outcome Content References:**

Fischman, S. (1993). Self-care: Practical periodontal care in today's practice. *International Dental Journal, 43*, 179-183.

Jones, J.A. (1989). Integrating the oral examination into clinical practice. *Hospital Practice, 24*(10A), 23-24, 26-27, 30.

+Kayser-Jones, J., Bird, W.F., Paul, S.M., Long, L. & Schell, E.S. (1995). An instrument to assess the oral health status of nursing home residents. *The Gerontologist, 35*(6), 814-824.

Matteson, M.A., McConnell E.S., & Linton, A.D. (1997). *Gerontological nursing: Concepts & practice* (2nd ed.). Philadelphia: W.B. Saunders.

Raybould, T.P., Carpenter, A.D., Ferretti, G.A., Brown, A.T., Lillich, T.T., & Henslee, J. (1994). Emergence of gram-negative bacilli in the mouths of bone marrow transplant recipients using chlorhexidine mouth rinse. *Oncology Nursing Forum, 21*(4), 691-696.

Richardson, A. (1987). A process standard for oral care. *Nursing Times, 83*(32), 38-40.

Speedie, G. (1983). Nursology of mouth care: Preventing, comforting and seeking activities related to mouth care. *Journal of Advanced Nursing, 8*(1), 33-40.

# *Ostomy Self-Care (1615)*

Domain-Health Knowledge & Behavior (IV)

Class-Health Behavior (Q)

Scale(s)-Never demonstrated to Consistently demonstrated (m)

Care Recipient:

Data Source:

**Definition:** Personal actions to maintain ostomy for elimination

OUTCOME TARGET RATING:    Maintain at_____    Increase to_____

| Ostomy Self-Care Overall Rating | | Never demonstrated 1 | Rarely demonstrated 2 | Sometimes demonstrated 3 | Often demonstrated 4 | Consistently demonstrated 5 | |
|---|---|---|---|---|---|---|---|
| 161501 | Describes functioning of ostomy | 1 | 2 | 3 | 4 | 5 | NA |
| 161502 | Describes purpose of ostomy | 1 | 2 | 3 | 4 | 5 | NA |
| 161503 | Appears comfortable viewing stoma | 1 | 2 | 3 | 4 | 5 | NA |
| 161504 | Measures stoma for proper appliance fit | 1 | 2 | 3 | 4 | 5 | NA |
| 161505 | Demonstrates skin care around ostomy | 1 | 2 | 3 | 4 | 5 | NA |
| 161506 | Demonstrates irrigation technique | 1 | 2 | 3 | 4 | 5 | NA |
| 161507 | Empties ostomy pouch | 1 | 2 | 3 | 4 | 5 | NA |
| 161508 | Changes ostomy pouch | 1 | 2 | 3 | 4 | 5 | NA |
| 161509 | Monitors for complications related to stoma | 1 | 2 | 3 | 4 | 5 | NA |
| 161510 | Monitors amount and consistency of stool | 1 | 2 | 3 | 4 | 5 | NA |
| 161511 | Follows schedule for changing ostomy pouch | 1 | 2 | 3 | 4 | 5 | NA |
| 161512 | Obtains supplies to care for ostomy | 1 | 2 | 3 | 4 | 5 | NA |
| 161513 | Avoids flatus-producing food and drink | 1 | 2 | 3 | 4 | 5 | NA |
| 161514 | Maintains adequate fluid intake | 1 | 2 | 3 | 4 | 5 | NA |
| 161515 | Follows recommended diet | 1 | 2 | 3 | 4 | 5 | NA |
| 161516 | Avoids odor producing foods | 1 | 2 | 3 | 4 | 5 | NA |
| 161517 | Modifies daily activities as needed | 1 | 2 | 3 | 4 | 5 | NA |
| 161518 | Seeks professional assistance as needed | 1 | 2 | 3 | 4 | 5 | NA |
| 161519 | Expresses acceptance of ostomy | 1 | 2 | 3 | 4 | 5 | NA |

O

*3rd edition*

Outcome Content References:

Bryant, D., & Fleischer, I. (2000). Changing an ostomy appliance. *Nursing, 30*(11), 51-53.

Lee, J. (2001). Nurse prescribing in practice: Patient choice in stoma care. *British Journal of Community Nursing, 6*(1), 33-34, 36-37.

Martins, M.L., & Cardoso, M. (2001). Group participative education for persons with an ostomy. *World Council of Enterostomal Therapists Journal, 21*(4), 8-17.

Metcalf, C. (1999). Clinical stoma care: Empowering patients through teaching practical skills. *British Journal of Nursing, 8*(9), 593-600.

Sage, S.J. (1991). Nephrostomy dressing change procedure. *Ostomy Wound Management, 32*, 32-33, 35-36.

Secord, C., Jackman, M., Wright, L., & Winton, S. (2001). Adjusting to life with an ostomy. *Canadian Nurse, 97*(1), 29-32.

Thompson, J. (2000). A practical ostomy guide. *RN, 63*(11), 61-68.

**O**

# Pain: Adverse Psychological Response (1306)

*Domain-Perceived Health (V)*

*Class-Symptom Status (V)*

*Scale(s)-Severe to None (n)*

*Care Recipient:*

*Data Source:*

---

**Definition:** Severity of observed or reported adverse cognitive and emotional responses to physical pain

OUTCOME TARGET RATING:     Maintain at_____     Increase to_____

| Pain: Adverse Psychological Response Overall Rating | Severe 1 | Substantial 2 | Moderate 3 | Mild 4 | None 5 | |
|---|---|---|---|---|---|---|
| **INDICATORS:** | | | | | | |
| 130601  Slowing of thought processes | 1 | 2 | 3 | 4 | 5 | NA |
| 130602  Memory impairment | 1 | 2 | 3 | 4 | 5 | NA |
| 130603  Interference with concentration | 1 | 2 | 3 | 4 | 5 | NA |
| 130604  Indecision | 1 | 2 | 3 | 4 | 5 | NA |
| 130605  Pain distress level | 1 | 2 | 3 | 4 | 5 | NA |
| 130606  Concern about tolerating the pain | 1 | 2 | 3 | 4 | 5 | NA |
| 130607  Concern about burdening others | 1 | 2 | 3 | 4 | 5 | NA |
| 130608  Concern about abandonment | 1 | 2 | 3 | 4 | 5 | NA |
| 130609  Depression | 1 | 2 | 3 | 4 | 5 | NA |
| 130610  Anxiety | 1 | 2 | 3 | 4 | 5 | NA |
| 130611  Sadness | 1 | 2 | 3 | 4 | 5 | NA |
| 130612  Helplessness | 1 | 2 | 3 | 4 | 5 | NA |
| 130613  Hopelessness | 1 | 2 | 3 | 4 | 5 | NA |
| 130614  Worthlessness | 1 | 2 | 3 | 4 | 5 | NA |
| 130615  Sense of isolation | 1 | 2 | 3 | 4 | 5 | NA |
| 130616  Fear of procedures and equipment | 1 | 2 | 3 | 4 | 5 | NA |
| 130617  Fear of unbearable pain | 1 | 2 | 3 | 4 | 5 | NA |
| 130618  Annoyance with disrupting effects of pain | 1 | 2 | 3 | 4 | 5 | NA |
| 130619  Suicidal thoughts | 1 | 2 | 3 | 4 | 5 | NA |
| 130620  Pessimistic thoughts | 1 | 2 | 3 | 4 | 5 | NA |
| 130621  Bitterness toward others | 1 | 2 | 3 | 4 | 5 | NA |
| 130622  Anger over disabling effects of pain | 1 | 2 | 3 | 4 | 5 | NA |

*2nd edition 2000; Revised 3rd edition (formerly Pain: Psychological Response)*

### Outcome Content References:

Copp, L.A. (1974). The spectrum of suffering. *American Journal of Nursing, 74*(3), 491-495.

Kalfoss, M.H. (1992). The assessment of psychological distress. *Scandinavian Journal of Caring Science, 6*(1), 23-28.

Price, D.D., & Harkins, S. W. (1992). Psychophysical approaches to pain measurement and assessment. In D. C. Turk & R. Melzack (Eds.), *Handbook of pain assessment* (pp. 111-134). New York: The Guilford Press.

Puntillo, K.A., & Wilkie, D. J. (1991). Assessment of pain in the critically ill. In K. A. Puntillo (Ed.), *Pain in the critically ill* (pp. 45-64). Gaithersburg, MD: Aspen Publishers.

P

# *Pain Control (1605)*

*Domain-Health Knowledge & Behavior (IV)*

*Class-Health Behavior (Q)*

*Scale(s)-Never demonstrated to Consistently demonstrated (m)*

*Care Recipient:*

*Data Source:*

**Definition:** Personal actions to control pain

OUTCOME TARGET RATING:     Maintain at_____     Increase to_____

| Pain Control Overall Rating | Never demonstrated 1 | Rarely demonstrated 2 | Sometimes demonstrated 3 | Often demonstrated 4 | Consistently demonstrated 5 | |
|---|---|---|---|---|---|---|
| INDICATORS: | | | | | | |
| 160502 Recognizes pain onset | 1 | 2 | 3 | 4 | 5 | NA |
| 160501 Describes causal factors | 1 | 2 | 3 | 4 | 5 | NA |
| 160510 Uses diary to monitor symptoms over time | 1 | 2 | 3 | 4 | 5 | NA |
| 160503 Uses preventive measures | 1 | 2 | 3 | 4 | 5 | NA |
| 160504 Uses non-analgesic relief measures | 1 | 2 | 3 | 4 | 5 | NA |
| 160505 Uses analgesics appropriately | 1 | 2 | 3 | 4 | 5 | NA |
| 160513 Reports changes in pain symptoms or sites to health care professional | 1 | 2 | 3 | 4 | 5 | NA |
| 160507 Reports uncontrolled symptoms to health care professional | 1 | 2 | 3 | 4 | 5 | NA |
| 160508 Uses available resources | 1 | 2 | 3 | 4 | 5 | NA |
| 160509 Recognizes associated symptoms of pain | 1 | 2 | 3 | 4 | 5 | NA |
| 160511 Reports pain controlled | 1 | 2 | 3 | 4 | 5 | NA |

*1st edition 1997; Revised 2nd edition 2000; Revised 3rd edition*

## Outcome Content References:

Acute Pain Management Guideline Panel. (1992). *Acute pain management: Operative or medical procedures and trauma. Clinical practice guideline* (AHCPR Publication No. 92-0032). Rockville, MD: Agency for Health Care Policy and Research, Public Health Service, U.S. Department of Health and Human Services.

Howe, C.J. (1993). A new standard of care for pediatric pain management. *American Journal of Maternal Child Nursing, 18*(6), 325-329.

+Hurley, A.C., Volicer, B.J., Hanrahan, P.A., Houde, S., & Volicer, L. (1992). Assessment of discomfort in advanced Alzheimer's patients. *Research in Nursing and Health, 15*(5), 369-377.

Jacox, A., Carr, D.B., Payne, R., et al. (1994). *Management of cancer pain. Clinical practice guideline* No. 9 (AHCPR Publication No. 94-0592). Rockville, MD: Agency for Health Care Policy and Research, U.S. Department of Health and Human Services, Public Health Service.

Mobily, P., & Herr, K.A. (2001). Pain. In M. Maas, K. Buckwalter, M. Hardy, T. Tripp-Reimer, M. Titler, & J. Specht (Eds.), *Nursing care of older adults: Diagnoses, outcomes & interventions* (pp. 455-475). St. Louis: Mosby.

Puntillo, K., & Weiss, S.J. (1994). Pain: Its mediators and associated morbidity in critically ill cardiovascular surgical patients. *Nursing Research, 43*(1), 31-36.

Sherbourne, C.D. (1992). Pain measures. In A.L. Stewart & J.E. Ware, Jr. (Eds.), *Measuring functioning and well-being* (pp. 220-234). Durham, NC: Duke University Press.

+ Walker, S.N., Sechrist, K.R., & Pender, N.J. (1995). *The Health-Promoting Lifestyle profile II.* Omaha, NE: University of Nebraska at Omaha.

+Walker, S.N., Sechrist, K.R., & Pender, N.J. (1987). The Health Promoting Lifestyle profile: Development and psychometric characteristics. *Nursing Research, 36*(2), 76-81.

P

# Pain: Disruptive Effects (2101)

*Domain-Perceived Health (V)*

*Class-Symptom Status (V)*

*Scale(s)-Severe to None (n) and Severely compromised to Not compromised (a)*

*Care Recipient:*

*Data Source:*

**Definition**: Severity of observed or reported disruptive effects of chronic pain on daily functioning

OUTCOME TARGET RATING:      Maintain at_____      Increase to_____

| Pain: Disruptive Effects Overall Rating | Severe 1 | Substantial 2 | Moderate 3 | Mild 4 | None 5 | |
|---|---|---|---|---|---|---|

INDICATORS:

| | | Severe 1 | Substantial 2 | Moderate 3 | Mild 4 | None 5 | |
|---|---|---|---|---|---|---|---|
| 210101 | Disruption of interpersonal relationships | 1 | 2 | 3 | 4 | 5 | NA |
| 210102 | Impaired role performance | 1 | 2 | 3 | 4 | 5 | NA |
| 210108 | Impaired concentration | 1 | 2 | 3 | 4 | 5 | NA |
| 210110 | Impaired mood | 1 | 2 | 3 | 4 | 5 | NA |
| 210111 | Lack of patience | 1 | 2 | 3 | 4 | 5 | NA |
| 210112 | Disruption of sleep | 1 | 2 | 3 | 4 | 5 | NA |
| 210119 | Disruption of routine | 1 | 2 | 3 | 4 | 5 | NA |
| 210113 | Impaired physical mobility | 1 | 2 | 3 | 4 | 5 | NA |
| 210114 | Impaired self-care | 1 | 2 | 3 | 4 | 5 | NA |
| 210115 | Loss of appetite | 1 | 2 | 3 | 4 | 5 | NA |
| 210117 | Impaired urinary elimination | 1 | 2 | 3 | 4 | 5 | NA |
| 210120 | Impaired bowel elimination | 1 | 2 | 3 | 4 | 5 | NA |
| 210121 | Absenteeism from work or school | 1 | 2 | 3 | 4 | 5 | NA |
| 210122 | Difficulty maintaining employment | 1 | 2 | 3 | 4 | 5 | NA |

| | | Severely compromised | Substantially compromised | Moderately compromised | Mildly compromised | Not compromised | |
|---|---|---|---|---|---|---|---|
| 210103 | Play activities | 1 | 2 | 3 | 4 | 5 | NA |
| 210104 | Leisure activities | 1 | 2 | 3 | 4 | 5 | NA |
| 210105 | Work or school productivity | 1 | 2 | 3 | 4 | 5 | NA |
| 210106 | Life enjoyment | 1 | 2 | 3 | 4 | 5 | NA |
| 210107 | Sense of control | 1 | 2 | 3 | 4 | 5 | NA |
| 210109 | Sense of hope | 1 | 2 | 3 | 4 | 5 | NA |

*1st edition 1997; Revised 3rd edition*

Outcome Content References:

Howe, C.J. (1993). A new standard of care for pediatric pain management. *American Journal of Maternal Child Nursing, 18*(6), 325-329.

Jacox, A., Carr, D.B., Payne, R., et al. (1994). *Management of cancer pain. Clinical practice guideline* No. 9 (AHCPR Publication No. 94-0592). Rockville, MD: Agency for Health Care Policy and Research, U.S. Department of Health and Human Services, Public Health Service.

Mobily, P., & Herr, K.A. (2001). Pain. In M. Maas, K. Buckwalter, M. Hardy, T. Tripp-Reimer, M. Titler, & J. Specht (Eds.), *Nursing care of older adults: Diagnoses, outcomes & interventions* (pp. 455-475). St. Louis: Mosby.

Puntillo, K., & Weiss, S.J. (1994). Pain: Its mediators and associated mobility in critically ill cardiovascular surgical patients. *Nursing Research, 43*(1), 31-36.

Sherbourne, C.D. (1992). Pain measures. In A.L. Stewart & J.E. Ware, Jr. (Eds.), *Measuring functioning and well-being* (pp. 220-234). Durham, NC: Duke University Press.

+Von Korff, M., Ormel, J., Keefe, F.J., & Dworkin, S.F. (1992). Grading the severity of chronic pain. *Pain, 50*(2), 133-149.

# *Pain Level (2102)*

Domain-Perceived Health (V)                     Care Recipient:

Class-Symptom Status (V)                         Data Source:

Scale(s)-Severe to None (n) and Severely compromised to Not compromised (a)

**Definition:** Severity of observed or reported pain

OUTCOME TARGET RATING:   Maintain at_____   Increase to_____

| Pain Level Overall Rating | Severe 1 | Substantial 2 | Moderate 3 | Mild 4 | None 5 | |
|---|---|---|---|---|---|---|
| **INDICATORS:** | | | | | | |
| 210201 Reported pain | 1 | 2 | 3 | 4 | 5 | NA |
| 210204 Length of pain episodes | 1 | 2 | 3 | 4 | 5 | NA |
| 210217 Moaning and crying | 1 | 2 | 3 | 4 | 5 | NA |
| 210206 Facial expressions of pain | 1 | 2 | 3 | 4 | 5 | NA |
| 210208 Restlessness | 1 | 2 | 3 | 4 | 5 | NA |
| 210218 Pacing | 1 | 2 | 3 | 4 | 5 | NA |
| 210219 Narrowed focus | 1 | 2 | 3 | 4 | 5 | NA |
| 210209 Muscle tension | 1 | 2 | 3 | 4 | 5 | NA |
| 210215 Loss of appetite | 1 | 2 | 3 | 4 | 5 | NA |

| | Severely compromised | Substantially compromised | Moderately compromised | Mildly compromised | Not compromised | |
|---|---|---|---|---|---|---|
| 210210 Respiratory rate | 1 | 2 | 3 | 4 | 5 | NA |
| 210211 Apical heart rate | 1 | 2 | 3 | 4 | 5 | NA |
| 210220 Radial pulse rate | 1 | 2 | 3 | 4 | 5 | NA |
| 210212 Blood pressure | 1 | 2 | 3 | 4 | 5 | NA |
| 210214 Perspiration | 1 | 2 | 3 | 4 | 5 | NA |

Site of pain _____

*1st edition 1997; Revised 3rd edition*

Outcome Content References:

+Acute Pain Management Guideline Panel. (1992). *Acute pain management: Operative or medical procedures and trauma. Clinical practice guideline* (AHCPR Publication No. 92-0032). Rockville, MD: Agency for Health Care Policy and Research, Public Health Service, U.S. Department of Health and Human Services.

Howe, C.J. (1993). A new standard of care for pediatric pain management. *American Journal of Maternal Child Nursing, 18*(6), 325-329.

+Hurley, A.C., Volicer, B.J., Hanrahan, P.A., Houde, S., & Volicer, L. (1992). Assessment of discomfort in advanced Alzheimer's patients. *Research in Nursing and Health, 15*(5), 369-377.

Jacox, A., Carr, D.B., Payne, R., et al. (1994). *Management of cancer pain. Clinical practice guideline* No. 9 (AHCPR Publication No. 94-0592). Rockville, MD: Agency for Health Care Policy and Research, U.S. Department of Health and Human Services, Public Health Service.

Mayer, D.M., Torma, L., Byock, I., & Norris, K. (2001). Speaking the language of pain. *American Journal of Nursing, 101*(2), 44-50.

Melzack, R. (1975). The McGill Pain Questionnaire: Major properties and scoring methods. *Pain, 30*(1), 277-299.

Merkel, S. (2002). Pain assessment in infants and young children: The Finger Span Scale. *American Journal of Nursing, 102*(11), 55-56.

Mobily, P., & Herr, K.A. (2001). Pain. In M. Maas, K. Buckwalter, M. Hardy, T. Tripp-Reimer, M. Titler, & J. Specht (Eds.), *Nursing care of older adults: Diagnoses, outcomes & interventions* (pp. 455-475). St. Louis: Mosby.

Puntillo, K., & Weiss, S.J. (1994). Pain: Its mediators and associated morbidity in critically ill cardiovascular surgical patients. *Nursing Research, 43*(1), 31-36.

Sherbourne, C.D. (1992). Pain measures. In A.L. Stewart, & J.E. Ware, Jr. (Eds.), *Measuring functioning and well-being* (pp. 220-234). Durham, NC: Duke University Press.

+Wong, D., & Baker, C.M. (1988). Pain in children: Comparison of assessment scales. *Pediatric Nursing, 14*(1), 9-17.

P

# Parent-Infant Attachment (1500)

*Domain-Psychosocial Health (III)*  
*Class-Social Interaction (P)*  
*Scale(s)-Never demonstrated to Consistently demonstrated (m)*

*Care Recipient:*  
*Data Source:*

**Definition:** Parent and infant behaviors that demonstrate an enduring affectionate bond

OUTCOME TARGET RATING:    Maintain at_____    Increase to_____

| Parent-Infant Attachment Overall Rating | Never demonstrated 1 | Rarely demonstrated 2 | Sometimes demonstrated 3 | Often demonstrated 4 | Consistently demonstrated 5 | |
|---|---|---|---|---|---|---|
| INDICATORS: | | | | | | |
| 150001 Parent(s) practice healthy behaviors during pregnancy | 1 | 2 | 3 | 4 | 5 | NA |
| 150002 Parent(s) assign specific attributes to fetus | 1 | 2 | 3 | 4 | 5 | NA |
| 150003 Parent(s) prepare for infant prior to birth | 1 | 2 | 3 | 4 | 5 | NA |
| 150004 Parent(s) verbalize positive feelings toward infant | 1 | 2 | 3 | 4 | 5 | NA |
| 150005 Parent(s) hold infant close | 1 | 2 | 3 | 4 | 5 | NA |
| 150006 Parent(s) touch, stroke, pat infant | 1 | 2 | 3 | 4 | 5 | NA |
| 150007 Parent(s) kiss infant | 1 | 2 | 3 | 4 | 5 | NA |
| 150008 Parent(s) smile at infant | 1 | 2 | 3 | 4 | 5 | NA |
| 150009 Parent(s) visit nursery | 1 | 2 | 3 | 4 | 5 | NA |
| 150010 Parent(s) talk to infant | 1 | 2 | 3 | 4 | 5 | NA |
| 150011 Parent(s) use en face position | 1 | 2 | 3 | 4 | 5 | NA |
| 150012 Parent(s) use eye contact | 1 | 2 | 3 | 4 | 5 | NA |
| 150013 Parent(s) smile and vocalize to infant | 1 | 2 | 3 | 4 | 5 | NA |
| 150014 Parent(s) play with infant | 1 | 2 | 3 | 4 | 5 | NA |
| 150015 Parent(s) respond to infant cues | 1 | 2 | 3 | 4 | 5 | NA |
| 150016 Parent(s) console/ soothe infant | 1 | 2 | 3 | 4 | 5 | NA |
| 150017 Parent(s) feed infant | 1 | 2 | 3 | 4 | 5 | NA |
| 150018 Parent(s) keep infant dry, clean, and warm | 1 | 2 | 3 | 4 | 5 | NA |
| 150019 Infant looks at parent(s) | 1 | 2 | 3 | 4 | 5 | NA |
| 150020 Infant responds to parent(s)' cues | 1 | 2 | 3 | 4 | 5 | NA |

P

| Parent-Infant<br>Attachment—cont'd | | Never<br>demonstrated | Rarely<br>demonstrated | Sometimes<br>demonstrated | Often<br>demonstrated | Consistently<br>demonstrated | |
|---|---|---|---|---|---|---|---|
| 150021 | Infant seeks<br>proximity with<br>parent(s) | 1 | 2 | 3 | 4 | 5 | NA |
| 150022 | Infant explores<br>environment | 1 | 2 | 3 | 4 | 5 | NA |

*1st edition 1997; Revised 3rd edition*

### Outcome Content References:

Ainsworth, M.S., & Wittig, B.A. (1969). Attachment and exploratory behavior of one-year olds in a strange situation. In B.M. Foss (Ed.), *Determinants of infant behavior* (pp. 111-133). London: Methuen.

Kennell, J., Jerauld, R., Wolfe, H., Chesler, D., Kreger, N.C., McAlpine, W., Steffa, M., & Klaus, M.H. (1974). Maternal behavior one year after early and extended post-partum contact. *Developmental Medicine and Child Neurology, 16(2)*, 172-279.

Koniak-Griffin, D. (1988). The relationship between social support, self-esteem, and maternal-fetal attachment in adolescents. *Research in Nursing and Health, 11*(4), 269-278.

+Müller, M. (1994). A questionnaire to measure mother-to-infant attachment. *Journal of Nursing Measurements, 2*(2), 129-141.

Norr, K.F., Roberts, J.E., & Freese, U. (1989). Early postpartum rooming-in and maternal attachment behaviors in a group of medically indigent primiparas. *Journal of Nurse-Midwifery, 34*(2), 85-91.

P

# *Parenting: Adolescent Physical Safety (2902)*

*Domain-Family Health (VI)*

*Class-Parenting (d)*

*Scale(s)-Never demonstrated to Consistently demonstrated (m)*

*Care Recipient:*

*Data Source:*

**Definition**: Parental actions to prevent physical injury in an adolescent from 12 years through 17 years of age

OUTCOME TARGET RATING:   Maintain at_____   Increase to_____

| Parenting: Adolescent Physical Safety Overall Rating | Never demonstrated 1 | Rarely demonstrated 2 | Sometimes demonstrated 3 | Often demonstrated 4 | Consistently demonstrated 5 | |
|---|---|---|---|---|---|---|
| INDICATORS: | | | | | | |
| 290201 Uses strategies to protect from sun exposure | 1 | 2 | 3 | 4 | 5 | NA |
| 290202 Uses strategies to encourage wearing of appropriate clothing for activity | 1 | 2 | 3 | 4 | 5 | NA |
| 290203 Maintains warning devices | 1 | 2 | 3 | 4 | 5 | NA |
| 290204 Practices family fire escape plan | 1 | 2 | 3 | 4 | 5 | NA |
| 290205 Maintains smoke free environment | 1 | 2 | 3 | 4 | 5 | NA |
| 290206 Monitors use of sport and recreational equipment | 1 | 2 | 3 | 4 | 5 | NA |
| 290207 Uses strategies to increase use of protective helmet and gear during high-risk activities | 1 | 2 | 3 | 4 | 5 | NA |
| 290208 Uses strategies to increase use of seatbelt | 1 | 2 | 3 | 4 | 5 | NA |
| 290209 Uses strategies to encourage observance of speed limits/rules of the road | 1 | 2 | 3 | 4 | 5 | NA |
| 290210 Uses strategies to prevent water accidents | 1 | 2 | 3 | 4 | 5 | NA |
| 290211 Uses strategies to prevent firearm injuries | 1 | 2 | 3 | 4 | 5 | NA |
| 290212 Uses strategies to prevent violence exposure/ involvement | 1 | 2 | 3 | 4 | 5 | NA |
| 290213 Uses strategies to prevent tobacco use | 1 | 2 | 3 | 4 | 5 | NA |

P

| Parenting: Adolescent Physical Safety—cont'd | | Never demonstrated | Rarely demonstrated | Sometimes demonstrated | Often demonstrated | Consistently demonstrated | |
|---|---|---|---|---|---|---|---|
| 290214 | Uses strategies to prevent alcohol use | 1 | 2 | 3 | 4 | 5 | NA |
| 290215 | Uses strategies to prevent recreational drug use | 1 | 2 | 3 | 4 | 5 | NA |
| 290216 | Uses strategies to prevent misuse of prescription drugs | 1 | 2 | 3 | 4 | 5 | NA |
| 290217 | Uses strategies to prevent inhaling/ exposure to toxic chemicals | 1 | 2 | 3 | 4 | 5 | NA |
| 290218 | Uses strategies to prevent exposure to excessive noise levels | 1 | 2 | 3 | 4 | 5 | NA |
| 290219 | Uses strategies to prevent sexual activity | 1 | 2 | 3 | 4 | 5 | NA |
| 290220 | Uses strategies to prevent unsafe sexual activity | 1 | 2 | 3 | 4 | 5 | NA |
| 290221 | Uses strategies to prevent unpro-tected sexual activity | 1 | 2 | 3 | 4 | 5 | NA |
| 290222 | Protects from phys-ical abuse | 1 | 2 | 3 | 4 | 5 | NA |
| 290223 | Protects from sexual abuse | 1 | 2 | 3 | 4 | 5 | NA |
| 290224 | Monitors for warning signs of self-harm | 1 | 2 | 3 | 4 | 5 | NA |
| 290225 | Seeks training to prepare for emergencies | 1 | 2 | 3 | 4 | 5 | NA |

*3rd edition*

Outcome Content References:

Bernardo, L., Garnder, J.J., & Seibel, K. (2001). Playground injuries in children: A review and Pennsylvania trauma center experience. *Journal of the Society of Pediatrics Nurses, 6*(1), 11-20.

Gresham, L.S., Zirkle, D.L., Tolchin, S., Jones, C., Maroufi, A., & Miranda, J. (2001). Partnering for injury prevention: Evaluation of a curriculum-based intervention program among elementary school children. *Journal of Pediatric Nursing, 16*(2), 79-87.

Hall-Long, B.A., Schell, K., & Corrigan, V. (2001). Youth safety education and injury prevention program. *Pediatric Nursing, 27*(2), 141-148.

Polivka, B.J., & Ryan-Wenger, N. (1999). Health promotion and injury prevention behaviors of elementary school children. *Pediatric Nursing 25*(2), 127-134.

P

## *Parenting: Early/Middle Childhood Physical Safety (2901)*

*Domain-Family Health (VI)*

*Class-Parenting (d)*

*Scale(s)-Never demonstrated to Consistently demonstrated (m)*

Care Recipient:

Data Source:

| Definition: Parental actions to avoid physical injury of a child from 3 years through 11 years of age |
|---|

OUTCOME TARGET RATING:     Maintain at_____     Increase to_____

| Parenting: Early/Middle Childhood Physical Safety Overall Rating | Never demonstrated 1 | Rarely demonstrated 2 | Sometimes demonstrated 3 | Often demonstrated 4 | Consistently demonstrated 5 | |
|---|---|---|---|---|---|---|
| **INDICATORS:** | | | | | | |
| 290101 Selects safe, age appropriate toys | 1 | 2 | 3 | 4 | 5 | NA |
| 290102 Provides supervision around pets and animals | 1 | 2 | 3 | 4 | 5 | NA |
| 290103 Provides supervision around water | 1 | 2 | 3 | 4 | 5 | NA |
| 290104 Avoids leaving child in motor vehicle unsupervised | 1 | 2 | 3 | 4 | 5 | NA |
| 290105 Monitors proper use of car seat/ seatbelt | 1 | 2 | 3 | 4 | 5 | NA |
| 290106 Supervises selection of weather appropriate clothing | 1 | 2 | 3 | 4 | 5 | NA |
| 290107 Protects from sun exposure | 1 | 2 | 3 | 4 | 5 | NA |
| 290108 Maintains environment to prevent harmful falls | 1 | 2 | 3 | 4 | 5 | NA |
| 290109 Maintains environment to prevent burns, electrical shock, and chemical exposure | 1 | 2 | 3 | 4 | 5 | NA |
| 290110 Maintains environment to prevent poisoning | 1 | 2 | 3 | 4 | 5 | NA |
| 290111 Practices family fire escape plan | 1 | 2 | 3 | 4 | 5 | NA |
| 290112 Keeps medications out of reach | 1 | 2 | 3 | 4 | 5 | NA |
| 290113 Maintains warning devices | 1 | 2 | 3 | 4 | 5 | NA |
| 290114 Locks or removes doors from unused appliances | 1 | 2 | 3 | 4 | 5 | NA |
| 290115 Maintains smoke free environment | 1 | 2 | 3 | 4 | 5 | NA |

P

| Parenting: Early/Middle Childhood Physical Safety—cont'd | | Never demonstrated | Rarely demonstrated | Sometimes demonstrated | Often demonstrated | Consistently demonstrated | |
|---|---|---|---|---|---|---|---|
| 290116 | Insures home play-ground equipment meets safety guidelines* | 1 | 2 | 3 | 4 | 5 | NA |
| 290117 | Provides supervision while on play-ground equipment | 1 | 2 | 3 | 4 | 5 | NA |
| 290118 | Selects appropriate clothing for activity | 1 | 2 | 3 | 4 | 5 | NA |
| 290119 | Uses strategies to increase the use of bicycle helmets | 1 | 2 | 3 | 4 | 5 | NA |
| 290120 | Uses strategies to increase use of protective helmet and gear during high-risk activities | 1 | 2 | 3 | 4 | 5 | NA |
| 290121 | Eliminates access to firearms | 1 | 2 | 3 | 4 | 5 | NA |
| 290122 | Protects from expo-sure to violence | 1 | 2 | 3 | 4 | 5 | NA |
| 290123 | Monitors use of sport and recreational equipment | 1 | 2 | 3 | 4 | 5 | NA |
| 290124 | Uses strategies to pre-vent tobacco use | 1 | 2 | 3 | 4 | 5 | NA |
| 290125 | Uses strategies to pre-vent alcohol use | 1 | 2 | 3 | 4 | 5 | NA |
| 290126 | Uses strategies to prevent recre-ational drug use | 1 | 2 | 3 | 4 | 5 | NA |
| 290127 | Uses strategies to prevent misuse of prescription drugs | 1 | 2 | 3 | 4 | 5 | NA |
| 290128 | Uses strategies to prevent inhaling/exposure to toxic chemicals | 1 | 2 | 3 | 4 | 5 | NA |
| 290129 | Uses strategies to prevent expo-sure to excessive noise levels | 1 | 2 | 3 | 4 | 5 | NA |
| 290130 | Uses strategies to prevent child from precocious sexual behavior | 1 | 2 | 3 | 4 | 5 | NA |
| 290131 | Protects from physical abuse | 1 | 2 | 3 | 4 | 5 | NA |
| 290132 | Protects from sexual abuse | 1 | 2 | 3 | 4 | 5 | NA |
| 290133 | Seeks training to prepare for emergencies | 1 | 2 | 3 | 4 | 5 | NA |

*US Consumer Product Safety Commission and National Program for Playground Safety Guidelines

*3rd edition*

*Continued*

Outcome Content References:

Bernardo, L., Garnder, J.J., & Seibel, K. (2001). Playground injuries in children: A review and Pennsylvania trauma center experience. *Journal of the Society of Pediatrics Nurses, 6*(1), 11-20.

Gresham, L.S., Zirkle, D.L., Tolchin, S., Jones, C., Maroufi, A., & Miranda, J. (2001). Partnering for injury prevention: Evaluation of a curriculum-based intervention program among elementary school children. *Journal of Pediatric Nursing, 16*(2), 79-87.

Hall-Long, B.A., Schell, K., & Corrigan, V. (2001). Youth safety education and injury prevention program. *Pediatric Nursing, 27*(2), 141-148.

Polivka, B.J., & Ryan-Wenger, N. (1999). Health promotion and injury prevention behaviors of elementary school children. *Pediatric Nursing, 25*(2), 127-134.

**P**

# *Parenting: Infant/Toddler Physical Safety (2900)*

Domain-Family Health (VI)

Class-Parenting (d)

Scale(s)-Never demonstrated to Consistently demonstrated (m)

Care Recipient:

Data Source:

**Definition:** Parental actions to avoid physical injury of a child from birth through 2 years of age

OUTCOME TARGET RATING:    Maintain at_____    Increase to_____

| Parenting: Infant/Toddler Physical Safety Overall Rating | Never demonstrated 1 | Rarely demonstrated 2 | Sometimes demonstrated 3 | Often demonstrated 4 | Consistently demonstrated 5 | |
|---|---|---|---|---|---|---|
| INDICATORS: | | | | | | |
| 290001 Handles infant/ toddler properly | 1 | 2 | 3 | 4 | 5 | NA |
| 290002 Uses crib that meets federal regulations | 1 | 2 | 3 | 4 | 5 | NA |
| 290003 Positions on back for sleep | 1 | 2 | 3 | 4 | 5 | NA |
| 290004 Selects safe, age appropriate toys | 1 | 2 | 3 | 4 | 5 | NA |
| 290005 Keeps sharp pointed objects out of reach | 1 | 2 | 3 | 4 | 5 | NA |
| 290006 Chooses foods that prevent choking | 1 | 2 | 3 | 4 | 5 | NA |
| 290007 Stores formula/ breastmilk appropriately | 1 | 2 | 3 | 4 | 5 | NA |
| 290008 Provides constant supervision around pets and animals | 1 | 2 | 3 | 4 | 5 | NA |
| 290009 Provides constant supervision around water | 1 | 2 | 3 | 4 | 5 | NA |
| 290010 Avoids leaving infant/toddler in motor vehicle unsupervised | 1 | 2 | 3 | 4 | 5 | NA |
| 290011 Uses car seat properly | 1 | 2 | 3 | 4 | 5 | NA |
| 290012 Selects weather appropriate clothing | 1 | 2 | 3 | 4 | 5 | NA |
| 290013 Protects from sun exposure | 1 | 2 | 3 | 4 | 5 | NA |
| 290014 Maintains environ- ment to prevent suffocation | 1 | 2 | 3 | 4 | 5 | NA |
| 290015 Maintains environ- ment to prevent harmful falls | 1 | 2 | 3 | 4 | 5 | NA |

*Continued*

| Parenting: Infant/Toddler Physical Safety—cont'd | | Never demonstrated | Rarely demonstrated | Sometimes demonstrated | Often demonstrated | Consistently demonstrated | |
|---|---|---|---|---|---|---|---|
| 290016 | Maintains environment to prevent burns, electrical shock, and chemical exposure | 1 | 2 | 3 | 4 | 5 | NA |
| 290017 | Maintains environment to prevent poisoning | 1 | 2 | 3 | 4 | 5 | NA |
| 290018 | Keeps medications out of reach | 1 | 2 | 3 | 4 | 5 | NA |
| 290019 | Maintains smoke free environment | 1 | 2 | 3 | 4 | 5 | NA |
| 290020 | Uses strategies to prevent exposure to excessive noise levels | 1 | 2 | 3 | 4 | 5 | NA |
| 290021 | Maintains warning devices | 1 | 2 | 3 | 4 | 5 | NA |
| 290022 | Seeks training to prepare for emergencies | 1 | 2 | 3 | 4 | 5 | NA |
| 290023 | Insures home playground equipment meets safety guidelines* | 1 | 2 | 3 | 4 | 5 | NA |
| 290024 | Provides supervision while on playground equipment | 1 | 2 | 3 | 4 | 5 | NA |
| 290025 | Insures that infant/toddler wears bike helmet properly | 1 | 2 | 3 | 4 | 5 | NA |
| 290026 | Protects from physical abuse | 1 | 2 | 3 | 4 | 5 | NA |
| 290027 | Protects from sexual abuse | 1 | 2 | 3 | 4 | 5 | NA |

*US Consumer Product Safety Commission and National Program for Playground Safety Guidelines

*3rd edition*

### Outcome Content References:

Kendrick, D., & Marsh, P. (1998). Babywalkers: Prevalence of use and relationship with other safety practices. *Injury Prevention, 4*(4), 295-298.

Kotch, J., et al (1997). Injuries among children in home and out-of-home care. *Injury Prevention, 3*(4), 267-271.

McBrien, M. (1997). Regency home care pediatric checklist. *Home Care Manager, 1*(2), 17.

Murphy, J. (1999). Pediatric occupant care safety: Clinical implications based on recent literature. *Pediatric Nursing, 25*(2), 137-144, 147-148.

O,Dea, T., Saly, G., & Holte, J. (1998). Safety investigation: Interaction of infant radiant warmers and bilirubin phototherapy lights in the regulation of temperature of newborn infants. *Biomedical Instrument Technology, 32*(4), 355-369.

Showers, J. (1992). "Don't shake the baby": The effectiveness of a prevention program. *Child Abuse & Neglect, 16*(1), 11-18.

Thompson, R., & Emslie, A. (2000). Young children and the risk of accidental injury: Running an audit at nine months. *Community Practitioner, 73*(10), 799-800.

Wong, D., Hockenberry-Eaton, M., Wilson, D., Winkelstein, M.L., & Schwartz, P. (2001). *Wong's essentials of pediatric nursing* (6th ed). St. Louis: Mosby.

# Parenting Performance (2211)

Domain-Family Health (VI)

Class-Parenting (d)

Scale(s)-Never demonstrated to Consistently demonstrated (m)

Care Recipient:

Data Source:

**Definition:** Parental actions to provide a child a nurturing and constructive physical, emotional, and social environment

OUTCOME TARGET RATING:  Maintain at_____  Increase to_____

| Parenting Performance Overall Rating | Never demonstrated 1 | Rarely demonstrated 2 | Sometimes demonstrated 3 | Often demonstrated 4 | Consistently demonstrated 5 | |
|---|---|---|---|---|---|---|
| INDICATORS: | | | | | | |
| 221101 Provides for child's physical needs | 1 | 2 | 3 | 4 | 5 | NA |
| 221122 Provides age-appropriate nutrition | 1 | 2 | 3 | 4 | 5 | NA |
| 221102 Eliminates controllable environmental hazards | 1 | 2 | 3 | 4 | 5 | NA |
| 221103 Provides regular preventative and episodic health care | 1 | 2 | 3 | 4 | 5 | NA |
| 221123 Provides structure for child | 1 | 2 | 3 | 4 | 5 | NA |
| 221104 Stimulates cognitive development | 1 | 2 | 3 | 4 | 5 | NA |
| 221105 Stimulates social development | 1 | 2 | 3 | 4 | 5 | NA |
| 221106 Stimulates emotional growth | 1 | 2 | 3 | 4 | 5 | NA |
| 221107 Stimulates spiritual growth | 1 | 2 | 3 | 4 | 5 | NA |
| 221124 Stimulates moral growth | 1 | 2 | 3 | 4 | 5 | NA |
| 221125 Imparts values that promote functioning in society | 1 | 2 | 3 | 4 | 5 | NA |
| 221126 Provides appropriate supervision for child | 1 | 2 | 3 | 4 | 5 | NA |
| 221127 Selects appropriate supplemental caregiver(s) | 1 | 2 | 3 | 4 | 5 | NA |
| 221128 Monitors supplemental caregiver(s) | 1 | 2 | 3 | 4 | 5 | NA |
| 221108 Uses community and other resources as appropriate | 1 | 2 | 3 | 4 | 5 | NA |
| 221110 Uses interactions appropriate for child's temperament | 1 | 2 | 3 | 4 | 5 | NA |

P

*Continued*

| Parenting Performance—cont'd | | Never demonstrated | Rarely demonstrated | Sometimes demonstrated | Often demonstrated | Consistently demonstrated | |
|---|---|---|---|---|---|---|---|
| 221111 | Uses behavior management if indicated | 1 | 2 | 3 | 4 | 5 | NA |
| 221112 | Uses appropriate discipline | 1 | 2 | 3 | 4 | 5 | NA |
| 221113 | Provides for child's special needs | 1 | 2 | 3 | 4 | 5 | NA |
| 221114 | Interacts positively with child | 1 | 2 | 3 | 4 | 5 | NA |
| 221115 | Empathizes with child | 1 | 2 | 3 | 4 | 5 | NA |
| 221129 | Maintains open communication | 1 | 2 | 3 | 4 | 5 | NA |
| 221116 | Verbalizes positive attributes of child | 1 | 2 | 3 | 4 | 5 | NA |
| 221117 | Exhibits a loving relationship | 1 | 2 | 3 | 4 | 5 | NA |
| 221118 | Expresses realistic expectations of parental role | 1 | 2 | 3 | 4 | 5 | NA |
| 221119 | Expresses satis-faction with parental role | 1 | 2 | 3 | 4 | 5 | NA |
| 221120 | Expresses positive self-esteem | 1 | 2 | 3 | 4 | 5 | NA |

*1st edition 1997; Revised 3rd edition (formerly Parenting)*

### Outcome Content References:

Causby, V., Nixon, C., & Bright, J.M. (1991). Influences on adolescent mother-infant interactions. *Adolescence, 26*(103), 619-630.

+Clarke, M., & Hornick, J. (1984). The development of the Nurturance Inventory: An instrument for assessing parenting practices. *Child Psychiatry & Human Development, 15*(1), 49-63.

Fulton, A.M., Murphy, K.R., & Anderson, S.L. (1991). Increasing adolescent mothers' knowledge of child development: An intervention program. *Adolescence, 26*(101), 73-81.

Greaves, P., Glik, D.C., Kronenfeld, J.J., & Jackson, K. (1994). Determinants of controllable in-home child safety hazards. *Health Education Research, 9*(3), 307-315.

Mercer, R.T., & Ferketich, S.L. (1994). Predictors of maternal role competence by risk status. *Nursing Research, 43*(1), 38-43.

Ohashi, J.P. (1992). Maternal role satisfaction: A new approach to assessing parenting. *Scholarly Inquiry for Nursing Practice: An International Journal, 6*(2), 135-149.

Reece, S.M. (1995). Stress and maternal adaptation in first-time mothers more than 35 years old. *Applied Nursing Research, 8*(2), 61-66.

Thompson, P.J., Powell, M.J., Patterson, R.J., & Ellerbee, S.M. (1995). Adolescent parenting: Outcomes and maternal perceptions. *Journal of Obstetric, Gynecologic, and Neonatal Nursing, 24*(8), 713-718.

P

# Parenting: Psychosocial Safety (1901)

Domain-Family Health (VI)

Class-Parenting (d)

Scale(s)-Never demonstrated to Consistently demonstrated (m)

Care Recipient:

Data Source:

**Definition:** Parental actions to protect a child from social contacts that might cause harm or injury

OUTCOME TARGET RATING:     Maintain at_____     Increase to_____

| Parenting: Psychosocial Safety Overall Rating | Never demonstrated 1 | Rarely demonstrated 2 | Sometimes demonstrated 3 | Often demonstrated 4 | Consistently demonstrated 5 | |
|---|---|---|---|---|---|---|

INDICATORS:

| | | | | | | | |
|---|---|---|---|---|---|---|---|
| 190101 | Monitors playmates | 1 | 2 | 3 | 4 | 5 | NA |
| 190102 | Monitors social contacts | 1 | 2 | 3 | 4 | 5 | NA |
| 190115 | Fosters open communication | 1 | 2 | 3 | 4 | 5 | NA |
| 190104 | Selects appropriate supplemental caregiver(s) | 1 | 2 | 3 | 4 | 5 | NA |
| 190103 | Monitors supplemental caregiver(s) | 1 | 2 | 3 | 4 | 5 | NA |
| 190105 | Recognizes risk(s) of abuse | 1 | 2 | 3 | 4 | 5 | NA |
| 190106 | Uses strategies to eliminate risk(s) of abuse | 1 | 2 | 3 | 4 | 5 | NA |
| 190107 | Actions to eliminate abuse | 1 | 2 | 3 | 4 | 5 | NA |
| 190109 | Provides needed level of supervision | 1 | 2 | 3 | 4 | 5 | NA |
| 190112 | Uses strategies to prevent high-risk social behaviors | 1 | 2 | 3 | 4 | 5 | NA |
| 190113 | Prevents gang participation | 1 | 2 | 3 | 4 | 5 | NA |
| 190116 | Fosters mutually interactive communication about sex | 1 | 2 | 3 | 4 | 5 | NA |
| 190117 | Sets clear rules for behavior | 1 | 2 | 3 | 4 | 5 | NA |
| 190118 | Maintains structure and daily routine in child's life | 1 | 2 | 3 | 4 | 5 | NA |

1st edition 1997; Revised 3rd edition (formerly Parenting: Social Safety)

**Outcome Content References:**

Glick, D., Kronenfeld, J., & Jackson, K. (1993). Safety behaviors among parents of preschoolers. *Health Values, 17*(1), 18-27.

Howell, J.C., & Lynch, J.P. (2000). *Youth gangs in schools.* YGS Bulletin. Washington, DC: U.S. Department of Justice, Office of Justice Programs, Office of Juvenile Justice and Delinquency Prevention.

*Continued*

P

Jackson, C., & Foshee, V.A. (1998). Violence-related behaviors of adolescents: Relations with responsive and demanding parenting. *Journal of Adolescent Research 13*(3), 343-359.

Jensen, L.R., Williams, S.D., Thurman, D.J., & Keller, P.A. (1992). Submersion injuries for children less than 5 years in urban Utah. *Western Journal of Medicine, 157*(6), 641-644.

Quan, L., Gore, E.J., Wentz, K., Allen, J., & Novack, A.H. (1989). Ten year study of pediatric drownings and near-drownings in King County, Washington: Lessons in injury prevention. *Pediatrics, 83*(6), 1035-1040.

Rosenthal, D.A., Feldman, S.S., & Edwards, D. (1998). Mum's the word: Mother's perspectives on communication about sexuality with adolescents. *Journal of Adolescence, 21*(6), 727-743.

Walker, M., Schmidt, L., & Lunghofer, L. (1993). Youth gangs. In M.I. Singer, L.T. Singer, & T.M. Anglin (Eds.). *Handbook for screening adolescents at psychosocial risk* (pp. 504-522). New York: Lexington Books.

**P**

# Participation in Health Care Decisions (1606)

Domain-Health Knowledge & Behavior (IV)

Class-Health Behavior (Q)

Scale(s)-Never demonstrated to Consistently demonstrated (m)

Care Recipient:

Data Source:

**Definition:** Personal involvement in selecting and evaluating health care options to achieve desired outcome

OUTCOME TARGET RATING:      Maintain at_____      Increase to_____

| Participation in Health Care Decisions Overall Rating | Never demonstrated 1 | Rarely demonstrated 2 | Sometimes demonstrated 3 | Often demonstrated 4 | Consistently demonstrated 5 | |
|---|---|---|---|---|---|---|
| INDICATORS: | | | | | | |
| 160601 Claims decision making responsibility | 1 | 2 | 3 | 4 | 5 | NA |
| 160602 Demonstrates self-direction in decision making | 1 | 2 | 3 | 4 | 5 | NA |
| 160603 Seeks relevant information | 1 | 2 | 3 | 4 | 5 | NA |
| 160604 Defines available options | 1 | 2 | 3 | 4 | 5 | NA |
| 160605 Specifies health outcome preferences | 1 | 2 | 3 | 4 | 5 | NA |
| 160606 Identifies health outcome priorities | 1 | 2 | 3 | 4 | 5 | NA |
| 160607 Identifies barriers to desired outcome achievement | 1 | 2 | 3 | 4 | 5 | NA |
| 160608 Uses problem solving techniques to achieve desired outcomes | 1 | 2 | 3 | 4 | 5 | NA |
| 160609 States intent to act on decision | 1 | 2 | 3 | 4 | 5 | NA |
| 160610 Identifies available support for achieving desired outcomes | 1 | 2 | 3 | 4 | 5 | NA |
| 160611 Seeks services to meet desired outcomes | 1 | 2 | 3 | 4 | 5 | NA |
| 160612 Negotiates for care preferences | 1 | 2 | 3 | 4 | 5 | NA |
| 160613 Monitors barriers to outcome achievement | 1 | 2 | 3 | 4 | 5 | NA |
| 160614 Identifies level of outcome achievement | 1 | 2 | 3 | 4 | 5 | NA |
| 160615 Evaluates satisfaction with health care outcomes | 1 | 2 | 3 | 4 | 5 | NA |

1st edition 1997; Revised 3rd edition (formerly Participation: Health Care Decisions)

P

Continued

Outcome Content References:

Conn, V., Taylor S., & Casey, B. (1992). Cardiac rehabilitation program participation and outcomes after myocardial infarction. *Rehabilitation Nursing, 17*(2), 58-62.

+Ende, J., Kazis, L., Ash, A., & Moskowitz, M.A. (1989). Measuring patient's desire for autonomy: Decision making and information-seeking preferences among medical patients. *Journal of General Internal Medicine, 4*(1), 23-30.

Hegyvary, S.T. (1993). Patient care outcomes related to management of symptoms. In J.J. Fitzpatrick & J.J. Stevenson (Eds.), *Annual review of nursing research.* (Vol. 11, pp. 145-168). New York: Springer.

Weiler, K. & Moorhead, S.A. (2001). Self-determination. In M. Maas, K. Buckwalter, M. Hardy, T. Tripp-Reimer, M. Titler, & J. Specht (Eds.), *Nursing care of older adults: Diagnoses, outcomes & interventions* (pp. 706-718). St. Louis: Mosby.

P

# *Personal Autonomy (1614)*

Domain-Health Knowledge & Behavior (IV)

Class-Health Behavior (Q)

Scale(s)-Never demonstrated to Consistently demonstrated (m)

Care Recipient:

Data Source:

**Definition:** Personal actions of a competent individual to exercise governance in life decisions

OUTCOME TARGET RATING:     Maintain at_____     Increase to_____

| Personal Autonomy Overall Rating | Never demonstrated 1 | Rarely demonstrated 2 | Sometimes demonstrated 3 | Often demonstrated 4 | Consistently demonstrated 5 | |
|---|---|---|---|---|---|---|
| INDICATORS: | | | | | | |
| 161401 Makes informed life decisions | 1 | 2 | 3 | 4 | 5 | NA |
| 161402 Considers other opinions when making choices | 1 | 2 | 3 | 4 | 5 | NA |
| 161403 Expresses independence with decision-making process | 1 | 2 | 3 | 4 | 5 | NA |
| 161404 Makes decisions free from undo pressure by parents | 1 | 2 | 3 | 4 | 5 | NA |
| 161405 Makes decisions free from undo pressure by spouse | 1 | 2 | 3 | 4 | 5 | NA |
| 161406 Makes decisions free from undo pressure by children | 1 | 2 | 3 | 4 | 5 | NA |
| 161407 Makes decisions free from undo pressure by extended family | 1 | 2 | 3 | 4 | 5 | NA |
| 161408 Makes decisions free from undo pressure by friends | 1 | 2 | 3 | 4 | 5 | NA |
| 161409 Makes decisions free from undo pressure by health care provider | 1 | 2 | 3 | 4 | 5 | NA |
| 161410 Asserts personal preferences | 1 | 2 | 3 | 4 | 5 | NA |
| 161411 Participates in health care decisions | 1 | 2 | 3 | 4 | 5 | NA |
| 161412 Expresses satisfaction with life choices | 1 | 2 | 3 | 4 | 5 | NA |

3rd edition

*Continued*

Outcome Content References:

Aveyard, H. (2000). Is there a concept of autonomy that can usefully inform nursing practice? *Journal of Advanced Nursing, 32*(2), 352-358.

Brennan, M. (1997). A concept analysis of consent. *Journal of Advanced Nursing, 25*(3), 477-484.

Dworkin, G. (1988). *The theory and practice of autonomy*. Cambridge: Cambridge University Press.

Valimaki, M., & Leino-Kilpi, H. (1998). Preconditions for and consequences of self-determination: The psychiatric patient's point of view. *Journal of Advanced Nursing, 27(1)*, 204-212.

Wiens, A. G. (1993). Patient autonomy: A theoretical framework for nursing. *Journal of Professional Nursing, 9*(2), 95-103.

**P**

# *Personal Health Status (2006)*

Domain-Perceived Health (V)

Class-Health & Life Quality (U)

Scale-Severely compromised to Not compromised (a)

Care Recipient:

Data Source:

**Definition:** Overall physical, psychological, social, and spiritual functioning of an adult 18 years or older

OUTCOME TARGET RATING:     Maintain at_____     Increase to_____

| Personal Health Status Overall Rating | Severely compromised 1 | Substantially compromised 2 | Moderately compromised 3 | Mildly compromised 4 | Not compromised 5 | |
|---|---|---|---|---|---|---|
| **INDICATORS:** | | | | | | |
| 200601 Physical fitness | 1 | 2 | 3 | 4 | 5 | NA |
| 200602 Mobility level | 1 | 2 | 3 | 4 | 5 | NA |
| 200603 Energy level | 1 | 2 | 3 | 4 | 5 | NA |
| 200604 Comfort level | 1 | 2 | 3 | 4 | 5 | NA |
| 200605 Performance of ADLs* | 1 | 2 | 3 | 4 | 5 | NA |
| 200606 Performance of IADLs* | 1 | 2 | 3 | 4 | 5 | NA |
| 200607 Resistance to infection | 1 | 2 | 3 | 4 | 5 | NA |
| 200608 Tissue healing | 1 | 2 | 3 | 4 | 5 | NA |
| 200609 Sleep-rest pattern | 1 | 2 | 3 | 4 | 5 | NA |
| 200610 Gastrointestinal function | 1 | 2 | 3 | 4 | 5 | NA |
| 200611 Cardiac function | 1 | 2 | 3 | 4 | 5 | NA |
| 200612 Peripheral tissue perfusion | 1 | 2 | 3 | 4 | 5 | NA |
| 200613 Neurologic function | 1 | 2 | 3 | 4 | 5 | NA |
| 200614 Pulmonary function | 1 | 2 | 3 | 4 | 5 | NA |
| 200615 Kidney function | 1 | 2 | 3 | 4 | 5 | NA |
| 200616 Weight in normal range | 1 | 2 | 3 | 4 | 5 | NA |
| 200617 Nutritional status | 1 | 2 | 3 | 4 | 5 | NA |
| 200618 Cognitive function | 1 | 2 | 3 | 4 | 5 | NA |
| 200619 Mental health | 1 | 2 | 3 | 4 | 5 | NA |
| 200620 Mood equilibrium | 1 | 2 | 3 | 4 | 5 | NA |
| 200621 Spiritual life | 1 | 2 | 3 | 4 | 5 | NA |
| 200622 Ability to cope | 1 | 2 | 3 | 4 | 5 | NA |
| 200623 Adjustment to chronic conditions | 1 | 2 | 3 | 4 | 5 | NA |
| 200624 Ability to express emotions | 1 | 2 | 3 | 4 | 5 | NA |
| 200625 Social relationships | 1 | 2 | 3 | 4 | 5 | NA |

*ADLs = Activities of daily living; IADLs = Instrumental activities of daily living.

*3rd edition*

## Outcome Content References:

Bergner, M., Bobbit, R.A., Carter, W.B., & Gilson, B.S. (1981). The sickness impact profile: Development and final revision of a health status measure. *Medical Care 19*(8), 787-805.

Kline, N.W. (1988). *Psychophysiological process of stress in people with a chronic physical illness.* Doctoral dissertation. The University of Michigan, Ann Arbor, MI.

Mossberg, K. & McFarland, C. (2001). A patient-oriented health status measure in outpatient rehabilitation. *American Journal of Physical Medicine & Rehabilitation, 80*(12), 896-902.

Radosevich, D., & Pruit, M. (1995). *Twelve-item Health Status Questionnaire.* Bloomington, MN: Health Outcomes Institute.

Ware, J.E., & Sherbourne, C.D. (1992). The MOS 36-item short-form health survey (SF-36). I. Conceptual framework and item selection. *Medical Care, 30*(6), 473-483.

P

# Personal Safety Behavior (1911)

*Domain-Health Knowledge & Behavior (IV)*

*Class-Risk Control & Safety (T)*

*Scale(s)-Never demonstrated to Consistently demonstrated (m)*

Care Recipient:

Data Source:

**Definition:** Personal actions of an adult to control behaviors that can cause physical injury

OUTCOME TARGET RATING:    Maintain at_____    Increase to_____

| Personal Safety Behavior Overall Rating | Never demonstrated 1 | Rarely demonstrated 2 | Sometimes demonstrated 3 | Often demonstrated 4 | Consistently demonstrated 5 | |
|---|---|---|---|---|---|---|
| **INDICATORS:** | | | | | | |
| 191102 Stores food to minimize spoilage | 1 | 2 | 3 | 4 | 5 | NA |
| 191103 Prepares food to minimize contamination | 1 | 2 | 3 | 4 | 5 | NA |
| 191104 Uses protective helmet and gear during high-risk activities | 1 | 2 | 3 | 4 | 5 | NA |
| 191105 Uses seatbelt | 1 | 2 | 3 | 4 | 5 | NA |
| 191106 Chooses appropriate clothing for activity | 1 | 2 | 3 | 4 | 5 | NA |
| 191122 Uses sunscreen | 1 | 2 | 3 | 4 | 5 | NA |
| 191107 Uses assistive devices correctly | 1 | 2 | 3 | 4 | 5 | NA |
| 191108 Practices safe leisure activities | 1 | 2 | 3 | 4 | 5 | NA |
| 191109 Practices safe sexual behaviors | 1 | 2 | 3 | 4 | 5 | NA |
| 191110 Uses tools correctly | 1 | 2 | 3 | 4 | 5 | NA |
| 191111 Uses machinery correctly | 1 | 2 | 3 | 4 | 5 | NA |
| 191113 Avoids recreational drugs | 1 | 2 | 3 | 4 | 5 | NA |
| 191115 Uses recommended precautions with prescription drugs | 1 | 2 | 3 | 4 | 5 | NA |
| 191117 Avoids tobacco use | 1 | 2 | 3 | 4 | 5 | NA |
| 191123 Avoids smoking in bed | 1 | 2 | 3 | 4 | 5 | NA |
| 191124 Uses precautions with flammable material | 1 | 2 | 3 | 4 | 5 | NA |
| 191118 Avoids alcohol misuse | 1 | 2 | 3 | 4 | 5 | NA |
| 191125 Avoids operating motor vehicle when using alcohol | 1 | 2 | 3 | 4 | 5 | NA |
| 191119 Avoids high-risk behaviors | 1 | 2 | 3 | 4 | 5 | NA |
| 191120 Observes speed limits/ rules of the road | 1 | 2 | 3 | 4 | 5 | NA |
| 191126 Protects self from injury | 1 | 2 | 3 | 4 | 5 | NA |

*1st edition 1997; Revised 3rd edition (formerly Safety Behavior: Personal)*

**Outcome Content References:**

+Hettler, B. (1982). Wellness promotion and risk reduction on a university campus. In M. Faber & A. Reinhardt (Eds.), *Promoting health through risk reduction*. New York: Macmillan.

Sorock, G.S. (1988). Falls among the elderly: Epidemiology and prevention. *American Journal of Preventive Medicine, 4*(5), 252-255.

Weitzel, E. (2001). Unilateral neglect. In M. Maas, K. Buckwalter, M. Hardy, T. Tripp-Reimer, M. Titler, & J. Specht (Eds.), *Nursing care of older adults: Diagnoses, outcomes & interventions* (pp. 492-502). St. Louis: Mosby.

P

# *Personal Well-Being (2002)*

Domain-Perceived Health (V)

Class-Health & Life Quality (U)

Scale(s)-Not at all satisfied to Completely satisfied (s)

Care Recipient:

Data Source:

**Definition:** Extent of positive perception of one's health status and life circumstances

OUTCOME TARGET RATING:    Maintain at_____    Increase to_____

| Personal Well-Being Overall Rating | Not at all satisfied 1 | Somewhat satisfied 2 | Moderately satisfied 3 | Very satisfied 4 | Completely satisfied 5 | |
|---|---|---|---|---|---|---|
| **INDICATORS:** | | | | | | |
| 200201 Performance of activities of daily living | 1 | 2 | 3 | 4 | 5 | NA |
| 200212 Performance of usual roles | 1 | 2 | 3 | 4 | 5 | NA |
| 200202 Psychological health | 1 | 2 | 3 | 4 | 5 | NA |
| 200203 Social relationships | 1 | 2 | 3 | 4 | 5 | NA |
| 200204 Spiritual life | 1 | 2 | 3 | 4 | 5 | NA |
| 200205 Physical health | 1 | 2 | 3 | 4 | 5 | NA |
| 200206 Cognitive function | 1 | 2 | 3 | 4 | 5 | NA |
| 200207 Ability to cope | 1 | 2 | 3 | 4 | 5 | NA |
| 200208 Ability to relax | 1 | 2 | 3 | 4 | 5 | NA |
| 200209 Level of happiness | 1 | 2 | 3 | 4 | 5 | NA |
| 200210 Ability to express emotions | 1 | 2 | 3 | 4 | 5 | NA |
| 200213 Ability to control activities | 1 | 2 | 3 | 4 | 5 | NA |
| 200214 Opportunities for health care choice(s) | 1 | 2 | 3 | 4 | 5 | NA |

*1st edition 1997; Revised 3rd edition (formerly Well-Being)*

Outcome Content References:

Davidhizar, R.E., & Giger, J.N. (2001). Powerlessness. In M. Maas, K. Buckwalter, M. Hardy, T. Tripp-Reimer, M. Titler, & J. Specht (Eds.), *Nursing care of older adults: Diagnoses, outcomes & interventions* (pp. 562-570). St. Louis: Mosby.

+Dupuy, H. (1984). The Psychological General Well-Being (PCWB) Index. In N.K. Wenger, ME. Mattson, C.D. Furberg, & J. Elinson (Eds.)., *Assessment of quality of life in clinical trials of cardiovascular therapies* (pp. 170-183, 353-356). Greenwich, CT: Le Jacq Publishing.

Ferrell, B., Grant, M., Schmidt, G.M., Rhiner, M., Whitehead, C.P., & Forman, S.J. (1992). The meaning of quality of life for bone marrow transplant survivors. Part 1. *Cancer Nursing, 15*(3), 153-160.

Ferrell, B.R., Dow, K.H., Leigh, S., Ly, J., & Gulasekaram, P. (1995). Quality of life in long-term cancer survivors. *Oncology Nursing Forum, 22*(6), 915-922.

Kozier, B., Erb, G., & Blais, K. (1992). *Concepts and issues in nursing practice* (2nd ed.). Redwood City, CA: Addison-Wesley Nursing.

+Revicki, D.A., Leidy, N.K., & Howland, L. (1996). Evaluating the psychometric characteristics of the Psychological General Well-Being Index with a new response scale. *Quality of Life Research, 5*(4), 419-425.

Stewart, A., Ware, J., Jr., Sherbourne, C., & Wells, K. (1992). Psychological distress/well-being and cognitive functioning measures. In A. Stewart & J. Ware, Jr. (Eds.), *Measuring functioning and well-being: The medical outcomes study approach* (pp. 102-142). Durham, NC: Duke University Press.

Waterman, J.D., Blegen, M., Clinton, P. & Specht, J.P. (2001). Social isolation. In M. Maas, K. Buckwalter, M. Hardy, T. Tripp-Reimer, M. Titler, & J. Specht (Eds.), *Nursing care of older adults: Diagnoses, outcomes & interventions* (pp. 651-663). St. Louis: Mosby.

Whedon, M., & Ferrell, B.R. (1994). Quality of life in adult bone marrow transplant patients: Beyond the first year. *Seminars in Oncology Nursing, 10*(1), 42-57.

P

# *Physical Aging (0113)*

*Domain-Functional Health (I)*

*Class-Growth & Development (B)*

*Scale(s)-Severe deviation from normal range to No deviation from normal range (b)*

*Care Recipient:*

*Data Source:*

**Definition**: Normal physical changes that occur with the natural aging process

OUTCOME TARGET RATING:     Maintain at_____     Increase to_____

| Physical Aging Overall Rating | Severe deviation from normal range 1 | Substantial deviation from normal range 2 | Moderate deviation from normal range 3 | Mild deviation from normal range 4 | No deviation from normal range 5 | |
|---|---|---|---|---|---|---|
| **INDICATORS:** | | | | | | |
| 011318 Memory | 1 | 2 | 3 | 4 | 5 | NA |
| 011319 Cognitive ability | 1 | 2 | 3 | 4 | 5 | NA |
| 011301 Mean body mass | 1 | 2 | 3 | 4 | 5 | NA |
| 011302 Bone density | 1 | 2 | 3 | 4 | 5 | NA |
| 011303 Cardiac output | 1 | 2 | 3 | 4 | 5 | NA |
| 011304 Vital capacity | 1 | 2 | 3 | 4 | 5 | NA |
| 011305 Blood pressure | 1 | 2 | 3 | 4 | 5 | NA |
| 011306 Skin elasticity | 1 | 2 | 3 | 4 | 5 | NA |
| 011307 Muscle strength | 1 | 2 | 3 | 4 | 5 | NA |
| 011320 Joint mobility | 1 | 2 | 3 | 4 | 5 | NA |
| 011321 Sensory acuity | 1 | 2 | 3 | 4 | 5 | NA |
| 011322 Bladder muscle tone | 1 | 2 | 3 | 4 | 5 | NA |
| 011323 Resistance to infection | 1 | 2 | 3 | 4 | 5 | NA |
| 011308 Hearing acuity | 1 | 2 | 3 | 4 | 5 | NA |
| 011309 Visual acuity | 1 | 2 | 3 | 4 | 5 | NA |
| 011310 Olfactory acuity | 1 | 2 | 3 | 4 | 5 | NA |
| 011311 Taste acuity | 1 | 2 | 3 | 4 | 5 | NA |
| 011312 Basal metabolic rate | 1 | 2 | 3 | 4 | 5 | NA |
| 011313 Fat distribution pattern | 1 | 2 | 3 | 4 | 5 | NA |
| 011314 Hair distribution pattern | 1 | 2 | 3 | 4 | 5 | NA |
| 011315 Menstrual pattern | 1 | 2 | 3 | 4 | 5 | NA |
| 011316 Sexual functioning | 1 | 2 | 3 | 4 | 5 | NA |

*1st edition 1997; Revised 3rd edition (formerly Physical Aging Status)*

Outcome Content References:

Bemben, M.G., & McCalip, G.A. (1999). Strength and power relationships as a function of age. *Journal of Strength & Conditioning Research, 13*(4), 330-338.

Kennedy-Malone, L., Fletcher, K.R., & Plank, L.M. (Eds.). (2000). *Management guidelines for gerontological nurse practitioners* (pp. 3-24, 536-553). Philadelphia: F.A. Davis.

McWhorter, J.W., & Schuerman, S.E. (2002). Balance and aging. *Orthopaedic Physical Therapy Clinics of North America, 11*(1), 111-130.

Rice, F.P. (2001). *Human development: A life-span approach.* Upper Saddle River, New Jersey: Prentice Hall.

Schuster, C., & Ashburn, S. (1992). *The process of human development: A holistic approach* (3rd ed.). Philadelphia: J.B. Lippincott.

Wong, A.M., Lin, Y., Chou, S., Tang, F., & Wong, P. (2001). Coordination exercise and postural stability in elderly people: Effect of Tai Chi Chuan. *Archives of Physical Medicine & Rehabilitation, 82*(5), 608-612.

# *Physical Fitness (2004)*

Domain-Perceived Health (V)

Class-Health & Life Quality (U)

Scale(s)-Severely compromised to Not compromised (a)

Care Recipient:

Data Source:

**Definition: Performance of physical activities with vigor**

OUTCOME TARGET RATING:    Maintain at_____    Increase to_____

| Physical Fitness Overall Rating | Severely compromised 1 | Substantially compromised 2 | Moderately compromised 3 | Mildly compromised 4 | Not compromised 5 | |
|---|---|---|---|---|---|---|
| INDICATORS: | | | | | | |
| 200401  Muscle strength | 1 | 2 | 3 | 4 | 5 | NA |
| 200402  Muscle endurance | 1 | 2 | 3 | 4 | 5 | NA |
| 200403  Joint flexibility | 1 | 2 | 3 | 4 | 5 | NA |
| 200404  Performance of physical activities | 1 | 2 | 3 | 4 | 5 | NA |
| 200405  Performance of routine exercise | 1 | 2 | 3 | 4 | 5 | NA |
| 200406  Cardiovascular function | 1 | 2 | 3 | 4 | 5 | NA |
| 200407  Respiratory function | 1 | 2 | 3 | 4 | 5 | NA |
| 200408  Aerobic fitness | 1 | 2 | 3 | 4 | 5 | NA |
| 200409  Body mass index | 1 | 2 | 3 | 4 | 5 | NA |
| 200410  Waist-to-hip ratio | 1 | 2 | 3 | 4 | 5 | NA |
| 200411  Blood pressure | 1 | 2 | 3 | 4 | 5 | NA |
| 200412  Target heart rate | 1 | 2 | 3 | 4 | 5 | NA |
| 200414  Resting heart rate | 1 | 2 | 3 | 4 | 5 | NA |

*2nd edition 2000; Revised 3rd edition*

Outcome Content References:

American College of Sports Medicine. (2000). *Guidelines for exercise testing and prescription* (6th ed.). Baltimore: Williams & Wilkins.

Brown, M., Sinacore, D.R., Ehsani, A.A., Binder, E.F., Holloszy, J.O., & Kohrt, W.M. (2000). Low-intensity exercise as a modifier of physical frailty in older adults. *Archives of Physical Medicine & Rehabilitation, 81*(7), 960-965.

Cauderay, M., Narring, F., & Michaud, P. (2000). A cross-sectional survey assessing physical fitness of 9 to 19 year old girls and boys in Switzerland. *Pediatric Exercise Science, 12*(4), 398-412.

NIH Consensus Development Panel on Physical Activity and Cardiovascular Health. (1996). Physical activity and cardiovascular health. *Journal of the American Medical Association, 276*(3), 241-246.

Pate, R., et al. (1995). Physical activity and public health. A recommendation from the Centers for Disease Control and the American College of Sports Medicine. *Journal of the American Medical Association, 273*(5), 402-407.

U.S. Department of Health and Human Services. (2000). *Healthy people 2010*. Washington, DC: Government Printing Office.

U.S. Department of Health and Human Services. (1991). *Healthy people 2000: National health promotion and disease prevention objectives*. (DHHS Pub No (PHS) 91-50012). Washington DC: Government Printing Office.

P

# *Physical Injury Severity (1913)*

Domain-Health Knowledge & Behavior (IV)

Class-Risk Control & Safety (T)

Scale(s)-Severe to None (n)

Care Recipient:

Data Source:

**Definition:** Severity of injuries from accidents and trauma

OUTCOME TARGET RATING:    Maintain at_____    Increase to_____

| Physical Injury Severity Overall Rating | Severe 1 | Substantial 2 | Moderate 3 | Mild 4 | None 5 | |
|---|---|---|---|---|---|---|
| INDICATORS: | | | | | | |
| 191301 Skin abrasions | 1 | 2 | 3 | 4 | 5 | NA |
| 191302 Bruises | 1 | 2 | 3 | 4 | 5 | NA |
| 191303 Lacerations | 1 | 2 | 3 | 4 | 5 | NA |
| 191304 Burns | 1 | 2 | 3 | 4 | 5 | NA |
| 191305 Extremity sprains | 1 | 2 | 3 | 4 | 5 | NA |
| 191306 Back sprains | 1 | 2 | 3 | 4 | 5 | NA |
| 191307 Extremity fractures | 1 | 2 | 3 | 4 | 5 | NA |
| 191308 Pelvic fractures | 1 | 2 | 3 | 4 | 5 | NA |
| 191309 Hip fractures | 1 | 2 | 3 | 4 | 5 | NA |
| 191310 Spinal fractures | 1 | 2 | 3 | 4 | 5 | NA |
| 191311 Cranial fractures | 1 | 2 | 3 | 4 | 5 | NA |
| 191312 Facial fractures | 1 | 2 | 3 | 4 | 5 | NA |
| 191313 Dental injuries | 1 | 2 | 3 | 4 | 5 | NA |
| 191314 Open head injuries | 1 | 2 | 3 | 4 | 5 | NA |
| 191315 Closed head injuries | 1 | 2 | 3 | 4 | 5 | NA |
| 191316 Impaired mobility | 1 | 2 | 3 | 4 | 5 | NA |
| 191317 Impaired consciousness | 1 | 2 | 3 | 4 | 5 | NA |

*1st edition 1997; Revised 3rd edition (formerly Safety Status: Physical Injury)*

Outcome Content References:

Lawrence, J.I., & Maher, P.L. (1992). An interdisciplinary falls consult team: A collaborative approach to patient falls. *Journal of Nursing Care Quality, 6*(3), 21-29.

Llewellyn, J., Martin, B., Shekleton, M., & Firlit, S. (1988). Analysis of falls in the acute surgical and cardiovascular surgical patient. *Applied Nursing Research, 1*(3), 116-121.

+Maas, M., Swanson, E., Buckwalter, K.C., Specht, J.P., Tripp-Reimer, T., Lenth, R., Tranel, D., Reed, D., Broffit, B., Brenneman, D., Peters, J., Rose, D., Kelley, L., Schutte, D.L., & Sun, C. (1999). *Final report: Nursing Interventions for Alzheimer's: Family Role Trials* (NINR R01-NRO1689). Rockville, MD: National Institutes of Health.

P

# Physical Maturation: Female (0114)

*Domain-Functional Health (I)*

*Class-Growth & Development (B)*

*Scale(s)-Severe deviation from normal range to No deviation from normal range (b)*

*Care Recipient:*

*Data Source:*

**Definition:** Normal physical changes in the female that occur with the transition from childhood to adulthood

OUTCOME TARGET RATING:  Maintain at_____  Increase to_____

| Physical Maturation: Female Overall Rating | Severe deviation from normal range 1 | Substantial deviation from normal range 2 | Moderate deviation from normal range 3 | Mild deviation from normal range 4 | No deviation from normal range 5 | |
|---|---|---|---|---|---|---|
| **INDICATORS:** | | | | | | |
| 011401 Growth spurt between 9.5-14.5 years of age | 1 | 2 | 3 | 4 | 5 | NA |
| 011402 Bone closure | 1 | 2 | 3 | 4 | 5 | NA |
| 011403 Voice changes | 1 | 2 | 3 | 4 | 5 | NA |
| 011404 Adult hair distribution | 1 | 2 | 3 | 4 | 5 | NA |
| 011405 Breast development | 1 | 2 | 3 | 4 | 5 | NA |
| 011406 Menstruation onset | 1 | 2 | 3 | 4 | 5 | NA |
| 011407 Increased muscle mass | 1 | 2 | 3 | 4 | 5 | NA |
| 011408 Decreased body fat | 1 | 2 | 3 | 4 | 5 | NA |
| 011409 Increased sebaceous secretions | 1 | 2 | 3 | 4 | 5 | NA |
| 011410 Increased perspiration | 1 | 2 | 3 | 4 | 5 | NA |

*1st edition 1997; Revised 3rd edition*

Outcome Content References:

Hockenberry, M.J., Wilson, D., Winkelstein, M.L., & Kline, N.E. (2003). *Wong's nursing care of infants and children* (7th ed.). St. Louis: Mosby.

Rice, F.P. (2001). *Human development: A life-span approach.* Upper Saddle River, New Jersey: Prentice Hall.

Schuster, C., & Ashburn, S. (1992). *The process of human development: A holistic approach* (3rd ed.). Philadelphia: J.B. Lippincott.

P

# Physical Maturation: Male (0115)

Domain-Functional Health (I)

Class-Growth & Development (B)

Scale(s)-Severe deviation from normal range to No deviation from normal range (b)

Care Recipient:

Data Source:

**Definition**: Normal physical changes in the male that occur with the transition from childhood to adulthood

OUTCOME TARGET RATING:    Maintain at_____    Increase to_____

| Physical Maturation: Male Overall Rating | Severe deviation from normal range 1 | Substantial deviation from normal range 2 | Moderate deviation from normal range 3 | Mild deviation from normal range 4 | No deviation from normal range 5 | |
|---|---|---|---|---|---|---|

**INDICATORS:**

| | | | | | | | |
|---|---|---|---|---|---|---|---|
| 011501 | Growth spurt between 10.5-16 years of age | 1 | 2 | 3 | 4 | 5 | NA |
| 011502 | Bone closure | 1 | 2 | 3 | 4 | 5 | NA |
| 011503 | Voice changes | 1 | 2 | 3 | 4 | 5 | NA |
| 011504 | Adult hair distribution | 1 | 2 | 3 | 4 | 5 | NA |
| 011505 | Testicular descent | 1 | 2 | 3 | 4 | 5 | NA |
| 011506 | Penis enlargement | 1 | 2 | 3 | 4 | 5 | NA |
| 011507 | First ejaculation of sperm (wet dream) | 1 | 2 | 3 | 4 | 5 | NA |
| 011508 | Increased muscle mass | 1 | 2 | 3 | 4 | 5 | NA |
| 011509 | Decreased body fat | 1 | 2 | 3 | 4 | 5 | NA |
| 011510 | Increased sebaceous secretions | 1 | 2 | 3 | 4 | 5 | NA |
| 011511 | Increased perspiration | 1 | 2 | 3 | 4 | 5 | NA |

*1st edition 1997; Revised 3rd edition*

P

Outcome Content References:

Hockenberry, M.J., Wilson, D., Winkelstein, M.L., & Kline, N.E. (2003). *Wong's nursing care of infants and children* (7th ed.). St. Louis: Mosby.

Rice, F.P. (2001). *Human development: A life-span approach.* Upper Saddle River, New Jersey: Prentice Hall.

Schuster, C., & Ashburn, S. (1992). *The process of human development: A holistic approach* (3rd ed.). Philadelphia: J.B. Lippincott.

# Play Participation (0116)

*Domain-Functional Health (I)*

*Class-Growth & Development (B)*

*Scale(s)-Never demonstrated to Consistently demonstrated (m)*

*Care Recipient:*

*Data Source:*

**Definition**: Use of activities by a child from 1 year through 11 years of age to promote enjoyment, entertainment, and development

OUTCOME TARGET RATING:    Maintain at_____    Increase to_____

| Play Participation Overall Rating | Never demonstrated 1 | Rarely demonstrated 2 | Sometimes demonstrated 3 | Often demonstrated 4 | Consistently demonstrated 5 | |
|---|---|---|---|---|---|---|
| **INDICATORS:** | | | | | | |
| 011601 Participates in play activities | 1 | 2 | 3 | 4 | 5 | NA |
| 011610 Expresses satis-faction with play activities | 1 | 2 | 3 | 4 | 5 | NA |
| 011603 Enjoys play activities | 1 | 2 | 3 | 4 | 5 | NA |
| 011604 Uses social skills during play activities | 1 | 2 | 3 | 4 | 5 | NA |
| 011605 Uses physical skills during play activities | 1 | 2 | 3 | 4 | 5 | NA |
| 011606 Uses imagination during play activities | 1 | 2 | 3 | 4 | 5 | NA |
| 011607 Expresses emotions during play activities | 1 | 2 | 3 | 4 | 5 | NA |
| 011608 Uses role playing | 1 | 2 | 3 | 4 | 5 | NA |

*1st edition 1997; Revised 3rd edition*

**P**

Outcome Content References:

Gillis, A.J. (1989). The effect of play on immobilized children in hospital. *International Journal of Nursing Studies, 26*(3), 261-269.

Gray, E. (1989). The emotional and play needs of the dying child. *Issues in Comprehensive Pediatric Nursing, 12*(2/3), 207-224.

Jack, L.W. (1987). Using play in psychiatric rehabilitation. *Journal of Psychosocial Nursing, 25*(7), 17-20.

Post, C. (1990). Play therapy with an abused child: A case study. *Journal of Child and Adolescent Psychiatric and Mental Health Nursing, 2*(2), 48-51.

# Post Procedure Recovery Status (2303)

Domain-Physiologic Health (II)  
Class-Therapeutic Response (a)  
Scale(s)-Severe deviation from normal range to No deviation from normal range (b) and Severe to None (n)

Care Recipient:  
Data Source:

**Definition:** Extent to which an individual returns to baseline function following a procedure(s) requiring anesthesia or sedation

OUTCOME TARGET RATING:    Maintain at_____    Increase to_____

| Post Procedure Recovery Status Overall Rating | Severe deviation from normal range 1 | Substantial deviation from normal range 2 | Moderate deviation from normal range 3 | Mild deviation from normal range 4 | No deviation from normal range 5 | |
|---|---|---|---|---|---|---|
| INDICATORS: | | | | | | |
| 230301 Patent airway | 1 | 2 | 3 | 4 | 5 | NA |
| 230302 Spontaneous respirations | 1 | 2 | 3 | 4 | 5 | NA |
| 230303 Respiratory rate | 1 | 2 | 3 | 4 | 5 | NA |
| 230304 Depth of inspiration | 1 | 2 | 3 | 4 | 5 | NA |
| 230305 Forceful cough | 1 | 2 | 3 | 4 | 5 | NA |
| 230306 $O_2$ saturation 92%-94% room air | 1 | 2 | 3 | 4 | 5 | NA |
| 230307 Systolic blood pressure within 20 mmHg of baseline | 1 | 2 | 3 | 4 | 5 | NA |
| 230308 Aldrete score | 1 | 2 | 3 | 4 | 5 | NA |
| 230309 Gag reflex | 1 | 2 | 3 | 4 | 5 | NA |
| 230310 Swallowing ability | 1 | 2 | 3 | 4 | 5 | NA |
| 230311 Retains oral fluids | 1 | 2 | 3 | 4 | 5 | NA |
| 230312 Answers questions | 1 | 2 | 3 | 4 | 5 | NA |
| 230313 Fully awake | 1 | 2 | 3 | 4 | 5 | NA |
| 230314 Moves extremities on command | 1 | 2 | 3 | 4 | 5 | NA |
| 230315 Ambulation tolerance | 1 | 2 | 3 | 4 | 5 | NA |
| 230316 Thermoregulation | 1 | 2 | 3 | 4 | 5 | NA |
| 230317 Urine output | 1 | 2 | 3 | 4 | 5 | NA |
| 230318 Voiding | 1 | 2 | 3 | 4 | 5 | NA |

| | Severe | Substantial | Moderate | Mild | None | |
|---|---|---|---|---|---|---|
| 230319 Drainage from tube/drain | 1 | 2 | 3 | 4 | 5 | NA |
| 230320 Drainage on dressing | 1 | 2 | 3 | 4 | 5 | NA |
| 230321 Nausea | 1 | 2 | 3 | 4 | 5 | NA |
| 230322 Vomiting | 1 | 2 | 3 | 4 | 5 | NA |
| 230323 Shivering | 1 | 2 | 3 | 4 | 5 | NA |
| 230324 Pain | 1 | 2 | 3 | 4 | 5 | NA |

3rd edition

P

Outcome Content References:

Aldrete, J.A. (1998). Modifications to the postanesthesia score for use in ambulatory surgery. *Journal of PeriAnesthesia Nursing, 13*(3), 148-155.

Aldrete J.A., & Kroulik, D. (1970). A postanesthetic recovery score. *Anesthesia & Analgesia, 49*(6), 924-934.

Cohen, S.E., Hamilton, C.L., Riley, E.T., Walker, D.S., Macario, A., & Halpern, J.W. (1998). Obstetric postanesthesia care unit stays: Reevaluation of discharge criteria after regional anesthesia. *Anesthesiology, 89*(6), 1559-1565.

Craney, J.M., & Gorman, L.N. (1997). Conscious sedation and implantable devices. Safe and effective sedation during pacemaker and implantable cardioverter defibrillator placement. *Critical Care Nursing Clinics of North America, 9*(3), 325-334.

Gross, J.B., et al. (1996). Practice guidelines for sedation and analgesia by non-anesthesiologists. *Anesthesiology, 84*(2), 459-471.

Joint Commission on Accreditation of Healthcare Organizations. (2001). *Comprehensive accreditation manual for hospitals: The official handbook.* Oakbrook Terrace (IL): Author.

Piper, S.N., Suttner, S.W., Schmidt, C.C., Maleck, W.H., Kumle, B., & Boldt, J. (1999). Nefopam and clonidine in the prevention of post anesthetic shivering. *Anaesthesia, 54*(7), 695-699.

P

# *Prenatal Health Behavior (1607)*

Domain-Health Knowledge & Behavior (IV)　　　　Care Recipient:

Class-Health Behavior (Q)　　　　Data Source:

Scale(s)-Never demonstrated to Consistently demonstrated (m)

| **Definition:** Personal actions to promote a healthy pregnancy and a healthy newborn |

OUTCOME TARGET RATING:　　Maintain at_____　Increase to_____

| Prenatal Health Behavior Overall Rating | Never demonstrated 1 | Rarely demonstrated 2 | Sometimes demonstrated 3 | Often demonstrated 4 | Consistently demonstrated 5 | |
|---|---|---|---|---|---|---|
| **INDICATORS:** | | | | | | |
| 160701 Maintains healthy preconceptual state | 1 | 2 | 3 | 4 | 5 | NA |
| 160702 Uses proper body mechanics | 1 | 2 | 3 | 4 | 5 | NA |
| 160703 Keeps appointments for prenatal care | 1 | 2 | 3 | 4 | 5 | NA |
| 160704 Maintains healthy weight gain pattern | 1 | 2 | 3 | 4 | 5 | NA |
| 160705 Receives proper dental care | 1 | 2 | 3 | 4 | 5 | NA |
| 160706 Uses seat belt appropriately | 1 | 2 | 3 | 4 | 5 | NA |
| 160707 Attends childbirth education classes | 1 | 2 | 3 | 4 | 5 | NA |
| 160709 Participates in regular exercise | 1 | 2 | 3 | 4 | 5 | NA |
| 160710 Maintains adequate nutrient intake for pregnancy | 1 | 2 | 3 | 4 | 5 | NA |
| 160711 Practices safe sex | 1 | 2 | 3 | 4 | 5 | NA |
| 160721 Uses medications as prescribed | 1 | 2 | 3 | 4 | 5 | NA |
| 160712 Consults health care professional concerning use of non-prescription drugs | 1 | 2 | 3 | 4 | 5 | NA |
| 160713 Avoids environmental hazards | 1 | 2 | 3 | 4 | 5 | NA |
| 160714 Avoids exposure to infectious diseases | 1 | 2 | 3 | 4 | 5 | NA |
| 160715 Avoids recreational drugs | 1 | 2 | 3 | 4 | 5 | NA |
| 160716 Abstains from alcohol | 1 | 2 | 3 | 4 | 5 | NA |
| 160717 Abstains from tobacco use | 1 | 2 | 3 | 4 | 5 | NA |
| 160718 Avoids teratogenic agents | 1 | 2 | 3 | 4 | 5 | NA |
| 160719 Avoids abusive situations | 1 | 2 | 3 | 4 | 5 | NA |

*2nd edition 2000; Revised 3rd edition*

Outcome Content References:

Bell, R., & O'Neill M. (1994). Exercise and pregnancy: A review. *Birth, 21*(2), 85-95.

Crowell, D.T. (1995). Weight change in the postpartum period. A review of the literature. *Journal of Nurse Midwifery, 40*(5), 418-23.

Freda, M.C., et al. (1993). What pregnant women want to know: A comparison of client and provider perceptions. *Journal of Obstetric, Gynecologic, and Neonatal Nursing, 22*(3), 237.

Kearney, M.H., Murphy, S., Irwin, K., & Rosenbaum, M. (1995). Salvaging self: A grounded theory of pregnancy on crack cocaine. *Nursing Research, 44*(4), 208-213.

McFarlane, J., et al. (1996). Abuse during pregnancy: Associations with maternal health and infant birth weight. *Nursing Research, 45*(1), 37-42.

Olds, S., et al. (1996). *Maternal-newborn nursing: A family-centered approach* (5th ed.). Menlo Park, CA: Addison-Wesley.

Shapiro, H.R. (1993). Prenatal education in the work place. *AWHONNS Clinical Issues in Perinatal & Women's Health Nursing, 4*(1), 113-121.

Summers, L. (1993). Preconception care: An opportunity to maximize health in pregnancy. *Journal of Nurse Midwifery, 38*(4), 188-198.

P

# *Preterm Infant Organization (0117)*

Domain-Functional Health (I)

Class-Growth & Development (B)

Scale(s)-Severely compromised to Not compromised (a)

Care Recipient:

Data Source:

---

**Definition:** Extrauterine integration of physiologic and behavioral function by the infant born 24 to 37 (term) weeks gestation

---

OUTCOME TARGET RATING:   Maintain at_____   Increase to_____

| Preterm Infant Organization Overall Rating | Severely compromised 1 | Substantially compromised 2 | Moderately compromised 3 | Mildly compromised 4 | Not compromised 5 | |
|---|---|---|---|---|---|---|
| **INDICATORS:** | | | | | | |
| 011701 Apical heart rate (120-160) | 1 | 2 | 3 | 4 | 5 | NA |
| 011702 Gestational age index | 1 | 2 | 3 | 4 | 5 | NA |
| 011703 Respiratory rate (30-60) | 1 | 2 | 3 | 4 | 5 | NA |
| 011704 Oxygen saturation >85% | 1 | 2 | 3 | 4 | 5 | NA |
| 011705 Thermoregulation | 1 | 2 | 3 | 4 | 5 | NA |
| 011706 Skin color | 1 | 2 | 3 | 4 | 5 | NA |
| 011707 Feeding tolerance | 1 | 2 | 3 | 4 | 5 | NA |
| 011708 Relaxed muscle tone | 1 | 2 | 3 | 4 | 5 | NA |
| 011709 Smooth synchronous movement | 1 | 2 | 3 | 4 | 5 | NA |
| 011710 Flexed posture | 1 | 2 | 3 | 4 | 5 | NA |
| 011711 Hands brought to mouth | 1 | 2 | 3 | 4 | 5 | NA |
| 011712 Deep sleep | 1 | 2 | 3 | 4 | 5 | NA |
| 011713 Light sleep | 1 | 2 | 3 | 4 | 5 | NA |
| 011714 Quiet-alert | 1 | 2 | 3 | 4 | 5 | NA |
| 011715 Active-alert | 1 | 2 | 3 | 4 | 5 | NA |
| 011716 Attentiveness to stimuli | 1 | 2 | 3 | 4 | 5 | NA |
| 011717 Response to stimuli | 1 | 2 | 3 | 4 | 5 | NA |
| 011718 Appropriate time-out signals | 1 | 2 | 3 | 4 | 5 | NA |
| 011719 Sustained alertness during interaction | 1 | 2 | 3 | 4 | 5 | NA |
| 011720 Interaction with caregiver | 1 | 2 | 3 | 4 | 5 | NA |
| 011721 Self-consolability | 1 | 2 | 3 | 4 | 5 | NA |

*2nd edition 2000; Revised 3rd edition*

Outcome Content References:

Blackburn, S. (1978). Sleep and wake states of the newborn. In K.E. Barnard, et al. (Eds.), *Early parent-infant relationships, module 3-A. A staff development program in perinatal nursing.* (pp. 22-32). White Plains, NY: The National Foundation: March of Dimes.

Blackburn S.T., &. VanderBerg K.A. (1993). Assessment and management of neurodevelopmental behavior development. In C. Kenner, A. Bueggenmeyer, & L.P. Gunderson (Eds.), *Comprehensive neonatal nursing* (pp. 1094-1121). Philadelphia: W. B. Saunders.

D'Apolito K. (1991). What is an organized infant? *Neonatal Network, 2*(1), 23-29.

Deacon, J., & O'Neill, P. (Eds.). (1999). *Core curriculum for neonatal intensive care nursing* (2nd ed.). Philadelphia: W.B. Saunders.

Jorgensen, K.M. (1993). *Developmental care of the preterm infant.* South Weymouth, MA: Children's Medical Ventures.

Mattson, S., & Smith, J.E. (Eds.). (2000). *Core curriculum for maternal-newborn nursing* (2nd ed.). Philadelphia: W.B. Saunders.

McGrath J.M., & Conliffe-Torres, S. (1996). Integrating family centered developmental assessment and interventions with routine cares in the neonatal intensive care unit. *Nursing Clinics of North America, 31*(2), 367-385.

National Association of Neonatal Nurses. (1993). *Infant developmental care guidelines.* Petaluma, CA: Author.

# *Psychomotor Energy (0006)*

Domain-Functional Health (I)                                Care Recipient:

Class-Energy Maintenance (A)                              Data Source:

Scale(s)-Never demonstrated to Consistently demonstrated (m) and Consistently demonstrated to Never demonstrated (t)

**Definition:** Personal drive and energy to maintain activities of daily living, nutrition, and personal safety

OUTCOME TARGET RATING:     Maintain at_____     Increase to_____

| Psychomotor Energy Overall Rating | Never demonstrated 1 | Rarely demonstrated 2 | Sometimes demonstrated 3 | Often demonstrated 4 | Consistently demonstrated 5 | |
|---|---|---|---|---|---|---|
| **INDICATORS:** | | | | | | |
| 000601 Exhibits appropriate affect | 1 | 2 | 3 | 4 | 5 | NA |
| 000602 Exhibits concentration | 1 | 2 | 3 | 4 | 5 | NA |
| 000603 Exhibits appropriate grooming and hygiene | 1 | 2 | 3 | 4 | 5 | NA |
| 000604 Exhibits normal appetite | 1 | 2 | 3 | 4 | 5 | NA |
| 000605 Complies with medication and therapeutic regimen | 1 | 2 | 3 | 4 | 5 | NA |
| 000606 Shows interest in surroundings | 1 | 2 | 3 | 4 | 5 | NA |
| 000608 Exhibits appropriate energy level | 1 | 2 | 3 | 4 | 5 | NA |
| 000609 Exhibits ability to accomplish daily tasks | 1 | 2 | 3 | 4 | 5 | NA |

| | Consistently demonstrated | Often demonstrated | Sometimes demonstrated | Rarely demonstrated | Never demonstrated | |
|---|---|---|---|---|---|---|
| 000607 Suicide ideation | 1 | 2 | 3 | 4 | 5 | NA |
| 000611 Lethargy | 1 | 2 | 3 | 4 | 5 | NA |
| 000612 Depression | 1 | 2 | 3 | 4 | 5 | NA |

*2nd edition 2000; Revised 3rd edition*

Outcome Content References:

American Psychiatric Association. (2000). *Diagnostic and statistical manual of mental disorders* (4th ed., text revision). Washington DC: Author.

U.S. Department of Health and Human Services. (1993). *Depression and primary care: Detection and diagnosis.* (Vol. 1) (AHCPR publication No. 93-0550). Rockville, MD: Government Printing Office.

U.S. Department of Health and Human Services. (1993). *Depression and primary care: Treatment of major depression.* (Vol. 2) (AHCPR publication No. 93-0551). Rockville, MD: Government Printing Office.

P

# Psychosocial Adjustment: Life Change (1305)

*Domain-Psychosocial Health (III)*

*Class-Psychosocial Adaptation (N)*

*Scale(s)-Never demonstrated to Consistently demonstrated (m)*

*Care Recipient:*

*Data Source:*

**Definition:** Adaptive psychosocial response of an individual to a significant life change

OUTCOME TARGET RATING:    Maintain at_____    Increase to_____

| Psychosocial Adjustment: Life Change Overall Rating | Never demonstrated 1 | Rarely demonstrated 2 | Sometimes demonstrated 3 | Often demonstrated 4 | Consistently demonstrated 5 | |
|---|---|---|---|---|---|---|
| **INDICATORS:** | | | | | | |
| 130501 Sets realistic goals | 1 | 2 | 3 | 4 | 5 | NA |
| 130502 Maintains self-esteem | 1 | 2 | 3 | 4 | 5 | NA |
| 130503 Maintains productivity | 1 | 2 | 3 | 4 | 5 | NA |
| 130504 Reports feeling useful | 1 | 2 | 3 | 4 | 5 | NA |
| 130505 Verbalizes optimism about present | 1 | 2 | 3 | 4 | 5 | NA |
| 130506 Verbalizes optimism about future | 1 | 2 | 3 | 4 | 5 | NA |
| 130507 Reports feeling empowered | 1 | 2 | 3 | 4 | 5 | NA |
| 130508 Identifies multiple coping strategies | 1 | 2 | 3 | 4 | 5 | NA |
| 130509 Uses effective coping strategies | 1 | 2 | 3 | 4 | 5 | NA |
| 130510 Uses effective financial management | 1 | 2 | 3 | 4 | 5 | NA |
| 130513 Uses available social support | 1 | 2 | 3 | 4 | 5 | NA |
| 130514 Participates in leisure activities | 1 | 2 | 3 | 4 | 5 | NA |
| 130511 Expresses satisfaction with living arrangements | 1 | 2 | 3 | 4 | 5 | NA |
| 130512 Reports feeling socially engaged | 1 | 2 | 3 | 4 | 5 | NA |

*1st edition 1997; Revised 3rd edition*

## Outcome Content References:

Hernan, J.A. (1984). Exploding aging myths through retirement counseling. *Journal of Gerontological Nursing, 10*(4), 31-33.

Johnson, R.A. (2001). Relocation stress syndrome. In M. Maas, K. Buckwalter, M. Hardy, T. Tripp-Reimer, M. Titler, & J. Specht (Eds.), *Nursing care of older adults: Diagnoses, outcomes & interventions* (pp. 619-630). St. Louis: Mosby.

+Liang, J. (1984). Dimensions of the Life Satisfaction Index A: A structural formulation. *Journal of Gerontology, 39*(5), 613-622.

+Neugarten, B.L., Havighurst, R.J., & Tobin, S. (1961). The measurement of life satisfaction. *Journal of Gerontology, 16*, 134-143.

Neuhs, H.P. (1991). Ready for retirement? *Geriatric Nursing, 12*(5), 240-241.

Rosenkoetter, M.M. (1985). Is your older client ready for a role change after retirement? *Journal of Gerontological Nursing, 11*(9), 21-24.

Tincher, B.J.V. (1992). Retirement: Perspectives and theory. *Physical & Occupational Therapy in Geriatrics, 11*(1), 55-62.

# *Quality of Life (2000)*

Domain-Perceived Health (V)

Class-Health & Life Quality (U)

Scale(s)-Not at all satisfied to Completely satisfied (s)

Care Recipient:

Data Source:

**Definition:** Extent of positive perception of current life circumstances

OUTCOME TARGET RATING:        Maintain at_____        Increase to_____

| Quality of Life Overall Rating | Not at all satisfied 1 | Somewhat satisfied 2 | Moderately satisfied 3 | Very satisfied 4 | Completely satisfied 5 | |
|---|---|---|---|---|---|---|
| **INDICATORS:** | | | | | | |
| 200001 Health status | 1 | 2 | 3 | 4 | 5 | NA |
| 200002 Social circumstances | 1 | 2 | 3 | 4 | 5 | NA |
| 200003 Environmental circumstances | 1 | 2 | 3 | 4 | 5 | NA |
| 200004 Economic status | 1 | 2 | 3 | 4 | 5 | NA |
| 200005 Education level | 1 | 2 | 3 | 4 | 5 | NA |
| 200006 Occupation | 1 | 2 | 3 | 4 | 5 | NA |
| 200007 Close relationships | 1 | 2 | 3 | 4 | 5 | NA |
| 200008 Achievement of life goals | 1 | 2 | 3 | 4 | 5 | NA |
| 200009 Ability to cope | 1 | 2 | 3 | 4 | 5 | NA |
| 200010 Self-concept | 1 | 2 | 3 | 4 | 5 | NA |
| 200011 Pervasive mood | 1 | 2 | 3 | 4 | 5 | NA |

*1st edition 1997; Revised 3rd edition*

Outcome Content References:

Andrews, F., & Withey, S. (1976). *Social indicators of well-being: Americans' perceptions of life quality.* New York: Plenum Press.

Davidhizar, R.E., & Giger, J.N. (2001). Powerlessness. In M. Maas, K. Buckwalter, M. Hardy, T. Tripp-Reimer, M. Titler, & J. Specht (Eds.), *Nursing care of older adults: Diagnoses, outcomes & interventions* (pp. 562-570). St. Louis: Mosby.

+Diener, E., Emmons, R.A., Larsen, R.J., & Griffin, S. (1985). The Satisfaction with Life Scale. *Journal of Personality Assessment, 49*(1), 71-75.

Gill, L., & Flenstein, A.R. (1994). A critical appraisal of the quality of quality-of-life measurements. *Journal of the American Medical Association, 272*(8), 619-626.

Padilla, G., Ferrell, B., Grant, M., & Rhiner, M. (1990). Defining the content domain of quality of life for cancer patients with pain. *Cancer Nursing, 13*(2), 108-115.

Ragsdale, D., Kotarba, J., & Morrow, J. (1992). Quality of life of hospitalized persons with AIDS. *Image - the Journal of Nursing Scholarship, 24*(4), 259-265.

Stewart, A., Ware, J., Sherbourne, C., & Wells, K. (1992). Psychological distress/well-being and cognitive functioning measures. In A. Stewart & J. Ware, Jr. (Eds.), *Measuring functioning and well-being: The medical outcomes study approach* (pp. 102-142). Durham, NC: Duke University Press.

**Q**

# Respiratory Status: Airway Patency (0410)

*Domain-Physiologic Health (II)*                          *Care Recipient:*

*Class-Cardiopulmonary (E)*                               *Data Source:*

*Scale(s)-Severely compromised to Not compromised (a) and Severe to None (n)*

**Definition:** Open, clear tracheobronchial passages for air exchange

OUTCOME TARGET RATING:    Maintain at_____    Increase to_____

| Respiratory Status: Airway Patency Overall Rating | Severely compromised 1 | Substantially compromised 2 | Moderately compromised 3 | Mildly compromised 4 | Not compromised 5 | |
|---|---|---|---|---|---|---|
| **INDICATORS:** | | | | | | |
| 041009  Ease of breathing | 1 | 2 | 3 | 4 | 5 | NA |
| 041004  Respiratory rate | 1 | 2 | 3 | 4 | 5 | NA |
| 041005  Respiratory rhythm | 1 | 2 | 3 | 4 | 5 | NA |
| 041006  Moves sputum out of airway | 1 | 2 | 3 | 4 | 5 | NA |
| 041010  Moves blockage out of airway | 1 | 2 | 3 | 4 | 5 | NA |
| | **Severe** | **Substantial** | **Moderate** | **Mild** | **None** | |
| 041002  Anxiety | 1 | 2 | 3 | 4 | 5 | NA |
| 041011  Fear | 1 | 2 | 3 | 4 | 5 | NA |
| 041003  Choking | 1 | 2 | 3 | 4 | 5 | NA |
| 041007  Adventitious breath sounds | 1 | 2 | 3 | 4 | 5 | NA |

*2nd edition 2000; Revised 3rd edition*

**Outcome Content References:**

Clochesy, J.M., Brey, C., Cardin, S., Whittaker, A.A., & Rudy, E.B. (1996). *Critical care nursing* (2nd ed.) Philadelphia: W.B. Saunders.

Lewis, S.M., Collier, I.C., Heitkermper, M.M., & Dirksen, S.R. (2000). *Medical-surgical nursing: Assessment & management of clinical problems* (5th ed.). St. Louis: Mosby.

McCance, K.L., & Huether, S.E. (2002). *Pathophysiology: The biologic basis for disease in adults and children* (4th ed.). St. Louis: Mosby.

Smeltzer, S.C., & Bare, B.G. (Eds.). (2003). *Brunner and Suddarth's textbook of medical-surgical nursing* (10th ed.). Philadelphia: Lippincott, Williams, & Wilkins.

**R**

# Respiratory Status: Gas Exchange (0402)

*Domain-Physiologic Health (II)*

*Class-Cardiopulmonary (E)*

*Scale(s)-Severely compromised to Not compromised (a) and Severe to None (n)*

*Care Recipient:*

*Data Source:*

> **Definition:** Alveolar exchange of carbon dioxide and oxygen to maintain arterial blood gas concentrations

OUTCOME TARGET RATING:    Maintain at_____    Increase to_____

| Respiratory Status: Gas Exchange Overall Rating | Severely compromised 1 | Substantially compromised 2 | Moderately compromised 3 | Mildly compromised 4 | Not compromised 5 | |
|---|---|---|---|---|---|---|
| **INDICATORS:** | | | | | | |
| 040201  Cognitive status | 1 | 2 | 3 | 4 | 5 | NA |
| 040202  Ease of breathing | 1 | 2 | 3 | 4 | 5 | NA |
| 040208  $PaO_2$* | 1 | 2 | 3 | 4 | 5 | NA |
| 040209  $PaCO_2$* | 1 | 2 | 3 | 4 | 5 | NA |
| 040210  Arterial pH | 1 | 2 | 3 | 4 | 5 | NA |
| 040211  Oxygen saturation | 1 | 2 | 3 | 4 | 5 | NA |
| 040212  End tidal carbon dioxide | 1 | 2 | 3 | 4 | 5 | NA |
| 040213  Chest x-ray findings | 1 | 2 | 3 | 4 | 5 | NA |
| 040214  Ventilation perfusion balance | 1 | 2 | 3 | 4 | 5 | NA |

| | Severe | Substantial | Moderate | Mild | None | |
|---|---|---|---|---|---|---|
| 040203  Dyspnea at rest | 1 | 2 | 3 | 4 | 5 | NA |
| 040204  Dyspnea with exertion | 1 | 2 | 3 | 4 | 5 | NA |
| 040205  Restlessness | 1 | 2 | 3 | 4 | 5 | NA |
| 040206  Cyanosis | 1 | 2 | 3 | 4 | 5 | NA |
| 040207  Somnolence | 1 | 2 | 3 | 4 | 5 | NA |

*$PaO_2$ = partial pressure of oxygen in arterial blood; $PaCO_2$= partial pressure of carbon dioxide in arterial blood.

*1st edition 1997; Revised 2nd edition 2000; Revised 3rd edition*

**R**

## Outcome Content References:

Ahrens, T. (1993). Changing perspectives in the assessment of oxygenation. *Critical Care Nurse, 13*(4), 78-83.

Berry, B.E., & Pinard, A.E. (2002). Assessing tissue oxygenation. *Critical Care Nurse, 22*(3), 22-36.

Hayden, R. (1992). What keeps oxygenation on track? *American Journal of Nursing, 92*(12), 32-40.

Janson-Bjerklie, S. (1993). Predicting the outcomes of living with asthma. *Research in Nursing and Health, 16*(4), 241-249.

McCarty, K., & Wilkins, R. (1990). Synopsis of clinical findings in respiratory disorders. In R. Wilkins, et al. (Eds.), *Clinical assessment in respiratory care*, (2nd ed., pp. 294-302). St. Louis: Mosby.

Morton, P. (1989). Respiratory systems. In P. Morton (Ed.), *Health assessment in nursing* (pp. 243-281). Springhouse, PA: Springhouse.

Patrick, M., et al. (1991). *Medical-surgical nursing: Pathophysiological concepts* (2nd ed.). Philadelphia: J.B. Lippincott.

Potter, P., & Perry, A. (1991). *Oxygenation: Basic nursing theory and practice*. St. Louis: Mosby.

# Respiratory Status: Ventilation (0403)

*Domain-Physiologic Health (II)*

*Class-Cardiopulmonary (E)*

*Scale(s)-Severely compromised to Not compromised (a) and Severe to None (n)*

*Care Recipient:*

*Data Source:*

**Definition:** Movement of air in and out of the lungs

OUTCOME TARGET RATING:   Maintain at_____   Increase to_____

| **Respiratory Status: Ventilation Overall Rating** | Severely compromised 1 | Substantially compromised 2 | Moderately compromised 3 | Mildly compromised 4 | Not compromised 5 | |
|---|---|---|---|---|---|---|
| **INDICATORS:** | | | | | | |
| 040301 Respiratory rate | 1 | 2 | 3 | 4 | 5 | NA |
| 040302 Respiratory rhythm | 1 | 2 | 3 | 4 | 5 | NA |
| 040303 Depth of inspiration | 1 | 2 | 3 | 4 | 5 | NA |
| 040304 Symmetrical chest expansion | 1 | 2 | 3 | 4 | 5 | NA |
| 040305 Ease of breathing | 1 | 2 | 3 | 4 | 5 | NA |
| 040306 Moves sputum out of airway | 1 | 2 | 3 | 4 | 5 | NA |
| 040307 Vocalization | 1 | 2 | 3 | 4 | 5 | NA |
| 040308 Expulsion of air | 1 | 2 | 3 | 4 | 5 | NA |
| 040318 Percussed sounds | 1 | 2 | 3 | 4 | 5 | NA |
| 040319 Ausculated breath sounds | 1 | 2 | 3 | 4 | 5 | NA |
| 040320 Ausculated vocalizations | 1 | 2 | 3 | 4 | 5 | NA |
| 040321 Bronchophony | 1 | 2 | 3 | 4 | 5 | NA |
| 040322 Egophony | 1 | 2 | 3 | 4 | 5 | NA |
| 040323 Whispered pectoriloquy | 1 | 2 | 3 | 4 | 5 | NA |
| 040324 Tidal volume | 1 | 2 | 3 | 4 | 5 | NA |
| 040325 Vital capacity | 1 | 2 | 3 | 4 | 5 | NA |
| 040326 Chest x-ray findings | 1 | 2 | 3 | 4 | 5 | NA |
| 040327 Pulmonary function tests | 1 | 2 | 3 | 4 | 5 | NA |

| | Severe | Substantial | Moderate | Mild | None | |
|---|---|---|---|---|---|---|
| 040309 Accessory muscle use | 1 | 2 | 3 | 4 | 5 | NA |
| 040310 Adventitious breath sounds | 1 | 2 | 3 | 4 | 5 | NA |
| 040311 Chest retraction | 1 | 2 | 3 | 4 | 5 | NA |
| 040312 Pursed lips breathing | 1 | 2 | 3 | 4 | 5 | NA |
| 040313 Dyspnea at rest | 1 | 2 | 3 | 4 | 5 | NA |
| 040314 Dyspnea with exertion | 1 | 2 | 3 | 4 | 5 | NA |
| 040315 Orthopnea | 1 | 2 | 3 | 4 | 5 | NA |
| 040316 Shortness of breath | 1 | 2 | 3 | 4 | 5 | NA |
| 040317 Tactile fremitus | 1 | 2 | 3 | 4 | 5 | NA |

*1st edition 1997; Revised 3rd edition*

Outcome Content References:

Ahrens, T. (1993). Changing perspectives in the assessment of oxygenation. *Critical Care Nurse, 13*(4), 78-83.

+Guyatt, G.H., Berman, L.B., Townsend, M., Pugsley, S.O., & Chambers, L. W. (1987). A measure of quality of life for clinical trials in chronic lung disease. *Thorax, 42*(10), 773-778.

Hayden, R. (1992). What keeps oxygenation on track? *American Journal of Nursing, 92*(12), 32-40.

Janson-Bjerklie, S. (1993). Predicting the outcomes of living with asthma. *Research in Nursing and Health, 16*(4), 241-249.

McCarty, K., & Wilkins, R. (1990). Synopsis of clinical findings in respiratory disorders. In R. Wilkins, et al. (Eds.), *Clinical assessment in respiratory care*, (2nd ed., pp. 294-302). St. Louis: Mosby.

Morton, P. (1989). Respiratory systems. In P. Morton (Ed.), *Health assessment in nursing* (pp. 243-281). Springhouse, PA: Springhouse.

Patrick, M., et al. (1991). *Medical-surgical nursing: Pathophysiological concepts* (2nd ed.). Philadelphia: J.B. Lippincott.

Potter, P., & Perry, A. (1991). *Oxygenation: Basic nursing theory and practice*. St. Louis: Mosby.

Wakefield, B. (2001). Ineffective breathing pattern. In M. Maas, K. Buckwalter, M. Hardy, T. Tripp-Reimer, M. Titler, & J. Specht (Eds.), *Nursing care of older adults: Diagnoses, outcomes & interventions* (pp. 313-323). St. Louis: Mosby.

R

# Rest (0003)

*Domain-Functional Health (I)*

*Class-Energy Maintenance (A)*

*Scale(s)-Extremely compromised to Not compromised (a)*

*Care Recipient:*

*Data Source:*

**Definition:** Quantity and pattern of diminished activity for mental and physical rejuvenation

OUTCOME TARGET RATING:    Maintain at_____    Increase to_____

| Rest Overall Rating | Extremely compromised 1 | Substantially compromised 2 | Moderately compromised 3 | Mildly compromised 4 | Not compromised 5 | |
|---|---|---|---|---|---|---|
| **INDICATORS:** | | | | | | |
| 000301 Amount of rest | 1 | 2 | 3 | 4 | 5 | NA |
| 000302 Rest pattern | 1 | 2 | 3 | 4 | 5 | NA |
| 000303 Rest quality | 1 | 2 | 3 | 4 | 5 | NA |
| 000304 Physically rested | 1 | 2 | 3 | 4 | 5 | NA |
| 000305 Mentally rested | 1 | 2 | 3 | 4 | 5 | NA |
| 000308 Emotionally rested | 1 | 2 | 3 | 4 | 5 | NA |
| 000306 Feelings of rejuve-nation after rest | 1 | 2 | 3 | 4 | 5 | NA |

*1st edition 1997; Revised 3rd edition*

Outcome Content References:

Brown, D.R., Morgan, W.P., & Raglin, J.S. (1993). Effects of exercise and rest on the state anxiety and blood pressure of physically challenged college students. *Journal of Sports Medicine and Physical Fitness, 33*(3), 300-305.

Ellis, J.R., & Nowlis, E.A. (1994). *Providing nursing care within the nursing process* (5th ed.). Philadelphia: J.B. Lippincott.

+Lee, K.A., Hicks, G., & Nino-Murcia, G. (1991). Validity and reliability of a scale to assess fatigue. *Psychiatry Research, 36*(3), 291-298.

Potter, P.A., & Perry, A.G. (2001). *Fundamentals of nursing* (5th ed.). St. Louis: Mosby.

Smeltzer, S.C., & Bare, B.G. (Eds.). (2003). *Brunner and Suddarth's textbook of medical-surgical nursing* (10th ed.). Philadelphia: Lippincott, Williams, & Wilkins.

R

# Risk Control (1902)

*Domain-Health Knowledge & Behavior (IV)*

*Class-Risk Control & Safety (T)*

*Scale(s)-Never demonstrated to Consistently demonstrated (m)*

*Care Recipient:*

*Data Source:*

**Definition:** Personal actions to prevent, eliminate, or reduce modifiable health threats

OUTCOME TARGET RATING:    Maintain at_____    Increase to_____

| Risk Control Overall Rating | Never demonstrated 1 | Rarely demonstrated 2 | Sometimes demonstrated 3 | Often demonstrated 4 | Consistently demonstrated 5 | |
|---|---|---|---|---|---|---|

INDICATORS:

| | | | | | | | |
|---|---|---|---|---|---|---|---|
| 190201 | Acknowledges risk factors | 1 | 2 | 3 | 4 | 5 | NA |
| 190202 | Monitors environ-mental risk factors | 1 | 2 | 3 | 4 | 5 | NA |
| 190203 | Monitors personal behavior risk factors | 1 | 2 | 3 | 4 | 5 | NA |
| 190204 | Develops effective risk control strategies | 1 | 2 | 3 | 4 | 5 | NA |
| 190205 | Adjusts risk control strategies as needed | 1 | 2 | 3 | 4 | 5 | NA |
| 190206 | Commits to risk control strategies | 1 | 2 | 3 | 4 | 5 | NA |
| 190207 | Follows selected risk control strategies | 1 | 2 | 3 | 4 | 5 | NA |
| 190208 | Modifies lifestyle to reduce risk | 1 | 2 | 3 | 4 | 5 | NA |
| 190209 | Avoids exposure to health threats | 1 | 2 | 3 | 4 | 5 | NA |
| 190210 | Participates in screening for associated health problems | 1 | 2 | 3 | 4 | 5 | NA |
| 190211 | Participates in screening for identified risks | 1 | 2 | 3 | 4 | 5 | NA |
| 190212 | Obtains appropriate immunizations | 1 | 2 | 3 | 4 | 5 | NA |
| 190213 | Uses health care services congru-ent with need | 1 | 2 | 3 | 4 | 5 | NA |
| 190214 | Uses personal support systems to control risk | 1 | 2 | 3 | 4 | 5 | NA |
| 190215 | Uses community resources to control risk | 1 | 2 | 3 | 4 | 5 | NA |
| 190216 | Recognizes changes in health status | 1 | 2 | 3 | 4 | 5 | NA |
| 190217 | Monitors health status changes | 1 | 2 | 3 | 4 | 5 | NA |

*1st edition 1997; Revised 3rd edition*

**R**

*Continued*

Outcome Content References:

+Hettler, B. (1982). Wellness promotion and risk reduction on a university campus. In M. Faber & A. Reinhardt (Eds.), *Promoting health through risk reduction*. New York: Macmillan.

Nease, R. (1994). Risk attitudes in gambles involving length of life: Aspirations, variations, and ruminations. *Medical Decision Making, 14*(2), 210-213.

Perez-Stable, E., Marin, G., & Marin, B. (1994). Behavioral risk factors: A comparison of Latinos and non-Latino whites in San Francisco. *American Journal of Public Health, 84*(6), 971-976.

Rost, K., Burnam, M., & Smith, G. (1993). Development of screeners for depressive disorders and substance abuse history. *Medical Care, 31*(3), 189-200.

Ryan, P. (1983). Altered health maintenance. In J.M. Thompston, et al. (Eds.), *Mosby's clinical nursing*. (3rd ed., pp. 1425-1427). St. Louis: Mosby.

Sickle Cell Disease Guideline Panel. (1993). *Sickle cell disease: Screening, diagnosis, management, and counseling in newborn and infants, clinical practice guideline*, No. 6. (AHCPR Publication No. 93-0562). Rockville, MD: U.S. Department of Health and Human Services. Public Health Services, Agency for Health Care Policy and Research.

Simons-Morton, D.G., Mullen, P.D., Mains, D.A., Tabak, E.R., & Green, L.W. (1992). Characteristics of controlled studies of patient education and counseling for preventive health behaviors. *Patient Education and Counseling, 19*(2), 174-204.

Tandy, L., & Malan, S. (2001). Impaired swallowing. In M. Maas, K. Buckwalter, M. Hardy, T. Tripp-Reimer, M. Titler, & J. Specht (Eds.), *Nursing care of older adults: Diagnoses, outcomes & interventions* (pp. 158-171). St. Louis: Mosby.

U.S. Department of Health and Human Services. (1998). *Clinician's handbook of preventive services: Put prevention into practice*. (2nd ed.). Washington, DC: Government Printing Office.

R

# Risk Control: Alcohol Use (1903)

Domain-Health Knowledge & Behavior (IV)

Class-Risk Control & Safety (T)

Scale(s)-Never demonstrated to Consistently demonstrated (m)

Care Recipient:

Data Source:

**Definition:** Personal actions to prevent, eliminate, or reduce alcohol use that poses a threat to health

OUTCOME TARGET RATING:     Maintain at_____     Increase to_____

| Risk Control: Alcohol Use Overall Rating | Never demonstrated 1 | Rarely demonstrated 2 | Sometimes demonstrated 3 | Often demonstrated 4 | Consistently demonstrated 5 | |
|---|---|---|---|---|---|---|
| INDICATORS: | | | | | | |
| 190301 Acknowledges risk for alcohol misuse | 1 | 2 | 3 | 4 | 5 | NA |
| 190302 Acknowledges personal consequences associated with alcohol misuse | 1 | 2 | 3 | 4 | 5 | NA |
| 190303 Monitors environ-ment for factors encouraging alcohol abuse | 1 | 2 | 3 | 4 | 5 | NA |
| 190304 Monitors personal alcohol use patterns | 1 | 2 | 3 | 4 | 5 | NA |
| 190305 Develops effective alcohol use control strategies | 1 | 2 | 3 | 4 | 5 | NA |
| 190306 Adjusts alcohol use control strategies as needes | 1 | 2 | 3 | 4 | 5 | NA |
| 190307 Commits to alcohol use control strategies | 1 | 2 | 3 | 4 | 5 | NA |
| 190308 Follows selected alcohol use control strategies | 1 | 2 | 3 | 4 | 5 | NA |
| 190309 Participates in screening for associated health problems | 1 | 2 | 3 | 4 | 5 | NA |
| 190310 Uses health care services con-gruent with needs | 1 | 2 | 3 | 4 | 5 | NA |
| 190311 Uses personal support systems to control alcohol misuse | 1 | 2 | 3 | 4 | 5 | NA |
| 190312 Uses support groups to control alcohol misuse | 1 | 2 | 3 | 4 | 5 | NA |

R

*Continued*

| Risk Control: Alcohol Use—cont'd | | Never demonstrated | Rarely demonstrated | Sometimes demonstrated | Often demonstrated | Consistently demonstrated | |
|---|---|---|---|---|---|---|---|
| 190313 | Uses community resources to control alcohol misuse | 1 | 2 | 3 | 4 | 5 | NA |
| 190314 | Recognizes changes in general health status | 1 | 2 | 3 | 4 | 5 | NA |
| 190315 | Monitors health status changes | 1 | 2 | 3 | 4 | 5 | NA |
| 190316 | Controls alcohol intake | 1 | 2 | 3 | 4 | 5 | NA |

*1st edition 1997; Revised 3rd edition*

**Outcome Content References:**

+MacNeil, G. (1991). A short-form scale to measure alcohol abuse. *Research on Social Work Practice, 1*(1), 68-75.

McCuster, J., Stoddard, A.M., Zapka, J.G., & Lewis, B.F. (1993). Behavioral outcomes of AIDS educational interventions for drug users in short term treatment, *American Journal of Public Health, 83*(10), 1463-1466.

Simons-Morton, D.G., Mullen, P.D., Mains, D.A., Tabek, E.R., & Green, L.W. (1992). Characteristics of controlled studies of patient education and counseling for preventive health behaviors. *Patient Education and Counseling, 19*(2), 174-204.

Talashek, M.L., Gerace, L.M., & Starr, K.L. (1994). The substance abuse pandemic: Determinants to guide interventions. *Public Health Nursing, 11*(2), 131-139.

U.S. Department of Health and Human Services. (1998). *Clinician's handbook of preventive services: Put prevention into practice* (2nd ed.). Washington: DC: Government Printing Office.

R

# *Risk Control: Cancer (1917)*

Domain-Health Knowledge & Behavior (IV)                    Care Recipient:

Class-Risk Control & Safety (T)                              Data Source:

Scale(s)-Never demonstrated to Consistently demonstrated (m)

**Definition:** Personal actions to detect or reduce the threat of cancer

OUTCOME TARGET RATING:    Maintain at_____    Increase to_____

| Risk Control: Cancer Overall Rating | Never demonstrated 1 | Rarely demonstrated 2 | Sometimes demonstrated 3 | Often demonstrated 4 | Consistently demonstrated 5 | |
|---|---|---|---|---|---|---|
| INDICATORS: | | | | | | |
| 191701 Seeks additional information about cancer prevention | 1 | 2 | 3 | 4 | 5 | NA |
| 191702 Avoids exposure to known or suspected carcinogens | 1 | 2 | 3 | 4 | 5 | NA |
| 191703 Protects self from known or suspected carcinogens | 1 | 2 | 3 | 4 | 5 | NA |
| 191704 Modifies environ-ment to decrease or eliminate exposure to known or suspected carcinogens | 1 | 2 | 3 | 4 | 5 | NA |
| 191705 Follows dietary recommenda-tions for reducing risk | 1 | 2 | 3 | 4 | 5 | NA |
| 191706 Performs recom-mended self-assessments for cancer detection | 1 | 2 | 3 | 4 | 5 | NA |
| 191707 Participates in recommended cancer screening | 1 | 2 | 3 | 4 | 5 | NA |
| 191708 Seeks health care services follow-ing abnormal screening results | 1 | 2 | 3 | 4 | 5 | NA |

*2nd edition 2000; Revised 3rd edition*

R

Outcome Content References:

American Nurses Association. (1994). *Clinicians handbook of preventive services*. Waldorf, MD: American Nurses Publishing.

Bassett, L.W., Hendrick, R.E., Bassford, T.L., et al. (1994). *Quality determinants of mammography*, No. 13. (AHCPR Publication No. 95-0632). Rockville, MD: U.S. Department of Health and Human Services. Public Health Services, Agency for Health Care Policy and Research.

Machia, J. (2001). Breast cancer: Risk, prevention, & tamoxifen. *American Journal of Nursing, 101*(4), 26-36.

U.S. Department of Health and Human Services. (1998). *Clinician's handbook of preventive services: Put prevention into practice* (2nd ed.). Washington: DC: Government Printing Office.

U.S. Preventive Services Task Force. (1996). *Guide to clinical preventive services* (2nd ed.). Baltimore: Williams & Wilkins.

# Risk Control: Cardiovascular Health (1914)

*Domain-Health Knowledge & Behavior (IV)*

*Class-Risk Control & Safety (T)*

*Scale(s)-Never demonstrated to Consistently demonstrated (m)*

*Care Recipient:*

*Data Source:*

**Definition:** Personal actions to eliminate or reduce threats to cardiovascular health

OUTCOME TARGET RATING:    Maintain at_____    Increase to_____

| Risk Control: Cardiovascular Health Overall Rating | Never demonstrated 1 | Rarely demonstrated 2 | Sometimes demonstrated 3 | Often demonstrated 4 | Consistently demonstrated 5 | |
|---|---|---|---|---|---|---|
| INDICATORS: | | | | | | |
| 191401 Acknowledges risk for cardio-vascular disease | 1 | 2 | 3 | 4 | 5 | NA |
| 191402 Acknowledges ability to change behavior | 1 | 2 | 3 | 4 | 5 | NA |
| 191403 Avoids tobacco use | 1 | 2 | 3 | 4 | 5 | NA |
| 191404 Monitors blood pressure | 1 | 2 | 3 | 4 | 5 | NA |
| 191405 Monitors radial pulse rate | 1 | 2 | 3 | 4 | 5 | NA |
| 191406 Uses stress management techniques | 1 | 2 | 3 | 4 | 5 | NA |
| 191407 Uses effective weight control strategies | 1 | 2 | 3 | 4 | 5 | NA |
| 191408 Follows recom-mended diet | 1 | 2 | 3 | 4 | 5 | NA |
| 191409 Uses health care services congru-ent with needs | 1 | 2 | 3 | 4 | 5 | NA |
| 191410 Follows recom-mended precautions concerning non-prescription drugs | 1 | 2 | 3 | 4 | 5 | NA |
| 191411 Seeks information about methods to maintain cardiovascular health | 1 | 2 | 3 | 4 | 5 | NA |
| 191412 Monitors effects of stimulants | 1 | 2 | 3 | 4 | 5 | NA |
| 191413 Participates in screening for cholesterol | 1 | 2 | 3 | 4 | 5 | NA |
| 191414 Uses medications as prescribed | 1 | 2 | 3 | 4 | 5 | NA |
| 191415 Participates in regular exercise | 1 | 2 | 3 | 4 | 5 | NA |
| 191416 Participates in aerobic exercise | 1 | 2 | 3 | 4 | 5 | NA |

*2nd edition 2000; Revised 3rd edition*

R

Outcome Content References:

Gomel, M., Oldenburg, B., Simpson, J.M., & Owen, N. (1993). Work-site cardiovascular risk reduction: A randomized trial of health risk assessment, education, counseling, and incentives. *American Journal of Public Health, 83*(9), 1231-1238.

Wenger, N.K., Froelicher, E.S., Smith, L.K., et al. (1995). *Cardiac rehabilitation, Clinical practice guideline*, No. 17. (AHCPR Publication No. 96-0672). Rockville, MD: U.S. Department of Health and Human Services. Public Health Services, Agency for Health Care Policy and Research and the National Heart, Lung, and Blood Institute.

Winkleby, M.A., Flora, J.A., & Kraemer, H.C. (1994). A community-based heart disease intervention: Predictors of change. *American Journal of Public Health, 84*(5), 767-771.

R

# Risk Control: Drug Use (1904)

Domain-Health Knowledge & Behavior (IV)

Class-Risk Control & Safety (T)

Scale(s)-Never demonstrated to Consistently demonstrated (m)

Care Recipient:

Data Source:

**Definition:** Personal actions to prevent, eliminate, or reduce drug use that poses a threat to health

OUTCOME TARGET RATING:   Maintain at_____   Increase to_____

| Risk Control: Drug Use Overall Rating | Never demonstrated 1 | Rarely demonstrated 2 | Sometimes demonstrated 3 | Often demonstrated 4 | Consistently demonstrated 5 | |
|---|---|---|---|---|---|---|
| INDICATORS: | | | | | | |
| 190401 Acknowledges risk for drug misuse | 1 | 2 | 3 | 4 | 5 | NA |
| 190402 Acknowledges personal consequences associated with drug misuse | 1 | 2 | 3 | 4 | 5 | NA |
| 190403 Monitors environment for factors encouraging drug misuse | 1 | 2 | 3 | 4 | 5 | NA |
| 190404 Monitors personal drug use patterns | 1 | 2 | 3 | 4 | 5 | NA |
| 190405 Develops effective drug use control strategies | 1 | 2 | 3 | 4 | 5 | NA |
| 190406 Adjusts drug use control strategies as needed | 1 | 2 | 3 | 4 | 5 | NA |
| 190407 Commits to drug use control strategies | 1 | 2 | 3 | 4 | 5 | NA |
| 190408 Follows selected drug use control strategies | 1 | 2 | 3 | 4 | 5 | NA |
| 190409 Participates in screening for associated health problems | 1 | 2 | 3 | 4 | 5 | NA |
| 190410 Uses health care services congruent with needs | 1 | 2 | 3 | 4 | 5 | NA |
| 190411 Uses personal support systems to control drug misuse | 1 | 2 | 3 | 4 | 5 | NA |
| 190412 Uses support groups to control drug misuse | 1 | 2 | 3 | 4 | 5 | NA |
| 190413 Uses community resources to control drug misuse | 1 | 2 | 3 | 4 | 5 | NA |

R

| Risk Control: Drug Use—cont'd | | Never demonstrated | Rarely demonstrated | Sometimes demonstrated | Often demonstrated | Consistently demonstrated | |
|---|---|---|---|---|---|---|---|
| 190414 | Recognizes changes in general health status | 1 | 2 | 3 | 4 | 5 | NA |
| 190415 | Monitors health status changes | 1 | 2 | 3 | 4 | 5 | NA |
| 190416 | Eliminates drug use | 1 | 2 | 3 | 4 | 5 | NA |

*1st edition 1997; Revised 3rd edition*

## Outcome Content References:

Brown, N.K. (2000). Clinical judgments of high-risk behavior during recovery. *Journal of Psychoactive Drugs, 32*(3), 299-304.

McCuster, J., Stoddard, A.M., Zapka, J.G., & Lewis, B.F. (1993). Behavioral outcomes of AIDS educational interventions for drug users in short term treatment. *American Journal of Public Health, 83*(10), 1463-1466.

Simons-Morton, D.G., Mullen, P.D., Mains, D.A., Tabek, E.R., & Green, L.W. (1992). Characteristics of controlled studies of patient education and counseling for preventive health behaviors. *Patient Education and Counseling, 19*(2), 174-204.

+Skinner, H.A. (1982). The drug abuse screening test. *Addictive Behaviors, 7*(4), 363-371.

Talashek, M.L., Gerace, L.M., & Starr, K.L. (1994). The substance abuse pandemic: Determinants to guide interventions. *Public Health Nursing, 11*(2), 131-139.

U.S. Department of Health and Human Services. (1998). *Clinician's handbook of preventive services: Put prevention into practice* (2nd ed.). Washington: DC: Government Printing Office.

Weitzel, E.A. (2001). Risk for poisoning: Drug toxicity. In M. Maas, K. Buckwalter, M. Hardy, T. Tripp-Reimer, M. Titler, & J. Specht (Eds.), *Nursing care of older adults: Diagnoses, outcomes & interventions* (pp. 34-46). St. Louis: Mosby.

R

# Risk Control: Hearing Impairment (1915)

*Domain-Health Knowledge & Behavior (IV)*

*Class-Risk Control & Safety (T)*

*Scale(s)-Never demonstrated to Consistently demonstrated (m)*

Care Recipient:

Data Source:

**Definition:** Personal actions to prevent, eliminate, or reduce threats to hearing function

OUTCOME TARGET RATING:　　Maintain at_____　　Increase to_____

| Risk Control: Hearing Impairment Overall Rating | Never demonstrated 1 | Rarely demonstrated 2 | Sometimes demonstrated 3 | Often demonstrated 4 | Consistently demonstrated 5 | |
|---|---|---|---|---|---|---|
| **INDICATORS:** | | | | | | |
| 191501 Monitors symptoms of hearing deterioration | 1 | 2 | 3 | 4 | 5 | NA |
| 191502 Protects eardrum integrity | 1 | 2 | 3 | 4 | 5 | NA |
| 191503 Avoids trauma to the ear | 1 | 2 | 3 | 4 | 5 | NA |
| 191504 Reduces noise exposure | 1 | 2 | 3 | 4 | 5 | NA |
| 191505 Maintains normal amount of cerumen | 1 | 2 | 3 | 4 | 5 | NA |
| 191506 Manages ear infections | 1 | 2 | 3 | 4 | 5 | NA |
| 191507 Uses hearing protective devices | 1 | 2 | 3 | 4 | 5 | NA |
| 191508 Obtains periodic ear examinations | 1 | 2 | 3 | 4 | 5 | NA |
| 191509 Obtains periodic hearing tests | 1 | 2 | 3 | 4 | 5 | NA |
| 191510 Uses ear medications correctly | 1 | 2 | 3 | 4 | 5 | NA |
| 191511 Avoids placing foreign objects in ear canal | 1 | 2 | 3 | 4 | 5 | NA |

*2nd edition 2000; Revised 3rd edition*

Outcome Content References:

Burrell, L.O. (Ed.) (1992). *Adult nursing in hospital and community settings*. Norwalk, CT: Appleton & Lange.

Phipps, W.J., Monahan, F.D., Sands J.K., Marek, J., & Neighbors, M. (Eds.). (2003). *Medical-surgical nursing: Concepts and clinical practice* (7th ed). St. Louis: Mosby.

Smeltzer, S.C., & Bare, B.G. (Eds.). (2003). *Brunner and Suddarth's textbook of medical-surgical nursing* (10th ed.). Philadelphia: Lippincott, Williams, & Wilkins.

Stool, S.E., Berg, A.O., Berman, S., Carney, C.J., Cooley, J.R., Culpepper, L., Eavey, R.D., Feagans, L.V., Finitzo, T., Friedman, E., et al. (1994). *Otitis media with effusion in young children*, No. 12 (AHCPR Publication No. 94-0622). Rockville, MD: U.S. Department of Health and Human Services. Public Health Services, Agency for Health Care Policy and Research.

U.S. Department of Health and Human Services. (1998). *Clinician's handbook of preventive services: Put prevention into practice* (2nd ed.). Washington: DC: Government Printing Office.

**R**

# Risk Control: Sexually Transmitted Diseases (STD) (1905)

Domain-Health Knowledge & Behavior (IV)

Class-Risk Control & Safety (T)

Scale(s)-Never demonstrated to Consistently demonstrated (m)

Care Recipient:

Data Source:

**Definition:** Personal actions to prevent, eliminate, or reduce behaviors associated with sexually transmitted disease

OUTCOME TARGET RATING:    Maintain at_____    Increase to_____

| Risk Control: Sexually Transmitted Diseases (STD) Overall Rating | Never demonstrated 1 | Rarely demonstrated 2 | Sometimes demonstrated 3 | Often demonstrated 4 | Consistently demonstrated 5 | |
|---|---|---|---|---|---|---|
| INDICATORS: | | | | | | |
| 190501 Acknowledges individual risk for STD* | 1 | 2 | 3 | 4 | 5 | NA |
| 190502 Acknowledges personal consequences associated with STDs | 1 | 2 | 3 | 4 | 5 | NA |
| 190503 Monitors contacts for STD exposure risks | 1 | 2 | 3 | 4 | 5 | NA |
| 190504 Monitors personal behaviors for STD exposure risk | 1 | 2 | 3 | 4 | 5 | NA |
| 190505 Develops effective strategies to reduce STD exposure | 1 | 2 | 3 | 4 | 5 | NA |
| 190506 Adjusts exposure control strategies as needed | 1 | 2 | 3 | 4 | 5 | NA |
| 190507 Commits to exposure control strategies | 1 | 2 | 3 | 4 | 5 | NA |
| 190508 Follows selected exposure control strategies | 1 | 2 | 3 | 4 | 5 | NA |
| 190509 Inquires of partner's STD status before sexual activity | 1 | 2 | 3 | 4 | 5 | NA |
| 190510 Uses methods to control STD transmission | 1 | 2 | 3 | 4 | 5 | NA |
| 190511 Recognizes STD signs and symptoms | 1 | 2 | 3 | 4 | 5 | NA |
| 190512 Participates in screening for STD | 1 | 2 | 3 | 4 | 5 | NA |
| 190513 Participates in screening for associated health problems | 1 | 2 | 3 | 4 | 5 | NA |
| 190514 Uses community health services for STD treatment | 1 | 2 | 3 | 4 | 5 | NA |

R

*Continued*

| Risk Control: Sexually Trasmitted Diseases (STD)—cont'd | | Never demonstrated | Rarely demonstrated | Sometimes demonstrated | Often demonstrated | Consistently demonstrated | |
|---|---|---|---|---|---|---|---|
| 190515 | Complies with recommended treatment for STDs | 1 | 2 | 3 | 4 | 5 | NA |
| 190516 | Notifies sexual partner(s) in event of STD infection | 1 | 2 | 3 | 4 | 5 | NA |
| 190517 | Maintains absence of STDs | 1 | 2 | 3 | 4 | 5 | NA |

*STD = Sexually transmitted disease.

*1st edition 1997; Revised 3rd edition*

Outcome Content References:

+Card, J.J. (Ed.). (1993). *Handbook of adolescent sexuality and pregnancy: Research and evaluation instruments.* Newbury Park: Sage Publications.

Miller, K.E., & Graves, J.C. (2000). Update on the prevention and treatment of sexually transmitted diseases. *American Family Physician, 61*(2), 379-386.

Rotheram-Borus, M.J., Reid, M.A., & Rosario, M. (1994). Factors mediating changes in sexual HIV risk behaviors among gay and bisexual male adolescents. *American Journal of Public Health, 84*(12), 1938-1946.

Simons-Morton, D.G., Mullen, P.D., Mains, D.A., Tabak, E.R., & Green, L.W. (1992). Characteristics of controlled studies of patient education and counseling for preventive health behaviors. *Patient Education and Counseling, 19*(2), 174-204.

U.S. Department of Health and Human Services. (1998). *Clinician's handbook of preventive services: Put prevention into practice* (2nd ed.). Washington: DC: Government Printing Office.

U.S. Department of Health and Human Services. (1994). *Evaluation and management of early HIV infection* (AHCPR Publication No. 94-0572). Rockville, MD: Public Health Service Agency for Health Care Policy and Research.

R

# Risk Control: Tobacco Use (1906)

*Domain-Health Knowledge & Behavior (IV)*

*Class-Risk Control & Safety (T)*

*Scale(s)-Never demonstrated to Consistently demonstrated (m)*

*Care Recipient:*

*Data Source:*

| **Definition:** Personal actions to prevent, eliminate, or reduce tobacco use |
|---|

OUTCOME TARGET RATING:      Maintain at_____      Increase to_____

| Risk Control: Tobacco Use Overall Rating | Never demonstrated 1 | Rarely demonstrated 2 | Sometimes demonstrated 3 | Often demonstrated 4 | Consistently demonstrated 5 | |
|---|---|---|---|---|---|---|
| INDICATORS: | | | | | | |
| 190601 Acknowledges risk for tobacco use | 1 | 2 | 3 | 4 | 5 | NA |
| 190602 Acknowledges personal consequences associated with tobacco use | 1 | 2 | 3 | 4 | 5 | NA |
| 190603 Monitors environment for factors encouraging tobacco use | 1 | 2 | 3 | 4 | 5 | NA |
| 190604 Monitors personal behaviors for tobacco use patterns | 1 | 2 | 3 | 4 | 5 | NA |
| 190605 Develops effective strategies to eliminate tobacco use | 1 | 2 | 3 | 4 | 5 | NA |
| 190606 Adjusts tobacco use control strategies as needed | 1 | 2 | 3 | 4 | 5 | NA |
| 190607 Commits to tobacco use control strategies | 1 | 2 | 3 | 4 | 5 | NA |
| 190608 Follows selected tobacco use control strategies | 1 | 2 | 3 | 4 | 5 | NA |
| 190609 Participates in screening for associated health problems | 1 | 2 | 3 | 4 | 5 | NA |
| 190610 Uses health services congruent with needs | 1 | 2 | 3 | 4 | 5 | NA |
| 190611 Complies with recommended tobacco use monitoring | 1 | 2 | 3 | 4 | 5 | NA |
| 190612 Uses personal support systems to eliminate tobacco use | 1 | 2 | 3 | 4 | 5 | NA |
| 190613 Uses support group to eliminate tobacco use | 1 | 2 | 3 | 4 | 5 | NA |

**R**

*Continued*

| Risk Control: Tobacco Use—cont'd | | Never demonstrated | Rarely demonstrated | Sometimes demonstrated | Often demonstrated | Consistently demonstrated | |
|---|---|---|---|---|---|---|---|
| 190614 | Uses community resources to eliminate tobacco use | 1 | 2 | 3 | 4 | 5 | NA |
| 190615 | Monitors health status changes | 1 | 2 | 3 | 4 | 5 | NA |
| 190616 | Eliminates tobacco use | 1 | 2 | 3 | 4 | 5 | NA |
| 190618 | Recognizes changes in general health status | 1 | 2 | 3 | 4 | 5 | NA |

*1st edition 1997; Revised 3rd edition*

### Outcome Content References:

+Fagerstrom, K.O., (1978). Measuring degree of physical dependence in tobacco smoking with reference to individualization. *Addiction Behavior*, 3, 235-241.

Hirdes, J.P., & Maxwell, M.A. (1994). Smoking cessation and quality of life outcomes among older adults in the Campbell's survey on well-being. *Canadian Journal of Public Health, 85*(2), 99-102.

Simons-Morton, D.G., Mullen, P.D., Mains, D.A., Tabak, E.R., & Green, L.W. (1992). Characteristics of controlled studies of patient education and counseling for preventive health behaviors. *Patient Education and Counseling, 19*(2), 174-204.

Sussman, S., Dent, C.W., Stacy, A.W., Sun, P., Craig, S., Simon, T.R., Burton, D., & Flay, B.R. (1993). Project towards no tobacco use: 1-year behavioral outcomes, *American Journal of Public Health, 83*(9), 1245-1250.

Talashek, M.L., Gerace, L.M., & Starr, K.L. (1994). The substance abuse pandemic: Determinants to guide interventions. *Public Health Nursing, 11*(2), 131-139.

U.S. Department of Health and Human Services. (1998). *Clinician's handbook of preventive services: Put prevention into practice* (2nd ed.). Washington: DC: Government Printing Office.

U.S. Department of Health and Human Services. (1996). *Smoking cessation* (AHCPR Publication No. 96-0692). Rockville, MD: Public Health Service Agency for Health Care Policy and Research.

Winsor, R.A., Lowe, J.B., Perkins, L.L., Smith-Yoder, D., Artz, L., Crawford, M., Amburgy, K., & Boyd, N.R. (1993). Health education for pregnant smokers: Its behavioral impact and cost benefit. *American Journal of Public Health, 83*(2), 201-206.

R

# *Risk Control: Unintended Pregnancy (1907)*

Domain-Health Knowledge & Behavior (IV)

Class-Risk Control & Safety (T)

Scale(s)-Never demonstrated to Consistently demonstrated (m)

Care Recipient:

Data Source:

**Definition:** Personal actions to prevent or reduce the possibility of unintended pregnancy

OUTCOME TARGET RATING:    Maintain at_____    Increase to_____

| Risk Control: Unintended Pregnancy Overall Rating | Never demonstrated 1 | Rarely demonstrated 2 | Sometimes demonstrated 3 | Often demonstrated 4 | Consistently demonstrated 5 | |
|---|---|---|---|---|---|---|
| INDICATORS: | | | | | | |
| 190701 Acknowledges risk for unintended pregnancy | 1 | 2 | 3 | 4 | 5 | NA |
| 190703 Describes personal consequences associated with unintended pregnancy | 1 | 2 | 3 | 4 | 5 | NA |
| 190705 Understands physiological processes of conception | 1 | 2 | 3 | 4 | 5 | NA |
| 190706 Develops effective pregnancy prevention strategies | 1 | 2 | 3 | 4 | 5 | NA |
| 190707 Adjusts pregnancy prevention strategies as needed | 1 | 2 | 3 | 4 | 5 | NA |
| 190708 Commits to pregnancy prevention strategies | 1 | 2 | 3 | 4 | 5 | NA |
| 190709 Follows selected pregnancy prevention strategies | 1 | 2 | 3 | 4 | 5 | NA |
| 190710 Uses support systems to enhance prevention strategies | 1 | 2 | 3 | 4 | 5 | NA |
| 190711 Uses community resources for information/ services | 1 | 2 | 3 | 4 | 5 | NA |
| 190712 Identifies appropriate birth control method for self | 1 | 2 | 3 | 4 | 5 | NA |
| 190713 Obtains contraceptive supplies and devices | 1 | 2 | 3 | 4 | 5 | NA |
| 190714 Uses contraceptive methods correctly | 1 | 2 | 3 | 4 | 5 | NA |

R

*Continued*

| Risk Control: Unintended Pregnancy—cont'd | | Never demonstrated | Rarely demonstrated | Sometimes demonstrated | Often demonstrated | Consistently demonstrated | |
|---|---|---|---|---|---|---|---|
| 190715 | Uses health care services congruent with need | 1 | 2 | 3 | 4 | 5 | NA |

*1st edition 1997; Revised 3rd edition*

Outcome Content References:

+Card, J.J. (Ed.). (1993). *Handbook of adolescent sexuality and pregnancy: Research and evaluation instruments.* Newbury Park: Sage Publications.

Simons-Morton, D.G., Mullen, P.D., Mains, D.A., Tabak, E.R., & Green, L.W. (1992). Characteristics of controlled studies of patient education and counseling for preventive health behaviors. *Patient Education and Counseling, 19*(2), 174-204.

U.S. Department of Health and Human Services. (1998). *Clinician's handbook of preventive services: Put prevention into practice* (2nd ed.). Washington: DC: Government Printing Office.

R

# Risk Control: Visual Impairment (1916)

Domain-Health Knowledge & Behavior (IV)

Class-Risk Control & Safety (T)

Scale(s)-Never demonstrated to Consistently demonstrated (m)

Care Recipient:

Data Source:

**Definition:** Personal actions to prevent, eliminate, or reduce threats to visual function

OUTCOME TARGET RATING:  Maintain at_____  Increase to_____

| Risk Control: Visual Impairment Overall Rating | Never demonstrated 1 | Rarely demonstrated 2 | Sometimes demonstrated 3 | Often demonstrated 4 | Consistently demonstrated 5 | |
|---|---|---|---|---|---|---|
| INDICATORS: | | | | | | |
| 191601 Monitors symptoms of vision deterioration | 1 | 2 | 3 | 4 | 5 | NA |
| 191602 Monitors environment for eye hazards | 1 | 2 | 3 | 4 | 5 | NA |
| 191603 Avoids eye hazards | 1 | 2 | 3 | 4 | 5 | NA |
| 191604 Uses adequate lighting for activity being performed | 1 | 2 | 3 | 4 | 5 | NA |
| 191605 Takes breaks from activity causing eye strain | 1 | 2 | 3 | 4 | 5 | NA |
| 191606 Monitors symptoms of eye disease | 1 | 2 | 3 | 4 | 5 | NA |
| 191607 Uses prescribed eye medications correctly | 1 | 2 | 3 | 4 | 5 | NA |
| 191608 Uses devices to protect eyes | 1 | 2 | 3 | 4 | 5 | NA |
| 191609 Obtains eye exams | 1 | 2 | 3 | 4 | 5 | NA |
| 191611 Obtains screening for glaucoma | 1 | 2 | 3 | 4 | 5 | NA |
| 191612 Obtains screening for macular degeneration | 1 | 2 | 3 | 4 | 5 | NA |

*2nd edition 2000; Revised 3rd edition*

Outcome Content References:

Burrell, L. O. (Ed). (1992). *Adult nursing in hospital and community settings.* Norwalk, CT: Appleton & Lange.

Cataract Management Guideline Panel. (1993). *Cataracts in adults: Management of functional impairment. Clinical practice guideline,* No.4 (AHCPR Publication No. 93-0542). Rockville, MD: U.S. Department of Health and Human Services. Public Health Services, Agency for Health Care Policy and Research.

Phipps, W.J., Monahan, F.D., Sands J.K., Marek, J., & Neighbors, M. (Eds.). (2003). *Medical-surgical nursing: Concepts and clinical practice* (7th ed). St. Louis: Mosby.

Smeltzer, S.C., & Bare, B.G. (Eds.). (2003). *Brunner and Suddarth's textbook of medical-surgical nursing* (10th ed.). Philadelphia: Lippincott, Williams, & Wilkins.

U.S. Department of Health and Human Services. (1998). *Clinician's handbook of preventive services: Put prevention into practice* (2nd ed.). Washington: DC: Government Printing Office.

R

# Risk Detection (1908)

*Domain-Health Knowledge & Behavior (IV)*

*Class-Risk Control & Safety (T)*

*Scale(s)-Never demonstrated to Consistently demonstrated (m)*

Care Recipient:

Data Source:

**Definition:** Personal actions to identify personal health threats

OUTCOME TARGET RATING:     Maintain at_____     Increase to_____

| Risk Detection Overall Rating | | Never demonstrated 1 | Rarely demonstrated 2 | Sometimes demonstrated 3 | Often demonstrated 4 | Consistently demonstrated 5 | |
|---|---|---|---|---|---|---|---|
| INDICATORS: | | | | | | | |
| 190801 | Recognizes signs and symptoms that indicate risks | 1 | 2 | 3 | 4 | 5 | NA |
| 190802 | Identifies potential health risks | 1 | 2 | 3 | 4 | 5 | NA |
| 190803 | Seeks validation of perceived risks | 1 | 2 | 3 | 4 | 5 | NA |
| 190804 | Performs self-examinations at recommended intervals | 1 | 2 | 3 | 4 | 5 | NA |
| 190805 | Participates in screening at recommended intervals | 1 | 2 | 3 | 4 | 5 | NA |
| 190806 | Acquires knowledge of family history | 1 | 2 | 3 | 4 | 5 | NA |
| 190807 | Maintains updated knowledge of family history | 1 | 2 | 3 | 4 | 5 | NA |
| 190808 | Maintains updated knowledge of personal history | 1 | 2 | 3 | 4 | 5 | NA |
| 190809 | Uses resources to stay informed about potential risks | 1 | 2 | 3 | 4 | 5 | NA |
| 190810 | Uses health care services congru-ent with needs | 1 | 2 | 3 | 4 | 5 | NA |
| 190812 | Obtains current information about changes in health care recommendations | 1 | 2 | 3 | 4 | 5 | NA |

*1st edition 1997; Revised 3rd edition*

Outcome Content References:

Bamberg, R., Acton, R.T., Goodson, L., Go, R., Struempler, B., & Roseman, J.M. (1989). The effect of risk assessment in conjunction with health promotion education on compliance with preventive behaviors. *Journal of Allied Health, 18*(1), 271-281.

Bassett, L.W., Hendrick, R.E., Bassford, T.L., et al. (1994). *Quality determinants of mammography*, No. 13. (AHCPR Publication No. 95-0632). Rockville, MD: U.S. Department of Health and Human Services. Public Health Services, Agency for Health Care Policy and Research.

R

+Hettler, B. (1982). Wellness promotion and risk reduction on a university campus. In M. Faber & A. Reinhardt (Eds.), *Promoting health through risk reduction*. New York: Macmillan.

*Sickle Cell Disease Guideline Panel. (1993).* Sickle Cell Disease: Screening, diagnosis, management, and counseling in newborn and infants, Clinical practice guideline, *No. 6. (AHCPR Publication No. 93-0562). Rockville, MD: U.S. Department of Health and Human Services. Public Health Services, Agency for Health Care Policy and Research.*

Simons-Morton, D.G., Mullen, P.D., Mains, D.A., Tabak, E.R., & Green, L.W. (1992). Characteristics of controlled studies of patient education and counseling for preventive health behaviors. *Patient Education and Counseling, 19*(2), 174-204.

U.S. Department of Health and Human Services. (1998). *Clinician's handbook of preventive services: Put prevention into practice* (2nd ed.). Washington: DC: Government Printing Office.

R

# Role Performance (1501)

Domain-Psychosocial Health (III)

Class-Social Interaction (P)

Scale(s)-Not adequate to Totally adequate (f)

Care Recipient:

Data Source:

**Definition:** Congruence of an individual's role behavior with role expectations

OUTCOME TARGET RATING:      Maintain at_____      Increase to_____

| Role Performance Overall Rating | Not adequate 1 | Slightly adequate 2 | Moderately adequate 3 | Substantially adequate 4 | Totally adequate 5 | |
|---|---|---|---|---|---|---|
| **INDICATORS:** | | | | | | |
| 150101 Ability to meet role expectations | 1 | 2 | 3 | 4 | 5 | NA |
| 150102 Knowledge of role transition periods | 1 | 2 | 3 | 4 | 5 | NA |
| 150103 Performance of family role behaviors | 1 | 2 | 3 | 4 | 5 | NA |
| 150115 Performance of parental role behaviors | 1 | 2 | 3 | 4 | 5 | NA |
| 150113 Performance of intimate role behaviors | 1 | 2 | 3 | 4 | 5 | NA |
| 150104 Performance of community role behaviors | 1 | 2 | 3 | 4 | 5 | NA |
| 150105 Performance of work role behaviors | 1 | 2 | 3 | 4 | 5 | NA |
| 150106 Performance of friendship role behaviors | 1 | 2 | 3 | 4 | 5 | NA |
| 150112 Reported comfort with role expectations | 1 | 2 | 3 | 4 | 5 | NA |
| 150107 Description of role changes with illness or disability | 1 | 2 | 3 | 4 | 5 | NA |
| 150108 Description of role changes with elderly dependents | 1 | 2 | 3 | 4 | 5 | NA |
| 150109 Description of role changes with new family member | 1 | 2 | 3 | 4 | 5 | NA |
| 150110 Description of role changes when family member leaves home | 1 | 2 | 3 | 4 | 5 | NA |
| 150111 Reported strategies for role change(s) | 1 | 2 | 3 | 4 | 5 | NA |
| 150116 Reported comfort with role change(s) | 1 | 2 | 3 | 4 | 5 | NA |

*1st edition 1997; Revised 3rd edition*

Outcome Content References:

Knutson, A.L. (1965). *The individual, society, and health behavior*. New York: Sage.

Moorhead, S.A. (1985). Role supplementation. In G.M. Bulechek, & J.C. McCloskey (Eds.), *Nursing interventions: Treatments for nursing diagnoses*. Philadelphia: W.B. Saunders.

+Weissman, M.M., & Bothwell, S. (1976). Assessment of social adjustment by patient self-report. *Archives of General Psychiatry*, 33(9), 1111-1115.

R

# Safe Home Environment (1910)

Domain-Health Knowledge & Behavior (IV)

Class-Risk Control & Safety (T)

Scale(s)-Not adequate to Totally adequate (f)

Care Recipient:

Data Source:

**Definition:** Physical arrangements to minimize environmental factors that might cause physical harm or injury in the home

OUTCOME TARGET RATING: Maintain at _____ Increase to _____

| Safe Home Environment Overall Rating | Not adequate 1 | Slightly adequate 2 | Moderately adequate 3 | Substantially adequate 4 | Totally adequate 5 | |
|---|---|---|---|---|---|---|
| INDICATORS: | | | | | | |
| 191001 Provision of lighting | 1 | 2 | 3 | 4 | 5 | NA |
| 191002 Placement of handrails | 1 | 2 | 3 | 4 | 5 | NA |
| 191023 Carbon monoxide detector maintenance | 1 | 2 | 3 | 4 | 5 | NA |
| 191003 Smoke detector maintenance | 1 | 2 | 3 | 4 | 5 | NA |
| 191004 Use of personal alarm system | 1 | 2 | 3 | 4 | 5 | NA |
| 191005 Provision of accessible telephone | 1 | 2 | 3 | 4 | 5 | NA |
| 191006 Placement of appropriate hazard warning labels | 1 | 2 | 3 | 4 | 5 | NA |
| 191024 Safe storage of medications to prevent accidental use | 1 | 2 | 3 | 4 | 5 | NA |
| 191007 Disposal of unused medications | 1 | 2 | 3 | 4 | 5 | NA |
| 191008 Provision of assistive devices in accessible location | 1 | 2 | 3 | 4 | 5 | NA |
| 191009 Provision of equipment that meets safety standards | 1 | 2 | 3 | 4 | 5 | NA |
| 191010 Safe storage of firearms to prevent accidents | 1 | 2 | 3 | 4 | 5 | NA |
| 191011 Safe storage of hazardous materials to prevent injury | 1 | 2 | 3 | 4 | 5 | NA |
| 191012 Safe disposal of hazardous materials | 1 | 2 | 3 | 4 | 5 | NA |
| 191025 Safe storage of matches/lighters | 1 | 2 | 3 | 4 | 5 | NA |
| 191013 Arrangement of furniture to reduce risks | 1 | 2 | 3 | 4 | 5 | NA |
| 191014 Provision of safe play area | 1 | 2 | 3 | 4 | 5 | NA |
| 191015 Removal of unused refrigerator and freezer doors | 1 | 2 | 3 | 4 | 5 | NA |
| 191016 Correction of lead hazard risks | 1 | 2 | 3 | 4 | 5 | NA |
| 191017 Provision of age-appropriate toys | 1 | 2 | 3 | 4 | 5 | NA |
| 191018 Use of electrical outlet covers | 1 | 2 | 3 | 4 | 5 | NA |
| 191019 Room temperature regulation | 1 | 2 | 3 | 4 | 5 | NA |
| 191020 Elimination of harmful noise levels | 1 | 2 | 3 | 4 | 5 | NA |
| 191021 Placement of window guards as needed | 1 | 2 | 3 | 4 | 5 | NA |

*1st edition 1997; Revised 3rd edition (formerly Safety Behavior: Home Physical Environment)*

S

*Continued*

Outcome Content References:

Black, S. (2002). Safe home. *Nursing Standard, 16*(25), 16-17.

Halperin, S.F., Bass, J.L., & Mehta, K.A., (1983). Knowledge of accident prevention among parents of young children in nine Massachusetts towns. *Public Health Reports, 98*(6), 548-552.

Head, B.J. (2001). Impaired home maintenance management. In M. Maas, K. Buckwalter, M. Hardy, T. Tripp-Reimer, M. Titler, & J. Specht (Eds.), *Nursing care of older adults: Diagnoses, outcomes & interventions* (pp. 64-74). St. Louis: Mosby.

Mayhew, M.S. (1991). Strategies for promoting safety and preventing injury. *Nursing Clinics of North America, 26*(1), 885-893.

+Tymchuk, A.J. (1997). Home dangers and precautions: Interview/observation. *The UCLA Parent/Child Health & Wellness Project.*

Wasserman, R.C., Dameron, D.O., Brozicevic, M.M., & Aronson, R.A. (1989). Injury hazards in home day care. *The Journal of Pediatrics, 114*(4), 591-593.

Weitzel, E. (2001). Unilateral neglect. In M. Maas, K. Buckwalter, M. Hardy, T. Tripp-Reimer, M. Titler, & J. Specht (Eds.), *Nursing care of older adults: Diagnoses, outcomes & interventions* (pp. 492-502). St. Louis: Mosby.

**S**

# *Seizure Control (1620)*

Domain-Health Knowledge & Behavior (IV)

Class-Health Behavior (Q)

Scale(s)-Never demonstrated to Consistently demonstrated (m)

Care Recipient:

Data Source:

**Definition:** Personal actions to reduce or minimize the occurrence of seizure episodes

OUTCOME TARGET RATING:     Maintain at _____     Increase to _____

| Seizure Control Overall Rating | | Never demonstrated 1 | Rarely demonstrated 2 | Sometimes demonstrated 3 | Often demonstrated 4 | Consistently demonstrated 5 | |
|---|---|---|---|---|---|---|---|
| INDICATORS: | | | | | | | |
| 162001 | Describes precipitating seizure factors | 1 | 2 | 3 | 4 | 5 | NA |
| 162002 | Self-administers medications accurately | 1 | 2 | 3 | 4 | 5 | NA |
| 162003 | Maintains adequate supply of medications | 1 | 2 | 3 | 4 | 5 | NA |
| 162004 | Contacts health care professional when medication side effects occur | 1 | 2 | 3 | 4 | 5 | NA |
| 162005 | Maintains proper balance between medication dosing schedule and nutritional intake | 1 | 2 | 3 | 4 | 5 | NA |
| 162006 | Avoids seizure triggers/risk factors | 1 | 2 | 3 | 4 | 5 | NA |
| 162007 | Seeks medical attention immediately if seizure frequency increases | 1 | 2 | 3 | 4 | 5 | NA |
| 162008 | Uses effective stress reduction techniques to decrease seizure occurrence | 1 | 2 | 3 | 4 | 5 | NA |
| 162109 | Maintains positive attitude toward seizure disorder | 1 | 2 | 3 | 4 | 5 | NA |
| 162010 | Maintains role performance | 1 | 2 | 3 | 4 | 5 | NA |
| 162011 | Maintains social relationships | 1 | 2 | 3 | 4 | 5 | NA |
| 162012 | Maintains consistent sleep-wake pattern | 1 | 2 | 3 | 4 | 5 | NA |
| 162013 | Follows prescribed physical exercise program | 1 | 2 | 3 | 4 | 5 | NA |

S

*Continued*

| Seizure Control—cont'd | | Never demonstrated | Rarely demonstrated | Sometimes demonstrated | Often demonstrated | Consistently demonstrated | |
|---|---|---|---|---|---|---|---|
| 162014 | Balances physical activities and other daily activities | 1 | 2 | 3 | 4 | 5 | NA |
| 162015 | Implements safety practices in home/work environment | 1 | 2 | 3 | 4 | 5 | NA |

*3rd edition*

Outcome Content References:

Dilorio, C., Faherty, B., & Manteuffel, B. (1993). Learning needs of persons with epilepsy: A comparison of perceptions of persons with epilepsy, nurses and physicians. *Journal of Neuroscience Nursing, 25*(1), 22-29.

Santilli, N. (Ed.). (1996). *Managing seizure disorders: A handbook for health care professionals.* Philadelphia: Lippincott-Raven.

S

# *Self-Care Status (0313)*

Domain-Functional Health (I)                          Care Recipient:

Class-Self-Care (D)                                   Data Source:

Scale(s)-Severely compromised to Not compromised (a)

**Definition:** Ability to perform basic personal care activities and household tasks

OUTCOME TARGET RATING:    Maintain at _____    Increase to _____

| Self-Care Status Overall Rating | Severely compromised 1 | Substantially compromised 2 | Moderately compromised 3 | Mildly compromised 4 | Not compromised 5 | |
|---|---|---|---|---|---|---|
| **INDICATORS:** | | | | | | |
| 031301 Bathes self | 1 | 2 | 3 | 4 | 5 | NA |
| 031302 Dresses self | 1 | 2 | 3 | 4 | 5 | NA |
| 031303 Prepares food and fluid for eating | 1 | 2 | 3 | 4 | 5 | NA |
| 031304 Feeds self | 1 | 2 | 3 | 4 | 5 | NA |
| 031305 Maintains personal cleanliness | 1 | 2 | 3 | 4 | 5 | NA |
| 031306 Maintains oral hygiene | 1 | 2 | 3 | 4 | 5 | NA |
| 031307 Toilets self independently | 1 | 2 | 3 | 4 | 5 | NA |
| 031308 Manages oral and topical medications to meet therapeutic goals | 1 | 2 | 3 | 4 | 5 | NA |
| 031309 Manages parenteral medications to meet therapeutic goals | 1 | 2 | 3 | 4 | 5 | NA |
| 031310 Performs household tasks | 1 | 2 | 3 | 4 | 5 | NA |
| 031311 Maintains household finances | 1 | 2 | 3 | 4 | 5 | NA |
| 031312 Arranges for own transportation | 1 | 2 | 3 | 4 | 5 | NA |
| 031313 Obtains needed household items | 1 | 2 | 3 | 4 | 5 | NA |
| 031314 Recognizes safety needs in the home | 1 | 2 | 3 | 4 | 5 | NA |

*3rd edition*

S

Outcome Content References:

Armer, J.M., Conn, V.S., Decker, S.A., & Tripp-Reimer, T. (2001). Self-care deficit. In M. Maas, K. Buckwalter, M. Hardy, T. Tripp-Reimer, M. Titler, & J. Specht (Eds.), *Nursing care of older adults: Diagnoses, outcomes & interventions* (pp. 366-384). St. Louis: Mosby.

Head, B.J. (2001). Impaired home maintenance management. In M. Maas, K. Buckwalter, M. Hardy, T. Tripp-Reimer, M. Titler, & J. Specht (Eds.), *Nursing care of older adults: Diagnoses, outcomes & interventions* (pp. 64-74). St. Louis: Mosby.

Hickey, T. (1988). Self-care behavior of older adults. *Family and Community Health, 11*(3), 22-35.

Katz, S. & Akpom, C.A. (1976). A measure of primary sociobiological functions. *International Journal of Health Services, 6*(3), 493-507.

Katz, S., Ford, A.B., Moskowitz, R.W., Jackson, B.A., & Jaffe, M.W. (1963). Studies of illness in the aged. The Index of ADL: A standardized measure of biological and psychosocial function. *Journal of the American Medical Association, 185*(12), 914-919.

Klein, R.M., & Bell, B. (1982). Self-care skills: Behavioral measurement with Klein-Bell ADL Scale. *Archives of Physical Medicine and Rehabilitation, 63*(7), 335-338.

Leenerts, M.H., Teel, C.S., & Pendleton, M.K. (2002). Building a model of self-care for health promotion in aging. *Journal of Nursing Scholarship, 34*(4), 355-361.

Resnick, B. (2001). Motivating older adults to engage in self-care. *Patient Care for the Nurse Practitioner, 4*(9), 13-14, 16, 19.

# Self-Care: Activities of Daily Living (ADL) (0300)

Domain-Functional Health (I)

Class-Self-Care (D)

Scale(s)-Severely compromised to Not compromised (a)

Care Recipient:

Data Source:

**Definition:** Ability to perform the most basic physical tasks and personal care activities independently with or without assistive device

OUTCOME TARGET RATING:      Maintain at _____      Increase to _____

| Self Care: Activities of Daily Living (ADL) Overall Rating | Severely compromised 1 | Substantially compromised 2 | Moderately compromised 3 | Mildly compromised 4 | Not compromised 5 | |
|---|---|---|---|---|---|---|
| INDICATORS: | | | | | | |
| 030001   Eating | 1 | 2 | 3 | 4 | 5 | NA |
| 030002   Dressing | 1 | 2 | 3 | 4 | 5 | NA |
| 030003   Toileting | 1 | 2 | 3 | 4 | 5 | NA |
| 030004   Bathing | 1 | 2 | 3 | 4 | 5 | NA |
| 030005   Grooming | 1 | 2 | 3 | 4 | 5 | NA |
| 030006   Hygiene | 1 | 2 | 3 | 4 | 5 | NA |
| 030007   Oral hygiene | 1 | 2 | 3 | 4 | 5 | NA |
| 030008   Walking | 1 | 2 | 3 | 4 | 5 | NA |
| 030009   Wheelchair mobility | 1 | 2 | 3 | 4 | 5 | NA |
| 030010   Transfer performance | 1 | 2 | 3 | 4 | 5 | NA |
| 030012   Positions self | 1 | 2 | 3 | 4 | 5 | NA |

*1st edition 1997; Revised 3rd edition*

## Outcome Content References:

Armer, J.M., Conn, V.S., Decker, S.A., & Tripp-Reimer, T. (2001). Self-care deficit. In M. Maas, K. Buckwalter, M. Hardy, T. Tripp-Reimer, M. Titler, & J. Specht (Eds.), *Nursing care of older adults: Diagnoses, outcomes & interventions* (pp. 366-384). St. Louis: Mosby.

Hickey, T. (1988). Self-care behavior of older adults. *Family and Community Health, 11*(3), 22-35.

Katz, S. & Akpom, C.A. (1976). A measure of primary sociobiological functions. *International Journal of Health Services, 6*(3), 493-507.

+Katz, S., Ford, A.B., Moskowitz, R.W., Jackson, B.A., & Jaffe, M.W. (1963). Studies of illness in the aged. The Index of ADL: A standardized measure of biological and psychosocial function. *Journal of the American Medical Association, 185*(12), 914-919.

Klein, R.M., & Bell, B. (1982). Self-care skills: Behavioral measurement with Klein-Bell ADL Scale. *Archives of Physical Medicine and Rehabilitation, 63*(7), 335-338.

Leenerts, M.H., Teel, C.S., & Pendleton, M.K. (2002). Building a model of self-care for health promotion in aging. *Journal of Nursing Scholarship, 34*(4), 355-361.

Resnick, B. (2001). Motivating older adults to engage in self-care. *Patient Care for the Nurse Practitioner, 4*(9), 13-14, 16, 19.

Weitzel, E. (2001). Unilateral neglect. In M. Maas, K. Buckwalter, M. Hardy, T. Tripp-Reimer, M. Titler, & J. Specht (Eds.), *Nursing care of older adults: Diagnoses, outcomes & interventions* (pp. 492-502). St. Louis: Mosby.

**S**

# Self-Care: Bathing (0301)

*Domain-Functional Health (I)*

*Class-Self-Care (D)*

*Scale(s)-Severely compromised to Not compromised (a)*

*Care Recipient:*

*Data Source:*

**Definition**: Ability to cleanse own body independently with or without assistive device

OUTCOME TARGET RATING:     Maintain at ＿＿＿＿     Increase to ＿＿＿＿

| Self-Care: Bathing Overall Rating | Severely compromised 1 | Substantially compromised 2 | Moderately compromised 3 | Mildly compromised 4 | Not compromised 5 | |
|---|---|---|---|---|---|---|
| INDICATORS: | | | | | | |
| 030101  Gets in and out of bathroom | 1 | 2 | 3 | 4 | 5 | NA |
| 030102  Gets bath supplies | 1 | 2 | 3 | 4 | 5 | NA |
| 030103  Obtains water | 1 | 2 | 3 | 4 | 5 | NA |
| 030104  Turns on water | 1 | 2 | 3 | 4 | 5 | NA |
| 030105  Regulates water temperature | 1 | 2 | 3 | 4 | 5 | NA |
| 030106  Regulates water flow | 1 | 2 | 3 | 4 | 5 | NA |
| 030107  Bathes at sink | 1 | 2 | 3 | 4 | 5 | NA |
| 030108  Bathes in tub | 1 | 2 | 3 | 4 | 5 | NA |
| 030109  Bathes in shower | 1 | 2 | 3 | 4 | 5 | NA |
| 030113  Washes face | 1 | 2 | 3 | 4 | 5 | NA |
| 030114  Washes upper body | 1 | 2 | 3 | 4 | 5 | NA |
| 030115  Washes lower body | 1 | 2 | 3 | 4 | 5 | NA |
| 030116  Cleans perineal area | 1 | 2 | 3 | 4 | 5 | NA |
| 030111  Dries body | 1 | 2 | 3 | 4 | 5 | NA |

*1st edition 1997; Revised 3rd edition*

Outcome Content References:

Armer, J.M., Conn, V.S., Decker, S.A., & Tripp-Reimer, T. (2001). Self-care deficit. In M. Maas, K. Buckwalter, M. Hardy, T. Tripp-Reimer, M. Titler, & J. Specht (Eds.), *Nursing care of older adults: Diagnoses, outcomes & interventions* (pp. 366-384). St. Louis: Mosby.

+*Guide for the Uniform Data Set for Medical Rehabilitation* (including the FIM™ instrument), (version 5.1) (1997). Buffalo, NY: University at Buffalo.

Gulick, E.E. (1990). The self-administered ADL scale for persons with multiple sclerosis. In C.F. Waltz, & O.L. Strickland (Eds.), *Measurement of nursing outcomes* (pp. 128-147). New York: Springer.

Hickey, T. (1988). Self-care behavior of older adults. *Family and Community Health, 11*(3), 22-35.

Klein, R.M., & Bell, B. (1982). Self-care skills: Behavioral measurement with Klein-Bell ADL Scale. *Archives of Physical Medicine and Rehabilitation, 63*(7), 335-338.

Leenerts, M.H., Teel, C.S., & Pendleton, M.K. (2002). Building a model of self-care for health promotion in aging. *Journal of Nursing Scholarship, 34*(4), 355-361.

McKeighten, R.J., Mehmert, P.A., & Dickel, C.A. (1990). Bathing/hygiene self-care deficit: Defining characteristics and related factors across age groups and diagnosis-related groups in an acute care setting. *Nursing Diagnosis, 1*(4), 155-161.

Resnick, B. (2001). Motivating older adults to engage in self-care. *Patient Care for the Nurse Practitioner, 4*(9), 13-14, 16, 19.

Shillam, L.L., & Beeman, C., & Loshin, P. (1983). Effect of occupational therapy intervention on bathing independence of disabled persons. *The American Journal of Occupational Therapy, 37*(11), 744-748.

S

# Self-Care: Dressing (0302)

*Domain-Functional Health (I)*

*Class-Self-Care (D)*

*Scale(s)-Severely compromised to Not compromised (a)*

*Care Recipient:*

*Data Source:*

> **Definition:** Ability to dress self independently with or without assistive device

OUTCOME TARGET RATING:    Maintain at _____    Increase to _____

| Self-Care: Dressing Overall Rating | Severely compromised 1 | Substantially compromised 2 | Moderately compromised 3 | Mildly compromised 4 | Not compromised 5 | |
|---|---|---|---|---|---|---|

INDICATORS:

| | | | | | | |
|---|---|---|---|---|---|---|
| 030201 | Selects clothing | 1 | 2 | 3 | 4 | 5 | NA |
| 030202 | Gets clothing from drawer and closet | 1 | 2 | 3 | 4 | 5 | NA |
| 030203 | Picks up clothing | 1 | 2 | 3 | 4 | 5 | NA |
| 030204 | Puts clothing on upper body | 1 | 2 | 3 | 4 | 5 | NA |
| 030205 | Puts clothing on lower body | 1 | 2 | 3 | 4 | 5 | NA |
| 030206 | Buttons clothing | 1 | 2 | 3 | 4 | 5 | NA |
| 030207 | Uses fasteners | 1 | 2 | 3 | 4 | 5 | NA |
| 030208 | Uses zippers | 1 | 2 | 3 | 4 | 5 | NA |
| 030209 | Puts on socks | 1 | 2 | 3 | 4 | 5 | NA |
| 030210 | Puts on shoes | 1 | 2 | 3 | 4 | 5 | NA |
| 030213 | Ties shoes | 1 | 2 | 3 | 4 | 5 | NA |
| 030211 | Removes clothes from upper body | 1 | 2 | 3 | 4 | 5 | NA |
| 030214 | Removes clothes from lower body | 1 | 2 | 3 | 4 | 5 | NA |

*1st edition 1997; Revised 3rd edition*

## Outcome Content References:

Armer, J.M., Conn, V.S., Decker, S.A., & Tripp-Reimer, T. (2001). Self-care deficit. In M. Maas, K. Buckwalter, M. Hardy, T. Tripp-Reimer, M. Titler, & J. Specht (Eds.), *Nursing care of older adults: Diagnoses, outcomes & interventions* (pp. 366-384). St. Louis: Mosby.

Beck, C. (1988). Measurement of dressing performance in persons with dementia. *American Journal of Alzheimer's Care and Related Disorders and Research, 3*(3), 21-25.

Cole, S.L. (1992). Dress for success: A nurse's knowledge of simple clothing adaptations and dressing aids may make the difference between rehabilitation success and failure. *Geriatric Nursing, 13*(4), 217-221.

Cook, E.A., Luschen, L., & Sikes, S. (1991). Dressing training for an elderly woman with cognitive and perceptual impairments. *The American Journal of Occupational Therapy, 45*(7), 652-654.

Dudgeon, B.J., DeLisa, J.A., & Miller, R.M. (1984). Optokinetic nystagmus and upper extremity dressing independence after stroke. *Archives of Physical Medicine & Rehabilitation, 66*(3), 164-167.

Ford, L.J. (1975). Teaching dressing skills to a severely retarded child. *The American Journal of Occupational Therapy, 2*(29), 87-92.

+*Guide for the Uniform Data Set for Medical Rehabilitation* (including the FIM™ instrument), (version 5.1) (1997). Buffalo, NY: University at Buffalo.

Hickey, T. (1988). Self-care behavior of older adults. *Family and Community Health, 11*(3), 22-35.

Leenerts, M.H., Teel, C.S., & Pendleton, M.K. (2002). Building a model of self-care for health promotion in aging. *Journal of Nursing Scholarship, 34*(4), 355-361.

Panikoff, L.B. (1983). Recovery trends of functional skills in the head injured adult. *The American Journal of Occupational Therapy, 37*(11), 735-743.

Resnick, B. (2001). Motivating older adults to engage in self-care. *Patient Care for the Nurse Practitioner, 4*(9), 13-14, 16, 19.

Runge, M. (1967). Self-dressing techniques for patients with spinal cord injury. *The American Journal of Occupational Therapy, 21*(6), 367-375.

S

# Self-Care: Eating (0303)

Domain-Functional Health (I)

Class-Self-Care (D)

Scale(s)-Severely compromised to Not compromised (a)

Care Recipient:

Data Source:

**Definition:** Ability to prepare and ingest food and fluid independently with or without assistive device

OUTCOME TARGET RATING:　　Maintain at _____　　Increase to _____

| Self-Care: Eating Overall Rating | Severely compromised 1 | Substantially compromised 2 | Moderately compromised 3 | Mildly compromised 4 | Not compromised 5 | |
|---|---|---|---|---|---|---|

INDICATORS:

| | | | | | | | |
|---|---|---|---|---|---|---|---|
| 030301 | Prepares food for ingestion | 1 | 2 | 3 | 4 | 5 | NA |
| 030302 | Opens containers | 1 | 2 | 3 | 4 | 5 | NA |
| 030316 | Cuts up food | 1 | 2 | 3 | 4 | 5 | NA |
| 030303 | Uses utensils | 1 | 2 | 3 | 4 | 5 | NA |
| 030304 | Gets food onto the utensil | 1 | 2 | 3 | 4 | 5 | NA |
| 030305 | Picks up cup or glass | 1 | 2 | 3 | 4 | 5 | NA |
| 030306 | Brings food to mouth with fingers | 1 | 2 | 3 | 4 | 5 | NA |
| 030307 | Brings food to mouth with container | 1 | 2 | 3 | 4 | 5 | NA |
| 030308 | Brings food to mouth with utensil | 1 | 2 | 3 | 4 | 5 | NA |
| 030309 | Drinks from a cup or glass | 1 | 2 | 3 | 4 | 5 | NA |
| 030310 | Places food in mouth | 1 | 2 | 3 | 4 | 5 | NA |
| 030311 | Manipulates food in mouth | 1 | 2 | 3 | 4 | 5 | NA |
| 030312 | Chews food | 1 | 2 | 3 | 4 | 5 | NA |
| 030313 | Swallows food | 1 | 2 | 3 | 4 | 5 | NA |
| 030317 | Swallows fluid | 1 | 2 | 3 | 4 | 5 | NA |
| 030314 | Completes a meal | 1 | 2 | 3 | 4 | 5 | NA |

*1st edition 1997; Revised 3rd edition*

**S**

Outcome Content References:

Armer, J.M., Conn, V.S., Decker, S.A., & Tripp-Reimer, T. (2001). Self-care deficit. In M. Maas, K. Buckwalter, M. Hardy, T. Tripp-Reimer, M. Titler, & J. Specht (Eds.), *Nursing care of older adults: Diagnoses, outcomes & interventions* (pp. 366-384). St. Louis: Mosby.

Athlin, E., Norberg, A., Axelson, K., Moller, A., & Nordstrom, G. (1989). Aberrant eating behavior in elderly parkinsonian patients with and without dementia: Analysis of video-recorded meals. *Research in Nursing and Health, 12*(1), 41-51.

+*Guide for the Uniform Data Set for Medical Rehabilitation* (including the FIM™ instrument), (version 5.1) (1997). Buffalo, NY: University at Buffalo.

Hickey, T. (1988). Self-care behavior of older adults. *Family and Community Health, 11*(3), 22-35.

Leenerts, M.H., Teel, C.S., & Pendleton, M.K. (2002). Building a model of self-care for health promotion in aging. *Journal of Nursing Scholarship, 34*(4), 355-361.

Luiselli, J.K. (1993). Training self-feeding skills in children who are deaf and blind. *Behavior Modification, 17*(4), 457-473.

Piazza, C.C., Anderson, C., & Fisher, W. (1993). Teaching self-feeding skills to patients with Rett Syndrome. *Developmental Medicine and Child Neurology, 35*(11), 991-996.

Resnick, B. (2001). Motivating older adults to engage in self-care. *Patient Care for the Nurse Practitioner, 4*(9), 13-14, 16, 19.

Tandy, L., & Malan, S. (2001). Impaired swallowing. In M. Maas, K. Buckwalter, M. Hardy, T. Tripp-Reimer, M. Titler, & J. Specht (Eds.), *Nursing care of older adults: Diagnoses, outcomes & interventions* (pp. 158-171). St. Louis: Mosby.

# Self-Care: Hygiene (0305)

Domain-Functional Health (I)

Class-Self-Care (D)

Scale(s)-Severely compromised to Not compromised (a)

Care Recipient:

Data Source:

**Definition:** Ability to maintain own personal cleanliness and kempt appearance independently with or without assistive device

OUTCOME TARGET RATING:    Maintain at _____    Increase to _____

| Self-Care: Hygiene Overall Rating | Severely compromised 1 | Substantially compromised 2 | Moderately compromised 3 | Mildly compromised 4 | Not compromised 5 | |
|---|---|---|---|---|---|---|
| **INDICATORS:** | | | | | | |
| 030501 Washes hands | 1 | 2 | 3 | 4 | 5 | NA |
| 030503 Cleans perineal area | 1 | 2 | 3 | 4 | 5 | NA |
| 030504 Cleans ears | 1 | 2 | 3 | 4 | 5 | NA |
| 030505 Keeps nose blown and clean | 1 | 2 | 3 | 4 | 5 | NA |
| 030506 Maintains oral hygiene | 1 | 2 | 3 | 4 | 5 | NA |
| 030508 Shampoos hair | 1 | 2 | 3 | 4 | 5 | NA |
| 030509 Combs or brushes hair | 1 | 2 | 3 | 4 | 5 | NA |
| 030510 Shaves | 1 | 2 | 3 | 4 | 5 | NA |
| 030511 Applies makeup | 1 | 2 | 3 | 4 | 5 | NA |
| 030512 Cares for nails | 1 | 2 | 3 | 4 | 5 | NA |
| 030513 Uses a mirror | 1 | 2 | 3 | 4 | 5 | NA |
| 030514 Maintains neat appearance | 1 | 2 | 3 | 4 | 5 | NA |

*1st edition 1997; Revised 3rd edition*

## Outcome Content References:

Armer, J.M., Conn, V.S., Decker, S.A., & Tripp-Reimer, T. (2001). Self-care deficit. In M. Maas, K. Buckwalter, M. Hardy, T. Tripp-Reimer, M. Titler, & J. Specht (Eds.), *Nursing care of older adults: Diagnoses, outcomes & interventions* (pp. 366-384). St. Louis: Mosby.

Cole, G. (1991). Hygiene and care of the patient's environment. In G. Cole (Ed.), *Basic nursing skills and concepts* (pp. 261-290). St. Louis: Mosby.

*Guide for the Uniform Data Set for Medical Rehabilitation* (including the FIM™ instrument), (version 5.1) (1997). Buffalo, NY: University at Buffalo.

Hallstrom, R., & Beck, S.L. (1993). Implementation of the AORN skin shaving standard: Evaluation of a planned change. *AORN Journal, 58*(3), 498-506.

Hickey, T. (1988). Self-care behavior of older adults. *Family and Community Health, 11*(3), 22-35.

Leenerts, M.H., Teel, C.S., & Pendleton, M.K. (2002). Building a model of self-care for health promotion in aging. *Journal of Nursing Scholarship, 34*(4), 355-361.

McKeighten, R.J., Mehmert, P.A., & Dickel, C.A. (1990). Bathing/hygiene self-care deficit: Defining characteristics and related factors across age groups and diagnosis-related groups in an acute care setting. *Nursing Diagnosis, 1*(4), 155-161.

Ney, D.F. (1993). Cerumen impaction, ear hygiene practices, and hearing acuity. *Geriatric Nursing—American Journal of Care for the Aging, 14*(2), 70-73.

Resnick, B. (2001). Motivating older adults to engage in self-care. *Patient Care for the Nurse Practitioner, 4*(9), 13-14, 16, 19.

Wong, S.E., Flanagan, S.G., Kuehnel, T.G., Liberman, R.P., Hunnicut, R., & Adams-Badgett, J. (1988). Training chronic mental patients to independently practice personal grooming skills, *Hospital and Community Psychiatry, 39*(8), 874-879.

S

## Self-Care: Instrumental Activities of Daily Living (IADL) (0306)

*Domain-Functional Health (I)*

*Class-Self-Care (D)*

*Scale(s)-Severely compromised to Not compromised (a)*

*Care Recipient:*

*Data Source:*

**Definition:** Ability to perform activities needed to function in the home or community independently with or without assistive device

OUTCOME TARGET RATING:    Maintain at _____    Increase to_____

| Self-Care: Instrumental Activities of Daily Living (IADL) Overall Rating | Severely compromised 1 | Substantially compromised 2 | Moderately compromised 3 | Mildly compromised 4 | Not compromised 5 | |
|---|---|---|---|---|---|---|

INDICATORS:

| | | | | | | | |
|---|---|---|---|---|---|---|---|
| 030601 | Shops for groceries | 1 | 2 | 3 | 4 | 5 | NA |
| 030602 | Shops for clothing | 1 | 2 | 3 | 4 | 5 | NA |
| 030603 | Shops for household needs | 1 | 2 | 3 | 4 | 5 | NA |
| 030604 | Prepares meals | 1 | 2 | 3 | 4 | 5 | NA |
| 030605 | Serves meals | 1 | 2 | 3 | 4 | 5 | NA |
| 030606 | Uses phone | 1 | 2 | 3 | 4 | 5 | NA |
| 030607 | Handles written communication | 1 | 2 | 3 | 4 | 5 | NA |
| 030608 | Opens containers | 1 | 2 | 3 | 4 | 5 | NA |
| 030609 | Performs housework | 1 | 2 | 3 | 4 | 5 | NA |
| 030610 | Performs household repairs | 1 | 2 | 3 | 4 | 5 | NA |
| 030611 | Performs yard work | 1 | 2 | 3 | 4 | 5 | NA |
| 030612 | Manages money | 1 | 2 | 3 | 4 | 5 | NA |
| 030613 | Manages business affairs | 1 | 2 | 3 | 4 | 5 | NA |
| 030614 | Travels on public transportation | 1 | 2 | 3 | 4 | 5 | NA |
| 030615 | Drives own car | 1 | 2 | 3 | 4 | 5 | NA |
| 030616 | Does own laundry | 1 | 2 | 3 | 4 | 5 | NA |
| 030617 | Manages medications | 1 | 2 | 3 | 4 | 5 | NA |

*1st edition 1997; Revised 3rd edition*

Outcome Content References:

Armer, J.M., Conn, V.S., Decker, S.A., & Tripp-Reimer, T. (2001). Self-care deficit. In M. Maas, K. Buckwalter, M. Hardy, T. Tripp-Reimer, M. Titler, & J. Specht (Eds.), *Nursing care of older adults: Diagnoses, outcomes & interventions* (pp. 366-384). St. Louis: Mosby.

Fillenbaum, G.G., & Smyer, M.A. (1981). The development, validity, and reliability of the OARS Multidimensional Functional Assessment Questionnaire. *Journal of Gerontology, 36*(4), 428-434.

Head, B.J. (2001). Impaired home maintenance management. In M. Maas, K. Buckwalter, M. Hardy, T. Tripp-Reimer, M. Titler, & J. Specht (Eds.), *Nursing care of older adults: Diagnoses, outcomes & interventions* (pp. 64-74). St. Louis: Mosby.

Hickey, T. (1988). Self-care behavior of older adults. *Family and Community Health, 11*(3), 22-35.

Jette, A.M. (1980). Functional status index: Reliability of a chronic disease evaluation instrument. *Archives of Physical Medicine & Rehabilitation, 61*(9), 395-401.

+Katz, S., Ford, A.B., Moskowitz, R.W., Jackson, B.A., & Jaffe, M.W. (1963). Studies of illness in the aged. The Index of ADL: A standardized measure of biological and psychosocial function. *Journal of the American Medical Association, 185*(12), 914-919.

Lawton, M.P. (1983). Assessment of behaviors required to maintain residence in the community. In T. Crook, S. Ferris, & R. Bartus (Eds.), *Assessment in geriatric psychopharmacology* (pp. 119-135). New Canaan, CT: Mark Powley Associates.

Lawton, M.P., & Brody, E.M. (1969). Assessment of older people: Self-maintaining and instrumental activities of daily living. *Gerontologist, 9*(3), 179-186.

*Continued*

S

Leenerts, M.H., Teel, C.S., & Pendleton, M.K. (2002). Building a model of self-care for health promotion in aging. *Journal of Nursing Scholarship, 34*(4), 355-361.

Linn, M.W., & Linn, B.S. (1982). The Rapid Disability Rating Scale-2. *Journal of the American Geriatric Society, 30*(6), 378-382.

Meenan, R.F., Gertman, P.M., & Mason, J.H. (1980). Measuring health status in arthritis: The arthritis impact measurement scales. *Arthritis Rheumatism, 23*(2), 146-152.

Pearlman, R. (1987). Development of a functional assessment questionnaire for geriatric patients: The Comprehensive Older Persons' Evaluation (COPE). *Journal of Chronic Disease, 40*(56), 85S-94S.

Resnick, B. (2001). Motivating older adults to engage in self-care. *Patient Care for the Nurse Practitioner, 4*(9), 13-14, 16, 19.

Shanas, E., Townsend, P., Wedderburn, D., Friis, H., Milhoj, P., & Stehouwer, J. (1968). *Old people in three industrial societies.* New York: Atherton Press.

S

## Self-Care: Non-Parenteral Medication (0307)

Domain-Functional Health (I)

Class-Self-Care (D)

Scale(s)-Severely compromised to Not compromised (a)

Care Recipient:

Data Source:

**Definition:** Ability to administer oral and topical medications to meet therapeutic goals independently with or without assistive device

OUTCOME TARGET RATING:    Maintain at _____    Increase to_____

| Self-Care: Non-Parenteral Medication Overall Rating | Severely compromised 1 | Substantially compromised 2 | Moderately compromised 3 | Mildly compromised 4 | Not compromised 5 | |
|---|---|---|---|---|---|---|
| INDICATORS: | | | | | | |
| 030701 Identifies medication | 1 | 2 | 3 | 4 | 5 | NA |
| 030702 Administers correct dose | 1 | 2 | 3 | 4 | 5 | NA |
| 030716 Monitors therapeutic response | 1 | 2 | 3 | 4 | 5 | NA |
| 030704 Adjusts dose appropriately | 1 | 2 | 3 | 4 | 5 | NA |
| 030705 Follows medication precautions | 1 | 2 | 3 | 4 | 5 | NA |
| 030706 Monitors side effects of medication | 1 | 2 | 3 | 4 | 5 | NA |
| 030707 Uses memory aids | 1 | 2 | 3 | 4 | 5 | NA |
| 030708 Performs self-monitoring activities | 1 | 2 | 3 | 4 | 5 | NA |
| 030709 Uses monitoring equipment accurately | 1 | 2 | 3 | 4 | 5 | NA |
| 030710 Maintains needed supplies | 1 | 2 | 3 | 4 | 5 | NA |
| 030711 Administers topical medication correctly | 1 | 2 | 3 | 4 | 5 | NA |
| 030712 Stores medication properly | 1 | 2 | 3 | 4 | 5 | NA |
| 030713 Disposes of medication appropriately | 1 | 2 | 3 | 4 | 5 | NA |
| 030714 Obtains needed laboratory tests | 1 | 2 | 3 | 4 | 5 | NA |

*1st edition 1997; Revised 3rd edition*

Outcome Content References:

Armer, J.M., Conn, V.S., Decker, S.A., & Tripp-Reimer, T. (2001). Self-care deficit. In M. Maas, K. Buckwalter, M. Hardy, T. Tripp-Reimer, M. Titler, & J. Specht (Eds.), *Nursing care of older adults: Diagnoses, outcomes & interventions* (pp. 366-384). St. Louis: Mosby.

Barry, K. (1993). Patient self-medication: An innovative approach to medication teaching. *Journal of Nursing Care Quality, 8*(1), 75-82.

Felsenthal, G., Glomski, N., & Jones, D. (1986). Medication education program in an inpatient geriatric rehabilitation unit. *Archives of Physical Medication and Rehabilitation, 67*(1), 27-29.

Hickey, T. (1988). Self-care behavior of older adults. *Family and Community Health, 11*(3), 22-35.

Leenerts, M.H., Teel, C.S., & Pendleton, M.K. (2002). Building a model of self-care for health promotion in aging. *Journal of Nursing Scholarship, 34*(4), 355-361.

Lorish, D.D., Richards, B., & Brown, S. (1990). Perspective of the patient with rheumatoid arthritis on issues related to missed medication. *Arthritis Care and Research, 3*(2), 78-84.

Resnick, B. (2001). Motivating older adults to engage in self-care. *Patient Care for the Nurse Practitioner, 4*(9), 13-14, 16, 19.

S

# Self-Care: Oral Hygiene (0308)

Domain-Functional Health (I)                         Care Recipient:

Class-Self-Care (D)                                  Data Source:

Scale(s)-Severely compromised to Not compromised (a)

**Definition:** Ability to care for own mouth and teeth independently with or without assistive device

OUTCOME TARGET RATING:      Maintain at _____      Increase to_____

| Self-Care: Oral Hygiene Overall Rating | Severely compromised 1 | Substantially compromised 2 | Moderately compromised 3 | Mildly compromised 4 | Not compromised 5 | |
|---|---|---|---|---|---|---|
| **INDICATORS:** | | | | | | |
| 030801 Brushes teeth | 1 | 2 | 3 | 4 | 5 | NA |
| 030802 Flosses teeth | 1 | 2 | 3 | 4 | 5 | NA |
| 030810 Uses mouthwash | 1 | 2 | 3 | 4 | 5 | NA |
| 030803 Cleans mouth, gums, and tongue | 1 | 2 | 3 | 4 | 5 | NA |
| 030804 Cleans dentures or dental appliances | 1 | 2 | 3 | 4 | 5 | NA |
| 030806 Uses fluoridation | 1 | 2 | 3 | 4 | 5 | NA |
| 030807 Obtains regular dental care | 1 | 2 | 3 | 4 | 5 | NA |

*1st edition 1997; Revised 3rd edition*

Outcome Content References:

Armer, J.M., Conn, V.S., Decker, S.A., & Tripp-Reimer, T. (2001). Self-care deficit. In M. Maas, K. Buckwalter, M. Hardy, T. Tripp-Reimer, M. Titler, & J. Specht (Eds.), (Eds.), *Nursing care of older adults: Diagnoses, outcomes & interventions* (pp. 366-384). St. Louis: Mosby.

Fischman, S. (1993). Self-care: Practical periodontal care in today's practice. *International Dental Journal, 43*(2 Suppl. 1), 179-183.

Hickey, T. (1988). Self-care behavior of older adults. *Family and Community Health, 11*(3), 22-35.

Horowitz, L.G. (1990). Dental patient education: Self-care to healthy human development. *Patient Education and Counseling, 15*(1), 65-71.

Leenerts, M.H., Teel, C.S., & Pendleton, M.K. (2002). Building a model of self-care for health promotion in aging. *Journal of Nursing Scholarship, 34*(4), 355-361.

+Niederman, R., & Sullivan, T.M. (1981). Oral Hygiene Skill Achievement Index I. *Journal of Periodontology, 52*(3), 143-149.

+Niederman, R., Sullivan, T.M., Weiss, D., Morhart, R., Robbins, W., & Maier, D. (1981). Oral hygiene skill achievement index II. *Journal of Periodontology. 52*(3), 150-154.

Rayant, G.A., & Sheiham, A. (1980). An analysis of factors affecting compliance with tooth-cleaning recommendations. *Journal of Clinical Periodontology, 7*(4), 289-299.

Resnick, B. (2001). Motivating older adults to engage in self-care. *Patient Care for the Nurse Practitioner, 4*(9), 13-14, 16, 19.

Richardson, A. (1987). A process standard for oral care. *Nursing Times, 83*(32), 38-40.

S

# Self-Care: Parenteral Medication (0309)

*Domain-Functional Health (I)*

*Class-Self-Care (D)*

*Scale(s)-Severely compromised to Not compromised (a)*

*Care Recipient:*

*Data Source:*

**Definition:** Ability to administer parenteral medications to meet therapeutic goals independently with or without assistive device

OUTCOME TARGET RATING:    Maintain at _____    Increase to_____

| Self-Care:<br>Parenteral Medication<br>Overall Rating | Severely<br>compromised<br>1 | Substantially<br>compromised<br>2 | Moderately<br>compromised<br>3 | Mildly<br>compromised<br>4 | Not<br>compromised<br>5 | |
|---|---|---|---|---|---|---|
| INDICATORS: | | | | | | |
| 030901 Identifies medication | 1 | 2 | 3 | 4 | 5 | NA |
| 030902 Administers correct dose | 1 | 2 | 3 | 4 | 5 | NA |
| 030918 Monitors therapeutic response | 1 | 2 | 3 | 4 | 5 | NA |
| 030904 Adjusts dose appropriately | 1 | 2 | 3 | 4 | 5 | NA |
| 030905 Follows medication precautions | 1 | 2 | 3 | 4 | 5 | NA |
| 030906 Monitors side effects of medication | 1 | 2 | 3 | 4 | 5 | NA |
| 030907 Uses memory aids | 1 | 2 | 3 | 4 | 5 | NA |
| 030908 Performs self-monitoring activities | 1 | 2 | 3 | 4 | 5 | NA |
| 030909 Uses monitoring equipment accurately | 1 | 2 | 3 | 4 | 5 | NA |
| 030910 Maintains needed supplies | 1 | 2 | 3 | 4 | 5 | NA |
| 030911 Administers medication correctly | 1 | 2 | 3 | 4 | 5 | NA |
| 030912 Stores medication properly | 1 | 2 | 3 | 4 | 5 | NA |
| 030913 Disposes of medication appropriately | 1 | 2 | 3 | 4 | 5 | NA |
| 030914 Maintains asepsis | 1 | 2 | 3 | 4 | 5 | NA |
| 030915 Monitors injection sites | 1 | 2 | 3 | 4 | 5 | NA |
| 030916 Obtains needed laboratory tests | 1 | 2 | 3 | 4 | 5 | NA |

*1st edition 1997; Revised 3rd edition*

Outcome Content References:

Armer, J.M., Conn, V.S., Decker, S.A., & Tripp-Reimer, T. (2001). Self-care deficit. In M. Maas, K. Buckwalter, M. Hardy, T. Tripp-Reimer, M. Titler, & J. Specht (Eds.), *Nursing care of older adults: Diagnoses, outcomes & interventions* (pp. 366-384). St. Louis: Mosby.

Gilbert, D.N., Dworkin, R.J., Raber, S.R., & Leggett, J.E. (1997). Outpatient parenteral antimicrobial-drug therapy. *New England Journal of Medicine, 337*(12), 829-838.

Hickey, T. (1988). Self-care behavior of older adults. *Family and Community Health, 11*(3), 22-35.

*Continued*

Leenerts, M.H., Teel, C.S., & Pendleton, M.K. (2002). Building a model of self-care for health promotion in aging. *Journal of Nursing Scholarship, 34*(4), 355-361.

Resnick, B. (2001). Motivating older adults to engage in self-care. *Patient Care for the Nurse Practitioner, 4*(9), 13-14, 16, 19.

Robinson, J., Gould, M.A., Burrows-Hudson, S., Baltz, P., Currier, H., Piwkiewicz, D., & Smith, L.J. (1991). A care plan for self-administration of epoetin alpha. *ANNA Journal, 18*(6), 573-580.

Sarisley, C. (1987). Designing a teaching program for outpatient antibiotic therapy. *Journal of Nursing Staff Development, 3*(3), 128-135.

S

# Self-Care: Toileting (0310)

Domain-Functional Health (I)

Care Recipient:

Class-Self-Care (D)

Data Source:

Scale(s)-Severely compromised to Not compromised (a)

**Definition:** Ability to toilet self independently with or without assistive device

OUTCOME TARGET RATING:     Maintain at _____     Increase to_____

| Self-Care: Toileting Overall Rating | Severely compromised 1 | Substantially compromised 2 | Moderately compromised 3 | Mildly compromised 4 | Not compromised 5 | |
|---|---|---|---|---|---|---|
| INDICATORS: | | | | | | |
| 031001 Responds to full bladder in timely manner | 1 | 2 | 3 | 4 | 5 | NA |
| 031002 Responds to urge to have a bowel movement in timely manner | 1 | 2 | 3 | 4 | 5 | NA |
| 031003 Gets to and from toilet | 1 | 2 | 3 | 4 | 5 | NA |
| 031004 Removes clothing | 1 | 2 | 3 | 4 | 5 | NA |
| 031005 Positions self on toilet or commode | 1 | 2 | 3 | 4 | 5 | NA |
| 031006 Empties bladder | 1 | 2 | 3 | 4 | 5 | NA |
| 031011 Empties bowel | 1 | 2 | 3 | 4 | 5 | NA |
| 031007 Wipes self after urinating | 1 | 2 | 3 | 4 | 5 | NA |
| 031012 Wipes self after bowel movement | 1 | 2 | 3 | 4 | 5 | NA |
| 031008 Gets up from toilet | 1 | 2 | 3 | 4 | 5 | NA |
| 031009 Adjusts clothing after toileting | 1 | 2 | 3 | 4 | 5 | NA |

*1st edition 1997; Revised 3rd edition*

Outcome Content References:

Armer, J.M., Conn, V.S., Decker, S.A., & Tripp-Reimer, T. (2001). Self-care deficit. In M. Maas, K. Buckwalter, M. Hardy, T. Tripp-Reimer, M. Titler, & J. Specht (Eds.), *Nursing care of older adults: Diagnoses, outcomes & interventions* (pp. 366-384). St. Louis: Mosby.

Burgio, K.L., Burgio, L.D., McCormick, K.A., & Engel, B.T. (1991). Assessing toileting skills and habits in an adult day care center. *Journal of Gerontological Nursing, 17*(12), 32-35.

+*Guide for the Uniform Data Set for Medical Rehabilitation* (including the FIM™ instrument), (version 5.1) (1997). Buffalo, NY: University at Buffalo.

Hickey, T. (1988). Self-care behavior of older adults. *Family and Community Health, 11*(3), 22-35.

+Katz, S., Ford, A.B., Moskowitz, R.W., Jackson, B.A., & Jaffe, M.W. (1963). Studies of illness in the aged. The Index of ADL: A standardized measure of biological and psychosocial function. *Journal of the American Medical Association, 185*(12), 914-919.

Leenerts, M.H., Teel, C.S., & Pendleton, M.K. (2002). Building a model of self-care for health promotion in aging. *Journal of Nursing Scholarship, 34*(4), 355-361.

Okamoto, G.A., Sousa, J., Telzrow, R.W., Holm, R.A., McCartin, R., & Shurtleff, D.B. (1984). Toileting skills in children with myelomeningocele: Rates of learning. *Archives of Physical Medicine and Rehabilitation, 65*(4), 182-185.

Resnick, B. (2001). Motivating older adults to engage in self-care. *Patient Care for the Nurse Practitioner, 4*(9), 13-14, 16, 19.

Seim, H.C. (1989). Toilet training in first children. *The Journal of Family Practice, 29*(6), 633-636.

**S**

# Self-Direction of Care (1613)

*Domain-Health Knowledge & Behavior (IV)*

*Class-Health Behavior (Q)*

*Scale(s)-Never demonstrated to Consistently demonstrated (m)*

Care Recipient:

Data Source:

**Definition:** Care recipient actions taken to direct others who assist with or perform physical tasks and personal health care

OUTCOME TARGET RATING:   Maintain at _____   Increase to_____

| Self-Direction of Care Overall Rating | Never demonstrated 1 | Rarely demonstrated 2 | Sometimes demonstrated 3 | Often demonstrated 4 | Consistently demonstrated 5 | |
|---|---|---|---|---|---|---|
| **INDICATORS:** | | | | | | |
| 161301 Sets health care goals | 1 | 2 | 3 | 4 | 5 | NA |
| 161302 Describes appropriate care | 1 | 2 | 3 | 4 | 5 | NA |
| 161303 Obtains resources as necessary | 1 | 2 | 3 | 4 | 5 | NA |
| 161304 Instructs others in appropriate care behaviors | 1 | 2 | 3 | 4 | 5 | NA |
| 161305 Evaluates the care given by others | 1 | 2 | 3 | 4 | 5 | NA |
| 161306 Determines that care is completed appropriately | 1 | 2 | 3 | 4 | 5 | NA |
| 161307 Expresses confidence in problem solving | 1 | 2 | 3 | 4 | 5 | NA |
| 161308 Takes corrective action when care is not appropriate | 1 | 2 | 3 | 4 | 5 | NA |
| 161309 Instructs others in appropriate health maintenance activities | 1 | 2 | 3 | 4 | 5 | NA |

*2nd edition 2000; Revised 3rd edition*

Outcome Content References:

Edwards, P.A. (Ed.). (2000). *The specialty practice of rehabilitation nursing: A core curriculum* (4th ed.). Glenview, IL: Association of Rehabilitation Nurses.

Orem, D. E. (1985). A concept of self-care for the rehabilitation client. *Rehabilitation Nursing, 10*(3), 33-36.

Rehabilitation Nursing Foundation. (1995). *Twenty-one rehabilitation nursing diagnoses: A guide to interventions and outcomes.* Glenview, IL: Author.

S

# Self-Esteem (1205)

Domain-Psychosocial Health (III)

Class-Psychological Well-Being (M)

Scale(s)-Never positive to Consistently positive (k)

Care Recipient:

Data Source:

**Definition:** Personal judgment of self-worth

OUTCOME TARGET RATING:        Maintain at _____    Increase to_____

| Self-Esteem Overall Rating | Never positive 1 | Rarely positive 2 | Sometimes positive 3 | Often positive 4 | Consistently positive 5 | |
|---|---|---|---|---|---|---|
| **INDICATORS:** | | | | | | |
| 120501 Verbalizations of self-acceptance | 1 | 2 | 3 | 4 | 5 | NA |
| 120502 Acceptance of self-limitations | 1 | 2 | 3 | 4 | 5 | NA |
| 120503 Maintenance of erect posture | 1 | 2 | 3 | 4 | 5 | NA |
| 120504 Maintenance of eye contact | 1 | 2 | 3 | 4 | 5 | NA |
| 120505 Description of self | 1 | 2 | 3 | 4 | 5 | NA |
| 120506 Regard for others | 1 | 2 | 3 | 4 | 5 | NA |
| 120507 Open communication | 1 | 2 | 3 | 4 | 5 | NA |
| 120508 Fulfillment of personally significant roles | 1 | 2 | 3 | 4 | 5 | NA |
| 120509 Maintenance of grooming/ hygiene | 1 | 2 | 3 | 4 | 5 | NA |
| 120510 Balance of participation and listening in groups | 1 | 2 | 3 | 4 | 5 | NA |
| 120511 Confidence level | 1 | 2 | 3 | 4 | 5 | NA |
| 120512 Acceptance of compliments from others | 1 | 2 | 3 | 4 | 5 | NA |
| 120513 Expected response from others | 1 | 2 | 3 | 4 | 5 | NA |
| 120514 Acceptance of constructive criticism | 1 | 2 | 3 | 4 | 5 | NA |
| 120515 Willingness to confront others | 1 | 2 | 3 | 4 | 5 | NA |
| 120516 Description of success in work or school | 1 | 2 | 3 | 4 | 5 | NA |
| 120517 Description of success in social groups | 1 | 2 | 3 | 4 | 5 | NA |
| 120518 Description of pride in self | 1 | 2 | 3 | 4 | 5 | NA |
| 120519 Feelings about self-worth | 1 | 2 | 3 | 4 | 5 | NA |

1st edition 1997

**S**

**Outcome Content References:**

Bonham, P., & Cheney, A. (1982). Concept of self: A framework for nursing assessment. In P.L. Chinn (Ed.), *Advances in nursing theory development* (pp. 173-189). Rockville, MD: Aspen.

Coopersmith, S. (1967). *The antecedents of self-esteem.* San Francisco: W.H. Freeman.

Crandall, R. (1973). The measurement of self-esteem and related constructs. In J.P. Robinson & P.R. Shaver (Eds.), *Measures of social psychological attitudes.* Ann Arbor, MI: Institute for Social Research, University of Michigan.

Fitts, W. (1965). *Manual for the Tennessee Self-Concept Scale.* Nashville, TN: Counselor Recordings & Tests.

Groh, C.J., & Whall, A.L. (2001). Self-esteem disturbance. In M. Maas, K. Buckwalter, M. Hardy, T. Tripp-Reimer, M. Titler, & J. Specht (Eds.), *Nursing care of older adults: Diagnoses, outcomes & interventions* (pp. 593-600). St. Louis: Mosby.

Larson, J. (1989). Validation of the defining characteristics of disturbance in self-esteem in patients with anorexia nervosa. In Carroll-Johnson, R. (Ed.) *Classification of nursing diagnoses: Proceedings of the eighth conference* (North American Nursing Diagnosis Association) (pp. 307-312). Philadelphia: J.B. Lippincott.

+Nugent, W.R., & Thomas, J.W. (1993). Validation of a clinical measure of self-esteem. *Research on Social Work Practice, 3*(2), 191-207.

Roid, G., & Fitts, W. (1988). *Tennessee Self-Concept Scale: Revised manual.* Los Angeles: Western Psychological Services.

Rosenberg, M. (1965). *Society & adolescent self image.* Princeton, NJ: Princeton University Press.

Stanwyck, D. (1983). Self-esteem through the life span. *Family & Community Health, 6*(2), 11-28.

# Self-Mutilation Restraint (1406)

*Domain-Psychosocial Health (III)*

*Class-Self-Control (O)*

*Scale(s)-Never demonstrated to Consistently demonstrated (m)*

Care Recipient:

Data Source:

---

**Definition:** Personal actions to refrain from intentional self-inflicted injury (non-lethal)

OUTCOME TARGET RATING:    Maintain at _____    Increase to _____

| Self-Mutilation Restraint Overall Rating | Never demonstrated 1 | Rarely demonstrated 2 | Sometimes demonstrated 3 | Often demonstrated 4 | Consistently demonstrated 5 | |
|---|---|---|---|---|---|---|

INDICATORS:

| | | | | | | | |
|---|---|---|---|---|---|---|---|
| 140601 | Refrains from gathering means for self-injury | 1 | 2 | 3 | 4 | 5 | NA |
| 140602 | Seeks help when feeling urge to injure self | 1 | 2 | 3 | 4 | 5 | NA |
| 140604 | Upholds contract to not harm self | 1 | 2 | 3 | 4 | 5 | NA |
| 140605 | Maintains self-control without supervision | 1 | 2 | 3 | 4 | 5 | NA |
| 140606 | Refrains from injuring self | 1 | 2 | 3 | 4 | 5 | NA |

*1st edition 1997; Revised 3rd edition*

Outcome Content References:

Burrow, S. (1994). Nursing management of self-mutilation. *British Journal of Nursing, 3*(8), 382-386.

Coler, M.S., & Vincent, K.G. (1995). Psychiatric mental health nursing. In K.V. Gettrust (Series Ed.), *Plans of care for specialty practice*. Albany, NY: Delmar Publishers.

Faye, P. (1995). Addictive characteristics of the behavior of self-mutilation. *Journal of Psychosocial Nursing and Mental Health Services, 33*(2), 19-22.

+Rojahn, J., Polster, L.M., Mulick, J.A., & Wisniewski, J.J. (1989). Reliability of the Behavior Problems Inventory. *Journal of the Multihandicapped Person, 2*, 283-293.

Stuart, G.W., & Laraia, M.T. (2001). *Principles and practice of psychiatric nursing* (7th ed.). St. Louis: Mosby.

Valente, S.M. (1991). Deliberate self-injury management in a psychiatric setting. *Journal of Psychosocial Nursing and Mental Health Services, 29*(12), 19-25.

Winchel, R.M. (1991). Self-injurious behavior. A review of the behavior and biology of self-mutilation. *American Journal of Psychiatry, 148*(3), 306-17.

**S**

# Sensory Function Status (2405)

*Domain-Physiologic Health (II)*               *Care Recipient:*

*Class-Sensory (Y)*                            *Data Source:*

*Scale(s)-Severe deviation from normal range to No deviation from normal range (b)*

**Definition:** Extent to which an individual correctly perceives skin stimulation, sounds, proprioception, taste and smell, and visual images

OUTCOME TARGET RATING:      Maintain at _____    Increase to _____

| Sensory Function Status Overall Rating | Severe deviation from normal range 1 | Substantial deviation from normal range 2 | Moderate deviation from normal range 3 | Mild deviation from normal range 4 | No deviation from normal range 5 | |
|---|---|---|---|---|---|---|
| **INDICATORS:** | | | | | | |
| 240501 Ability to sense skin stimulation | 1 | 2 | 3 | 4 | 5 | NA |
| 240502 Ability to hear and interpret sounds | 1 | 2 | 3 | 4 | 5 | NA |
| 240503 Ability to sense position changes of the head and body | 1 | 2 | 3 | 4 | 5 | NA |
| 240504 Ability to discriminate odors | 1 | 2 | 3 | 4 | 5 | NA |
| 240505 Ability to discriminate taste | 1 | 2 | 3 | 4 | 5 | NA |
| 240506 Ability to see and interpret images | 1 | 2 | 3 | 4 | 5 | NA |

*3rd edition*

Outcome Content References:

Cataract Management Guideline Panel. (1993). *Cataracts in adults: Management of functional impairment. Clinical practice guideline*, No.4 (AHCPR Publication No. 93-0542). Rockville, MD: U.S. Department of Health and Human Services. Public Health Services, Agency for Health Care Policy and Research.

McCance, K.L., & Huether, S.E. (2002). *Pathophysiology: The biologic basis for disease in adults and children* (4th ed.). St. Louis: Mosby.

Phipps, W.J., Monahan, F.D., Sands J.K., Marek, J., & Neighbors, M. (Eds.). (2003). *Medical-surgical nursing: Concepts and clinical practice* (7th ed). St. Louis: Mosby.

Swanson, E.A., & Drury, J. (2001). Sensory/perceptual alterations. In M. Maas, K. Buckwalter, M. Hardy, T. Tripp-Reimer, M. Titler, & J. Specht (Eds.), *Nursing care of older adults: Diagnoses, outcomes & interventions* (pp. 476-491). St. Louis: Mosby.

**S**

# Sensory Function: Cutaneous (2400)

*Domain-Physiologic Health (II)*

*Class-Sensory (Y)*

*Scale(s)-Severe deviation from normal range to No deviation from normal range (b) and Severe to None (n)*

Care Recipient:

Data Source:

**Definition:** Extent to which stimulation of the skin is correctly sensed

OUTCOME TARGET RATING:     Maintain at _____     Increase to _____

| Sensory Function: Cutaneous Overall Rating | Severe deviation from normal range 1 | Substantial deviation from normal range 2 | Moderate deviation from normal range 3 | Mild deviation from normal range 4 | No deviation from normal range 5 | |
|---|---|---|---|---|---|---|
| **INDICATORS:** | | | | | | |
| 240001 Sharp versus dull discrimination | 1 | 2 | 3 | 4 | 5 | NA |
| 240002 2-point discrimination | 1 | 2 | 3 | 4 | 5 | NA |
| 240003 Vibration discrimination | 1 | 2 | 3 | 4 | 5 | NA |
| 240004 Warmth discrimination | 1 | 2 | 3 | 4 | 5 | NA |
| 240005 Cold discrimination | 1 | 2 | 3 | 4 | 5 | NA |
| 240006 Tickle and itch discrimination | 1 | 2 | 3 | 4 | 5 | NA |
| 240007 Noxious stimulus discrimination | 1 | 2 | 3 | 4 | 5 | NA |

| | Severe | Substantial | Moderate | Mild | None | |
|---|---|---|---|---|---|---|
| 240008 Paresthesia | 1 | 2 | 3 | 4 | 5 | NA |
| 240009 Hyperparesthesia | 1 | 2 | 3 | 4 | 5 | NA |
| 240011 Tingling | 1 | 2 | 3 | 4 | 5 | NA |
| 240012 Loss of sensation | 1 | 2 | 3 | 4 | 5 | NA |

*2nd edition 2000; Revised 3rd edition*

## Outcome Content References:

Lewis, S.M., Collier, I.C., Heitkermper, M.M., & Dirksen, S.R. (2000). *Medical-surgical nursing: Assessment & management of clinical problems* (5th ed.). St. Louis: Mosby.

McCance, K.L., & Huether, S.E. (2002). *Pathophysiology: The biologic basis for disease in adults and children* (4th ed.). St. Louis: Mosby.

Swanson, E.A., & Drury, J. (2001). Sensory/perceptual alterations. In M. Maas, K. Buckwalter, M. Hardy, T. Tripp-Reimer, M. Titler, & J. Specht (Eds.), *Nursing care of older adults: Diagnoses, outcomes & interventions* (pp. 476-491). St. Louis: Mosby.

**S**

# Sensory Function: Hearing (2401)

Domain-Physiologic Health (II)

Class-Sensory (Y)

Scale(s)-Severe deviation from normal range to No deviation from normal range (b) and Severe to None (n)

Care Recipient:

Data Source:

**Definition:** Extent to which sounds are correctly sensed

OUTCOME TARGET RATING:    Maintain at _____    Increase to _____

| Sensory Function: Hearing Overall Rating | Severe deviation from normal range 1 | Substantial deviation from normal range 2 | Moderate deviation from normal range 3 | Mild deviation from normal range 4 | No deviation from normal range 5 | |
|---|---|---|---|---|---|---|
| INDICATORS: | | | | | | |
| 240101 Auditory acuity (left) | 1 | 2 | 3 | 4 | 5 | NA |
| 240102 Auditory acuity (right) | 1 | 2 | 3 | 4 | 5 | NA |
| 240103 Air conduction of sound (left) | 1 | 2 | 3 | 4 | 5 | NA |
| 240112 Air conduction of sound (right) | 1 | 2 | 3 | 4 | 5 | NA |
| 240104 Bone conduction of sound (left) | 1 | 2 | 3 | 4 | 5 | NA |
| 240113 Bone conduction of sound (right) | 1 | 2 | 3 | 4 | 5 | NA |
| 240105 Ratio of air and bone conduction | 1 | 2 | 3 | 4 | 5 | NA |
| 240107 Auditory discrimination of discrete sounds | 1 | 2 | 3 | 4 | 5 | NA |
| 240108 Hears a whisper 6 inches from left ear (voice test) | 1 | 2 | 3 | 4 | 5 | NA |
| 240114 Hears a whisper 6 inches from right ear (voice test) | 1 | 2 | 3 | 4 | 5 | NA |
| 240109 Turns to sound | 1 | 2 | 3 | 4 | 5 | NA |
| 240110 Shows interest in auditory stimuli | 1 | 2 | 3 | 4 | 5 | NA |

| | Severe | Substantial | Moderate | Mild | None | |
|---|---|---|---|---|---|---|
| 240106 Tinnitus (left) | 1 | 2 | 3 | 4 | 5 | NA |
| 240115 Tinnitus (right) | 1 | 2 | 3 | 4 | 5 | NA |
| 240116 Loss of high pitch tones | 1 | 2 | 3 | 4 | 5 | NA |
| 240117 Loss of ability to distinguish conversation from background environmental noise | 1 | 2 | 3 | 4 | 5 | NA |

Assistive device YES / NO

*2nd edition 2000; Revised 3rd edition*

## Outcome Content References:

Burrell, L.O. (Ed.) (1992). *Adult nursing in hospital and community settings*. Norwalk, CT: Appleton & Lange.

May, J.J. (2000). Occupational hearing loss. *American Journal of Industrial Medicine, 37*(1), 112-120.

Phipps, W.J., Monahan, F.D., Sands J.K., Marek, J., & Neighbors, M. (Eds.). (2003). *Medical-surgical nursing: Concepts and clinical practice* (7th ed.). St. Louis: Mosby.

*Continued*

**S**

Sataloff, J, & Roberts, B. (1999). Differential diagnosis in occupation hearing loss compensation claims. *Journal of Occupation Hearing Loss, 2*(4), 183-189.

Smeltzer, S.C., & Bare, B.G. (Eds.). (2003). *Brunner and Suddarth's textbook of medical-surgical nursing* (10th ed.). Philadelphia: Lippincott, Williams, & Wilkins.

Stool, S.E., Berg, A.O., Berman, S., Carney, C.J., Cooley, J.R., Culpepper, L., Eavey, R.D., Feagans, L.V., Finitzo, T., Friedman, E., et al. (1994). *Otitis media with effusion in young children*, No. 12 (AHCPR Publication No. 94-0622). Rockville, MD: U.S. Department of Health and Human Services. Public Health Services, Agency for Health Care Policy and Research.

Swanson, E.A., & Drury, J. (2001). Sensory/perceptual alterations. In M. Maas, K. Buckwalter, M. Hardy, T. Tripp-Reimer, M. Titler, & J. Specht (Eds.), *Nursing care of older adults: Diagnoses, outcomes & interventions* (pp. 476-491). St. Louis: Mosby.

**S**

# Sensory Function: Proprioception (2402)

*Domain-Physiologic Health (II)*

*Class-Sensory (Y)*

*Scale(s)-Severe deviation from normal range to No deviation from normal range (b) and Severe to None (n)*

Care Recipient:

Data Source:

> **Definition:** Extent to which the position and movement of the head and body are correctly sensed

OUTCOME TARGET RATING:    Maintain at _____    Increase to _____

| Sensory Function: Proprioception Overall Rating | Severe deviation from normal range 1 | Substantial deviation from normal range 2 | Moderate deviation from normal range 3 | Mild deviation from normal range 4 | No deviation from normal range 5 | |
|---|---|---|---|---|---|---|
| **INDICATORS:** | | | | | | |
| 240201 Head position discrimination | 1 | 2 | 3 | 4 | 5 | NA |
| 240202 Head movement discrimination | 1 | 2 | 3 | 4 | 5 | NA |
| 240203 Upper limb movement discrimination | 1 | 2 | 3 | 4 | 5 | NA |
| 240210 Lower limb movement discrimination | 1 | 2 | 3 | 4 | 5 | NA |
| 240204 Upper limb position discrimination | 1 | 2 | 3 | 4 | 5 | NA |
| 240211 Lower limb position discrimination | 1 | 2 | 3 | 4 | 5 | NA |
| 240212 Trunk movement discrimination | 1 | 2 | 3 | 4 | 5 | NA |
| 240213 Trunk position discrimination | 1 | 2 | 3 | 4 | 5 | NA |
| 240205 Sense of balance | 1 | 2 | 3 | 4 | 5 | NA |
| | **Severe** | **Substantial** | **Moderate** | **Mild** | **None** | |
| 240206 Vertigo | 1 | 2 | 3 | 4 | 5 | NA |
| 240207 Lightheadedness | 1 | 2 | 3 | 4 | 5 | NA |
| 240208 Nystagmus | 1 | 2 | 3 | 4 | 5 | NA |

*2nd edition 2000; Revised 3rd edition*

Outcome Content References:

Lewis, S.M., Collier, I.C., Heitkermper, M.M., & Dirksen, S.R. (2000). *Medical-surgical nursing: Assessment & management of clinical problems* (5th ed.). St. Louis: Mosby.

McCance, K.L., & Huether, S.E. (2002). *Pathophysiology: The biologic basis for disease in adults and children* (4th ed.). St. Louis: Mosby.

Swanson, E.A., & Drury, J. (2001). Sensory/perceptual alterations. In M. Maas, K. Buckwalter, M. Hardy, T. Tripp-Reimer, M. Titler, & J. Specht (Eds.), *Nursing care of older adults: Diagnoses, outcomes & interventions* (pp. 476-491). St. Louis: Mosby.

S

# Sensory Function: Taste & Smell (2403)

Domain-Physiologic Health (II)

Class-Sensory (Y)

Scale(s)-Severe deviation from normal range to No deviation from normal range (b) and Severe to None (n)

Care Recipient:

Data Source:

**Definition**: Extent to which chemicals inhaled or dissolved in saliva are correctly sensed

OUTCOME TARGET RATING:  Maintain at _____  Increase to _____

| Sensory Function: Taste & Smell Overall Rating | Severe deviation from normal range 1 | Substantial deviation from normal range 2 | Moderate deviation from normal range 3 | Mild deviation from normal range 4 | No deviation from normal range 5 | |
|---|---|---|---|---|---|---|
| **INDICATORS:** | | | | | | |
| 240301 Discriminates odors | 1 | 2 | 3 | 4 | 5 | NA |
| 240304 Recognizes sweet flavor | 1 | 2 | 3 | 4 | 5 | NA |
| 240305 Recognizes salty flavor | 1 | 2 | 3 | 4 | 5 | NA |
| 240306 Recognizes bitter flavor | 1 | 2 | 3 | 4 | 5 | NA |
| 240307 Recognizes sour flavor | 1 | 2 | 3 | 4 | 5 | NA |
| | Severe | Substantial | Moderate | Mild | None | |
| 240302 Odor distortion | 1 | 2 | 3 | 4 | 5 | NA |
| 240308 Taste distortion | 1 | 2 | 3 | 4 | 5 | NA |
| 240310 Metallic taste | 1 | 2 | 3 | 4 | 5 | NA |
| 240311 Hemianosmia | 1 | 2 | 3 | 4 | 5 | NA |

*2nd edition 2000; Revised 3rd edition*

Outcome Content References:

Burrell, L. O. (Ed). (1992). *Adult nursing in hospital and community settings*. Norwalk, CT: Appleton & Lange.

Phipps, W.J., Monahan, F.D., Sands J.K., Marek, J., & Neighbors, M. (Eds.). (2003). *Medical-surgical nursing: Concepts and clinical practice* (7th ed). St. Louis: Mosby.

Smeltzer, S.C., & Bare, B.G. (Eds.). (2003). *Brunner and Suddarth's textbook of medical-surgical nursing* (10th ed.). Philadelphia: Lippincott, Williams, & Wilkins.

Swanson, E.A., & Drury, J. (2001). Sensory/perceptual alterations. In M. Maas, K. Buckwalter, M. Hardy, T. Tripp-Reimer, M. Titler, & J. Specht (Eds.), *Nursing care of older adults: Diagnoses, outcomes & interventions* (pp. 476-491). St. Louis: Mosby.

S

# Sensory Function: Vision (2404)

*Domain-Physiologic Health (II)*

*Class-Sensory (Y)*

*Scale(s)-Severe deviation from normal range to No deviation from normal range (b) and Severe to None (n)*

*Care Recipient:*

*Data Source:*

**Definition:** Extent to which visual images are correctly sensed

OUTCOME TARGET RATING:    Maintain at _____    Increase to _____

| Sensory Function: Vision Overall Rating | Severe deviation from normal range 1 | Substantial deviation from normal range 2 | Moderate deviation from normal range 3 | Mild deviation from normal range 4 | No deviation from normal range 5 | |
|---|---|---|---|---|---|---|
| **INDICATORS:** | | | | | | |
| 240401 Central visual acuity (left) | 1 | 2 | 3 | 4 | 5 | NA |
| 240421 Central visual acuity (right) | 1 | 2 | 3 | 4 | 5 | NA |
| 240402 Peripheral visual acuity (left) | 1 | 2 | 3 | 4 | 5 | NA |
| 240422 Peripheral visual acuity (right) | 1 | 2 | 3 | 4 | 5 | NA |
| 240403 Central visual fields (left) | 1 | 2 | 3 | 4 | 5 | NA |
| 240423 Central visual fields (right) | 1 | 2 | 3 | 4 | 5 | NA |
| 240404 Peripheral visual fields (left) | 1 | 2 | 3 | 4 | 5 | NA |
| 240424 Peripheral visual fields (right) | 1 | 2 | 3 | 4 | 5 | NA |
| 240416 Response to visual stimuli | 1 | 2 | 3 | 4 | 5 | NA |

| | Severe | Substantial | Moderate | Mild | None | |
|---|---|---|---|---|---|---|
| 240405 Hemianopia | 1 | 2 | 3 | 4 | 5 | NA |
| 240406 Floaters | 1 | 2 | 3 | 4 | 5 | NA |
| 240407 Flashes of light | 1 | 2 | 3 | 4 | 5 | NA |
| 240408 Halos around lights | 1 | 2 | 3 | 4 | 5 | NA |
| 240409 Spiderwebs | 1 | 2 | 3 | 4 | 5 | NA |
| 240410 Double vision | 1 | 2 | 3 | 4 | 5 | NA |
| 240411 Blurred vision | 1 | 2 | 3 | 4 | 5 | NA |
| 240412 Distorted vision | 1 | 2 | 3 | 4 | 5 | NA |
| 240413 Color vision distortions | 1 | 2 | 3 | 4 | 5 | NA |
| 240414 Night blindness | 1 | 2 | 3 | 4 | 5 | NA |
| 240415 Day blindness | 1 | 2 | 3 | 4 | 5 | NA |
| 240417 Headaches | 1 | 2 | 3 | 4 | 5 | NA |
| 240418 Dizziness | 1 | 2 | 3 | 4 | 5 | NA |
| 240419 Eye strain | 1 | 2 | 3 | 4 | 5 | NA |

Assistive device YES/NO

*2nd edition 2000; Revised 3rd edition*

Outcome Content References:

Burrell, L. O. (Ed). (1992). *Adult nursing in hospital and community settings*. Norwalk, CT: Appleton & Lange.

Cataract Management Guideline Panel. (1993). *Cataracts in adults: Management of functional impairment. Clinical practice guideline*, No.4 (AHCPR Publication No. 93-0542). Rockville, MD: U.S. Department of Health and Human Services. Public Health Services, Agency for Health Care Policy and Research.

*Continued*

Phipps, W.J., Monahan, F.D., Sands J.K., Marek, J., & Neighbors, M. (Eds.). (2003). *Medical-surgical nursing: Concepts and clinical practice* (7th ed). St. Louis: Mosby.

Smeltzer, S.C., & Bare, B.G. (Eds.). (2003). *Brunner and Suddarth's textbook of medical-surgical nursing* (10th ed.). Philadelphia: Lippincott, Williams, & Wilkins.

Swanson, E.A., & Drury, J. (2001). Sensory/perceptual alterations. In M. Maas, K. Buckwalter, M. Hardy, T. Tripp-Reimer, M. Titler, & J. Specht (Eds.), *Nursing care of older adults: Diagnoses, outcomes & interventions* (pp. 476-491). St. Louis: Mosby.

S

# *Sexual Functioning (0119)*

Domain-Functional Health (I)

Class-Growth & Development (B)

Scale(s)-Never demonstrated to Consistently demonstrated (m)

Care Recipient:

Data Source:

**Definition:** Integration of physical, socioemotional, and intellectual aspects of sexual expression and performance

OUTCOME TARGET RATING:    Maintain at _____    Increase to _____

| Sexual Functioning Overall Rating | Never demonstrated 1 | Rarely demonstrated 2 | Sometimes demonstrated 3 | Often demonstrated 4 | Consistently demonstrated 5 | |
|---|---|---|---|---|---|---|

INDICATORS:

| | | | | | | | |
|---|---|---|---|---|---|---|---|
| 011901 | Attains sexual arousal | 1 | 2 | 3 | 4 | 5 | NA |
| 011902 | Sustains penile/ clitoral erection through orgasm | 1 | 2 | 3 | 4 | 5 | NA |
| 011903 | Sustains arousal through orgasm | 1 | 2 | 3 | 4 | 5 | NA |
| 011904 | Performs sexually with assistive device as needed | 1 | 2 | 3 | 4 | 5 | NA |
| 011905 | Adapts sexual technique as needed | 1 | 2 | 3 | 4 | 5 | NA |
| 011906 | Refrains from alcohol/drug use that adversely affects sexual function | 1 | 2 | 3 | 4 | 5 | NA |
| 011907 | Expresses ability to perform sexually despite physical imperfections | 1 | 2 | 3 | 4 | 5 | NA |
| 011908 | Expresses comfort with sexual expression | 1 | 2 | 3 | 4 | 5 | NA |
| 011909 | Expresses self-esteem | 1 | 2 | 3 | 4 | 5 | NA |
| 011910 | Expresses comfort with body | 1 | 2 | 3 | 4 | 5 | NA |
| 011911 | Expresses sexual interest | 1 | 2 | 3 | 4 | 5 | NA |
| 011912 | Expresses ability to be intimate | 1 | 2 | 3 | 4 | 5 | NA |
| 011913 | Expresses willing-ness to be sexual | 1 | 2 | 3 | 4 | 5 | NA |
| 011914 | Reports available consenting partner | 1 | 2 | 3 | 4 | 5 | NA |
| 011915 | Expresses respect for partner | 1 | 2 | 3 | 4 | 5 | NA |
| 011916 | Expresses acceptance of partner | 1 | 2 | 3 | 4 | 5 | NA |
| 011917 | Expresses knowledge of partner's sexual capabilities | 1 | 2 | 3 | 4 | 5 | NA |

S

*Continued*

| Sexual Functioning—cont'd | | Never demonstrated | Rarely demonstrated | Sometimes demonstrated | Often demonstrated | Consistently demonstrated | |
|---|---|---|---|---|---|---|---|
| 011918 | Expresses knowledge of personal sexual capabilities | 1 | 2 | 3 | 4 | 5 | NA |
| 011919 | Expresses knowledge of partner's sexual needs | 1 | 2 | 3 | 4 | 5 | NA |
| 011920 | Expresses knowledge of personal sexual needs | 1 | 2 | 3 | 4 | 5 | NA |
| 011921 | Communicates comfortably with partner | 1 | 2 | 3 | 4 | 5 | NA |
| 011922 | Communicates sexual needs with partner | 1 | 2 | 3 | 4 | 5 | NA |
| 011923 | Communicates sexual preferences with partner | 1 | 2 | 3 | 4 | 5 | NA |
| 011924 | Performs sexually if environment conducive | 1 | 2 | 3 | 4 | 5 | NA |
| 011925 | Performs sexually without coercion of partner | 1 | 2 | 3 | 4 | 5 | NA |

*2nd edition 2000; Revised 3rd edition*

Outcome Content References:

Clark, J.C. (1993). Psychosocial responses of the patient: Altered sexual health. In S.I. Groenwald, M.H., Frogge, M. Goodman, & C.H. Yarbro (Eds.), *Cancer nursing principles and practice* (3rd ed., pp. 449-467). Boston: Jones & Bartlett.

Dobkin, P.L., & Bradley, I. (1991). Assessment of sexual dysfunction in oncology patients: Review, critique, and suggestions. *Journal of Psychosocial Oncology, 9*(1), 43-71.

Dunning, P. (1993). Sexuality and women with diabetes. *Patient Education and Counseling, 21*(1-2), 5-14.

Masters, W.H., & Johnson, V.E. (1970). *Human sexual inadequacy.* Boston: Little, Brown and Company.

Tuttle, B. (1984). Adult sexual response. In L.P. Higgins, & J.W. Hawkins (Eds.), *Human sexuality across the life span: Implications for nursing practice* (pp. 39-76). Monterey, CA: Wadsworth Health Sciences Division.

S

# *Sexual Identity (1207)*

*Domain-Psychosocial Health (III)*

*Class-Psychological Well-Being (M)*

*Scale(s)-Never demonstrated to Consistently demonstrated (m)*

*Care Recipient:*

*Data Source:*

**Definition:** Acknowledgment and acceptance of own sexual identity

OUTCOME TARGET RATING:     Maintain at _____          Increase to _____

| Sexual Identity Overall Rating | Never demonstrated 1 | Rarely demonstrated 2 | Sometimes demonstrated 3 | Often demonstrated 4 | Consistently demonstrated 5 | |
|---|---|---|---|---|---|---|
| INDICATORS: | | | | | | |
| 120701 Affirms self as a sexual being | 1 | 2 | 3 | 4 | 5 | NA |
| 120702 Exhibits clear sense of sexual orientation | 1 | 2 | 3 | 4 | 5 | NA |
| 120703 Exhibits comfort with sexual orientation | 1 | 2 | 3 | 4 | 5 | NA |
| 120704 Integrates sexual orientation into life roles | 1 | 2 | 3 | 4 | 5 | NA |
| 120705 Sets resilient boundaries with respect to societal prejudice/ discrimination | 1 | 2 | 3 | 4 | 5 | NA |
| 120706 Uses healthy coping behaviors to resolve sexual identity crises | 1 | 2 | 3 | 4 | 5 | NA |
| 120707 Challenges negative images of sexual self | 1 | 2 | 3 | 4 | 5 | NA |
| 120708 Seeks support of peers | 1 | 2 | 3 | 4 | 5 | NA |
| 120709 Reports healthy intimate relation- ships | 1 | 2 | 3 | 4 | 5 | NA |
| 120710 Reports healthy sexual functioning | 1 | 2 | 3 | 4 | 5 | NA |
| 120711 Describes risks associated with sexual activity | 1 | 2 | 3 | 4 | 5 | NA |
| 120712 Uses precautions to minimize risks associated with sexual activity | 1 | 2 | 3 | 4 | 5 | NA |
| 120713 Describes personal sexual value system | 1 | 2 | 3 | 4 | 5 | NA |
| 120714 Sets personal sexual boundaries | 1 | 2 | 3 | 4 | 5 | NA |

*2nd edition 2000; Revised 3rd edition (formerly Sexual Identity: Acceptance)*

S

*Continued*

Outcome Content References:

Bohan, J.S. (1996). *Psychology and sexual orientation: Coming to terms*. New York: Routledge.

Cain, R. (1991). Stigma management and gay identity development. *Social Work, 36*(1), 67-73.

Cass, V.E. (1984). Homosexual identity formation: Testing a theoretical model. *The Journal of Sex Research, 20*(2), 143-167.

Eliason, M.J. (1996). *Who cares? Institutional barriers to health care for lesbian, gay, and bisexual persons*. New York: NLN Press.

Kinsey, A.C., Pomeroy, W.B., & Martin, C.E. (1948). *Sexual behavior in the human male*. Philadelphia: W.B. Saunders.

Nass, G., Libby, R., & Fischer, M.P. (1989). *Sexual choices: An introduction to human sexuality* (2nd ed.). Montery, CA: Wadsworth Health Sciences.

Troiden, R.R. (1989). The formation of homosexual identities. *Journal of Homosexuality, 17*(1-2), 43-73.

Tuttle, B. (1984). Adult sexual response. In L.P. Higgins, & J.W. Hawkins (Eds.), *Human sexuality across the life span: Implications for nursing practice* (pp. 39-76). Monterey, CA: Wadsworth Health Sciences Division.

S

# *Skeletal Function (0211)*

*Domain-Functional Health (I)*

*Class-Mobility (C)*

*Scale(s)-Severely compromised to Not compromised (a)*

*Care Recipient:*

*Data Source:*

**Definition:** Ability of the bones to support the body and facilitate movement

OUTCOME TARGET RATING:    Maintain at _____    Increase to _____

| Skeletal Function<br>Overall Rating | Severely<br>compromised<br>1 | Substantially<br>compromised<br>2 | Moderately<br>compromised<br>3 | Mildly<br>compromised<br>4 | Not<br>compromised<br>5 | |
|---|---|---|---|---|---|---|
| INDICATORS: | | | | | | |
| 021101    Bone integrity | 1 | 2 | 3 | 4 | 5 | NA |
| 021102    Bone density | 1 | 2 | 3 | 4 | 5 | NA |
| 021103    Joint movement | 1 | 2 | 3 | 4 | 5 | NA |
| 021104    Weight bearing | 1 | 2 | 3 | 4 | 5 | NA |
| 021105    Skeletal alignment | 1 | 2 | 3 | 4 | 5 | NA |
| 021106    Joint stability | 1 | 2 | 3 | 4 | 5 | NA |

*2nd edition 2000; Revised 3rd edition*

## Outcome Content References:

Bouxsein, M.L., Myers, E.R., & Hayes, W.C. (1996). Biomechanics of age–related fractures. In R. Marcus, D. Feldman, & J. Kelsey (Eds.), *Osteoporosis*. San Diego: Academic Press.

Carter, D.R., Van Der Meulen, M.C.H., & Beaupre, G.S. (1996). Skeletal development: Mechanical consequences of growth, aging, and disease. In R. Marcus, D. Feldman, & J. Kelsey (Eds.), *Osteoporosis*. San Diego: Academic Press.

Krahl, H., Michaelis, U., Peiper, H., Quack, G., & Montag, M. (1994) Stimulation of bone growth through sports: A radiologic investigation of the upper extremities in professional tennis players. *The American Journal of Sports Medicine, 22*(6), 751-8.

Melton, L.J (1997). Epidemiology of spinal osteoporosis. *Spine, 22*(Suppl. 24), 2S-11S.

Mourad, L. (1991). *Orthopedic Disorders*. St. Louis: Mosby.

Sowers, M. (1997). Clinical epidemiology and osteoporosis: Measures and their interpretation. *Epidemiology and Clinical Decision Making 26*(1), 219-231.

S

# Sleep (0004)

*Domain-Functional Health (I)*

*Class-Energy Maintenance (A)*

*Scale(s)-Severely compromised to Not compromised (a) and Severe to None (n)*

*Care Recipient:*

*Data Source:*

> **Definition:** Natural periodic suspension of consciousness during which the body is restored

OUTCOME TARGET RATING:     Maintain at _____     Increase to _____

| Sleep<br>Overall Rating | Severely compromised<br>1 | Substantially compromised<br>2 | Moderately compromised<br>3 | Mildly compromised<br>4 | Not compromised<br>5 | |
|---|---|---|---|---|---|---|
| **INDICATORS:** | | | | | | |
| 000401 Hours of sleep (at least 5 hr/24 hr.)* | 1 | 2 | 3 | 4 | 5 | NA |
| 000402 Observed hours of sleep | 1 | 2 | 3 | 4 | 5 | NA |
| 000403 Sleep pattern | 1 | 2 | 3 | 4 | 5 | NA |
| 000404 Sleep quality | 1 | 2 | 3 | 4 | 5 | NA |
| 000405 Sleep efficiency (ratio of sleep time/total time trying) | 1 | 2 | 3 | 4 | 5 | NA |
| 000407 Sleep routine | 1 | 2 | 3 | 4 | 5 | NA |
| 000418 Sleeps through the night consistently | 1 | 2 | 3 | 4 | 5 | NA |
| 000408 Feels rejuvenated after sleep | 1 | 2 | 3 | 4 | 5 | NA |
| 000410 Wakeful at appropriate times | 1 | 2 | 3 | 4 | 5 | NA |
| 000411 Electroencephalogram findings | 1 | 2 | 3 | 4 | 5 | NA |
| 000412 Electromyogram findings | 1 | 2 | 3 | 4 | 5 | NA |
| 000413 Electro-oculogram findings | 1 | 2 | 3 | 4 | 5 | NA |

| | Severe | Substantial | Moderate | Mild | None | |
|---|---|---|---|---|---|---|
| 000406 Interrupted sleep | 1 | 2 | 3 | 4 | 5 | NA |
| 000409 Inappropriate napping | 1 | 2 | 3 | 4 | 5 | NA |
| 000416 Sleep apnea | 1 | 2 | 3 | 4 | 5 | NA |
| 000417 Dependence on sleep aids | 1 | 2 | 3 | 4 | 5 | NA |

*Appropriate for adults

*1st edition 1997; Revised 2nd edition 2000; Revised 3rd edition*

Outcome Content References:

+Buysse, D.J., Reynolds, C.F, III, Monk, T.H., Berman, S.R., & Kupfer, D.J. (1989). The Pittsburgh Sleep Quality Index: A new instrument for psychiatric practice and research. *Psychiatry Research, 28*(2), 193-213.

Ellis, J.R., & Nowlis, E.A. (1994). *Providing nursing care within the nursing process* (5th ed.). Philadelphia: J.B. Lippincott.

Hoch, C.C., Reynolds, C.F., & Houck, P. (1988). Sleep patterns in Alzheimer, depressed, and healthy elderly. *Western Journal of Nursing Research, 10*(3), 239-256.

Mead-Bennet, E. (1989). The relationship of primigravid sleep experience and select moods on the first postpartum day. *Journal of Obstetric, Gynecologic, & Neonatal Nursing, 19*(2), 146-152.

S

Paulsen, V.M., & Shaver, J.L. (1991). Stress, support, psychological states and sleep. *Social Science and Medicine, 32*(11), 1237-1243.

Porth, C.M. (2002). *Pathophysiology: Concepts of altered health states* (6th ed.). Philadelphia: Lippincott Williams & Wilkins.

Potter, P.A., & Perry, A.G. (2001). *Fundamentals of nursing* (5th ed.). St. Louis: Mosby.

Redeker, N.S. (2000). Sleep in acute care settings: An integrative review. *Journal of Nursing Scholarship, 32*(1), 31-38.

Schoenfelder, D.P., & Culp, K.R. (2001). Sleep pattern disturbance. In M. Maas, K. Buckwalter, M. Hardy, T. Tripp-Reimer, M. Titler, & J. Specht (Eds.), *Nursing care of older adults: Diagnoses, outcomes & interventions* (pp. 401-413). St. Louis: Mosby.

Topf, M. (1992). Effects of personal control over hospital noise on sleep. *Research in Nursing and Health, 15*(1), 19-28.

Topf, M., & Davis, J.E. (1993). Critical care unit noise and rapid eye movement sleep. *Heart & Lung, 22*(3), 252-258.

Williams, P.D., White, M.A., Powell, G.M., Alexander, D.J., & Conlon, M. (1988). Activity level in hospitalized children during sleep onset latency. *Computers in Nursing, 6*(2), 70-76.

**S**

# Social Interaction Skills (1502)

*Domain-Psychosocial Health (III)*                                    Care Recipient:

*Class-Social Interaction (P)*                                        Data Source:

*Scale(s)-Never demonstrated to Consistently demonstrated (m)*

**Definition:** Personal behaviors that promote effective relationships

OUTCOME TARGET RATING:      Maintain at _____      Increase to _____

| Social Interaction Skills Overall Rating | Never demonstrated 1 | Rarely demonstrated 2 | Sometimes demonstrated 3 | Often demonstrated 4 | Consistently demonstrated 5 | |
|---|---|---|---|---|---|---|
| **INDICATORS:** | | | | | | |
| 150201 Uses disclosure as appropriate | 1 | 2 | 3 | 4 | 5 | NA |
| 150202 Exhibits receptiveness | 1 | 2 | 3 | 4 | 5 | NA |
| 150203 Cooperates with others | 1 | 2 | 3 | 4 | 5 | NA |
| 150204 Exhibits sensitivity to others | 1 | 2 | 3 | 4 | 5 | NA |
| 150205 Uses assertive behaviors as appropriate | 1 | 2 | 3 | 4 | 5 | NA |
| 150206 Uses confrontation as appropriate | 1 | 2 | 3 | 4 | 5 | NA |
| 150207 Exhibits consideration | 1 | 2 | 3 | 4 | 5 | NA |
| 150208 Exhibits genuineness | 1 | 2 | 3 | 4 | 5 | NA |
| 150209 Exhibits warmth | 1 | 2 | 3 | 4 | 5 | NA |
| 150210 Exhibits poise | 1 | 2 | 3 | 4 | 5 | NA |
| 150211 Appears relaxed | 1 | 2 | 3 | 4 | 5 | NA |
| 150212 Engages others | 1 | 2 | 3 | 4 | 5 | NA |
| 150213 Exhibits trust | 1 | 2 | 3 | 4 | 5 | NA |
| 150214 Uses compromise | 1 | 2 | 3 | 4 | 5 | NA |
| 150216 Uses conflict resolution methods | 1 | 2 | 3 | 4 | 5 | NA |

*1st edition 1997; Revised 3rd edition*

Outcome Content References:

Erickson, D.H., Beiser, M., Iacono, W.G., Fleming, J.A.E., & Lin, T. (1989). The role of social relationships in the course of first-episode schizophrenia and affective psychosis. *American Journal of Psychiatry, 146*(11), 1456-1461.

Gotcher, J.M. (1992). Interpersonal communication and psychosocial adjustment. *Journal of Psychosocial Oncology, 10*(3), 21-39.

Heltsley, M.E., & Powers, R.C. (1975). Social interaction and perceived adequacy of interaction of the rural aged. *The Gerontologist, 15*(6), 533-536.

Levin, J., & Levin, W.C. (1981). Willingness to interact with an old person. *Research on Aging, 3*(2), 211-217.

Nussbaum, J.F. (1983). Relational closeness of elderly interaction: Implications for life satisfaction. *Western Journal of Speech Communication, 47*, 229-243.

+Ruehlman, L.S., & Karoly, P. (1991). With a little flak from my friends: Development and preliminary validation of the Test of Negative Social Exchange (TENSE). *Psychological Assessment: A Journal of Consulting and Clinical Psychology, 3*(1), 97-104.

Richter, G., & Richter, J. (1989). Social relationships reflected by depressive inpatients. *Acta Psychiatrica Scandinavica, 80*(6), 573-578.

Sheppard, M. (1993). Client satisfaction, extended intervention and interpersonal skills in community mental health. *Journal of Advanced Nursing, 18*(2), 246-259.

Waterman, J.D., Blegen, M., Clinton, P., & Specht, J.P. (2001). Social isolation. In M. Maas, K. Buckwalter, M. Hardy, T. Tripp-Reimer, M. Titler, & J. Specht (Eds.), *Nursing care of older adults: Diagnoses, outcomes & interventions* (pp. 651-663). St. Louis: Mosby.

Webb, L., Delaney, J.J., & Young, L.R. (1989). Age, interpersonal attraction, and social interaction. *Research on Aging, 11*(1), 107-123.

**S**

# *Social Involvement (1503)*

Domain-Psychosocial Health (III)                                  Care Recipient:

Class-Social Interaction (P)                                      Data Source:

Scale(s)-Never demonstrated to Consistently demonstrated (m)

**Definition:** Social interactions with persons, groups, or organizations

OUTCOME TARGET RATING:     Maintain at _____    Increase to _____

| Social Involvement Overall Rating | Never demonstrated 1 | Rarely demonstrated 2 | Sometimes demonstrated 3 | Often demonstrated 4 | Consistently demonstrated 5 | |
|---|---|---|---|---|---|---|
| **INDICATORS:** | | | | | | |
| 150301 Interacts with close friends | 1 | 2 | 3 | 4 | 5 | NA |
| 150302 Interacts with neighbors | 1 | 2 | 3 | 4 | 5 | NA |
| 150303 Interacts with family members | 1 | 2 | 3 | 4 | 5 | NA |
| 150304 Interacts with members of work group(s) | 1 | 2 | 3 | 4 | 5 | NA |
| 150305 Participates as member of church | 1 | 2 | 3 | 4 | 5 | NA |
| 150306 Participates in active church work | 1 | 2 | 3 | 4 | 5 | NA |
| 150307 Participates in organized activity | 1 | 2 | 3 | 4 | 5 | NA |
| 150308 Participates as officer in organization | 1 | 2 | 3 | 4 | 5 | NA |
| 150309 Participates as a volunteer | 1 | 2 | 3 | 4 | 5 | NA |
| 150311 Participates in leisure activities with others | 1 | 2 | 3 | 4 | 5 | NA |
| 150313 Participates in team sports | 1 | 2 | 3 | 4 | 5 | NA |

*1st edition 1997; Revised 3rd edition*

Outcome Content References:

Erickson, D.H., Beiser, M., Iacono, W.G., Fleming, J.A.E., & Lin, T. (1989). The role of social relationships in the course of first-episode schizophrenia and affective psychosis. *American Journal of Psychiatry, 146*(11), 1456-1461.

Gotcher, J.M. (1992). Interpersonal communication and psychosocial adjustment. *Journal of Psychosocial Oncology, 10*(3), 21-39.

Heltsley, M.E., & Powers, R.C. (1975). Social interaction and perceived adequacy of interaction of the rural aged. *The Gerontologist, 15*(6), 533-536.

Jylha, M., & Aro, S. (1989). Social ties and survival among the elderly in Tampere, Finland. *International Journal of Epidemiology, 18*(1) 158-164.

Levin, J., & Levin, W.C. (1981). Willingness to interact with an old person. *Research on Aging, 3*(2), 211-217.

Nussbaum, J.F. (1983). Relational closeness of elderly interaction: Implications for life satisfaction. *Western Journal of Speech Communication, 47*, 229-243.

Richter, G., & Richter, J. (1989). Social relationships reflected by depressive inpatients. *Acta Psychiatrica Scandinavica, 80*(6), 573-578.

Sheppard, M. (1993). Client satisfaction, extended intervention and interpersonal skills in community mental health. *Journal of Advanced Nursing, 18*(2), 246-259.

Waterman, J.D., Blegen, M., Clinton, P., & Specht, J.P. (2001). Social isolation. In M. Maas, K. Buckwalter, M. Hardy, T. Tripp-Reimer, M. Titler, & J. Specht (Eds.), *Nursing care of older adults: Diagnoses, outcomes & interventions* (pp. 651-663). St. Louis: Mosby.

Webb, L., Delaney, J.J., & Young, L.R. (1989). Age, interpersonal attraction, and social interaction. *Research on Aging, 11*(1), 107-123.

S

# Social Support (1504)

*Domain-Psychosocial Health (III)*

*Class-Social Interaction (P)*

*Scale(s)-Not adequate to Totally adequate (f)*

*Care Recipient:*

*Data Source:*

**Definition:** Perceived availability and actual provision of reliable assistance from others

OUTCOME TARGET RATING:    Maintain at _____    Increase to _____

| Social Support Overall Rating | Not adequate 1 | Slightly adequate 2 | Moderately adequate 3 | Substantially adequate 4 | Totally adequate 5 | |
|---|---|---|---|---|---|---|

INDICATORS:

| | | | | | | | |
|---|---|---|---|---|---|---|---|
| 150401 | Money available from others if needed | 1 | 2 | 3 | 4 | 5 | NA |
| 150412 | Help offered by others | 1 | 2 | 3 | 4 | 5 | NA |
| 150402 | Time provided by others | 1 | 2 | 3 | 4 | 5 | NA |
| 150403 | Labor provided by others | 1 | 2 | 3 | 4 | 5 | NA |
| 150404 | Information provided by others | 1 | 2 | 3 | 4 | 5 | NA |
| 150405 | Emotional assistance provided by others | 1 | 2 | 3 | 4 | 5 | NA |
| 150406 | Confidant relationship(s) | 1 | 2 | 3 | 4 | 5 | NA |
| 150407 | Persons who can help when needed | 1 | 2 | 3 | 4 | 5 | NA |
| 150408 | Willingness to call on others for help | 1 | 2 | 3 | 4 | 5 | NA |
| 150409 | Assistive social network | 1 | 2 | 3 | 4 | 5 | NA |
| 150410 | Supportive social contacts | 1 | 2 | 3 | 4 | 5 | NA |
| 150411 | Stable social network | 1 | 2 | 3 | 4 | 5 | NA |

*1st edition 1997; Revised 3rd edition*

Outcome Content References:

Akister, J., & Johnson, K. (2002). Parenting issues that may be addressed through a confidential helpline. *Health & Social Care in the Community, 10*(2), 106-111.

Dimond, M., & Jones, S.L. (1983). Social support: A review and theoretical integration. In P.L. Chinn (Ed.), *Advances in nursing theory development* (pp. 235-249). Rockville, MD: Aspen.

Gleeson-Kreig, J., Bernal, H., & Woolley, S. (2002). The role of social support in the self-management of diabetes mellitus among a Hispanic population. *Public Health Nursing, 19*(3), 215-222.

Hutchison, C. (1999). Social support: Factors to consider when designing studies that measure social support. *Journal of Advanced Nursing, 29*(6), 1520-1526.

Martire, L.M., Schulz, R., Mittelmark, M.B., & Newsom, J.T. (1999). Stability and change in older adults' social contact and social support: The cardiovascular health study. *Journals of Gerontology Series B-Psychological Sciences & Social Sciences, 54*(5), S302-311.

+Sarason, I.G., Sarason, B.R., Shearin, E.N., & Pierce, G.R. (1987). A brief measure of social support: Practical and theoretical implications. *Journal of Social and Personal Relationships, 4,* 497-510.

Tilden, V.P. (1985). Issues of conceptualization and measurement of social support in the construction of nursing theory. *Research in Nursing and Health, 8*(2), 199-206.

Travis, S., & Hunt, P. (2001). Supportive and palliative care networks: A new model for integrated care. *International Journal of Palliative Nursing, 7*(10), 501-504.

van Tilburg, T. (1998). Losing and gaining in old age: Changes in personal network size and social support in a four-year longitudinal study. *Journals of Gerontology Series B-Psychological Sciences & Social Sciences, 53*(6), S313-S323.

Warren, B.J. (1997). Depression, stressful life events, social support, and self-esteem in middle class African American women. *Archives of Psychiatric Nursing, 11*(3), 107-117.

Waterman, J.D., Blegen, M., Clinton, P., & Specht, J.P. (2001). Social isolation. In M. Maas, K. Buckwalter, M. Hardy, T. Tripp-Reimer, M. Titler, & J. Specht (Eds.), *Nursing care of older adults: Diagnoses, outcomes & interventions* (pp. 651-663). St. Louis: Mosby.

Wellisch, D., Kagawa-Singer, M., Reid, S.L., & Lin, Y., Nishikawa-Lee, S., & Wellisch, M. (1999). An exploratory study of social support: A cross-cultural comparison of Chinese, Japanese, and Anglo-American breast cancer patients. *Psycho-Oncology, 8*(3), 207-219.

S

# *Spiritual Health (2001)*

Domain-Perceived Health (V)

Class-Health & Life Quality (U)

Scale(s)-Severely compromised to Not compromised (a)

Care Recipient:

Data Source:

> **Definition:** Connectedness with self, others, higher power, all life, nature, and the universe that transcends and empowers the self

OUTCOME TARGET RATING:    Maintain at _____    Increase to _____

| Spiritual Health Overall Rating | Severely compromised 1 | Substantially compromised 2 | Moderately compromised 3 | Mildly compromised 4 | Not compromised 5 | |
|---|---|---|---|---|---|---|

INDICATORS:

| | | | | | | |
|---|---|---|---|---|---|---|
| 200101 | Quality of faith | 1 | 2 | 3 | 4 | 5 | NA |
| 200102 | Quality of hope | 1 | 2 | 3 | 4 | 5 | NA |
| 200103 | Meaning and purpose in life | 1 | 2 | 3 | 4 | 5 | NA |
| 200104 | Achievement of spiritual world view | 1 | 2 | 3 | 4 | 5 | NA |
| 200105 | Feelings of peacefulness | 1 | 2 | 3 | 4 | 5 | NA |
| 200106 | Ability to love | 1 | 2 | 3 | 4 | 5 | NA |
| 200107 | Ability to forgive | 1 | 2 | 3 | 4 | 5 | NA |
| 200109 | Ability to pray | 1 | 2 | 3 | 4 | 5 | NA |
| 200110 | Ability to worship | 1 | 2 | 3 | 4 | 5 | NA |
| 200108 | Spiritual experiences | 1 | 2 | 3 | 4 | 5 | NA |
| 200111 | Participation in spiritual rites and passages | 1 | 2 | 3 | 4 | 5 | NA |
| 200113 | Participation in meditation | 1 | 2 | 3 | 4 | 5 | NA |
| 200115 | Participation in spiritual reading | 1 | 2 | 3 | 4 | 5 | NA |
| 200112 | Interaction with spiritual leaders | 1 | 2 | 3 | 4 | 5 | NA |
| 200114 | Expression through song/music | 1 | 2 | 3 | 4 | 5 | NA |
| 200119 | Expression through art | 1 | 2 | 3 | 4 | 5 | NA |
| 200120 | Expression through writing | 1 | 2 | 3 | 4 | 5 | NA |
| 200116 | Connectedness with inner-self | 1 | 2 | 3 | 4 | 5 | NA |
| 200117 | Connectedness with others | 1 | 2 | 3 | 4 | 5 | NA |
| 200121 | Interaction with others to share thoughts, feelings, and beliefs | 1 | 2 | 3 | 4 | 5 | NA |

*1st edition 1997; Revised 3rd edition (formerly Spiritual Well-Being)*

S

*Continued*

Outcome Content References:

Burkhardt, M.A. (1989). Spirituality: An analysis of the concept. *Holistic Nursing Practice, 3*(3), 69-77.

Burkhart, L., & Solari-Twadell, P. A. (2001). Spirituality and religiousness: Differentiating the diagnoses through a review of the nursing literature. Nursing Diagnosis: *The International Journal of Nursing Language and Classification, 12*(2), 45-54.

Emblen, J.D. (1992). Religion and spirituality defined according to current use in nursing literature. *Journal of Professional Nursing, 8*(1), 41-47.

Haase, J.E., et al. (1992). Simultaneous concept analysis of spiritual perspective, hope, acceptance and self-transcendence. *Image - the Journal of Nursing Scholarship, 24*(2), 141-146.

Labun, E. (1988). Spiritual care: An element in nursing care planning. *Journal of Advanced Nursing, 13*(3), 314-320.

LeMone, P. (2001). Spiritual distress. In M. Maas, K. Buckwalter, M. Hardy, T. Tripp-Reimer, M. Titler, & J. Specht (Eds.), *Nursing care of older adults: Diagnoses, outcomes & interventions* (pp. 782-793). St. Louis: Mosby.

Pender, N., Murdaugh, C., & Parsons, M.A. (2001). *Health promotion in nursing practice* (4th ed.). Upper Saddle River, New Jersey: Prentice Hall.

Reed, P.G. (1992). An emerging paradigm for the investigation of spirituality in nursing. *Research in Nursing and Health, 15*(5), 349-357.

+Roberts, K.T., & Aspy, C.B. (1993). Development of the Serenity Scale. *Journal of Nursing Measurement, 1*(2), 145-164.

S

# Stress Level (1212)

Domain-Psychosocial Health (III)

Class-Psychological Well-Being (M)

Scale(s)-Severe to None (n)

Care Recipient:

Data Source:

**Definition:** Severity of manifested physical or mental tension resulting from factors that alter an existing equilibrium

OUTCOME TARGET RATING:     Maintain at _____   Increase to _____

| Stress Level Overall Rating | Severe 1 | Substantial 2 | Moderate 3 | Mild 4 | None 5 | |
|---|---|---|---|---|---|---|

INDICATORS:

| | | Severe 1 | Substantial 2 | Moderate 3 | Mild 4 | None 5 | |
|---|---|---|---|---|---|---|---|
| 121201 | Elevated blood pressure | 1 | 2 | 3 | 4 | 5 | NA |
| 121202 | Increased radial pulse rate | 1 | 2 | 3 | 4 | 5 | NA |
| 121203 | Increased respiratory rate | 1 | 2 | 3 | 4 | 5 | NA |
| 121204 | Dilated pupils | 1 | 2 | 3 | 4 | 5 | NA |
| 121205 | Increased muscle tension in neck, shoulders and/or back | 1 | 2 | 3 | 4 | 5 | NA |
| 121206 | Tension headache | 1 | 2 | 3 | 4 | 5 | NA |
| 121207 | Sweaty palms | 1 | 2 | 3 | 4 | 5 | NA |
| 121208 | Dry mouth and throat | 1 | 2 | 3 | 4 | 5 | NA |
| 121209 | Diarrhea | 1 | 2 | 3 | 4 | 5 | NA |
| 121210 | Urinary frequency | 1 | 2 | 3 | 4 | 5 | NA |
| 121211 | Change in food intake | 1 | 2 | 3 | 4 | 5 | NA |
| 121212 | Upset stomach | 1 | 2 | 3 | 4 | 5 | NA |
| 121213 | Restlessness | 1 | 2 | 3 | 4 | 5 | NA |
| 121214 | Sleep disturbance | 1 | 2 | 3 | 4 | 5 | NA |
| 121215 | Forgetfulness and blocking | 1 | 2 | 3 | 4 | 5 | NA |
| 121216 | Frequent mental mistakes | 1 | 2 | 3 | 4 | 5 | NA |
| 121217 | Diminished attention to detail | 1 | 2 | 3 | 4 | 5 | NA |
| 121218 | Inability to concentrate on tasks | 1 | 2 | 3 | 4 | 5 | NA |
| 121219 | Emotional outbursts | 1 | 2 | 3 | 4 | 5 | NA |
| 121220 | Irritability | 1 | 2 | 3 | 4 | 5 | NA |
| 121221 | Depression | 1 | 2 | 3 | 4 | 5 | NA |
| 121222 | Anxiety | 1 | 2 | 3 | 4 | 5 | NA |
| 121223 | Suspiciousness | 1 | 2 | 3 | 4 | 5 | NA |
| 121224 | Oppressive thoughts | 1 | 2 | 3 | 4 | 5 | NA |
| 121225 | Flashback episodes | 1 | 2 | 3 | 4 | 5 | NA |
| 121226 | Dissociation | 1 | 2 | 3 | 4 | 5 | NA |
| 121227 | Compulsive behavior | 1 | 2 | 3 | 4 | 5 | NA |
| 121228 | Increased alcohol use | 1 | 2 | 3 | 4 | 5 | NA |
| 121229 | Increased psychotropic drug(s) use | 1 | 2 | 3 | 4 | 5 | NA |
| 121230 | Increased smoking | 1 | 2 | 3 | 4 | 5 | NA |
| 121231 | Absenteeism | 1 | 2 | 3 | 4 | 5 | NA |
| 121232 | Decreased productivity | 1 | 2 | 3 | 4 | 5 | NA |
| 121233 | Increased frequency of accidents | 1 | 2 | 3 | 4 | 5 | NA |
| 121234 | Change in libido | 1 | 2 | 3 | 4 | 5 | NA |

*3rd edition*

Outcome Content References:

American Psychiatric Association. (2000). *Diagnostic and statistical manual of mental disorders* (4th ed., text revision). Washington DC: Author.

Campbell, R.J. (1989). *Psychiatric dictionary* (6th ed.). New York: Oxford University.

Lazarus, R. S., & Folkman, S. (1984). *Stress, appraisal, and coping.* New York: Springer.

Stanhope, M., & Lancaster, J. (1988). Community health nursing: Process and practice for promoting health (2nd ed.). St. Louis: Mosby.

Tasman, A., Kay, J., & Lieberman, J.A. (1997). *Psychiatry* (Vol. 2). Philadelphia: Saunders.

S

# Student Health Status (2005)

*Domain-Perceived Health (V)*

*Class-Health & Life Quality (U)*

*Scale-Severely compromised to Not compromised (a) and Severe to None (n)*

*Care Recipient:*

*Data Source:*

**Definition:** Physical, cognitive/emotional, and social status of school age children that contribute to school attendance, participation in school activities, and ability to learn

OUTCOME TARGET RATING:    Maintain at_____    Increase to_____

| Student Health Status Overall Rating | | Severely compromised 1 | Substantially compromised 2 | Moderately compromised 3 | Mildly compromised 4 | Not compromised 5 | |
|---|---|---|---|---|---|---|---|
| 200501 | Physical health | 1 | 2 | 3 | 4 | 5 | NA |
| 200502 | Mental/emotional health | 1 | 2 | 3 | 4 | 5 | NA |
| 200503 | School attendance | 1 | 2 | 3 | 4 | 5 | NA |
| 200504 | Readiness to learn | 1 | 2 | 3 | 4 | 5 | NA |
| 200505 | Academic performance at grade level or higher | 1 | 2 | 3 | 4 | 5 | NA |
| 200506 | Standardized test performance at grade level or higher | 1 | 2 | 3 | 4 | 5 | NA |
| 200507 | Progression to graduation on expected schedule | 1 | 2 | 3 | 4 | 5 | NA |
| 200508 | Return to class after visit to health office | 1 | 2 | 3 | 4 | 5 | NA |
| 200509 | Physician office visits minimized | 1 | 2 | 3 | 4 | 5 | NA |
| 200510 | Emergency room visits minimized | 1 | 2 | 3 | 4 | 5 | NA |
| 200511 | Reports to the health office for medications at appropriate time | 1 | 2 | 3 | 4 | 5 | NA |
| 200512 | Participation in mandated screenings | 1 | 2 | 3 | 4 | 5 | NA |
| 200513 | Family follow up of referrals | 1 | 2 | 3 | 4 | 5 | NA |
| 200514 | Participation in self-care activities appropriate to age and ability | 1 | 2 | 3 | 4 | 5 | NA |
| 200515 | Students with chronic illness or special needs managed according to IHP*/IEP* | 1 | 2 | 3 | 4 | 5 | NA |

S

| Student Health Status—cont'd | | Severely compromised | Substantially compromised | Moderately compromised | Mildly compromised | Not compromised | |
|---|---|---|---|---|---|---|---|
| 200516 | Financial resources for health care needs | 1 | 2 | 3 | 4 | 5 | NA |
| 200517 | Participation in curricular school activities | 1 | 2 | 3 | 4 | 5 | NA |
| 200518 | Participation in extracurricular school activities | 1 | 2 | 3 | 4 | 5 | NA |
| 200519 | Participation in physical activities | 1 | 2 | 3 | 4 | 5 | NA |
| 200520 | Normal growth for age | 1 | 2 | 3 | 4 | 5 | NA |
| 200521 | Normal development for age | 1 | 2 | 3 | 4 | 5 | NA |
| 200522 | Normal weight for age | 1 | 2 | 3 | 4 | 5 | NA |
| 200523 | Healthy dietary habits | 1 | 2 | 3 | 4 | 5 | NA |
| 200524 | Postponement of sexual activity | 1 | 2 | 3 | 4 | 5 | NA |
| 200525 | Avoidance of sexual activity | 1 | 2 | 3 | 4 | 5 | NA |
| 200526 | Avoidance of pregnancy | 1 | 2 | 3 | 4 | 5 | NA |

| | | Severe | Substantial | Moderate | Mild | None | |
|---|---|---|---|---|---|---|---|
| 200527 | Alcohol use | 1 | 2 | 3 | 4 | 5 | NA |
| 200528 | Drug use | 1 | 2 | 3 | 4 | 5 | NA |
| 200529 | Tobacco use | 1 | 2 | 3 | 4 | 5 | NA |
| 200530 | Occurrence of accidents | 1 | 2 | 3 | 4 | 5 | NA |
| 200531 | Disruptive behavior | 1 | 2 | 3 | 4 | 5 | NA |
| 200532 | Occurrence of sexually transmitted disease | 1 | 2 | 3 | 4 | 5 | NA |

*IHP = Individualized Healthcare Plan, IEP = Individualized Educational Plan.

*3rd edition*

Outcome Content References:

Council of Chief State School Officers. (1998). *Incorporating health-related indicators in education accountability systems*. Washington, DC: Author.

Howard, M. (1991). *How to help your teenager postpone sexual involvement*. Lexington, NY: Continuum Publishing Co.

Marx, E., & Wooley, S.F. (Eds). (1998). *Health is academic: A guide to coordinated school health programs*. New York: Teachers College Columbia University.

Miller, B., Card, J., Paikoff, R.J., & Peterson, J. (1992). *Preventing adolescent pregnancy*. Newbury Park, CA: Sage Publications.

Novello, A.C., DeGraw, C., & Kleinman, D.V. (1992). Healthy children ready to learn: An essential collaboration between health and education. *Public Health Reports, 107*(1), 3-10.

Tyson, H. (1999). A load off the teachers' backs: Coordinated school health programs. *Phi Delta Kappan, 80*(5), K1-K8.

Washington State Office of Superintendent of Public Instruction. (2001). *School nurse outcome measures*, Olympia, WA: Author.

# Substance Addiction Consequences (1407)

*Domain-Psychosocial Health (III)*

*Class-Self-Control (O)*

*Scale(s)-Severe to None (n)*

*Care Recipient:*

*Data Source:*

| **Definition:** Severity of change in health status and social functioning due to substance addiction |
|---|

OUTCOME TARGET RATING:     Maintain at _____     Increase to_____

| Substance Addiction Consequences Overall Rating | Severe 1 | Substantial 2 | Moderate 3 | Mild 4 | None 5 | |
|---|---|---|---|---|---|---|
| **INDICATORS:** | | | | | | |
| 140701 Sustained decrease in physical activity | 1 | 2 | 3 | 4 | 5 | NA |
| 140702 Chronic impaired motor function | 1 | 2 | 3 | 4 | 5 | NA |
| 140703 Chronic decreased endurance | 1 | 2 | 3 | 4 | 5 | NA |
| 140704 Chronic fatigue | 1 | 2 | 3 | 4 | 5 | NA |
| 140705 Chronic impaired cognitive function | 1 | 2 | 3 | 4 | 5 | NA |
| 140706 Chronic impaired breathing | 1 | 2 | 3 | 4 | 5 | NA |
| 140707 Prolonged recovery from illnesses | 1 | 2 | 3 | 4 | 5 | NA |
| 140708 Absenteeism from work or school | 1 | 2 | 3 | 4 | 5 | NA |
| 140709 Difficulty maintaining employment | 1 | 2 | 3 | 4 | 5 | NA |
| 140710 Difficulty maintaining adequate housing | 1 | 2 | 3 | 4 | 5 | NA |
| 140711 Difficulty supporting self financially | 1 | 2 | 3 | 4 | 5 | NA |

S

| | | Severe (4+ occurrences) | Substantial (3 occurrences) | Moderate (2 occurrences) | Mild (1 occurrence) | None (no occurrence) | |
|---|---|---|---|---|---|---|---|
| 140712 | Traffic accidents within the last year | 1 | 2 | 3 | 4 | 5 | NA |
| 140717 | Traffic tickets within the last year | 1 | 2 | 3 | 4 | 5 | NA |
| 140713 | Arrests within the last year | 1 | 2 | 3 | 4 | 5 | NA |
| 140714 | Emergency room visits within the last year | 1 | 2 | 3 | 4 | 5 | NA |
| 140715 | Hospitalizations within the last year | 1 | 2 | 3 | 4 | 5 | NA |

*1st edition 1997; Revised 3rd edition*

Outcome Content References:

McCuster, J., Stoddard, A.M., Zapka, J.G., & Lewis, B.F. (1993). Behavioral outcomes of AIDS educational interventions for drug users in short term treatment. *American Journal of Public Health, 83*(10), 1463-1466.

+McLellan, A.T., Luborsky, L., Woody, G.E., & O'Brien, C.P. (1980). An improved diagnostic evaluation instrument for substance abuse patients. *Journal of Nervous and Mental Disease, 168*, 26-33.

Simons-Morton, D.G., Mullen, P.D., Mains, D.A., Tabak, E.R., & Green, L.W. (1992). Characteristics of controlled studies of patient education and counseling for preventive health behaviors. *Patient Education and Counseling, 19*(2), 174-204.

Talashek, M.L., Gerace, L.M., & Starr, K.L. (1994). The substance abuse pandemic: Determinants to guide interventions. *Public Health Nursing, 11*(2), 131-139.

S

# Suffering Severity (2003)

Domain-Perceived Health (V)

Class-Symptom Status (V)

Scale(s)-Severe to None (n)

Care Recipient:

Data Source:

**Definition:** Severity of anguish associated with a distressing symptom, injury or loss that has potential long-term effects

OUTCOME TARGET RATING:    Maintain at _____    Increase to _____

| Suffering Severity Overall Rating | Severe 1 | Substantial 2 | Moderate 3 | Mild 4 | None 5 | |
|---|---|---|---|---|---|---|
| INDICATORS: | | | | | | |
| 200301    Self-absorption | 1 | 2 | 3 | 4 | 5 | NA |
| 200302    Depression | 1 | 2 | 3 | 4 | 5 | NA |
| 200303    Sadness | 1 | 2 | 3 | 4 | 5 | NA |
| 200304    Powerlessness | 1 | 2 | 3 | 4 | 5 | NA |
| 200305    Grief | 1 | 2 | 3 | 4 | 5 | NA |
| 200306    Guilt | 1 | 2 | 3 | 4 | 5 | NA |
| 200307    Hopelessness | 1 | 2 | 3 | 4 | 5 | NA |
| 200308    Helplessness | 1 | 2 | 3 | 4 | 5 | NA |
| 200309    Worthlessness | 1 | 2 | 3 | 4 | 5 | NA |
| 200314    Vulnerability | 1 | 2 | 3 | 4 | 5 | NA |
| 200315    Spiritual distress | 1 | 2 | 3 | 4 | 5 | NA |
| 200316    Despair | 1 | 2 | 3 | 4 | 5 | NA |
| 200319    Loneliness | 1 | 2 | 3 | 4 | 5 | NA |
| 200310    Fear of reoccurrence | 1 | 2 | 3 | 4 | 5 | NA |
| 200311    Fear of unbearable pain | 1 | 2 | 3 | 4 | 5 | NA |
| 200312    Fear of unknown circumstances | 1 | 2 | 3 | 4 | 5 | NA |
| 200313    Fear of being alone | 1 | 2 | 3 | 4 | 5 | NA |
| 200317    Bitterness toward others | 1 | 2 | 3 | 4 | 5 | NA |

*2nd edition 2000; Revised 3rd edition (formerly Suffering Level)*

### Outcome Content References:

Cherny, N.I., Coyle, N., & Foley, K.M. (1994). The treatment of suffering when patients request elective death. *Journal of Palliative Care, 10*(2), 71-79.

Copp, L.A. (1974). The spectrum of suffering. *American Journal of Nursing, 74*(3), 491-495.

Duffy, M.E. (1992). A theoretical and empirical review of the concept of suffering. In P.L. Starck & J.P. McGovern (Eds.), *The hidden dimension of illness: Human suffering* (Pub. No. 15-2451, pp. 291-303). New York: National League for Nursing Press.

Jacob, S.R. & Scandrett-Hobdon, S. (1994). Mothers grieving the death of a child: case reports of maternal grief. *The Nurse Practitioner, 19*(7), 60-65.

Mount, B.M. (1984). Psychological and social aspects of cancer pain. In P. D. Wall & R. Melzack (Eds.), *Textbook of pain* (pp. 460-471). New York: Churchill Livingstone.

Price, D.D., & Harkins, S.W. (1992). Psychophysical approaches to pain measurement and assessment. In D.C. Turk & R. Melzack (Eds.), *Handbook of pain assessment* (pp. 111-134). New York: The Guilford Press.

Steeves, R.H., Kahn, D.L., & Benoliel, J.Q. (1990). Nurses' interpretation of the suffering of their patients. *Western Journal of Nursing Research, 12*(6), 714-731.

S

# Suicide Self-Restraint (1408)

*Domain-Psychosocial Health (III)*

*Class-Self-Control (O)*

*Scale(s)-Never demonstrated to Consistently demonstrated (m)*

*Care Recipient:*

*Data Source:*

**Definition:** Personal actions to refrain from gestures and attempts at killing self

OUTCOME TARGET RATING:    Maintain at _____    Increase to _____

| Suicide Self-Restraint Overall Rating | Never demonstrated 1 | Rarely demonstrated 2 | Sometimes demonstrated 3 | Often demonstrated 4 | Consistently demonstrated 5 | |
|---|---|---|---|---|---|---|
| **INDICATORS:** | | | | | | |
| 140801 Expresses feelings | 1 | 2 | 3 | 4 | 5 | NA |
| 140815 Expresses sense of hope | 1 | 2 | 3 | 4 | 5 | NA |
| 140802 Maintains connectedness in relationships | 1 | 2 | 3 | 4 | 5 | NA |
| 140803 Seeks help when feeling self-destructive | 1 | 2 | 3 | 4 | 5 | NA |
| 140804 Verbalizes suicidal ideas | 1 | 2 | 3 | 4 | 5 | NA |
| 140805 Controls impulses | 1 | 2 | 3 | 4 | 5 | NA |
| 140806 Refrains from gathering means for suicide | 1 | 2 | 3 | 4 | 5 | NA |
| 140807 Refrains from giving away possessions | 1 | 2 | 3 | 4 | 5 | NA |
| 140816 Refrains from inflicting serious injury | 1 | 2 | 3 | 4 | 5 | NA |
| 140809 Refrains from using non-prescribed mood-altering substance(s) | 1 | 2 | 3 | 4 | 5 | NA |
| 140810 Discloses plan for suicide if present | 1 | 2 | 3 | 4 | 5 | NA |
| 140811 Upholds suicide contract | 1 | 2 | 3 | 4 | 5 | NA |
| 140812 Maintains self-control without supervision | 1 | 2 | 3 | 4 | 5 | NA |
| 140813 Refrains from attempting suicide | 1 | 2 | 3 | 4 | 5 | NA |
| 140817 Seeks treatment for depression | 1 | 2 | 3 | 4 | 5 | NA |
| 140818 Seeks treatment for substance abuse | 1 | 2 | 3 | 4 | 5 | NA |

**S**

*Continued*

| Suicide Self-Restraint—cont'd | | Never demonstrated | Rarely demonstrated | Sometimes demonstrated | Often demonstrated | Consistently demonstrated | |
|---|---|---|---|---|---|---|---|
| 140819 | Reports adequate pain control for chronic pain | 1 | 2 | 3 | 4 | 5 | NA |
| 140820 | Uses suicide prevention resources and social support groups within the community | 1 | 2 | 3 | 4 | 5 | NA |
| 140821 | Uses available mental health services | 1 | 2 | 3 | 4 | 5 | NA |
| 140822 | Plans for future | 1 | 2 | 3 | 4 | 5 | NA |

*1st edition 1997; Revised 2nd edition 2000; Revised 3rd edition*

Outcome Content References:

Conwell, Y. (1997). Management of suicidal behavior in the elderly. *The Psychiatric Clinics of North America, 20*(3), 667-683.

Cugino, A., Markovich, E.I., Rosenblatt, S., Jarjoura, D., Blend, D., & Whittier, F.C. (1992). Searching for a pattern: Repeat suicide attempts. *Journal of Psychosocial Nursing, 30*(3), 23-25.

Forster, P. (1994). Accurate assessment of short-term suicide risk in a crisis. *Psychiatric Annals, 24*(11), 571-578.

Hirschfeld, R.M.A., & Russell, J.M. (1997). Assessment and treatment of suicidal patients. *The New England Journal of Medicine, 337*(13), 910-915.

Ingram, T.N. (2001). Risk for violence: Self-directed or directed at others. In M. Maas, K. Buckwalter, M. Hardy, T. Tripp-Reimer, M. Titler, & J. Specht (Eds.), *Nursing care of older adults: Diagnoses, outcomes & interventions* (pp. 696-705). St. Louis: Mosby.

+Ivanoff, A., Joon Jang, S., Smyth, N.J., & Linehan, M.M. (1994). Fewer reasons for staying alive when you are thinking of killing yourself: The Brief Reasons for Living Inventory. *Journal of Psychopathology and Behavioral Assessment, 16*(1), 1-13.

Josepho, S.A., & Plutchek, R. (1994). Stress, coping, and suicide risk in psychiatric inpatients. *Suicide and Life-Threatening Behavior, 24*(1), 48-57.

+Linehan, M.M., Goodstein, J.L., Nielsen, S.L., Chiles, J.A. (1983). Reasons for staying alive when you are thinking of killing yourself: The Reasons for Living Inventory. *Journal of Consulting and Clinical Psychology, 51*(2), 276-286, 484-485.

Lipshitz, A. (1995). Suicide prevention in young adults (age 18-30). *Suicide and Life-Threatening Behavior, 25*(1), 155-169.

Mellick, E., Buckwalter, K.C., & Stolley, J.M. (1992). Suicide among elderly white men: Development of a profile. *Journal of Psychosocial Nursing, 30*(2), 29-34.

Robie, D., Edgemon-Hill, E.J., Phelps, B., Schmitz, C., & Laughlin, J.A. (1999). Suicide prevention protocol: One hospital's nursing protocol for identification and intervention. *American Journal of Nursing, 99*(12), 53, 55, 57.

Valente, S.M., & Trainor, D. (1998). Rational suicide among patients who are terminally ill. *Official Journal of the Association of Operating Room Nurses, 68*(2), 252-255, 257-258, 260-264.

S

# *Swallowing Status (1010)*

Domain-Physiologic Health (II)                          Care Recipient:

Class-Nutrition (K)                                      Data Source:

Scale(s)-Severely compromised to Not compromised (a) and Severe to None (n)

**Definition:** Safe passage of fluids and/or solids from the mouth to the stomach

OUTCOME TARGET RATING:    Maintain at _____    Increase to _____

| Swallowing Status Overall Rating | | Severely compromised 1 | Substantially compromised 2 | Moderately compromised 3 | Mildly compromised 4 | Not compromised 5 | |
|---|---|---|---|---|---|---|---|
| INDICATORS: | | | | | | | |
| 101001 | Maintains food in mouth | 1 | 2 | 3 | 4 | 5 | NA |
| 101002 | Handles oral secretions | 1 | 2 | 3 | 4 | 5 | NA |
| 101003 | Saliva production | 1 | 2 | 3 | 4 | 5 | NA |
| 101004 | Chewing ability | 1 | 2 | 3 | 4 | 5 | NA |
| 101005 | Delivery of bolus to hypopharynx is timed with swallow reflex | 1 | 2 | 3 | 4 | 5 | NA |
| 101006 | Ability to clear oral cavity | 1 | 2 | 3 | 4 | 5 | NA |
| 101007 | Timely bolus formation | 1 | 2 | 3 | 4 | 5 | NA |
| 101008 | Number of swallows appropriate for bolus size/texture | 1 | 2 | 3 | 4 | 5 | NA |
| 101009 | Meal duration with respect to amount consumed | 1 | 2 | 3 | 4 | 5 | NA |
| 101010 | Timely swallow reflex | 1 | 2 | 3 | 4 | 5 | NA |
| 101015 | Maintains neutral head and trunk position | 1 | 2 | 3 | 4 | 5 | NA |
| 101016 | Food acceptance | 1 | 2 | 3 | 4 | 5 | NA |
| 101018 | Swallow study findings | 1 | 2 | 3 | 4 | 5 | NA |

| | | Severe | Substantial | Moderate | Mild | None | |
|---|---|---|---|---|---|---|---|
| 101011 | Changes in voice quality | 1 | 2 | 3 | 4 | 5 | NA |
| 101012 | Choking | 1 | 2 | 3 | 4 | 5 | NA |
| 101020 | Coughing | 1 | 2 | 3 | 4 | 5 | NA |
| 101021 | Gagging | 1 | 2 | 3 | 4 | 5 | NA |
| 101013 | Increased swallow effort | 1 | 2 | 3 | 4 | 5 | NA |
| 101014 | Gastric reflux | 1 | 2 | 3 | 4 | 5 | NA |
| 101017 | Discomfort with swallowing | 1 | 2 | 3 | 4 | 5 | NA |

*2nd edition 2000; Revised 3rd edition*

S

*Continued*

Outcome Content References:

Arvedson, J., & Brodsky, L., (Eds.). (2002). *Pediatric swallowing and feeding: Assessment and management* (2nd ed.). San Diego: Singular Publishing Group.

Bosch, J., Van Dyke, D., Smith, S., & Poulton, S. (1997). The role of medical condition in the exacerbation of self-injurious behavior: An exploratory study. *Mental Retardation, 35*(2), 124-130.

Christensen, J.R. (1989). Developmental approach to pediatric neurogenic dysphagia. *Dysphagia, 3*(3), 131-134.

Feinberg, M. (1997). The effects of medication on swallowing. In B. Sonies (Ed.), *Dysphagia: A Continuum of Care* (pp. 107-120). Gaithersburg, MD: Aspen

Gresham, G.E., Duncan, P.W., Stason, W.B., et al. (1995). *Post-stroke rehabilitation. Clinical practice guideline*, No. 16. (AHCPR Publication No. 95-0062). Rockville, MD: U.S. Department of Health and Human Services. Public Health Services, Agency for Health Care Policy and Research.

Hendrix, T.R. (1993). Art and science of history taking in the patient with difficulty swallowing. *Dysphagia, 8*(2), 69-73.

The Joanna Briggs Institute for Evidence Based Nursing and Midwifery. (2000). Identification and nursing management of dysphagia in adults with neurological impairment. *Best Practice, 4*(2), Blackwell Science-Asia, Australia.

Kramer, S.S., & Eicher, P. M. (1993). The evaluation of pediatric feeding abnormalities. *Dysphagia, 8*(3), 215-24.

Langmore, S. (2000). *Endoscopic evaluation and treatment of swallowing disorders.* New York: Thieme Medical Publishers.

Lespargot, A., Langevin, M., Muller, S., & Guillemont, S. (1993). Swallowing disturbances associated with drooling in cerebral-palsied children. *Developmental Medicine and Child Neurology, 35*(4), 298-304.

Morris, S.E. (1989) Development of oral-motor skills in the neurologically impaired child receiving non-oral feedings. *Dysphagia, 3*(3), 135-154.

Ramsay, M., Gisel, E.G., & Boutry, M. (1993). Non-organic failure to thrive: Growth failure secondary to feeding skills disorder. *Developmental Medicine and Child Neurology, 35*(4), 285-297.

Tuchman, D., & Walter, R. (Eds.). (1994). *Disorders of feeding and swallowing in infants and children.* San Diego: Singular Publishing Group.

Wolf, L.S., & Glass, R.P. (1992). *Feeding and swallowing disorders in infancy.* Tucson: Therapy Skill Builders.

S

# Swallowing Status: Esophageal Phase (1011)

*Domain-Physiologic Health (II)*                              *Care Recipient:*

*Class-Nutrition (K)*                                          *Data Source:*

*Scale(s)-Severely compromised to Not compromised (a) and Severe to None (n)*

**Definition:** Safe passage of fluids and/or solids from the pharynx to the stomach

OUTCOME TARGET RATING:    Maintain at _____    Increase to _____

| Swallowing Status: Esophageal Phase Overall Rating | Severely compromised 1 | Substantially compromised 2 | Moderately compromised 3 | Mildly compromised 4 | Not compromised 5 | |
|---|---|---|---|---|---|---|
| **INDICATORS:** | | | | | | |
| 101106  Maintains neutral head and neck position | 1 | 2 | 3 | 4 | 5 | NA |
| 101114  Food acceptance | 1 | 2 | 3 | 4 | 5 | NA |
| 101115  Volume acceptance | 1 | 2 | 3 | 4 | 5 | NA |
| 101116  Swallow study findings: esophageal phase | 1 | 2 | 3 | 4 | 5 | NA |
| | **Severe** | **Substantial** | **Moderate** | **Mild** | **None** | |
| 101101  Choking with swallowing | 1 | 2 | 3 | 4 | 5 | NA |
| 101118  Coughing with swallowing | 1 | 2 | 3 | 4 | 5 | NA |
| 101102  Gastric reflux | 1 | 2 | 3 | 4 | 5 | NA |
| 101103  Epigastric pain | 1 | 2 | 3 | 4 | 5 | NA |
| 101104  Discomfort with swallowing | 1 | 2 | 3 | 4 | 5 | NA |
| 101108  Nighttime coughing | 1 | 2 | 3 | 4 | 5 | NA |
| 101109  Nighttime vomiting | 1 | 2 | 3 | 4 | 5 | NA |
| 101119  Nighttime choking | 1 | 2 | 3 | 4 | 5 | NA |
| 101110  Repetitive swallowing | 1 | 2 | 3 | 4 | 5 | NA |
| 101111  Hematemesis | 1 | 2 | 3 | 4 | 5 | NA |
| 101112  Acidic breath odor | 1 | 2 | 3 | 4 | 5 | NA |
| 101113  Bruxism | 1 | 2 | 3 | 4 | 5 | NA |

*2nd edition 2000; Revised 3rd edition*

Outcome Content References:

Arvedson, J., & Brodsky, L., (Eds.). 2002. *Pediatric swallowing and feeding: Assessment and management* (2nd ed.). San Diego: Singular Publishing Group.

Bosch, J., Van Dyke, D., Smith, S., & Poulton, S. (1997). The role of medical condition in the exacerbation of self injurious behavior: An exploratory study. *Mental Retardation, 35*(2), 124-130.

Christensen, J.R. (1989). Developmental approach to neurogenic pediatric dysphagia. *Dysphagia, 3*(3), 131-134.

Feinberg, M. (1997). The effects of medication on swallowing. In B. Sonies (Ed.), *Dysphagia: A Continuum of Care* (pp. 107-120). Gaithersburg, MD: Aspen.

Hendrix, T.R. (1993). Art and science of history taking in the patient with difficulty swallowing. *Dysphagia, 8*(2), 69-73.

Kramer, S., & Eicher, P. M. (1993). The evaluation of pediatric feeding abnormalities. *Dysphagia, 8*(3), 215-24.

Langmore, S. (2000). *Endoscopic evaluation and treatment of swallowing disorders.* New York: Thieme Medical Publishers.

*Continued*

S

Lespargot, A., Langevin, M., Muller, S., & Guillemont, S. (1993). Swallowing disturbances associated with drooling in cerebral-palsied children. *Developmental Medicine and Child Neurology, 35*(4), 298-304.

Morris, S. (1989). Development of oral-motor skills in the neurologically impaired child receiving non-oral feedings. *Dysphagia, 3*(3), 135-154.

Ramsay, M., Gisel, E.G., & Boutry, M. (1993). Non-organic failure to thrive: Growth failure secondary to feeding skills disorder. *Developmental Medicine and Child Neurology, 35*(4), 285-297.

Tuchman, D., & Walter, R. (Eds.). (1994). *Disorders of feeding and swallowing in infants and children.* San Diego: Singular Publishing.

Wolf, L.S., & Glass, R.P. (1992). *Feeding and swallowing disorders in infancy.* Tucson: Therapy Skill Builders.

S

# Swallowing Status: Oral Phase (1012)

*Domain-Physiologic Health (II)*

*Class-Nutrition (K)*

*Scale(s)-Severely compromised to Not compromised (a) and Severe to None (n)*

*Care Recipient:*

*Data Source:*

**Definition:** Preparation, containment and posterior movement of fluids and/or solids in the mouth

OUTCOME TARGET RATING:    Maintain at _____    Increase to _____

| Swallowing Status: Oral Phase Overall Rating | Severely compromised 1 | Substantially compromised 2 | Moderately compromised 3 | Mildly compromised 4 | Not compromised 5 | |
|---|---|---|---|---|---|---|
| INDICATORS: | | | | | | |
| 101201 Maintains food in mouth | 1 | 2 | 3 | 4 | 5 | NA |
| 101202 Handles oral secretions | 1 | 2 | 3 | 4 | 5 | NA |
| 101203 Bolus formation | 1 | 2 | 3 | 4 | 5 | NA |
| 101204 Timely bolus formation | 1 | 2 | 3 | 4 | 5 | NA |
| 101205 Chewing ability | 1 | 2 | 3 | 4 | 5 | NA |
| 101206 Delivery of bolus to hypopharynx timed with swallow reflex | 1 | 2 | 3 | 4 | 5 | NA |
| 101207 Ability to clear oral cavity | 1 | 2 | 3 | 4 | 5 | NA |
| 101209 Lip closure | 1 | 2 | 3 | 4 | 5 | NA |
| 101210 Number of swallows appropriate for bolus size/texture | 1 | 2 | 3 | 4 | 5 | NA |
| 101211 Nippling efficiency | 1 | 2 | 3 | 4 | 5 | NA |
| 101212 Rate of food consumption | 1 | 2 | 3 | 4 | 5 | NA |
| 101214 Gag reflex | | | | | | NA |
| 101215 Swallow study findings: oral phase | 1 | 2 | 3 | 4 | 5 | NA |

| | Severe | Substantial | Moderate | Mild | None | |
|---|---|---|---|---|---|---|
| 101208 Coughing before swallowing | 1 | 2 | 3 | 4 | 5 | NA |
| 101217 Choking before swallowing | 1 | 2 | 3 | 4 | 5 | NA |
| 101218 Gagging before swallowing | 1 | 2 | 3 | 4 | 5 | NA |
| 101213 Nasal reflux | 1 | 2 | 3 | 4 | 5 | NA |

*2nd edition 2000; Revised 3rd edition*

S

*Continued*

Outcome Content References:

Arvedson, J., & Brodsky, L., (Eds.). (2002). *Pediatric swallowing and feeding: Assessment and management* (2nd ed.). San Diego: Singular Publishing Group.

Bosch, J., Van Dyke, D., Smith, S., & Poulton, S. (1997). The role of medical condition in the exacerbation of self injurious behavior: An exploratory study. *Mental Retardation, 35*(2), 124-130.

Christensen, J.R. (1989). Developmental approach to neurogenic pediatric dysphagia. *Dysphagia, 3*(3), 131-134.

Feinberg, M. (1997). The effects of medication on swallowing. In B. Sonies (Ed.), *Dysphagia: A Continuum of Care* (pp. 107-120). Gaithersburg, MD: Aspen.

Hendrix, T.R. (1993). Art and science of history taking in the patient with difficulty swallowing. *Dysphagia, 8*(2), 69-73.

Kramer, S., & Eicher, P.M. (1993). The evaluation of pediatric feeding abnormalities. *Dysphagia, 8*(3), 215-24.

Langmore, S. (2000). *Endoscopic evaluation and treatment of swallowing disorders.* New York: Thieme Medical Publishers.

Lespargot, A., Langevin, M., Muller, S., & Guillemont, S. (1993). Swallowing disturbances associated with drooling in cerebral-palsied children. *Developmental Medicine and Child Neurology, 35*(4), 298-304.

Morris, S., (1989) Development of oral-motor skills in the neurologically impaired child receiving non-oral feedings. *Dysphagia, 3*(3), 135-154.

Ramsay, M., Gisel, E.G., & Boutry, M. (1993). Non-organic failure to thrive: Growth failure secondary to feeding skills disorder. *Developmental Medicine and Child Neurology, 35*(4), 285-297.

Tuchman, D., & Walter, R. (Eds.). (1994). *Disorders of feeding and swallowing in infants and children.* San Diego: Singular Publishing Group.

Wolf, L.S., & Glass, R. P. (1992). *Feeding and swallowing disorders in infancy.* Tucson: Therapy Skill Builders.

S

# Swallowing Status: Pharyngeal Phase (1013)

*Domain-Physiologic Health (II)*

*Class-Nutrition (K)*

*Scale(s)-Severely compromised to Not compromised (a) and Severe to None (n)*

*Care Recipient:*

*Data Source:*

**Definition:** Safe passage of fluids and/or solids from the mouth to the esophagus

OUTCOME TARGET RATING:    Maintain at _____    Increase to _____

| Swallowing Status: Pharyngeal Phase Overall Rating | Severely compromised 1 | Substantially compromised 2 | Moderately compromised 3 | Mildly compromised 4 | Not compromised 5 | |
|---|---|---|---|---|---|---|
| INDICATORS: | | | | | | |
| 101301 Timely swallow reflex | 1 | 2 | 3 | 4 | 5 | NA |
| 101304 Number of swallows appropriate for bolus size/texture | 1 | 2 | 3 | 4 | 5 | NA |
| 101305 Maintains neutral head and neck position | 1 | 2 | 3 | 4 | 5 | NA |
| 101307 Laryngeal elevation | 1 | 2 | 3 | 4 | 5 | NA |
| 101311 Food acceptance | 1 | 2 | 3 | 4 | 5 | NA |
| 101312 Swallow study findings: pharyngeal phase | 1 | 2 | 3 | 4 | 5 | NA |

| | Severe | Substantial | Moderate | Mild | None | |
|---|---|---|---|---|---|---|
| 101302 Changes in voice quality | 1 | 2 | 3 | 4 | 5 | NA |
| 101303 Choking | 1 | 2 | 3 | 4 | 5 | NA |
| 101314 Coughing | 1 | 2 | 3 | 4 | 5 | NA |
| 101315 Gagging | 1 | 2 | 3 | 4 | 5 | NA |
| 101306 Increased swallow effort | 1 | 2 | 3 | 4 | 5 | NA |
| 101310 Nasal reflux | 1 | 2 | 3 | 4 | 5 | NA |
| 101316 Aspirations | 1 | 2 | 3 | 4 | 5 | NA |

*2nd edition 2000; Revised 3rd edition*

Outcome Content References:

Arvedson, J., & Brodsky, L., (Eds.). (2002). *Pediatric swallowing and feeding: Assessment and management* (2nd ed.). San Diego: Singular Publishing Group.

Bosch, J., Van Dyke, D., Smith, S., & Poulton, S. (1997). The role of medical condition in the exacerbation of self injurious behavior: An exploratory study. *Mental Retardation, 35*(2), 124-130.

Christensen, J.R. (1989). Developmental approach to neurogenic pediatric dysphagia. *Dysphagia, 3*(3), 131-134.

Feinberg, M. (1997). The effects of medication on swallowing. In B. Sonies (Ed.), *Dysphagia: A Continuum of Care* (pp. 107-120). Gaithersburg, MD: Aspen.

Hendrix, T.R. (1993). Art and science of history taking in the patient with difficulty swallowing. *Dysphagia, 8*(2), 69-73.

Kramer, S., & Eicher, P.M. (1993). The evaluation of pediatric feeding abnormalities. *Dysphagia, 8*(3), 215-24.

Langmore, S. (2000). *Endoscopic evaluation and treatment of swallowing disorders.* New York: Thieme Medical Publishers.

Lespargot, A., Langevin, M., Muller, S., & Guillemont, S. (1993). Swallowing disturbances associated with drooling in cerebral-palsied children. *Developmental Medicine and Child Neurology, 35*(4), 298-304.

Morris, S., (1989) Development of oral-motor skills in the neurologically impaired child receiving non-oral feedings. *Dysphagia, 3*(3), 135-154.

Ramsay, M., Gisel, E.G., & Boutry, M. (1993). Non-organic failure to thrive: Growth failure secondary to feeding skills disorder. *Developmental Medicine and Child Neurology, 35*(4), 285-297.

Tuchman, D., & Walter, R. (Eds.). (1994). *Disorders of feeding and swallowing in infants and children.* San Diego: Singular Publishing Group.

Wolf, L.S., & Glass, R. P. (1992). *Feeding and swallowing disorders in infancy.* Tucson: Therapy Skill Builders.

S

# *Symptom Control (1608)*

*Domain-Health Knowledge & Behavior (IV)*

*Class-Health Behavior (Q)*

*Scale(s)-Never demonstrated to Consistently demonstrated (m)*

Care Recipient:

Data Source:

> **Definition:** Personal actions to minimize perceived adverse changes in physical and emotional functioning

OUTCOME TARGET RATING:   Maintain at_____   Increase to_____

| Symptom Control Overall Rating | Never demonstrated 1 | Rarely demonstrated 2 | Sometimes demonstrated 3 | Often demonstrated 4 | Consistently demonstrated 5 | |
|---|---|---|---|---|---|---|
| **INDICATORS:** | | | | | | |
| 160801   Monitors symptom onset | 1 | 2 | 3 | 4 | 5 | NA |
| 160802   Monitors symptom persistence | 1 | 2 | 3 | 4 | 5 | NA |
| 160803   Monitors symptom severity | 1 | 2 | 3 | 4 | 5 | NA |
| 160804   Monitors symptom frequency | 1 | 2 | 3 | 4 | 5 | NA |
| 160805   Monitors symptom variation | 1 | 2 | 3 | 4 | 5 | NA |
| 160806   Uses preventive measures | 1 | 2 | 3 | 4 | 5 | NA |
| 160807   Uses relief measures | 1 | 2 | 3 | 4 | 5 | NA |
| 160808   Uses warning signs to seek health care | 1 | 2 | 3 | 4 | 5 | NA |
| 160809   Uses available resources | 1 | 2 | 3 | 4 | 5 | NA |
| 160810   Uses diary to monitor symptoms over time | 1 | 2 | 3 | 4 | 5 | NA |
| 160811   Reports symptoms controlled | 1 | 2 | 3 | 4 | 5 | NA |

*1st edition 1997; Revised 2nd edition 2000; Revised 3rd edition*

## Outcome Content References:

Epstein, L., & Cluss, P.A. (1982). A behavioral medicine perspective on adherence to long-term medical regimens. *Journal of Consulting and Clinical Psychology, 50*(6), 950-971.

Hardy, M.D. (2001). Impaired skin integrity: Dry skin. In M. Maas, K. Buckwalter, M. Hardy, T. Tripp-Reimer, M. Titler, & J. Specht (Eds.), *Nursing care of older adults: Diagnoses, outcomes & interventions* (pp. 137-144). St. Louis: Mosby.

Hartford, M., Karlson, B.W., Sjolin, M., Holmberg, S., & Herlitz, J. (1993). Symptoms, thoughts, and environmental factors in suspected acute myocardial infarction. *Heart & Lung, 22*(1), 64-70.

Hegyvary, S.T. (1993). Patient care outcomes related to management of symptoms. In J.J. Fitzpatrick & J.S. Stevenson (Eds.), *Annual review of nursing research*, (Vol. 11, pp. 145-168). New York: Springer.

+McCorkle, R., & Benoliel, J.Q. (1983). Symptom distress, current concerns, and mood disturbances after diagnosis of life-threatening disease. *Social Science Medicine, 17*(7), 431-438.

+McCorkle, R., & Young, K. (1978). Development of a Symptom Distress Scale. *Cancer Nursing, 1*(5), 373-378.

Sherbourne, C.D., Allen, H.M., Kamberg, C.J., & Wells, K.B. (1992). Physical/psychophysiological symptoms measure. In A.L. Stewart & J.E. Ware, Jr. (Eds.), *Measuring functioning and well-being* (pp. 261-272). Durham, NC: Duke University Press.

Sickle Cell Disease Guideline Panel. (1993). *Sickle cell disease: Screening, diagnosis, management, and counseling in newborn and infants, Clinical practice guideline*, No. 6. (AHCPR Publication No. 93-0562). Rockville, MD: U.S. Department of Health and Human Services. Public Health Services, Agency for Health Care Policy and Research.

Strauss, A.L., Corbin, J., Fagerhaugh, S., Glaser, B.G., Maines, D., Suczek, B., & Wiener, C.L. (1984). Symptom control. In *Chronic illness and the quality of life* (2nd ed., pp. 49-59). St. Louis: Mosby.

Wright, L.K. (2001). Sexual dysfunction. In M. Maas, K. Buckwalter, M. Hardy, T. Tripp-Reimer, M. Titler, & J. Specht (Eds.), *Nursing care of older adults: Diagnoses, outcomes & interventions* (pp. 733-749). St. Louis: Mosby.

**S**

# *Symptom Severity (2103)*

*Domain-Perceived Health (V)*

*Class-Symptom Status (V)*

*Scale(s)-Severe to None (n)*

Care Recipient:

Data Source:

**Definition:** Severity of perceived adverse changes in physical, emotional, and social functioning

OUTCOME TARGET RATING:      Maintain at_____      Increase to_____

| Symptom Severity<br>Overall Rating | Severe<br>1 | Substantial<br>2 | Moderate<br>3 | Mild<br>4 | None<br>5 | |
|---|---|---|---|---|---|---|
| **INDICATORS:** | | | | | | |
| 210301   Symptom intensity | 1 | 2 | 3 | 4 | 5 | NA |
| 210302   Symptom frequency | 1 | 2 | 3 | 4 | 5 | NA |
| 210303   Symptom persistence | 1 | 2 | 3 | 4 | 5 | NA |
| 210304   Associated discomfort | 1 | 2 | 3 | 4 | 5 | NA |
| 210305   Associated restlessness | 1 | 2 | 3 | 4 | 5 | NA |
| 210306   Associated fear | 1 | 2 | 3 | 4 | 5 | NA |
| 210307   Associated anxiety | 1 | 2 | 3 | 4 | 5 | NA |
| 210308   Impaired physical mobility | 1 | 2 | 3 | 4 | 5 | NA |
| 210309   Impaired role performance | 1 | 2 | 3 | 4 | 5 | NA |
| 210310   Impaired interpersonal<br>            relationships | 1 | 2 | 3 | 4 | 5 | NA |
| 210311   Impaired mood | 1 | 2 | 3 | 4 | 5 | NA |
| 210312   Impaired life enjoyment | 1 | 2 | 3 | 4 | 5 | NA |
| 210313   Inadequate sleep | 1 | 2 | 3 | 4 | 5 | NA |
| 210316   Loss of sleep | 1 | 2 | 3 | 4 | 5 | NA |
| 210314   Loss of appetite | 1 | 2 | 3 | 4 | 5 | NA |

*1st edition 1997; Revised 3rd edition*

Outcome Content References:

Hartford, M., Karlson, B.W., Sjolin, M., Holmberg, S., & Herlitz, J. (1993). Symptoms, thoughts, and environmental factors in suspected acute myocardial infarction. *Heart & Lung, 22*(1), 64-70.

Hegyvary, S.T. (1993). Patient care outcomes related to management of symptoms. In J.J. Fitzpatrick & J.S. Stevenson (Eds.), *Annual review of nursing research*, (Vol. 11, pp. 145-168). New York: Springer.

+McCorkle, R., & Benoliel, J.Q. (1983). Symptom distress, current concerns, and mood disturbances after diagnosis of life-threatening disease. *Social Science Medicine, 17*(7), 431-438.

+McCorkle, R., & Young, K. (1978). Development of a Symptom Distress Scale. *Cancer Nursing, 1*(5), 373-378.

Sherbourne, C.D., Allen, H.M., Kamberg, C.J., & Wells, K.B. (1992). Physical/psychophysiologic symptoms measure. In A.L. Stewart & J.E. Ware, Jr. (Eds.), *Measure functioning and well-being* (pp. 261-272). Durham, NC: Duke University Press.

Strauss, A.L., Corbin, J., Fagerhaugh, S., Glaser, B.G., Maines, D., Suczek, B., & Wiener, C.L. (1984). Symptom control. In *Chronic illness and the quality of life* (2nd ed., pp. 49-59). St. Louis: Mosby.

S

# Symptom Severity: Perimenopause (2104)

| | |
|---|---|
| *Domain-Perceived Health (V)* | *Care Recipient:* |
| *Class-Symptom Status (V)* | *Data Source:* |
| *Scale(s)-Severe to None (n)* | |

**Definition:** Severity of symptoms caused by declining hormonal levels

OUTCOME TARGET RATING:    Maintain at_____    Increase to_____

| Symptom Severity: Perimenopause<br>Overall Rating | Severe<br>1 | Substantial<br>2 | Moderate<br>3 | Mild<br>4 | None<br>5 | |
|---|---|---|---|---|---|---|
| **INDICATORS:** | | | | | | |
| 210401 Menstrual irregularity | 1 | 2 | 3 | 4 | 5 | NA |
| 210402 Abdominal cramps | 1 | 2 | 3 | 4 | 5 | NA |
| 210403 Hot flashes | 1 | 2 | 3 | 4 | 5 | NA |
| 210404 Night sweats | 1 | 2 | 3 | 4 | 5 | NA |
| 210405 Vaginal dryness | 1 | 2 | 3 | 4 | 5 | NA |
| 210406 Mood swings | 1 | 2 | 3 | 4 | 5 | NA |
| 210407 Menstrual flow | 1 | 2 | 3 | 4 | 5 | NA |
| 210408 Insomnia | 1 | 2 | 3 | 4 | 5 | NA |
| 210409 Fatigue | 1 | 2 | 3 | 4 | 5 | NA |
| 210410 Musculoskeletal pain | 1 | 2 | 3 | 4 | 5 | NA |
| 210411 Weight gain | 1 | 2 | 3 | 4 | 5 | NA |
| 210412 Decreased libido | 1 | 2 | 3 | 4 | 5 | NA |
| 210413 Heart palpitations | 1 | 2 | 3 | 4 | 5 | NA |
| 210414 Vertigo | 1 | 2 | 3 | 4 | 5 | NA |
| 210415 Memory changes | 1 | 2 | 3 | 4 | 5 | NA |

*2nd edition 2000; Revised 3rd edition*

## Outcome Content References:

Alexander, L.L. & LaRosa, J. (1994). *New Dimensions in Women's Health*. Boston: Jones & Bartlett.

Andrews, G. *Women's sexual health* (2nd ed.). London: Bailliere Tindall.

Clark, A.J., Flowers, J. Boots, L., & Shettar, S. (1995). Sleep disturbance in mid-life women. *Journal of Advanced Nursing 22*(3), 562-568.

Fogel, C.I., & Woods, N.F. (Eds.). (1995). *Women's health care: A comprehensive handbook*. Thousand Oaks: Sage Publications.

Logothetis, M.L. (1991). Women's decisions about estrogen replacement therapy. *Western Journal of Nursing Research, 13*(4), 458-474.

Woods, N.F., & Mitchell, E.S. (1996). Patterns of depressed mood in midlife women: Observations from the Seattle Midlife Women's Health Study. *Research in Nursing and Health, 19*(2), 111-123.

S

# Symptom Severity: Premenstrual Syndrome (PMS) (2105)

*Domain-Perceived Health (V)*

*Class-Symptom Status (V)*

*Scale(s)-Severe to None (n)*

*Care Recipient:*

*Data Source:*

**Definition:** Severity of symptoms caused by cyclic hormonal fluctuations

OUTCOME TARGET RATING:    Maintain at_____    Increase to_____

| Symptom Severity: Premenstrual Syndrome (PMS) Overall Rating | Severe 1 | Substantial 2 | Moderate 3 | Mild 4 | None 5 | |
|---|---|---|---|---|---|---|
| INDICATORS: | | | | | | |
| 210501  Abdominal bloating | 1 | 2 | 3 | 4 | 5 | NA |
| 210502  Abdominal cramps | 1 | 2 | 3 | 4 | 5 | NA |
| 210503  Disrupted bowel patterns | 1 | 2 | 3 | 4 | 5 | NA |
| 210504  Decreased urine output | 1 | 2 | 3 | 4 | 5 | NA |
| 210505  Acne | 1 | 2 | 3 | 4 | 5 | NA |
| 210506  Anxiety | 1 | 2 | 3 | 4 | 5 | NA |
| 210507  Backache | 1 | 2 | 3 | 4 | 5 | NA |
| 210508  Breast tenderness | 1 | 2 | 3 | 4 | 5 | NA |
| 210509  Decreased energy | 1 | 2 | 3 | 4 | 5 | NA |
| 210510  Depression | 1 | 2 | 3 | 4 | 5 | NA |
| 210511  Fluid retention | 1 | 2 | 3 | 4 | 5 | NA |
| 210512  Food cravings | 1 | 2 | 3 | 4 | 5 | NA |
| 210513  Headaches | 1 | 2 | 3 | 4 | 5 | NA |
| 210514  Insomnia | 1 | 2 | 3 | 4 | 5 | NA |
| 210515  Irritability | 1 | 2 | 3 | 4 | 5 | NA |
| 210516  Mood swings | 1 | 2 | 3 | 4 | 5 | NA |
| 210517  Nausea | 1 | 2 | 3 | 4 | 5 | NA |
| 210518  Vertigo | 1 | 2 | 3 | 4 | 5 | NA |
| 210519  Vomiting | 1 | 2 | 3 | 4 | 5 | NA |

*2nd edition 2000; Revised 3rd edition*

Outcome Content References:

Alexander, L.L., & LaRosa, J. (1994). *New dimensions in women's health.* Boston: Jones & Bartlett.

Carter, J., & Verhoef, M.J. (1994). Efficacy of self-help and alternative treatments of premenstrual syndrome. *Women's Health Issues, 4*(3), 130-137.

Fogel, C.I., & Woods, N.F. (Eds.). (1995). *Women's health care: A comprehensive handbook.* Thousand Oaks: Sage Publications.

Lewis, L.L. (1995). One year in the life of a woman with premenstrual syndrome: A case study. *Nursing Research, 44*(2), 111-116.

Mitchell, E.S., Woods, N.F., & Lentz, M.J. (1994). Differentiation of women with three premenstrual symptom patterns. *Nursing Research, 43*(1), 25-30.

Taylor, D.L. (1994). Evaluating therapeutic change in symptom severity at the level of the individual woman experiencing severe PMS. *Image -the Journal of Nursing Scholarship 26*(1), 25-33.

Woods, N.F., Lentz, M., Mitchell, E., Taylor, D, & Lee, K. (1986). *The daily health diary. The prevalence of PMS: Final report* (NV01054). Washington, DC: Division of Nursing U.S. Public Health Services, U.S. Department of Health and Human Services.

Woods, N.F., Mitchell E.S., & Lentz, M.F. (1995). Social pathways to premenstrual symptoms. *Research in Nursing & Health, 18*(3), 225-237.

S

# *Systemic Toxin Clearance: Dialysis (2302)*

Domain-Physiologic Health (II)

Class-Therapeutic Response (a)

Scale(s)-Severely compromised to Not compromised (a) and Severe to None (n)

Care Recipient:

Data Source:

**Definition:** Clearance of toxins from the body with peritoneal or hemodialysis

OUTCOME TARGET RATING:    Maintain at_____    Increase to_____

| Systemic Toxin Clearance: Dialysis Overall Rating | Severely compromised 1 | Substantially compromised 2 | Moderately compromised 3 | Mildly compromised 4 | Not compromised 5 | |
|---|---|---|---|---|---|---|
| INDICATORS: | | | | | | |
| 230201 Complies with treatment schedule | 1 | 2 | 3 | 4 | 5 | NA |
| 230202 Concentration | 1 | 2 | 3 | 4 | 5 | NA |
| 230212 Urea reduction ratio (URR) ≥ 65% | 1 | 2 | 3 | 4 | 5 | NA |
| 230213 Weight | 1 | 2 | 3 | 4 | 5 | NA |
| 230214 Serum potassium | 1 | 2 | 3 | 4 | 5 | NA |
| 230216 Blood pressure | 1 | 2 | 3 | 4 | 5 | NA |
| 230217 Serum sodium | 1 | 2 | 3 | 4 | 5 | NA |
| | **Severe** | **Substantial** | **Moderate** | **Mild** | **None** | |
| 230203 Nausea | 1 | 2 | 3 | 4 | 5 | NA |
| 230204 Vomiting | 1 | 2 | 3 | 4 | 5 | NA |
| 230205 Weakness | 1 | 2 | 3 | 4 | 5 | NA |
| 230206 Malaise | 1 | 2 | 3 | 4 | 5 | NA |
| 230207 Anorexia | 1 | 2 | 3 | 4 | 5 | NA |
| 230208 Insomnia | 1 | 2 | 3 | 4 | 5 | NA |
| 230209 Edema | 1 | 2 | 3 | 4 | 5 | NA |
| 230210 Dizziness | 1 | 2 | 3 | 4 | 5 | NA |
| 230211 Pruritus | 1 | 2 | 3 | 4 | 5 | NA |
| 230218 Ascites | 1 | 2 | 3 | 4 | 5 | NA |
| 230219 Muscle cramps | 1 | 2 | 3 | 4 | 5 | NA |

*2nd edition 2000; Revised 3rd edition*

Outcome Content References:

Brundage, D.J. (1992). *Renal disorders*. St. Louis: Mosby.

Gutch, C.F., Stoner, M.H., & Corea, A.L. (1999). *Review of hemodialysis for nurses and dialysis personnel* (6th ed.). St. Louis: Mosby.

Guzman, N.J., & Peterson, J.C. (1993). In C.C. Tisher, & C.S. Wilcox (Eds.). *House officers series: Nephrology* (2nd ed., pp. 60-87). Baltimore, MD: Wilkins & Wilkins.

Lancaster, L.E. (Ed.). (1995). *ANNA's core curriculum for nephrology nurses* (3rd ed.) (Section X.). Pitman, NJ: Janetti.

S

# Thermoregulation (0800)

*Domain-Physiologic Health (II)*

*Class-Metabolic Regulation (I)*

*Scale(s)-Severely compromised to Not compromised (a) and Severe to None (n)*

Care Recipient:

Data Source:

**Definition:** Balance among heat production, heat gain, and heat loss

OUTCOME TARGET RATING:     Maintain at_____     Increase to_____

| Thermoregulation Overall Rating | Severely compromised 1 | Substantially compromised 2 | Moderately compromised 3 | Mildly compromised 4 | Not compromised 5 | |
|---|---|---|---|---|---|---|
| **INDICATORS:** | | | | | | |
| 080009 Presence of goose bumps when cold | 1 | 2 | 3 | 4 | 5 | NA |
| 080010 Sweating when hot | 1 | 2 | 3 | 4 | 5 | NA |
| 080011 Shivering when cold | 1 | 2 | 3 | 4 | 5 | NA |
| 080017 Apical heart rate | 1 | 2 | 3 | 4 | 5 | NA |
| 080012 Radial pulse rate | 1 | 2 | 3 | 4 | 5 | NA |
| 080013 Respiratory rate | 1 | 2 | 3 | 4 | 5 | NA |
| 080015 Reported thermal comfort | 1 | 2 | 3 | 4 | 5 | NA |

| | Severe | Substantial | Moderate | Mild | None | |
|---|---|---|---|---|---|---|
| 080001 Increased skin temperature | 1 | 2 | 3 | 4 | 5 | NA |
| 080018 Decreased skin temperature | 1 | 2 | 3 | 4 | 5 | NA |
| 080019 Hyperthermia | 1 | 2 | 3 | 4 | 5 | NA |
| 080020 Hypothermia | 1 | 2 | 3 | 4 | 5 | NA |
| 080003 Headache | 1 | 2 | 3 | 4 | 5 | NA |
| 080004 Muscle aches | 1 | 2 | 3 | 4 | 5 | NA |
| 080005 Irritability | 1 | 2 | 3 | 4 | 5 | NA |
| 080006 Drowsiness | 1 | 2 | 3 | 4 | 5 | NA |
| 080007 Skin color changes | 1 | 2 | 3 | 4 | 5 | NA |
| 080008 Muscle twitching | 1 | 2 | 3 | 4 | 5 | NA |
| 080014 Dehydration | 1 | 2 | 3 | 4 | 5 | NA |

*1st edition 1997; Revised 3rd edition*

**Outcome Content References:**

Caruso, C., Hadley, B., Shuklou, R., & Frame, P. (1992). Cooling effects and comfort of four cooling blanket temperatures in humans with fever. *Nursing Research, 41*(2), 68-72.

Erickson, R., & Kerklin, S. (1992). Comparison of methods for core temperature measurement. *Heart & Lung, 21*(3), 297.

Finke, C. (1991). Measurement of the thermoregulatory response: A review. *Focus on Critical Care, 18*(5), 408-412.

Franceschl, V. (1991). Accuracy and feasibility of measuring oral temperature in critically ill adults. *Focus on Critical Care, 18*(3), 221-228.

Hollander, H. (1993). Neurological and febrile syndromes in HIV. *Emergency Medicine, 25*(4), 26-40.

Holtzclaw, B.J. (2001). Risk for altered body temperature. In M. Maas, K. Buckwalter, M. Hardy, T. Tripp-Reimer, M. Titler, & J. Specht (Eds.), *Nursing care of older adults: Diagnoses, outcomes & interventions* (pp. 201-216). St. Louis: Mosby.

Holtzclaw, B.J. (1992). The febrile response in critical care: State of the science. *Heart & Lung, 21*(5), 482-501.

Kluger, M. (1978). Fever versus hyperthermia. *New England Journal of Medicine, 299*(10), 555.

Murphy, K. (1992). Acetaminophen and ibuprofen: Finer control and overdose. *Pediatric Nursing, 18*(4), 428-431.

Segatore, M. (1992). Fever after traumatic brain injury. *American Association of Neuroscience Nurse, 24*(2), 104-109.

Stewart, G., & Webster, D. (1992). Re-evaluation of the tympanic thermometer in the emergency department. *Annals of Emergency Medicine, 21*(2), 158-161.

Summers, S., Dudgeon, N., Byram, K., & Zingsheim, K. (1990). The effects of two warming methods on core and surface temperatures, hemoglobin oxygen saturation, blood pressure, and perceived comfort of hypothermic postanesthesia patients. *Journal of Post Anesthesia Nursing, 5*(5), 354-364.

T

# Thermoregulation: Newborn (0801)

Domain-Physiologic Health (II)

Class-Metabolic Regulation (I)

Scale(s)-Severely compromised to Not compromised (a) and Severe to None (n)

Care Recipient:

Data Source:

**Definition:** Balance among heat production, heat gain, and heat loss during the first 28 days of life

OUTCOME TARGET RATING:    Maintain at _____    Increase to _____

| Thermoregulation: Newborn Overall Rating | Severely compromised 1 | Substantially compromised 2 | Moderately compromised 3 | Mildly compromised 4 | Not compromised 5 | |
|---|---|---|---|---|---|---|
| INDICATORS: | | | | | | |
| 080106 Weight gain | 1 | 2 | 3 | 4 | 5 | NA |
| 080107 Non-shivering thermogenesis | 1 | 2 | 3 | 4 | 5 | NA |
| 080108 Assumes heat retention posture with hypothermia | 1 | 2 | 3 | 4 | 5 | NA |
| 080109 Assumes heat dissipation posture with hyperthermia | 1 | 2 | 3 | 4 | 5 | NA |
| 080110 Weaning from Isolette to crib | 1 | 2 | 3 | 4 | 5 | NA |
| 080113 Acid/base balance | 1 | 2 | 3 | 4 | 5 | NA |
| | **Severe** | **Substantial** | **Moderate** | **Mild** | **None** | |
| 080116 Temperature instability | 1 | 2 | 3 | 4 | 5 | NA |
| 080117 Hyperthermia | 1 | 2 | 3 | 4 | 5 | NA |
| 080118 Hypothermia | 1 | 2 | 3 | 4 | 5 | NA |
| 080119 Irregular respirations | 1 | 2 | 3 | 4 | 5 | NA |
| 080120 Tachypnea | 1 | 2 | 3 | 4 | 5 | NA |
| 080103 Restlessness | 1 | 2 | 3 | 4 | 5 | NA |
| 080104 Lethargy | 1 | 2 | 3 | 4 | 5 | NA |
| 080105 Skin color changes | 1 | 2 | 3 | 4 | 5 | NA |
| 080111 Dehydration | 1 | 2 | 3 | 4 | 5 | NA |
| 080112 Blood glucose instability | 1 | 2 | 3 | 4 | 5 | NA |
| 080114 Hyperbilirubinemia | 1 | 2 | 3 | 4 | 5 | NA |

*1st edition 1997; Revised 3rd edition (formerly Thermoregulation: Neonate)*

Outcome Content References:

Bliss-Holtz, J. (1992). Temperature relationships in cold-stressed infants. *Neonatal Network, 11*(2), 72.

Deacon, J., & O'Neill, P. (Eds.) (1999). *Core curriculum for neonatal intensive care nursing* (2nd ed.). Philadelphia: W.B. Saunders.

Greer, P. (1988). Head coverings for newborns under radiant warmers. *Journal of Obstetric, Gynecologic, and Neonatal Nursing, 17*(4), 265-270.

Keeling, E.B. (1992). Thermoregulation and axillary temperature measurements in neonates: A review of the literature. *Maternal-Child Nursing Journal, 20*(3-4), 124-140.

Konrad, C. (1980). *Nursing interventions to assess and control fever in infants and small children.* Unpublished master's thesis, The University of Iowa, Iowa City.

Mattson, S., & Smith, J.E. (Eds.) (2000). *Core curriculum for maternal-newborn nursing* (2nd ed.). Philadelphia: W.B. Saunders.

T

# Tissue Integrity: Skin & Mucous Membranes (1101)

*Domain-Physiologic Health (II)*

*Class-Tissue Integrity (L)*

*Scale(s)-Severely compromised to Not compromised (a) and Severe to None (n)*

*Care Recipient:*

*Data Source:*

**Definition:** Structural intactness and normal physiological function of skin and mucous membranes

OUTCOME TARGET RATING:    Maintain at _____    Increase to _____

| Tissue Integrity: Skin & Mucous Membranes Overall Rating | Severely compromised 1 | Substantially compromised 2 | Moderately compromised 3 | Mildly compromised 4 | Not compromised 5 | |
|---|---|---|---|---|---|---|
| **INDICATORS:** | | | | | | |
| 110101 Skin temperature | 1 | 2 | 3 | 4 | 5 | NA |
| 110102 Sensation | 1 | 2 | 3 | 4 | 5 | NA |
| 110103 Elasticity | 1 | 2 | 3 | 4 | 5 | NA |
| 110104 Hydration | 1 | 2 | 3 | 4 | 5 | NA |
| 110106 Perspiration | 1 | 2 | 3 | 4 | 5 | NA |
| 110108 Texture | 1 | 2 | 3 | 4 | 5 | NA |
| 110109 Thickness | 1 | 2 | 3 | 4 | 5 | NA |
| 110111 Tissue perfusion | 1 | 2 | 3 | 4 | 5 | NA |
| 110112 Hair growth on skin | 1 | 2 | 3 | 4 | 5 | NA |
| 110113 Skin intactness | 1 | 2 | 3 | 4 | 5 | NA |
| | **Severe** | **Substantial** | **Moderate** | **Mild** | **None** | |
| 110105 Abnormal pigmentation | 1 | 2 | 3 | 4 | 5 | NA |
| 110115 Skin lesions | 1 | 2 | 3 | 4 | 5 | NA |
| 110116 Mucous membrane lesions | 1 | 2 | 3 | 4 | 5 | NA |
| 110117 Scar tissue | 1 | 2 | 3 | 4 | 5 | NA |
| 110118 Skin cancers | 1 | 2 | 3 | 4 | 5 | NA |
| 110119 Skin flaking | 1 | 2 | 3 | 4 | 5 | NA |
| 110120 Skin scaling | 1 | 2 | 3 | 4 | 5 | NA |
| 110121 Erythema | 1 | 2 | 3 | 4 | 5 | NA |
| 110122 Blanching | 1 | 2 | 3 | 4 | 5 | NA |
| 110123 Necrosis | 1 | 2 | 3 | 4 | 5 | NA |
| 110124 Induration | 1 | 2 | 3 | 4 | 5 | NA |

*1st edition 1997; Revised 3rd edition*

**T**

Outcome Content References:

+Bergstrom, N., Braden, B.J., Laguzza, A., & Holman, V. (1987). The Braden Scale for predicting pressure sore risk. *Nursing Research, 36*(4), 205-210.

Cohen, I.K., Diegelmann, R.F., & Lindblad, W.L. (1992). *Wound healing: Biochemical and clinical aspects.* Philadelphia: W.B. Saunders.

Hardy, M.D. (2001). Impaired skin integrity: Dry skin. In M. Maas, K. Buckwalter, M. Hardy, T. Tripp-Reimer, M. Titler, & J. Specht (Eds.), *Nursing care of older adults: Diagnoses, outcomes & interventions* (pp. 137-144). St. Louis: Mosby.

Lazarus, G.S., Cooper, D.M., Knighton, D.R., Margohs, D.J., Pecoraro, R.E., Rodeheaver, G., & Robson, M.C. (1994). Definitions and guidelines for assessment of wounds and evaluation of healing. *Archives of Dermatology, 130*(4), 489-493.

Maklebust, J., & Sieggreen, M., (1996). *Pressure ulcers: Guidelines for prevention and nursing management.* (2nd ed.) Springhouse, PA: Springhouse.

Potter, P.A., & Perry, A.G. (2001). *Fundamentals of nursing* (5th ed.). St. Louis: Mosby.

Rijswijk, L., et al. (1993). Full-thickness leg ulcers: Patient demographics and predictors of healing. *The Journal of Family Practice, 36*(6), 625-632.

U.S. Department of Health and Human Services. (1992). *Pressure ulcers in adults: Prediction and prevention* (AHCPR Publication No. 92-0047). Rockville, MD: Public Health Service Agency for Health Care Policy and Research.

U.S. Department of Health and Human Services. (1994). *Treatment of pressure ulcers* (AHCPR Publication No. 95-0652). Rockville, MD: Public Health Service Agency for Health Care Policy and Research.

# *Tissue Perfusion: Abdominal Organs (0404)*

Domain-Physiologic Health (II)

Class-Cardiopulmonary (E)

Scale(s)-Severely compromised to Not compromised (a) and Severe to None (n)

Care Recipient:

Data Source:

**Definition:** Adequacy of blood flow through the small vessels of the abdominal viscera to maintain organ function

OUTCOME TARGET RATING:    Maintain at _____    Increase to _____

| Tissue Perfusion: Abdominal Organs Overall Rating | Severely compromised 1 | Substantially compromised 2 | Moderately compromised 3 | Mildly compromised 4 | Not compromised 5 | |
|---|---|---|---|---|---|---|
| INDICATORS: | | | | | | |
| 040424 Diastolic blood pressure | 1 | 2 | 3 | 4 | 5 | NA |
| 040425 Systolic blood pressure | 1 | 2 | 3 | 4 | 5 | NA |
| 040402 Urine output | 1 | 2 | 3 | 4 | 5 | NA |
| 040403 Electrolyte and acid/base balance | 1 | 2 | 3 | 4 | 5 | NA |
| 040404 Fluid balance | 1 | 2 | 3 | 4 | 5 | NA |
| 040405 Bowel sounds | 1 | 2 | 3 | 4 | 5 | NA |
| 040406 Appetite | 1 | 2 | 3 | 4 | 5 | NA |
| 040418 Urine specific gravity | 1 | 2 | 3 | 4 | 5 | NA |
| 040419 Blood urea nitrogen | 1 | 2 | 3 | 4 | 5 | NA |
| 040420 Plasma crea- tinine | 1 | 2 | 3 | 4 | 5 | NA |
| 040421 Liver function test findings | 1 | 2 | 3 | 4 | 5 | NA |
| 040422 Pancreatic enzymes | 1 | 2 | 3 | 4 | 5 | NA |

| | Severe | Substantial | Moderate | Mild | None | |
|---|---|---|---|---|---|---|
| 040407 Abnormal thirst | 1 | 2 | 3 | 4 | 5 | NA |
| 040408 Abdominal pain | 1 | 2 | 3 | 4 | 5 | NA |
| 040409 Nausea | 1 | 2 | 3 | 4 | 5 | NA |
| 040410 Vomiting | 1 | 2 | 3 | 4 | 5 | NA |
| 040411 Malabsorption deficiencies | 1 | 2 | 3 | 4 | 5 | NA |
| 040412 Chronic gastritis | 1 | 2 | 3 | 4 | 5 | NA |
| 040413 Abdominal distention | 1 | 2 | 3 | 4 | 5 | NA |
| 040414 Ascites | 1 | 2 | 3 | 4 | 5 | NA |
| 040415 Gastrointestinal varices | 1 | 2 | 3 | 4 | 5 | NA |
| 040416 Constipation | 1 | 2 | 3 | 4 | 5 | NA |
| 040417 Diarrhea | 1 | 2 | 3 | 4 | 5 | NA |

*1st edition 1997; Revised 3rd edition*

Outcome Content References:

Lewis, S.M., Collier, I.C., Heitkermper, M.M., & Dirksen, S.R. (2000). *Medical-surgical nursing: Assessment & management of clinical problems* (5th ed.). St. Louis: Mosby.

McCance, K.L., & Huether, S.E. (2002). *Pathophysiology: The biologic basis for disease in adults and children* (4th ed.). St. Louis: Mosby.

T

# Tissue Perfusion: Cardiac (0405)

Domain-Physiologic Health (II)

Class-Cardiopulmonary (E)

Scale(s)-Severely compromised to Not compromised (a) and Severe to None (n)

Care Recipient:

Data Source:

**Definition:** Adequacy of blood flow through the coronary vasculature to maintain heart function

OUTCOME TARGET RATING:    Maintain at _____    Increase to _____

| Tissue Perfusion: Cardiac Overall Rating | Severely compromised 1 | Substantially compromised 2 | Moderately compromised 3 | Mildly compromised 4 | Not compromised 5 | |
|---|---|---|---|---|---|---|
| INDICATORS: | | | | | | |
| 040501  Ejection fraction | 1 | 2 | 3 | 4 | 5 | NA |
| 040502  Pulmonary wedge pressure | 1 | 2 | 3 | 4 | 5 | NA |
| 040503  Cardiac index | 1 | 2 | 3 | 4 | 5 | NA |
| 040509  Electrocardiogram findings | 1 | 2 | 3 | 4 | 5 | NA |
| 040510  Cardiac enzymes | 1 | 2 | 3 | 4 | 5 | NA |
| 040511  Coronary angiogram findings | 1 | 2 | 3 | 4 | 5 | NA |
| 040512  Exercise stress test findings | 1 | 2 | 3 | 4 | 5 | NA |
| 040513  Thallium scan findings | 1 | 2 | 3 | 4 | 5 | NA |
| 040515  Apical heart rate | 1 | 2 | 3 | 4 | 5 | NA |
| 040516  Radial pulse rate | 1 | 2 | 3 | 4 | 5 | NA |
| 040517  Systolic blood pressure | 1 | 2 | 3 | 4 | 5 | NA |
| 040518  Diastolic blood pressure | 1 | 2 | 3 | 4 | 5 | NA |

| | Severe | Substantial | Moderate | Mild | None | |
|---|---|---|---|---|---|---|
| 040504  Angina | 1 | 2 | 3 | 4 | 5 | NA |
| 040505  Profuse diaphoresis | 1 | 2 | 3 | 4 | 5 | NA |
| 040506  Nausea | 1 | 2 | 3 | 4 | 5 | NA |
| 040507  Vomiting | 1 | 2 | 3 | 4 | 5 | NA |

*1st edition 1997; Revised 2nd edition 2000; Revised 3rd edition*

**T**

Outcome Content References:

Lewis, S.M., Collier, I.C., Heitkermper, M.M., & Dirksen, S.R. (2000). *Medical-surgical nursing: Assessment & management of clinical problems* (5th ed.). St. Louis: Mosby.

McCance, K.L., & Huether, S.E. (2002). *Pathophysiology: The biologic basis for disease in adults and children* (4th ed.). St. Louis: Mosby.

Wenger, N.K., Froelicher, E.S., Smith, L.K., et al. (1995). *Cardiac rehabilitation, Clinical practice guideline*, No. 17. (AHCPR Publication No. 96-0672). Rockville, MD: U.S. Department of Health and Human Services. Public Health Services, Agency for Health Care Policy and Research and the National Heart, Lung, and Blood Institute.

# *Tissue Perfusion: Cerebral (0406)*

Domain-Physiologic Health (II)

Class-Cardiopulmonary (E)

Scale(s)-Severely compromised to Not compromised (a) and Severe to None (n)

Care Recipient:

Data Source:

**Definition:** Adequacy of blood flow through the cerebral vasculature to maintain brain function

OUTCOME TARGET RATING:    Maintain at _____    Increase to _____

| Tissue Perfusion: Cerebral Overall Rating | Severely compromised 1 | Substantially compromised 2 | Moderately compromised 3 | Mildly compromised 4 | Not compromised 5 | |
|---|---|---|---|---|---|---|
| **INDICATORS:** | | | | | | |
| 040601 Neurological function | 1 | 2 | 3 | 4 | 5 | NA |
| 040602 Intracranial pressure | 1 | 2 | 3 | 4 | 5 | NA |
| 040613 Systolic blood pressure | 1 | 2 | 3 | 4 | 5 | NA |
| 040614 Diastolic blood pressure | 1 | 2 | 3 | 4 | 5 | NA |
| 040615 Cerebral angiogram findings | 1 | 2 | 3 | 4 | 5 | NA |
| | Severe | Substantial | Moderate | Mild | None | |
| 040603 Headache | 1 | 2 | 3 | 4 | 5 | NA |
| 040604 Carotid bruit | 1 | 2 | 3 | 4 | 5 | NA |
| 040605 Restlessness | 1 | 2 | 3 | 4 | 5 | NA |
| 040606 Listlessness | 1 | 2 | 3 | 4 | 5 | NA |
| 040607 Unexplained anxiety | 1 | 2 | 3 | 4 | 5 | NA |
| 040608 Agitation | 1 | 2 | 3 | 4 | 5 | NA |
| 040609 Vomiting | 1 | 2 | 3 | 4 | 5 | NA |
| 040610 Hiccoughs | 1 | 2 | 3 | 4 | 5 | NA |
| 040611 Syncope | 1 | 2 | 3 | 4 | 5 | NA |
| 040616 Fever | 1 | 2 | 3 | 4 | 5 | NA |

*1st edition 1997; Revised 3rd edition*

Outcome Content References:

Lewis, S.M., Collier, I.C., Heitkermper, M.M., & Dirksen, S.R. (2000). *Medical-surgical nursing: Assessment & management of clinical problems* (5th ed.). St. Louis: Mosby.

McCance, K.L., & Huether, S.E. (2002). *Pathophysiology: The biologic basis for disease in adults and children* (4th ed.). St. Louis: Mosby.

T

# Tissue Perfusion: Peripheral (0407)

Domain-Physiologic Health (II)                                  Care Recipient:

Class-Cardiopulmonary (E)                                       Data Source:

Scale(s)-Severely compromised to Not compromised (a) and Severe to None (n)

**Definition:** Adequacy of blood flow through the small vessels of the extremities to maintain tissue function

OUTCOME TARGET RATING:    Maintain at _____    Increase to _____

| Tissue Perfusion: Peripheral Overall Rating | Severely compromised 1 | Substantially compromised 2 | Moderately compromised 3 | Mildly compromised 4 | Not compromised 5 | |
|---|---|---|---|---|---|---|
| **INDICATORS:** | | | | | | |
| 040715 | Capillary refill fingers | 1 | 2 | 3 | 4 | 5 | NA |
| 040716 | Capillary refill toes | 1 | 2 | 3 | 4 | 5 | NA |
| 040706 | Sensation | 1 | 2 | 3 | 4 | 5 | NA |
| 040707 | Skin color | 1 | 2 | 3 | 4 | 5 | NA |
| 040708 | Muscle function | 1 | 2 | 3 | 4 | 5 | NA |
| 040709 | Skin integrity | 1 | 2 | 3 | 4 | 5 | NA |
| 040710 | Extremity skin temperature | 1 | 2 | 3 | 4 | 5 | NA |
| 040717 | Carotid pulse rate (right) | 1 | 2 | 3 | 4 | 5 | NA |
| 040718 | Carotid pulse rate (left) | 1 | 2 | 3 | 4 | 5 | NA |
| 040719 | Brachial pulse rate (right) | 1 | 2 | 3 | 4 | 5 | NA |
| 040720 | Brachial pulse rate (left) | 1 | 2 | 3 | 4 | 5 | NA |
| 040721 | Radial pulse rate (right) | 1 | 2 | 3 | 4 | 5 | NA |
| 040722 | Radial pulse rate (left) | 1 | 2 | 3 | 4 | 5 | NA |
| 040723 | Femoral pulse rate (right) | 1 | 2 | 3 | 4 | 5 | NA |
| 040724 | Femoral pulse rate (left) | 1 | 2 | 3 | 4 | 5 | NA |
| 040725 | Pedal pulse rate (right) | 1 | 2 | 3 | 4 | 5 | NA |
| 040726 | Pedal pulse rate (left) | 1 | 2 | 3 | 4 | 5 | NA |
| 040727 | Systolic blood pressure | 1 | 2 | 3 | 4 | 5 | NA |
| 040728 | Diastolic blood pressure | 1 | 2 | 3 | 4 | 5 | NA |

| | Severe | Substantial | Moderate | Mild | None | |
|---|---|---|---|---|---|---|
| 040711 | Extremity bruits | 1 | 2 | 3 | 4 | 5 | NA |
| 040712 | Peripheral edema | 1 | 2 | 3 | 4 | 5 | NA |
| 040713 | Localized extremity pain | 1 | 2 | 3 | 4 | 5 | NA |
| 040729 | Necrosis | 1 | 2 | 3 | 4 | 5 | NA |

*1st edition 1997; Revised 3rd edition*

Outcome Content References:

Cohen, I.K., Diegelmann, R.F., & Lindblad, W.L. (1992). *Wound healing: Biochemical and clinical aspects*. Philadelphia: W.B. Saunders.

Lazarus, G.S., Cooper, D.M., Knighton, D.R., Margohs, D.J., Pecoraro, R.E., Rodeheaver, G., & Robson, M.C. (1994). Definitions and guidelines for assessment of wounds and evaluation of healing. *Archives of Dermatology, 130*(4), 489-493.

Maklebust, J., & Sieggreen, M. (1996). *Pressure ulcers: Guidelines for prevention and nursing management* (2nd ed.). Springhouse, PA: Springhouse.

Potter, P.A., & Perry, A.G. (2001). *Fundamentals of nursing* (5th ed.). St. Louis: Mosby.

Rijswijk, L., et al. (1993). Full-thickness leg ulcers: Patient demographics and predictors of healing. *The Journal of Family Practice, 36*(6), 625-632.

T

# Tissue Perfusion: Pulmonary (0408)

*Domain-Physiologic Health (II)*

*Class-Cardiopulmonary (E)*

*Scale(s)-Severely compromised to Not compromised (a) and Severe to None (n)*

*Care Recipient:*

*Data Source:*

**Definition:** Adequacy of blood flow through pulmonary vasculature to perfuse alveoli/capillary unit

OUTCOME TARGET RATING:    Maintain at _____    Increase to _____

| Tissue Perfusion: Pulmonary Overall Rating | Severely compromised 1 | Substantially compromised 2 | Moderately compromised 3 | Mildly compromised 4 | Not compromised 5 | |
|---|---|---|---|---|---|---|
| **INDICATORS:** | | | | | | |
| 040810 Ventilation-perfusion scan | 1 | 2 | 3 | 4 | 5 | NA |
| 040811 Pulmonary artery pressure (PAP) | 1 | 2 | 3 | 4 | 5 | NA |
| 040814 Respiratory function | 1 | 2 | 3 | 4 | 5 | NA |
| 040815 Respiratory rate | 1 | 2 | 3 | 4 | 5 | NA |
| 040816 Systolic blood pressure | 1 | 2 | 3 | 4 | 5 | NA |
| 040817 Diastolic blood pressure | 1 | 2 | 3 | 4 | 5 | NA |
| 040818 $PaO_2$* | 1 | 2 | 3 | 4 | 5 | NA |
| 040819 $PaCO_2$* | 1 | 2 | 3 | 4 | 5 | NA |
| 040820 Arterial pH | 1 | 2 | 3 | 4 | 5 | NA |
| 040821 Oxygen saturation | 1 | 2 | 3 | 4 | 5 | NA |
| | **Severe** | **Substantial** | **Moderate** | **Mild** | **None** | |
| 040805 Chest pain | 1 | 2 | 3 | 4 | 5 | NA |
| 040806 Pleural friction rub | 1 | 2 | 3 | 4 | 5 | NA |
| 040807 Hemoptysis | 1 | 2 | 3 | 4 | 5 | NA |
| 040808 Unexplained anxiety | 1 | 2 | 3 | 4 | 5 | NA |

*$PaO_2$= Partial pressure of oxygen in arterial blood; $PaCO_2$= partial pressure of carbon dioxide in arterial blood.

*1st edition 1997; Revised 3rd edition*

Outcome Content References:

Lewis, S.M., Collier, I.C., Heitkermper, M.M., & Dirksen, S.R. (2000). *Medical-surgical nursing: Assessment & management of clinical problems* (5th ed.). St. Louis: Mosby.

McCance, K.L., & Huether, S.E. (2002). *Pathophysiology: The biologic basis for disease in adults and children* (4th ed.). St. Louis: Mosby.

T

# *Transfer Performance (0210)*

*Domain-Functional Health (I)*

*Class-Mobility (C)*

*Scale(s)-Severely compromised to Not compromised (a)*

*Care Recipient:*

*Data Source:*

**Definition:** Ability to change body location independently with or without assistive device

OUTCOME TARGET RATING:  Maintain at _____  Increase to _____

| Transfer Performance Overall Rating | Severely compromised 1 | Substantially compromised 2 | Moderately compromised 3 | Mildly compromised 4 | Not compromised 5 | |
|---|---|---|---|---|---|---|

INDICATORS:

| | | | | | | | |
|---|---|---|---|---|---|---|---|
| 021001 | Transfers from bed to chair | 1 | 2 | 3 | 4 | 5 | NA |
| 021002 | Transfers from chair to bed | 1 | 2 | 3 | 4 | 5 | NA |
| 021003 | Transfers from chair to chair | 1 | 2 | 3 | 4 | 5 | NA |
| 021004 | Transfers from wheelchair to vehicle | 1 | 2 | 3 | 4 | 5 | NA |
| 021005 | Transfers from vehicle to wheelchair | 1 | 2 | 3 | 4 | 5 | NA |
| 021007 | Transfers from wheelchair to toilet | 1 | 2 | 3 | 4 | 5 | NA |
| 021008 | Transfers from toilet to wheelchair | 1 | 2 | 3 | 4 | 5 | NA |

*1st edition 1997; Revised 3rd edition*

Outcome Content References:

+*Guide for the Uniform Data Set for Medical Rehabilitation* (including the FIM™ instrument), (version 5.1) (1997). Buffalo, NY: University at Buffalo.

Kane, R.L., & Kane, R.A. (2000). *Assessing older persons: Measures, meaning, and practical applications.* New York: Oxford University Press.

Mikulic, M.A., Griffith, E.R., & Jebsen, R.H. (1976). Clinical application of a standardized mobility test. *Archives of Physical Medicine and Rehabilitation, 57*(3), 143-146.

T

# Treatment Behavior: Illness or Injury (1609)

Domain-Health Knowledge & Behavior (IV)

Class-Health Behavior (Q)

Scale-Never demonstrated to Consistently demonstrated (m)

Care Recipient:

Data Source:

**Definition:** Personal actions to palliate or eliminate pathology

OUTCOME TARGET RATING:    Maintain at _____    Increase to _____

| Treatment Behavior: Illness Or Injury Overall Rating | Never demonstrated 1 | Rarely demonstrated 2 | Sometimes demonstrated 3 | Often demonstrated 4 | Consistently demonstrated 5 | |
|---|---|---|---|---|---|---|
| INDICATORS: | | | | | | |
| 160901 Follows recommended precautions | 1 | 2 | 3 | 4 | 5 | NA |
| 160902 Follows recommended treatment regimen | 1 | 2 | 3 | 4 | 5 | NA |
| 160903 Follows prescribed treatments | 1 | 2 | 3 | 4 | 5 | NA |
| 160904 Follows prescribed activities | 1 | 2 | 3 | 4 | 5 | NA |
| 160905 Follows medication regimen | 1 | 2 | 3 | 4 | 5 | NA |
| 160906 Avoids behaviors that potentiate pathology | 1 | 2 | 3 | 4 | 5 | NA |
| 160907 Performs self-care consistent with ability | 1 | 2 | 3 | 4 | 5 | NA |
| 160908 Monitors treatment effects | 1 | 2 | 3 | 4 | 5 | NA |
| 160909 Monitors treatment side effects | 1 | 2 | 3 | 4 | 5 | NA |
| 160910 Monitors disease side effects | 1 | 2 | 3 | 4 | 5 | NA |
| 160911 Monitors changes in disease status | 1 | 2 | 3 | 4 | 5 | NA |
| 160912 Uses treatment devices correctly | 1 | 2 | 3 | 4 | 5 | NA |
| 160913 Alters role functions to meet treatment requirements | 1 | 2 | 3 | 4 | 5 | NA |
| 160914 Balances treatment, exercise, work, leisure, rest, and nutrition | 1 | 2 | 3 | 4 | 5 | NA |
| 160915 Seeks advice from health care professional as needed | 1 | 2 | 3 | 4 | 5 | NA |
| 160916 Schedules appoint- ments with health care professional as needed | 1 | 2 | 3 | 4 | 5 | NA |

*1st edition 1997; Revised 3rd edition*

Outcome Content References:

Conn, V., Taylor, S., & Casey, B. (1992). Cardiac rehabilitation program participation and outcomes after myocardial infarction. *Rehabilitation Nursing, 17*(2), 58-62.

Wenger, N.K., Froelicher, E.S., Smith, L.K., et al. (1995). *Cardiac rehabilitation, Clinical practice guideline*, No. 17. (AHCPR Publication No. 96-0672). Rockville, MD: U.S. Department of Health and Human Services. Public Health Services, Agency for Health Care Policy and Research and the National Heart, Lung, and Blood Institute.

Woods, N. (1989). Conceptualizations of self-care: Toward health-oriented models. *Advances in Nursing Science, 12*(1), 1-13.

T

# Urinary Continence (0502)

Domain-Physiologic Health (II)                                       Care Recipient:

Class-Elimination (F)                                                Data Source:

Scale(s)-Never demonstrated to Consistently demonstrated (m) and Consistently demonstrated to Never demonstrated (t)

**Definition:** Control of elimination of urine from the bladder

OUTCOME TARGET RATING:    Maintain at _____    Increase to _____

| Urinary Continence Overall Rating | Never demonstrated 1 | Rarely demonstrated 2 | Sometimes demonstrated 3 | Often demonstrated 4 | Consistently demonstrated 5 | |
|---|---|---|---|---|---|---|
| INDICATORS: | | | | | | |
| 050201 Recognizes urge to void | 1 | 2 | 3 | 4 | 5 | NA |
| 050202 Maintains predictable pattern of voiding | 1 | 2 | 3 | 4 | 5 | NA |
| 050203 Responds to urge in timely manner | 1 | 2 | 3 | 4 | 5 | NA |
| 050204 Voids in appropriate receptacle | 1 | 2 | 3 | 4 | 5 | NA |
| 050205 Gets to toilet between urge and passage of urine | 1 | 2 | 3 | 4 | 5 | NA |
| 050218 Maintains barrier-free environment for independent toileting | 1 | 2 | 3 | 4 | 5 | NA |
| 050206 Voids >150 cc each time | 1 | 2 | 3 | 4 | 5 | NA |
| 050208 Starts and stops stream | 1 | 2 | 3 | 4 | 5 | NA |
| 050209 Empties bladder completely | 1 | 2 | 3 | 4 | 5 | NA |
| 050215 Ingests adequate amount of fluid | 1 | 2 | 3 | 4 | 5 | NA |
| 050216 Manages clothing independently | 1 | 2 | 3 | 4 | 5 | NA |
| 050217 Toilets independently | 1 | 2 | 3 | 4 | 5 | NA |
| 050219 Identifies medications that interfere with urinary control | 1 | 2 | 3 | 4 | 5 | NA |

U

| Urinary Continence—cont'd | | Consistently demonstrated | Often demonstrated | Sometimes demonstrated | Rarely demonstrated | Never demonstrated | |
|---|---|---|---|---|---|---|---|
| 050207 | Urine leakage between voidings | 1 | 2 | 3 | 4 | 5 | NA |
| 050210 | Post void residual >100-200 cc | 1 | 2 | 3 | 4 | 5 | NA |
| 050211 | Urine leakage with increased abdominal pressure (e.g., sneezing, laughing, lifting) | 1 | 2 | 3 | 4 | 5 | NA |
| 050212 | Wets underclothing during day | 1 | 2 | 3 | 4 | 5 | NA |
| 050213 | Wets underclothing or bedding during night | 1 | 2 | 3 | 4 | 5 | NA |
| 050214 | Urinary tract infection (<100,000 white blood count) | 1 | 2 | 3 | 4 | 5 | NA |

*1st edition 1997; Revised 3rd edition*

## Outcome Content References:

+Morris, J.N., Hawes, C., et al. (1990). Designing the national resident assessment instrument for nursing homes. *Gerontologist* 30(3), 293-307.

+O'Donnell, P.D., & Calandro, V.J. (1991). Incontinence Management Scale for elderly inpatient men. *Urology, 37*(3), 220-223.

Palmer, M.H., McCormick, K.A., Langford, A., Langlais, J., & Alvaran, M. (1992). Continence outcomes: Documentation on medical records in the nursing home environment. *Journal of Nursing Care Quality, 6*(3), 36-43.

Specht, J.P., & Maas, M.L. (2001). Urinary incontinence: Functional, iatrogenic, overflow, reflex, stress, total, and urge. In M. Maas, K. Buckwalter, M. Hardy, T. Tripp-Reimer, M. Titler, & J. Specht (Eds.), *Nursing care of older adults: Diagnoses, outcomes & interventions* (pp. 252-278). St. Louis: Mosby.

Urinary Incontinence Guideline Panel. (1992). *Urinary incontinence in adults: Clinical practice guideline* (AHCPR Publication No. 92-0038). Rockville, MD: Agency for Health Care Policy and Research, Public Health Service, U.S. Department of Health and Human Services.

U

# *Urinary Elimination (0503)*

*Domain-Physiologic Health (II)*                    *Care Recipient:*

*Class-Elimination (F)*                              *Data Source:*

*Scale(s)-Severely compromised to Not compromised (a) and Severe to None (n)*

## *Definition:* Collection and discharge of urine

OUTCOME TARGET RATING:     Maintain at _____   Increase to _____

| Urinary Elimination Overall Rating | Severely compromised 1 | Substantially compromised 2 | Moderately compromised 3 | Mildly compromised 4 | Not compromised 5 | |
|---|---|---|---|---|---|---|
| **INDICATORS:** | | | | | | |
| 050301 Elimination pattern | 1 | 2 | 3 | 4 | 5 | NA |
| 050302 Urine odor | 1 | 2 | 3 | 4 | 5 | NA |
| 050303 Urine amount | 1 | 2 | 3 | 4 | 5 | NA |
| 050304 Urine color | 1 | 2 | 3 | 4 | 5 | NA |
| 050306 Urine clarity | 1 | 2 | 3 | 4 | 5 | NA |
| 050307 Adequate fluid intake | 1 | 2 | 3 | 4 | 5 | NA |
| 050313 Empties bladder completely | 1 | 2 | 3 | 4 | 5 | NA |
| 050314 Recognition of urge | 1 | 2 | 3 | 4 | 5 | NA |

| | Severe | Substantial | Moderate | Mild | None | |
|---|---|---|---|---|---|---|
| 050305 Visible urine particles | 1 | 2 | 3 | 4 | 5 | NA |
| 050329 Visible blood in urine | 1 | 2 | 3 | 4 | 5 | NA |
| 050309 Pain with urination | 1 | 2 | 3 | 4 | 5 | NA |
| 050330 Burning with urination | | | | | | |
| 050310 Hesitancy with urination | 1 | 2 | 3 | 4 | 5 | NA |
| 050331 Urinary frequency | 1 | 2 | 3 | 4 | 5 | NA |
| 050311 Urgency with urination | 1 | 2 | 3 | 4 | 5 | NA |
| 050332 Urinary retention | 1 | 2 | 3 | 4 | 5 | NA |
| 050333 Nocturia | 1 | 2 | 3 | 4 | 5 | NA |
| 050312 Urinary incontinence | 1 | 2 | 3 | 4 | 5 | NA |
| 050334 Stress incontinence | 1 | 2 | 3 | 4 | 5 | NA |
| 050335 Urge incontinence | 1 | 2 | 3 | 4 | 5 | NA |
| 050336 Functional incontinence | 1 | 2 | 3 | 4 | 5 | NA |

*1st edition 1997; Revised 3rd edition*

Outcome Content References:

Brundage, D.J., & Linton, A.D. (1997). Age related changes in the genitourinary system. In M.A. Matteson, E.S. McConnell, & A.D. Linton (Eds.), *Gerontological nursing: Concepts in practice* (2nd ed.). Philadelphia, W.B. Saunders.

Fantl J.A., Newman, D.K., Colling, J., et al. (1996). *Urinary incontinence in adults: Acute and chronic management. Clinical practice guideline*, No. 2, 1996 update. (AHCPR Publication No. 96-0682). Rockville, MD: U.S. Department of Health and Human Services. Public Health Service, Agency for Health Care and Policy Research.

McConnell, J.D., Barry, M.J., Brusketwitz, R.C., et al. (1994). *Benign prostatic hyperplasia: Diagnosis and treatment. Clinical practice guideline*, No. 8. (AHCPR Publication No. 94-0582). Rockville, MD: Agency for Health Care Policy and Research, Public Health Service, U.S. Department of Health and Human Services.

Morton, P.G. (1989). *Health assessment in nursing*. Springhouse, PA: Springhouse.

U

Palmer, M.H., McCormick, K.A., Langford, A., Langlais, J., & Alvaran, M. (1992). Continence outcomes: Documentation on medical records in the nursing home environment. *Journal of Nursing Care Quality, 6*(3), 36-43.

Potter, P.A., & Perry, A.G. (2001). *Fundamentals of nursing* (5th ed.). St. Louis: Mosby.

Urinary Incontinence Guideline Panel. (1992). *Urinary incontinence in adults: clinical practice guidelines* (AHCPR Publication No. 92-0038). Rockville, MD: Agency for Health Care Policy and Research, Public Health Service, U.S. Department of Health and Human Services.

**U**

# *Vision Compensation Behavior (1611)*

*Domain-Health & Knowledge Behavior (IV)*

*Class-Health Behavior (Q)*

*Scale(s)-Never demonstrated to Consistently demonstrated (m)*

Care Recipient:

Data Source:

**Definition:** Personal actions to compensate for visual impairment

OUTCOME TARGET RATING:     Maintain at _____     Increase to _____

| Vision Compensation Behavior Overall Rating | Never demonstrated 1 | Rarely demonstrated 2 | Sometimes demonstrated 3 | Often demonstrated 4 | Consistently demonstrated 5 | |
|---|---|---|---|---|---|---|
| **INDICATORS:** | | | | | | |
| 161101 Monitors symptoms of vision deterioration | 1 | 2 | 3 | 4 | 5 | NA |
| 161102 Positions self to advantage vision | 1 | 2 | 3 | 4 | 5 | NA |
| 161103 Reminds others to use techniques that advantage vision | 1 | 2 | 3 | 4 | 5 | NA |
| 161104 Uses adequate lighting for activity being performed | 1 | 2 | 3 | 4 | 5 | NA |
| 161105 Wears eyeglasses correctly | 1 | 2 | 3 | 4 | 5 | NA |
| 161106 Wears contact lenses correctly | 1 | 2 | 3 | 4 | 5 | NA |
| 161107 Cares for eyewear correctly | 1 | 2 | 3 | 4 | 5 | NA |
| 161108 Uses vision assistive devices | 1 | 2 | 3 | 4 | 5 | NA |
| 161109 Uses computer assistive devices | 1 | 2 | 3 | 4 | 5 | NA |
| 161113 Uses animal assistive devices | 1 | 2 | 3 | 4 | 5 | NA |
| 161110 Uses support services for low-vision | 1 | 2 | 3 | 4 | 5 | NA |
| 161111 Uses braille | 1 | 2 | 3 | 4 | 5 | NA |

*2nd edition 2000; Revised 3rd edition*

Outcome Content References:

Burrell, L.O. (Ed.). (1992). *Adult nursing in hospital and community settings.* Norwalk, CT: Appleton & Lange.

Cataract Management Guideline Panel. (1993). *Cataracts in adults: Management of functional impairment. Clinical practice guideline,* No. 4 (AHCPR Publication No. 93-0542). Rockville, MD: U.S. Department of Health and Human Services. Public Health Services, Agency for Health Care Policy and Research.

Phipps, W.J., Monahan, F.D., Sands J.K., Marek, J., & Neighbors, M. (Eds.). (2003). *Medical-surgical nursing: Concepts and clinical practice* (7th ed). St. Louis: Mosby.

Smeltzer, S.C., & Bare, B.G. (Eds.). (2003). *Brunner and Suddarth's textbook of medical-surgical nursing* (10th ed.). Philadelphia: Lippincott, Williams, & Wilkins.

V

# Vital Signs (0802)

*Domain-Physiologic Health (II)*

*Class-Metabolic Regulation (I)*

*Scale(s)-Severe deviation from normal range to No deviation from normal range (b)*

*Care Recipient:*

*Data Source:*

**Definition:** Extent to which temperature, pulse, respiration, and blood pressure are within normal range

OUTCOME TARGET RATING:     Maintain at _____     Increase to _____

| Vital Signs Overall Rating | Severe deviation from normal range 1 | Substantial deviation from normal range 2 | Moderate deviation from normal range 3 | Mild deviation from normal range 4 | No deviation from normal range 5 | |
|---|---|---|---|---|---|---|
| INDICATORS: | | | | | | |
| 080201  Body temperature | 1 | 2 | 3 | 4 | 5 | NA |
| 080202  Apical heart rate | 1 | 2 | 3 | 4 | 5 | NA |
| 080208  Apical heart rhythm | 1 | 2 | 3 | 4 | 5 | NA |
| 080203  Radial pulse rate | 1 | 2 | 3 | 4 | 5 | NA |
| 080204  Respiratory rate | 1 | 2 | 3 | 4 | 5 | NA |
| 080205  Systolic blood pressure | 1 | 2 | 3 | 4 | 5 | NA |
| 080206  Diastolic blood pressure | 1 | 2 | 3 | 4 | 5 | NA |
| 080209  Pulse pressure | 1 | 2 | 3 | 4 | 5 | NA |

*1st edition 1997; Revised 3rd edition (formerly Vital Signs Status)*

Outcome Content References:

Caruso, C., Hadley, B., Shukla, R., & Frame, P. (1992). Cooling effects and comfort of four cooling blanket temperatures in humans with fever. *Nursing Research, 41*(2), 68-72.

Finke, C. (1991). Measurement of the thermoregulatory response: A review. *Focus on Critical Care, 18*(5), 408-412.

Summers, S., Dudgeon, N., Byram, K., & Zingsheim, K. (1990). The effects of two warming methods on core and surface temperatures, hemoglobin oxygen saturation, blood pressure, and perceived comfort of hypothermic postanesthesia patients. *Journal of Post Anesthesia Nursing, 5*(5), 354-364.

Thomas, S.A., Liehr, P., DeKeyser, F., Frazier, L., & Friedmann, E. (2002). A review of nursing research on blood pressure. *Journal of Nursing Scholarship, 34*(4), 313-321.

V

# Weight: Body Mass (1006)

*Domain-Physiologic Health (II)*

*Class-Metabolic Regulation (I)*

*Scale(s)-Severe deviation from normal range to No deviation from normal range (b)*

*Care Recipient:*

*Data Source:*

> **Definition**: Extent to which body weight, muscle, and fat are congruent to height, frame, gender and age

OUTCOME TARGET RATING:     Maintain at _____     Increase to _____

| Weight: Body Mass Overall Rating | Severe deviation from normal range 1 | Substantial deviation from normal range 2 | Moderate deviation from normal range 3 | Mild deviation from normal range 4 | No deviation from normal range 5 | |
|---|---|---|---|---|---|---|
| **INDICATORS:** | | | | | | |
| 100601 Weight | 1 | 2 | 3 | 4 | 5 | NA |
| 100602 Triceps skinfold thickness | 1 | 2 | 3 | 4 | 5 | NA |
| 100603 Subscapular skinfold thickness | 1 | 2 | 3 | 4 | 5 | NA |
| 100604 Waist/hip circumference ratio (women) | 1 | 2 | 3 | 4 | 5 | NA |
| 100605 Neck/waist circumference ratio (men) | 1 | 2 | 3 | 4 | 5 | NA |
| 100606 Body fat percentage | 1 | 2 | 3 | 4 | 5 | NA |
| 100607 Head circumference percentile (child) | 1 | 2 | 3 | 4 | 5 | NA |
| 100608 Height percentile (child) | 1 | 2 | 3 | 4 | 5 | NA |
| 100609 Weight percentile (child) | 1 | 2 | 3 | 4 | 5 | NA |

*1st edition 1997; Revised 3rd edition (formerly Nutritional Status: Body Mass)*

Outcome Content References:

Collinsworth, R., & Boyle, K. (1989). Nutritional assessment of the elderly. *Journal of Gerontological Nursing, 15*(12), 17-21.

Curtas, S., Chapman, G., & Meguid, M. (1989). Evaluation of nutritional status. *Nursing Clinics of North America, 24*(2), 301-313.

Folsom, A.R., Kaye, S.A., Sellers, T.A., Hang, C.P., Cerhan, J.R., Potter, J.D., & Prineas, R.J. (1993). Body fat distribution and five year risk of death in older women. *Journal of the American Medical Association, 269*(4), 483-487.

Gianino, S., & St. John, R.E. (1993). Nutritional assessment of the patient in the intensive care unit. *Critical Care Nursing Clinics of North America, 5*(1), 1-16.

**W**

# *Weight Control (1612)*

*Domain-Health Knowledge & Behavior (IV)*

*Class-Health Behavior (Q)*

*Scale(s)-Never demonstrated to Consistently demonstrated (m)*

*Care Recipient:*

*Data Source:*

**Definition:** Personal actions to achieve and maintain optimum body weight

OUTCOME TARGET RATING:    Maintain at _____    Increase to _____

| Weight Control Overall Rating | Never demonstrated 1 | Rarely demonstrated 2 | Sometimes demonstrated 3 | Often demonstrated 4 | Consistently demonstrated 5 | |
|---|---|---|---|---|---|---|
| INDICATORS: | | | | | | |
| 161201 Monitors body weight | 1 | 2 | 3 | 4 | 5 | NA |
| 161202 Maintains optimal daily caloric intake | 1 | 2 | 3 | 4 | 5 | NA |
| 161203 Balances exercise with caloric intake | 1 | 2 | 3 | 4 | 5 | NA |
| 161204 Selects nutritious meals and snacks | 1 | 2 | 3 | 4 | 5 | NA |
| 161205 Uses nutrient supplements as needed | 1 | 2 | 3 | 4 | 5 | NA |
| 161206 Eats in response to hunger | 1 | 2 | 3 | 4 | 5 | NA |
| 161207 Maintains recommended eating pattern | 1 | 2 | 3 | 4 | 5 | NA |
| 161208 Retains ingested foods | 1 | 2 | 3 | 4 | 5 | NA |
| 161209 Maintains fluid balance | 1 | 2 | 3 | 4 | 5 | NA |
| 161210 Recognizes signs and symptoms of electrolyte imbalance | 1 | 2 | 3 | 4 | 5 | NA |
| 161211 Seeks treatment for electrolyte imbalance | 1 | 2 | 3 | 4 | 5 | NA |
| 161212 Seeks professional assistance as needed | 1 | 2 | 3 | 4 | 5 | NA |
| 161213 Uses personal support systems to help change dietary pattern | 1 | 2 | 3 | 4 | 5 | NA |
| 161214 Identifies social situations that affect food intake | 1 | 2 | 3 | 4 | 5 | NA |
| 161215 Identifies emotional states that affect food intake | 1 | 2 | 3 | 4 | 5 | NA |
| 161216 Plans strategies for situations that affect food intake | 1 | 2 | 3 | 4 | 5 | NA |

W

*Continued*

| Weight Control—cont'd | | Never demonstrated | Rarely demonstrated | Sometimes demonstrated | Often demonstrated | Consistently demonstrated | |
|---|---|---|---|---|---|---|---|
| 161217 | Controls preoccupation with food | 1 | 2 | 3 | 4 | 5 | NA |
| 161218 | Controls preoccupation with weight | 1 | 2 | 3 | 4 | 5 | NA |
| 161219 | Expresses realistic body image | 1 | 2 | 3 | 4 | 5 | NA |
| 161220 | Demonstrates progress toward target weight | 1 | 2 | 3 | 4 | 5 | NA |
| 161221 | Achieves optimum weight | 1 | 2 | 3 | 4 | 5 | NA |
| 161222 | Maintains optimum weight | 1 | 2 | 3 | 4 | 5 | NA |

*2nd edition 2000; Revised 3rd edition*

Outcome Content References:

American Psychiatric Association. (1993). Practice guideline for eating disorders. *American Journal of Psychiatry, 150*(2), 212-223.

Bruce, B., & Wilfley, D. (1996). Binge eating among the overweight population: A serious and prevalent problem. *Journal of the American Dietetic Association, 96*(1), 58-62.

Chang, B.L. Uman, G.C., Linn, L.S., Ware, J.E.,& Kane, R.L. (1985). Adherence to healthcare regimens among elderly women. *Nursing Research, 34*(1) 27-31.

Curtas, S., Chapman, G., & Meguid, M. (1989). Evaluation of nutritional status. *Nursing Clinics of North America, 24*(2), 301-313.

Farrow, J. (1992). The adolescent male with an eating disorder. *Pediatric Annals, 21*(11), 769-774.

Fisher, M., et.al. (1995). Eating disorders in adolescents: A background paper. *Journal of Adolescent Health, 16*(6), 420-437.

Halmi, K. (1994). A multimodal model for understanding and treating eating disorders. *Journal of Women's Health, 3*(6), 487-493.

Hawks, S.R., & Richins, P. (1994). Toward a new paradigm for the management of obesity. *Journal of Health Education, 25*(3), 147-153.

Wilson, P., et al. (1991). Eating strategies used by persons with head and neck cancer during and after radiotherapy. *Cancer Nursing, 14*(2), 98-104.

Yates, A. (1992). Biologic considerations in the etiology of eating disorders. *Pediatric Annals, 21*(11), 739-744.

W

# *Will to Live (1206)*

*Domain-Psychosocial Health (III)*         *Care Recipient:*

*Class-Psychological Well-Being (M)*         *Data Source:*

*Scale(s)-Severely compromised to Not compromised (a) and Severe to None (n)*

**Definition:** Desire, determination, and effort to survive

OUTCOME TARGET RATING:     Maintain at _____     Increase to _____

| Will To Live Overall Rating | Severely compromised 1 | Substantially compromised 2 | Moderately compromised 3 | Mildly compromised 4 | Not compromised 5 | |
|---|---|---|---|---|---|---|

**INDICATORS:**

| | | Severely compromised 1 | Substantially compromised 2 | Moderately compromised 3 | Mildly compromised 4 | Not compromised 5 | |
|---|---|---|---|---|---|---|---|
| 120601 | Expression of determination to live | 1 | 2 | 3 | 4 | 5 | NA |
| 120602 | Expression of hope | 1 | 2 | 3 | 4 | 5 | NA |
| 120603 | Expression of optimism | 1 | 2 | 3 | 4 | 5 | NA |
| 120604 | Expression of sense of control | 1 | 2 | 3 | 4 | 5 | NA |
| 120605 | Expression of feelings | 1 | 2 | 3 | 4 | 5 | NA |
| 120606 | Inquires about one's illness/ treatment | 1 | 2 | 3 | 4 | 5 | NA |
| 120607 | Seeks information about one's illness/ treatment | 1 | 2 | 3 | 4 | 5 | NA |
| 120608 | Use of strategies to compensate for problems associated with disease | 1 | 2 | 3 | 4 | 5 | NA |
| 120612 | Use of treatments to compensate for problems associated with disease | 1 | 2 | 3 | 4 | 5 | NA |
| 120613 | Use of treatments to lengthen life | 1 | 2 | 3 | 4 | 5 | NA |
| 120609 | Use of strategies to enhance health | 1 | 2 | 3 | 4 | 5 | NA |
| 120610 | Use of strategies to lengthen life | 1 | 2 | 3 | 4 | 5 | NA |

| | | Severe | Substantial | Moderate | Mild | None | |
|---|---|---|---|---|---|---|---|
| 120614 | Depression | 1 | 2 | 3 | 4 | 5 | NA |
| 120615 | Suicidal thoughts | 1 | 2 | 3 | 4 | 5 | NA |
| 120616 | Pessimistic thoughts | 1 | 2 | 3 | 4 | 5 | NA |

*1st edition 1997; Revised 3rd edition*

**W**

*Continued*

Outcome Content References:

Gaskins, S., & Brown, K. (1992). Psychosocial responses among individuals with human immunodeficiency virus infection. *Applied Nursing Research, 5*(3), 111-121.

Greer, S., Morris, T., & Pettingale, K. (1979). Psychological response to breast cancer: Effect on outcome. *The Lancet, 2*(8146), 785-787.

Hagopian, G. (1993). Cognitive strategies used in adapting to a cancer diagnosis. *Oncology Nursing Forum, 20*(5), 759-763.

+Ivanoff, A., Joon Jang, S., Smyth, N.J., & Linehan, M.M. (1994). Fewer reasons for staying alive when you are thinking of killing yourself: The Brief Reasons for Living Inventory. *Journal of Psychopathology and Behavioral Assessment, 16*(1), 1-13.

Katz, R., & Lowe, L. (1989). The "will to live" as perceived by nurses and physicians. *Issues in Mental Health Nursing, 10*(1), 15-22.

+Linehan, M.M., Goodstein, J.L., Nielsen, S.L., & Chiles, J.A. (1983). Reasons for staying alive when you are thinking of killing yourself: The Reasons for Living Inventory. *Journal of Consulting and Clinical Psychology, 51*(2), 276-286, 484-485.

Weisman, A. (1972). *On death and denying: A psychiatric study of terminality*. New York: Behavioral Publications.

**W**

# Wound Healing: Primary Intention (1102)

*Domain-Physiologic Health (II)*

*Class-Tissue Integrity (L)*

*Scale(s)-None to Extensive (i) and Extensive to None (h)*

*Care Recipient:*

*Data Source:*

**Definition:** Extent of regeneration of cells and tissues following intentional closure

OUTCOME TARGET RATING:    Maintain at _____    Increase to _____

| Wound Healing: Primary Intention Overall Rating | None 1 | Limited 2 | Moderate 3 | Substantial 4 | Extensive 5 | |
|---|---|---|---|---|---|---|

INDICATORS:

| | | None 1 | Limited 2 | Moderate 3 | Substantial 4 | Extensive 5 | |
|---|---|---|---|---|---|---|---|
| 110201 | Skin approximation | 1 | 2 | 3 | 4 | 5 | NA |
| 110213 | Wound edge approximation | 1 | 2 | 3 | 4 | 5 | NA |
| 110214 | Scar formation | 1 | 2 | 3 | 4 | 5 | NA |

| | | Extensive | Substantial | Moderate | Limited | None | |
|---|---|---|---|---|---|---|---|
| 110202 | Purulent drainage | 1 | 2 | 3 | 4 | 5 | NA |
| 110203 | Serous drainage | 1 | 2 | 3 | 4 | 5 | NA |
| 110204 | Sanguineous drainage | 1 | 2 | 3 | 4 | 5 | NA |
| 110205 | Serosanguineous drainage | 1 | 2 | 3 | 4 | 5 | NA |
| 110206 | Sanguineous drainage from drain | 1 | 2 | 3 | 4 | 5 | NA |
| 110207 | Serosanguineous drainage from drain | 1 | 2 | 3 | 4 | 5 | NA |
| 110208 | Surrounding skin erythema | 1 | 2 | 3 | 4 | 5 | NA |
| 110215 | Surrounding skin bruising | 1 | 2 | 3 | 4 | 5 | NA |
| 110209 | Periwound edema | 1 | 2 | 3 | 4 | 5 | NA |
| 110210 | Skin temperature elevation | 1 | 2 | 3 | 4 | 5 | NA |
| 110211 | Foul wound odor | 1 | 2 | 3 | 4 | 5 | NA |

Location of wound (# from picture): _____

*1st edition 1997; Revised 3rd edition*

1. Front of head
2. Right ear
3. Left ear
4. Front of Neck
5. Right Chest
6. Left Chest
7. Sternum
8. Right upper quadrant
9. Left upper quadrant
10. Right lower quadrant
11. Left lower quadrant
12. Abdominal midline
13. Navel
14. Pubic and perineal area
15. Right trochanter (hip)
16. Left trochanter (hip)
17. Right anterior thigh
18. Right knee
19. Right lower anterior leg
20. Right ankle (inner/outer)

21. Right foot
22. Right toes
23. Left anterior thigh
24. Left knee
25. Left lower anterior leg
26. Left ankle (inner/outer)
27. Left foot
28. Left toes
29. Right upper interior arm
30. Right interior forearm
31. Right wrist
32. Right palm
33. Right fingers _____(specify)
34. Left upper interior arm
35. Left interior forearm
36. Left wrist
37. Left palm
38. Left fingers _____(specify)
39. Back of head
40. Back of neck
41. Left scapula
42. Right scapula

43. Spine
44. Left back
45. Right back
46. Left buttock
47. Right buttock
48. Sacrum
49. Left posterior thigh
50. Left lower posterior leg
51. Left heel
52. Left bottom foot
53. Right posterior thigh
54. Right lower posterior leg
55. Right heel
56. Right bottom foot
57. Left upper posterior arm
58. Left elbow
59. Left posterior forearm
60. Left dorsal hand
61. Right upper posterior arm
62. Right elbow
63. Right posterior forearm
64. Right dorsal hand

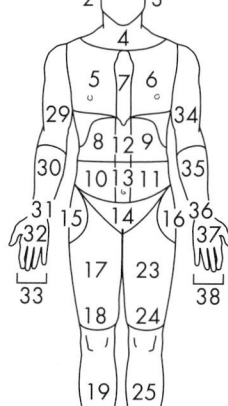
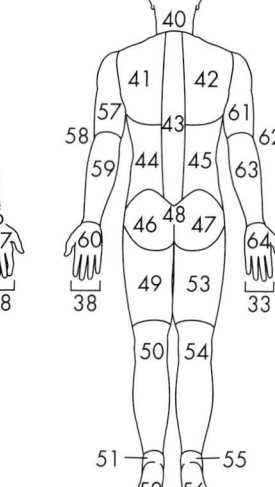
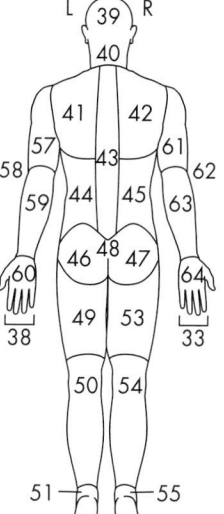

**W**

*Continued*

Outcome Content References:

Cohen, I.K., Diegelmann, R.F., & Lindblad, W.L. (1992). *Wound healing: Biochemical and clinical aspects*. Philadelphia: W.B. Saunders.

+Holden-Lund, C. (1988). Effects of relaxation with guided imagery on surgical stress and wound healing. *Research in Nursing & Health, 11*(4), 235-244.

Lazarus, G.S., Cooper, D.M., Knighton, D.R., Margohs, D.J., Pecoraro, R.E., Rodeheaver, G., & Robson, M.C. (1994). Definitions and guidelines for assessment of wounds and evaluation of healing. *Archives of Dermatology, 130*(4), 489-493.

Potter, P.A., & Perry, A.G. (2001). *Fundamentals of nursing* (5th ed.). St. Louis: Mosby.

**W**

# *Wound Healing: Secondary Intention (1103)*

Domain-Physiologic Health (II)

Class-Tissue Integrity (L)

Scale(s)-None to Extensive (i) and Extensive to None (h)

Care Recipient:

Data Source:

**Definition:** Extent of regeneration of cells and tissues in an open wound

OUTCOME TARGET RATING:    Maintain at _____    Increase to _____

| Wound Healing: Secondary Intention Overall Rating | None 1 | Limited 2 | Moderate 3 | Substantial 4 | Extensive 5 | |
|---|---|---|---|---|---|---|
| **INDICATORS:** | | | | | | |
| 110301 Granulation | 1 | 2 | 3 | 4 | 5 | |
| 110320 Scar formation | 1 | 2 | 3 | 4 | 5 | |
| 110321 Decreased wound size | 1 | 2 | 3 | 4 | 5 | |
| | Extensive | Substantial | Moderate | Limited | None | |
| 110303 Purulent drainage | 1 | 2 | 3 | 4 | 5 | NA |
| 110304 Serous drainage | 1 | 2 | 3 | 4 | 5 | NA |
| 110305 Sanguineous drainage | 1 | 2 | 3 | 4 | 5 | NA |
| 110306 Serosanguineous drainage | 1 | 2 | 3 | 4 | 5 | NA |
| 110307 Surrounding skin erythema | 1 | 2 | 3 | 4 | 5 | NA |
| 110322 Wound inflammation | 1 | 2 | 3 | 4 | 5 | NA |
| 110308 Periwound edema | 1 | 2 | 3 | 4 | 5 | NA |
| 110310 Blistered skin | 1 | 2 | 3 | 4 | 5 | NA |
| 110311 Macerated skin | 1 | 2 | 3 | 4 | 5 | NA |
| 110312 Necrosis | 1 | 2 | 3 | 4 | 5 | NA |
| 110313 Sloughing | 1 | 2 | 3 | 4 | 5 | NA |
| 110314 Tunneling | 1 | 2 | 3 | 4 | 5 | NA |
| 110315 Undermining | 1 | 2 | 3 | 4 | 5 | NA |
| 110316 Sinus tract formation | 1 | 2 | 3 | 4 | 5 | NA |
| 110317 Foul wound odor | 1 | 2 | 3 | 4 | 5 | NA |

Location of wound (# from picture) _____

*1st edition 1997; Revised 3rd edition*

1. Front of head
2. Right ear
3. Left ear
4. Front of Neck
5. Right Chest
6. Left Chest
7. Sternum
8. Right upper quadrant
9. Left upper quadrant
10. Right lower quadrant
11. Left lower quadrant
12. Abdominal midline
13. Navel
14. Pubic and perineal area
15. Right trochanter (hip)
16. Left trochanter (hip)
17. Right anterior thigh
18. Right knee
19. Right lower anterior leg
20. Right ankle (inner/outer)
21. Right foot
22. Right toes
23. Left anterior thigh
24. Left knee
25. Left lower anterior leg
26. Left ankle (inner/outer)
27. Left foot
28. Left toes
29. Right upper interior arm
30. Right interior forearm
31. Right wrist
32. Right palm
33. Right fingers _____(specify)
34. Left upper interior arm
35. Left interior forearm
36. Left wrist
37. Left palm
38. Left fingers _____(specify)
39. Back of head
40. Back of neck
41. Left scapula
42. Right scapula
43. Spine
44. Left back
45. Right back
46. Left buttock
47. Right buttock
48. Sacrum
49. Left posterior thigh
50. Left lower posterior leg
51. Left heel
52. Left bottom foot
53. Right posterior thigh
54. Right lower posterior leg
55. Right heel
56. Right bottom foot
57. Left upper posterior arm
58. Left elbow
59. Left posterior forearm
60. Left dorsal hand
61. Right upper posterior arm
62. Right elbow
63. Right posterior forearm
64. Right dorsal hand

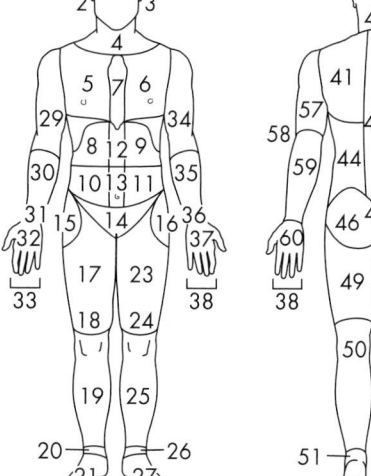
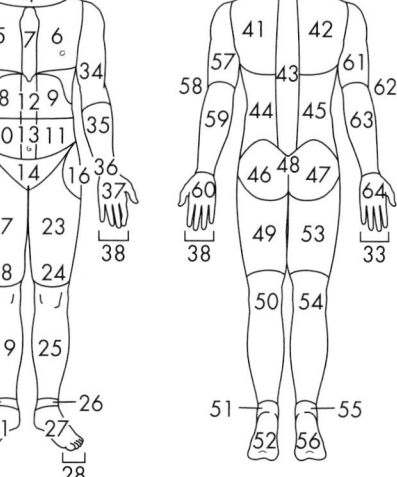

*Continued*

W

Outcome Content References:

Bergstrom, N., Bennett, M.A., Carlson, C.E., et al. (1994). *Treatment of pressure ulcers. Clinical practice guideline*, No. 15 (AHCPR Publication No. 95-0652). Rockville, MD: U.S. Department of Health and Human Services, Agency for Health Care Policy and Research.

Cohen, I.K., Diegelmann, R.F., & Lindblad, W.L. (1992). *Wound healing: Biochemical and clinical aspects.* Philadelphia: W.B. Saunders.

Flanagan, M. (1994). Assessment criteria. *Nursing Times, 90*(35), 76-88.

Frantz, R.A. (2001). Impaired skin integrity: Pressure ulcer. In M. Maas, K. Buckwalter, M. Hardy, T. Tripp-Reimer, M. Titler, & J. Specht (Eds.), *Nursing care of older adults: Diagnoses, outcomes & interventions* (pp. 121-136). St. Louis: Mosby.

Frantz, R.A., & Gardner, S. (1994). Elderly skin care: Principles of chronic wound care. *Journal of Gerontological Nursing, 20*(9), 35-44.

Lazarus, G.S., Cooper, D.M., Knighton, D.R., Margohs, D.J., Pecoraro, R.E., Rodeheaver, G., & Robson, M.C. (1994). Definitions and guidelines for assessment of wounds and evaluation of healing. *Archives of Dermatology, 130*(4), 489-493.

Maklebust, J., & Sieggreen, M. (1996). *Pressure ulcers: Guidelines for prevention and nursing management* (2nd ed.). Springhouse, PA: Springhouse.

Potter, P.A., & Perry, A.G. (2001). *Fundamentals of nursing* (5th ed.). St. Louis: Mosby.

Rijswijk, L., et al. (1993). Full-thickness leg ulcers: Patient demographics and predictors of healing. *The Journal of Family Practice, 36*(6), 625-632.

+Thomas, D.R., et al. (1997). Pressure ulcer scale for healing: Derivation and validation of the PUSH tool. *Advances in Wound Care 10*(5) 96-101.

W

# PART FOUR

# Health Patterns—
# NOC Linkages
# NANDA International—
# NOC Linkages

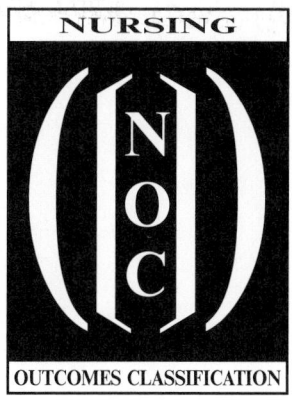

# Health Patterns—NOC Linkages

This section provides updated linkages among the Health Patterns identified by Gordon[1] and the NOC outcomes developed to date at three levels of abstraction: the individual, family, and community. These linkages were first published in the second edition of NOC. Early work by Gordon suggests the importance of the nurse assessing 11 health concepts using patterns of behavior over time rather than isolated patient events. This approach examines the *sequence of behavior* over time, incorporating a broad view of behavior as physiological, psychological, or sociological in nature. The patterns were proposed by Gordon to serve as a means of identifying nursing diagnoses during the early development of patient problem statements that were standardized for use in clinical practice. The patterns areas provide a structured framework for the assessment of a client. The nurse uses an interview approach and performs a physical examination for each patient receiving nursing care to assess each of the 11 health patterns.

Due to the popularity and long history of use of these health patterns in nursing, linkages among the NOC outcomes and the 11 health patterns were developed to assist nurses who routinely use the health patterns as an assessment structure in practice. In addition, many educational institutions use the patterns as an assessment tool to teach the assessment phase of the nursing process to nursing students. The linkages provide one way of identifying relevant outcomes for nurses using the NOC in education, practice, and research. Each outcome is placed under a specific pattern based on the pattern name and definition developed by Gordon. Outcomes that describe the actual health status of a more general nature were placed in the Health-Perception–Health-Management Pattern when they did not fit into a more specific pattern. Many of these outcomes would be assessed primarily by physical examination rather than by interviewing the client about his or her perceptions of health.

Several specific outcomes could not be easily placed in this structure and appear as a list at the end of the linkages. Linkages of the NOC to the 11 health patterns are important for: (1) assisting individuals to learn and use the NOC, (2) improving diagnostic reasoning skills in nursing, (3) identifying new outcomes for development of the NOC, especially as the family and community level outcomes are further developed, and (4) emphasizing the effectiveness of nursing interventions with the current emphasis in health care on outcomes. Current use of this pattern focus by nurses is predominant in the United States as well as in many countries worldwide.

## Reference

1. Gordon, M. (1994). *Nursing diagnosis: Process and application* (3rd ed.). New York: McGraw-Hill.

# Nursing Outcomes Classification (NOC) Organized by the 11 Health Patterns (Gordon, 1994)

**HEALTH-PERCEPTION–HEALTH-MANAGEMENT PATTERN:** Describes client's perceived pattern of health and well-being and how health is managed.

### INDIVIDUAL LEVEL

Acceptance: Health Status
Adherence Behavior
Aspiration Prevention
Caregiver Emotional Health
Caregiver Home Care Readiness
Caregiver Performance: Direct Care
Caregiver Performance: Indirect Care
Caregiver Physical Health
Caregiver Well-Being
Child Development: 1 Month
Child Development: 2 Months
Child Development: 4 Months
Child Development: 6 Months
Child Development: 12 Months
Child Development: 2 Years
Child Development: 3 Years
Child Development: 4 Years
Child Development: Preschool
Child Development: Middle Childhood
Child Development: Adolescence
Compliance Behavior
Diabetes Self-Management
Discharge Readiness: Independent Living
Discharge Readiness: Supported Living
Fall Prevention Behavior
Falls Occurrence
Fetal Status: Antepartum
Fetal Status: Intrapartum
Health Promoting Behavior
Health Seeking Behavior
Immune Hypersensitivity Response
Immune Status
Immunization Behavior
Infection Severity
Infection Severity: Newborn
Maternal Status: Antepartum

Maternal Status: Intrapartum
Maternal Status: Postpartum
Medication Response
Participation in Health Care Decisions
Personal Health Status
Personal Safety Behavior
Personal Well-Being
Physical Aging
Physical Injury Severity
Prenatal Health Behavior
Preterm Infant Organization
Quality of Life
Risk Control
Risk Control: Alcohol Use
Risk Control: Cancer
Risk Control: Cardiovascular Health
Risk Control: Drug Use
Risk Control: Hearing Impairment
Risk Control: Sexually Transmitted Diseases
Risk Control: Tobacco Use
Risk Control: Unintended Pregnancy
Risk Control: Visual Impairment
Risk Detection
Safe Home Environment
Seizure Control
Self-Care: Non-Parenteral Medication
Self-Care: Parenteral Medication
Self-Direction of Care
Student Health Status
Symptom Control
Thermoregulation
Thermoregulation: Newborn
Treatment Behavior: Illness or Injury
Vital Signs
Will to Live

**FAMILY LEVEL**
Family Health Status
Family Participation in Professional Care
Family Physical Environment

**COMMUNITY LEVEL**
Community Disaster Readiness
Community Health Status
Community Health Status: Immunity
Community Risk Control: Chronic Disease
Community Risk Control: Communicable Disease
Community Risk Control: Lead Exposure
Community Risk Control: Violence
Community Violence Level

**NUTRITION-METABOLIC PATTERN:** Describes pattern of food and fluid consumption relative to metabolic need and pattern indicators of local nutrient supply.

**INDIVIDUAL LEVEL**

Appetite
Blood Glucose Level
Breastfeeding Establishment: Infant
Breastfeeding Establishment: Maternal
Breastfeeding Maintenance
Breastfeeding Weaning
Electrolyte & Acid/Base Balance
Fluid Balance
Fluid Overload Severity
Growth
Hydration
Nausea & Vomiting Control
Nausea & Vomiting: Disruptive Effects
Nausea & Vomiting Severity
Nutritional Status

Nutritional Status: Biochemical Measures
Nutritional Status: Energy
Nutritional Status: Food & Fluid Intake
Nutritional Status: Nutrient Intake
Oral Hygiene
Swallowing Status
Swallowing Status: Esophageal Phase
Swallowing Status: Oral Phase
Swallowing Status: Pharyngeal Phase
Tissue Integrity: Skin & Mucous Membranes
Weight: Body Mass
Weight Control
Wound Healing: Primary Intention
Wound Healing: Secondary Intention

**ELIMINATION PATTERN:** Describes patterns of excretory function (bowel, bladder, and skin).

**INDIVIDUAL LEVEL:**

Bowel Continence
Bowel Elimination
Kidney Function
Ostomy Self-Care

Systemic Toxin Clearance: Dialysis
Urinary Continence
Urinary Elimination

---

**ACTIVITY-EXERCISE PATTERN:** Describes pattern of exercise, activity, leisure, and recreation.

---

**INDIVIDUAL LEVEL**

Activity Tolerance
Ambulation
Ambulation: Wheelchair
Asthma Self-Management
Balance
Body Mechanics Performance
Body Positioning: Self-Initiated
Bone Healing
Cardiac Disease Self-Management
Cardiac Pump Effectiveness
Circulation Status
Coordinated Movement
Endurance
Energy Conservation
Hyperactivity Level
Immobility Consequences: Physiological
Immobility Consequences: Psycho-Cognitive
Joint Movement: Ankle
Joint Movement: Elbow
Joint Movement: Fingers
Joint Movement: Hip
Joint Movement: Knee
Joint Movement: Neck
Joint Movement: Shoulder
Joint Movement: Spine
Joint Movement: Wrist

Joint Movement: Passive
Leisure Participation
Mobility
Physical Fitness
Play Participation
Psychomotor Energy
Respiratory Status: Airway Patency
Respiratory Status: Gas Exchange
Respiratory Status: Ventilation
Self-Care Status
Self-Care: Activities of Daily Living (ADL)
Self-Care: Bathing
Self-Care: Dressing
Self-Care: Eating
Self-Care: Hygiene
Self-Care: Instrumental Activities of Daily Living (IADL)
Self Care: Oral Hygiene
Self Care: Tolieting
Skeletal Function
Tissue Perfusion: Abdominal Organs
Tissue Perfusion: Cardiac
Tissue Perfusion: Peripheral
Tissue Perfusion: Pulmonary
Transfer Performance

**COGNITIVE-PERCEPTUAL PATTERN:** Describes sensory and perceptual and cognitive pattern.

**INDIVIDUAL LEVEL**

Cognition
Cognitive Orientation
Concentration
Decision-Making
Distorted Thought Self-Control
Hearing Compensation Behavior
Information Processing
Knowledge: Body Mechanics
Knowledge: Breastfeeding
Knowledge: Cardiac Disease Management
Knowledge: Child Physical Safety
Knowledge: Conception Prevention
Knowledge: Diabetes Management
Knowledge: Diet
Knowledge: Disease Process
Knowledge: Energy Conservation
Knowledge: Fall Prevention
Knowledge: Fertility Promotion
Knowledge: Health Behavior
Knowledge: Health Promotion
Knowledge: Health Resources
Knowledge: Illness Care
Knowledge: Infant Care
Knowledge: Infection Control
Knowledge: Labor & Delivery
Knowledge: Medication
Knowledge: Ostomy Care
Knowledge: Parenting

Knowledge: Personal Safety
Knowledge: Postpartum Maternal Health
Knowledge: Preconception Maternal Health
Knowledge: Pregnancy
Knowledge: Prescribed Activity
Knowledge: Sexual Functioning
Knowledge: Substance Use Control
Knowledge: Treatment Procedure(s)
Knowledge: Treatment Regimen
Memory
Neurological Status
Neurological Status: Autonomic
Neurological Status: Central Motor Control
Neurological Status: Consciousness
Neurological Status: Cranial Sensory/Motor
    Function
Neurological Status: Spinal Sensory/Motor
    Function
Pain: Disruptive Effects
Sensory Function Status
Sensory Function: Cutaneous
Sensory Function: Hearing
Sensory Function: Proprioception
Sensory Function: Taste & Smell
Sensory Function: Vision
Tissue Perfusion: Cerebral
Vision Compensation Behavior

**COMMUNITY LEVEL**

Community Competence

**SLEEP-REST PATTERN:** Describes pattern of sleep, rest, and relaxation.

**INDIVIDUAL LEVEL**

Rest
Sleep

**SELF-PERCEPTION–SELF-CONCEPT PATTERN:** Describes self-concept pattern and perceptions of self.

**INDIVIDUAL LEVEL**

Body Image
Comfort Level
Hope
Identity
Mood Equilibrium
Motivation
Pain: Adverse Psychological Response

Pain Level
Personal Autonomy
Self-Esteem
Suffering Severity
Symptom Severity

**Role-Relationship Pattern:** Describes pattern of role-engagements and relationships.

**Individual Level**

Abuse Cessation
Abuse Protection
Abusive Behavior Self-Restraint
Caregiver-Patient Relationship
Communication
Communication: Expressive
Communication: Receptive
Loneliness Severity
Neglect Cessation
Neglect Recovery
Parent-Infant Attachment

Parenting: Adolescent Physical Safety
Parenting: Early/Middle Childhood Physical Safety
Parenting: Infant/Toddler Physical Safety
Parenting Performance
Parenting: Psychosocial Safety
Role Performance
Social Interaction Skills
Social Involvement
Social Support

**Family Level**

Family Functioning
Family Integrity
Family Social Climate
Family Support During Treatment

**Sexuality-Reproductive Pattern:** Describes client's patterns of satisfaction and dissatisfaction with sexuality pattern; describes reproductive patterns.

**Individual Level**

Abuse Recovery: Sexual
Physical Maturation: Female
Physical Maturation: Male
Sexual Functioning

Sexual Identity
Symptom Severity: Perimenopause
Symptom Severity: Premenstrual Syndrome (PMS)

**Coping–Stress-Tolerance Pattern:** Describes general coping pattern and effectiveness of the pattern in terms of stress tolerance.

**Individual Level**

Abuse Recovery Status
Abuse Recovery: Emotional
Abuse Recovery: Financial
Abuse Recovery: Physical
Adaptation to Physical Disability
Aggression Self-Control
Anxiety Level
Anxiety Self-Control
Caregiver Adaptation To Patient
   Institutionalization
Caregiver Lifestyle Disruption
Caregiver Stressors
Caregiving Endurance Potential
Child Adaptation to Hospitalization
Comfortable Death
Coping

Depression Level
Depression Self-Control
Dignified Life Closure
Fear Level
Fear Level: Child
Fear Self-Control
Grief Resolution
Impulse Self-Control
Newborn Adaptation
Pain Control
Psychosocial Adjustment: Life Change
Self-Mutilation Restraint
Stress Level
Substance Addiction Consequences
Suicide Self-Restraint

**Family Level**

Family Coping
Family Normalization
Family Resiliency

**Value-Belief Pattern:** Describes patterns of values, beliefs (including spiritual), or goals that guide choices and decisions.

**Individual Level**

Health Beliefs
Health Beliefs: Perceived Ability to Perform
Health Beliefs: Perceived Control
Health Beliefs: Perceived Resources

Health Beliefs: Perceived Threat
Health Orientation
Spiritual Health

**Outcomes Not Placed Within a Pattern**

Allergic Response: Localized
Allergic Response: Systemic
Blood Coagulation
Blood Loss Severity
Blood Transfusion Reaction
Client Satisfaction: Access to Care Resources
Client Satisfaction: Caring
Client Satisfaction: Communication
Client Satisfaction: Continuity of Care
Client Satisfaction: Cultural Needs
   Fulfillment
Client Satisfaction: Functional Assistance
Client Satisfaction: Physical Care

Client Satisfaction: Physical Environment
Client Satisfaction: Protection of Rights
Client Satisfaction: Psychological Care
Client Satisfaction: Safety
Client Satisfaction: Symptom Control
Client Satisfaction: Teaching
Client Satisfaction: Technical Aspects of Care
Hemodialysis Access
Mechanical Ventilation Response: Adult
Mechanical Ventilation Weaning Response:
   Adult
Post Procedure Recovery Status

# NANDA International—NOC Linkages

## OVERVIEW

This section of the book contains suggested linkages between the NANDA International classification[1] published in 2003 and the current edition of NOC. The terms and definitions in this section reflect the 2003 edition of the diagnoses and are organized alphabetically by key terms. The 330 NOC outcomes in this edition are linked to 176 nursing diagnoses. A linkage is an association or relationship that exists between a patient problem (nursing diagnosis) and a desired outcome (resolution or improvement of the problem). The change in outcome is usually a result of an intervention by a nurse or other health care provider. Treatments for a diagnosis will vary, depending on the outcome selected. Linkages among NANDA, NOC, and NIC are available in a separate publication.[2] Linkages assist the nurse to select an outcome for a specific patent problem, thus facilitating clinical decision-making and diagnostic reasoning. The linkages also assist in the development of standardized care plans for specific populations and efforts to computerize nursing data in electronic health records. The linkage work supports the continuing refinement of the classification by helping to identify missing outcomes for future development.

The linkages identified in this section are options from which the nurse can select. Other outcomes may also be appropriate for a specific clinical problem. The linkages are based on expert judgment, and in a few cases actual clinical data were used to identify NANDA-NOC linkages from our test sites. This section is organized by NANDA diagnoses, and each problem has the NANDA definition included. Two categories of outcomes are available for each diagnosis. Outcomes considered to be the closest match to the diagnosis are listed under the category Suggested Outcomes. Outcomes closely associated to the diagnosis are listed under the category Additional Associated Outcomes. For the Risk Diagnoses only suggested outcomes are included. There have been substantial changes in the linkages between NANDA and NOC since these were first published in the second edition. This is largely due to the addition of 76 new outcomes in this edition, some of which provided a better match for specific nursing diagnoses.

## References

1. NANDA International. (2003). NANDA nursing diagnoses: Definition and classification 2003-2004. Philadelphia: Author.
2. Johnson, M., Bulechek, G., McCloskey Dochterman, J. Maas, M. & Moorhead, S. (2001). *Nursing diagnoses, outcomes and interventions: NANDA, NOC and NIC Linkages.* St. Louis: Mosby.

A

## *Activity Intolerance*

DEFINITION: Insufficient physiological or psychological energy to endure or complete required or desired daily activities

SUGGESTED OUTCOMES:

Activity Tolerance
Endurance
Energy Conservation
Psychomotor Energy

Self-Care Status
Self-Care: Activities of Daily Living (ADL)
Self-Care: Instrumental Activities of Daily
    Living (IADL)

ADDITIONAL ASSOCIATED OUTCOMES:

Ambulation
Ambulation: Wheelchair
Asthma Self-Management
Cardiac Disease Self-Management
Cardiac Pump Effectiveness
Coordinated Movement
Circulation Status
Client Satisfaction: Functional Assistance
Client Satisfaction: Symptom Control
Discharge Readiness: Independent Living
Health Beliefs: Perceived Ability to Perform

Immobility Consequences: Physiological
Mobility
Mood Equilibrium
Nutritional Status: Energy
Pain: Disruptive Effects
Physical Fitness
Respiratory Status: Gas Exchange
Respiratory Status: Ventilation
Symptom Severity
Vital Signs

## *Activity Intolerance, Risk for*

DEFINITION: At risk for experiencing insufficient physiological or psychological energy to endure or complete required or desired daily activities

SUGGESTED OUTCOMES:

Activity Tolerance
Asthma Self-Management
Cardiac Disease Self-Management
Cardiac Pump Effectiveness
Circulation Status
Coordinated Movement
Depression Level
Endurance
Energy Conservation
Health Beliefs: Perceived Control
Knowledge: Diet
Knowledge: Disease Process

Knowledge: Prescribed Activity
Mood Equilibrium
Nutritional Status: Energy
Pain: Disruptive Effects
Pain Level
Physical Fitness
Respiratory Status: Gas Exchange
Respiratory Status: Ventilation
Risk Control
Risk Detection
Symptom Control
Symptom Severity

A

## Adjustment, Impaired

**DEFINITION:** Inability to modify life style/behavior in a manner consistent with a change in health status

**SUGGESTED OUTCOMES:**

Acceptance: Health Status
Adaptation to Physical Disability
Compliance Behavior
Coping

Health Seeking Behavior
Motivation
Psychosocial Adjustment: Life Change
Treatment Behavior: Illness or Injury

**ADDITIONAL ASSOCIATED OUTCOMES:**

Adherence Behavior
Cardiac Disease Self-Management
Child Adaptation to Hospitalization
Cognition
Diabetes Self-Management
Discharge Readiness: Independent Living
Family Resiliency
Grief Resolution

Health Belief: Perceived Ability to Perform
Health Belief: Perceived Control
Impulse Self-Control
Mood Equilibrium
Participation in Health Care Decisions
Self-Esteem
Social Support
Stress Level

## Airway Clearance, Ineffective

**DEFINITION:** Inability to clear secretions or obstructions from the respiratory tract to maintain a clear airway

**SUGGESTED OUTCOMES:**

Aspiration Prevention
Mechanical Ventilation Response: Adult
Respiratory Status: Airway Patency
Respiratory Status: Ventilation

**ADDITIONAL ASSOCIATED OUTCOMES:**

Allergic Response: Systemic
Anxiety Level
Asthma Self-Management
Cognition
Endurance
Immune Hypersensitivity Response
Infection Severity
Mechanical Ventilation Weaning
  Response: Adult

Neurological Status
Pain Level
Post Procedure Recovery Status
Respiratory Status: Gas Exchange
Risk Control: Tobacco Use
Symptom Control
Treatment Behavior: Illness or Injury
Vital Signs

A

## *Anxiety*

**DEFINITION:** Vague uneasy feeling of discomfort or dread accompanied by an autonomic response (the source often nonspecific or unknown to the individual); a feeling of apprehension caused by anticipation of danger. It is an altering signal that warns of impending danger and enables the individual to take measures to deal with threat.

**SUGGESTED OUTCOMES:**

Anxiety Level
Anxiety Self-Control
Concentration

Coping
Hyperactivity Level

**ADDITIONAL ASSOCIATED OUTCOMES:**

Acceptance: Health Status
Aggression Self-Control
Child Adaptation to Hospitalization
Client Satisfaction: Caring
Client Satisfaction: Psychological Care
Grief Resolution
Impulse Self-Control
Information Processing

Neurological Status: Autonomic
Parent-Infant Attachment
Psychosocial Adjustment: Life Change
Self-Mutilation Restraint
Social Interaction Skills
Stress Level
Symptom Control
Vital Signs

## *Aspiration, Risk for*

**DEFINITION:** At risk for entry of gastrointestinal secretions, oropharyngeal secretions, solids or fluids into tracheobronchial passages

**SUGGESTED OUTCOMES:**

Aspiration Prevention
Body Positioning: Self-Initiated
Cognition
Cognitive Orientation
Immobility Consequences: Physiological
Knowledge: Treatment Procedure(s)
Mechanical Ventilation Response: Adult
Nausea & Vomiting Severity
Neurological Status

Post Procedure Recovery Status
Respiratory Status: Airway Patency
Respiratory Status: Ventilation
Risk Control
Risk Detection
Seizure Control
Self Care: Non-Parenteral Medication
Swallowing Status

A

## *Autonomic Dysreflexia*

DEFINITION: Life-threatening, uninhibited sympathetic response of the nervous system to a noxious stimulus after a spinal cord injury at T7 or above

SUGGESTED OUTCOMES:
Neurological Status: Autonomic
Sensory Function: Cutaneous
Vital Signs

ADDITIONAL ASSOCIATED OUTCOMES:

Circulation Status
Knowledge: Disease Process
Neurological Status
Sensory Function Status

Sensory Function: Vision
Symptom Severity
Tissue Integrity: Skin & Mucous Membranes
Treatment Behaviors: Illness or Injury

## *Autonomic Dysreflexia, Risk for*

DEFINITION: At risk for life-threatening, uninhibited response of the sympathetic nervous system, post spinal shock, in an individual with a spinal cord injury or lesion at T6 or above (has been demonstrated in patients with injuries at T7 and T8)

SUGGESTED OUTCOMES:

Bowel Elimination
Caregiver Home Care Readiness
Comfort Level
Infection Severity
Knowledge: Disease Process
Knowledge: Medication
Medication Response
Neurological Status: Autonomic
Pain Level

Risk Control
Risk Detection
Symptom Severity
Thermoregulation
Tissue Integrity: Skin & Mucous Membranes
Treatment Behavior: Illness or Injury
Urinary Elimination
Vital Signs

**B**

## Body Image, Disturbed

DEFINITION: Confusion in mental picture of one's physical self

SUGGESTED OUTCOMES:
Adaptation to Physical Disability
Body Image
Child Development: Adolescence
Self-Esteem

ADDITIONAL ASSOCIATED OUTCOMES:
Acceptance: Health Status
Child Development: 2 Years
Child Development: 3 Years
Child Development: 4 Years
Child Development: Preschool
Child Development: Middle Childhood

Coping
Distorted Thought Self-Control
Identity
Sexual Functioning
Sexual Identity
Weight: Body Mass

## Body Temperature, Risk for Imbalanced

DEFINITION: At risk for failure to maintain body temperature within normal range

SUGGESTED OUTCOMES:
Hydration
Immune Status
Infection Severity
Infection Severity: Newborn
Medication Response
Neglect Recovery

Neurological Status: Autonomic
Post Procedure Recovery Status
Risk Control
Risk Detection
Thermoregulation
Thermoregulation: Newborn

## Bowel Incontinence

DEFINITION: Change in normal bowel habits characterized by involuntary passage of stool

SUGGESTED OUTCOMES:
Bowel Continence
Bowel Elimination
Tissue Integrity: Skin & Mucous Membranes

ADDITIONAL ASSOCIATED OUTCOMES:
Cognition
Knowledge: Ostomy Care
Neurological Status: Autonomic
Neurological Status: Spinal Sensory/Motor
    Function

Nutritional Status: Food & Fluid Intake
Ostomy Self-Care
Self-Care: Hygiene
Self-Care: Toileting

## *Breastfeeding, Effective*

**DEFINITION:** Mother-infant dyad/family exhibits adequate proficiency and satisfaction with breastfeeding process

**SUGGESTED OUTCOMES:**
Breastfeeding Establishment: Infant
Breastfeeding Establishment: Maternal
Breastfeeding Maintenance
Breastfeeding Weaning

**ADDITIONAL ASSOCIATED OUTCOMES:**

Anxiety Self-Control
Child Development: 1 Month
Child Development: 2 Months
Cognition
Fluid Balance
Growth
Hydration

Knowledge: Breastfeeding
Nutritional Status: Food & Fluid Intake
Parent-Infant Attachment
Social Support
Swallowing Status
Urinary Elimination
Weight: Body Mass

## *Breastfeeding, Ineffective*

**DEFINITION:** Dissatisfaction or difficulty a mother, infant, or child experiences with the breast-feeding process

**SUGGESTED OUTCOMES:**

Breastfeeding Establishment: Infant
Breastfeeding Establishment: Maternal
Breastfeeding Maintenance

Breastfeeding Weaning
Knowledge: Breastfeeding

**ADDITIONAL ASSOCIATED OUTCOMES:**

Anxiety Self-Control
Child Development: 1 Month
Child Development: 2 Months
Cognition
Family Integrity
Fluid Balance
Growth
Hydration
Knowledge: Infant Care

Nutritional Status: Food & Fluid Intake
Pain Level
Parent-Infant Attachment
Personal Health Status
Social Support
Swallowing Status
Urinary Elimination
Weight: Body Mass

**B**

## *Breastfeeding, Interrupted*

**DEFINITION:** Break in the continuity of the breastfeeding process as a result of inability or inadvisability to put baby to breast for feeding

**SUGGESTED OUTCOMES:**
Breastfeeding Maintenance
Breastfeeding Weaning
Knowledge: Breastfeeding
Parent-Infant Attachment

**ADDITIONAL ASSOCIATED OUTCOMES:**

Infection Severity
Medication Response
Motivation
Parenting Performance
Personal Health Status

Risk Control: Alcohol Use
Risk Control: Drug Use
Role Performance
Stress Level


## *Breathing Pattern, Ineffective*

**DEFINITION:** Inspiration and/or expiration which does not provide adequate ventilation

**SUGGESTED OUTCOMES:**
Allergic Response: Systemic
Mechanical Ventilation Response: Adult
Respiratory Status: Airway Patency

Respiratory Status: Gas Exchange
Respiratory Status: Ventilation
Vital Signs

**ADDITIONAL ASSOCIATED OUTCOMES:**
Anxiety Level
Asthma Self-Management
Cognition
Comfort Level
Electrolyte & Acid/Base Balance
Energy Conservation
Fluid Overload Severity

Infection Severity
Neurological Status: Autonomic
Neurological Status: Central Motor Control
Pain Level
Weight: Body Mass
Weight Control

## Cardiac Output, Decreased

**DEFINITION:** Inadequate blood pumped by the heart to meet the metabolic demands of the body

**SUGGESTED OUTCOMES:**

Blood Loss Severity
Cardiac Pump Effectiveness
Circulation Status
Tissue Perfusion: Abdominal Organs

Tissue Perfusion: Cardiac
Tissue Perfusion: Cerebral
Tissue Perfusion: Peripheral
Tissue Perfusion: Pulmonary
Vital Signs

**ADDITIONAL ASSOCIATED OUTCOMES:**

Blood Coagulation
Cardiac Disease Self-Management
Cognition
Electrolyte & Acid/Base Balance
Endurance
Energy Conservation
Fluid Balance

Fluid Overload Severity
Hydration
Neurological Status: Autonomic
Respiratory Status: Gas Exchange
Respiratory Status: Ventilation
Urinary Elimination

## Caregiver Role Strain

**DEFINITION:** Difficulty in performing caregiver role

**SUGGESTED OUTCOMES:**

Caregiver Emotional Health
Caregiver Endurance Potential
Caregiver Lifestyle Disruption
Caregiver-Patient Relationship
Caregiver Performance: Direct Care
Caregiver Performance: Indirect Care
Caregiver Physical Health

Caregiver Stressors
Caregiver Well-Being
Family Resiliency
Family Support During Treatment
Parenting Performance
Role Performance

**Additional Associated Outcomes:**

Caregiver Home Care Readiness
Depression Level
Depression Self-Control
Family Coping
Family Functioning

Knowledge: Health Resources
Leisure Participation
Social Involvement
Social Support
Stress Level

C

## Caregiver Role Strain, Risk for

**DEFINITION:** Caregiver is vulnerable for felt difficulty in performing the family caregiver role

**SUGGESTED OUTCOMES:**

Caregiver Emotional Health
Caregiver Home Care Readiness
Caregiver Lifestyle Disruption
Caregiver-Patient Relationship
Caregiver Performance: Direct Care
Caregiver Performance: Indirect Care
Caregiver Physical Health
Caregiver Stressors
Caregiving Endurance Potential
Coping
Discharge Readiness: Supported Living
Family Coping
Family Functioning

Family Resiliency
Family Support During Treatment
Knowledge: Energy Conservation
Knowledge: Health Behavior
Knowledge: Health Resources
Parenting Performance
Rest
Risk Control
Risk Detection
Role Performance
Sleep
Stress Level

## Communication, Impaired Verbal

**DEFINITION:** Decreased, delayed, or absent ability to receive, process, transmit, and use a system of symbols

**SUGGESTED OUTCOMES:**

Communication
Communication: Expressive
Communication: Receptive
Information Processing

**ADDITIONAL ASSOCIATED OUTCOMES:**

Client Satisfaction: Communication
Cognition
Cognitive Orientation
Distorted Thought Self-Control
Neurological Status

Neurological Status: Cranial Sensory/Motor
   Function
Sensory Function Status
Sensory Function: Hearing
Sensory Function: Vision
Tissue Perfusion: Cerebral

## *Communication, Readiness for Enhanced*

**DEFINITION:** A pattern of exchanging information and ideas with others that is sufficient for meeting one's needs and life's goals and can be strengthened

**SUGGESTED OUTCOMES:**
Communication
Communication: Expressive
Communication: Receptive

**ADDITIONAL ASSOCIATED OUTCOMES:**
Client Satisfaction: Communication
Hearing Compensation Behavior
Social Interaction Skills

## *Community Coping, Ineffective*

**DEFINITION:** Pattern of community activities (for adaptation and problem solving) that is unsatisfactory for meeting the demands or needs of the community

**SUGGESTED OUTCOMES:**
Community Competence
Community Disaster Readiness
Community Risk Control: Chronic Disease
Community Risk Control: Communicable Disease
Community Risk Control: Lead Exposure
Community Risk Control: Violence

**ADDITIONAL ASSOCIATED OUTCOMES:**
Community Health Status
Community Health Status: Immunity
Community Violence Level

C

**C**

## *Community Coping, Readiness for Enhanced*

**DEFINITION:** Pattern of community activities for adaptation and problem solving that is satisfactory for meeting the demands or needs of the community but can be improved for management of current and future problems/stressors

**SUGGESTED OUTCOMES:**
Community Competence
Community Disaster Readiness

**ADDITIONAL ASSOCIATED OUTCOMES:**
Community Risk Control: Chronic Disease
Community Risk Control: Communicable Disease
Community Risk Control: Lead Exposure
Community Risk Control: Violence

## *Community Therapeutic Regimen Management, Ineffective*

**DEFINITION:** Pattern of regulating and integrating into community processes programs for treatment of illness and the sequelae of illness that are unsatisfactory for meeting health-related goals

**SUGGESTED OUTCOMES:**
Community Risk Control: Chronic Disease
Community Risk Control: Communicable Disease
Community Risk Control: Lead Exposure

**ADDITIONAL ASSOCIATED OUTCOMES:**
Community Health Status
Community Health Status: Immunity

## Confusion, Acute

**DEFINITION:** Abrupt onset of a cluster of global, transient changes and disturbances in attention, cognition, psychomotor activity, level of consciousness, and/or sleep/wake cycle

**SUGGESTED OUTCOMES:**
Cognitive Orientation
Distorted Thought Self-Control
Information Processing
Neurological Status: Consciousness

**ADDITIONAL ASSOCIATED OUTCOMES:**
Abuse Protection
Anxiety Level
Blood Glucose Level
Cognition
Concentration
Electrolyte & Acid/Base Balance
Fluid Balance
Infection Severity

Memory
Respiratory Status: Gas Exchange
Risk Control: Alcohol Use
Risk Control: Drug Use
Safe Home Environment
Sleep
Thermoregulation

## Confusion, Chronic

**DEFINITION:** Irreversible, long-standing and/or progressive deterioration of intellect and personality characterized by decreased ability to interpret environmental stimuli; decreased capacity for intellectual thought processes and manifested by disturbances of memory, orientation, and behavior

**SUGGESTED OUTCOMES:**
Cognition
Cognitive Orientation
Concentration
Decision-Making
Distorted Thought Self-Control

Identity
Information Processing
Memory
Neurological Status: Consciousness

**ADDITIONAL ASSOCIATED OUTCOMES:**
Client Satisfaction: Access to Care Resources
Client Satisfaction: Continuity of Care
Client Satisfaction: Protection of Rights
Client Satisfaction: Safety
Communication

Personal Autonomy
Risk Control: Alcohol Use
Risk Control: Drug Use
Safe Home Environment
Social Interaction Skills

C

# Constipation

**DEFINITION:** Decrease in normal frequency of defecation accompanied by difficult or incomplete passage of stool and/or passage of excessively hard, dry stool

**SUGGESTED OUTCOMES:**
Bowel Elimination
Hydration
Symptom Control

**ADDITIONAL ASSOCIATED OUTCOMES:**
Appetite
Comfort Level
Medication Response
Mobility
Nutritional Status: Food & Fluid Intake
Self-Care: Non-Parenteral Medication
Self-Care: Toileting

# Constipation, Perceived

**DEFINITION:** Self-diagnosis of constipation and abuse of laxatives, enemas, and suppositories to ensure a daily bowel movement

**SUGGESTED OUTCOMES:**
Bowel Elimination
Health Beliefs
Knowledge: Health Behavior

**ADDITIONAL ASSOCIATED OUTCOMES:**
Adherence Behavior
Health Beliefs: Perceived Threat
Hydration
Knowledge: Ostomy Care
Medication Response
Mobility
Nutritional Status: Food & Fluid Intake
Treatment Behavior: Illness or Injury

## *Constipation, Risk for*

**DEFINITION:** At risk for a decrease in normal frequency of defecation accompanied by difficult or incomplete passage of stool and/or passage of excessively hard, dry stool

**SUGGESTED OUTCOMES:**
Appetite
Bowel Elimination
Hydration
Immobility Consequences: Physiological
Knowledge: Medication
Medication Response
Mobility
Nutritional Status: Food & Fluid Intake
Risk Control
Risk Detection
Self-Care: Non-Parenteral Medication
Self-Care: Toileting
Symptom Control
Treatment Behavior: Illness or Injury

## *Coping, Defensive*

**DEFINITION:** Repeated projection of falsely positive self-evaluation based on a self-protective pattern that defends against underlying perceived threats to positive self-regard

**SUGGESTED OUTCOMES:**
Acceptance: Health Status
Adaptation to Physical Disability
Child Development: Adolescence

Coping
Self-Esteem
Social Interaction Skills

**ADDITIONAL ASSOCIATED OUTCOMES:**
Grief Resolution
Impulse Self-Control
Psychosocial Adjustment: Life Change
Risk Control: Alcohol Use

Risk Control: Drug Use
Risk Control: Tobacco Use
Social Involvement
Social Support

C

## Coping, Ineffective

**DEFINITION:** Inability to form a valid appraisal of the stressors, inadequate choices of practiced responses, and/or inability to use available resources

**SUGGESTED OUTCOMES:**

Acceptance: Health Status
Adaptation to Physical Disability
Child Adaptation to Hospitalization
Coping
Decision-Making

Impulse Self-Control
Knowledge: Health Resources
Psychosocial Adjustment: Life Change
Role Performance
Stress Level

**ADDITIONAL ASSOCIATED OUTCOMES:**

Abusive Behavior Self-Restraint
Aggression Self-Control
Anxiety Self-Control
Caregiver Stressors
Depression Self-Control
Grief Resolution
Information Processing
Personal Well-Being
Quality of Life

Risk Control: Alcohol Use
Risk Control: Drug Use
Risk Control: Tobacco Use
Self-Esteem
Self-Mutilation Restraint
Sleep
Social Interaction Skills
Social Support
Suicide Self-Restraint

## Coping, Readiness for Enhanced

**DEFINITION:** A pattern of cognitive and behavioral efforts to manage demands that is sufficient for well-being and can be strengthened

**SUGGESTED OUTCOMES:**

Acceptance: Health Status
Adaptation to Physical Disability
Coping

Personal Well-Being
Role Performance
Stress Level

**ADDITIONAL ASSOCIATED OUTCOMES:**

Caregiver Emotional Health
Caregiver Stressors
Child Adaptation to Hospitalization

Quality of Life
Self-Esteem
Social Interaction Skills

## Death Anxiety

**DEFINITION:** Apprehension, worry, or fear related to death or dying

**SUGGESTED OUTCOMES:**

Acceptance: Health Status

Anxiety Self-Control

Comfortable Death

Dignified Life Closure

Fear Self-Control

Psychosocial Adjustment: Life Change

Spiritual Health

**ADDITIONAL ASSOCIATED OUTCOMES:**

Anxiety Level

Coping

Depression Level

Depression Self-Control

Fear Level

Health Beliefs: Perceived Threat

Hope

Pain Control

Participation in Health Care Decisions

Personal Autonomy

Social Support

Stress Level

## Decisional Conflict (Specify)

**DEFINITION:** Uncertainty about course of action to be taken when choice among competing actions involves risk, loss, or challenge to personal life values

**SUGGESTED OUTCOMES:**

Decision-Making

Information Processing

Participation in Health Care Decisions

Personal Autonomy

**ADDITIONAL ASSOCIATED OUTCOMES:**

Coping

Family Coping

Family Functioning

Family Social Climate

Health Beliefs

Health Orientation

Knowledge: Disease Process

Knowledge: Treatment Regimen

Psychosocial Adjustment: Life Change

Social Support

**D**

## Denial, Ineffective

**DEFINITION:** Conscious or unconscious attempt to disavow the knowledge or meaning of an event to reduce anxiety/fear, but leading to the detriment of health

**SUGGESTED OUTCOMES:**
Acceptance: Health Status
Anxiety Self-Control
Fear Self-Control
Health Beliefs: Perceived Threat
Symptom Severity

**ADDITIONAL ASSOCIATED OUTCOMES:**

Anxiety Level
Coping
Fear Level
Health Beliefs
Health Seeking Behavior

Mood Equilibrium
Psychosocial Adjustment: Life Change
Stress Level
Symptom Control

## Dentition, Impaired

**DEFINITION:** Disruption in tooth development/eruption patterns or structural integrity of individual teeth

**SUGGESTED OUTCOMES:**
Oral Hygiene
Self-Care: Oral Hygiene

**ADDITIONAL ASSOCIATED OUTCOMES:**

Health Beliefs: Perceived Resources
Infection Severity
Knowledge: Health Behavior
Knowledge: Health Resources
Medication Response

Nausea & Vomiting Severity
Nutritional Status: Nutrient Intake
Pain Level
Risk Control: Drug Use
Risk Control: Tobacco Use

## Development, Risk for Delayed

**DEFINITION:** At risk for delay of 25% or more in one or more of the areas of social or self-regulatory behavior, or cognitive, language, gross or fine motor skills

**SUGGESTED OUTCOMES:**

Abuse Recovery Status
Abuse Recovery: Physical
Abusive Behavior Self-Restraint
Caregiver Emotional Health
Caregiver Physical Health
Child Development: 1 Month
Child Development: 2 Months
Child Development: 4 Months
Child Development: 6 Months
Child Development: 12 Months
Child Development: 2 Years
Child Development: 3 Years
Child Development: 4 Years
Child Development: Preschool
Child Development: Middle Childhood
Child Development: Adolescence
Family Functioning
Family Integrity
Family Physical Environment
Family Social Climate
Fetal Status: Antepartum
Fetal Status: Intrapartum
Growth
Knowledge: Infant Care

Knowledge: Parenting
Maternal Status: Antepartum
Maternal Status: Intrapartum
Neglect Recovery
Newborn Adaptation
Parent-Infant Attachment
Parenting: Adolescent Physical Safety
Parenting: Early/Middle Childhood Physical
  Safety
Parenting: Infant/Toddler Physical Safety
Parenting Performance
Parenting: Psychosocial Safety
Personal Autonomy
Play Participation
Prenatal Health Behavior
Preterm Infant Organization
Risk Control
Risk Control: Alcohol Use
Risk Control: Drug Use
Risk Detection
Social Interaction Skills
Student Health Status
Substance Addiction Consequences

## Diarrhea

**DEFINITION:** Passage of loose, unformed stools

**SUGGESTED OUTCOMES:**

Bowel Continence
Bowel Elimination
Electrolyte & Acid/Base Balance
Fluid Balance

Hydration
Ostomy Self-Care
Symptom Severity

**ADDITIONAL ASSOCIATED OUTCOMES:**

Anxiety Level
Anxiety Self-Control
Infection Severity
Medication Response
Nutritional Status: Biochemical Measures
Nutritional Status: Food & Fluid Intake

Risk Control: Alcohol Use
Risk Control: Drug Use
Self-Care: Non-Parenteral Medication
Stress Level
Symptom Control
Treatment Behavior: Illness or Injury

**D**

## Disuse Syndrome, Risk for

**DEFINITION:** At risk for deterioration of body systems as the result of prescribed or unavoidable musculoskeletal inactivity

**Suggested Outcomes:**

Comfort Level
Coordinated Movement
Endurance
Immobility Consequences: Physiological
Immobility Consequences: Psycho-Cognitive
Joint Movement: Ankle
Joint Movement: Elbow
Joint Movement: Fingers
Joint Movement: Hip
Joint Movement: Knee
Joint Movement: Neck

Joint Movement: Passive
Joint Movement: Shoulder
Joint Movement: Spine
Joint Movement: Wrist
Mobility
Neurological Status: Consciousness
Pain Level
Risk Control
Risk Detection
Transfer Performance

## Diversional Activity, Deficient

**DEFINITION:** Decreased stimulation from (or interest or engagement in) recreational or leisure activities

**SUGGESTED OUTCOMES:**

Family Physical Environment
Leisure Participation
Motivation

Play Participation
Social Involvement

**ADDITIONAL ASSOCIATED OUTCOMES:**

Child Development: 2 Years
Child Development: 3 Years
Child Development: 4 Years
Child Development: Preschool
Child Development: Middle Childhood

Child Development: Adolescence
Health Promoting Behavior
Loneliness Severity
Personal Well-Being
Social Interaction Skills

## Energy Field, Disturbed

**DEFINITION:** Disruption of the flow of energy surrounding a person's being that results in disharmony of the body, mind, and/or spirit

**SUGGESTED OUTCOMES:**
Personal Health Status
Personal Well-Being
Spiritual Health

**ADDITIONAL ASSOCIATED OUTCOMES:**
Comfort Level
Health Beliefs
Health Orientation
Pain Level
Suffering Severity

E

## Environmental Interpretation Syndrome, Impaired

**DEFINITION:** Consistent lack of orientation to person, place, time, or circumstances over more than 3 to 6 months, necessitating a protective environment

**SUGGESTED OUTCOMES:**
Cognitive Orientation
Concentration
Fall Prevention Behavior
Memory
Neurological Status: Consciousness
Safe Home Environment

**ADDITIONAL ASSOCIATED OUTCOMES:**

| | |
|---|---|
| Anxiety Level | Depression Self-Control |
| Cognition | Family Resiliency |
| Communication | Information Processing |
| Decision-Making | Loneliness Severity |
| Depression Level | |

F

## Failure to Thrive, Adult

**DEFINITION:** Progressive functional deterioration of a physical and cognitive nature. The individual's ability to live with multisystem diseases, cope with ensuing problems, and manage his/her care are remarkably diminished.

**SUGGESTED OUTCOMES:**

Appetite
Cognition
Endurance
Nutritional Status
Nutritional Status: Food & Fluid Intake

Physical Aging
Self-Care: Activities of Daily Living (ADL)
Weight: Body Mass
Will to Live

**ADDITIONAL ASSOCIATED OUTCOMES:**

Acceptance Health Status
Bowel Continence
Communication
Decision-Making
Depression Level
Depression Self-Control
Discharge Readiness: Independent Living
Hydration
Infection Severity
Information Processing
Leisure Participation
Mood Equilibrium

Nausea & Vomiting Severity
Neglect Cessation
Neglect Recovery
Nutritional Status: Nutrient Intake
Personal Health Status
Psychosocial Adjustment: Life Change
Self-Care: Instrumental Activities of Daily
   Living (IADL)
Social Involvement
Treatment Behavior: Illness or Injury
Urinary Continence
Weight Control

## Falls, Risk for

**DEFINITION:** Increased susceptibility to falling that may cause physical harm

**SUGGESTED OUTCOMES:**

Ambulation
Balance
Blood Glucose Level
Cognition
Coordinated Movement
Endurance
Fall Prevention Behavior
Falls Occurrence
Knowledge: Child Physical Safety
Knowledge: Fall Prevention
Mobility
Neurological Status: Central Motor Control
Nutritional Status
Pain Level

Parenting: Infant/Toddler Physical Safety
Parenting: Early/Middle Childhood Physical
   Safety
Physical Injury Severity
Post Procedure Recovery Status
Risk Control
Risk Detection
Seizure Control
Sensory Function Status
Sensory Function: Hearing
Sensory Function: Vision
Transfer Performance
Vision Compensation Behavior

## Family Coping, Compromised

**DEFINITION:** Usually supportive primary person (family member or close friend) provides insufficient, ineffective or compromised support, comfort, assistance or encouragement that may be needed by the client to manage or master adaptive tasks related to his/her health challenge

**SUGGESTED OUTCOMES:**

Caregiver Emotional Health
Caregiver-Patient Relationship
Caregiver Performance: Direct Care
Caregiver Performance: Indirect Care

Caregiving Endurance Potential
Family Coping
Family Normalization

**ADDITIONAL ASSOCIATED OUTCOMES:**

Caregiver Stressors
Family Participation in Professional Care
Family Resiliency
Family Support During Treatment
Neglect Cessation
Parent-Infant Attachment
Parenting Performance

## Family Coping, Disabled

**DEFINITION:** Behavior of significant person (family member or other primary person) that disables his/her capacities and the client's capacities to effectively address tasks essential to either person's adaptation to the health challenge

**SUGGESTED OUTCOMES:**

Caregiver-Patient Relationship
Caregiver Performance: Direct Care
Caregiver Performance: Indirect Care
Caregiver Well-Being

Caregiving Endurance Potential
Family Coping
Family Normalization

**ADDITIONAL ASSOCIATED OUTCOMES:**

Adaptation to Physical Disability
Caregiver Emotional Health
Caregiver Stressors
Coping
Depression Level
Depression Self-Control

Family Health Status
Family Resiliency
Family Social Climate
Family Support During Treatment
Neglect Recovery

**F**

## Family Coping, Readiness for Enhanced

DEFINITION: Effective management of adaptive tasks by family member involved with the client's health challenge, who now exhibits desire and readiness for enhanced health and growth in regard to self and in relation to the client

SUGGESTED OUTCOMES:

Caregiver-Patient Relationship
Caregiver Well-Being
Family Coping
Family Normalization

Health Promoting Behavior
Health Seeking Behavior
Participation in Health Care Decisions

ADDITIONAL ASSOCIATED OUTCOMES:

Caregiver Emotional Health
Caregiver Lifestyle Disruption
Caregiver Performance: Indirect Care
Family Functioning
Family Health Status

Family Participation in Professional Care
Family Resiliency
Family Support During Treatment
Parent-Infant Attachment
Parenting Performance

## Family Processes, Dysfunctional: Alcoholism

DEFINITION: Psychosocial, spiritual, and physiological functions of the family unit are chronically disorganized, which leads to conflict, denial of problems, resistance to change, ineffective problem-solving, and a series of self-perpetuating crises

SUGGESTED OUTCOMES:

Family Coping
Family Functioning
Family Resiliency
Family Social Climate

Parenting Performance
Role Performance
Substance Addiction Consequences

ADDITIONAL ASSOCIATED OUTCOMES:

Aggression Self-Control
Compliance Behavior
Decision-Making
Depression Level
Depression Self-Control
Family Health Status
Family Integrity

Family Normalization
Family Support During Treatment
Knowledge: Substance Use Control
Social Interaction Skills
Social Involvement
Stress Level
Treatment Behavior: Illness or Injury

## Family Processes, Interrupted

**DEFINITION:** Change in family relationships and/or functioning

**SUGGESTED OUTCOMES:**

Adaptation to Physical Disability
Family Coping
Family Functioning
Family Normalization

Family Resiliency
Family Social Climate
Parenting Performance

**ADDITIONAL ASSOCIATED OUTCOMES:**

Abuse Protection
Coping
Decision-Making
Family Health Status
Family Participation in Professional Care
Grief Resolution
Parent-Infant Attachment

Psychosocial Adjustment: Life Change
Role Performance
Social Interaction Skills
Social Involvement
Social Support
Stress Level

F

## Family Processes, Readiness for Enhanced

**DEFINITION:** A pattern of family functioning that is sufficient to support the well-being of family members and can be strengthened

**SUGGESTED OUTCOMES:**

Family Coping
Family Functioning
Family Resiliency
Family Social Climate

**ADDITIONAL ASSOCIATED OUTCOMES:**

Family Health Status
Family Integrity
Family Normalization
Family Participation in Professional Care
Family Support During Treatment

F

## *Family Therapeutic Regimen Management, Ineffective*

**DEFINITION:** Pattern of regulating and integrating into family processes a program for treatment of illness and the sequelae of illness that is unsatisfactory for meeting specific health goals

**SUGGESTED OUTCOMES:**

Caregiver Performance: Direct Care
Caregiver Performance: Indirect Care
Family Coping
Family Functioning

Family Normalization
Family Participation in Professional Care
Family Resiliency
Knowledge: Treatment Regimen

**ADDITIONAL ASSOCIATED OUTCOMES:**

Adherence Behavior
Compliance Behavior
Family Health Status

Family Integrity
Family Social Climate
Family Support During Treatment


## *Fatigue*

**DEFINITION:** An overwhelming sustained sense of exhaustion and decreased capacity for physical and mental work at usual level

**SUGGESTED OUTCOMES:**

Activity Tolerance
Endurance
Energy Conservation

Nutritional Status: Energy
Psychomotor Energy

**ADDITIONAL ASSOCIATED OUTCOMES:**

Blood Glucose Level
Comfort Level
Concentration
Mobility
Mood Equilibrium
Pain Level
Personal Health Status
Personal Well-Being

Quality of Life
Rest
Self-Care Status
Self-Care: Activities of Daily Living (ADL)
Self-Care: Instrumental Activities of Daily
   Living (IADL)
Sleep
Stress Level

# *Fear*

**DEFINITION:** Response to a perceived threat that is consciously recognized as a danger

**SUGGESTED OUTCOMES:**
Fear Level
Fear Level: Child
Fear Self-Control

**ADDITIONAL ASSOCIATED OUTCOMES:**

Anxiety Self-Control
Comfort Level
Comfortable Death

Coping
Health Beliefs: Perceived Threat
Pain Level

# *Fluid Balance, Readiness for Enhanced*

**DEFINITION:** A pattern of equilibrium between fluid volume and chemical composition of body fluids that is sufficient for meeting physical needs and can be strengthened

**SUGGESTED OUTCOMES:**
Fluid Balance
Fluid Overload Severity
Hydration
Kidney Function

**ADDITIONAL ASSOCIATED OUTCOMES:**

Appetite
Blood Loss Severity
Cardiac Pump Effectiveness
Knowledge: Disease Process
Knowledge: Treatment Regimen
Nausea & Vomiting Severity

Nutritional Status: Food & Fluid Intake
Thermoregulation
Thermoregulation: Newborn
Vital Signs
Weight: Body Mass

F

## Fluid Volume, Deficient

**DEFINITION:** Decreased intravascular, interstitial and/or intracellular fluid. This refers to dehydration, water loss alone without change in sodium.

**SUGGESTED OUTCOMES:**
Electrolyte & Acid/Base Balance
Fluid Balance
Hydration
Nutritional Status: Food & Fluid Intake

**ADDITIONAL ASSOCIATED OUTCOMES:**
Appetite
Blood Loss Severity
Bowel Elimination
Breastfeeding Establishment: Infant
Breastfeeding Maintenance
Cognition

Knowledge: Medication
Nausea & Vomiting Severity
Thermoregulation
Thermoregulation: Newborn
Urinary Elimination

## Fluid Volume, Excess

**DEFINITION:** Increased isotonic fluid retention.

**SUGGESTED OUTCOMES:**
Electrolyte & Acid/Base Balance
Fluid Balance
Fluid Overload Severity
Kidney Function

**ADDITIONAL ASSOCIATED OUTCOMES:**
Cardiac Pump Effectiveness
Knowledge: Disease Process
Knowledge: Treatment Regimen
Nutritional Status: Food & Fluid Intake
Respiratory Status: Gas Exchange

Self-Care: Parenteral Medication
Urinary Elimination
Vital Signs
Weight: Body Mass

## Fluid Volume, Risk for Deficient

**DEFINITION:** At risk of experiencing vascular, cellular, or intracellular dehydration

**SUGGESTED OUTCOMES:**

Appetite
Blood Loss Severity
Bowel Elimination
Breastfeeding Maintenance
Electrolyte & Acid/Base Balance
Fluid Balance
Hydration
Knowledge: Disease Process
Knowledge: Health Behavior
Knowledge: Medication

Knowledge: Treatment Regimen
Nausea & Vomiting Severity
Nutritional Status: Food & Fluid Intake
Risk Control
Risk Detection
Self-Care Status
Swallowing Status
Thermoregulation
Thermoregulation: Newborn
Urinary Elimination

F

## Fluid Volume, Risk for Imbalanced

**DEFINITION:** A risk of a decrease, increase, or rapid shift from one to the other of intravascular, interstitial, and/or intracellular fluid. This refers to body fluid loss, gain, or both.

**SUGGESTED OUTCOMES:**

Appetite
Blood Loss Severity
Bowel Elimination
Breastfeeding Establishment: Infant
Breastfeeding Maintenance
Cardiac Pump Effectiveness
Electrolyte & Acid/Base Balance
Fluid Balance
Fluid Overload Severity
Hydration
Kidney Function
Knowledge: Disease Process
Knowledge: Health Behavior
Knowledge: Medication

Knowledge: Treatment Regimen
Nausea & Vomiting Severity
Nutritional Status: Food & Fluid Intake
Physical Aging
Post Procedure Recovery Status
Risk Control
Risk Detection
Self-Care Status
Thermoregulation
Thermoregulation: Newborn
Urinary Elimination
Vital Signs
Wound Healing: Secondary Intention

## Gas Exchange, Impaired

**DEFINITION:** Excess or deficit in oxygenation and/or carbon dioxide elimination at the alveolar-capillary membrane

**SUGGESTED OUTCOMES:**

Allergic Response: Systemic
Electrolyte & Acid/Base Balance
Mechanical Ventilation Response: Adult
Respiratory Status: Gas Exchange

Respiratory Status: Ventilation
Tissue Perfusion: Pulmonary
Vital Signs

**ADDITIONAL ASSOCIATED OUTCOMES:**

Asthma Self-Management
Cognition
Cognitive Orientation

Tissue Perfusion: Abdominal Organs
Tissue Perfusion: Cardiac
Tissue Perfusion: Peripheral

## Grieving, Anticipatory

**DEFINITION:** Intellectual and emotional responses and behaviors by which individuals, families, communities work through the process of modifying self-concept based on the perception of potential loss

**SUGGESTED OUTCOMES:**

Adaptation to Physical Disability
Coping
Family Coping

Family Social Climate
Grief Resolution
Psychosocial Adjustment: Life Change

**ADDITIONAL ASSOCIATED OUTCOMES:**

Aggression Self-Control
Caregiver Adaptation to Patient
    Institutionalization
Caregiver Emotional Health
Communication
Depression Level
Depression Self-Control

Dignified Life Closure
Family Resiliency
Hope
Role Performance
Sleep
Spiritual Health

## Grieving, Dysfunctional

**DEFINITION:** Extended, unsuccessful use of intellectual and emotional responses by which individuals, families, communities attempt to work through the process of modifying self-concept based upon the perception of loss

**SUGGESTED OUTCOMES:**

Coping

Family Coping

Family Resiliency

Grief Resolution

Psychosocial Adjustment: Life Change

Role Performance

**ADDITIONAL ASSOCIATED OUTCOMES:**

Aggression Self-Control

Appetite

Communication

Depression Level

Depression Self-Control

Mood Equilibrium

Motivation

Personal Health Status

Self-Esteem

Sleep

## Growth and Development, Delayed

**DEFINITION:** Deviations from age-group norms

**SUGGESTED OUTCOMES:**

Child Development: 1 Month

Child Development: 2 Months

Child Development: 4 Months

Child Development: 6 Months

Child Development: 12 Months

Child Development: 2 Years

Child Development: 3 Years

Child Development: 4 Years

Child Development: Preschool

Child Development: Middle Childhood

Child Development: Adolescence

Growth

Physical Aging

Physical Maturation: Female

Physical Maturation: Male

**ADDITIONAL ASSOCIATED OUTCOMES:**

Abuse Recovery Status

Abuse Recovery: Emotional

Abuse Recovery: Physical

Knowledge: Parenting

Neglect Recovery

Parenting Performance

Personal Autonomy

Psychosocial Adjustment: Life Change

Weight: Body Mass

H

## *Growth, Risk for Disproportionate*

**DEFINITION:** At risk for growth above the 97th percentile or below the 3rd percentile for age, crossing two percentile channels, disproportionate growth

**SUGGESTED OUTCOMES:**

Appetite
Body Image
Child Development: 1 Month
Child Development: 2 Months
Child Development: 4 Months
Child Development: 6 Months
Child Development: 12 Months
Child Development: 2 Years
Child Development: 3 Years
Child Development: 4 Years
Child Development: Preschool
Child Development: Middle Childhood
Child Development: Adolescence

Growth
Infection Severity: Newborn
Knowledge: Infant Care
Knowledge: Preconception Maternal Health
Knowledge: Pregnancy
Parenting Performance
Physical Maturation: Female
Physical Maturation: Male
Prenatal Health Behavior
Risk Control
Risk Detection
Weight: Body Mass

## *Health Maintenance, Ineffective*

**DEFINITION:** Inability to identify, manage, and/or seek out help to maintain health

**SUGGESTED OUTCOMES:**

Health Beliefs: Perceived Resources
Health Promoting Behavior
Health Seeking Behavior
Knowledge: Health Behavior
Knowledge: Health Promotion
Knowledge: Health Resources

Knowledge: Treatment Regimen
Participation in Health Care Decisions
Personal Health Status
Risk Detection
Self-Care Status
Student Health Status

**ADDITIONAL ASSOCIATED OUTCOMES:**

Adaptation to Physical Disability
Anxiety Self-Control
Cognition
Communication
Community Risk Control: Chronic Disease
Coping
Decision-Making
Grief Resolution
Information Processing

Motivation
Psychosocial Adjustment: Life Change
Risk Control
Self-Direction of Care
Social Support
Spiritual Health
Symptom Control
Treatment Behavior: Illness or Injury

## *Health Seeking Behaviors (Specify)*

**DEFINITION:** Active seeking (by a person in stable health) of ways to alter personal health habits and/or the environment in order to move toward a higher level of health

**SUGGESTED OUTCOMES:**

Adherence Behavior
Health Beliefs
Health Orientation
Health Promoting Behavior
Health Seeking Behavior

Knowledge: Health Promotion
Knowledge: Health Resources
Personal Health Status
Personal Well-Being

**ADDITIONAL ASSOCIATED OUTCOMES:**

Adaptation to Physical Disability
Body Mechanics Performance
Energy Conservation
Motivation
Participation in Health Care Decisions
Personal Safety Behavior
Psychosocial Adjustment: Life Change
Quality of Life
Risk Control
Risk Control: Alcohol Use

Risk Control: Cancer
Risk Control: Cardiovascular Health
Risk Control: Drug Use
Risk Control: Hearing Impairment
Risk Control: Sexually Transmitted Diseases
  (STD)
Risk Control: Tobacco Use
Risk Control: Unintended Pregnancy
Risk Control: Visual Impairment
Safe Home Environment

## *Home Maintenance, Impaired*

**DEFINITION:** Inability to independently maintain a safe growth-promoting immediate environment

**SUGGESTED OUTCOMES:**

Family Functioning
Family Physical Environment
Parenting Performance
Parenting: Psychosocial Safety

Role Performance
Safe Home Environment
Self Care: Instrumental Activities of Daily
  Living (IADL)

**ADDITIONAL ASSOCIATED OUTCOMES:**

Caregiver Emotional Health
Caregiver Physical Health
Client Satisfaction: Physical Environment
Cognition
Discharge Readiness: Independent Living
Mobility

H

## Hopelessness

**DEFINITION:** Subjective state in which an individual sees limited or no alternatives or personal choices available and is unable to mobilize energy on own behalf

**SUGGESTED OUTCOMES:**

Depression Self-Control
Hope
Mood Equilibrium

Psychomotor Energy
Quality of Life
Will to Live

**ADDITIONAL ASSOCIATED OUTCOMES:**

Acceptance: Health Status
Adaptation to Physical Disability
Comfort Level
Coping
Decision-Making
Depression Level
Fear Self-Control
Grief Resolution
Immobility Consequences: Psycho-Cognitive

Motivation
Pain: Adverse Psychological Response
Pain Control
Pain: Disruptive Effects
Sleep
Spiritual Health
Suffering Severity
Symptom Severity

## Hyperthermia

**DEFINITION:**  Body temperature elevated above normal range

**SUGGESTED OUTCOMES:**

Thermoregulation
Thermoregulation: Newborn
Vital Signs

**ADDITIONAL ASSOCIATED OUTCOMES:**

Blood Transfusion Reaction
Comfort Level
Hydration
Immune Status
Infection Severity
Neurological Status: Autonomic

# Hypothermia

**DEFINITION:** Body temperature below normal range

**SUGGESTED OUTCOMES:**
Thermoregulation
Thermoregulation: Newborn
Vital Signs

**ADDITIONAL ASSOCIATED OUTCOMES:**
Comfort Level
Neurological Status: Autonomic

# Infant Behavior, Disorganized

**DEFINITION:** Disintegrated physiological and neurobehavioral responses to the environment

**SUGGESTED OUTCOMES:**

Child Development: 1 Month
Child Development: 2 Months
Neurological Status

Preterm Infant Organization
Sleep
Thermoregulation: Newborn

**ADDITIONAL ASSOCIATED OUTCOMES:**

Breastfeeding Establishment: Infant
Child Development: 4 Months
Child Development: 6 Months
Child Development: 12 Months

Comfort Level
Knowledge: Infant Care
Nutritional Status: Food & Fluid Intake
Vital Signs

# Infant Behavior, Risk for Disorganized

**DEFINITION:** Risk for alteration in integrating and modulation of the physiological and behavioral systems of functioning (i.e., autonomic, motor, state, organizational, self-regulatory, and attentional-interactional systems)

**SUGGESTED OUTCOMES:**

Child Development: 1 Month
Child Development: 2 Months
Child Development: 4 Months
Child Development: 6 Months
Child Development: 12 Months
Coordinated Movement
Knowledge: Infant Care

Knowledge: Parenting
Neurological Status
Preterm Infant Organization
Risk Control
Risk Detection
Sleep
Thermoregulation: Newborn

I

## *Infant Behavior: Organized, Readiness for Enhanced*

DEFINITION: A pattern of modulation of the physiologic and behavioral systems of functioning (i.e., autonomic, motor, state-organizational, self-regulatory, and attentional-interactional systems) in an infant that is satisfactory but that can be improved, resulting in higher levels of integration in response to environmental stimuli

SUGGESTED OUTCOMES:
Child Development: 1 Month
Child Development: 2 Months
Neurological Status
Sleep
Thermoregulation: Newborn

ADDITIONAL ASSOCIATED OUTCOMES:
Child Development: 4 Months
Child Development: 6 Months
Child Development: 12 Months
Knowledge: Infant Care

Knowledge: Parenting
Pain Level
Parent-Infant Attachment

## *Infant Feeding Pattern, Ineffective*

DEFINITION: Impaired ability to suck or coordinate the suck swallow response

SUGGESTED OUTCOMES:
Aspiration Prevention
Breastfeeding Establishment: Infant
Breastfeeding: Maintenance
Hydration
Nutritional Status: Food & Fluid Intake
Swallowing Status

ADDITIONAL ASSOCIATED OUTCOMES:
Bowel Elimination
Breastfeeding Establishment: Maternal
Knowledge: Breastfeeding
Neurological Status
Nutritional Status: Biochemical Measures

Swallowing Status: Esophageal Phase
Swallowing Status: Oral Phase
Swallowing Status: Pharyngeal Phase
Urinary Elimination
Weight: Body Mass

## Infection, Risk for

**DEFINITION:** At increased risk for being invaded by pathogenic organisms

**SUGGESTED OUTCOMES:**

Aspiration Prevention
Community Risk Control: Communicable
    Disease
Health Beliefs
Hemodialysis Access
Immobility Consequences: Physiological
Immune Status
Immunization Behavior
Infection Severity
Infection Severity: Newborn
Knowledge: Infection Control

Knowledge: Treatment Procedure(s)
Nutritional Status
Risk Control
Risk Control: Sexually Transmitted Diseases
    (STD)
Risk Detection
Self-Care: Hygiene
Tissue Integrity: Skin & Mucous Membranes
Treatment Behavior: Illness or Injury
Wound Healing: Primary Intention
Wound Healing: Secondary Intention

## Injury, Risk for

**DEFINITION:** At risk of injury as a result of environmental conditions interacting with the individual's adaptive and defensive resources

**SUGGESTED OUTCOMES:**

Abuse Protection
Allergic Response: Systemic
Aspiration Prevention
Balance
Blood Glucose Level
Blood Loss Severity
Coordinated Movement
Fall Prevention Behavior
Falls Occurrence
Knowledge: Body Mechanics
Knowledge: Child Physical Safety
Knowledge: Fall Prevention
Knowledge: Personal Safety
Maternal Status: Postpartum

Parenting: Infant/Toddler Physical Safety
Parenting: Early/Middle Childhood Physical
    Safety
Parenting: Psychosocial Safety
Personal Safety Behavior
Physical Injury Severity
Risk Control
Risk Control: Hearing Impairment
Risk Control: Visual Impairment
Risk Detection
Safe Home Environment
Seizure Control
Self-Care Status

I

## Intracranial Adaptive Capacity, Decreased

**DEFINITION:** Intracranial fluid dynamic mechanisms that normally compensate for increases in intracranial volumes are comprised, resulting in repeated disproportionate increases in intracranial pressure (ICP) in response to a variety of noxious and non-noxious stimuli

**SUGGESTED OUTCOMES:**
Neurological Status
Neurological Status: Consciousness
Seizure Control
Tissue Perfusion: Cerebral

**ADDITIONAL ASSOCIATED OUTCOMES:**

Cognition
Cognitive Orientation
Communication
Electrolyte & Acid/Base Balance
Fluid Balance
Neurological Status: Autonomic

Neurological Status: Central Motor Control
Neurological Status: Cranial Sensory/Motor
   Function
Neurological Status: Spinal Sensory/Motor
   Function

**K**

## Knowledge, Deficient (Specify)

**DEFINITION:** Absence or deficiency of cognitive information related to specific topic

**SUGGESTED OUTCOMES:**

Knowledge: Body Mechanics
Knowledge: Breastfeeding
Knowledge: Cardiac Disease Management
Knowledge: Child Physical Safety
Knowledge: Conception Prevention
Knowledge: Diabetes Management
Knowledge: Diet
Knowledge: Disease Process
Knowledge: Energy Conservation
Knowledge: Fall Prevention
Knowledge: Fertility Promotion
Knowledge: Health Behavior
Knowledge: Health Promotion
Knowledge: Health Resources
Knowledge: Illness Care

Knowledge: Infant Care
Knowledge: Infection Control
Knowledge: Labor & Delivery
Knowledge: Medication
Knowledge: Ostomy Care
Knowledge: Parenting
Knowledge: Personal Safety
Knowledge: Postpartum Maternal Health
Knowledge: Preconception Maternal Health
Knowledge: Pregnancy
Knowledge: Prescribed Activity
Knowledge: Sexual Functioning
Knowledge: Substance Use Control
Knowledge: Treatment Procedure(s)
Knowledge: Treatment Regimen

**ADDITIONAL ASSOCIATED OUTCOMES:**

Client Satisfaction: Teaching
Cognition
Communication: Receptive
Concentration

Information Processing
Memory
Motivation
Stress Level

## Knowledge (Specify), Readiness for Enhanced

**DEFINITION:** The presence or acquisition of cognitive information related to a specific topic is sufficient for meeting health-related goals and can be strengthened

**SUGGESTED OUTCOMES:**

Knowledge: Body Mechanics
Knowledge: Breastfeeding
Knowledge: Cardiac Disease Management
Knowledge: Child Physical Safety
Knowledge: Conception Prevention
Knowledge: Diabetes Management
Knowledge: Diet
Knowledge: Disease Process
Knowledge: Energy Conservation
Knowledge: Fall Prevention
Knowledge: Fertility Promotion
Knowledge: Health Behavior
Knowledge: Health Promotion
Knowledge: Health Resources
Knowledge: Illness Care

Knowledge: Infant Care
Knowledge: Infection Control
Knowledge: Labor & Delivery
Knowledge: Medication
Knowledge: Ostomy Care
Knowledge: Parenting
Knowledge: Personal Safety
Knowledge: Postpartum Maternal Health
Knowledge: Preconception Maternal Health
Knowledge: Pregnancy
Knowledge: Prescribed Activity
Knowledge: Sexual Functioning
Knowledge: Substance Use Control
Knowledge: Treatment Procedure(s)
Knowledge: Treatment Regimen

**ADDITIONAL ASSOCIATED OUTCOMES:**

Client Satisfaction: Teaching
Cognition
Communication: Receptive
Concentration
Information Processing
Memory
Motivation
Stress Level

## Latex Allergy Response

**DEFINITION:** An allergic response to natural latex rubber products

**SUGGESTED OUTCOMES:**

Allergic Response: Localized
Immune Hypersensitivity Response
Tissue Integrity: Skin & Mucous Membranes

**ADDITIONAL ASSOCIATED OUTCOMES:**

Comfort Level
Infection Severity
Knowledge: Infection Control
Knowledge: Treatment Regimen
Symptom Severity

## Latex Allergy Response, Risk for

**DEFINITION:** At risk for allergic response to natural latex rubber products

**SUGGESTED OUTCOMES:**

Allergic Response: Localized
Immune Hypersensitivity Response
Knowledge: Health Behavior

Risk Control
Risk Detection
Tissue Integrity: Skin & Mucous Membranes

## Loneliness, Risk for

**DEFINITION:** At risk for experiencing vague dysphoria

**SUGGESTED OUTCOMES:**

Adaptation to Physical Disability
Communication
Family Functioning
Family Integrity
Family Social Climate
Grief Resolution
Immobility Consequences: Psycho-Cognitive
Leisure Participation

Loneliness Severity
Neglect Cessation
Psychosocial Adjustment: Life Change
Risk Control
Risk Detection
Social Interaction Skills
Social Involvement
Social Support

## Memory, Impaired

**DEFINITION:** Inability to remember or recall bits of information or behavioral skills.*
May be attributed to pathophysiological or situational causes that are either temporary or permanent.

**SUGGESTED OUTCOMES:**

Cognition
Cognitive Orientation
Concentration

Memory
Neurological Status
Neurological Status: Consciousness

**ADDITIONAL ASSOCIATED OUTCOMES:**

Anxiety Level
Cardiac Pump Effectiveness
Circulation Status
Depression Level
Discharge Readiness: Supported Living
Electrolyte & Acid/Base Balance

Hydration
Medication Response
Physical Aging
Respiratory Status: Gas Exchange
Respiratory Status: Ventilation
Stress Level

## Mobility: Bed, Impaired

**DEFINITION:** Limitation of independent movement from one bed position to another

**SUGGESTED OUTCOMES:**

Body Mechanics Performance
Body Positioning: Self-Initiated
Coordinated Movement

Immobility Consequences: Physiological
Mobility

**ADDITIONAL ASSOCIATED OUTCOMES:**

Cognition
Endurance
Immobility Consequences: Psycho-Cognitive
Joint Movement: Ankle
Joint Movement: Elbow
Joint Movement: Fingers
Joint Movement: Hip
Joint Movement: Knee
Joint Movement: Neck

Joint Movement: Shoulder
Joint Movement: Spine
Joint Movement: Wrist
Knowledge: Body Mechanics
Neurological Status
Neurological Status: Central Motor Control
Pain Level
Rest
Skeletal Function

**M**

## Mobility: Physical, Impaired

**DEFINITION:** Limitation in independent, purposeful physical movement of the body or of one or more extremities

**SUGGESTED OUTCOMES:**

Ambulation
Ambulation: Wheelchair
Balance
Body Mechanics Performance

Body Positioning: Self-Initiated
Coordinated Movement
Mobility
Transfer Performance

**ADDITIONAL ASSOCIATED OUTCOMES:**

Cognition
Endurance
Energy Conservation
Fall Prevention Behavior
Health Beliefs: Perceived Ability to Perform
Health Orientation
Immobility Consequences: Physiological
Immobility Consequences: Psycho-Cognitive
Joint Movement: Ankle
Joint Movement: Elbow
Joint Movement: Hip
Joint Movement: Knee
Joint Movement: Shoulder

Joint Movement: Spine
Knowledge: Prescribed Activity
Motivation
Neurological Status: Spinal Sensory/Motor
    Function
Nutritional Status: Energy
Pain Level
Psychomotor Energy
Self Care: Activities of Daily Living (ADL)
Sensory Function Status
Sensory Function: Cutaneous
Sensory Function: Proprioception
Sensory Function: Vision

## *Mobility: Wheelchair, Impaired*

**DEFINITION:** Limitation of independent operation of wheelchair within environment

**SUGGESTED OUTCOMES:**

Adaptation to Physical Disability
Ambulation: Wheelchair
Balance

Coordinated Movement
Mobility
Transfer Performance

**ADDITIONAL ASSOCIATED OUTCOMES:**

Body Mechanics Performance
Cognition
Endurance
Fall Prevention Behavior
Immobility Consequences: Physiological
Immobility Consequences: Psycho-Cognitive
Joint Movement: Elbow

Joint Movement: Fingers
Joint Movement: Shoulder
Joint Movement: Wrist
Knowledge: Body Mechanics
Neurological Status
Physical Fitness

## *Nausea*

**DEFINITION:** A subjective unpleasant, wavelike sensation in the back of the throat, epigastrium, or abdomen that may lead to the urge or need to vomit

**SUGGESTED OUTCOMES:**

Appetite
Comfort Level
Hydration
Nausea & Vomiting Control
Nausea & Vomiting: Disruptive Effects
Nausea & Vomiting Severity
Nutritional Status: Food & Fluid Intake

**ADDITIONAL ASSOCIATED OUTCOMES:**

Client Satisfaction: Symptom Control
Electrolyte & Acid/Base Balance
Fluid Balance
Infection Severity
Kidney Function
Maternal Status: Antepartum

Medication Response
Pain Level
Suffering Severity
Symptom Control
Symptom Severity

**M**

## *Noncompliance*

**DEFINITION:** Behavior of person and/or caregiver that fails to coincide with a health-promoting or therapeutic plan agreed on by the person (and/or family and/or community) and healthcare professional. In the presence of an agreed-on, health-promoting or therapeutic plan, person's or caregiver's behavior is fully or partially nonadherent and may lead to clinically ineffective or partially ineffective outcomes.

**SUGGESTED OUTCOMES:**

Adherence Behavior
Caregiver Performance: Direct Care
Caregiver Performance: Indirect Care
Compliance Behavior

Motivation
Symptom Control
Treatment Behaviors: Illness or Injury

**ADDITIONAL ASSOCIATED OUTCOMES:**

Acceptance: Health Status
Adaptation to Physical Disability
Caregiver-Patient Relationship
Caregiver Stressors
Family Coping
Family Participation in Professional Care
Family Resiliency
Health Beliefs
Health Beliefs: Perceived Ability to Perform
Health Beliefs: Perceived Control

Health Beliefs: Perceived Resources
Health Beliefs: Perceived Threat
Health Orientation
Knowledge: Disease Process
Knowledge: Treatment Regimen
Participation in Health Care Decisions
Self-Care: Non-Parenteral Medication
Self-Care: Parenteral Medication
Will to Live

**N**

## *Nutrition: Imbalanced, Less than Body Requirements*

**DEFINITION:** Intake of nutrients insufficient to meet metabolic needs

**SUGGESTED OUTCOMES:**

Appetite
Breastfeeding Establishment: Infant
Nutritional Status
Nutritional Status: Food & Fluid Intake

Nutritional Status: Nutrient Intake
Self-Care: Eating
Weight: Body Mass

**ADDITIONAL ASSOCIATED OUTCOMES:**

Adherence Behavior
Body Image
Bowel Elimination
Compliance Behavior
Depression Level
Endurance
Health Beliefs
Hydration

Knowledge: Diet
Nausea & Vomiting Severity
Nutritional Status: Biochemical Measures
Nutritional Status: Energy
Sensory Function: Taste & Smell
Symptom Control
Symptom Severity
Weight Control

## Nutrition: Imbalanced, More than Body Requirements

DEFINITION: Intake of nutrients that exceeds metabolic needs

SUGGESTED OUTCOMES:

Nutritional Status                       Weight: Body Mass
Nutritional Status: Food & Fluid Intake  Weight Control
Nutritional Status: Nutrient Intake

ADDITIONAL ASSOCIATED OUTCOMES:

Adherence Behavior          Health Beliefs: Perceived Ability to Perform
Body Image                  Knowledge: Diet
Compliance Behavior         Motivation
Depression Level            Stress Level
Health Beliefs

## Nutrition: Imbalanced, Risk for More Than Body Requirements

DEFINITION: At risk for an intake of nutrients that exceeds metabolic needs

SUGGESTED OUTCOMES:

Knowledge: Diet                          Risk Detection
Nutritional Status                       Stress Level
Nutritional Status: Food & Fluid Intake  Weight: Body Mass
Nutritional Status: Nutrient Intake      Weight Control
Risk Control

## Nutrition, Readiness for Enhanced

DEFINITION: A pattern of nutrient intake that is sufficient for meeting metabolic needs and can be strengthened

SUGGESTED OUTCOMES:

Knowledge: Diet
Nutritional Status
Nutritional Status: Food & Fluid Intake
Nutritional Status: Nutrient Intake

ADDITIONAL ASSOCIATED OUTCOMES:

Appetite                                 Symptom Control
Breastfeeding Establishment: Infant      Symptom Severity
Sensory Function: Taste & Smell          Weight Control
Stress Level

## Oral Mucous Membrane, Impaired

**DEFINITION:** Disruption of the lips and soft tissue of the oral cavity

**SUGGESTED OUTCOMES:**
Oral Hygiene
Tissue Integrity: Skin & Mucous Membrane

**ADDITIONAL ASSOCIATED OUTCOMES:**
Allergic Response: Localized
Hydration
Immune Status
Infection Severity
Infection Severity: Newborn
Nausea & Vomiting Severity
Nutritional Status
Nutritional Status: Food & Fluid Intake
Pain Level
Self-Care: Oral Hygiene
Swallowing Status
Swallowing Status: Oral Phase

## Pain, Acute

**DEFINITION:** Unpleasant sensory and emotional experience arising from actual or potential tissue damage or described in terms of such damage (International Association for the Study of Pain); sudden or slow onset of any intensity from mild to severe with an anticipated or predictable end and a duration of less than 6 months

**SUGGESTED OUTCOMES:**
Comfort Level
Pain Control
Pain Level
Stress Level

**P**

**ADDITIONAL ASSOCIATED OUTCOMES:**
Anxiety Level
Client Satisfaction: Symptom Control
Fear Level
Fear Level: Child
Nausea & Vomiting Severity
Personal Well-Being
Rest
Sleep
Symptom Control
Symptom Severity
Symptom Severity: Perimenopause
Symptom Severity: Premenstrual Syndrome
(PMS)
Vital Signs

## *Pain, Chronic*

**DEFINITION:** Unpleasant sensory and emotional experience arising from actual or potential tissue damage or described in terms of such damage (International Association for the Study of Pain); sudden or slow onset of any intensity from mild to severe, constant or recurring without an anticipated or predictable end and a duration of greater than 6 months

**SUGGESTED OUTCOMES:**

Comfort Level

Depression Level

Pain: Adverse Psychological Response

Pain Control

Pain: Disruptive Effects

Pain Level

**ADDITIONAL ASSOCIATED OUTCOMES:**

Client Satisfaction: Symptom Control

Depression Self-Control

Personal Well-Being

Quality of Life

Rest

Sleep

Stress Level

Symptom Control

Symptom Severity

Will to Live

## *Parent/Infant/Child Attachment, Risk for Impaired*

**DEFINITION:** Disruption of the interactive process between parent/significant other, child, and infant that fosters the development of a protective and nurturing reciprocal relationship

**SUGGESTED OUTCOMES:**

Caregiver Adaptation to Patient
    Institutionalization

Caregiver Performance: Direct Care

Child Development: 1 Month

Child Development: 2 Months

Child Development: 4 Months

Child Development: 6 Months

Child Development: 12 Months

Cognition

Coping

Depression Self-Control

Family Functioning

Family Social Climate

Knowledge: Parenting

Parent-Infant Attachment

Parenting Performance

Risk Control

Risk Detection

Role Performance

Social Interaction Skills

Stress Level

Substance Addiction Consequences

## *Parental Role Conflict*

DEFINITION: Parent experience of role confusion and conflict in response to crisis

SUGGESTED OUTCOMES:

Caregiver Adaptation to Patient
   Institutionalization
Caregiver Home Care Readiness
Caregiver Lifestyle Disruption
Coping

Family Functioning
Family Social Climate
Parenting Performance
Psychosocial Adjustment: Life Change
Role Performance

ADDITIONAL ASSOCIATED OUTCOMES:

Anxiety Self-Control
Caregiver Performance: Direct Care
Caregiver Performance: Indirect Care
Caregiver Physical Health
Caregiver Stressors
Family Coping

Family Health Status
Family Normalization
Family Resiliency
Knowledge: Infant Care
Parent-Infant Attachment

## *Parenting, Impaired*

DEFINITION: Inability of the primary caretaker to create, maintain, or regain an environment that promotes the optimum growth and development of the child

SUGGESTED OUTCOMES:

Child Development: 1 Month
Child Development: 2 Months
Child Development: 4 Months
Child Development: 6 Months
Child Development: 12 Months
Child Development: 2 Years
Child Development: 3 Years
Child Development: 4 Years
Child Development: Preschool

Child Development: Middle Childhood
Child Development: Adolescence
Family Coping
Family Functioning
Family Social Climate
Parent-Infant Attachment
Parenting Performance
Parenting: Psychosocial Safety
Role Performance

ADDITIONAL ASSOCIATED OUTCOMES:

Abuse Cessation
Abuse Protection
Abuse Recovery Status
Abusive Behavior Self-Restraint
Anxiety Level
Anxiety Self-Control
Caregiver Performance: Direct Care
Caregiver Performance: Indirect Care
Cognition
Coping
Depression Level
Depression Self-Control
Family Physical Environment

Knowledge: Child Physical Safety
Knowledge: Infant Care
Knowledge: Parenting
Motivation
Neglect Recovery
Parenting: Adolescent Physical Safety
Parenting: Early/Middle Childhood Physical
   Safety
Parenting: Infant/Toddler Physical Safety
Psychosocial Adjustment: Life Change
Social Interaction Skills
Social Support
Stress Level

P

## Parenting, Readiness for Enhanced

**DEFINITION:** A pattern of providing an environment for children or other dependent person(s) that is sufficient to nurture growth and development and can be strengthened

**SUGGESTED OUTCOMES:**

Family Functioning
Knowledge: Child Physical Safety
Knowledge: Infant Care

Knowledge: Parenting
Parenting Performance
Parenting: Psychosocial Safety

**ADDITIONAL ASSOCIATED OUTCOMES:**

Child Development: 1 Month
Child Development: 2 Months
Child Development: 4 Months
Child Development: 6 Months
Child Development: 12 Months
Child Development: 2 Years
Child Development: 3 Years
Child Development: 4 Years
Child Development: Preschool
Child Development: Middle Childhood

Child Development: Adolescence
Family Coping
Family Normalization
Family Physical Environment
Family Social Climate
Parenting: Adolescent Physical Safety
Parenting: Early/Middle Childhood Physical
   Safety
Parenting: Infant/Toddler Physical Safety

## Parenting, Risk for Impaired

**DEFINITION:** Risk for inability of the primary caretaker to create, maintain, or regain an environment that promotes the optimum growth and development of the child

**SUGGESTED OUTCOMES:**

Abuse Recovery Status
Abuse Recovery: Emotional
Abuse Recovery: Physical
Abuse Recovery: Sexual
Abusive Behavior Self-Restraint
Aggression Self-Control
Caregiver Emotional Health
Caregiver Physical Health
Caregiver Stressors
Caregiver Well-Being
Cognition
Coping
Decision-Making
Distorted Thought Self-Control
Family Coping
Family Health Status

Family Normalization
Family Resiliency
Family Social Climate
Knowledge: Health Resources
Knowledge: Infant Care
Knowledge: Parenting
Parent-Infant Attachment
Parenting Performance
Risk Control
Risk Control: Alcohol Use
Risk Control: Drug Use
Risk Control: Tobacco Use
Risk Detection
Role Performance
Social Interaction Skills
Social Support

## Perioperative Positioning Injury, Risk for

**DEFINITION:** At risk for injury as a result of the environmental conditions found in the perioperative setting

**SUGGESTED OUTCOMES:**

Allergic Response: Systemic
Aspiration Prevention
Blood Coagulation
Blood Loss Severity
Circulation Status
Cognition
Cognitive Orientation
Fluid Overload Severity
Immune Status
Medication Response

Neurological Status: Spinal Sensory/Motor
    Function
Respiratory Status: Gas Exchange
Respiratory Status: Ventilation
Risk Control
Risk Detection
Thermoregulation
Tissue Integrity: Skin & Mucous Membranes
Tissue Perfusion: Peripheral

## Peripheral Neurovascular Dysfunction, Risk for

**DEFINITION:** At risk for disruption in circulation, sensation or motion of an extremity

**SUGGESTED OUTCOMES:**

Blood Coagulation
Body Positioning: Self-Initiated
Bone Healing
Circulation Status
Coordinated Movement
Joint Movement: Ankle
Joint Movement: Elbow
Joint Movement: Hip
Joint Movement: Knee
Mobility

Neurological Status
Neurological Status: Cranial Sensory/Motor
    Function
Neurological Status: Spinal Sensory/Motor
    Function
Physical Injury Severity
Risk Control
Risk Detection
Tissue Perfusion: Peripheral

**P**

## Personal Identity, Disturbed

**DEFINITION:** Inability to distinguish between self and nonself

**SUGGESTED OUTCOMES:**

Distorted Thought Self-Control
Identity
Self-Mutilation Restraint

**ADDITIONAL ASSOCIATED OUTCOMES:**

Anxiety Level
Anxiety Self-Control
Depression Level

Depression Self-Control
Sexual Identity

## Poisoning, Risk for

**DEFINITION:** Accentuated risk of accidental exposure to, or ingestion of, drugs or dangerous products in doses sufficient to cause poisoning

**SUGGESTED OUTCOMES:**

Caregiver Performance: Direct Care
Cognition
Community Risk Control: Lead Exposure
Family Physical Environment
Knowledge: Medication
Parenting: Adolescent Physical Safety
Parenting: Early/Middle Childhood Physical Safety
Parenting: Infant/Toddler Physical Safety

Personal Safety Behavior
Risk Control
Risk Control: Alcohol Use
Risk Control: Drug Use
Risk Detection
Safe Home Environment
Self-Care: Non-Parenteral Medication
Self-Care: Parental Medication

## Post-Trauma Syndrome

**DEFINITION:** Sustained maladaptive response to a traumatic, overwhelming event

**SUGGESTED OUTCOMES:**

Abuse Recovery: Emotional
Abuse Recovery: Financial
Abuse Recovery: Physical
Abuse Recovery: Sexual
Anxiety Level
Coping
Depression Level

Fear Level
Fear Level: Child
Impulse Self-Control
Self-Mutilation Restraint
Stress Level
Suicide Self-Restraint

**ADDITIONAL ASSOCIATED OUTCOMES:**

Abuse Cessation
Abuse Protection
Abuse Recovery Status
Adaptation to Physical Disability
Aggression Self-Control
Anxiety Self-Control
Body Image
Cognition
Concentration
Depression Self-Control
Distorted Thought Self-Control
Fear Self-Control

Grief Resolution
Hope
Information Processing
Personal Safety Behavior
Psychosocial Adjustment: Life Change
Quality of Life
Risk Detection
Self-Esteem
Sleep
Social Support
Will to Live

P

## Post-Trauma Syndrome, Risk for

**DEFINITION:** At risk for sustained maladaptive response to a traumatic, overwhelming event

**SUGGESTED OUTCOMES:**

Abuse Cessation
Abuse Protection
Abuse Recovery Status
Abuse Recovery: Emotional
Abuse Recovery: Sexual
Adaptation to Physical Disability
Aggression Self-Control
Anxiety Level
Anxiety Self-Control
Body Image
Cognition
Coping
Depression Level
Depression Self-Control
Distorted Thought Self-Control
Grief Resolution

Impulse Self-Control
Information Processing
Mood Equilibrium
Psychosocial Adjustment: Life Change
Quality of Life
Risk Control
Risk Control: Drug Use
Risk Detection
Self-Esteem
Self-Mutilation Restraint
Sleep
Social Support
Spiritual Health
Stress Level
Suicide Self-Restraint

## Powerlessness

**DEFINITION:** Perception that one's own action will not significantly affect an outcome; a perceived lack of control over a current situation or immediate happening

**P**

**SUGGESTED OUTCOMES:**

Family Participation in Professional Care
Health Beliefs
Health Beliefs: Perceived Ability to Perform
Health Beliefs: Perceived Control
Health Beliefs: Perceived Resources

Hope
Participation in Health Care Decisions
Personal Autonomy
Self-Esteem

**ADDITIONAL ASSOCIATED OUTCOMES:**

Abuse Recovery Status
Anxiety Level
Anxiety Self-Control
Client Satisfaction: Access to Care Resources
Client Satisfaction: Protection of Rights
Decision-Making
Depression Level
Depression Self-Control

Family Resiliency
Health Orientation
Information Processing
Social Interaction Skills
Social Involvement
Social Support
Stress Level

## Powerlessness, Risk for

**DEFINITION:** At risk for perceived lack of control over a situation and/or one's ability to significantly affect an outcome

**SUGGESTED OUTCOMES:**

Abuse Recovery Status
Anxiety Level
Anxiety Self-Control
Decision-Making
Depression Level
Depression Self-Control
Fear Level
Fear Self-Control
Health Beliefs
Health Beliefs: Perceived Ability to Perform
Health Beliefs: Perceived Control
Health Beliefs: Perceived Resources
Immobility Consequences: Psycho-Cognitive
Information Processing
Participation in Health Care Decisions
Personal Autonomy
Risk Control
Risk Detection
Self-Esteem
Social Interaction Skills
Social Involvement
Social Support
Stress Level

## Protection, Ineffective

**DEFINITION:** Decrease in the ability to guard the self from internal or external threats such as illness or injury

**SUGGESTED OUTCOMES:**

Abuse Protection
Community Violence Level
Health Beliefs: Perceived Ability to Perform
Health Promoting Behavior
Immune Status
Immunization Behavior
Knowledge: Personal Safety
Personal Autonomy

**ADDITIONAL ASSOCIATED OUTCOMES:**

Blood Coagulation
Client Satisfaction: Safety
Cognition
Cognitive Orientation
Community Health Status: Immunity
Community Risk Control: Violence
Coping
Endurance
Infection Severity
Infection Severity: Newborn
Information Processing
Knowledge: Body Mechanics
Knowledge: Health Promotion
Knowledge: Health Resources
Knowledge: Infection Control
Neurological Status: Consciousness
Nutritional Status
Participation in Health Care Decisions
Respiratory Status: Ventilation
Risk Control
Risk Detection
Self-Direction of Care
Sleep
Stress Level
Symptom Severity
Tissue Integrity: Skin & Mucous Membranes
Wound Healing: Primary Intention
Wound Healing: Secondary Intention

P

# Rape-Trauma Syndrome

**DEFINITION:** Sustained maladaptive response to a forced, violent sexual penetration against the victim's will and consent

**SUGGESTED OUTCOMES:**

Abuse Protection
Abuse Recovery: Emotional
Abuse Recovery: Sexual

Coping
Sexual Functioning
Stress Level

**ADDITIONAL ASSOCIATED OUTCOMES:**

Abuse Cessation
Abuse Recovery Status
Anxiety Level
Anxiety Self-Control
Body Image
Cognition
Depression Level
Depression Self-Control
Distorted Thought Self-Control
Fear Level
Fear Self-Control

Grief Resolution
Impulse Self-Control
Personal Autonomy
Personal Well-Being
Quality of Life
Self-Esteem
Self-Mutilation Restraint
Sleep
Social Involvement
Will to Live

# Rape-Trauma Syndrome: Compound Reaction

**DEFINITION:** Forced violent sexual penetration against the victim's will and consent. The trauma syndrome that develops from this attack or attempted attack includes an acute phase of disorganization of the victim's lifestyle and a long-term process of reorganization of lifestyle.

**SUGGESTED OUTCOMES:**

Abuse Recovery: Emotional
Abuse Recovery: Sexual
Personal Autonomy
Psychosocial Adjustment: Life Change

Self-Esteem
Sexual Functioning
Stress Level

**ADDITIONAL ASSOCIATED OUTCOMES:**

Abuse Cessation
Abuse Protection
Abuse Recovery Status
Anxiety Level
Anxiety Self-Control
Decision-Making
Depression Level
Depression Self-Control
Family Coping
Family Normalization
Fear Level

Fear Self-Control
Mood Equilibrium
Personal Well-Being
Quality of Life
Risk Control: Alcohol Use
Risk Control: Drug Use
Sleep
Social Interaction Skills
Social Involvement
Will to Live

R

## Rape-Trauma Syndrome: Silent Reaction

DEFINITION: Forced violent sexual penetration against the victim's will and consent. The trauma syndrome that develops from this attack or attempted attack includes an acute phase of disorganization of the victim's lifestyle and a long-term process of reorganization of lifestyle.

SUGGESTED OUTCOMES:

Abuse Protection
Abuse Recovery: Emotional
Abuse Recovery: Sexual
Anxiety Level

Anxiety Self-Control
Fear Control
Sexual Functioning

ADDITIONAL ASSOCIATED OUTCOMES:

Abuse Cessation
Abuse Recovery Status
Depression Level
Depression Self-Control
Fear Level
Fear Self-Control
Mood Equilibrium

Personal Autonomy
Personal Well-Being
Self-Esteem
Social Interaction Skills
Social Involvement
Stress Level

## Relocation Stress Syndrome

DEFINITION: Physiological and/or psychosocial disturbance following transfer from one environment to another

SUGGESTED OUTCOMES:

Anxiety Level
Child Adaptation to Hospitalization
Coping
Depression Level

Loneliness Severity
Psychosocial Adjustment: Life Change
Quality of Life
Stress Level

ADDITIONAL ASSOCIATED OUTCOMES:

Anxiety Self-Control
Caregiver Adaptation to Patient
    Institutionalization
Caregiver Home Care Readiness
Cognition
Depression Self-Control
Discharge Readiness: Independent Living
Discharge Readiness: Supported Living
Family Participation in Professional Care
Grief Resolution

Information Processing
Memory
Mood Equilibrium
Participation in Health Care Decisions
Self-Care: Activities of Daily Living (ADL)
Self-Direction of Care
Sleep
Social Involvement
Social Support

R

# Relocation Stress Syndrome, Risk for

**DEFINITION:** At risk for physiological and/or psychosocial disturbance following transfer from one environment to another

**SUGGESTED OUTCOMES:**

Acceptance: Health Status
Adaptation to Physical Disability
Anxiety Level
Anxiety Self-Control
Child Adaptation to Hospitalization
Cognition
Discharge Readiness: Supported Living
Family Participation in Professional Care
Information Processing
Knowledge: Health Resources
Leisure Participation
Memory
Mobility

Participation in Health Care Decisions
Personal Health Status
Risk Control
Risk Detection
Role Performance
Self-Care: Activities of Daily Living (ADL)
Self-Care: Instrumental Activities of Daily Living (IADL)
Self-Direction of Care
Social Interaction Skills
Social Involvement
Stress Level

# Role Performance, Ineffective

**DEFINITION:** Patterns of behavior and self-expression that do not match the environmental context, norms, and expectations

**SUGGESTED OUTCOMES:**

Anxiety Level
Caregiver Lifestyle Disruption
Cognition
Coping
Depression Level

Parenting Performance
Psychosocial Adjustment: Life Change
Role Performance
Stress Level

**ADDITIONAL ASSOCIATED OUTCOMES:**

Anxiety Self-Control
Caregiver Adaptation to Patient Institutionalization
Caregiver Home Care Readiness
Caregiver Performance: Direct Care
Caregiver Performance: Indirect Care
Depression Self-Control
Family Functioning
Information Processing

Knowledge: Parenting
Memory
Motivation
Parent-Infant Attachment
Parenting: Adolescent Physical Safety
Parenting: Early/Middle Childhood Physical Safety
Parenting: Infant/Toddler Physical Safety
Psychomotor Energy

**R**

## Self-Care Deficit: Bathing/Hygiene

**DEFINITION:** Impaired ability to perform or complete bathing/hygiene activities for oneself

**SUGGESTED OUTCOMES:**
Ostomy Self-Care
Self-Care: Activities of Daily Living (ADL)
Self-Care: Bathing
Self-Care: Hygiene
Self-Care: Oral Hygiene

**ADDITIONAL ASSOCIATED OUTCOMES:**
Adaptation to Physical Disability
Anxiety Self-Control
Body Mechanics Performance
Client Satisfaction: Functional Assistance
Client Satisfaction: Physical Care
Cognition
Comfort Level
Coordinated Movement
Endurance
Energy Conservation
Knowledge: Body Mechanics
Knowledge: Ostomy Care
Mobility
Neurological Status
Pain Level
Psychomotor Energy
Self-Care Status
Self-Direction of Care

## Self-Care Deficit: Dressing/Grooming

**DEFINITION:** Impaired ability to perform or complete dressing and grooming activities for self

**SUGGESTED OUTCOMES:**
Self-Care: Activities of Daily Living (ADL)
Self-Care: Dressing
Self-Care: Hygiene

**ADDITIONAL ASSOCIATED OUTCOMES:**
Adaptation to Physical Disability
Anxiety Self-Control
Body Mechanics Performance
Client Satisfaction: Functional Assistance
Client Satisfaction: Physical Care
Cognition
Comfort Level
Coordinated Movement
Endurance
Energy Conservation
Knowledge: Body Mechanics
Mobility
Motivation
Neurological Status
Pain Level
Psychomotor Energy
Self-Care Status
Self-Direction of Care

S

## Self-Care Deficit: Feeding

DEFINITION: Impaired ability to perform or complete feeding activities

**SUGGESTED OUTCOMES:**
Nutritional Status
Nutritional Status: Food & Fluid Intake
Self-Care: Activities of Daily Living (ADL)
Self-Care: Eating
Swallowing Status

**ADDITIONAL ASSOCIATED OUTCOMES:**
Adaptation to Physical Disability
Anxiety Self-Control
Appetite
Client Satisfaction: Functional Assistance
Client Satisfaction: Physical Care
Cognition
Endurance
Joint Movement: Elbow
Joint Movement: Fingers
Joint Movement: Shoulder
Joint Movement: Wrist
Nausea & Vomiting Control
Neurological Status: Central Motor Control
Pain Control
Psychomotor Energy
Self-Care Status
Self-Direction of Care

## Self-Care Deficit: Toileting

DEFINITION: Impaired ability to perform or complete own toileting activities

**SUGGESTED OUTCOMES:**
Knowledge: Ostomy Care
Ostomy Self-Care
Self-Care: Activities of Daily Living (ADL)
Self Care: Hygiene
Self-Care: Toileting

**ADDITIONAL ASSOCIATED OUTCOMES:**
Ambulation
Anxiety Self-Control
Balance
Client Satisfaction: Functional Assistance
Client Satisfaction: Physical Care
Cognition
Comfort Level
Coordinated Movement
Endurance
Energy Conservation
Mobility
Neurological Status
Pain Level
Self-Care Status
Self-Direction of Care
Skeletal Function
Transfer Performance

S

## *Self-Concept, Readiness for Enhanced*

**DEFINITION:** A pattern of perceptions or ideas about the self that is sufficient for well-being and can be strengthened

**SUGGESTED OUTCOMES:**
Abuse Recovery Status
Body Image
Personal Autonomy
Self-Esteem

**ADDITIONAL ASSOCIATED OUTCOMES:**

Abuse Recovery: Emotional
Abuse Recovery: Financial
Abuse Recovery: Physical
Abuse Recovery: Sexual
Adaptation to Physical Disability

Child Development: Adolescence
Depression Self-Control
Neglect Recovery
Personal Well-Being
Psychosocial Adjustment: Life Change

## *Self-Esteem: Chronic Low*

**DEFINITION:** Long-standing negative self-evaluation/feelings about self or self-capabilities

**SUGGESTED OUTCOMES:**
Depression Level
Personal Autonomy
Quality of Life
Self-Esteem

**ADDITIONAL ASSOCIATED OUTCOMES:**

Body Image
Depression Self-Control
Hope
Mood Equilibrium

Motivation
Role Performance
Social Interaction Skills
Stress Level

S

# Self-Esteem: Situational Low

**DEFINITION:** Development of a negative perception of self-worth in response to a current situation (specify)

**SUGGESTED OUTCOMES:**
Adaptation to Physical Disability
Grief Resolution
Psychosocial Adjustment: Life Change
Self-Esteem

**ADDITIONAL ASSOCIATED OUTCOMES:**

Abuse Recovery Status
Abuse Recovery: Emotional
Abuse Recovery: Physical
Abuse Recovery: Sexual
Anxiety Level
Coping

Fear Level
Fear Level: Child
Neglect Recovery
Personal Autonomy
Role Performance
Stress Level

# Self-Esteem: Situational Low, Risk for

**DEFINITION:** At risk for developing negative perception of self-worth in response to a current situation (specify)

**SUGGESTED OUTCOMES:**

Abuse Recovery Status
Abuse Recovery: Emotional
Abuse Recovery: Financial
Abuse Recovery: Physical
Abuse Recovery: Sexual
Adaptation to Physical Disability
Body Image
Child Development: Adolescence

Coping
Grief Resolution
Neglect Recovery
Psychosocial Adjustment: Life Change
Risk Control
Risk Detection
Role Performance
Self-Esteem

**S**

## Self-Mutilation

DEFINITION: Deliberate self-injurious behavior causing tissue damage with the intent of causing nonfatal injury to attain relief of tension

SUGGESTED OUTCOMES:
Identity
Impulse Self-Control
Self-Mutilation Restraint

ADDITIONAL ASSOCIATED OUTCOMES:
Abuse Recovery Status
Abuse Recovery: Emotional
Abuse Recovery: Physical
Abuse Recovery: Sexual

Anxiety Level
Body Image
Distorted Thought Self-Control
Self-Esteem

## Self-Mutilation, Risk for

DEFINITION: At risk for deliberate self-injurious behavior causing tissue damage with the intent of causing nonfatal injury to attain relief of tension

SUGGESTED OUTCOMES:
Abuse Recovery Status
Abuse Recovery: Emotional
Abuse Recovery: Physical
Abuse Recovery: Sexual
Anxiety Level
Distorted Thought Self-Control

Impulse Self-Control
Mood Equilibrium
Risk Control
Risk Detection
Self-Mutilation Restraint
Substance Addiction Consequences

## Sensory Perception: Auditory, Disturbed

DEFINITION: Change in the amount or patterning of incoming stimuli accompanied by a diminished, exaggerated, distorted, or impaired response to such stimuli

SUGGESTED OUTCOMES:
Communication: Receptive
Hearing Compensation Behavior
Sensory Function: Hearing

ADDITIONAL ASSOCIATED OUTCOMES:
Cognitive Orientation
Distorted Thought Self-Control
Neurological Status: Cranial Sensory/Motor Function
Risk Control: Hearing Impairment

## Sensory Perception: Gustatory, Disturbed

**DEFINITION:** Change in the amount or patterning of incoming stimuli accompanied by a diminished, exaggerated, distorted, or impaired response to such stimuli

**SUGGESTED OUTCOMES:**
Appetite
Nutritional Status: Food & Fluid Intake
Sensory Function: Taste & Smell

**ADDITIONAL ASSOCIATED OUTCOMES:**
Cognitive Orientation
Distorted Thought Self-Control
Nausea & Vomiting Severity

Neurological Status: Cranial Sensory/Motor
  Function
Stress Level

## Sensory Perception: Kinesthetic, Disturbed

**DEFINITION:** Change in the amount or patterning of incoming stimuli accompanied by a diminished, exaggerated, distorted, or impaired response to such stimuli

**SUGGESTED OUTCOMES:**
Balance
Body Positioning: Self-Initiated
Coordinated Movement
Sensory Function: Proprioception

**ADDITIONAL ASSOCIATED OUTCOMES:**
Ambulation
Body Mechanics Performance
Cognitive Orientation

Distorted Thought Self-Control
Neurological Status: Central Motor Control

**S**

## Sensory Perception: Olfactory, Disturbed

**DEFINITION:** Change in the amount or patterning of incoming stimuli accompanied by a diminished, exaggerated, distorted, or impaired response to such stimuli

**SUGGESTED OUTCOMES:**
Appetite
Nutritional Status: Food & Fluid Intake
Sensory Function: Taste & Smell

**ADDITIONAL ASSOCIATED OUTCOMES:**
Cognitive Orientation
Distorted Thought Self-Control
Nausea & Vomiting Severity
Neurological Status: Cranial Sensory/Motor Function

## Sensory Perception: Tactile, Disturbed

**DEFINITION:** Change in the amount or patterning of incoming stimuli accompanied by a diminished, exaggerated, distorted, or impaired response to such stimuli

**SUGGESTED OUTCOMES:**
Sensory Function: Cutaneous

**ADDITIONAL ASSOCIATED OUTCOMES:**
Cognitive Orientation
Distorted Thought Self-Control
Neurological Status: Spinal Sensory/Motor Function
Tissue Integrity: Skin & Mucous Membranes

## Sensory Perception: Visual, Disturbed

**DEFINITION:** Change in the amount or patterning of incoming stimuli accompanied by a diminished, exaggerated, distorted, or impaired response to such stimuli

**SUGGESTED OUTCOMES:**
Sensory Function: Vision
Vision Compensation Behavior

**ADDITIONAL ASSOCIATED OUTCOMES:**
Cognitive Orientation
Distorted Thought Self-Control
Neurological Status: Cranial Sensory/Motor Function
Risk Control: Visual Impairment

S

# Sexual Dysfunction

**DEFINITION:** Change in sexual function that is viewed as unsatisfying, unrewarding, inadequate

**SUGGESTED OUTCOMES:**

Abuse Recovery: Sexual
Physical Aging
Risk Control: Sexually Transmitted
   Disease (STD)

Sexual Functioning
Sexual Identity

**ADDITIONAL ASSOCIATED OUTCOMES:**

Abuse Cessation
Abuse Recovery Status
Abuse Recovery: Emotional
Abuse Recovery: Physical
Adaptation to Physical Disability
Anxiety Level
Body Image
Fear Level

Knowledge: Cardiac Disease Management
Physical Maturation: Female
Physical Maturation: Male
Role Performance
Self-Esteem
Social Interaction Skills
Stress Level

# Sexuality Patterns, Ineffective

**DEFINITION:** Expressions of concern regarding own sexuality

**SUGGESTED OUTCOMES:**

Abuse Recovery: Sexual
Body Image
Physical Maturation: Female
Physical Maturation: Male

Role Performance
Self-Esteem
Sexual Identity

**ADDITIONAL ASSOCIATED OUTCOMES:**

Abuse Cessation
Abuse Recovery Status
Anxiety Level
Anxiety Self-Control
Child Development: Middle Childhood
Child Development: Adolescence
Personal Well-Being
Physical Aging
Psychosocial Adjustment: Life Change
Risk Control: Sexually Transmitted Disease
   (STD)
Risk Control: Unintended Pregnancy
Stress Level

S

## Skin Integrity, Impaired

**DEFINITION:** Altered epidermis and/or dermis

**SUGGESTED OUTCOMES:**

Allergic Response: Localized
Hemodialysis Access
Tissue Integrity: Skin & Mucous Membranes

Wound Healing: Primary Intention
Wound Healing: Secondary Intention

**ADDITIONAL ASSOCIATED OUTCOMES:**

Fluid Balance
Fluid Overload Severity
Immobility Consequences: Physiological
Infection Severity
Infection Severity: Newborn
Nutritional Status

Ostomy Self-Care
Self-Care: Hygiene
Thermoregulation
Thermoregulation: Newborn
Tissue Perfusion: Peripheral
Treatment Behavior: Illness or Injury

## Skin Integrity, Risk for Impaired

**DEFINITION:** At risk for skin being adversely altered

**SUGGESTED OUTCOMES:**

Allergic Response: Localized
Child Development: Adolescence
Fluid Overload Severity
Hemodialysis Access
Immobility Consequences: Physiological
Infection Severity
Infection Severity: Newborn
Nutritional Status
Nutritional Status: Biochemical Measures

Ostomy Self-Care
Physical Aging
Risk Control
Risk Detection
Self-Mutilation Restraint
Tissue Integrity: Skin & Mucous Membranes
Tissue Perfusion: Peripheral
Wound Healing: Primary Intention
Wound Healing: Secondary Intention

S

## *Sleep Deprivation*

**DEFINITION:** Prolonged periods of time without sleep (sustained natural, periodic suspension of relative consciousness)

**SUGGESTED OUTCOMES:**
Concentration
Mood Equilibrium
Rest
Sleep

**ADDITIONAL ASSOCIATED OUTCOMES:**
Anxiety Level
Anxiety Self-Control
Cognition
Distorted Thought Self-Control
Endurance
Energy Conservation
Information Processing
Memory
Pain Control
Psychomotor Energy
Stress Level
Symptom Severity

## *Sleep Pattern, Disturbed*

**DEFINITION:** Time limited disruption of sleep (natural, periodic, suspension of consciousness) amount and quality

**SUGGESTED OUTCOMES:**
Mood Equilibrium
Personal Well-Being
Rest
Sleep

**ADDITIONAL ASSOCIATED OUTCOMES:**
Anxiety Level
Anxiety Self-Control
Bowel Elimination
Comfort Level
Depression Level
Fear Level
Fear Level: Child
Leisure Participation
Medication Response
Pain Level
Respiratory Status: Ventilation
Stress Level
Urinary Continence
Urinary Elimination

**S**

## *Sleep, Readiness for Enhanced*

**DEFINITION:** A pattern of natural, periodic suspension of consciousness that provides adequate rest, sustains desired a lifestyle, and can be strengthened

**SUGGESTED OUTCOMES:**
Comfort Level
Pain Control
Rest
Sleep

**ADDITIONAL ASSOCIATED OUTCOMES:**
Depression Self-Control
Leisure Participation
Mood Equilibrium
Stress Level

## *Social Interaction, Impaired*

**DEFINITION:** Insufficient or excessive quantity or ineffective quality of social exchange

**SUGGESTED OUTCOMES:**
Child Development: Middle Childhood
Child Development: Adolescence
Family Social Climate
Leisure Participation

Play Participation
Social Interaction Skills
Social Involvement

**ADDITIONAL ASSOCIATED OUTCOMES:**
Adaptation to Physical Disability
Body Image
Communication
Distorted Thought Self-Control
Family Functioning
Family Integrity
Fear Level
Fear Level: Child

Hyperactivity Level
Immobility Consequences: Psycho-Cognitive
Psychomotor Energy
Role Performance
Self-Esteem
Stress Level
Student Health Status

S

## Social Isolation

**DEFINITION:** Aloneness experienced by the individual and perceived as imposed by others and as a negative or threatening state

**SUGGESTED OUTCOMES:**

Family Social Climate
Leisure Participation
Loneliness Severity
Personal Well-Being

Play Participation
Social Interaction Skills
Social Involvement
Social Support

**ADDITIONAL ASSOCIATED OUTCOMES:**

Adaptation to Physical Disability
Aggression Self-Control
Body Image
Client Satisfaction: Communication
Communication
Depression Level
Fear Level

Fear Level: Child
Mobility
Mood Equilibrium
Self-Esteem
Sensory Function Status
Sensory Function: Hearing
Sensory Function: Vision

## Sorrow: Chronic

**DEFINITION:** Cyclical, recurring, and potentially progressive pattern of pervasive sadness experienced (by a parent, caregiver, individual with chronic illness or disability) in response to continual loss, throughout the trajectory of an illness or disability

**SUGGESTED OUTCOMES:**

Acceptance: Health Status
Depression Level
Depression Self-Control
Grief Resolution

Hope
Loneliness Severity
Mood Equilibrium
Psychosocial Adjustment: Life Change

**ADDITIONAL ASSOCIATED OUTCOMES:**

Adaptation to Physical Disability
Coping
Fear Level
Physical Aging
Quality of Life

Self-Esteem
Social Involvement
Spiritual Health
Suffering Severity

S

## *Spiritual Distress*

**DEFINITION:** Impaired ability to experience and integrate meaning and purpose in life through a person's connectedness with self, others, art, music, literature, nature, or a power greater than oneself

**SUGGESTED OUTCOMES:**
Dignified Life Closure
Hope
Spiritual Health

**ADDITIONAL ASSOCIATED OUTCOMES:**

Anxiety Level
Comfortable Death
Grief Resolution
Personal Autonomy
Personal Well-Being

Psychosocial Adjustment: Life Change
Quality of Life
Stress Level
Suicide Self-Restraint
Will to Live

## *Spiritual Distress, Risk for*

**DEFINITION:** At risk for an altered sense of harmonious connectedness with all of life and the universe in which dimensions that transcend and empower the self may be disrupted

**SUGGESTED OUTCOMES:**

Anxiety Level
Client Satisfaction: Cultural Needs
Fulfillment
Comfortable Death
Coping
Dignified Life Closure
Grief Resolution
Hope
Loneliness Severity

Mood Equilibrium
Personal Autonomy
Personal Well-Being
Psychosocial Adjustment: Life Change
Quality of Life
Risk Control
Risk Detection
Social Interaction Skills
Spiritual Health

S

## Spiritual Well-Being, Readiness for Enhanced

DEFINITION: Ability to experience and integrate meaning and purpose in life through connectedness with self, others, art, music, literature, nature, or a power greater than oneself

SUGGESTED OUTCOMES:
Hope
Personal Well-Being
Quality of Life
Spiritual Health

ADDITIONAL ASSOCIATED OUTCOMES:
Client Satisfaction: Cultural Needs
   Fulfillment
Dignified Life Closure
Grief Resolution

Personal Health Status
Psychosocial Adjustment: Life Change

## Sudden Infant Death Syndrome, Risk for

DEFINITION: Presence of risk factors for sudden death of an infant under 1 year of age

SUGGESTED OUTCOMES:
Knowledge: Infant Care
Knowledge: Parenting
Parenting: Infant/Toddler Physical Safety
Parenting Performance
Prenatal Health Behavior
Preterm Infant Organization

Risk Control
Risk Control: Tobacco Use
Risk Detection
Thermoregulation: Newborn

## Suffocation, Risk for

DEFINITION: Accentuated risk of accidental suffocation (inadequate air available for inhalation)

SUGGESTED OUTCOMES:
Aspiration Prevention
Asthma Self-Management
Body Positioning: Self-Initiated
Knowledge: Child Physical Safety
Knowledge: Infant Care
Knowledge: Personal Safety
Neurological Status: Consciousness
Parenting: Infant/Toddler Physical Safety

Personal Safety Behavior
Post Procedure Recovery Status
Respiratory Status: Airway Patency
Respiratory Status: Ventilation
Risk Control
Risk Detection
Substance Addiction Consequences

**S**

## Suicide, Risk for

**DEFINITION:** At risk for self-inflicted, life-threatening injury

**SUGGESTED OUTCOMES:**

Abuse Recovery Status
Abuse Recovery: Emotional
Abuse Recovery: Financial
Abuse Recovery: Physical
Abuse Recovery: Sexual
Client Satisfaction: Psychological Care
Depression Level
Impulse Self-Control
Loneliness Severity
Mood Equilibrium
Pain: Adverse Psychological Response
Pain Control

Personal Well-Being
Psychomotor Energy
Risk Control
Risk Control: Alcohol Use
Risk Control: Drug Use
Risk Detection
Social Interaction Skills
Social Support
Stress Level
Substance Addiction Consequences
Suicide Self-Restraint
Will to Live

## Surgical Recovery, Delayed

**DEFINITION:** Extension of the number of postoperative days required to initiate and perform activities that maintain life, health, and well-being

**SUGGESTED OUTCOMES:**

Ambulation
Blood Loss Severity
Endurance
Fluid Overload Severity
Hydration
Immobility Consequences: Physiological

Infection Severity
Nausea & Vomiting Severity
Pain Level
Post Procedure Recovery Status
Self-Care: Activities of Daily Living (ADL)
Wound Healing: Primary Intention

**ADDITIONAL ASSOCIATED OUTCOMES:**

Allergic Response: Systemic
Appetite
Client Satisfaction: Physical Care
Client Satisfaction: Safety
Client Satisfaction: Technical Aspects of Care
Discharge Readiness: Independent Living
Discharge Readiness: Supported Living
Health Beliefs
Immobility Consequences: Psycho-Cognitive
Infection Severity: Newborn
Kidney Function
Maternal Status: Postpartum
Mechanical Ventilation Weaning Response: Adult
Medication Response

Mobility
Nutritional Status: Energy
Nutritional Status: Food & Fluid Intake
Nutritional Status: Nutrient Intake
Pain Control
Pain: Disruptive Effects
Role Performance
Self-Care Status
Self-Care: Bathing
Self-Care: Dressing
Self-Care: Eating
Self-Care: Hygiene
Self-Care: Instrumental Activities of Daily Living (IADL)
Transfer Performance

S

# Swallowing, Impaired

**DEFINITION:** Abnormal functioning of the swallowing mechanism associated with deficits in oral, pharyngeal, or esophageal structure or function

**SUGGESTED OUTCOMES:**

Aspiration Prevention
Swallowing Status
Swallowing Status: Esophageal Phase

Swallowing Status: Oral Phase
Swallowing Status: Pharyngeal Phase

**ADDITIONAL ASSOCIATED OUTCOMES:**

Appetite
Cognition
Endurance
Energy Conservation
Neurological Status: Consciousness
Neurological Status: Cranial Sensory/Motor
   Function

Nutritional Status: Food & Fluid Intake
Respiratory Status: Airway Patency
Self-Care: Eating

# Therapeutic Regimen Management, Effective

**DEFINITION:** Pattern of regulating and integrating into daily living a program for treatment of illness and its sequelae that are satisfactory for meeting specific health goals

**SUGGESTED OUTCOMES:**

Adherence Behavior
Compliance Behavior
Family Participation in Professional Care
Knowledge: Treatment Regimen

Participation in Health Care Decisions
Risk Control
Symptom Control
Treatment Behavior: Illness or Injury

**ADDITIONAL ASSOCIATED OUTCOMES:**

Energy Conservation
Health Beliefs: Perceived Ability to Perform
Health Promoting Behavior
Knowledge: Cardiac Disease Management
Knowledge: Diabetes Management
Knowledge: Diet
Knowledge: Disease Process

Knowledge: Energy Conservation
Knowledge: Illness Care
Knowledge: Medication
Knowledge: Prescribed Activity
Knowledge: Treatment Procedure(s)
Self-Care: Non-Parenteral Medication
Self-Care: Parenteral Medication

T

## *Therapeutic Regimen Management, Ineffective*

DEFINITION: Pattern of regulating and integrating into daily living a program for treatment of illness and the sequelae of illness that is unsatisfactory for meeting specific health goals

SUGGESTED OUTCOMES:

Compliance Behavior
Knowledge: Diet
Knowledge: Treatment Regimen

Participation in Health Care Decisions
Symptom Control
Treatment Behavior: Illness or Injury

ADDITIONAL ASSOCIATED OUTCOMES:

Adherence Behavior
Cardiac Disease Self-Management
Diabetes Self-Management
Discharge Readiness: Independent Living
Family Support During Treatment
Health Beliefs
Health Beliefs: Perceived Ability to Perform
Health Beliefs: Perceived Control
Health Beliefs: Perceived Resources

Health Beliefs: Perceived Threat
Health Orientation
Knowledge: Disease Process
Knowledge: Illness Care
Knowledge: Treatment Procedure(s)
Motivation
Self-Care: Non-Parenteral Medication
Self-Care: Parenteral Medication
Self-Direction of Care

## *Therapeutic Regimen Management, Readiness for Enhanced*

DEFINITION: A pattern of regulating and integrating into daily living a program(s) for treatment of illness and its sequelae that is sufficient for meeting health-related goals and can be strengthened

SUGGESTED OUTCOMES:

Adherence Behavior
Compliance Behavior
Family Participation in Professional Care
Knowledge: Treatment Regimen

Participation in Health Care Decisions
Risk Control
Symptom Control
Treatment Behavior: Illness or Injury

ADDITIONAL ASSOCIATED OUTCOMES:

Energy Conservation
Health Beliefs: Perceived Ability to Perform
Health Promoting Behavior
Knowledge: Cardiac Disease Management
Knowledge: Diabetes Management
Knowledge: Diet
Knowledge: Disease Process

Knowledge: Energy Conservation
Knowledge: Illness Care
Knowledge: Medication
Knowledge: Prescribed Activity
Knowledge: Treatment Procedure(s)
Self-Care: Non-Parenteral Medication
Self-Care: Parenteral Medication

T

## Thermoregulation, Ineffective

DEFINITION: Temperature fluctuation between hypothermia and hyperthermia

SUGGESTED OUTCOMES:
Thermoregulation
Thermoregulation: Newborn

ADDITIONAL ASSOCIATED OUTCOMES:

Hydration
Neurological Status: Autonomic
Newborn Adaptation

Preterm Infant Organization
Symptom Severity: Perimenopause
Vital Signs

## Thought Processes, Disturbed

DEFINITION: Disruption in cognitive operations and activities

SUGGESTED OUTCOMES:

Cognition
Cognitive Orientation
Concentration
Decision-Making
Distorted Thought Self-Control

Identity
Information Processing
Memory
Neurological Status: Consciousness

ADDITIONAL ASSOCIATED OUTCOMES

Blood Glucose Level
Blood Loss Severity
Communication
Communication: Expressive
Communication: Receptive
Electrolyte & Acid/Base Balance
Fall Prevention Behavior
Fluid Balance

Hydration
Medication Response
Personal Safety Behavior
Respiratory Status: Gas Exchange
Risk Control: Alcohol Use
Risk Control: Drug Use
Safe Home Environment

T

## *Tissue Integrity, Impaired*

**DEFINITION:** Damage to mucous membrane, corneal, integumentary, or subcutaneous tissues

**SUGGESTED OUTCOMES:**

Allergic Response: Localized
Ostomy Self-Care
Tissue Integrity: Skin & Mucous Membranes

Wound Healing: Primary Intention
Wound Healing: Secondary Intention

**ADDITIONAL ASSOCIATED OUTCOMES:**

Fluid Overload Severity
Hydration
Immobility Consequences: Physiological
Infection Severity
Infection Severity: Newborn
Knowledge: Treatment Regimen

Nutritional Status
Self-Care: Hygiene
Sensory Function: Cutaneous
Thermoregulation
Thermoregulation: Newborn
Tissue Perfusion: Peripheral

## *Tissue Perfusion: Cardiopulmonary, Ineffective*

**DEFINITION:** Decrease in oxygen resulting in the failure to nourish the tissues at the capillary level

**SUGGESTED OUTCOMES:**

Cardiac Pump Effectiveness
Circulation Status
Respiratory Status: Gas Exchange

Tissue Perfusion: Cardiac
Tissue Perfusion: Pulmonary
Vital Signs

**ADDITIONAL ASSOCIATED OUTCOMES:**

Blood Coagulation
Blood Loss Severity
Electrolyte & Acid/Base Balance

Fluid Balance
Pain Level
Tissue Perfusion: Peripheral

T

## *Tissue Perfusion: Cerebral, Ineffective*

**DEFINITION:** Decrease in oxygen resulting in the failure to nourish the tissues at the capillary level

**SUGGESTED OUTCOMES:**

Cognition
Neurological Status
Neurological Status: Consciousness

Neurological Status: Central Motor Control
Seizure Control
Tissue Perfusion: Cerebral

**ADDITIONAL ASSOCIATED OUTCOMES:**

Blood Coagulation
Circulation Status
Cognitive Orientation
Communication
Communication: Expressive
Communication: Receptive

Concentration
Coordinated Movement
Information Processing
Memory
Swallowing Status
Tissue Perfusion: Peripheral

## *Tissue Perfusion: Gastrointestinal, Ineffective*

**DEFINITION:** Decrease in oxygen resulting in the failure to nourish the tissues at the capillary level

**SUGGESTED OUTCOMES:**

Electrolyte & Acid/Base Balance
Fluid Balance
Hydration
Tissue Perfusion: Abdominal Organ

**ADDITIONAL ASSOCIATED OUTCOMES:**

Appetite
Blood Coagulation
Blood Loss Severity
Bowel Elimination
Circulation Status
Nausea & Vomiting Severity

Nutritional Status
Nutritional Status: Biochemical Measures
Nutritional Status: Energy
Nutritional Status: Food & Fluid Intake
Pain Level

T

## *Tissue Perfusion: Peripheral, Ineffective*

DEFINITION: Decrease in oxygen resulting in the failure to nourish the tissues at the capillary level

SUGGESTED OUTCOMES:
Circulation Status
Fluid Overload Severity
Tissue Integrity: Skin & Mucous Membranes
Tissue Perfusion: Peripheral

ADDITIONAL ASSOCIATED OUTCOMES:
Blood Coagulation
Electrolyte & Acid/Base Balance
Fluid Balance
Sensory Function Status

Vital Signs
Wound Healing: Primary Intention
Wound Healing: Secondary Intention

## *Tissue Perfusion: Renal, Ineffective*

DEFINITION: Decrease in oxygen resulting in the failure to nourish the tissues at the capillary level

SUGGESTED OUTCOMES:
Circulation Status
Electrolyte & Acid/Base Balance
Fluid Balance

Fluid Overload Severity
Kidney Function
Tissue Perfusion: Abdominal Organs

ADDITIONAL ASSOCIATED OUTCOMES:
Blood Coagulation
Blood Transfusion Reaction
Cardiac Pump Effectiveness
Hydration
Urinary Elimination
Vital Signs

T

# Transfer Ability, Impaired

**DEFINITION:** Limitation of independent movement between two nearby surfaces

**SUGGESTED OUTCOMES:**

Balance
Body Mechanics Performance
Body Positioning: Self-Initiated

Coordinated Movement
Mobility
Transfer Performance

**ADDITIONAL ASSOCIATED OUTCOMES:**

Ambulation
Ambulation: Wheelchair
Cognition
Endurance
Immobility Consequences: Physiological
Immobility Consequences: Psycho-Cognitive
Joint Movement: Hip
Joint Movement: Knee

Joint Movement: Shoulder
Joint Movement: Spine
Knowledge: Body Mechanics
Knowledge: Fall Prevention
Neurological Status
Self-Care: Bathing
Self-Care: Toileting
Skeletal Function

# Trauma, Risk for

**DEFINITION:** Accentuated risk of accidental tissue injury (e.g., wound, burn, fracture)

**SUGGESTED OUTCOMES:**

Abuse Protection
Balance
Community Risk Control: Violence
Community Violence Level
Coordinated Movement
Fall Prevention Behavior
Falls Occurrence
Family Physical Environment
Knowledge: Child Physical Safety
Knowledge: Fall Prevention
Knowledge: Personal Safety
Parenting: Adolescent Physical Safety

Parenting: Early/Middle Childhood Physical
  Safety
Parenting: Infant/Toddler Physical Safety
Personal Safety Behavior
Physical Injury Severity
Risk Control
Risk Control: Alcohol Use
Risk Control: Drug Use
Risk Detection
Safe Home Environment
Tissue Integrity: Skin & Mucous Membranes

T

## Unilateral Neglect

**DEFINITION:** Lack of awareness and attention to one side of the body

**SUGGESTED OUTCOMES:**
Adaptation to Physical Disability
Body Positioning: Self-Initiated
Coordinated Movement

**ADDITIONAL ASSOCIATED OUTCOMES:**

Balance
Body Image
Body Mechanics Performance
Client Satisfaction: Functional Assistance
Client Satisfaction: Safety
Joint Movement: Passive
Knowledge: Fall Prevention

Neurological Status
Personal Safety Behavior
Safe Home Environment
Self Care: Activities of Daily Living (ADL)
Self Care: Instrumental Activities of Daily
    Living (IADL)
Transfer Performance

## Urinary Elimination, Impaired

**DEFINITION:** Disturbance in urine elimination

**SUGGESTED OUTCOMES:**
Urinary Continence
Urinary Elimination

**ADDITIONAL ASSOCIATED OUTCOMES:**

Hydration
Infection Severity
Kidney Function
Knowledge: Disease Process
Knowledge: Medication
Knowledge: Treatment Regimen
Neurological Status

Pain Level
Self-Care: Toileting
Symptom Control
Symptom Severity
Systemic Toxin Clearance: Dialysis
Tissue Integrity: Skin & Mucous Membranes

**U**

## Urinary Elimination, Readiness for Enhanced

**DEFINITION:** A pattern of urinary functions that is sufficient for meeting eliminatory needs and can be strengthened

**SUGGESTED OUTCOMES:**
Kidney Function
Self-Care: Toileting
Urinary Continence
Urinary Elimination

**ADDITIONAL ASSOCIATED OUTCOMES:**

Hydration
Infection Severity
Knowledge: Disease Process
Knowledge: Medication

Neurological Status
Symptom Control
Symptom Severity

## Urinary Incontinence: Functional

**DEFINITION:** Inability of usually continent person to reach toilet in time to avoid unintentional loss of urine

**SUGGESTED OUTCOMES:**
Medication Response
Self-Care: Toileting
Urinary Continence
Urinary Elimination

**ADDITIONAL ASSOCIATED OUTCOMES:**

Ambulation
Ambulation: Wheelchair
Cognition
Coordinated Movement
Infection Severity
Mobility

Stress Level
Symptom Control
Symptom Severity
Tissue Integrity: Skin & Mucous Membranes
Transfer Performance

U

## *Urinary Incontinence: Reflex*

**DEFINITION:** Involuntary loss of urine at somewhat predictable intervals when a specific bladder volume is reached

**SUGGESTED OUTCOMES:**
Neurological Status: Autonomic
Tissue Integrity: Skin & Mucous Membranes
Urinary Continence
Urinary Elimination

**ADDITIONAL ASSOCIATED OUTCOMES:**

Caregiver Performance: Direct Care
Knowledge: Disease Process
Knowledge: Treatment Regimen
Neurological Status
Nutritional Status: Food & Fluid Intake
Quality of Life

Self Care: Hygiene
Self-Care: Toileting
Symptom Control
Symptom Severity
Treatment Behavior: Illness or Injury

## *Urinary Incontinence: Stress*

**DEFINITION:** Loss of less than 50 ml of urine occurring with increased abdominal pressure

**SUGGESTED OUTCOMES:**
Urinary Continence
Urinary Elimination

**ADDITIONAL ASSOCIATED OUTCOMES:**

Client Satisfaction: Symptom Control
Knowledge: Treatment Procedure(s)
Knowledge: Treatment Regimen
Self-Care: Hygiene
Self-Care: Toileting

Self-Esteem
Symptom Control
Symptom Severity
Tissue Integrity: Skin & Mucous Membranes

U

## Urinary Incontinence: Total

DEFINITION:  Continuous and unpredictable loss of urine

SUGGESTED OUTCOMES:
Tissue Integrity: Skin & Mucous Membranes
Urinary Continence
Urinary Elimination

ADDITIONAL ASSOCIATED OUTCOMES:
Adaptation to Physical Disability
Client Satisfaction: Symptom Control
Cognition
Infection Severity
Knowledge: Treatment Procedure(s)
Neurological Status: Autonomic

Self-Care: Hygiene
Self-Care: Toileting
Self-Esteem
Symptom Control
Symptom Severity
Treatment Behavior: Illness or Injury

## Urinary Incontinence: Urge

DEFINITION:  Involuntary passage of urine occurring soon after a strong sense of urgency to void

SUGGESTED OUTCOMES:
Self-Care: Toileting
Urinary Continence
Urinary Elimination

ADDITIONAL ASSOCIATED OUTCOMES:
Cognition
Knowledge: Disease Process
Knowledge: Treatment Regimen
Mobility
Self-Care: Hygiene

Self-Esteem
Symptom Control
Tissue Integrity: Skin & Mucous Membranes
Treatment Behavior: Illness or Injury

## Urinary Incontinence: Urge, Risk for

U

DEFINITION:  At risk for involuntary loss of urine associated with a sudden, strong sensation or urinary urgency

SUGGESTED OUTCOMES:
Infection Severity
Knowledge: Medication
Knowledge: Treatment Regimen
Medication Response
Neurological Status: Autonomic

Risk Control
Risk Detection
Stress Level
Urinary Continence
Urinary Elimination

## Urinary Retention

**DEFINITION:** Incomplete emptying of the bladder

**SUGGESTED OUTCOMES:**
Urinary Continence
Urinary Elimination

**ADDITIONAL ASSOCIATED OUTCOMES:**

Infection Severity
Knowledge: Disease Process
Knowledge: Medication
Knowledge: Treatment Regimen

Medication Response
Neurological Status
Symptom Control
Symptom Severity

## Ventilation, Impaired Spontaneous

**DEFINITION:** Decreased energy reserves result in an individual's inability to maintain breathing adequate to support life

**SUGGESTED OUTCOMES:**
Allergic Response: Systemic
Mechanical Ventilation Response: Adult
Respiratory Status: Gas Exchange

Respiratory Status: Ventilation
Vital Signs

**ADDITIONAL ASSOCIATED OUTCOMES:**

Anxiety Level
Anxiety Self-Control
Electrolyte & Acid/Base Balance
Endurance
Energy Conservation

Mechanical Ventilation Weaning Response:
   Adult
Neurological Status: Central Motor Control
Neurological Status: Consciousness
Post Procedure Recovery Status

U

## *Ventilatory Weaning Response, Dysfunctional*

**DEFINITION:** Inability to adjust to lowered levels of mechanical ventilator support that interrupts and prolongs the weaning process

**SUGGESTED OUTCOMES:**

Anxiety Self-Control
Mechanical Ventilation Weaning Response:
   Adult

Respiratory Status: Gas Exchange
Respiratory Status: Ventilation
Vital Signs

**ADDITIONAL ASSOCIATED OUTCOMES:**

Anxiety Level
Client Satisfaction: Technical Aspects of Care
Cognition
Electrolyte & Acid/Base Balance
Knowledge: Treatment Procedures(s)
Mechanical Ventilation Response: Adult

Neurological Status: Consciousness
Pain Control
Post Procedure Recovery Status
Sleep
Symptom Severity

## *Violence: Other-Directed, Risk for*

**DEFINITION:** At risk for behaviors in which an individual demonstrates that he/she can be physically, emotionally, and/or sexually harmful to others

**SUGGESTED OUTCOMES:**

Abuse Cessation
Abuse Protection
Abusive Behavior Self-Restraint
Aggression Self-Control
Cognition
Community Risk Control: Violence
Community Violence Level
Depression Self-Control
Distorted Thought Self-Control

Fear Level
Fear Level: Child
Hyperactivity Level
Impulse Self-Control
Risk Control
Risk Control: Alcohol Use
Risk Control: Drug Use
Risk Detection
Stress Level

**V**

## *Violence: Self-Directed, Risk for*

**DEFINITION:** At risk for behaviors in which an individual demonstrates that he/she can be physically, emotionally, and/or sexually harmful to self

**SUGGESTED OUTCOMES:**

Adaptation to Physical Disability
Cognition
Coping
Depression Level
Depression Self-Control
Distorted Thought Self-Control
Impulse Self-Control
Loneliness Severity
Mood Equilibrium

Quality of Life
Risk Control
Risk Control: Alcohol Use
Risk Control: Drug Use
Risk Detection
Self-Mutilation Restraint
Stress Level
Suicide Self-Restraint
Will to Live

## *Walking, Impaired*

**DEFINITION:** Limitation of independent movement within the environment on foot

**SUGGESTED OUTCOMES:**

Ambulation
Balance
Coordinated Movement

Endurance
Mobility

**ADDITIONAL ASSOCIATED OUTCOMES:**

Body Mechanics Performance
Client Satisfaction: Functional Assistance
Client Satisfaction: Safety
Fall Prevention Behavior
Falls Occurrence
Joint Movement: Ankle
Joint Movement: Hip
Joint Movement: Knee
Joint Movement: Spine

Knowledge: Body Mechanics
Knowledge: Fall Prevention
Neurological Status: Central Motor Control
Pain Level
Physical Injury Severity
Safe Home Environment
Self Care: Activities of Daily Living (ADL)
Skeletal Function

W

## *Wandering*

**DEFINITION:** Meandering, aimless or repetitive locomotion that exposes the individual to harm; frequently incongruent with boundaries, limits, or obstacles

**SUGGESTED OUTCOMES:**
Fall Prevention Behavior
Safe Home Environment

**ADDITIONAL ASSOCIATED OUTCOMES:**
Anxiety Level
Hyperactivity Level
Rest
Sleep

W

# PART FIVE

# Core Outcomes for Nursing Specialty Areas

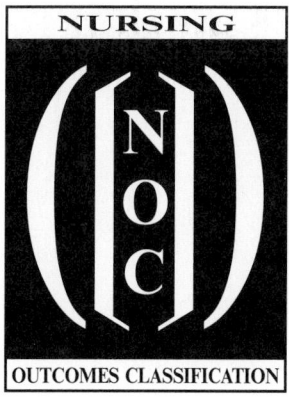

## IDENTIFYING CORE OUTCOMES

Core outcomes identified by 33 nursing organizations representing areas of nursing specialization and nurses representing eight areas of specialty practice are included in this section. Information was collected from the organizations and specialty nurses through surveys sent in 1999 and 2000. Only second edition NOC outcomes were included in the survey; thus new outcomes in this edition are not part of this research. Since the surveys were sent, 48 outcomes have had label changes; these are identified as label name changes and can be found in Appendix A. The outcomes from the surveys are listed in descending order of importance as identified by each organization and specialty nursing practice. Organizational responses are listed alphabetically by the area of specialization, followed by an alphabetical listing of the specializations of the nurses who responded to the survey. The organizations and specialty nurses that responded to the survey are listed at the end, with the area of specialization highlighted. It is important to note that this is the first attempt to identify core outcomes for specialty groups; further information is needed to validate these initial results.

### The Survey

The survey was conducted in two phases. In September 1999 questionnaires were mailed to 13 specialty organizations, specialty nurses who were members of these 13 organizations, and names of nurses from the American Nurses Credentialing Center (ANCC). The thirteen associations that received the questionnaire are identified by an asterisk in the list at the end of this introduction. Names of the specialty nurses were obtained from the organizations and from the ANCC for the following areas of specialization: (1) cardiac rehabilitation, (2) community health, (3) gerontology, (4) home heath, (5) medical surgical, (6) pediatrics, (7) psychiatric, and (8) school nurses. Questionnaires were mailed to 50 randomly selected nurses from the organizational lists and from the ANCC lists.

The second phase of the study took place in July 2000 when a questionnaire containing the 260 outcomes in the second edition of NOC were mailed to 27 specialty organizations. To ensure equity, the 13 organizations that completed the first questionnaire received a second questionnaire in July 2000 with the 32 outcomes not included in the initial survey. They also received a tabulated list of their responses from the first questionnaire. Individual nurses did not receive the additional list of 32 questions because the decision was made to approach the organizations rather than individual nurses who were members of specialty organizations.

The questionnaire asked the organizations to rate on a scale of 0% to 100% the percent of patients in the practice specialty for whom the outcome is important. The directions also included the example, for what percent of your patients is "Knowledge: Treatment Regimen" an important outcome? The directions to individual nurses asked them to think about the patients they have cared for in the last 3 months and rate the percent of patients for whom the outcome would be important. An example similar to the one given to organizations was given to the individual nurses.

Directions to organizations indicated that the president, the board, or other members could complete the questionnaire. The only requirement was that the individual or individuals who responded should be an expert nurse in the area of specialization represented by the organization. Reminder postcards, telephone calls, and mailing second questionnaires were techniques used to increase returns from the organizations. Only reminder postcards were used for the individual nurses.

### Survey Results

All of the first 13 organizations that received the questionnaire returned both the initial questionnaire and the follow-up 32-item questionnaire. Twenty of the 27 organizations from the second mailing returned usable questionnaires. Thirty-three of the 40 questionnaires were returned, for a response rate of 83%. Organizations that were sent questionnaires but did not respond or declined to participate were: American College of Nurse-Midwives; American Society of Plastic and Reconstructive Surgical Nurses, Inc.; Association for Professionals in Infection Control and Epidemiology, Inc.; Developmental Disabilities Nurses Association; Health Ministries Association; the International Society of Psychiatric-Mental Health Nurses; and the National Nurses Society on Addictions.

Response rates for the nurses from the specialty organizations varied from 10% to 38% (Table 5-1); the low response rate at a relatively high cost was one of the reasons we chose to continue only with specialty organizations. Although greatly appreciated, the returns from the nurses representing specialty organizations are not provided here but will appear in other publications. Although the response rate of nurses from the ANCC specialty groups was no higher, we are including these responses since some of the areas (i.e., gerontological; medical-surgical; cardiac rehabilitation; and school nurses) are not represented by the current specialty organizations.

The length of the core outcome lists varies. We had intended to take the top 20 items from each list but were unable to do so. The specialty organizations in Table 5-2 indicated that all of the outcomes we list in their core are important for 100% of the patients. Since we needed to go beyond a minimum of 20 for these organizations, we elected to cut off the core list for other organizations when there was a natural break of five or more points between the items on the core list and those not listed. Since the responses from the individual nurses were averaged, few natural breaks occurred in the percent of patients for whom the outcomes were important; therefore we elected to place the top-ranking 20 to 30 outcomes in the core list.

## Discussion

Although this is beginning work to identify core outcomes used in specialty practice, the results are an important step in enhancing the nursing profession's ability to clarify the outcomes nurses routinely address with specific populations of patients. The identification of core outcomes will enhance effectiveness research on patient populations and identify important content for educational programs in specialty areas of nursing. With further research in this area, core outcomes can be identified for educational programs for different levels of students. For example, there could be a core set of outcomes that all BSN students learn as part of their basic nursing education. These core outcomes should be determined by the combined efforts of nurses from educational and practice institutions to better prepare nurses for current and future roles in health care.

We have defined core outcomes as a concise set of outcomes that captures the essence of specialty practice by identifying the outcomes selected most frequently but is not comprehensive enough to include all outcomes used by nurses in that specialty. These outcomes provide a means to measure the effectiveness of practice and are one of the elements that direct the interventions

**Table 5-1**    RESPONSE RATE FOR SPECIALTY NURSES

| Association | Number Mailed | Number Returned | Percent |
| --- | --- | --- | --- |
| ANCC-Cardiac-Rehabilitation | 50 | 19 | 38% |
| ANCC-Community Health | 50 | 12 | 24% |
| ANCC-Gerontological | 50 | 11 | 22% |
| ANCC-Home Health | 50 | 19 | 38% |
| ANCC-Medical Surgical | 50 | 15 | 30% |
| ANCC-Pediatric | 50 | 10 | 20% |
| ANCC-Psychiatric | 50 | 9 | 10% |
| ANCC-School Nurse | 50 | 13 | 26% |

| **Table 5-2** | SPECIALTY ORGANIZATIONS WITH ALL OUTCOMES ON CORE LIST IDENTIFIED AS IMPORTANT FOR 100% OF THEIR PATIENTS |
| --- | --- |

American Association of Nurse **Anesthetists**
National Consortium of **Chemical Dependency** Nurses
**Hospice and Palliative** Nurses Association
**Intravenous** Nursing Society
National Association of **Neonatal** Nurses
American **Nephrology** Nurses Association
American Association of **Neuroscience** Nurses
Association of **Operating Room** Nurses, Inc.
American Society of **Pain Management** Nurses
Society of **Pediatric** Nurses
Association of **PeriOperative** Registered Nurses
American College of Nurse **Practitioners**
Society for Education and Research in **Psychiatric-Mental Health** Nursing
American **Radiological** Nurses Association
Association of **Rehabilitation** Nurses
American Association of **Spinal Cord Injury** Nurses

nurses use in the specialty. Examining the data from this survey is one way to approach the development of core outcomes of nursing care. In this study the NOC outcome Vital Signs Status was the most frequently identified outcome across the specialty practice organizations included in this study. Twenty-five specialty groups identified this outcome as core to their practice. The second most common outcome selected was Comfort Level. These are the only two outcomes selected by more than 50% of the organizations surveyed.

Table 5-3 shows the top core outcomes identified across specialties in this first attempt to identify core outcomes of specialty practice. Only 24 outcomes were selected by 13 or more specialty organizations as core to their practice. This list contains many basic outcomes that nurses could address in a variety of settings and with different populations. One is not surprised that this list of outcomes is considered core to nursing practice. Table 5-4 lists the 24 outcomes from the second edition of NOC that were not selected as core for any of the specialties that responded to the survey. There are many outcomes that are specific to maternity or women's health issues on this list that would have probably been core outcomes for organizations such as the American College of Nurse-Midwives. The second edition of NOC has many specific for maternal health and infant outcomes.

Refinement of this initial work on core outcomes for specialty practice is a worthwhile endeavor. Much work is needed on outcome identification and development for specialty practice in the future to improve both the education and quality of patient care delivered by nurses. The 76 new outcomes need to be examined for inclusion in this work. We need to debate and analyze the question: What is a reasonable number of core outcomes for each specialty to address? We need to identify methods to keep this work on core outcomes for specialty practice current and find ways to involve specialty organizations in the evolution and continued development of NOC outcomes. Efforts in this direction will allow for continued improvement in the effectiveness efforts involving standardized languages.

We would like to thank the following organizations and all individual nurses who responded to the questionnaire.

**Specialty Organizations Responding to Survey**
American Academy of Ambulatory Care Nursing
American Association of Nurse Anesthetists

| Table 5-3 | MOST FREQUENT NOC OUTCOMES IDENTIFIED AS CORE BY SPECIALTY ORGANIZATIONS |
| --- | --- |

| NOC Outcome | Number of Organizations |
| --- | --- |
| Vital Signs Status | 25 |
| Comfort Level | 24 |
| Medication Response | 19 |
| Respiratory Status: Airway Patency | 19 |
| Knowledge: Treatment Regimen | 18 |
| Nutritional Status | 17 |
| Knowledge: Medication | 17 |
| Communication Ability | 16 |
| Communication: Receptive Ability | 16 |
| Participation: Health Care Decisions | 16 |
| Pain Level | 15 |
| Respiratory Status: Gas Exchange | 15 |
| Tissue Perfusion: Cardiac | 15 |
| Cognitive Orientation | 14 |
| Communication: Expressive Ability | 14 |
| Knowledge: Treatment Procedure(s) | 14 |
| Pain: Psychological Response | 14 |
| Respiratory Status: Ventilation | 14 |
| Sleep | 14 |
| Symptom Severity | 14 |
| Tissue Perfusion: Pulmonary | 14 |
| Hydration | 13 |
| Neurological Status | 13 |
| Knowledge: Disease Process | 13 |

| Table 5-4 | OUTCOMES NOT SELECTED AS CORE |
| --- | --- |

| | |
| --- | --- |
| Abusive Behavior Self-Control | Knowledge: Preconception |
| Ambulation: Wheelchair | Knowledge: Pregnancy |
| Breastfeeding Establishment: Infant | Knowledge: Substance Use Control |
| Breastfeeding Establishment: Maternal | Maternal Status: Antepartum |
| Impulse Control | Maternal Status: Intrapartum |
| Knowledge: Breastfeeding | Maternal Status: Postpartum |
| Knowledge: Conception Prevention | Risk Control: Alcohol Use |
| Knowledge: Diabetes Management | Self-Mutilation Restraint |
| Knowledge: Fertility Promotion | Suicide Self-Restraint |
| Knowledge: Labor & Delivery | Symptom Severity: Perimenopause |
| Knowledge: Maternal-Child Health | Symptom Severity: Premenstrual Syndrome (PMS) |
| Knowledge: Postpartum | Weight Control |

National Consortium of Chemical Dependency Nurses
Association of Community Health Nursing Educators
*American Association of Critical-Care Nurses
Dermatology Nurses Association
*Emergency Nurses Association
Society of Gastroenterology Nurses and Associates, Inc.

International Society of Nurses in Genetics
Home Healthcare Nurses Association
Hospice and Palliative Nurses Association
Intravenous Nursing Society
*National Association of Neonatal Nurses
*American Nephrology Nurses Association
*American Association of Neuroscience Nurses
*Association of Operating Room Nurses, Inc.
*American Society of Ophthalmic Registered Nurses, Inc.
*National Association of Orthopaedic Nurses
Society of Otorhinolaryngology and Head-Neck Nurses, Inc.
American Society of Pain Management Nurses
Society of Pediatric Nurses
*Association of Pediatric Oncology Nurses
American Society of PeriAnesthesia Nurses
Association of PeriOperative Registered Nurses
American College of Nurse Practitioners
Society for Education and Research in Psychiatric-Mental Health Nursing
American Radiological Nurses Association
*Association of Rehabilitation Nurses
*American Association of Spinal Cord Injury Nurses
Air and Surface Transport Nurses Association
Society of Urologic Nurses & Associates, Inc.
*Society for Vascular Nursing
*Association of Women's Health, Obstetric and Neonatal Nurses

### Specialty Areas of Individual Nurses Responding to Survey
ANCC Cardiac Rehabilitation
ANCC Community Health
ANCC Gerontological
ANCC Home Health
ANCC Medical-Surgical
ANCC Pediatric
ANCC Psychiatric/Mental Health
ANCC School Nurse

## SPECIALTY ORGANIZATIONS

### *American Academy of Ambulatory Care Nursing*

Vital Signs Status
Knowledge: Health Promotion
Medication Response
Physical Aging Status
Health Seeking Behavior
Acceptance: Health Status
Compliance Behavior
Knowledge: Health Behaviors
Health Promoting Behavior
Knowledge: Health Resources

Nutritional Status: Body Mass
Adherence Behavior
Knowledge: Treatment Regimen
Self-Care: Activities of Daily Living (ADL)
Health Beliefs: Perceived Threat
Health Orientation
Knowledge: Treatment Procedure(s)
Nutritional Status
Health Beliefs: Perceived Resources

### *American Association of Nurse Anesthetists*

Balance
Blood Transfusion Reaction Control
Body Positioning: Self-Initiated
Cardiac Pump Effectiveness
Circulation Status
Coagulation Status
Cognitive Ability
Cognitive Orientation
Comfort Level
Communication Ability
Communication: Expressive Ability
Communication: Receptive Ability
Concentration
Decision Making
Electrolyte & Acid/Base Balance
Fetal Status: Antepartum
Fetal Status: Intrapartum
Fluid Balance
Growth
Hydration
Immune Hypersensitivity Control
Information Processing
Knowledge: Treatment Procedure(s)
Medication Response
Memory
Neurological Status

Neurological Status: Autonomic
Neurological Status: Central Motor
   Control
Neurological Status: Consciousness
Neurological Status: Cranial Sensory/Motor
   Function
Neurological Status: Spinal Sensory/Motor
   Function
Newborn Adaptation
Pain: Disruptive Effects
Pain Level
Pain: Psychological Response
Participation: Health Care Decisions
Respiratory Status: Airway Patency
Respiratory Status: Gas Exchange
Respiratory Status: Ventilation
Suffering Level
Symptom Severity
Thermoregulation
Thermoregulation: Neonate
Tissue Perfusion: Abdominal Organs
Tissue Perfusion: Cardiac
Tissue Perfusion: Cerebral
Tissue Perfusion: Peripheral
Tissue Perfusion: Pulmonary
Vital Signs Status

## *National Consortium of* Chemical Dependency *Nurses*

Abuse Protection
Abuse Recovery: Emotional
Abuse Recovery: Financial
Abuse Recovery: Physical
Abuse Recovery: Sexual
Caregiver Emotional Health
Caregiver Lifestyle Disruption
Caregiver Performance: Direct Care
Caregiver Performance: Indirect Care
Caregiver Physical Health
Caregiver Stressors
Caregiver-Patient Relationship
Caregiving Endurance Potential
Comfort Level
Health Beliefs: Perceived Threat

Health Orientation
Knowledge: Health Resources
Knowledge: Medication
Knowledge: Personal Safety
Pain: Disruptive Effects
Pain Level
Quality of Life
Risk Control: Sexually Transmitted Diseases
  (STD)
Risk Control: Unintended Pregnancy
Spiritual Well-Being
Substance Addiction Consequences
Suffering Level
Symptom Severity

## *Association of* Community Health *Nursing Educators*

Community Competence
Community Health Status
Community Health: Immunity
Family Coping
Family Environment: Internal
Family Functioning
Family Health Status
Family Integrity
Family Normalization
Family Participation in Professional Care
Knowledge: Health Promotion
Knowledge: Health Resources
Ambulation: Walking
Comfort Level
Community Risk Control: Chronic Disease
Community Risk Control: Communicable
  Disease
Community Risk Control: Lead Exposure
Health Beliefs

Health Beliefs: Perceived Ability to
  Perform
Health Beliefs: Perceived Control
Health Beliefs: Perceived Resources
Health Beliefs: Perceived Threat
Health Orientation
Knowledge: Health Behaviors
Self-Care: Activities of Daily Living (ADL)
Self-Care: Bathing
Self-Care: Dressing
Self-Care: Eating
Self-Care: Grooming
Self-Care: Hygiene
Self-Care: Instrumental Activities of Daily
  Living (IADL)
Self-Care: Non-Parenteral Medication
Self-Care: Oral Hygiene
Self-Care: Toileting
Vital Signs Status

## American Association of Critical-Care Nurses

Coagulation Status
Medication Response
Neurological Status: Consciousness
Newborn Adaptation
Nutritional Status
Pain: Disruptive Effects
Pain: Psychological Response
Preterm Infant Organization
Psychosocial Adjustment: Life Change
Symptom Severity
Tissue Perfusion: Cardiac
Tissue Perfusion: Cerebral
Tissue Perfusion: Pulmonary
Vital Signs Status

Cognitive Orientation
Electrolyte & Acid/Base Balance
Family Coping
Family Participation in Professional Care
Neurological Status: Autonomic
Neurological Status: Cranial Sensory/Motor
   Function
Neurological Status: Spinal Sensory/Motor
   Function
Nutritional Status: Biochemical Measures
Pain Level
Respiratory Status: Airway Patency
Risk Control: Cardiovascular Health
Swallowing Status

## Dermatology Nurses Association

Medication Response
Knowledge: Medication
Knowledge: Treatment Regimen
Tissue Integrity: Skin & Mucous Membranes
Body Image
Health Beliefs: Perceived Control
Comfort Level
Knowledge: Disease Process
Adherence Behavior
Compliance Behavior
Coping

Quality of Life
Symptom Severity
Well-Being
Suffering Level
Cognitive Ability
Communication Ability
Communication: Receptive Ability
Information Processing
Health Promoting Behavior
Health Seeking Behavior
Social Involvement

## Emergency Nurses Association

Community Health Status
Community Risk Control: Communicable
   Disease
Health Seeking Behavior
Knowledge: Health Promotion
Knowledge: Health Resources
Knowledge: Treatment Regimen
Participation: Health Care Decisions
Compliance Behavior
Treatment Behavior: Illness or Injury
Vital Signs Status

Knowledge: Health Behaviors
Knowledge: Medication
Pain Control
Knowledge: Illness Care
Skeletal Function
Adherence Behavior
Health Beliefs
Health Beliefs: Perceived Resources
Knowledge: Personal Safety
Knowledge: Treatment Procedure(s)

## *Society of* Gastroenterology *Nurses and Associates, Inc.*

Health Seeking Behavior
Nutritional Status
Nutritional Status: Biochemical Measures
Nutritional Status: Food & Fluid Intake
Nutritional Status: Nutrient Intake
Sensory Function: Hearing
Sensory Function: Proprioception
Swallowing Status
Swallowing Status: Esophageal Phase
Swallowing Status: Oral Phase
Swallowing Status: Pharyngeal Phase

Vital Signs Status
Acceptance: Health Status
Health Promoting Behavior
Knowledge: Health Promotion
Respiratory Status: Airway Patency
Communication Ability
Communication: Expressive Ability
Communication: Receptive Ability
Concentration
Decision Making
Participation: Health Care Decisions

## *International Society of Nurses in* Genetics

Family Coping
Family Participation in Professional Care
Knowledge: Disease Process
Coping
Family Environment: Internal
Cognitive Ability
Communication Ability
Social Support
Participation: Health Care Decisions
Well-Being
Sensory Function: Vision
Sleep
Concentration

Family Functioning
Family Health Status
Family Integrity
Quality of Life
Cognitive Orientation
Information Processing
Ambulation: Walking
Comfort Level
Health Beliefs
Nutritional Status
Risk Detection
Spiritual Well-Being
Will to Live

## Home Healthcare *Nurses Association*

Medication Response
Wound Healing: Secondary Intention
Self-Care: Non-Parenteral Medication
Treatment Behavior: Illness or Injury
Comfort Level
Community Risk Control: Communicable
   Disease
Health Beliefs
Health Beliefs: Perceived Ability to Perform

Health Beliefs: Perceived Control
Health Beliefs: Perceived Resources
Health Beliefs: Perceived Threat
Health Orientation
Knowledge: Disease Process
Knowledge: Illness Care
Knowledge: Medication
Knowledge: Prescribed Activity
Knowledge: Treatment Regimen

## Hospice & Palliative *Nurses Association*

Acceptance: Health Status
Comfort Level
Communication: Receptive Ability
Community Competence
Community Health Status
Coping
Dignified Dying
Family Coping
Family Environment: Internal
Family Health Status
Family Integrity
Family Normalization
Family Participation in Professional Care
Grief Resolution
Health Beliefs
Knowledge: Medication
Knowledge: Personal Safety
Medication Response

Oral Health
Pain: Disruptive Effects
Pain Level
Pain: Psychological Response
Participation: Health Care Decisions
Psychosocial Adjustment: Life Change
Quality of Life
Safety Behavior: Fall Prevention
Safety Behavior: Home Physical Environment
Safety Status: Falls Occurrence
Self-Esteem
Social Support
Spiritual Well-Being
Suffering Level
Symptom Control
Symptom Severity
Well-Being

## Intravenous *Nurses Society*

Blood Transfusion Reaction Control
Caregiver Home Care Readiness
Circulation Status
Coagulation Status
Comfort Level
Communication: Expressive Ability
Communication: Receptive Ability
Electrolyte & Acid/Base Balance
Family Participation in Professional Care
Fluid Balance
Hydration
Immobility Consequences: Physiological
Infection Status
Knowledge: Infection Control
Knowledge: Prescribed Activity

Knowledge: Treatment Procedure(s)
Medication Response
Nutritional Status: Biochemical Measures
Pain: Disruptive Effects
Pain Level
Pain: Psychological Response
Quality of Life
Self-Care: Hygiene
Self-Care: Non-Parenteral Medication
Self-Care: Parenteral Medication
Symptom Severity
Tissue Perfusion: Peripheral
Urinary Elimination
Vital Signs Status

## *National Association of* **Neonatal** *Nurses*

Blood Glucose Control
Bowel Elimination
Circulation Status
Coagulation Status
Electrolyte & Acid/Base Balance
Fluid Balance
Growth
Hydration
Immune Status
Newborn Adaptation
Nutritional Status
Nutritional Status: Biochemical Measures
Nutritional Status: Energy
Nutritional Status: Food & Fluid Intake
Nutritional Status: Nutrient Intake

Parent-Infant Attachment
Parenting
Preterm Infant Organization
Respiratory Status: Gas Exchange
Respiratory Status: Ventilation
Thermoregulation
Thermoregulation: Neonate
Tissue Integrity: Skin & Mucous Membranes
Tissue Perfusion: Abdominal Organs
Tissue Perfusion: Cardiac
Tissue Perfusion: Cerebral
Tissue Perfusion: Peripheral
Tissue Perfusion: Pulmonary
Urinary Elimination
Vital Signs Status

## *American* **Nephrology** *Nurses Association*

Adherence Behavior
Body Image
Caregiver Home Care Readiness
Caregiver Lifestyle Disruption
Caregiver-Patient Relationship
Caregiver Performance: Direct Care
Caregiver Stressors
Caregiving Endurance Potential
Comfort Level
Compliance Behavior
Health Beliefs
Health Beliefs: Perceived Control
Health Beliefs: Perceived Threat
Health Promoting Behavior
Health Seeking Behavior
Hearing Compensation Behavior
Identity
Knowledge: Diet
Knowledge: Disease Process
Knowledge: Energy Conservation
Knowledge: Health Resources
Knowledge: Personal Safety
Knowledge: Prescribed Activity
Knowledge: Treatment Procedure(s)
Knowledge: Treatment Regimen
Leisure Participation
Loneliness
Mood Equilibrium
Neurological Status

Neurological Status: Autonomic
Neurological Status: Central Motor
   Control
Neurological Status: Consciousness
Neurological Status: Cranial Sensory/Motor
   Function
Neurological Status: Spinal Sensory/Motor
   Function
Nutritional Status
Nutritional Status: Biochemical Measures
Nutritional Status: Body Mass
Nutritional Status: Energy
Nutritional Status: Food & Fluid Intake
Nutritional Status: Nutrient Intake
Participation: Health Care Decisions
Risk Control: Cardiovascular Health
Self-Care: Non-Parenteral Medication
Self-Esteem
Sensory Function: Cutaneous
Sexual Identity: Acceptance
Social Interaction Skills
Social Involvement
Spiritual Well-Being
Suffering Level
Symptom Control
Symptom Severity
Treatment Behavior: Illness or Injury
Well-Being
Wound Healing: Primary Intention

## *American Association of* Neuroscience Nurses

Activity Tolerance
Ambulation: Walking
Comfort Level
Coping
Family Coping
Family Normalization
Family Participation in Professional Care
Hope
Knowledge: Disease Process
Knowledge: Health Promotion

Knowledge: Illness Care
Knowledge: Treatment Regimen
Medication Response
Mobility Level
Neurological Status
Physical Fitness
Psychomotor Energy
Rest
Sleep

## *Association of* Operating Room *Nurses, Inc.*

Activity Tolerance
Ambulation: Walking
Aspiration Control
Circulation Status
Coagulation Status
Cognitive Ability
Cognitive Orientation
Comfort Level
Communication Ability
Communication: Expressive Ability
Communication: Receptive Ability
Community Health: Immunity
Electrolyte & Acid/Base Balance
Energy Conservation
Family Coping
Family Health Status
Family Participation in Professional Care
Fluid Balance
Health Beliefs: Perceived Control
Health Beliefs: Perceived Resources
Hydration
Immobility Consequences: Physiological
Infection Status
Joint Movement: Active
Knowledge: Health Promotion
Knowledge: Illness Care
Knowledge: Infection Control
Knowledge: Treatment Procedure(s)
Knowledge: Treatment Regimen
Medication Response

Mobility Level
Nutritional Status: Food & Fluid Intake
Nutritional Status: Nutrient Intake
Pain Control
Pain Level
Participation: Health Care Decisions
Physical Fitness
Psychomotor Energy
Respiratory Status: Airway Patency
Respiratory Status: Gas Exchange
Respiratory Status: Ventilation
Rest
Self-Care: Non-Parenteral Medication
Self-Direction of Care
Skeletal Function
Sleep
Swallowing Status
Swallowing Status: Esophageal Phase
Swallowing Status: Oral Phase
Swallowing Status: Pharyngeal Phase
Symptom Severity
Thermoregulation
Tissue Integrity: Skin & Mucous Membranes
Tissue Perfusion: Abdominal Organs
Tissue Perfusion: Cardiac
Tissue Perfusion: Cerebral
Tissue Perfusion: Peripheral
Tissue Perfusion: Pulmonary
Vital Signs Status
Wound Healing: Primary Intention

## American Society of Ophthalmic Registered Nurses, Inc.

Knowledge: Personal Safety
Neurological Status: Cranial Sensory
   Motor Function
Risk Control: Visual Impairment
Sensory Function: Vision
Vision Compensation Behavior
Knowledge: Health Behaviors
Knowledge: Treatment Regimen
Decision-Making

Knowledge: Disease Process
Neurological Status
Participation: Health Care Decisions
Risk Control
Knowledge: Health Resources
Physical Aging Status
Knowledge: Medication
Health Beliefs

## National Association of Orthopaedic Nurses

Joint Movement: Active
Joint Movement: Passive
Mobility Level
Muscle Function
Transfer Performance
Balance
Bone Healing:
Caregiver Home Care Readiness
Caregiver Lifestyle Disruption
Coagulation Status
Cognitive Ability
Cognitive Orientation
Comfort Level
Communication Ability
Communication: Expressive Ability
Communication: Receptive Ability
Depression Level
Infection Status
Knowledge: Infection Control
Neurological Status: Consciousness
Neurological Status: Cranial Sensory/Motor
   Function
Neurological Status: Spinal Sensory/Motor
   Function

Nutritional Status: Biochemical
   Measures
Nutritional Status: Food & Fluid
   Intake
Pain Control
Pain: Disruptive Effects
Pain Level
Pain: Psychological Response
Participation: Health Care Decisions
Respiratory Status: Airway Patency
Respiratory Status: Gas Exchange
Safety Behavior: Fall Prevention
Safety Behavior: Home Physical
   Environment
Safety Status: Physical Injury
Self-Care: Toileting
Symptom Severity
Tissue Perfusion: Abdominal Organs
Tissue Perfusion: Cardiac
Tissue Perfusion: Peripheral
Vital Signs Status
Well-Being
Wound Healing: Primary Intention
Wound Healing: Secondary Intention

## Society of Otorhinolaryngology and Head-Neck Nurses, Inc.

Acceptance: Health Status
Activity Tolerance
Ambulation: Walking
Aspiration Control
Asthma Control
Body Image
Comfort Level
Communication Ability
Communication: Expressive Ability
Communication: Receptive Ability
Community Health Status
Community Health: Immunity
Community Risk Control: Chronic Disease
Community Risk Control: Communicable
  Disease
Compliance Behavior
Coping
Electrolyte & Acid/Base Balance
Fluid Balance
Health Promoting Behavior
Health Seeking Behavior
Hearing Compensation Behavior
Hydration
Immobility Consequences: Physiological
Immobility Consequences: Psycho-Cognitive
Immune Status
Infection Status
Knowledge: Health Promotion
Knowledge: Health Resources
Knowledge: Infection Control
Knowledge: Treatment Procedure(s)
Knowledge: Treatment Regimen
Medication Response
Mobility Level

Neurological Status: Cranial Sensory/Motor
  Function
Nutritional Status
Nutritional Status: Biochemical Measures
Pain Control
Pain Level
Pain: Psychological Response
Participation: Health Care Decisions
Quality of Life
Respiratory Status: Airway Patency
Respiratory Status: Gas Exchange
Respiratory Status: Ventilation
Risk Control
Risk Control: Cancer
Risk Control: Hearing Impairment
Risk Control: Tobacco Use
Self-Care: Activities of Daily Living (ADL)
Self-Care: Bathing
Self-Care: Grooming
Sensory Function: Hearing
Sensory Function: Taste & Smell
Spiritual Well-Being
Swallowing Status
Swallowing Status: Esophageal Phase
Swallowing Status: Oral Phase
Swallowing Status: Pharyngeal Phase
Symptom Control
Tissue Integrity: Skin & Mucous Membranes
Tissue Perfusion: Pulmonary
Vital Signs Status
Well-Being
Will to Live
Wound Healing: Primary Intention
Wound Healing: Secondary Intention

## American Society of Pain Management Nurses

Ambulation: Walking
Cognitive Orientation
Communication Ability
Electrolyte & Acid/Base Balance
Fetal Status: Antepartum
Fetal Status: Intrapartum
Fluid Balance
Growth
Information Processing
Neurological Status: Consciousness

Respiratory Status: Airway Patency
Respiratory Status: Gas Exchange
Respiratory Status: Ventilation
Self-Care: Activities of Daily Living (ADL)
Self-Care: Bathing
Self-Care: Dressing
Skeletal Function
Thermoregulation
Tissue Perfusion: Cardiac
Vital Signs Status

## *Society of* **Pediatric Nurses**

Ambulation: Walking
Balance
Body Positioning: Self-Initiated
Breastfeeding Maintenance
Breastfeeding Weaning
Caregiver Adaptation to Patient
  Institutionalization
Caregiver Emotional Health
Caregiver Home Care Readiness
Caregiver Lifestyle Disruption
Caregiver-Patient Relationship
Caregiver Performance: Direct Care
Caregiver Performance: Indirect Care
Caregiver Physical Health
Caregiver Stressors
Caregiver Well-Being
Caregiving Endurance Potential
Child Adaptation to Hospitalization
Child Development: 2 Months
Child Development: 4 Months
Child Development: 6 Months
Child Development: 12 Months
Child Development: 2 Years
Child Development: 3 Years
Child Development: 4 Years
Child Development: 5 Years
Child Development: Adolescence (12-17 years)
Child Development: Middle Childhood
  (6-11 years)
Comfort Level
Coping
Dignified Dying
Family Coping
Family Environment: Internal
Family Functioning
Family Health Status
Family Integrity
Family Normalization
Family Participation in Professional Care
Grief Resolution
Growth
Health Promoting Behavior
Health Seeking Behavior
Immobility Consequences: Physiological
Immobility Consequences: Psycho-Cognitive
Immunization Behavior
Joint Movement: Active
Knowledge: Child Safety
Knowledge: Disease Process
Knowledge: Health Behaviors
Knowledge: Infant Care

Knowledge: Infection Control
Knowledge: Medication
Knowledge: Personal Safety
Knowledge: Treatment Procedure(s)
Knowledge: Treatment Regimen
Medication Response
Mobility Level
Newborn Adaptation
Nutritional Status
Nutritional Status: Body Mass
Oral Health
Pain Level
Pain: Disruptive Effects
Pain: Psychological Response
Parent-Infant Attachment
Parenting
Parenting: Social Safety
Physical Fitness
Physical Maturation: Female
Physical Maturation: Male
Play Participation
Preterm Infant Organization
Psychosocial Adjustment: Life Change
Respiratory Status: Airway Patency
Respiratory Status: Gas Exchange
Respiratory Status: Ventilation
Risk Control
Role Performance
Safety Status: Physical Injury
Self-Care: Activities of Daily Living (ADL)
Self-Care: Bathing
Self-Care: Dressing
Self-Care: Eating
Self-Care: Grooming
Self-Care: Hygiene
Self-Care: Non-Parenteral Medication
Self-Care: Oral Hygiene
Self-Care: Parenteral Medication
Self-Care: Toileting
Sexual Functioning
Skeletal Function
Social Interaction Skills
Social Support
Spiritual Well-Being
Symptom Severity
Thermoregulation: Neonate
Tissue Integrity: Skin & Mucous Membranes
Tissue Perfusion: Pulmonary
Transfer Performance
Vital Signs Status
Wound Healing: Secondary Intention

## Association of Pediatric Oncology Nurses

Knowledge: Disease Process
Knowledge: Health Promotion
Knowledge: Illness Care
Parenting
Psychomotor Energy
Skeletal Function
Swallowing Status
Swallowing Status: Esophageal Phase
Swallowing Status: Oral Phase
Swallowing Status: Pharyngeal Phase
Caregiver Performance: Direct Care
Caregiver Performance: Indirect Care

Child Adaptation to Hospitalization
Coping
Knowledge: Infection Control
Knowledge: Medication
Knowledge: Treatment Regimen
Activity Tolerance
Comfort Level
Family Normalization
Family Participation in Professional Care
Hope
Pain: Psychological Response
Will to Live

## American Society of Perianesthesia Nurses

Aspiration Control
Circulation Status
Respiratory Status: Gas Exchange
Spiritual Well-Being
Blood Transfusion Reaction Control
Bowel Continence
Bowel Elimination
Child Adaptation to Hospitalization
Coagulation Status
Health Beliefs
Health Beliefs: Perceived Control
Health Orientation
Hydration
Immune Hypersensitivity Control
Immune Status
Infection Status
Knowledge: Disease Process
Knowledge: Energy Conservation
Knowledge: Infection Control
Knowledge: Medication
Knowledge: Personal Safety
Knowledge: Treatment Procedure(s)
Knowledge: Treatment Regimen
Medication Response

Pain: Psychological Response
Parent-Infant Attachment
Participation: Health Care Decisions
Prenatal Health Behavior
Respiratory Status: Airway Patency
Risk Control: Cardiovascular Health
Risk Control: Sexually Transmitted Diseases
  (STD)
Role Performance
Safety Behavior: Fall Prevention
Safety Behavior: Home Physical
  Environment
Safety Behavior: Personal
Self-Direction of Care
Skeletal Function
Thermoregulation
Thermoregulation: Neonate
Tissue Perfusion: Abdominal Organs
Tissue Perfusion: Cardiac
Tissue Perfusion: Cerebral
Tissue Perfusion: Pulmonary
Well-Being
Wound Healing: Primary Intention
Wound Healing: Secondary Intention

## *Association of* **Perioperative** *Registered Nurses*

Abuse Cessation
Abuse Protection
Abuse Recovery: Physical
Abuse Recovery: Sexual
Aspiration Control
Asthma Control
Blood Glucose Control
Blood Transfusion Reaction Control
Bone Healing
Bowel Elimination
Cardiac Pump Effectiveness
Caregiver Emotional Health
Caregiver Physical Health
Circulation Status
Coagulation Status
Comfort Level
Communication Ability
Communication: Expressive Ability
Communication: Receptive Ability
Dialysis Access Integrity
Electrolyte & Acid/Base Balance
Family Coping
Family Environment: Internal
Family Functioning
Family Health Status
Family Integrity
Family Normalization
Family Participation in Professional Care
Fluid Balance
Hydration
Immune Hypersensitivity Control
Immune Status
Infection Status
Joint Movement: Active
Joint Movement: Passive
Knowledge: Infection Control
Knowledge: Medication
Knowledge: Treatment Procedure(s)
Knowledge: Treatment Regimen
Medication Response

Mobility Level
Muscle Function
Neglect Recovery
Neurological Status
Neurological Status: Autonomic
Neurological Status: Consciousness
Neurological Status: Cranial Sensory/Motor
    Function
Neurological Status: Spinal Sensory/Motor
    Function
Nutritional Status: Body Mass
Nutritional Status: Food & Fluid Intake
Nutritional Status: Nutrient Intake
Pain Control
Pain Level
Pain: Disruptive Effects
Pain: Psychological Response
Respiratory Status: Airway Patency
Respiratory Status: Gas Exchange
Respiratory Status: Ventilation
Risk Control: Cancer
Risk Control: Cardiovascular Health
Safety Status: Physical Injury
Sensory Function: Cutaneous
Skeletal Function
Symptom Severity
Systemic Toxin Clearance
Thermoregulation
Thermoregulation: Neonate
Tissue Integrity: Skin & Mucous
    Membranes
Tissue Perfusion: Abdominal Organs
Tissue Perfusion: Cardiac
Tissue Perfusion: Cerebral
Tissue Perfusion: Peripheral
Tissue Perfusion: Pulmonary
Urinary Elimination
Vital Signs Status
Wound Healing: Primary Intention
Wound Healing: Secondary Intention

## *American College of Nurse Practitioners*

Adherence Behavior
Blood Glucose Control
Bowel Elimination
Cardiac Pump Effectiveness
Circulation Status
Cognitive Ability
Cognitive Orientation
Comfort Level
Communication: Expressive Ability
Communication: Receptive Ability
Compliance Behavior
Family Coping
Family Environment: Internal
Family Functioning
Family Health Status
Family Integrity
Family Normalization
Family Participation in Professional Care
Fluid Balance
Health Beliefs
Health Beliefs: Perceived Ability to Perform
Health Beliefs: Perceived Control
Health Beliefs: Perceived Resources
Health Promoting Behavior
Health Seeking Behavior
Hydration
Identity
Immunization Behavior
Infection Status
Knowledge: Diet
Knowledge: Energy Conservation
Knowledge: Health Behaviors
Knowledge: Health Resources
Knowledge: Illness Care
Knowledge: Infection Control
Knowledge: Medication
Knowledge: Personal Safety
Knowledge: Prescribed Activity
Knowledge: Treatment Procedure(s)
Knowledge: Treatment Regimen
Medication Response
Mobility Level
Mood Equilibrium
Muscle Function

Neurological Status
Neurological Status: Autonomic
Neurological Status: Central Motor Control
Neurological Status: Consciousness
Neurological Status: Cranial Sensory/Motor Function
Neurological Status: Spinal Sensory/Motor Function
Nutritional Status
Nutritional Status: Body Mass
Nutritional Status: Energy
Nutritional Status: Nutrient Intake
Oral Health
Pain: Disruptive Effects
Pain Level
Physical Fitness
Quality of Life
Respiratory Status: Airway Patency
Respiratory Status: Gas Exchange
Respiratory Status: Ventilation
Risk Control
Risk Control: Cancer
Risk Control: Cardiovascular Health
Risk Control: Drug Use
Risk Control: Tobacco Use
Safety Behavior: Personal
Self-Care: Toileting
Self-Esteem
Sensory Function: Hearing
Sensory Function: Proprioception
Sensory Function: Vision
Skeletal Function
Symptom Severity
Thermoregulation
Tissue Integrity: Skin & Mucous Membranes
Tissue Perfusion: Abdominal Organs
Tissue Perfusion: Cardiac
Tissue Perfusion: Cerebral
Tissue Perfusion: Peripheral
Tissue Perfusion: Pulmonary
Urinary Elimination
Vital Signs Status
Well-Being

## Society for Education and Research in Psychiatric-Mental Health Nursing

Cognitive Ability
Cognitive Orientation
Communication Ability
Communication: Expressive Ability
Communication: Receptive Ability
Concentration
Coping
Decision-Making
Information Processing
Knowledge: Disease Process
Knowledge: Medication

Medication Response
Memory
Mood Equilibrium
Neurological Status: Consciousness
Nutritional Status
Nutritional Status: Food & Fluid Intake
Oral Health
Participation: Health Care Decisions
Self-Care: Activities of Daily Living (ADL)
Self-Care: Non-Parenteral Medication
Sleep

## American Radiological Nurses Association

Acceptance: Health Status
Aggression Control
Anxiety Control
Balance
Blood Transfusion Reaction Control
Body Positioning: Self-Initiated
Cardiac Pump Effectiveness
Circulation Status
Depression Control
Electrolyte & Acid/Base Balance
Fear Control
Fluid Balance
Hope
Hydration
Identity
Immune Hypersensitivity Control
Immune Status
Infection Status
Joint Movement: Active
Loneliness
Mobility Level
Neurological Status
Neurological Status: Autonomic
Neurological Status: Central Motor Control
Neurological Status: Consciousness
Neurological Status: Cranial Sensory/Motor
   Function
Neurological Status: Spinal Sensory/Motor
   Function
Nutritional Status

Nutritional Status: Biochemical Measures
Nutritional Status: Nutrient Intake
Pain Control
Pain: Psychological Response
Psychosocial Adjustment: Life Change
Respiratory Status: Airway Patency
Respiratory Status: Gas Exchange
Respiratory Status: Ventilation
Rest
Sensory Function: Hearing
Sensory Function: Proprioception
Sensory Function: Taste & Smell
Skeletal Function
Sleep
Social Support
Swallowing Status
Swallowing Status: Esophageal Phase
Swallowing Status: Oral Phase
Swallowing Status: Pharyngeal Phase
Thermoregulation
Tissue Integrity: Skin & Mucous
   Membranes
Tissue Perfusion: Abdominal Organs
Tissue Perfusion: Cardiac
Tissue Perfusion: Cerebral
Tissue Perfusion: Peripheral
Tissue Perfusion: Pulmonary
Transfer Performance
Vital Signs Status
Will to Live

## *Association of* **Rehabilitation** *Nurses*

Aspiration Control
Bowel Continence
Bowel Elimination
Cognitive Ability
Cognitive Orientation
Communication: Expressive Ability
Communication: Receptive Ability
Concentration
Decision-Making
Information Processing
Memory
Mobility Level
Neurological Status
Psychomotor Energy
Psychosocial Adjustment: Life Change
Safety Behavior: Fall Prevention

Self-Care: Activities of Daily Living (ADL)
Self-Care: Hygiene
Self-Care: Instrumental Activities of Daily
   Living (IADL)
Self-Care: Non-Parenteral Medication
Self-Care: Oral Hygiene
Self-Care: Toileting
Sleep
Swallowing Status
Swallowing Status: Esophageal Phase
Swallowing Status: Oral Phase
Swallowing Status: Pharyngeal Phase
Transfer Performance
Urinary Continence
Urinary Elimination

## *American Association of* **Spinal Cord Injury** *Nurses*

Activity Tolerance
Adherence Behavior
Bowel Continence
Community Risk Control: Communicable
   Disease
Community Risk Control: Lead Exposure
Compliance Behavior
Depression Control
Endurance
Energy Conservation
Family Coping
Family Environment: Internal
Family Functioning
Family Health Status
Family Integrity
Family Normalization

Grief Resolution
Health Beliefs: Perceived Ability to Perform
Health Beliefs: Perceived Control
Knowledge: Health Promotion
Knowledge: Health Resources
Knowledge: Illness Care
Knowledge: Medication
Knowledge: Personal Safety
Knowledge: Treatment Procedure(s)
Knowledge: Treatment Regimen
Leisure Participation
Medication Response
Psychomotor Energy
Psychosocial Adjustment: Life Change
Self-Direction of Care
Skeletal Function

## *Air and Surface* **Transport** *Nurses Association*

Electrolyte & Acid/Base Balance
Immune Status
Neurological Status: Spinal Sensory/Motor
    Function
Respiratory Status: Ventilation
Tissue Perfusion: Abdominal Organs
Tissue Perfusion: Pulmonary
Asthma Control
Blood Transfusion Reaction Control
Body Image
Caregiver Adaptation to Patient
    Institutionalization
Circulation Status
Coagulation Status
Cognitive Ability
Cognitive Orientation
Comfort Level
Communication Ability
Communication: Expressive Ability
Communication: Receptive Ability
Concentration
Coping
Decision-Making
Fluid Balance
Hope
Hydration

Identity
Immune Hypersensitivity Control
Infection Status
Information Processing
Medication Response
Memory
Neurological Status
Neurological Status: Autonomic
Neurological Status: Central Motor Control
Neurological Status: Cranial Sensory/Motor
    Function
Pain: Disruptive Effects
Pain Level
Pain: Psychological Response
Quality of Life
Respiratory Status: Airway Patency
Respiratory Status: Gas Exchange
Self-Esteem
Symptom Severity
Thermoregulation
Thermoregulation: Neonate
Tissue Perfusion: Cardiac
Tissue Perfusion: Cerebral
Tissue Perfusion: Peripheral
Vital Signs Status
Will to Live

## *Society of* **Urologic** *Nurses & Associates, Inc.*

Urinary Elimination
Bowel Continence
Bowel Elimination
Self-Care: Toileting
Urinary Continence
Neurological Status: Central Motor Control
Psychomotor Energy
Acceptance: Health Status
Sexual Identity: Acceptance

Sleep
Tissue Perfusion: Cerebral
Will to Live
Activity Tolerance
Knowledge: Prescribed Activity
Knowledge: Sexual Functioning
Knowledge: Treatment Procedure(s)
Knowledge: Treatment Regimen
Medication Response

## Society *for* Vascular *Nursing*

Activity Tolerance
Aggression Control
Anxiety Control
Blood Glucose Control
Blood Transfusion Reaction Control
Cardiac Pump Effectiveness
Circulation Status
Cognitive Ability
Cognitive Orientation
Communication Ability
Communication: Expressive Ability
Communication: Receptive Ability
Dignified Dying
Distorted Thought Control
Electrolyte & Acid/Base Balance
Fear Control
Fluid Balance
Grief Resolution
Hearing Compensation Behavior
Hope
Hydration
Infection Status
Knowledge: Health Promotion
Knowledge: Illness Care
Knowledge: Treatment Procedure(s)
Knowledge: Treatment Regimen
Neurological Status
Neurological Status: Autonomic
Neurological Status: Central Motor Control
Neurological Status: Consciousness
Neurological Status: Cranial Sensory/Motor
   Function
Neurological Status: Spinal Sensory/Motor
   Function
Nutritional Status
Nutritional Status: Biochemical Measures
Nutritional Status: Body Mass

Nutritional Status: Energy
Nutritional Status: Food & Fluid Intake
Nutritional Status: Nutrient Intake
Pain Control
Pain Level
Pain: Psychological Response
Participation: Health Care Decisions
Psychomotor Energy
Psychosocial Adjustment: Life Change
Quality of Life
Respiratory Status: Airway Patency
Respiratory Status: Gas Exchange
Respiratory Status: Ventilation
Rest
Self-Care: Eating
Sensory Function: Cutaneous
Sensory Function: Proprioception
Sensory Function: Hearing
Sensory Function: Taste & Smell
Sensory Function: Vision
Skeletal Function
Sleep
Spiritual Well-Being
Suffering Level
Symptom Severity
Thermoregulation
Tissue Integrity: Skin & Mucous Membranes
Tissue Perfusion: Abdominal Organs
Tissue Perfusion: Cardiac
Tissue Perfusion: Cerebral
Tissue Perfusion: Peripheral
Tissue Perfusion: Pulmonary
Treatment Behavior: Illness or Injury
Urinary Elimination
Vital Signs Status
Wound Healing: Primary Intention
Wound Healing: Secondary Intention

## *Association of* Women's Health, Obstetric, and Neonatal *Nurses*

Medication Response
Knowledge: Health Promotion
Physical Fitness
Family Coping
Family Environment: Internal
Family Functioning
Family Health Status
Family Integrity
Family Normalization
Family Participation in Professional Care
Comfort Level
Skeletal Function
Nutritional Status
Nutritional Status: Body Mass
Respiratory Status: Airway Patency
Rest
Sleep

Urinary Continence
Pain Level
Activity Tolerance
Bowel Elimination
Community Health: Immunity
Community Risk Control: Communicable
    Disease
Community Risk Control: Lead Exposure
Circulation Status
Coagulation Status
Respiratory Status: Gas Exchange
Respiratory Status: Ventilation
Tissue Perfusion: Cardiac
Tissue Perfusion: Cerebral
Tissue Perfusion: Peripheral
Tissue Perfusion: Pulmonary

## SPECIALTY AREAS OF INDIVIDUAL NURSES

### *American Nurses Credentialing Center*—Cardiac Rehabilitation

Vital Signs Status
Health Seeking Behavior
Health Promoting Behavior
Compliance Behavior
Knowledge: Medication
Knowledge: Health Behaviors
Knowledge: Disease Process
Circulation Status
Risk Control: Cardiovascular Health
Cardiac Pump Effectiveness
Knowledge: Prescribed Activity
Well-Being
Tissue Perfusion: Cardiac
Health Beliefs: Perceived Ability to Perform
Knowledge: Diet
Ambulation: Walking
Health Beliefs: Perceived Resources

Health Beliefs: Perceived Control
Health Beliefs
Health Orientation
Endurance
Quality of Life
Participation: Health Care Decisions
Comfort Level
Adherence Behavior
Acceptance: Health Status
Self-Care: Activities of Daily Living (ADL)
Psychosocial Adjustment: Life Change
Knowledge: Health Resources
Balance
Coping
Hope
Respiratory Status: Airway Patency
Self-Care: Non-Parenteral Medication

### *American Nurses Credentialing Center*—Community *Health*

Endurance
Social Support
Health Promoting Behavior
Comfort Level
Well-Being
Decision Making
Quality of Life
Nutritional Status
Participation: Health Care Decisions
Information Processing

Immunization Behavior
Spiritual Well-Being
Memory
Coping
Body Image
Ambulation: Walking
Health Seeking Behavior
Compliance Behavior
Knowledge: Health Resources
Vital Signs Status

## *American Nurses Credentialing Center—*Gerontological

Nutritional Status
Oral Health
Nutritional Status: Energy
Nutritional Status: Food & Fluid Intake
Urinary Elimination
Safety Behavior: Fall Prevention
Vital Signs Status
Tissue Integrity: Skin & Mucous Membranes
Sleep
Nutritional Status: Biochemical Measures
Sensory Function: Vision
Neurological Status
Nutritional Status: Nutrient Intake
Urinary Continence
Neurological Status: Spinal Sensory/Motor
   Function
Bowel Continence
Nutritional Status: Body Mass

Neurological Status: Cranial Sensory/Motor
   Function
Neurological Status: Autonomic
Endurance
Rest
Neurological Status: Consciousness
Neurological Status: Central Motor Control
Quality of Life
Energy Conservation
Respiratory Status: Airway Patency
Bowel Elimination
Muscle Function
Self-Care: Grooming
Comfort Level
Hydration
Social Involvement
Communication Ability
Sensory Function: Hearing

## *American Nurses Credentialing Center—*Home Health

Knowledge: Medication
Safety Behavior: Fall Prevention
Self-Care: Activities of Daily Living (ADL)
Self-Care: Toileting
Ambulation: Walking
Safety Behavior: Home Physical Environment
Knowledge: Disease Process
Endurance
Vital Signs Status
Self-Care: Dressing
Self-Care: Bathing

Comfort Level
Knowledge: Infection Control
Bowel Elimination
Knowledge: Personal Safety
Self-Care: Hygiene
Joint Movement: Active
Knowledge: Treatment Regimen
Self-Care: Eating
Mobility Level
Caregiver Performance: Direct Care

## American Nurses Credentialing Center—Medical-Surgical

Vital Signs Status
Self-Care: Toileting
Nutritional Status: Food & Fluid Intake
Knowledge: Medication
Sleep
Balance
Ambulation: Walking
Physical Aging Status
Cognitive Orientation
Knowledge: Disease Process
Self-Care: Activities of Daily Living (ADL)
Self-Care: Oral Hygiene
Respiratory Status: Ventilation
Communication Ability
Acceptance: Health Status
Body Positioning: Self-Initiated
Tissue Perfusion: Peripheral
Pain: Psychological Response
Pain Level

Self-Care: Hygiene
Rest
Tissue Integrity: Skin & Mucous Membranes
Wound Healing: Primary Intention
Endurance
Infection Status
Joint Movement: Active
Self-Care: Bathing
Transfer Performance
Self-Care: Instrumental Activities of Daily Living (IADL)
Self-Care: Non-Parenteral Medication
Self-Care: Eating
Self-Care: Grooming
Muscle Function
Comfort Level
Mobility Level
Participation: Health Care Decisions

## American Nurses Credentialing Center—Pediatric

Sleep
Vital Signs Status
Growth
Nutritional Status: Food & Fluid Intake
Hydration
Rest
Nutritional Status
Nutritional Status: Nutrient Intake
Child Development: Adolescence (12-17 Years)
Play Participation
Endurance
Muscle Function
Mobility Level
Bowel Elimination
Infection Status
Nutritional Status: Energy

Nutritional Status: Biochemical Measures
Tissue Perfusion: Pulmonary
Respiratory Status: Gas Exchange
Child Development: 5 Years
Urinary Elimination
Sensory Function: Vision
Neurological Status
Respiratory Status: Airway Patency
Child Development: 3 Years
Respiratory Status: Ventilation
Tissue Perfusion: Cardiac
Tissue Perfusion: Abdominal Organs
Social Support
Child Development: 4 Years
Child Development: 6 Months
Child Development: 2 Months

## *American Nurses Credentialing Center*—Psychiatric/Mental Health

Hope
Knowledge: Medication
Coping
Sleep
Decision-Making
Communication: Receptive Ability
Communication Ability
Communication: Expressive Ability
Mood Equilibrium
Information Processing
Concentration
Self-Care: Hygiene
Social Involvement
Self-Esteem
Cognitive Ability

Self-Care: Activities of Daily Living (ADL)
Cognitive Orientation
Self-Care: Grooming
Memory
Loneliness
Psychosocial Adjustment: Life Change
Rest
Self-Care: Bathing
Social Support
Will to Live
Self-Care: Dressing
Identity
Symptom Control
Acceptance: Health Status

## *American Nurses Credentialing Center*—School Nurse

Oral Health
Growth
Body Image
Cognitive Orientation
Sleep
Memory
Communication: Receptive Ability
Communication: Expressive Ability
Self-Esteem
Endurance
Child Development: Middle Childhood
   (6-11 Years)
Sensory Function: Vision
Communication Ability

Vital Signs Status
Play Participation
Ambulation: Walking
Sensory Function: Hearing
Information Processing
Neurological Status
Identity
Mood Equilibrium
Hope
Respiratory Status: Airway Patency
Nutritional Status
Social Involvement
Concentration
Neurological Status: Central Motor Control

# PART SIX

# Appendixes

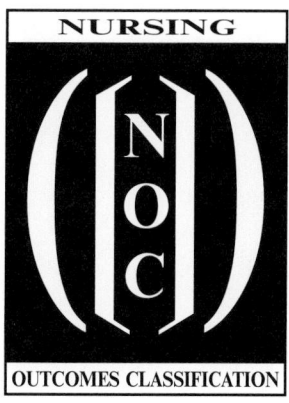

NURSING

NOC

OUTCOMES CLASSIFICATION

# Outcomes: New, Revised, and Retired Since the Second Edition

## Outcomes New to the Third Edition (n=76)

| | | | |
|---|---|---|---|
| 2514 | Abuse Recovery Status | 1213 | Fear Level: Child |
| 1308 | Adaptation to Physical Disability | 0603 | Fluid Overload Severity |
| 0705 | Allergic Response: Localized | 0915 | Hyperactivity Level |
| 0706 | Allergic Response: Systemic | 0707 | Immune Hypersensitivity Response |
| 1211 | Anxiety Level | 0708 | Infection Severity: Newborn |
| 1014 | Appetite | 0213 | Joint Movement: Ankle |
| 0413 | Blood Loss Severity | 0214 | Joint Movement: Elbow |
| 1616 | Body Mechanics Performance | 0215 | Joint Movement: Fingers |
| 1617 | Cardiac Disease Self-Management | 0216 | Joint Movement: Hip |
| 0120 | Child Development: 1 Month | 0217 | Joint Movement: Knee |
| 3000 | Client Satisfaction: Access to Care Resources | 0218 | Joint Movement: Neck |
| | | 0219 | Joint Movement: Shoulder |
| 3001 | Client Satisfaction: Caring | 0220 | Joint Movement: Spine |
| 3002 | Client Satisfaction: Communication | 0221 | Joint Movement: Wrist |
| 3003 | Client Satisfaction: Continuity of Care | 0504 | Kidney Function |
| 3004 | Client Satisfaction: Cultural Needs Fulfillment | 1827 | Knowledge: Body Mechanics |
| | | 1830 | Knowledge: Cardiac Disease Management |
| 3005 | Client Satisfaction: Functional Assistance | 1828 | Knowledge: Fall Prevention |
| 3006 | Client Satisfaction: Physical Care | 1829 | Knowledge: Ostomy Care |
| 3007 | Client Satisfaction: Physical Environment | 1826 | Knowledge: Parenting |
| 3008 | Client Satisfaction: Protection of Rights | 0411 | Mechanical Ventilation Response: Adult |
| 3009 | Client Satisfaction: Psychological Care | 0412 | Mechanical Ventilation Weaning Response: Adult |
| 3010 | Client Satisfaction: Safety | | |
| 3011 | Client Satisfaction: Symptom Control | 1209 | Motivation |
| | | 1618 | Nausea & Vomiting Control |
| 3012 | Client Satisfaction: Teaching | 2106 | Nausea & Vomiting: Disruptive Effects |
| 3013 | Client Satisfaction: Technical Aspects of Care | 2107 | Nausea & Vomiting Severity |
| | | 2513 | Neglect Cessation |
| 2007 | Comfortable Death | 1615 | Ostomy Self-Care |
| 2804 | Community Disaster Readiness | 2900 | Parenting: Infant/Toddler Physical Safety |
| 2805 | Community Risk Control: Violence | 2901 | Parenting: Early/Middle Childhood Physical Safety |
| 2702 | Community Violence Level | | |
| 0212 | Coordinated Movement | 2902 | Parenting: Adolescent Physical Safety |
| 1619 | Diabetes Self-Management | 1614 | Personal Autonomy |
| 1307 | Dignified Life Closure | 2006 | Personal Health Status |
| 0311 | Discharge Readiness: Independent Living | 2303 | Post Procedure Recovery Status |
| 0312 | Discharge Readiness: Supported Living | 1620 | Seizure Control |
| 2607 | Family Physical Environment | 0313 | Self-Care Status |
| 2608 | Family Resiliency | 2405 | Sensory Function Status |
| 2609 | Family Support During Treatment | 1212 | Stress Level |
| 1210 | Fear Level | 2005 | Student Health Status |

# Outcomes Revised for the Third Edition
## Label Name Changes (n=10)

Outcomes in this category have label name changes that affect the alphabetical listing.

| Second Edition Outcome | | Change for Third Edition Outcome | |
|---|---|---|---|
| 0409 | Coagulation Status | 0409 | Blood Coagulation |
| 1105 | Dialysis Access Integrity | 1105 | Hemodialysis Access |
| 2601 | Family Environment: Internal | 2601 | Family Social Climate |
| 1006 | Nutritional Status: Body Mass | 1006 | Weight: Body Mass |
| 1909 | Safety Behavior: Fall Prevention | 1909 | Fall Prevention Behavior |
| 1910 | Safety Behavior: Home Physical Environment | 1910 | Safe Home Environment |
| 1911 | Safety Behavior: Personal | 1911 | Personal Safety Behavior |
| 1912 | Safety Status: Falls Occurrence | 1912 | Falls Occurrence |
| 1913 | Safety Status: Physical Injury | 1913 | Physical Injury Severity |
| 2002 | Well-Being | 2002 | Personal Well-Being |

## Label Name Changes (n=38)

Outcomes in this category have minor changes in the label name.

| Second Edition Outcome | | Change for Third Edition Outcome | |
|---|---|---|---|
| 1400 | Abusive Behavior Self-Control | 1400 | Abusive Behavior Self-Restraint |
| 1401 | Aggression Control | 1401 | Aggression Self-Control |
| 0200 | Ambulation: Walking | 0200 | Ambulation |
| 1402 | Anxiety Control | 1402 | Anxiety Self-Control |
| 1918 | Aspiration Control | 1918 | Aspiration Prevention |
| 0704 | Asthma Control | 0704 | Asthma Self-Management |
| 2300 | Blood Glucose Control | 2300 | Blood Glucose Level |
| 0700 | Blood Transfusion Reaction Control | 0700 | Blood Transfusion Reaction |
| 0107 | Child Development: 5 Years | 0107 | Child Development: Preschool |
| 0108 | Child Development: Middle Childhood (6-11 Years) | 0108 | Child Development: Middle Childhood |
| 0109 | Child Development: Adolescence (12-17 Years) | 0109 | Child Development: Adolescence |
| 0900 | Cognitive Ability | 0900 | Cognition |
| 0902 | Communication Ability | 0902 | Communication |
| 0903 | Communication: Expressive Ability | 0903 | Communication: Expressive |
| 0904 | Communication: Receptive Ability | 0904 | Communication: Receptive |
| 2800 | Community Health: Immunity | 2800 | Community Health Status: Immunity |
| 1409 | Depression Control | 1409 | Depression Self-Control |
| 1403 | Distorted Thought Control | 1403 | Distorted Thought Self-Control |
| 1404 | Fear Control | 1404 | Fear Self-Control |
| 1405 | Impulse Control | 1405 | Impulse Self-Control |
| 0703 | Infection Status | 0703 | Infection Severity |
| 1801 | Knowledge: Child Safety | 1801 | Knowledge: Child Physical Safety |
| 1805 | Knowledge: Health Behaviors | 1805 | Knowledge: Health Behavior |
| 1818 | Knowledge: Postpartum | 1818 | Knowledge: Postpartum Maternal Health |
| 1822 | Knowledge: Preconception | 1822 | Knowledge: Preconception Maternal Health |
| 1203 | Loneliness | 1203 | Loneliness Severity |
| 0208 | Mobility Level | 0208 | Mobility |
| 1100 | Oral Health | 1100 | Oral Hygiene |
| 1306 | Pain: Psychological Response | 1306 | Pain: Adverse Psychological Response |
| 2211 | Parenting | 2211 | Parenting Performance |

| 1901 | Parenting: Social Safety | 1901 | Parenting: Psychosocial Safety |
| 1606 | Participation: Health Care Decisions | 1606 | Participation in Health Care Decisions |
| 0113 | Physical Aging Status | 0113 | Physical Aging |
| 1207 | Sexual Identity: Acceptance | 1207 | Sexual Identity |
| 2001 | Spiritual Well-Being | 2001 | Spiritual Health |
| 2003 | Suffering Level | 2003 | Suffering Severity |
| 0801 | Thermoregulation: Neonate | 0801 | Thermoregulation: Newborn |
| 0802 | Vital Signs Status | 0802 | Vital Signs |

# Definition Changes (n=184)

Outcomes in this category have minor changes in definition that clarifies the concept and improves definition consistency within each scale. For example, specifying "personal actions" rather than "actions," or the addition of "severity of" or "extent of" to previous definitions to be consistent with the scales.

| 2500 | Abuse Cessation | 0903 | Communication: Expressive |
| 2502 | Abuse Recovery: Emotional | 0904 | Communication: Receptive |
| 2503 | Abuse Recovery: Financial | 2700 | Community Competence |
| 2504 | Abuse Recovery: Physical | 2800 | Community Health Status: Immunity |
| 2505 | Abuse Recovery: Sexual | 1601 | Compliance Behavior |
| 1400 | Abusive Behavior Self-Restraint | 1302 | Coping |
| 1300 | Acceptance: Health Status | 0906 | Decision-Making |
| 0005 | Activity Tolerance | 0001 | Endurance |
| 1600 | Adherence Behavior | 0002 | Energy Conservation |
| 0200 | Ambulation | 1909 | Fall Prevention Behavior |
| 1402 | Anxiety Self-Control | 1912 | Falls Occurrence |
| 0409 | Blood Coagulation | 2602 | Family Functioning |
| 2300 | Blood Glucose Level | 2606 | Family Health Status |
| 0700 | Blood Transfusion Reaction | 2603 | Family Integrity |
| 1200 | Body Image | 2604 | Family Normalization |
| 0203 | Body Positioning: Self-Initiated | 2601 | Family Social Climate |
| 1104 | Bone Healing | 1404 | Fear Self-Control |
| 0501 | Bowel Elimination | 0111 | Fetal Status: Antepartum |
| 1000 | Breastfeeding Establishment: Infant | 0112 | Fetal Status: Intrapartum |
| 1001 | Breastfeeding Establishment: Maternal | 0601 | Fluid Balance |
| 1002 | Breastfeeding Maintenance | 0110 | Growth |
| 1003 | Breastfeeding Weaning | 1704 | Health Beliefs: Perceived Threat |
| 0400 | Cardiac Pump Effectiveness | 1705 | Health Orientation |
| 2200 | Caregiver Adaptation To Patient Institutionalization | 1602 | Health Promoting Behavior |
|  |  | 1603 | Health Seeking Behavior |
| 2506 | Caregiver Emotional Health | 1610 | Hearing Compensation Behavior |
| 2202 | Caregiver Home Care Readiness | 1105 | Hemodialysis Access |
| 2203 | Caregiver Lifestyle Disruption | 1201 | Hope |
| 2205 | Caregiver Performance: Direct Care | 0602 | Hydration |
| 2206 | Caregiver Performance: Indirect Care | 1202 | Identity |
| 2507 | Caregiver Physical Health | 0204 | Immobility Consequences: Physiological |
| 2208 | Caregiver Stressors | 0205 | Immobility Consequences: Psycho-Cognitive |
| 2508 | Caregiver Well-Being |  |  |
| 1301 | Child Adaptation to Hospitalization | 0702 | Immune Status |
| 0107 | Child Development: Preschool | 1900 | Immunization Behavior |
| 0108 | Child Development: Middle Childhood | 0703 | Infection Severity |
| 0109 | Child Development: Adolescence | 0207 | Joint Movement: Passive |
| 0401 | Circulation Status | 1801 | Knowledge: Child Physical Safety |
| 0901 | Cognitive Orientation | 1821 | Knowledge: Conception Prevention |
| 2100 | Comfort Level | 1820 | Knowledge: Diabetes Management |
| 0902 | Communication | 1802 | Knowledge: Diet |

| | | | |
|---|---|---|---|
| 1823 | Knowledge: Health Promotion | 1908 | Risk Detection |
| 1806 | Knowledge: Health Resources | 1910 | Safe Home Environment |
| 1824 | Knowledge: Illness Care | 0300 | Self-Care: Activities of Daily Living (ADL) |
| 1819 | Knowledge: Infant Care | | |
| 1817 | Knowledge: Labor & Delivery | 0301 | Self-Care: Bathing |
| 1809 | Knowledge: Personal Safety | 0302 | Self-Care: Dressing |
| 1810 | Knowledge: Pregnancy | 0303 | Self-Care: Eating |
| 1812 | Knowledge: Substance Use Control | 0305 | Self-Care: Hygiene |
| 1604 | Leisure Participation | 0306 | Self-Care: Instrumental Activities of Daily Living (IADL) |
| 1203 | Loneliness Severity | | |
| 2509 | Maternal Status: Antepartum | 0307 | Self-Care: Non-Parenteral Medication |
| 2510 | Maternal Status: Intrapartum | 0308 | Self-Care: Oral Hygiene |
| 2511 | Maternal Status: Postpartum | 0309 | Self-Care: Parenteral Medication |
| 0208 | Mobility | 0310 | Self-Care: Toileting |
| 2512 | Neglect Recovery | 1613 | Self-Direction of Care |
| 0909 | Neurological Status | 1406 | Self-Mutilation Restraint |
| 0910 | Neurological Status: Autonomic | 2400 | Sensory Function: Cutaneous |
| 0911 | Neurological Status: Central Motor Control | 2401 | Sensory Function: Hearing |
| | | 2402 | Sensory Function: Proprioception |
| 0912 | Neurological Status: Consciousness | 2403 | Sensory Function: Taste & Smell |
| 0913 | Neurological Status: Cranial Sensory/Motor Function | 2404 | Sensory Function: Vision |
| | | 0119 | Sexual Functioning |
| 0914 | Neurological Status: Spinal Sensory/Motor Function | 0211 | Skeletal Function |
| | | 0004 | Sleep |
| 0118 | Newborn Adaptation | 1502 | Social Interaction Skills |
| 1007 | Nutritional Status: Energy | 1503 | Social Involvement |
| 1009 | Nutritional Status: Nutrient Intake | 1504 | Social Support |
| 1306 | Pain: Adverse Psychological Response | 2001 | Spiritual Health |
| 2101 | Pain: Disruptive Effects | 1407 | Substance Addiction Consequences |
| 2102 | Pain Level | 2003 | Suffering Severity |
| 1500 | Parent-Infant Attachment | 1408 | Suicide Self-Restraint |
| 2211 | Parenting Performance | 1010 | Swallowing Status |
| 1901 | Parenting: Psychosocial Safety | 1011 | Swallowing Status: Esophageal Phase |
| 1606 | Participation in Health Care Decisions | 1012 | Swallowing Status: Oral Phase |
| 1911 | Personal Safety Behavior | 1013 | Swallowing Status: Pharyngeal Phase |
| 2002 | Personal Well-Being | 2103 | Symptom Severity |
| 0113 | Physical Aging | 2104 | Symptom Severity: Perimenopause |
| 2004 | Physical Fitness | 2105 | Symptom Severity: Premenstrual Syndrome (PMS) |
| 0116 | Play Participation | | |
| 1607 | Prenatal Health Behavior | 2302 | Systemic Toxin Clearance: Dialysis |
| 0006 | Psychomotor Energy | 0801 | Thermoregulation: Newborn |
| 1305 | Psychosocial Adjustment: Life Change | 0404 | Tissue Perfusion: Abdominal Organs |
| 2000 | Quality of Life | 0405 | Tissue Perfusion: Cardiac |
| 0410 | Respiratory Status: Airway Patency | 0406 | Tissue Perfusion: Cerebral |
| 0003 | Rest | 0407 | Tissue Perfusion: Peripheral |
| 1902 | Risk Control | 0408 | Tissue Perfusion: Pulmonary |
| 1903 | Risk Control: Alcohol Use | 0210 | Transfer Performance |
| 1917 | Risk Control: Cancer | 0502 | Urinary Continence |
| 1914 | Risk Control: Cardiovascular Health | 0503 | Urinary Elimination |
| 1904 | Risk Control: Drug Use | 1611 | Vision Compensation Behavior |
| 1915 | Risk Control: Hearing Impairment | 0802 | Vital Signs |
| 1905 | Risk Control: Sexually Transmitted Diseases (STD) | 1006 | Weight: Body Mass |
| | | 1612 | Weight Control |
| 1906 | Risk Control: Tobacco Use | 1102 | Wound Healing: Primary Intention |
| 1907 | Risk Control: Unintended Pregnancy | 1103 | Wound Healing: Secondary Intention |
| 1916 | Risk Control: Visual Impairment | | |

# Scale Changes (n=74)

| Code | Outcome | Old Scale | New Scale |
|------|---------|-----------|-----------|
| 2500 | Abuse Cessation | No evidence to Extensive evidence (o) | None to Extensive (i) |
| 1300 | Acceptance: Health Status | None to Extensive (i) | Never demonstrated to Consistently demonstrated (m) |
| 0200 | Ambulation | Dependent, does not participate to Completely independent (c) | Severely compromised to Not compromised (a) |
| 0201 | Ambulation: Wheelchair | Dependent, does not participate to Completely independent (c) | Severely compromised to Not compromised (a) |
| 0202 | Balance | Dependent, does not participate to Completely independent (c) | Severely compromised to Not compromised (a) and Severe to None (n) |
| 2300 | Blood Glucose Level | Not at all to To a very great extent (e) | Severe deviation from normal range to No deviation form normal range (b) |
| 0700 | Blood Transfusion Reaction | Not at all to To a very great extent (e) | Severe to None (n) |
| 0203 | Body Positioning: Self-Initiated | Dependent, does not participate to Completely independent (c) | Severely compromised to Not compromised (a) |
| 1104 | Bone Healing | None to Complete (j) | None to Extensive (i) and Extensive to None (h) |
| 2200 | Caregiver Adaptation to Patient Institutionalization | None to Extensive (i) | Never demonstrated to Consistently demonstrated (m) |
| 2202 | Caregiver Home Care Readiness | None to Extensive (i) | Not adequate to Totally adequate (f) |
| 2208 | Caregiver Stressors | Extensive to None (h) | Severe to None (n) |
| 2508 | Caregiver Well-Being | Extremely compromised to Not compromised (a) | Not at all satisfied to Completely satisfied (s) |

*Continued*

# Scale Changes (n=74)—cont'd

| Code | Outcome | Old Scale | New Scale |
|------|---------|-----------|-----------|
| 1301 | Child Adaptation to Hospitalization | None to Extensive (i) | Never demonstrated to Consistently demonstrated (m) and Consistently to Never demonstrated (t) |
| 0100 | Child Development: 2 Months | Extreme delay from expected range to No delay from expected range (p) | Never demonstrated to Consistently demonstrated (m) |
| 0101 | Child Development: 4 Months | Extreme delay from expected range to No delay from expected range (p) | Never demonstrated to Consistently demonstrated (m) |
| 0102 | Child Development: 6 Months | Extreme delay from expected range to No delay from expected range (p) | Never demonstrated to Consistently demonstrated (m) |
| 0103 | Child Development: 12 Months | Extreme delay from expected range to No delay from expected range (p) | Never demonstrated to Consistently demonstrated (m) |
| 0104 | Child Development: 2 Years | Extreme delay from expected range to No delay from expected range (p) | Never demonstrated to Consistently demonstrated (m) |
| 0105 | Child Development: 3 Years | Extreme delay from expected range to No delay from expected range (p) | Never demonstrated to Consistently demonstrated (m) |
| 0106 | Child Development: 4 Years | Extreme delay from expected range to No delay from expected range (p) | Never demonstrated to Consistently demonstrated (m) |
| 0107 | Child Development: Preschool | Extreme delay from expected range to No delay from expected range (p) | Never demonstrated to Consistently demonstrated (m) |
| 0108 | Child Development: Middle Childhood | Extreme delay from expected range to No delay from expected range (p) | Never demonstrated to Consistently demonstrated (m) |
| 0109 | Child Development: Adolescence | Extreme delay from expected range to No delay from expected range (p) | Never demonstrated to Consistently demonstrated (m) |
| 0901 | Cognitive Orientation | Never demonstrated to Consistently demonstrated (m) | Severely compromised to Not compromised (a) |

| Code | Outcome | Scale 1 | Scale 2 |
|---|---|---|---|
| 2100 | Comfort Level | None to Extensive (i) | Not at all satisfied to Completely satisfied (s) |
| 0905 | Concentration | Never demonstrated to Consistently demonstrated (m) | Severely compromised to Not compromised (a) |
| 0906 | Decision-Making | Never demonstrated to Consistently demonstrated (m) | Severely compromised to Not compromised (a) |
| 0002 | Energy Conservation | Not at all to To a very great extent (e) | Never demonstrated to Consistently demonstrated (m) |
| 1909 | Fall Prevention Behavior | Not adequate to Totally adequate (f) | Never demonstrated to Consistently demonstrated (m) |
| 1304 | Grief Resolution | Not at all to To a very great extent (e) | Never demonstrated to Consistently demonstrated (m) |
| 1105 | Hemodialysis Access | Extreme deviation from expected range to No deviation from expected range (b) | Severely compromised to Not compromised (a) and Severe to None (n) |
| 1201 | Hope | None to Extensive (i) | Never demonstrated to Consistently demonstrated (m) |
| 0907 | Information Processing | Never demonstrated to Consistently demonstrated (m) | Severely compromised to Not compromised (a) |
| 0207 | Joint Movement: Passive | No motion to Full motion (d) | Severe deviation from normal range to No deviation from normal range (b) |
| 1604 | Leisure Participation | Not adequate to Totally adequate (f) | Never demonstrated to Consistently demonstrated (m) |
| 1203 | Loneliness Severity | Extensive to None (h) | Severe to None (n) |
| 2301 | Medication Response | Not at all to To a very great extent (e) | Severely compromised to Not compromised (a) and Severe to None (n) |
| 0908 | Memory | Never demonstrated to Consistently demonstrated (m) | Severely compromised to Not compromised (a) |
| 0208 | Mobility | Dependent, does not participate to Completely independent (c) | Severely compromised to Not compromised (a) |
| 2512 | Neglect Recovery | No evidence to Extensive evidence (o) | None to Extensive (i) and Extensive to None (h) |

*Continued*

# Scale Changes (n=74)—cont'd

| Code | Outcome | Old Scale | New Scale |
|------|---------|-----------|-----------|
| 1004 | Nutritional Status | Extremely compromised to Not compromised (a) | Severe deviation from normal range to No deviation from normal range (b) |
| 1007 | Nutritional Status: Energy | Extremely compromised to Not compromised (a) | Severe deviation from normal range to No deviation from normal range (b) |
| 2211 | Parenting Performance | Not adequate to Totally adequate (f) | Never demonstrated to Consistently demonstrated (m) |
| 1901 | Parenting: Psychosocial Safety | Not adequate to Totally adequate (f) | Never demonstrated to Consistently demonstrated (m) |
| 1911 | Personal Safety Behavior | Not adequate to Totally adequate (f) | Never demonstrated to Consistently demonstrated (m) |
| 2002 | Personal Well-Being | Extremely compromised to Not compromised (a) | Not at all satisfied to Completely satisfied (s) |
| 2004 | Physical Fitness | Poor to Excellent (r) | Severely compromised to Not compromised (a) |
| 0116 | Play Participation | Not adequate to Totally adequate (f) | Never demonstrated to Consistently demonstrated (m) |
| 0117 | Preterm Infant Organization | Extreme deviation from expected range to No deviation from expected range (b) | Severely compromised to Not compromised (a) |
| 1305 | Psychosocial Adjustment: Life Change | None to Extensive (i) | Never demonstrated to Consistently demonstrated (m) |
| 2000 | Quality of Life | Extremely compromised to Not compromised (a) | Not at all satisfied to Completely satisfied (s) |
| 0300 | Self-Care: Activities of Daily Living | Dependent, does not participate to Completely independent (c) | Severely compromised to Not compromised (a) |
| 0301 | Self-Care: Bathing | Dependent, does not participate to Completely independent (c) | Severely compromised to Not compromised (a) |

| | | | |
|---|---|---|---|
| 0302 | Self-Care: Dressing | Dependent, does not participate to Completely independent (c) | Severely compromised to Not compromised (a) |
| 0303 | Self-Care: Eating | Dependent, does not participate to Completely independent (c) | Severely compromised to Not compromised (a) |
| 0305 | Self-Care: Hygiene | Dependent, does not participate to Completely independent (c) | Severely compromised to Not compromised (a) |
| 0306 | Self-Care: Instrumental Activities of Daily Living | Dependent, does not participate to Completely independent (c) | Severely compromised to Not compromised (a) |
| 0307 | Self-Care: Non-Parenteral Medication | Dependent, does not participate to Completely independent (c) | Severely compromised to Not compromised (a) |
| 0308 | Self-Care: Oral Hygiene | Dependent, does not participate to Completely independent (c) | Severely compromised to Not compromised (a) |
| 0309 | Self-Care: Parenteral Medication | Dependent, does not participate to Completely independent (c) | Severely compromised to Not compromised (a) |
| 0310 | Self-Care: Toileting | Dependent, does not participate to Completely independent (c) | Severely compromised to Not compromised (a) |
| 2400 | Sensory Function: Cutaneous | Extremely compromised to Not compromised (a) | Severe deviation from normal range to No deviation from normal range (b) and Severe to None (n) |
| 2401 | Sensory Function: Hearing | Extremely compromised to Not compromised (a) | Severe deviation from normal range to No deviation from normal range (b) and Severe to None (n) |
| 2402 | Sensory Function: Proprioception | Extremely compromised to Not compromised (a) | Severe deviation from normal range to No deviation from normal range (b) and Severe to None (n) |
| 2403 | Sensory Function: Taste & Smell | Extremely compromised to Not compromised (a) | Severe deviation from normal range to No deviation from normal range (b) and Severe to None (n) |

*Continued*

## Scale Changes (n=74)—cont'd

| Code | Outcome | Old Scale | New Scale |
|------|---------|-----------|-----------|
| 2404 | Sensory Function: Vision | Extremely compromised to Not compromised (a) | Severe deviation from normal range to No deviation from normal range (b) and Severe to None (n) |
| 1502 | Social Interaction Skills | None to Extensive (i) | Never demonstrated to Consistently demonstrated (m) |
| 1503 | Social Involvement | None to Extensive (i) | Never demonstrated to Consistently demonstrated (m) |
| 1504 | Social Support | None to Extensive (i) | Not adequate to Totally adequate (f) |
| 2302 | Systemic Toxin Clearance: Dialysis | Never demonstrated to Consistently demonstrated (m) | Severely compromised to Not compromised (a) and Severe to None (n) |
| 0210 | Transfer Performance | Dependent, does not participate to Completely independent (c) | Severely compromised to Not compromised (a) |
| 1102 | Wound Healing: Primary Intention | None to Complete (j) | None to Extensive (i) and Extensive to None (h) |
| 1103 | Wound Healing: Secondary Intention | None to Complete (j) | None to Extensive (i) and Extensive to None (h) |

# Second Scale Added (n=50)

| Code | Outcome | Scale Added |
|------|---------|-------------|
| 2502 | Abuse Recovery: Emotional | Extensive to None (h) |
| 2505 | Abuse Recovery: Sexual | Extensive to None (h) |
| 0704 | Asthma Self-Management | Consistently demonstrated to Never demonstrated (t) |
| 0409 | Blood Coagulation | Severe to None (n) |
| 0500 | Bowel Continence | Consistently demonstrated to Never demonstrated (t) |
| 0501 | Bowel Elimination | Severe to None (n) |
| 0400 | Cardiac Pump Effectiveness | Severe to None (n) |
| 2506 | Caregiver Emotional Health | Severe to None (n) |
| 2203 | Caregiver Lifestyle Disruption | Severely compromised to Not compromised (a) |
| 0401 | Circulation Status | Severe to None (n) |
| 0001 | Endurance | Severe to None (n) |
| 2606 | Family Health Status | Severe to None (n) |
| 0601 | Fluid Balance | Severe to None (n) |
| 0602 | Hydration | Severe to None (n) |
| 0204 | Immobility Consequences: Physiological | Severely compromised to Not compromised (a) |
| 0205 | Immobility Consequences: Psycho-Cognitive | Severely compromised to Not compromised (a) |
| 0702 | Immune Status | Severe to None (n) |
| 2509 | Maternal Status: Antepartum | Severe to None (n) |
| 2510 | Maternal Status: Intrapartum | Severe to None (n) |
| 2511 | Maternal Status: Postpartum | Severe to None (n) |
| 1204 | Mood Equilibrium | Consistently demonstrated to Never demonstrated (t) |
| 0909 | Neurological Status | Severe to None (n) |
| 0910 | Neurological Status: Autonomic | Severe to None (n) |
| 0911 | Neurological Status: Central Motor Control | Severe to None (n) |
| 0912 | Neurological Status: Consciousness | Severe to None (n) |
| 0913 | Neurological Status: Cranial Sensory/ Motor Function | Severe to None (n) |
| 0914 | Neurological Status: Spinal Sensory/ Motor Function | Severe to None (n) |
| 1100 | Oral Hygiene | Severe to None (n) |
| 2101 | Pain: Disruptive Effects | Severely compromised to Not compromised (a) |
| 2102 | Pain Level | Severely compromised to Not compromised (a) |
| 0006 | Psychomotor Energy | Consistently demonstrated to Never demonstrated (t) |
| 0410 | Respiratory Status: Airway Patency | Severe to None (n) |
| 0402 | Respiratory Status: Gas Exchange | Severe to None (n) |
| 0403 | Respiratory Status: Ventilation | Severe to None (n) |
| 0004 | Sleep | Severe to None (n) |
| 1010 | Swallowing Status | Severe to None (n) |
| 1011 | Swallowing Status: Esophageal Phase | Severe to None (n) |
| 1012 | Swallowing Status: Oral Phase | Severe to None (n) |
| 1013 | Swallowing Status: Pharyngeal Phase | Severe to None (n) |
| 0800 | Thermoregulation | Severe to None (n) |
| 0801 | Thermoregulation: Newborn | Severe to None (n) |
| 1101 | Tissue Integrity: Skin & Mucous Membranes | Severe to None (n) |
| 0404 | Tissue Perfusion: Abdominal Organs | Severe to None (n) |
| 0405 | Tissue Perfusion: Cardiac | Severe to None (n) |
| 0406 | Tissue Perfusion: Cerebral | Severe to None (n) |
| 0407 | Tissue Perfusion: Peripheral | Severe to None (n) |
| 0408 | Tissue Perfusion: Pulmonary | Severe to None (n) |

*Continued*

## Second Scale Added (n=50)—cont'd

| Code | Outcome | Scale Added |
|------|---------|-------------|
| 0502 | Urinary Continence | Consistently demonstrated to Never demonstrated (t) |
| 0503 | Urinary Elimination | Severe to None (n) |
| 1206 | Will to Live | Severe to None (n) |

## Reclassified in Taxonomy (n=8)

0704 Asthma Self-Management
    Reclassified Domain Health, Knowledge, & Behavior (IV); Class Health Behaviors (Q)
2100 Comfort Level
    Reclassified Class Health & Life Quality (U)
2800 Community Health Status: Immunity
    Reclassified Class Community Well-Being (b)
1306 Pain: Adverse Psychological Response
    Reclassified Domain Perceived Health (V); Class Symptom Status (V)
2211 Parenting Performance
    Reclassified Class Parenting (d)
1901 Parenting: Psychosocial Safety
    Reclassified Domain Family Health (VI); Class Parenting (d)
2003 Suffering Severity
    Reclassified Class Symptom Status (V)
1006 Weight: Body Mass
    Class Metabolic Regulation (I)

## Outcomes in the Second Edition That Were Deleted for This Edition (n=6)

1303 Dignified Dying
    Replaced with Dignified Life Closure and Comfortable Death
0701 Immune Hypersensitivity Control
    Replaced with Immune Hypersensitivity Response
0206 Joint Movement: Active
    Relabeled with specific joints
1825 Knowledge: Maternal-Child Health
    Deleted
0209 Muscle Function
    Subsumed under Coordinated Movement
0304 Self-Care: Grooming
    Subsumed under Self-Care: Hygiene

# NOC Outcomes Placed in the Taxonomy of Nursing Practice

## A COMMON STRUCTURE FOR NANDA, NIC, AND NOC

An invitational conference was convened in August 2001 to develop a common taxonomic structure for the nomenclature of NANDA International, Nursing Interventions Classification (NIC) and Nursing Outcomes Classification (NOC) (NNN). The purposes of the common structure are to facilitate linking nursing diagnoses, nursing interventions, and patient outcomes sensitive to nursing practice and to demonstrate the relationships between NANDA, NIC, and NOC terms and concepts. Although developed for the purpose of linking these three classifications, the common structure is in the public domain and can be used by all nursing classifications. The participants and methods used to develop the structure are discussed in a monograph published by the American Nurses Association.[1]

The taxonomy of nursing practice that appears in this section is the current structure, with NOC outcomes placed in the structure. As each of the languages is placed within the structure, it is anticipated that modifications of the structure might be necessary. To be able to place NOC outcomes in the common structure, some liberty was taken in interpreting the structure and the definitions. The following interpretations guided placement of the outcomes.

1. The class Values/Beliefs under the Functional Domain was interpreted to include perceptions such as client satisfaction, although this is not a value or belief per se.
2. The outcome Post Procedure Recovery Status includes indicators applicable to a number of the physiologic classes but was placed in the Pharmacological Function class to avoid repetition in a number of classes.
3. Behaviors that promote physical as well as mental and emotional health were placed under the classes Knowledge, Behavior, and Coping in the Psychosocial Domain. Although they do not fit with the domain definition, this was the only place available in the taxonomy to place these outcomes, and they are consistent with the class definitions.
4. All risk control outcomes were placed in the class Risk Management in the Environmental Domain. Again, this is not consistent with the domain name, but it is consistent with the definition for the class Risk Management. It should be noted that some of the risk control outcomes, such as Risk Control: Cardiovascular Disease, could also fit within the class Cardiac in the Functional Domain, but the decision was made to keep all risk control outcomes together at this time.
5. Parenting outcomes that were measures of safety were placed in the Risk Management class rather than in the Roles/Relationship Class in the Psychosocial Domain.

Although most of the outcomes were placed in the taxonomy of nursing practice, we found it problematic to place some of the outcomes. The following general health outcomes were not placed in the structure because they related to a number of domains and/or classes: 2507 Caregiver Physical Health, 2508 Caregiver Well-Being, 2606 Family Health Status, 2006 Personal Health Status, 2002 Personal Well-Being, 2005 Student Health Status. The outcome 1604 Leisure Participation was not placed in the common structure since it did not seem to fit any of the classes.

It is evident from the above comments that this is the first attempt to use the common structure for NOC outcomes. We anticipate that a number of changes will take place as the structure develops and the three languages reach some agreement on placement of terms within the structure. However, we wanted to share this beginning work with readers and would appreciate feedback on concerns or suggestions for this initial placement of NOC  outcomes.

1. Dochterman, J., & Jones, D. (2003). *Unifying nursing languages: The harmonization of NANDA, NIC and NOC*. Washington, D.C.: American Nurses Association.

| *Level 1* **Domains** | **I. Functional Domain**<br>Includes diagnoses, outcomes, and interventions to promote basic needs | |
|---|---|---|
| *Level 2* **Classes** | **Activity/Exercise**<br>Physical activity, including energy conservation and expenditure | **Comfort**<br>A sense of emotional, physical, and spiritual well-being and relative freedom from distress |
| *Level 3* **Outcomes** | 0005 Activity Tolerance<br>0200 Ambulation<br>0201 Ambulation: Wheelchair<br>0202 Balance<br>1616 Body Mechanics Performance<br>0212 Coordinated Movement<br>0001 Endurance<br>0002 Energy Conservation<br>0213 Joint Movement: Ankle<br>0214 Joint Movement: Elbow<br>0215 Joint Movement: Fingers<br>0216 Joint Movement: Hip<br>0217 Joint Movement: Knee<br>0218 Joint Movement: Neck<br>0207 Joint Movement: Passive<br>0219 Joint Movement: Shoulder<br>0220 Joint Movement: Spine<br>0221 Joint Movement: Wrist<br>0208 Mobility<br>2004 Physical Fitness<br>0006 Psychomotor Energy<br>0211 Skeletal Function | 2514 Abuse Recovery Status<br>2503 Abuse Recovery: Financial<br>2504 Abuse Recovery: Physical<br>2100 Comfort Level<br>2007 Comfortable Death<br>0204 Immobility Consequences:<br>    Physiological<br>0205 Immobility Consequences:<br>    Psycho-Cognitive<br>1618 Nausea & Vomiting Control<br>2106 Nausea & Vomiting: Disruptive<br>    Effects<br>2107 Nausea & Vomiting Severity<br>2512 Neglect Recovery<br>1605 Pain Control<br>2101 Pain: Disruptive Effects<br>2102 Pain Level<br>1913 Physical Injury Severity<br>2001 Spiritual Health<br>2003 Suffering Severity<br>1608 Symptom Control<br>2103 Symptom Severity<br>2104 Symptom Severity:<br>    Perimenopause<br>2105 Symptom Severity:<br>    Premenstrual Syndrome (PMS) |

| *Level 1* **Domains** | **I. Functional Domain—cont'd** Includes diagnoses, outcomes, and interventions to promote basic needs | |
|---|---|---|
| *Level 2* **Classes** | **Growth and Development** Physical, emotional, and social growth and development milestones | **Nutrition** Processes related to taking in, assimilating, and using nutrients |
| *Level 3* **Outcomes** | 0120 Child Development: 1 Month<br>0100 Child Development: 2 Months<br>0101 Child Development: 4 Months<br>0102 Child Development: 6 Months<br>0103 Child Development: 12 Months<br>0104 Child Development: 2 Years<br>0105 Child Development: 3 Years<br>0106 Child Development: 4 Years<br>0107 Child Development: Preschool<br>0108 Child Development: Middle Childhood<br>0109 Child Development: Adolescence<br>0110 Growth<br>0915 Hyperactivity Level<br>0118 Newborn Adaptation<br>0113 Physical Aging<br>0116 Play Participation<br>0117 Preterm Infant Organization<br>1305 Psychosocial Adjustment: Life Change | 1014 Appetite<br>1000 Breastfeeding Establishment: Infant<br>1001 Breastfeeding Establishment: Maternal<br>1002 Breastfeeding Maintenance<br>1003 Breastfeeding Weaning<br>1004 Nutritional Status<br>1005 Nutritional Status: Biochemical Measures<br>1007 Nutritional Status: Energy<br>1008 Nutritional Status: Food & Fluid Intake<br>1009 Nutritional Status: Nutrient Intake<br>1010 Swallowing Status<br>1011 Swallowing Status: Esophageal Phase<br>1012 Swallowing Status: Oral Phase<br>1013 Swallowing Status: Pharyngeal Phase<br>1006 Weight: Body Mass |

**I. Functional Domain**
Includes diagnoses, outcomes, and interventions to promote basic needs

| Level 1 Domains | Level 2 Classes | | | |
|---|---|---|---|---|
| | **Self-Care** Ability to accomplish basic and instrumental activities of daily living | **Sexuality** Maintenance or modification of sexual identity and patterns | **Sleep/Rest** The quantity and quality, sleep, rest, and relaxation patterns | **Values/Beliefs** Ideas, goals, perceptions, spiritual and other beliefs that influence choices or decisions |
| **Level 3 Outcomes** | 0203 Body Positioning: Self-Initiated<br>0311 Discharge Readiness: Independent Living<br>0312 Discharge Readiness: Supported Living<br>1615 Ostomy Self-Care<br>0313 Self-Care Status<br>0300 Self-Care: Activities of Daily Living (ADL)<br>0301 Self-Care: Bathing<br>0302 Self-Care: Dressing<br>0303 Self-Care: Eating<br>0305 Self-Care: Hygiene<br>0306 Self-Care: Instrumental Activities of Daily Living (IADL)<br>0307 Self-Care: Non-Parenteral Medication<br>0308 Self-Care: Oral Hygiene<br>0309 Self-Care: Parenteral Medication<br>0310 Self-Care: Toileting<br>1613 Self-Direction of Care<br>0210 Transfer Performance | 2505 Abuse Recovery: Sexual<br>0114 Physical Maturation: Female<br>0115 Physical Maturation: Male<br>0119 Sexual Functioning<br>1207 Sexual Identity | 0003 Rest<br>0004 Sleep | 3000 Client Satisfaction: Access to Care Resources<br>3001 Client Satisfaction: Caring<br>3002 Client Satisfaction: Communication<br>3003 Client Satisfaction: Continuity of Care<br>3004 Client Satisfaction: Cultural Needs Fulfillment<br>3005 Client Satisfaction: Functional Assistance<br>3006 Client Satisfaction: Physical Care<br>3007 Client Satisfaction: Physical Environment<br>3008 Client Satisfaction: Protection of Rights<br>3009 Client Satisfaction: Psychological Care<br>3010 Client Satisfaction: Safety<br>3011 Client Satisfaction: Symptom Control<br>3012 Client Satisfaction: Teaching<br>3013 Client Satisfaction: Technical Aspects of Care<br>1700 Health Beliefs<br>1701 Health Beliefs: Perceived Ability to Perform<br>1702 Health Beliefs: Perceived Control<br>1703 Health Beliefs: Perceived Resources<br>1704 Health Beliefs: Perceived Threat<br>1705 Health Orientation<br>1209 Motivation<br>2000 Quality of Life<br>1206 Will to Live |

714 Part Six   Appendixes

**Level 1 Domains**

**II. Physiological Domain**
Includes diagnoses, outcomes, and interventions to promote optimal biophysical health

**Level 2 Classes** / **Level 3 Outcomes**

| Cardiac Function | Elimination | Fluid & Electrolyte | Neurocognition |
|---|---|---|---|
| Cardiac mechanisms used to maintain tissue profusion | Processes related to secretion and excretion of body wastes | Regulation of fluid/electrolytes and acid base balance | Mechanisms related to the nervous system and neurocognitive functioning, including memory, thinking and judgment |
| 0409 Blood Coagulation<br>0413 Blood Loss Severity<br>0400 Cardiac Pump Effectiveness<br>0401 Circulation Status<br>0404 Tissue Perfusion: Abdominal Organs<br>0405 Tissue Perfusion: Cardiac<br>0406 Tissue Perfusion: Cerebral<br>0407 Tissue Perfusion: Peripheral<br>0408 Tissue Perfusion: Pulmonary | 0500 Bowel Continence<br>0501 Bowel Elimination<br>0504 Kidney Function<br>2302 Systemic Toxin Clearance: Dialysis<br>0502 Urinary Continence<br>0503 Urinary Elimination | 0600 Electrolyte & Acid/Base Balance<br>0601 Fluid Balance<br>0603 Fluid Overload Severity<br>0602 Hydration | 0900 Cognition<br>0901 Cognitive Orientation<br>0905 Concentration<br>0906 Decision-Making<br>0907 Information Processing<br>0908 Memory<br>0909 Neurological Status<br>0910 Neurological Status: Autonomic<br>0911 Neurological Status: Central Motor Control<br>0912 Neurological Status: Consciousness<br>0913 Neurological Status: Cranial Sensory/Motor Function<br>0914 Neurological Status: Spinal Sensory/Motor Function |

| *Level 1* **Domains** | **II. Physiological Domain** Includes diagnoses, outcomes, and interventions to promote optimal biophysical health | | |
|---|---|---|---|
| *Level 2* **Classes** | **Pharmacological Function** Effects (therapeutic and adverse) of medications or drugs and other pharmacologically active products | **Physical Regulation** Body temperature, endocrine, and immune system responses to regulate cellular processes | **Reproduction** Processes related to human procreation and birth | **Respiratory Function** Ventilation adequate to maintain arterial blood gases within normal limits |
| *Level 3* **Outcomes** | 2300 Blood Glucose Level 2301 Medication Response 2303 Post Procedure Recovery Status | 0705 Allergic Response: Localized 0706 Allergic Response: Systemic 0700 Blood Transfusion Reaction 0707 Immune Hypersensitivity Response 0702 Immune Status 0703 Infection Severity 0708 Infection Severity: Newborn 0800 Thermoregulation 0801 Thermoregulation: Newborn 0802 Vital Signs | 0111 Fetal Status: Antepartum 0112 Fetal Status: Intrapartum 2509 Maternal Status: Antepartum 2510 Maternal Status: Intrapartum 2511 Maternal Status: Postpartum 1607 Prenatal Health Behavior | 0411 Mechanical Ventilation Response: Adult 0412 Mechanical Ventilation Weaning Response: Adult 0410 Respiratory Status: Airway Patency 0402 Respiratory Status: Gas Exchange 0403 Respiratory Status: Ventilation |

| | | |
|---|---|---|
| **Level 1** **Domains** | **II. Physiological Domain** Includes diagnoses, outcomes, and interventions to promote optimal biophysical health | |
| **Level 2** **Classes** | **Sensation/Perception** Intake and interpretation of information through the senses, including seeing, hearing, touching, tasting, smelling | **Tissue Integrity** Skin and mucous membrane protection to support secretion, excretion, and healing |
| **Level 3** **Outcomes** | 1610 Hearing Compensation Behavior 2405 Sensory Function Status 2400 Sensory Function: Cutaneous 2401 Sensory Function: Hearing 2402 Sensory Function: Proprioception 2403 Sensory Function: Taste & Smell 2404 Sensory Function: Vision 1611 Vision Compensation Behavior | 1104 Bone Healing 1105 Hemodialysis Access 1100 Oral Hygiene 1101 Tissue Integrity: Skin & Mucous Membranes 1102 Wound Healing: Primary Intention 1103 Wound Healing: Secondary Intention |

| Level 1 Domains | III. Psychosocial Domain | | | |
|---|---|---|---|---|
| | Includes diagnoses, outcomes, and interventions to promote optimal mental and emotional health and social functioning | | | |
| Level 2 Classes | Behavior* Actions that promote, maintain, or restore health | Communication Receiving, interpreting, and expressing spoken, written, and non-verbal messages | Coping* Adjusting or adapting to stressful events | Emotional A mental state or feeling that may influence perceptions of the world |
| Level 3 Outcomes | 1600 Adherence Behavior<br>0704 Asthma Self-Management<br>1617 Cardiac Disease Self-Management<br>2205 Caregiver Performance: Direct Care<br>2206 Caregiver Performance: Indirect Care<br>1601 Compliance Behavior<br>1619 Diabetes Self-Management<br>2605 Family Participation in Professional Care<br>1602 Health Promoting Behavior<br>1603 Health Seeking Behavior<br>1900 Immunization Behavior<br>1606 Participation in Health Care Decisions<br>1614 Personal Autonomy<br>1609 Treatment Behavior: Illness or Injury<br>1612 Weight Control | 0902 Communication<br>0903 Communication: Expressive<br>0904 Communication: Receptive | 1400 Abusive Behavior Self-Restraint<br>1300 Acceptance: Health Status<br>1308 Adaptation to Physical Disability<br>1401 Aggression Self-Control<br>1402 Anxiety Self-Control<br>2200 Caregiver Adaptation to Patient Institutionalization<br>2210 Caregiving Endurance Potential<br>1301 Child Adaptation To Hospitalization<br>1302 Coping<br>1409 Depression Self-Control<br>1307 Dignified Life Closure<br>1403 Distorted Thought Self-Control<br>2600 Family Coping<br>2604 Family Normalization<br>2608 Family Resiliency<br>2609 Family Support During Treatment<br>1404 Fear Self-Control<br>1304 Grief Resolution<br>1405 Impulse Self-Control<br>1406 Self-Mutilation Restraint<br>1408 Suicide Self-Restraint | 2502 Abuse Recovery: Emotional<br>1211 Anxiety Level<br>2506 Caregiver Emotional Health<br>2203 Caregiver Lifestyle Disruption<br>2208 Caregiver Stressors<br>1208 Depression Level<br>1210 Fear Level<br>1213 Fear Level: Child<br>1201 Hope<br>1203 Loneliness Severity<br>1204 Mood Equilibrium<br>1306 Pain: Adverse Psychological Response<br>1212 Stress Level |

*Behaviors that promote physical health as well as mental and emotional health were placed in this domain, in spite of a poor match with the concept "psychosocial"

*Continued*

| Level 1 Domains | | |
|---|---|---|
| **III. Psychosocial Domain** Includes diagnoses, outcomes, and interventions to promote optimal mental and emotional health and social functioning | | |
| **Level 2 Classes** | | |
| **Knowledge** Understanding and skill in applying information to promote, maintain, and restore health | **Roles/Relationships** Maintenance and/or modification of expected social behaviors and emotional connectedness with others | **Self Perception** Awareness of one's body and personal identity |
| **Level 3 Outcomes** | | |
| 2202 Caregiver Home Care Readiness<br>1827 Knowledge: Body Mechanics<br>1800 Knowledge: Breastfeeding<br>1830 Knowledge: Cardiac Disease Management<br>1801 Knowledge: Child Physical Safety<br>1821 Knowledge: Conception Prevention<br>1820 Knowledge: Diabetes Management<br>1802 Knowledge: Diet<br>1803 Knowledge: Disease Process<br>1804 Knowledge: Energy Conservation<br>1828 Knowledge: Fall Prevention<br>1816 Knowledge: Fertility Promotion<br>1805 Knowledge: Health Behavior<br>1823 Knowledge: Health Promotion<br>1806 Knowledge: Health Resources<br>1824 Knowledge: Illness Care<br>1819 Knowledge: Infant Care<br>1807 Knowledge: Infection Control<br>1817 Knowledge: Labor & Delivery<br>1808 Knowledge: Medication<br>1829 Knowledge: Ostomy Care<br>1826 Knowledge: Parenting<br>1809 Knowledge: Personal Safety<br>1818 Knowledge: Postpartum Maternal Health<br>1822 Knowledge: Preconception Maternal Health<br>1810 Knowledge: Pregnancy<br>1811 Knowledge: Prescribed Activity<br>1815 Knowledge: Sexual Functioning<br>1812 Knowledge: Substance Use Control<br>1814 Knowledge: Treatment Procedure(s)<br>1813 Knowledge: Treatment Regimen | 2204 Caregiver-Patient Relationship<br>2602 Family Functioning<br>2603 Family Integrity<br>2601 Family Social Climate<br>1500 Parent-Infant Attachment<br>2211 Parenting Performance<br>1501 Role Performance<br>1502 Social Interaction Skills<br>1503 Social Involvement<br>1504 Social Support | 1200 Body Image<br>1202 Identity<br>1205 Self-Esteem |

| Level 1 Domains | IV. Environmental Domain<br>Includes diagnoses, outcomes, and interventions to promote and protect the environmental health and safety of individuals, systems, and communities | | |
| --- | --- | --- | --- |
| Level 2 Classes | **Health Care System**<br>Social, political, and economic structures and processes for the delivery of health care services | **Populations**<br>Aggregates of individuals or communities having characteristics in common | **Risk Management**<br>Avoidance or control of identifiable health threats |
| Level 3 Outcomes | 2804 Community Disaster Readiness | 2700 Community Competence<br>2701 Community Health Status<br>2800 Community Health Status: Immunity<br>2702 Community Violence Level | 2500 Abuse Cessation<br>2501 Abuse Protection<br>1918 Aspiration Prevention<br>2801 Community Risk Control: Chronic Disease<br>2802 Community Risk Control: Communicable Disease<br>2803 Community Risk Control: Lead Exposure<br>2805 Community Risk Control: Violence<br>1909 Fall Prevention Behavior<br>1912 Falls Occurrence<br>2607 Family Physical Environment<br>2513 Neglect Cessation<br>2900 Parenting: Infant/Toddler Physical Safety<br>2901 Parenting: Early/Middle Childhood Physical Safety<br>2902 Parenting: Adolescent Physical Safety<br>1901 Parenting: Psychosocial Safety<br>1911 Personal Safety Behavior<br>1902 Risk Control<br>1903 Risk Control: Alcohol Use<br>1917 Risk Control: Cancer<br>1914 Risk Control: Cardiovascular Health<br>1904 Risk Control: Drug Use<br>1915 Risk Control: Hearing Impairment<br>1905 Risk Control: Sexually Transmitted Diseases (STD)<br>1906 Risk Control: Tobacco Use<br>1907 Risk Control: Unintended Pregnancy<br>1916 Risk Control: Visual Impairment<br>1908 Risk Detection<br>1920 Safe Home Environment<br>1620 Seizure Control<br>1407 Substance Addiction Consequences |

# Selected Criterion Tools With Psychometrics for Evaluating NOC Outcomes Used in Test Sites

| Outcome | Measurement Tool Selected | Primary Source | Psychometrics* |
|---|---|---|---|
| Abuse Cessation | Abusive Behavior Inventory (ABI) Partner Form | Shepard, M.F., & Campbell, J.A. (1992). The abusive behavior inventory: A measure of psychological and physical abuse. *Journal of Interpersonal Violence, 7*(3), 291-305. | Internal consistency: α=0.80-0.91

Criterion validity: significant difference between subjects in abusive relationships & those in non-abusive relationships (p<0.001)

Construct validity: variables believed to be related to abusive relationships (clinical & self-assessment of abuse, previous arrest for domestic abuse) had stronger correlation to ABI than variables thought to be unrelated (age, size of household)

Tool limitation: sample drawn from drug treatment center population, not tested on general population. |
| Abuse Protection | Response to Violence Inventory | Dutton, M.A. (1992). *Empowering and healing the battered woman: A model for assessment and intervention.* New York: Springer. | Unable to find. Tool published as appendix in Dutton's book, but no psychometrics or testing included. |
| Abuse Recovery: Emotional | Trauma Symptom Checklist (TSC-33) | Briere, J., & Runtz, M. (1989). The trauma symptom checklist (TSC-33): Early data on a new scale. *Journal of Interpersonal Violence, 4*(2), 151-163. | Internal consistency: α=0.89

Discriminant analysis: TSC-33 score significantly higher for abused than nonabused subjects t(193)=6.22, p<0.0001 |
| Abuse Recovery: Financial | Effectiveness in Obtaining Resources Scale | Sullivan, C.M., Campbell, R., Angelique, H., Eby, K.K., & Davidson, W. S. II. (1994). An advocacy intervention program for women with abusive partners: Six-month follow-up. *American Journal of Community Psychology, 22,* 101-122. | Internal consistency: α=0.64

Item reliability (item-total correlations): R=0.27-0.52

(Psychometric information supplied by Dr. Sullivan via personal correspondence. Was not published in journal article referenced.) |

*Continued*

*Psychometrics are from primary source unless otherwise indicated.

| Outcome | Measurement Tool Selected | Primary Source | Psychometrics* |
|---|---|---|---|
| Abuse Recovery: Physical | Trauma Symptom Checklist (TSC-33) | Briere, J., & Runtz, M. (1989). The trauma symptom checklist (TSC-33): Early data on a new scale. *Journal of Interpersonal Violence, 4*(2), 151-163 | Internal consistency: $\alpha=0.89$<br><br>Discriminant analysis: TSC-33 score significantly higher for abused than nonabused subjects t(193)=6.22, p<0.0001 |
| Abuse Recovery: Sexual | Trauma Symptom Checklist (TSC-33) | Briere, J., & Runtz, M. (1989). The trauma symptom checklist (TSC-33): Early data on a new scale. *Journal of Interpersonal Violence, 4*(2), 151-163 | Internal consistency: $\alpha=0.89$<br><br>Discriminant analysis: TSC-33 score significantly higher for abused than nonabused subjects t(193)=6.22, p<0.0001 |
| Abusive Behavior Self-Control | The Aggression Questionnaire | Buss, A.H., & Perry, M. (1992). The Aggression questionnaire. *Journal of Personality and Social Psychology,* 63(3), 452-459. | Internal consistency: $\alpha=0.89$ total score<br>Test-retest coefficient = .80<br><br>Construct validity: Significant correlations (p<.05) found between peer nomination of others identified as "aggressive" and Aggression Q scores.<br><br>(Tool limitation: tested only on college students, not general population. May not be generalizable to abusive clients.) |
| Acceptance: Health Status | Acceptance of Self & Life Questionnaire (Subscale of Resilience Scale) | Wagnild, G.M., & Young, H.M. (1993). Development and psychometric evaluation of the resilience scale. *Journal of Nursing Measurement, 1*(2), 165-178. | *Psychometrics are from data obtained with entire 25-item Resilience Scale. Subscale data tested alone not available.<br><br>Test-retest coefficient = 0.81 (Killien & Jarrett work with population of 1st time mothers, as cited in Wagnild & Young, 1993)<br>Internal consistency: Cronbach $\alpha$ = 0.91<br>Item to total correlations range 0.37-0.75 (all significant at p<0.001)<br><br>Concurrent validity demonstrated by correlation with related measures: Beck Depression Inventory −0.37; Life Satisfaction Index 0.30; Philadelphia Geriatric Center Morale Scale 0.28; Health Status Self-Report −0.26. p<0.001 for all coefficients. |

| | | |
|---|---|---|
| Adherence Behavior | Wellness Inventory Section of Lifestyle Assessment Questionnaire (Exercise, Nutrition, & Self-Care Subscales) | Hettler, B. (1982). Wellness promotion and risk reduction on a university campus. In M. Faber & A. Reinhardt (Eds.), *Promoting health through risk reduction*. New York: Macmillan. | Internal consistency of subscales: Exercise Cronbach's α=0.67 (low-recommended is .7) Nutritional Cronbach's α=0.81 Self-care Cronbach's α=0.72<br><br>*Validity psychometrics are from data obtained with entire 173-item Wellness Inventory. Subscale data tested alone not available.<br><br>Test-retest reliability: r=0.81-0.97 (2-week interval)<br><br>Content validity: Index of Content Validity (CVI) used to quantify extent of agreement between expert judges. CVI=0.98<br><br>Predictive validity quasi-experimental study yielded insignificant results. |
| Aggression Control | The Aggression Questionnaire | Buss, A.H., & Perry, M. (1992). The Aggression Questionnaire. *Journal of Personality and Social Psychology, 63*(3), 452-459. | Richter, J.M. (1988). Reliability and validity of the Lifestyle Assessment Questionnaire. In C.F. Waltz & O.L. Strickland (Eds.), *Measurement of nursing outcomes: Measuring client outcomes* (Vol. 1, pp. 352-376). New York: Springer.<br>(Tool limitation: tested on college-age females only. May not be generalizable to NOC study population.)<br><br>Internal consistency: α=0.89 total score Test-retest coefficient=0.80<br><br>Construct Validity: Significant correlations (p<.05) found between peer nomination of others identified as "aggressive" and Aggression Q scores.<br><br>(Tool limitation: tested only on college students, not generalizable to NOC study population. May not be generalizable to NOC study population.) |

*Continued*

---

*Psychometrics are from primary source unless otherwise indicated.

| Outcome | Measurement Tool Selected | Primary Source | Psychometrics* |
|---|---|---|---|
| Ambulation: Walking | Functional Independence Measure (FIM) | *Guide for the Uniform Data Set for Medical Rehabilitation (including the FIM™ instrument), version 5.1.* Buffalo, NY 14214: University at Buffalo; 1997. | Interrater reliability=0.95<br><br>Face validity established by expert opinion in response to 4 assessment questions re: the FIM Ottenbacher, K.J., Hsu,Y., Granger, C.V., & Fielder, R.C. (1996). The reliability of the functional independence measure: A quantitative review. *Archives of Physical Medicine & Rehabilitation, 77*(12), 1226-1232.<br><br>Predictive validity: FIM scores improved between admission and discharge and reflected patient's discharge destination<br>Dodds, T.A., Martin, D.P., Stolov, W.C., & Deyo, R.A. (1993). A validation of the Functional Independence Measurement and its performance among rehabilitation inpatients. *Archives of Physical Medicine and Rehabilitation, 74*(5), 531-536. |
| Ambulation: Wheelchair | Functional Independence Measure (FIM) | *Guide for the Uniform Data Set for Medical Rehabilitation (including the FIM™ instrument), version 5.1.* Buffalo, NY 14214: University at Buffalo; 1997. | Interrater reliability=0.95<br><br>Face validity established by expert opinion in response to 4 assessment questions re: the FIM Ottenbacher, K.J., Hsu,Y., Granger, C.V., & Fielder, R.C. (1996). The reliability of the functional independence measure: A quantitative review. *Archives of Physical Medicine & Rehabilitation, 77*(12), 1226-1232.<br><br>Predictive validity: FIM scores improved between admission and discharge and reflected patient's discharge destination<br>Dodds, T.A., Martin, D.P., Stolov, W.C., & Deyo, R.A. (1993). A validation of the Functional Independence Measurement and its performance among rehabilitation inpatients. *Archives of Physical Medicine and Rehabilitation, 74*(5), 531-536. |

| Outcome | Tool | Citation | Psychometrics |
|---|---|---|---|
| Anxiety Control | Clinical Anxiety Scale (CAS) | Hudson, W.W. (1992). *The WALMYR assessment scales scoring manual.* Tempe, AZ: WALMYR Publishing Co. | Internal consistency: coefficient $\alpha = 0.94$ (Westhuis & Thyer, 1989)<br><br>Test-retest reliability: r=0.64-0.74 (2-week interval) Thyer, B.A., & Westhuis, D. (1989). Test-retest reliability of the clinical anxiety scale. *Phobia Practice and Research Journal, 2,* 111-113.<br><br>Discriminant analysis: Tool distinguishes between known groups of those with anxiety and control group, error rate 6.9%<br>Westhuis, D., & Thyer, B.A. (1989). Development and validation of the clinical anxiety scale: A rapid assessment instrument for empirical practice. *Education and Psychological Measurement, 49,* 153-163. |
| Balance | Balance Scale | Berg, K., Wood-Dauphinee, S., Williams, J.I., & Gayton, D. (1989). Measuring balance in the elderly: Preliminary development of an instrument. *Physiotherapy Canada, 41,* 304-311. | Interrater reliability=0.98; Intrarater reliability=0.99<br>Internal consistency: Cronbach's $\alpha$=0.96<br><br>Criterion validity:<br>Scores correlated strongly (r=0.81) with global ratings of balance made by treating therapists<br>Scores correlated significantly with caregiver's global rating (range 0.46-0.62) and self-ratings (range 0.39-0.42) at 4 evaluation points ($\alpha$<0.05).<br><br>Predictive validity: Balance Scale score, as well as visual deficits and a recent fall, were significant predictors of the occurrence of multiple falls over the next year<br>Berg, K., Wood-Dauphinee, S., Williams, J.I., & Maki, B. (1992). Measuring balance in the elderly: Validation of an instrument. *Canadian Journal of Public Health, 83*(Suppl. 2), S7-S11. |
| Blood Transfusion Reaction Control | | Data collected from clinical record | |

*Psychometrics are from primary source unless otherwise indicated.

*Continued*

| Outcome | Measurement Tool Selected | Primary Source | Psychometrics* |
|---|---|---|---|
| Body Image | Body Image Avoidance Questionnaire (BIAQ) | Rosen, J.C., Srebnik, D., Saltzberg, E., & Wendt, S. (1991). Development of a body image avoidance questionnaire. Psychological Assessment. A Journal of Consulting and Clinical Psychology, 3(1), 32-37. | Internal consistency: Cronbach's α=0.89 Test-retest reliability: r=0.87 (2-week interval) Concurrent validity: Correlation between scores and body size estimation test r=0.22 (p<0.01) Correlation between scores and "Body Shape Questionnaire" r=0.78 (p<0.0001) Correlation between scores and "Shape Concern and Weight Concern" scales r=00.68 (p<0.0001) High correlation between self-rating scores and independent ratings by female roommates (r=0.72, p<0.0001) (Tool limitation: tested on college-age females only, avg. age 19.7) |
| Body Positioning: Self Initiated | Balance Scale | Berg, K., Wood-Dauphinee, S., Williams, J.I., & Gayton, D. (1989). Measuring balance in the elderly: Preliminary development of an instrument. Physiotherapy Canada, 41, 304-311. | Interrater reliability=0.98; Intrarater reliability=0.99 Internal consistency: Cronbach's α=0.96 Criterion validity: Scores correlated strongly (r=0.81) with global ratings of balance made by treating therapists Scores correlated significantly with caregiver's global rating (range 0.46-0.62) and self-ratings (range 0.39-0.42) at 4 evaluation points (α<0.05) Predictive validity: Balance Scale score, as well as visual deficits and a recent fall, were significant predictors of the occurrence of multiple falls over the next year Berg, K., Wood-Dauphinee, S., Williams, J.I., & Maki, B. (1992). Measuring balance in the elderly: Validation of an instrument. Canadian Journal of Public Health, 83(Suppl. 2), S7-S11. |
| Bone Healing | | Data collected from clinical record | |

| Bowel Continence | MDS for Resident Assessment and Care Screening Score Section F | Morris, J.N., Hawes, C., et al. (1990). Designing the national resident assessment instrument for nursing homes. *Gerontologist, 30*(3), 293-307. | Interrater reliability using Spearman-Brown intraclass coefficient .91 Hawes, C., Morris, J.N., Phillips, C.D., Mor, V., Fries, B.E., & Nonemaker, S. (1995). Reliability estimates for the minimum data set for nursing home resident assessment and care screening. *The Gerontologist, 35*(2), 172-178. |
| --- | --- | --- | --- |
| Bowel Elimination | | Data collected from clinical record | |
| Breastfeeding Establishment: Infant | Mother-Baby Assessment Form (MBA) | Muldford, C. (1992). The mother-baby assessment (MBA): An "Apgar Score" for breastfeeding. *Journal of Human Lactation, 8*(2), 79-82. | Interrater reliability: range 0.33-0.66 (only 3 maternity nurses in sample) Test-retest reliability: average rater agreement 84% (2 of the 5 indicators scored <80%; only 3 maternity nurses in sample) Validity: Correlation between MBA and LATCH assessment tool=0.68; correlation between MBA and Infant Breastfeeding Assessment Tool (IBFAT)=0.78 Riordan, J.M., & Koehn, M. (1997). Reliability and validity testing of three breastfeeding assessment tools. *Journal of Obstetric, Gynecologic, and Neonatal Nursing, 26*(2), 181-187. |
| Breastfeeding Establishment: Maternal | Mother-Baby Assessment Form (MBA) | Muldford, C. (1992). The mother-baby assessment (MBA): An "Apgar Score" for breastfeeding. *Journal of Human Lactation, 8*(2), 79-82. | Interrater reliability: range 0.33-0.66 (only 3 maternity nurses in sample) Test-retest reliability: average rater agreement 84% (2 of the 5 indicators scored <80%; only 3 maternity nurses in sample) Validity: Correlation between MBA and LATCH assessment tool=0.68; correlation between MBA and Infant Breastfeeding Assessment Tool (IBFAT)=0.78 Riordan, J.M., & Koehn, M. (1997). Reliability and validity testing of three breastfeeding assessment tools. *Journal of Obstetric, Gynecologic, and Neonatal Nursing, 26*(2), 181-187. |
| Cardiac Pump Effectiveness | | Data collected from clinical record | Pulmonary Artery Wedge Pressure, Thermal Dilution Cardiac Output Measurement, Radiocardiograph-cardiac index, stroke index, LV ejection fraction |

*Continued*

| Outcome | Measurement Tool Selected | Primary Source | Psychometrics* |
|---|---|---|---|
| Caregiver Adaptation to Patient Institutionalization (2 instruments) | Picot's Caregiver Rewards Scale (2nd version) | Picot, S.J.F., Youngblut, J., & Zeller, R. (1997). Development and testing of a measure of perceived caregiver rewards in adults. *Journal of Nursing Measurement, 5*(1), 33-52. | Internal consistency: Cronbach's $\alpha=0.88$ Test-retest reliability: coefficient of stability=0.75 (2-4 weeks apart)

Construct validity: As hypothesized, higher levels of rewards were correlated with lower levels of depression (CES-D scores) (p<0.0001) and higher levels of rewards were correlated with lower levels of caregiver burden (Zarit Burden Interview scores) (p<0.0001) |
| Caregiver Adaptation to Patient Institutionalization (2 instruments) | Montgomery, Gonyea, & Hooyman Inventories | Montgomery, R.J.V., Gonyea, J.G., & Hooyman, N.R. (1985). Caregiving and the experience of subjective and objective burden. *Family Relations, 34*, 19-26. | Internal consistency: Cronbach's $\alpha=0.86$

Construct validity: correlated .34 with 2 measures of burden. |
| Caregiver Emotional Health | Caregiver Strain Index (CSI) | Robinson, B.C. (1983). Validation of a caregiver strain index. *Journal of Gerontology, 38*(3), 344-348. | Internal consistency: Cronbach's $\alpha=0.86$

Construct validity: variables believed to be related to caregiver stress (patient characteristics, caregivers' subjective perceptions of the caretaking relationship, and physical and emotional health of the caregiver) were examined for their relationships to overall CSI scores. Results showed the majority of the selected criterion variables had a significant correlation (see primary source for detailed statistical data; too complex to include here). |
| Caregiver Home Care Readiness | Picot's Caregiver Rewards Scale (2nd version) | Picot, S.J.F., Youngblut, J., & Zeller, R. (1997). Development and testing of a measure of perceived caregiver rewards in adults. *Journal of Nursing Measurement, 5*(1), 33-52. | Internal consistency: Cronbach's $\alpha=0.88$ Test-retest reliability: coefficient of stability=0.75 (2-4 weeks apart)

Construct validity: As hypothesized, higher levels of rewards were correlated with lower levels of depression (CES-D scores) (p<0.0001), and higher levels of rewards were correlated with lower levels of caregiver burden (Zarit Burden Interview scores) (p<0.0001) |

| | Tool | Citation | Psychometrics |
|---|---|---|---|
| Caregiver Lifestyle Disruption | Caregiver Strain Index | Robinson, B.C. (1983). Validation of a caregiver strain index. *Journal of Gerontology, 38*(3), 344-348. | Internal consistency: Cronbach's $\alpha$=0.86<br><br>Construct validity: variables believed to be related to caregiver stress (patient characteristics, caregiver's subjective perceptions of the caretaking relationship, and physical and emotional health of the caregiver) were examined for their relationships to overall CSI scores. Results showed the majority of the selected criterion variables had a significant correlation (see primary source for detailed statistical data; too complex to include here). |
| Caregiver Performance: Direct Care (2 instruments) | Sense of Competence Questionnaire (SCQ) | Vermooij-Dassen, M.J.F.J. (1993). *Dementia and home care: Determinants of the sense of competence of primary caregivers and the effect of professionally guided caregiver support* (in Dutch). Lisse, The Netherlands: Swets & Seitliger. | Internal consistency: Cronbach's $\alpha$=0.83 (total scale)<br>Intraclass correlation coefficient=0.93 (total scale)<br><br>Construct validity: principle component analysis showed that the SCQ contains 3 factors with a min. eigen-value of 2, 42% of total variance explained<br><br>Clinical validity: higher SCQ scores associated with impaired functional health (measured by Mini-Mental State Exam, Barthel Index, Rankin Scale & Sickness Impact Profile) — effect size range 0.37-0.72.<br><br>(Tool limitation: population for Scholte op Reimer et al. studies was stroke patients only.) Scholte op Reimer, W.J.M, de Hann, R.J., Limburg, M., Pijnenborg, J.M.A., & van den Bos, G.A.M. (1998). Assessment of burden in partners of stroke patients with the sense of competence questionnaire. *Stroke, 29,* 373-379. |
| Caregiver Performance: Direct Care (2 instruments) | Picot's Caregiver Rewards Scale (2nd version) | Picot, S.J.F., Youngblut, J., & Zeller, R. (1997). Development and testing of a measure of perceived caregiver rewards in adults. *Journal of Nursing Measurement, 5*(1), 33-52. | Internal consistency: Cronbach's $\alpha$=0.88<br>Test-retest reliability: coefficient of stability=0.75 (2-4 weeks apart)<br><br>Construct validity: As hypothesized, higher levels of rewards were correlated with lower levels of depression |

*Psychometrics are from primary source unless otherwise indicated.

*Continued*

| Outcome | Measurement Tool Selected | Primary Source | Psychometrics* |
|---|---|---|---|
| | | | (CES-D scores) (p<0.0001) and higher levels of rewards were correlated with lower levels of caregiver burden (Zarit Burden Interview scores) (p<0.0001) |
| Caregiver Performance: Indirect Care | Sense of Competence Questionnaire (SCQ) | Vermooij-Dassen, M.J.F.J. (1993). *Dementia and home care: Determinants of the sense of competence of primary caregivers and the effect of professionally guided caregiver support* (in Dutch). Lisse, The Netherlands: Swets & Seitliger. | Internal consistency: Cronbach's α=0.83 (total scale) Intraclass correlation coefficient=0.93 (total scale) Construct validity: principle component analysis showed that the SCQ contains 3 factors with a min. eigen-value of 2, 42% of total variance explained. Clinical validity: higher SCQ scores associated with impaired functional health (measured by Mini-Mental State Exam, Barthel Index, Rankin Scale & Sickness Impact Profile) — effect size range 0.37-0.72. (Tool limitation: population for Scholte op Reimer et al. studies was stroke patients only.) Scholte op Reimer, W.J.M, de Hann, R.J., Limburg, M., Pijnenborg, J.M.A., & van den Bos, G.A.M. (1998). Assessment of burden in partners of stroke patients with the sense of competence questionnaire. *Stroke, 29,* 373-379. |
| Caregiver Physical Health | Caregiver Strain Index | Robinson, B.C. (1983). Validation of a caregiver strain index. *Journal of Gerontology, 38*(3), 344-348. | Internal consistency: Cronbach's α=0.86 Construct validity: variables believed to be related to caregiver stress (patient characteristics, caregivers' subjective perceptions of the caretaking relationship, and physical and emotional health of the caregiver) were examined for their relationships to overall CSI scores. Results showed the majority of the selected criterion variables had a significant correlation (see primary source for detailed statistical data; too complex to include here). |

| | | | |
|---|---|---|---|
| Caregiver Stressors | Caregiver Strain Index | Robinson, B.C. (1983). Validation of a caregiver strain index. *Journal of Gerontology, 38*(3), 344-348. | Internal consistency: Cronbach's α=0.86<br><br>Construct validity: variables believed to be related to caregiver stress (patient characteristics, caregiver's subjective perceptions of the caretaking relationship, and physical and emotional health of the caregiver) were examined for their relationships to overall CSI scores. Results showed the majority of the selected criterion variables had a significant correlation (see primary source for detailed statistical data; too complex to include here). |
| Caregiver Well-Being | Picot's Caregiver Rewards Scale (2nd version) | Picot, S.J.F., Youngblut, J., & Zeller, R. (1997). Development and testing of a measure of perceived caregiver rewards in adults. *Journal of Nursing Measurement, 5*(1), 33-52. | Internal consistency: Cronbach's α=0.88<br>Test-retest reliability: coefficient of stability=0.75 (2-4 weeks apart)<br><br>Construct validity: As hypothesized, higher levels of rewards were correlated with lower levels of depression (CES-D scores) (p<0.0001) and higher levels of rewards were correlated with lower levels of caregiver burden (Zarit Burden Interview scores) (p<0.0001) |
| Caregiver-Patient Relationship (2 instruments) | Sense of Competence Questionnaire (SCQ) | Vermooij-Dassen, M.J.F.J. (1993). *Dementia and home care: Determinants of the sense of competence of primary caregivers and the effect of professionally guided caregiver support* (in Dutch). Lisse, The Netherlands: Swets & Seitliger. | Internal consistency: Cronbach's α=0.83 (total scale)<br>Intraclass correlation coefficient=0.93 (total scale)<br><br>Construct validity: principle component analysis showed that the SCQ contains 3 factors with a min. eigen-value of 2, 42% of total variance explained.<br><br>Clinical validity: higher SCQ scores associated with impaired functional health (measured by Mini-Mental State Exam, Barthel Index, Rankin Scale & Sickness Impact Profile) — effect size range 0.37-0.72.<br><br>(Tool limitation: population for Scholte op Reimer et al. studies was stroke patients only.)<br>Scholte op Reimer, W.J.M, de Hann, R.J., Limburg, M., Pijnenborg, J.M.A., & van den Bos, G.A.M. (1998). Assessment of burden in partners of stroke patients with the sense of competence questionnaire. *Stroke, 29,* 373-379. |

*Continued*

*Psychometrics are from primary source unless otherwise indicated.

| Outcome | Measurement Tool Selected | Primary Source | Psychometrics* |
|---|---|---|---|
| Caregiver-Patient Relationship (2 instruments) | Picot's Caregiver Rewards Scale (2nd version) | Picot, S.J.F., Youngblut, J., & Zeller, R. (1997). Development and testing of a measure of perceived caregiver rewards in adults. *Journal of Nursing Measurement, 5*(1), 33-52. | Internal consistency: Cronbach's α=0.88 Test-retest reliability: coefficient of stability=0.75 (2-4 weeks apart)<br><br>Construct validity: As hypothesized, higher levels of rewards were correlated with lower levels of depression (CES-D scores) (p<0.0001) and higher levels of rewards were correlated with lower levels of caregiver burden (Zarit Burden Interview scores) (p<0.0001) |
| Caregiving Endurance Potential | Picot's Caregiver Rewards Scale (2nd version) | Picot, S.J.F., Youngblut, J., & Zeller, R. (1997). Development and testing of a measure of perceived caregiver rewards in adults. *Journal of Nursing Measurement, 5*(1), 33-52. | Internal consistency: Cronbach's α=0.88 Test-retest reliability: coefficient of stability=0.75 (2-4 weeks apart)<br><br>Construct validity: As hypothesized, higher levels of rewards were correlated with lower levels of depression (CES-D scores) (p<0.0001) and higher levels of rewards were correlated with lower levels of caregiver burden (Zarit Burden Interview scores) (p<0.0001) |
| Circulation Status | | Data collected from clinical record | |
| Cognitive Ability | Mini-Mental State (MMS) | Folstein, M.F., Folstein, S.E., & McHugh, P.R. (1975). "Mini-Mental State": A practical method for grading the cognitive state of patients for the clinician. *Journal of Psychiatric Research, 12*(3), 189-195. | Test-retest reliability 0.89, interrater reliability 0.82 Anthony, J.C., LeResche, L., Niaz, U., VonKorff, M.R., & Folstein, M.F. (1982). Limits of the "Mini-Mental State" as a screening test for dementia and delirium among hospital patients. *Psychological Medicine, 12*(2), 397-408.<br><br>Concurrent validity demonstrated by correlation of MMS to Weschler Adult Intelligence Scale: Verbal IQ – Pearson r = 0.776 (p < 0.0001) Performance IQ – Pearson r = 0.660 (p < 0.001) (Folstein, Folstein, & McHugh, 1975) |
| Cognitive Orientation | Short Portable Mental Status Questionnaire | Pfeiffer, E. (1975). A short portable mental status questionnaire for the | Test-retest reliability >0.80 |

| Outcome | Tool / Reference | Psychometrics |
| --- | --- | --- |
| (SPMSQ) | assessment of organic brain deficit in elderly patients. *American Geriatrics Society, 23*(10), 433-441. | Interrater reliability range 0.62-0.87 (Fillenbaum, G.C., & Smyer, M. (1981). The development, validity, and reliability of the ORS multidimensional functional assessment questionnaire. *Journal of Gerontology 36,* 428-434.<br><br>Clinical validity: 92% agreement between SPMSQ score and clinical diagnosis when SPMSQ indicated definite impairment; 82% agreement when SPMSQ indicated no impairment/mild impairment in population of elderly community clients (n=133). |
| Comfort Level | General Comfort Questionnaire (Revised)<br><br>Kolcaba, K. (1992). Holistic comfort: Operationalizing the construct as a nurse-sensitive outcome. *Advances in Nursing Science, 15*(1), 1-10.<br><br>Kolcaba, K. (personal communication, December 15, 1994). | Cronbach's $\alpha=0.90$ (on original 35-item tool; no data available on revised tool of 28 items)<br><br>Validity supported by significant differences in expected directions on GCQ scores between several groups (i.e. med-surg and oncology; psych and community) |
| Communication Ability | Patient Evaluation and Conference System (PECS)<br><br>Harvey, R., & Jellinek, H. (1981). Functional Performance Assessment: A program approach. *Archives of Physical Medicine & Rehabilitation 62*(9), 456-460. | Interrater reliability 0.68 – 0.88 (range within various disciplines) (Harvey & Jellinek, 1981)<br><br>Validity supported by 0.84 correlation between PECS communication subscale items and Functional Independence Measure (FIM) Expression and Comprehension items<br><br>Silverstein, B., Fisher, W.P., Kilgore, K.M., Harley, J.P., & Harvey, R.F. (1992). Applying psychometric criteria to functional assessment in medical rehabilitation: II. Defining interval measures. *Archives of Physical Medicine & Rehabilitation, 73*(6), 507-518. |
| Communication: Expressive Ability | Patient Evaluation and Conference System (PECS) selection of items from section<br><br>Harvey, R. & Jellinek, H. (1981). Functional Performance Assessment: A program approach. *Archives of Physical Medicine & Rehabilitation 62*(9), 456-460. | Interrater reliability 0.68 – 0.88 (range within various disciplines) (Harvey & Jellinek, 1981)<br><br>Validity supported by 0.84 correlation between PECS communication subscale items and Functional Independence Measure (FIM) Expression and Comprehension items |

*Psychometrics are from primary source unless otherwise indicated.

*Continued*

| Outcome | Measurement Tool Selected | Primary Source | Psychometrics* |
|---|---|---|---|
| | | | Silverstein, B., Fisher, W.P., Kilgore, K.M., Harley, J.P., & Harvey, R.F. (1992). Applying psychometric criteria to functional assessment in medical rehabilitation: II. Defining interval measures. *Archives of Physical Medicine & Rehabilitation, 73*(6), 507-518. |
| Communication: Receptive Ability | Patient Evaluation and Conference System (PECS) selection of items from section | Harvey, R. & Jellinek, H. (1981). Functional Performance Assessment: A program approach. *Archives of Physical Medicine & Rehabilitation 62*(9), 456-460. | Interrater reliability 0.68 – 0.88 (range within various disciplines) (Harvey & Jellinek, 1981) |
| | | | Validity supported by 0.84 correlation between PECS communication subscale items and Functional Independence Measure (FIM) Expression and Comprehension items Silverstein, B., Fisher, W.P., Kilgore, K.M., Harley, J.P., & Harvey, R.F. (1992). Applying psychometric criteria to functional assessment in medical rehabilitation: II. Defining interval measures. *Archives of Physical Medicine & Rehabilitation, 73*(6), 507-518. |
| Compliance Behavior | Medical Outcome Study General Adherence Scale | DiMatteo, M.R., Hays, R.D., & Sherbourne, C.D. (1992). Adherence to cancer regimens: Implications for treating the older patient. *Oncology, 6*(2 Suppl.), 50-57. | Internal consistency: α=0.81 Test-retest reliability r=0.40 |
| Concentration | Mini-Mental State | Folstein, M.F., Folstein, S.E., & McHugh, P.R. (1975). "Mini-Mental State": A practical method for grading the cognitive state of patients for the clinician. *Journal of Psychiatric Research, 12*(3), 189-198. | Test-retest reliability 0.89, interrater reliability 0.82 Anthony, J.C., LeResche, L., Niaz, U., VonKorff, M.R., & Folstein, M.F. (1982). Limits of the "Mini-Mental State" as a screening test for dementia and delirium among hospital patients. *Psychological Medicine, 12*(2), 397-408. |
| | | | Concurrent validity demonstrated by correlation of MMS to Weschler Adult Intelligence Scale: Verbal IQ – Pearson r = 0.776 (p < 0.0001) Performance IQ – Pearson r = 0.660 (p < 0.001) (Folstein, Folstein, & McHugh, 1975). |

| | | |
|---|---|---|
| Coping | Brief COPE | Carver, C.S., Scheier, M.F., & Weintraub, J.K. (1989). Assessing coping strategies: A theoretically based approach. *Journal of Personality and Social Psychology, 56*(2), 267-283.<br><br>Carver, C.S. (1997). You want to measure coping but your protocol's too long: Consider the Brief COPE. *International Journal of Behavioral Medicine, 4*, 92-100. | Internal consistency: all 14 of the scales had item reliabilities of 0.50 or above (Carver, 1997)<br><br>Tool authors claim convergent and discriminant validity by a number of significant associations between scale items and selected personality measures. See Carver, et al. article (1989) for statistical details. Too complex for notation here.<br><br>(Tool limitation: testing population survivors of hurricane only) |
| Decision Making | Functional Independence Measure (FIM) | *Guide for the Uniform Data Set for Medical Rehabilitation (including the FIM™ instrument), version 5.1.* Buffalo, NY 14214: University at Buffalo; 1997. | Interrater reliability=0.95<br><br>Face validity established by expert opinion in response to 4 assessment questions re: the FIM<br>Ottenbacher, K.J., Hsu,Y., Granger, C.V., & Fielder, R.C. (1996). The reliability of the functional independence measure: a quantitative review. *Archives of Physical Medicine & Rehabilitation, 77*(12), 1226-1232.<br><br>Predictive validity: FIM scores improved between admission and discharge and reflected patient's discharge destination<br>Dodds, T.A., Martin, D.P., Stolov, W.C., & Deyo, R.A. (1993). A validation of the Functional Independence Measurement and its performance among rehabilitation inpatients. *Archives of Physical Medicine and Rehabilitation, 74*(5), 531-536. |
| Dignified Dying | The McCanse Readiness for Death Instrument (MRDI) | McCanse, R.P. (1995). The McCanse Readiness for Death Instrument (MRDI): A reliable and valid measure for hospice care. *Hospice Journal, 10*(1), 15-26. | Internal consistency: coefficient α=0.76<br><br>Discriminant validity (terminal vs. nonterminally ill) t=1.76, (p< .01) |
| Distorted Thought Control | Neuropsychiatric Inventory (NPI) (delusions and hallucinations disturbance sections only) | Cummings, J.L. (1997). The Neuropsychiatric Inventory: Assessing psychopathology in dementia patients. *Neurology, 48* (Suppl. 6), S10-S16. | Interrater reliability range 96%-100%<br>Test-retest reliability r=0.79 (frequency) and r=0.86 (severity) (at 3 weeks) |

*Psychometrics are from primary source unless otherwise indicated.

*Continued*

| Outcome | Measurement Tool Selected | Primary Source | Psychometrics* |
|---|---|---|---|
| | | | Concurrent validity: scores on NPI correlated significantly with BEHAVE-AD and Hamilton Rating Scale for Depression (p<0.05) |
| Electrolyte & Acid/Base Balance | | Data collected from clinical record | Lab results |
| Endurance | COOP Chart: Physical Condition | Dartmouth Primary Care Cooperative Information Project. (1987). COOP Charts. Hanover, NH: Department of Community and Family Medicine, Dartmouth Medical School. | Test-retest intraclass correlation coefficients 0.78-0.98 (elderly patient sample) and 0.73-0.98 (low income patient sample) Nelson, E.C., Wasson, J.H., Johnson, D.J., & Hayes, R.D. (2002). *Dartmouth COOP Functional Health Assessment Charts: Brief measures for clinical practice.* Retrieved February 20, 2002, from http://www.dartmouth.edu/~coopproj/more_charts.html. |
| | | | Convergent validity: correlation between COOP Chart: Physical Condition and RAND Physical scale significant at p<0.001 Nelson, E., Wasson, J., Kirk, J., Keller, A., Clark, D., Dietrich, A., & Zubkoff, M. (1987). Assessment of function in routine clinical practice: Description of the COOP chart method and preliminary findings. *Journal of Chronic Diseases, 40*(1), 55S-63S. |
| Energy Conservation | Visual Analogue Scale for Fatigue (VAS-F) | Lee, K.A., Hicks, G., & Nino-Murcia, G. (1991). Validity and reliability of a scale to assess fatigue. *Psychiatry Research, 36*(3), 291-298. | Reliability: fatigue subscale (am & pm data) Cronbach's α=0.91-0.96 (healthy subjects) Cronbach's α=0.96-0.95 (am & pm data) (sleep-disorder subjects) Reliability: energy subscale (am & pm data) Cronbach's α=0.94-0.95 (healthy subjects) Cronbach's α=0.96-0.94 (am & pm data) (sleep-disorder subjects) |
| | | | Concurrent validity: significant correlation (p<0.01) between VAS-F scores and Stanford Sleepiness Scale and the Profile of Mood States |

| | | |
|---|---|---|
| Fear Control | Fear Questionnaire — 4 Parts | Marks, I.M., & Matthews, A.M. (1979). Brief standard self-rating for phobic patients. *Behavior Research and Therapy, 17*(3), 263-267. | Good test-restest reliability Correlation 0.82 for one week period Subscales main target phobia (.93), global phobia rating (.79) and anxiety-depression (.82) Marks, I.M., & Mathews, A.M. (1994). Fear Questionnaire (FQ). In J. Fischer, & K. Corcoran, *Measures for clinical practice: A sourcebook* (2nd edition, Volume 2. Adults, pp. 221-223). New York The Free Press. |
| Fluid Balance | Data collected from clinical record | The following items collected from the chart: Intake and Output, Body Weight, Edema, Dehydration, Skin Turgor, Neuromuscular Irritability, Capillary Refill Time Test |
| Grief Resolution | Inventory of Complicated Grief (ICG) | Prigerson, H.G., Maciejewski, P.K., Reynolds, C.F., Bierhals, A., Newsom, J.T., Fasiczka, A., Frank, E., Doman, J., & Miller, M. (1995). Inventory of complicated grief: A scale to measure maladaptive symptoms of loss. *Psychiatry Research, 59*(1-2), 65-79. | Cronbach's $\alpha$=0.94 (19 item) Test-retest reliability 0.80 |
| Health Beliefs (2 instruments) | Osteoporosis Health Belief Scale (susceptibility & seriousness subscales only) | Kim, K.K., Horan, M.L., Gendler, P., & Patel, M.K. (1991). Development and evaluation of the osteoporosis health belief scale. *Research in Nursing & Health, 14*(2), 155-163. | Susceptibility subscale: Test-retest r=0.84; Cronbach's $\alpha$=0.82 Seriousness subscale: Test-retest r=0.79; Cronbach's $\alpha$=0.71 Construct validity determined by factor analysis of entire scale (Osteoporosis Health Belief Scale). Factor loadings of susceptibility items ranged from 0.56-0.84, seriousness items ranged from 0.46-0.73. Kim, K.K., Horan, M.L., & Gendler, P. (1991, May). *Refinement of the Osteoporosis Health Belief Scale.* Paper presented at Sigma Theta Tau International Research Conference, Columbus, OH. |

*Continued*

*Psychometrics are from primary source unless otherwise indicated.

| Outcome | Measurement Tool Selected | Primary Source | Psychometrics* |
|---|---|---|---|
| Health Beliefs (2 instruments) | Breast Self-Examination Health Belief Model Scale (all 6 subscales) | Champion, V.L. (1993). Instrument refinement for breast cancer screening behaviors. *Nursing Research, 42*(3), 139-143. | Test-retest reliability: 0.45-0.70 (up to 2 months) Cronbach's $\alpha$=0.80-0.93<br><br>Predictive validity demonstrated by regressing actual BSE behavior on the 6 subscales of the instrument. The combined independent variables accounted for 24% of the variance in BSE, and the F values were significant for each of the subscales and for the overall equation |
| Health Beliefs: Perceived Ability to Perform (2 instruments) | Perceived Health Competence Scale | Smith, M.S., Wallston, K.A., & Smith, C.A. (1995). The development and validation of the perceived health competence scale. *Health Education Research, 10*(1), 51-64. | Test-retest reliability .59-.82 Internal consistency $\alpha$=.82-.90<br><br>Construct validity statistically significant correlations in expected direction with health status and health beliefs. |
| Health Beliefs: Perceived Ability to Perform (2 instruments) | Breast Self-Examination Health Belief Model Scale (all 6 subscales) | Champion, V.L. (1993). Instrument refinement for breast cancer screening behaviors. *Nursing Research, 42*(3), 139-143. | Test-retest reliability: 0.45-0.70 (up to 2 months) Cronbach's $\alpha$=0.80-0.93<br><br>Predictive validity demonstrated by regressing actual BSE behavior on the 6 subscales of the instrument. The combined independent variables accounted for 24% of the variance in BSE and the F values were significant for each of the subscales and for the overall equation |
| Health Beliefs: Perceived Control (2 instruments) | Multidimensional Health Locus of Control Scales: Form A (3 separate subscales) | Wallston, K.A., Wallston, B.S., DeVellis, R. (1978). Development of the Multidimensional Health Locus of Control (MHLC) Scales. *Health Education Monographs, 6,* 160-170.<br><br>Wallston, K.A., & Wallston, B.S. (1981). Health locus of control scales. In H. Lefcourt (Ed.) *Research with the locus of control construct*, Volume 1. New York: Academic Press. | Alpha coefficient for 3 subscales were .767 for Internal Health Locus of Control; .673 for Powerful Others Health Locus of Control; and .753 for Chance Health Locus of Control. (Wallston, Wallston, DeVellis, 1978). |

| | | | |
|---|---|---|---|
| Health Beliefs: Perceived Control (2 instruments) | Breast Self-Examination Health Belief Model Scale (all 6 subscales) | Champion, V.L. (1993). Instrument refinement for breast cancer screening behaviors. *Nursing Research, 42*(3), 139-143. | Test-retest reliability: 0.45-0.70 (up to 2 months) Cronbach's α=0.80-0.93<br><br>Predictive validity demonstrated by regressing actual BSE behavior on the 6 subscales of the instrument. The combined independent variables accounted for 24% of the variance in BSE, and the F values were significant for each of the subscales and for the overall equation |
| Health Beliefs: Perceived Resources (2 instruments) | Barriers to Health Promotion Activities Among Persons with Disabilities (Barriers Scale) | Becker, H., Stuifbergen, A.K., & Sands, D. (1991). Development of a scale to measure barriers to health promotion activities among persons with disabilities. *American Journal of Health Promotion, 5*(6), 449-454. | Cronbach's α=0.82 Factor analysis — 3 factor solution accounted for 48% of the variance |
| Health Beliefs: Perceived Resources (2 instruments) | Breast Self-Examination Health Belief Model Scale (all 6 subscales) | Champion, V.L. (1993). Instrument refinement for breast cancer screening behaviors. *Nursing Research, 42*(3), 139-143. | Test-retest reliability: 0.45-0.70 (up to 2 months) Cronbach's α=0.80-0.93<br><br>Predictive validity demonstrated by regressing actual BSE behavior on the 6 subscales of the instrument. The combined independent variables accounted for 24% of the variance in BSE and the F values were significant for each of the subscales and for the overall equation |
| Health Beliefs: Perceived Threat (2 instruments) | Osteoporosis Health Belief Scale (susceptibility & seriousness subscales only) | Kim, K.K., Horan, M.L., Gendler, P., & Patel, M.K. (1991). Development and evaluation of the osteoporosis health belief scale. *Research in Nursing & Health, 14*(2), 155-163. | Susceptibility subscale: Test-retest r=0.84; Cronbach's α=0.82<br><br>Seriousness subscale: Test-retest r=0.79; Cronbach's α=0.71<br><br>Construct validity determined by factor analysis of entire scale (Osteoporosis Health Belief Scale). Factor loadings of susceptibility items ranged from 0.56-0.84, seriousness items ranged from 0.46-0.73.<br>Kim, K.K., Horan, M.L., & Gendler, P. (1991, May). *Refinement of the Osteoporosis Health Belief Scale.* Paper presented at Sigma Theta Tau International Research Conference, Columbus, OH. |

*Psychometrics are from primary source unless otherwise indicated.

*Continued*

| Outcome | Measurement Tool Selected | Primary Source | Psychometrics* |
|---|---|---|---|
| Health Beliefs: Perceived Threat (2 instruments) | Breast Self-Examination Health Belief Model Scale (all 6 subscales) | Champion, V.L. (1993). Instrument refinement for breast cancer screening behaviors. *Nursing Research, 42(3)*, 139-143. | Test-retest reliability: 0.45-0.70 (up to 2 months) Cronbach's α=0.80-0.93<br><br>Predictive validity demonstrated by regressing actual BSE behavior on the 6 subscales of the instrument. The combined independent variables accounted for 24% of the variance in BSE, and the F values were significant for each of the subscales and for the overall equation |
| Health Orientation | Health Promoting Lifestyle Profile II | Walker, S.N., Sechrist, K., & Pender, N. (1987). The Health-Promoting Lifestyle Profile: Development and psychometric characteristics. *Nursing Research, 36(2)*, 76-81.<br><br>Walker, S.N., Sechrist, K.R., & Pender, N. (1995). The Health-Promoting Lifestyle Profile II. Omaha, NE: University of Nebraska at Omaha. | *All psychometric data from Walker and Hill-Polerecky paper (as cited in Berger, A.M. & Walker, S.N. (1997). Measuring healthy lifestyle. In Frank-Stromborg, M., & Olsen, S.J. (Eds.), Instruments for clinical health care research* (3rd ed.) (pp. 363-377). Boston: Jones & Bartlett.)<br><br>Internal consistency α=0.94 (total scale); subscales ranged from 0.79-0.87. Test-retest r=0.89 (3-week interval).<br><br>Construct validity: Factor analysis of the 6 subscales showed the Spiritual Growth and Interpersonal Relations subscale items loading together, the remaining 4 subscales loaded on separate factors at 0.43 or >, and a nuisance factor with no significant loadings. Convergent validity: Compared to the Personal Lifestyle Questionnaire, correlation=0.68. Criterion validity: Correlation of the scale with the Medical Outcomes Study Short-Form General Health Survey general health perception scale=0.26; with the Quality of Life Index=0.46. |
| Health Promoting Behavior | Health Promoting Lifestyle Profile II | Walker, S.N., Sechrist, K., & Pender, N. (1987). The Health-Promoting Lifestyle Profile: Development and psychometric characteristics. *Nursing Research, 36(2)*, 76-81. | *All psychometric data from Walker and Hill-Polerecky paper (as cited in Berger, A.M. & Walker, S.N. (1997). Measuring healthy lifestyle. In Frank-Stromborg, M., & Olsen, S.J. (Eds.), Instruments for clinical health care research* (3rd ed.) (pp. 363-377). Boston: Jones & Bartlett.) |

| | | |
|---|---|---|
| | Walker, S.N., Sechrist, K.R., & Pender, N. (1995). The Health-Promoting Lifestyle Profile II. Omaha, NE: University of Nebraska at Omaha. | Internal consistency $\alpha$=0.94 (total scale); subscales ranged from 0.79-0.87. Test-retest r=0.89 (3-week interval). Construct validity: Factor analysis of the 6 subscales showed the Spiritual Growth and Interpersonal Relations subscale items loading together, the remaining 4 subscales loaded on separate factors at 0.43 or >, and a nuisance factor with no significant loadings. Convergent validity: Compared to the Personal Lifestyle Questionnaire, correlation=0.68. Criterion validity: Correlation of the scale with the Medical Outcomes Study Short-Form General Health Survey general health perception scale=0.26; with the Quality of Life Index=0.46. |
| Health Seeking Behavior | Health Promoting Lifestyle Profile II (Health Responsibility Subscale) | *All psychometric data from Walker and Hill-Polerecky paper (as cited in Berger, A.M., & Walker, S.N. (1997). Measuring healthy lifestyle. In Frank-Stromborg, M., & Olsen, S.J. (Eds.), Instruments for clinical health care research (3rd ed.) (pp.363-377). Boston: Jones & Bartlett.)* |
| | Walker, S.N., Sechrist, K., & Pender, N. (1987). The Health-Promoting Lifestyle Profile: Development and psychometric characteristics. *Nursing Research, 36*(2), 76-81. | Internal consistency $\alpha$=0.94 (total scale): Health Responsibility subscale 0.86. Test-retest r=0.89 (3-week interval). |
| | Walker, S.N., Sechrist, K.R., & Pender, N. (1995). The Health-Promoting Lifestyle Profile II. Omaha, NE: University of Nebraska at Omaha. | Construct validity: Factor analysis of the 6 subscales showed the Spiritual Growth and Interpersonal Relations subscale items loading together, the remaining 4 subscales loaded on separate factors at 0.43 or >, and a nuisance factor with no significant loadings. Convergent validity: Compared to the Personal Lifestyle Questionnaire, correlation=0.68. Criterion validity: Correlation of the scale with the Medical Outcomes Study Short-Form General Health Survey general health perception scale=0.26; with the Quality of Life Index=0.46. |

*Continued*

Psychometrics are from primary source unless otherwise indicated.

| Outcome | Measurement Tool Selected | Primary Source | Psychometrics* |
|---|---|---|---|
| Hope | Cognitive Triad Inventory (CTI) (10-item subscale "View of the Future") | Beckman, E.E., Leber, W.R., Watkins, J.T., Boyer, J.L., & Cook, J.B. (1986). Development of an instrument to measure Beck's cognitive triad: The cognitive triad inventory. *Journal of Consulting and Clinical Psychology, 54(4)*, 566-567. | Internal reliability: View of Future subscale Cronbach's α=.93, Overall scale α=.95<br><br>Criterion validity correlation with Hopelessness Scale .90<br><br>Overall scale: Convergent validity F 15.06 variance component 67%; Discriminant validity F 1.10 variance component 13% |
| Hydration | | Data collected from clinical record | |
| Identity | Ego Identity Scale | Tan, A.L., Kendis, R.J., Fine, J.T., & Porac, J. (1977). A short measure of Ericksonian ego identity. *Journal of Personality Assessment, 41*, 279-284. | Odd-even split half reliability=0.68 Average inter-item correlation=0.114<br><br>Construct validity: scores correlated to 5 other measures of personality variables reasoned to be present in those who have achieved successful resolution of psychosocial crises within Erickson's scheme (trust, internal control, intimacy, dogmatism, and extent to which an individual derives values from own life experiences). All were in expected direction, 4 of 5 statistically significant. |
| Immobility Consequences: Physiological | | Data collected from clinical record | |
| Immobility Consequences: Psycho-Cognitive | | Data collected from clinical record | |
| Immunization Behavior | | Data collected from clinical record | |
| Immune Hyper-sensitivity Control | | Data collected from clinical record | |
| Immune Status | | Data collected from clinical record | |

| Outcome | Tool/Method | Source | Psychometrics |
|---|---|---|---|
| Impulse Control | Self-Report Test of Impulse Control (STIC) (Factors II and III only) | Lazarro, T.A., Beggs, D.L., & McNeil, K.A. (1969). The development and validation of the Self-Report Test of Impulse Control. *Journal of Clinical Psychology, 25*(4), 434-438. | Test-retest reliability 0.89 at one month. Concurrent validity: correlations between STIC scale and the Barratt Impulsiveness Scale (−0.50) and the Self-control subscale of the California Psychological Inventory scale (0.62) significant at p<0.01. |
| Infection Status | | Data collected from clinical record | Retrieve from the chart the presence of an infection and the microorganisms causing it. Culture results and Colony Counts |
| Information Processing | Mini-Mental State | Folstein, M.F., Folstein, S.E., & McHugh, P.R. (1975). "Mini-Mental State": A practical method for grading the cognitive state of patients for the clinician. *Journal of Psychiatric Research, 12*(3), 189-198. | Test-retest reliability 0.89, interrater reliability 0.82 Anthony, J.C., LeResche, L., Niaz, U., VonKorff, M.R., & Folstein, M.F. (1982). Limits of the "Mini-Mental State" as a screening test for dementia and delirium among hospital patients. *Psychological Medicine, 12*(2), 397-408. Concurrent validity demonstrated by correlation of MMS to Weschler Adult Intelligence Scale: Verbal IQ – Pearson r=0.776 (p<0.0001) Performance IQ – Pearson r=0.660 (p<0.001) (Folstein, Folstein, & McHugh, 1975). |
| Joint Movement: Active | | Data collected from clinical record | |
| Joint Movement: Passive | | Data collected from clinical record | |
| Knowledge: Breastfeeding | | | Patient's self-rating compared to nurse's rating for this outcome. |
| Knowledge: Diet | | | Patient's self-rating compared to nurse's rating for this outcome. |
| Knowledge: Disease Process | | | Patient's self-rating compared to nurse's rating for this outcome. |

*Continued*

¹Psychometrics are from primary source unless otherwise indicated.

| Outcome | Measurement Tool Selected | Primary Source | Psychometrics* |
|---|---|---|---|
| Knowledge: Energy Conservation | | | Patient's self-rating compared to nurse's rating for this outcome. |
| Knowledge: Health Behaviors | | | Patient's self-rating compared to nurse's rating for this outcome. |
| Knowledge: Health Resources | | | Patient's self-rating compared to nurse's rating for this outcome. |
| Knowledge: Infection Control | | | Patient's self-rating compared to nurse's rating for this outcome. |
| Knowledge: Medication | | | Patient's self-rating compared to nurse's rating for this outcome. |
| Knowledge: Personal Safety | | | Patient's self-rating compared to nurse's rating for this outcome. |
| Knowledge: Prescribed Activity | | | Patient's self-rating compared to nurse's rating for this outcome. |
| Knowledge: Substance Use Control | | | Patient's self-rating compared to nurse's rating for this outcome. |
| Knowledge: Treatment Procedure | | | Patient's self-rating compared to nurse's rating for this outcome. |
| Knowledge: Treatment Regimen | | | Patient's self-rating compared to nurse's rating for this outcome. |
| Leisure Participation | Nottingham Leisure Questionnaire | Drummond, A.E.R., & Walker, M.F. (1994). The Nottingham Leisure Questionnaire for stroke patients. *British* | Interrater reliability range 0.76-1.00 for 40 categories; 0.65 for one (Meditation/Relaxation) Test-retest reliability ranged from poor (<0.40, |

| | | |
|---|---|---|
| | *Journal of Occupational Therapy, 57(11),* 414-418. | 6 categories) to excellent (> or = 0.75, 12 categories) at 2 weeks. After weighted kappa calculated on the 6 with poor agreement, all but two improved. |
| | | Instrument used in a randomized controlled clinical trial by Drummond, and "proved sensitive to treatment" (as cited in Drummond & Walker, 1994). |
| | | Tested on sample of patients who had had a stroke. No statistics on other populations available. |
| Loneliness | Russell, D., Peplau, L.A., & Ferguson, M. (1978). Developing a measure of loneliness. *Journal of Personality Assessment, 42(3),* 290-294. | Internal consistency of revised measure is high coefficient = 0.94 (Russell et al 1980). |
| | Russell, D., Peplau, L.A., & Cutrona, C.E. (1980). The Revised UCLA Loneliness Scale: Concurrent and discriminant validity evidence. *Journal of Personality and Social Psychology, 39(3),* 472-480. | |
| Memory | Pfeiffer, E. (1975). A short portable mental status questionnaire for the assessment of organic brain deficit in elderly patients. *American Geriatrics Society, 23(10),* 433-441. | Test-retest reliability > 0.80 |
| Short Portable Mental Status Questionnaire (SPMSQ) | | Interrater reliability range 0.62-0.87 Fillenbaum, G.C., & Smyer, M. (1981). The development, validity and reliability of the ORS multidimensional functional assessment questionnaire. *Journal of Gerontology, 36,* 428-434. |
| | | Clinical validity: 92% agreement between SPMSQ score and clinical diagnosis when SPMSQ indicated definite impairment; 82% agreement when SPMSQ indicated no impairment/mild impairment in population of elderly community clients (n=133). |

*Continued*

*Psychometrics are from primary source unless otherwise indicated.

| Outcome | Measurement Tool Selected | Primary Source | Psychometrics* |
|---|---|---|---|
| Mobility Level | Timed "Up and Go" | Podsiadlo, D., & Richardson, S. (1991). The timed "Up & Go": A test of basic functional mobility for frail elderly persons. *Journal of American Geriatrics Society, 39*(2), 142-148. | Interrater reliability coefficient=0.99<br><br>Validity supported by significant correlation between "Up & Go" scores and:<br>Balance (r=–0.72)<br>Gait Speed (r=–0.55)<br>Functional Capacity (r=–0.51) |
| Mood Equilibrium | Mood Survey | Underwood, B., & Froming, W.J. (1980). The Mood Survey: A personality measure of happy and sad moods. *Journal of Personality Assessment, 44*(4), 404-413. | Test-restest reliability 0.80-0.85 after 3 weeks<br><br>Concurrent validity: significant correlation with Beck Depression Inventory (r=0.47, p<0.001 for both subscales) and the Mood Adjective Checklist.<br><br>Tested on college students only. |
| Muscle Function | Muscle Grade Measurement Tool (from Alverno) | Cole, J.H., Furness, A.L., & Twomey, L.T. (1988). *Muscles in action.* New York: Churchill Livingstone.<br><br>Kendall, F.P., & McCreary, E.K. (1983). *Muscles: Testing and function* (2$^{nd}$ ed.). Baltimore: Williams & Wilkins. | Clinical evaluation tool, no psychometric data available. |
| Neglect Recovery | | Data collected from clinical record | |
| Neurological Status | Glasgow Coma Scale | Teasdale, G., & Jennett, B. (1974). Assessment of coma and impaired consciousness: A practical scale. *Lancet, 2*, 81-84. | Reliability mean coefficient (left eye, right eye, verbal, left motor, right motor) .91<br>Disagreement rate mean coefficient .37<br>Rowley, G., & Fielding, K. (1991). Reliability and accuracy of the Glasgow Coma Scale with experienced and inexperienced users. *The Lancet, 337*(8740), 535-538.<br><br>Acceptable criterion validity reported. Juarez, V.J., & Lyons, M. (1995). Interrater reliability of the Glasgow Coma Scale. *Journal of Neuroscience Nursing, 27*(5), 283-286. |

| | | | |
|---|---|---|---|
| Neurological Status: Autonomic | | Data collected from clinical record | |
| Neurological Status: Central Motor Control | | Data collected from clinical record | |
| Neurological Status: Consciousness | | Data collected from clinical record | |
| Neurological Status: Cranial Sensory/Motor Function | | Data collected from clinical record | |
| Neurological Status: Spinal Sensory/Motor Function | | Data collected from clinical record | |
| Nutritional Status | Mini Nutritional Assessment (MNA) | Guigoz, Y., Vallas, B.J., & Garry, P.J. (1994). Mini Nutritional Assessment: A practical assessment tool for grading the nutritional state of elderly patients. *Facts and Research in Gerontology, 4* (Suppl. 2), 15-59. | Discriminate analysis: MNA scores compared to clinical status (per physician assessment blinded to MNA scores). Identical nutrition status was obtained by the MNA test without biochemical indices for 89% of the subjects, while the MNA with biochemical indices classified 88% of the subjects identically with clinical status determination. |
| Nutritional Status: Biochemical Measures | | Data collected from clinical record | |
| Nutritional Status: Energy | COOP Chart: Physical Condition | Dartmouth Primary Care Cooperative Information Project (1987). COOP Charts. Hanover, NH: Department of Community and Family Medicine, Dartmouth Medical School. | Test-retest intraclass correlation coefficients 0.78-0.98 (elderly patient sample) and 0.73-0.98 (low income patient sample) (as cited in Nelson, E.C., Wasson, J.H., Johnson, D.J., & Hayes, R.D. (2002). *Dartmouth COOP Functional Health Assessment Charts: Brief measures for clinical practice.* Retrieved February 20, 2002, from http://www.dartmouth.edu/~coopproj/more_charts.html.) |

*Continued*

---

¹Psychometrics are from primary source unless otherwise indicated.

| Outcome | Measurement Tool Selected | Primary Source | Psychometrics* |
|---|---|---|---|
| | | | Convergent validity: correlation between COOP Chart: Physical Condition and RAND Physical Scale significant at p<0.001<br><br>Nelson, E., Wasson, J., Kirk, J., Keller, A., Clark, D., Dietrich, A., & Zubkoff, M. (1987). Assessment of function in routine clinical practice: Description of the COOP chart method and preliminary findings. *Journal of Chronic Diseases 40*(1), 55S-63S. |
| Nutritional Status: Food & Fluid Intake | | Data collected from clinical record | |
| Nutritional Status: Nutrient Intake | | Data collected from clinical record | |
| Oral Health | Kayser-Jones Brief Oral Health Status Examination | Kayser-Jones, J., Bird, W.F., Paul, S.M., Long, L., & Schell, E.S. (1995). An instrument to assess the oral health status of nursing home residents. *The Gerontologist, 35*(6), 814-824. | Interrater reliability coefficient ranges 0.40-0.68 between dentist and assorted other nursing home staff. Test-retest coefficients close to or above 0.80 for all staff examiners (time interval 1-2 days)<br><br>According to authors, concurrent validity not established due to lack of comparable oral health tool. |
| Pain Control (2 instruments) | Discomfort Scale for Patients with Dementia of the Alzheimer's Type (Used only with cognitively impaired patients) | Hurley, A.C., Volicer, B.J., Hanrahan, P.A., Houde, S., & Volicer, L. (1992). Assessment of discomfort in advanced Alzheimer patients. *Research in Nursing & Health, 15*(5), 369-377. | Interrater reliability r = 0.86-0.98, Internal Consistency α > 0.80<br><br>Construct validity demonstrated by statistically significant differences (p < 0.001) in peak mean DS-DAT scores during fever episodes versus baseline and resolution scores |
| Pain Control (2 instruments) | Health Promoting Lifestyle Profile II (Health Responsibility Subscale) | Walker, S.N., Sechrist, K., & Pender, N. (1987). The Health-Promoting Lifestyle Profile: Development and psychometric characteristics. *Nursing Research, 36*(2), 76-81. | *All psychometric data from Walker and Hill-Polerecky paper (as cited in Berger, A.M., & Walker, S.N. (1997). Measuring healthy lifestyle. In Frank-Stromborg, M., & Olsen, S.J. (Eds.), Instruments for clinical health care research (3rd ed.) (pp. 363-377). Boston: Jones & Bartlett.)* |

| | | |
|---|---|---|
| | Walker, S.N., Sechrist, K.R., & Pender, N. (1995). The Health-Promoting Lifestyle Profile II. Omaha, NE: University of Nebraska at Omaha. | Internal consistency $\alpha=0.94$ (total scale); Health Responsiblity subscale 0.86. Test-retest r=0.89 (3-week interval). Construct validity: Factor analysis of the 6 subscales showed the Spiritual Growth and Interpersonal Relations subscale items loading together, the remaining 4 subscales loaded on separate factors at 0.43 or >, and a nuisance factor with no significant loadings. Convergent validity: Compared to the Personal Lifestyle Questionnaire, correlation=0.68. Criterion validity: Correlation of the scale with the Medical Outcomes Study Short-Form General Health Survey general health perception scale=0.26; with the Quality of Life Index=0.46. |
| Pain Level (3 instruments) | Discomfort Scale for Patients With Dementia of the Alzheimer's Type (DS-DAT) (Used only with cognitively impaired patients) | Hurley, A.C., Volicer, B.J., Hanrahan, P.A., Houde, S., & Volicer, L. (1992). Assessment of discomfort in advanced Alzheimer's patients. *Research in Nursing and Health, 15*(5), 369-377. | Interrater reliability r = 0.86-0.98, Internal Consistency $\alpha > 0.80$ Construct validity demonstrated by statistically significant differences ($p < 0.001$) in peak mean DS-DAT scores during fever episodes versus baseline and resolution scores |
| Pain Level (3 instruments) | Numeric Pain Intensity Scale | U.S. Department of Health and Human Services (1992). *Acute pain management: Operative or medical procedures and trauma* (AHCPR Publication No. 92-0032). Rockville, Maryland: Public Health Service Agency for Health Care Policy and Research. | Content validity of numeric scales supported by significant correlation to simultaneous ratings on a visual analogue scale (gamma 0.888) Aradine, C.R., Beyer, J.E., & Tompkins, J.M. (1988). Children's pain perception before and after analgesia: A study of instrument construct validity and related issues. *Journal of Pediatric Nursing, 3*(1), 11-23. |
| Pain Level (3 instruments) | Wong Baker Faces Rating Scale (Used only for nonverbal patients) | Wong, D., & Baker, C. (1988). Pain in children: Comparison of assessment scales. *Pediatric Nursing, 14*, 9-17. | Test-retest reliability (elderly sample) r = 0.94 (p < 0.01) Herr, K.A., Mobily, P.R., Kohout, F.J., & Wagenaar, D. (1998). Evaluation of the Faces Pain Scale for use with the elderly. *Clinical Journal of Pain, 14*, 29-38. Test-retest reliability (pediatric sample) r = 0.90 (p < 0.001) |

*Continued*

Psychometrics are from primary source unless otherwise indicated.

| Outcome | Measurement Tool Selected | Primary Source | Psychometrics* |
|---|---|---|---|
| | | | Discriminant validity supported by significant differences between pre- and post-procedure scores ($p < 0.001$). |
| | | | Concurrent validity supported by significant ($p < 0.01$) correlations between the "Faces" scale and a visual analog scale (r = .71) and a numerical scale (r = .75) Keck, J.F., Gerkensmeyer, J.E., Joyce, B.A., & Schade, J.G. (1996). Reliability and validity of the faces and word descriptor scales to measure procedural pain. *Journal of Pediatric Nursing, 11*(6), 368-374. |
| Pain: Disruptive Effects | The Chronic Pain Grade Questionnaire (CPG) (used "disability points" score only, did not calculate "pain grade") | Von Korff, M, Ormel, J., Keefe, F.J., & Dworkin, S.F. (1992). Grading the severity of chronic pain. *Pain, 50*(2), 133-149. | Internal consistency: item total correlation range 0.69-0.83; Cronbach α=0.91 |
| | | | Convergent validity confirmed by Spearman correlation coefficients between the CPG score and scores from 8 comparable dimensions of the SF-36, range 0.38-0.84 ($p<0.001$) (Smith, et al., 1997) Confirmatory factor analysis: all items had factor loading > 0.75 Smith, B.H., Penny, K.I., Purves, A.M., Munro, C., Wilson, B., Grimshaw, J., Chambers, W.A., & Smith, W.C. (1997). The Chronic Grade Questionnaire: Validation and reliability in postal research. *Pain, 71*, 141-147. |
| Parent-Infant Attachment | Maternal Attachment Inventory (MAI) | Muller, M. (1994). A questionnaire to measure mother-to-infant attachment. *Journal of Nursing Measurement, 2*(2), 129-141. | Internal consistency: coefficient α=0.85 (Test-retest scores low, authors state scores are expected to change over time.) |
| | | | Construct validity quantified by submission to expert panel of "theoreticians, postpartum and neonatal nurses, and women with young infants" (Muller, p. 132) Concurrent validity: MAI scores correlated significantly with the How I Feel About My Baby Now scales (r=0.45, $p<0.001$), the Maternal Separation Anxiety Scale (r=0.46, $p<0.001$), and the Postnatal Maternal Attitudes and Maternal Adjustment Scale (r=0.30, $p<0.01$) |

| | | | |
|---|---|---|---|
| Parenting | The Nurturance Inventory | Clarke, M., & Hornick, J. (1984). The development of the Nurturance Inventory: An instrument for assessing parenting practices. *Child Psychiatry & Human Development, 15*(1), 49-63. | (Psychometric testing done on samples of mothers only; fathers were not tested.) Internal consistency: coefficient $\alpha$=0.88 Item-to-total correlations: range 0.39-0.77 Concurrent validity: correlations between mother self-report and observations of actual behavior by interviewer range from 0.07-0.58. Predictive validity: discriminant analysis showed that 88% of abusers correctly classified, 85% of non-abusers correctly classified. |
| Participation: Health Care Decisions | Autonomy Preference Index (API) | Ende, J., Kazis, L., Ash, A., & Moskowitz, M.A. (1989). Measuring patient's desire for autonomy: Decision making and information-seeking preferences among medical patients. *Journal of General Internal Medicine, 4*(1), 23-30. | Decision-making subscale: Test-retest r=0.84 (2-week interval) Cronbach's $\alpha$=0.82 Information-seeking subscale: Test-retest r=0.83 (2-week interval) Cronbach's $\alpha$=0.82 Concurrent validity established by significant correlation of scale score to single, global item asking opinion of who should control medical care, r=0.54, p<0.0001. Validity also tested by administering API to select population of patients with diabetes previously identified by clinic staff as "highly motivated to self-care & home monitoring," and scores compared to general population sample; diabetic patients scored significantly higher (p<0.01). |
| Psychosocial Adjustment: Life Change | Life Satisfaction Index A (revised version by Liang) | Neugarten, B.L., Havighurst, R.J., & Tobin, S. (1961). The measurement of life satisfaction. *Journal of Gerontology, 16*, 134-143. | Test-retest reliability at 2 weeks: r=0.81 (Neugarten, Havighurst, 1961) Internal consistency: Cronbach's $\alpha$=0.84 (Neugarten, Havighurst, 1961) |

*Continued*

*Psychometrics are from primary source unless otherwise indicated.

| Outcome | Measurement Tool Selected | Primary Source | Psychometrics* |
|---|---|---|---|
| | | Liang, J. (1984). Dimensions of the Life Satisfaction Index A: A structural formulation. *Journal of Gerontology*, 39, 613-622. | LISREL analysis identified 3 factors (mood tone, zest, and congruence) using 11 of original 20 tool items (Liang, 1984) |
| Quality of Life | Satisfaction with Life Scale (SWLS) | Diener, E., Emmons, R.A., Larsen, R.J., & Griffin, S. (1985). The satisfaction with life scale. *Journal of Personality Assessment*, 49(1), 71-75. | Internal Consistency $\alpha$=0.87<br>Test-retest reliability: r=0.82 (2-month period)<br><br>Concurrent validity:<br>SWLS scores of 2 samples of college students (total n=339) correlated with 9 measures of subjective well-being. SWLS scores of an elderly sample (n=53) correlated (0.46) with scores on Life Satisfaction Index and independent ratings of life satisfaction (0.43). |
| Respiratory Status: Gas Exchange | | Data collected from clinical record | |
| Respiratory Status: Ventilation | Chronic Respiratory Disease Questionnaire (CRQ) | Guyatt, G.H., Berman, L.B., Townsend, M., Pugsley, S.O., & Chambers, L.W. (1987). A measure of quality of life for clinical trials in chronic lung disease. *Thorax*, 42(10), 773-778. | Test-retest reliability: "mean scores were similar for all four dimensions at each administration" (p. 774) (administered at 2-week intervals)<br>Responsiveness demonstrated by administering tool to subjects at baseline and then again after treatment that was expected to result in improvement; CRQ scores were "substantially better" at follow-up (p. 774).<br><br>Validity: based on measures of FEV, Slow Vital Capacity, and other tests, agreement between predicted and observed CRQ scores was good (weighted kappa 0.51, p<0.05). |
| Rest | Visual Analogue Scale for Fatigue (VAS-F) | Lee, K.A., Hicks, G., & Nino-Murcia, G. (1991). Validity and reliability of a scale to assess fatigue. *Psychiatry Research*, 36(3), 291-298. | Reliability: fatigue subscale (am & pm data) Cronbach's $\alpha$=0.91-0.96 (healthy subjects)<br>Cronbach's $\alpha$=0.96-0.95 (am & pm data) (sleep-disorder subjects)<br>Reliability: energy subscale (am & pm data) Cronbach's $\alpha$=0.94-0.95 (healthy subjects) |

| | | |
|---|---|---|
| Risk Control | Lifestyle Assessment Questionnaire (Self-Care and Drug Usage subscales) | Cronbach's $\alpha$=0.96-0.94 (am & pm data) (sleep-disorder subjects) |
| | | Concurrent validity: significant correlation ($p<0.01$) between VAS-F scores and Stanford Sleepiness Scale and the Profile of Mood States |
| | Hettler, B. (1982). Wellness promotion and risk reduction on a university campus. In M. Faber and A. Reinhardt (Eds.), *Promoting health through risk reduction*. New York: Macmillan. | Internal consistency of subscales: Self-Care Cronbach's $\alpha$=0.72; Drug Use Cronbach's $\alpha$=0.82 |
| | | Validity psychometrics are from data obtained with entire 173-item Wellness Inventory section of the Lifestyle Assessment Questionnaire. Subscale data tested alone not available. |
| | | Test-retest reliability: r=0.81-0.97 (2-week interval) |
| | | Content validity: Index of Content Validity (CVI) used to quantify extent of agreement between expert judges. CVI=0.98 |
| | | Predictive validity quasi-experiemental study yielded insignificant results |
| | | Richter, J.M. (1988). Reliability and validity of the Lifestyle Assessment Questionnaire. In C.F. Waltz & O.L. Strickland (Eds.), *Measurement of nursing outcomes: Measuring client outcomes* (Vol. 1, pp. 352-376). New York: Springer. |
| | | (Tool limitation: tested on college-age females only. May not be generalizable to NOC study population.) |
| Risk Control: Alcohol Use | Index of Alcohol Involvement (IAI) | Coefficient alpha=0.90 |
| | MacNeil, G. (1991). A short-form scale to measure alcohol abuse. *Research on Social Work Practice, 1*(1), 68-75. | Factor analysis reported correlations with 8 criterion measures. |

*Continued*

| Outcome | Measurement Tool Selected | Primary Source | Psychometrics* |
|---|---|---|---|
| Risk Control: Drug Use | Drug Abuse Screening Test (DAST) | Skinner, H.A. (1982). The drug abuse screening test. *Addictive Behaviors, 7*(4), 363-371. | Coefficient alpha=0.92 Item scale correlations (.43-.78) Factor analysis reported |
| Risk Control: Sexually Transmitted Diseases | Prevention Minimum Evaluation Data Set (PMEDS) | Card, J.J. (Ed.). (1993). *Handbook of adolescent sexuality and pregnancy: Research and Evaluation Instruments.* Newbury Park: Sage Publications. | No psychometrics available |
| Risk Control: Tobacco Use | Fagerstrom Tolerance Questionnaire (FTQ) | Fagerstrom, K.O. (1978). Measuring degree of physical dependence in tobacco smoking with reference to individualization of treatment. *Addiction Behavior, 3,* 235-241. | Coefficient alpha=0.51-0.55 Item-total correlations for 5 items=0.40-0.60 In clinical trials, the FTQ predicted outcome in cessation attempts without use of nicotine replacement. The FTQ has widespread use Fagerstrom, K., & Schneider, N.G. (1989). Measuring nicotine dependence: A review of the Fagerstrom tolerance questionnaire. *Journal of Behavioral Medicine, 12*(2), 159-182. |
| Risk Control: Unintended Pregnancy | Prevention Minimum Evaluation Data Set (PMEDS) | Card, J.J. (Ed.). (1993). *Handbook of adolescent sexuality and pregnancy: Research and Evaluation Instruments.* Newbury Park: Sage Publications. | No psychometrics available |
| Risk Detection | Lifestyle Assessment Questionnaire (Self Care subscale) | Hettler, B. (1982). Wellness promotion and risk reduction on a university campus. In M. Faber and A. Reinhardt (Eds.), *Promoting health through risk reduction.* New York: Macmillan. | Internal consistency of subscale: Self-Care Cronbach's α=0.72 Validity psychometrics are from data obtained with entire 173-item Wellness Inventory section of the Lifestyle Assessment Questionnaire. Subscale data tested alone not available. Test-retest reliability: r=0.81-0.97 (2-week interval) Content validity: Index of Content Validity (CVI) used to quantify extent of agreement between expert judge CVI=0.98 |

| Outcome | Tool | Reference | Psychometrics* |
|---|---|---|---|
| Role Performance | Social Adjustment Scale | Weissman, M.M., & Bothwell, S. (1976). Assessment of social adjustment by patient self-report. *Archives of General Psychiatry, 33,* 1111-1115. | Predictive validity quasi-experimental study yielded insignificant results. Richter, J.M. (1988). Reliability and validity of the Lifestyle Assessment Questionnaire. In C.F. Waltz & O.L. Strickland (Eds.), *Measurement of nursing outcomes: Measuring client outcomes* (Vol. 1, pp. 352-376). New York: Springer. (Tool limitation: tested on college-age females only. May not be generalizable to NOC study population.) Alpha coefficient = 0.74 Test-retest reliability 0.74 after one month |
| Safety Behavior: Fall Prevention | Home Safety Checklist for Older Adults | National Safety Council (1982). *Home Safety Checklist for Older Adults.* Chicago: National Safety Council. | Developed for use as assessment tool, not as research instrument. No psychometric data available. |
| Safety Behavior: Home Physical Environment | Modified Home Dangers/Precautions: Interview/Observation | Tymchuk, A.J. (1997). Home Dangers and Precautions: Interview/observation. *The UCLA Parent/Child Health & Wellness Project.* | Instrument modified by NOC research team. The following psychometric data is from evaluation of the Home Inventory of Dangers and Safety Precautions-2 tool developed by Tymchuk and associates (Tymchuk, A.J., Lang, C.M., Dolyniuk, C.A., Berney-Ficklin, K., & Spitz, R. (1998). The Home Inventory of Dangers and Safety Precautions-2: Addressing critical needs for prescriptive assessment devices in child maltreatment and in healthcare. *Child Abuse & Neglect, 23*(1), 1-14). Test-retest reliability range 90%-100% at 1 week. Internal consistency Cronbach's α=0.96 for total dangers and α=0.98 for total dangers; Alphas for individual categories were low (0.62 or less). |
| Safety Behavior: Personal | Lifestyle Assessment Questionnaire (Vehicle Safety and Drug Use Subscales) | Hettler, B. (1982). Wellness promotion and risk reduction on a university campus. In M. Faber and A. Reinhardt (Eds.), *Promoting health through risk reduction.* New York: Macmillan. | Internal consistency of subscales: Vehicle Safety Cronbach's α=0.69; Drug Use Cronbach's α=0.82 Validity psychometrics are from data obtained with entire 173-item Wellness Inventory section of the Lifestyle Assessment Questionnaire. Subscale data tested alone not available. |

*Continued*

*Psychometrics are from primary source unless otherwise indicated.

| Outcome | Measurement Tool Selected | Primary Source | Psychometrics* |
|---|---|---|---|
| | | | Test-retest reliability: r=0.81-0.97 (2-week interval) |
| | | | Content validity: Index of Content Validity (CVI) used to quantify extent of agreement between expert judges. CVI=0.98 |
| | | | Predictive validity quasi-experimental study yielded insignificant results. Richter, J.M. (1988). Reliability and validity of the Lifestyle Assessment Questionnaire. In C.F. Waltz & O.L. Strickland (Eds.), *Measurement of nursing outcomes: Measuring client outcomes* (Vol. 1, pp. 352-376). New York: Springer. |
| | | | (Tool limitation: tested on college-age females only. May not be generalizable to NOC study population.) |
| Safety Status: Physical Injury | FIC Tool | Maas, M., Swanson, E., Buckwalter, K.C., Specht, J.P., Tripp-Reimer, T., Lenth, R. et al. (1999). *Final report: Nursing interventions for Alzheimer's: Family role trials (NINR R01-NRO1689)*. Rockville, MD: National Institutes of Health. | Correlations with 20 resident records (chart and incident reports) r=.82 Interrater reliability=.93 |
| Safety Status: Falls Occurrence | | Data collected from clinical record | Number of falls |
| Self-Care: Activities of Daily Living (ADL) | Index of Independence in Activities of Daily Living (Katz Index of ADL) | Katz, S., Ford, A.B., Moskowitz, R.W., Jackson, B.A., & Jaffe, M.W. (1963). Studies of illness in the aged. The Index of ADL: A standardized measure of biological and psychosocial function. *Journal of the American Medical Association, 185*(12), 914-919. | Interrater reliability: differences between observers doing simultaneous ratings resulted in differences occurring only once in 20 evaluations or less Predictive validity demonstrated by significant (p < 0.05) differences in Index of ADL scores between treatment and control groups in a rheumatoid arthritis treatment effectiveness study conducted by Katz and associates |

Katz, S., Vignos, P.J., Moskowitz, R.W., Thompson, H.M., & Svec, K.H. (1968). Comprehensive outpatient care in rheumatoid arthritis. *JAMA, 206*(6), 1249-1254.

The Index of ADL predicted long-term adaptation, in terms of mobility and home confinement, as well as or better than did selected measures of mental or physical function
Katz, S., Downs, T.D., Cash, H.R., & Grotz, R.C. (1970). Progress in development of the Index of ADL. *Gerontologist, 10*(1), 20-30.

| Self-Care: Bathing | Functional Independence Measure (FIM) | *Guide for the Uniform Data Set for Medical Rehabilitation (including the FIM™ instrument), version 5.1.* Buffalo, NY 14214: University at Buffalo; 1997. | Interrater reliability=0.95<br>Face validity established by expert opinion in response to 4 assessment questions re: the FIM<br>Ottenbacher, K.J., Hsu,Y., Granger, C.V., & Fielder, R.C. (1996). The reliability of the functional independence measure: a quantitative review. *Archives of Physical Medicine & Rehabilitation, 77*(12), 1226-1232.<br><br>Predictive validity: FIM scores improved between admission and discharge and reflected patient's discharge destination<br>Dodds, T.A., Martin, D.P., Stolov, W.C., & Deyo, R.A. (1993). A validation of the Functional Independence Measurement and its performance among rehabilitation inpatients. *Archives of Physical Medicine Rehabilitation, 74*(5), 531-536. |
| Self-Care: Dressing | Functional Independence Measure (FIM) | *Guide for the Uniform Data Set for Medical Rehabilitation (including the FIM™ instrument), version 5.1.* Buffalo, NY 14214: University at Buffalo; 1997. | Interrater reliability=0.95<br>Face validity established by expert opinion in response to 4 assessment questions re: the FIM<br>Ottenbacher, K.J., Hsu,Y., Granger, C.V., & Fielder, R.C. (1996). The reliability of the functional independence measure: A quantitative review. *Archives of Physical Medicine & Rehabilitation, 77*(12), 1226-1232. |

*Continued*

*Psychometrics are from primary source unless otherwise indicated.

| Outcome | Measurement Tool Selected | Primary Source | Psychometrics* |
|---|---|---|---|
| | | | Predictive validity: FIM scores improved between admission and discharge and reflected patient's discharge destination |
| | | | Dodds, T.A., Martin, D.P., Stolov, W.C., & Deyo, R.A. (1993). A validation of the Functional Independence Measurement and its performance among rehabilitation inpatients. *Archives of Physical Medicine and Rehabilitation, 74*(5), 531-536. |
| Self-Care: Eating | Functional Independence Measure (FIM) | *Guide for the Uniform Data Set for Medical Rehabilitation (including the FIM™ instrument), version 5.1.* Buffalo, NY 14214: University at Buffalo; 1997. | Interrater reliability=0.95 |
| | | | Face validity established by expert opinion in response to 4 assessment questions re: the FIM |
| | | | Ottenbacher, K.J., Hsu,Y., Granger, C.V., & Fielder, R.C. (1996). The reliability of the functional independence measure: a quantitative review. *Archives of Physical Medicine & Rehabilitation, 77*(12), 1226-1232. |
| | | | Predictive validity: FIM scores improved between admission and discharge and reflected patient's discharge destination |
| | | | Dodds, T.A., Martin, D.P., Stolov, W.C., & Deyo, R.A. (1993). A validation of the Functional Independence Measurement and its performance among rehabilitation inpatients. *Archives of Physical Medicine and Rehabilitation, 74*(5), 531-536. |
| Self-Care: Grooming | Functional Independence Measure (FIM) | *Guide for the Uniform Data Set for Medical Rehabilitation (including the FIM™ instrument), version 5.1.* Buffalo, NY 14214: University at Buffalo; 1997. | Interrater reliability=0.95 |
| | | | Face validity established by expert opinion in response to 4 assessment questions re: the FIM |
| | | | Ottenbacher, K.J., Hsu,Y., Granger, C.V., & Fielder, R.C. (1996). The reliability of the functional independence measure: a quantitative review. *Archives of Physical Medicine & Rehabilitation, 77*(12), 1226-1232. |

| | | | |
|---|---|---|---|
| Self-Care: Instrumental Activities of Daily Living (IADL) | Katz Self-Care ADL | Katz, S., Ford, A.B., Moskowitz, R.W., Jackson, B.S., & Jaffe, M.W. (1963). Studies of illness in the aged. The Index of ADL: A standardized measure of biological and psychosocial function. *Journal of the American Medical Association, 185*(12), 914-919. | Predictive validity: FIM scores improved between admission and discharge and reflected patient's discharge destination<br><br>Dodds, T.A., Martin, D.P., Stolov, W.C., & Deyo, R.A. (1993). A validation of the Functional Independence Measurement and its performance among rehabilitation inpatients. *Archives of Physical Medicine Rehabilitation, 74*(5), 531-536.<br><br>Interrater reliability: differences between observers doing simultaneous ratings resulted in differences occurring only once in 20 evaluations or less<br><br>Predictive validity demonstrated by significant (p<0.05) differences in Index of ADL scores between treatment and control groups in a rheumatoid arthritis treatment effectiveness study conducted by Katz and associates<br><br>Katz, S., Vignos, P.J., Moskowitz, R.W., Thompson, H.M., & Svec, K.H. (1968). Comprehensive outpatient care in rheumatoid arthritis. *JAMA, 206*(6), 1249-1254.<br><br>The Index of ADL predicted long-term adaptation, in terms of mobility and home confinement, as well as or better than did selected measures of mental or physical function<br><br>Katz, S., Downs, T.D., Cash, H.R., & Grotz, R.C. (1970). Progress in development of the Index of ADL. *Gerontologist, 10*(1), 20-30. |
| Self-Care: Non-Parenteral Medication | | Data collected from clinical record | |
| Self-Care: Oral Hygiene | Oral Hygiene Skill Achievement Index | Niederman, R. & Sullivan, T.M. (1981). Oral Hygiene skill achievement index I. *Journal of Periodontology, 52*(3), 143-149. | Reliability of the index was measured by subscales evaluating toothbrushing ≥0.91; evaluating flossing ≥ 0.91; total 0.91.<br>Reliability after 6 months ≥0.96 |

*Psychometrics are from primary source unless otherwise indicated.*

*Continued*

| Outcome | Measurement Tool Selected | Primary Source | Psychometrics* |
|---|---|---|---|
| Self-Care: Parenteral Medication | | Niederman, R., Sullivan, T.M., Weiss, D., Morhart, R., Robbins, W., & Maier, D. (1981). Oral hygiene skill achievement index II. *Journal of Periodontology, 52*(3), 150-154.<br><br>Data collected from clinical record | |
| Self-Care: Toileting (2 instruments) | Functional Independence Measure (FIM) | *Guide for the Uniform Data Set for Medical Rehabilitation (including the FIM™ instrument), version 5.1.* Buffalo, NY 14214: University at Buffalo; 1997. | Interrater reliability=0.95<br><br>Face validity established by expert opinion in response to 4 assessment questions re: the FIM Ottenbacher, K.J., Hsu,Y., Granger, C.V., & Fielder, R.C. (1996). The reliability of the functional independence measure: a quantitative review. *Archives of Physical Medicine & Rehabilitation, 77*(12), 1226-1232.<br><br>Predictive validity: FIM scores improved between admission and discharge and reflected patient's discharge destination Dodds, T.A., Martin, D.P., Stolov, W.C., & Deyo, R.A. (1993). A validation of the Functional Independence Measurement and its performance among rehabilitation inpatients. *Archives of Physical Medicine Rehabilitation, 74*(5), 531-536. |
| Self-Care: Toileting (2 instruments) | Katz Self-Care ADL | Katz, S., Ford, A.B., Moskowitz, R.W., Jackson, B.A., & Jaffe, M.W. (1963). Studies of illness in the aged. The Index of ADL: A standardized measure of biological and psychosocial function. *Journal of the American Medical Association, 185*(12), 914-919. | Interrater reliability: differences between observers doing simultaneous ratings resulted in differences occurring only once in 20 evaluations or less<br><br>Predictive validity demonstrated by significant ($p < 0.05$) differences in Index of ADL scores between treatment and control groups in a rheumatoid arthritis treatment effectiveness study conducted by Katz and associates |

| | | | |
|---|---|---|---|
| | | Katz, S., Vignos, P.J., Moskowitz, R.W., Thompson, H.M., & Svec, K.H. (1968). Comprehensive outpatient care in rheumatoid arthritis. *JAMA, 206*(6), 1249-1254. | |
| | | The Index of ADL predicted long-term adaptation, in terms of mobility and home confinement, as well as or better than did selected measures of mental or physical function | |
| | | Katz, S., Downs, T.D., Cash, H.R., & Grotz, R.C. (1970). Progress in development of the Index of ADL. *Gerontologist, 10*(1), 20-30. | |
| Self-Esteem | Self-Esteem Rating Scale (SERS) | Nugent, W.R. & Thomas, J.W. (1993). Validation of a clinical measure of self-esteem. *Research on Social Work Practice, 3*(2), 191-207. | Factor analysis confirmed a single common factor and that the scale is unidimensional. Positive findings ranged from 0.56 to 0.83. |
| | | | Alpha reliability 0.97 |
| Self-Mutilation Restraint | Behavior Problems Inventory (Self-Injurious Behavior Subscale) | Rojahn, J., Polster, L.M., Mulick, J.A. & Wisniewski, J.J. (1989). Reliability of the Behavior Problems Inventory. *Journal of the Multihandicapped Person, 2*, 283-293. | Reliability was calculated using Cohen's Kappa for each item and for global categories of self-injurious behavior (.84), stereotyped behavior (0.89), and aggression (0.83). |
| Sleep (2 instruments) | | Data collected from clinical record | |
| Sleep (2 instruments) | Pittsburgh Sleep Quality Index (PSQI) | Buysse, K.J., Reynolds, C.F., III, Monk, T.H., Berman, S.R., & Kupfer, D.J. (1989). The Pittsburgh Sleep Quality Index: A new instrument for psychiatric practice and research. *Psychiatry Research, 28*(2), 193-213. | Internal consistency $\alpha=0.83$ |
| | | | Items and total scores for 3 groups known to be "normal," "depressed," and "poor" sleepers remained stable over time. |
| | | | Post hoc PSQI cutoff score of 5 "correctly identified 88.5% of all patients and controls (kappa=0.75, $p<0.001$). This represents a sensitivity of 89.6% and a specificity of 86.5%" (p. 199). |

*Continued*

*Psychometrics are from primary source unless otherwise indicated.

| Outcome | Measurement Tool Selected | Primary Source | Psychometrics* |
|---|---|---|---|
| Social Interaction Skills | Test of Negative Social Exchange (TENSE) | Ruehlman, L.S. & Karoly, P. (1991). With a little flak from my friends: Development and preliminary validation of the Test of Negative Social Exchange (TENSE). *Psychological Assessment: A Journal of Consulting and Clinical Psychology, 3(1), 97-104.* | Test/retest for subscales hostility/impatience 0.80, insensitivity 0.72, interference 0.65, ridicule 0.70. Internal consistency subscales alpha coefficient: hostility/impatience 0.83, insensitivity 0.82, interference 0.75, and ridicule 0.70. |
| Social Involvement | Tool created/adapted based upon 2 articles: Palisi (1985) and Jylha & Aro (1989) | Jylha, M., & Aro, S. (1989). Socialties and survival among the elderly in Tampere, Finland. *International Journal of Epidemiology, 18(1), 158-164.*<br><br>Palisi, B.J. Formal and informal participation in urban areas. *The Journal of Social Psychology, 125(4), 429-447.* | Social participation scale strongly correlated with health status and survival (Jylha & Aro, 1989). |
| Social Support | Social Support Questionniare (Short Form) SSQSR | Sarason, I.G., Sarason, B.R., Shearin, E.N., & Pierce, G.R. (1987). A brief measure of social support: Practical and theoretical implications. *Journal of Social and Personal Relationships, 4, 497-510.* | Internal consistency: Cronbach's α range 0.90-0.93.<br><br>Validity measured by correlating SSQSR scores to the full SSQ (27-item Social Support Questionnaire) developed by authors. Results showed significant correlation between the two scale versions.<br><br>Testing administered to university students; no other populations were tested. |
| Spiritual Well-Being | Serenity Scale | Roberts, K.T. & Aspy, C.B. (1993). Development of the serenity scale. *Journal of Nursing Measurement, 1(2), 145-164.* | Internal consistency Cronbach's α=0.92<br><br>Content validity established by expert panel analysis during instrument development.<br>Factor analysis revealed 9 factors that explained 58.2% of variance. |
| Substance Addiction Consequences | Addiction Severity Index | McLellan, A.T., Luborsky, L., Woody, G.E., & O'Brien, C.P. (1980). An improved diagnostic evaluation instrument for substance abuse patients. *Journal of Nervous and Mental Disease, 168(1), 26-33.* | Extensive reliability data provided for several time frames of scale development.<br>Interrater reliability for substance abuse subscale .89 to .91; alpha coefficients for items range from .43 to .71 |

| | | |
|---|---|---|
| Suicide Self-Restraint | Linehan, M.M., Goodstein, J., Nielsen, S.L., & Chiles, J.A. (1983). Reasons for staying alive when you are thinking of killing yourself: The reasons for living inventory. *Journal of Consulting and Clinical Psychology, 51*(2), 276-286 & 484-485.<br><br>Ivanoff, A., Joon Jang, S., Smyth, N.J., & Linehan, M.M. (1994). Fewer reasons for staying alive when you are thinking of killing yourself: The brief reasons for living inventory. *Journal of Psychopathology and Behavioral Assessment, 16*(1), 1-13. | Inter-item coefficient α=0.86 (Ivanoff, Joon Jang, Smyth, & Linehan, 1994)<br><br>Strong positive correlation between Linehan Reasons for Living 48-item scale and BRFL scores (0.937) (Ivanoff, Joon Jang, Smyth, & Linehan, 1994)<br><br>Predictive validity: BRFL scores added significantly to prediction of suicidality ($R^2$ change not large, but statistically significant) (Ivanoff, Joon Jang, Smyth, & Linehan, 1994) |
| Brief Reasons for Living Inventory (BRFL) | | |
| Symptom Control | McCorkle, R., & Young, K. (1978). Development of a symptom distress scale. *Cancer Nursing, 1*(5), 373-378.<br><br>McCorkle, R., & Benoliel, J.Q. (1983). Symptom distress, current concerns, and mood disturbance after diagnosis of life-threatening disease. *Social Science Medicine, 17*(7), 431-438. | Coefficient α=0.82 (McCorkle & Young, 1978) (tested on patients with chronic illness)<br>Test-retest reliability 0.78 (McCorkle & Benoliel, 1983)<br>Internal consistency 0.78-0.79 (McCorkle & Benoliel, 1983)<br>Item total coefficients 0.37-0.73 (McCorkle & Benoliel, 1983)<br><br>Discriminant validity demonstrated by the tool discriminating between cancer and heart patients (McCorkle & Benoliel, 1983) |
| Symptom Distress Scale (SDS) | | |
| Symptom Severity | McCorkle, R., & Young, K. (1978). Development of a symptom distress scale. *Cancer Nursing, 1*(5), 373-378.<br><br>McCorkle, R., & Benoliel, J.Q. (1983). Symptom distress, current concerns, and mood disturbance after diagnosis of life-threatening disease. *Social Science Medicine, 17*(7), 431-438. | Coefficient α=0.82 (McCorkle & Young, 1978) (tested on patients with chronic illness)<br>Test-retest reliability 0.78 (McCorkle & Benoliel, 1983)<br>Internal consistency 0.78-0.79 (McCorkle & Benoliel, 1983)<br>Item total coefficients 0.37-0.73 (McCorkle & Benoliel, 1983)<br><br>Discriminant validity demonstrated by the tool discriminating between cancer and heart patients (McCorkle & Benoliel, 1983) |
| Symptom Distress Scale (SDS) | | |

*Continued*

*Psychometrics are from primary source unless otherwise indicated.

| Outcome | Measurement Tool Selected | Primary Source | Psychometrics* |
|---|---|---|---|
| Thermoregulation | | Data collected from clinical record | |
| Tissue Integrity: Skin & Mucous Membranes | Braden Scale for Predicting Pressure Sore Risk | Bergstrom, N., Braden, B.J., Laguzza, A., & Holman, V. (1987). The Braden Scale for predicting pressure sore risk. *Nursing Research, 36*(4), 205-210. | Interrater reliability 88% (RN raters)<br><br>Predictive validity: Sensitivity 79%, Specificity 74%, Predictive Value of (+) Test 54%, Predictive Value of (−) Test 90%, Correct Classification Rate 75% Braden, B.J., & Bergstrom, N. (1994). Predictive validity of the Braden Scale for pressure sore risk in a nursing home population. *Research in Nursing & Health, 17,* 459-470. |
| Tissue Perfusion: Abdominal Organs | | Data collected from clinical record | |
| Tissue Perfusion: Cardiac | | Data collected from clinical record | |
| Tissue Perfusion: Cerebral | | Data collected from clinical record | |
| Tissue Perfusion: Peripheral | | Data collected from clinical record | |
| Tissue Perfusion: Pulmonary | | Data collected from clinical record | |
| Transfer Performance | Functional Independence Measure (FIM) | *Guide for the Uniform Data Set for Medical Rehabilitation (including the FIM™ instrument), version 5.1.* Buffalo, NY 14214: University at Buffalo; 1997. | Interrater reliability=0.95<br><br>Face validity established by expert opinion in response to 4 assessment questions re: the FIM Ottenbacher, K.J., Hsu,Y., Granger, C.V., & Fielder, R.C. (1996). The reliability of the functional independence measure: A quantitative review. *Archives of Physical Medicine & Rehabilitation, 77*(12), 1226-1232. |

| NOC Outcome | Criterion Tool | Psychometrics |
|---|---|---|
| Treatment Behavior: Illness or Injury | NOC outcomes: Compliance Behavior, Health Seeking Behavior, Knowledge: Treatment Procedure, & Knowledge: Treatment Regimen | Predictive validity: FIM scores improved between admission and discharge and reflected patient's discharge destination<br>Dodds, T.A., Martin, D.P., Stolov, W.C., & Deyo, R.A. (1993). A validation of the Functional Independence Measurement and its performance among rehabilitation inpatients. *Archives of Physical Medicine & Rehabilitation, 74*(5), 531-536. |
| Urinary Continence (2 instruments) | Incontinence Management Scale | O'Donnell, P.D., & Calandro, V.J. (1991). Incontinence management scale for elderly inpatient men. *Urology, 37*(3), 220-223. | No reliability data available<br>Significant association between severity of incontinence (frequency of episodes and total urine loss volume) and incontinence management category on scale (p<0.01) |
| Urinary Continence (2 instruments) | MDS Score Section F | Morris, J.N., Hawes, C., et al. (1990). Designing the national resident assessment instrument for nursing homes. *Gerontologist, 30*(3), 293-307 | Interrater reliability using Spearman-Brown intraclass coefficient .91<br>Hawes, C., Morris, J.N., Phillips, C.D., Mor, V., Fries, B.E., & Nonemaker, S. (1995). Reliability estimates for the minimum data set for nursing home resident assessment and care screening. *The Gerontologist, 35*(2), 172-178. |
| Urinary Elimination | Data collected from clinical record | Documented urine characteristics, voiding characteristics, urinalysis results. |
| Vital Signs Status | Data collected from clinical record | |
| Well Being | Psychological General Well-Being Index — revised version (PGWB-R) | Dupuy, H. (1984). The Psychological General Well-Being (PCWB) Index. In N.K. Wenger, M.E. Mattson, C.D. Furberg, & J. Elinson (Eds.), *Assessment of quality of life in clinical trials of cardiovascular therapies* (pp. 170-183, 353-356). Greenwich, CT: Le Jacq Publishing, Inc. | Internal consistency Cronbach's $\alpha$=0.93 total for face-to-face interview, 0.95 total for telephone interview (Revicki, Leidy, & Howland, 1996)<br>Validity: mean subscale and total scale scores of the original PGWB and the PGWB-R not significantly different (Revicki, Leidy, & Howland, 1996) |

*Continued*

Psychometrics are from primary source unless otherwise indicated.

| Outcome | Measurement Tool Selected | Primary Source | Psychometrics* |
|---------|---------------------------|----------------|----------------|
| | | Revicki, D.A., Leidy, N.K. & Howland, L. (1996). Evaluating the psychometric characteristics of the Psychological General Well-Being Index with a new response scale. *Quality of Life Research, 5*(4), 419-425. | |
| Will to Live | Brief Reasons for Living Inventory (BRFL) | Linehan, M.M., Goodstein, J., Nielsen, S.L., & Chiles, J.A. (1983). Reasons for staying alive when you are thinking of killing yourself: The reasons for living inventory. *Journal of Consulting and Clinical Psychology, 51*(2), 276-286 & 484-485. | Inter-item coefficient α=0.86 (Ivanoff, Joon Jang, Smyth, & Linehan, 1994)

Strong positive correlation between Linehan Reasons for Living 48-item scale and BRFL scores (0.937) (Ivanoff, Joon Jang, Smyth, & Linehan, 1994) |
| | | Ivanoff, A., Joon Jang, S., Smyth, N.J., & Linehan, M.M. (1994). Fewer reasons for staying alive when you are thinking of killing yourself: The brief reasons for living inventory. *Journal of Psycho-pathology and Behavioral Assessment, 16*(1), 1-13. | Predictive validity: BRFL scores added significantly to prediction of suicidality ($R^2$ change not large, but statistically significant) (Ivanoff, Joon Jang, Smyth, & Linehan, 1994) |
| Wound Healing: Primary Intention | Wound Assessment Inventory | Holden-Lund, C. (1988). Effects of relaxation with guided imagery on surgical stress and wound healing. *Research in Nursing & Health, 11*, 235-244. | Interrater reliability r=0.70 (12 ratings done during pilot)

Content validity established by panel of judges (2 nurses, 2 surgeons). |
| Wound Healing: Secondary Intention | Pressure Ulcer Scale for Healing (PUSH Scale) | Thomas, D., et al. (1997). Pressure ulcer scale for healing: Derivation and validation of the PUSH tool. *Advances in Wound Care, 10*(5), 96-101. | Principal component analysis indicated 55%-60% of variance explained by scale model at weeks 0-8 of ulcer healing progression (p<0.01)

Sensitivity of scale shown by significant difference in baseline scores from scores at weeks 4, 6, and 8 |

# Summary Data for NOC Outcomes Tested in 10 Sites

RELIABILITY AND VALIDITY ESTIMATES FOR ALL NOC OUTCOMES TESTED IN 10 SITES

| NOC Outcomes | Patient N | IRR* Near Agreement† N | IRR* Near Agreement† % | IRR Absolute Agreement‡ N | IRR Absolute Agreement‡ % | Intra-Class Correlation N | Intra-Class Correlation ICC | Validity N | Validity r |
|---|---|---|---|---|---|---|---|---|---|
| **Outcomes With a Patient N of At Least 25** | | | | | | | | | |
| Acceptance: Health Status | 36 | 27 | 88 | 26 | 54 | 27 | .64 | 35 | .36 |
| Adherence Behavior | 32 | 28 | 90 | 25 | 68 | 25 | .72 | 27 | .65 |
| Aggression Control | 59 | 19 | 94 | 12 | 58 | 12 | .56 | 48 | -.12 |
| Ambulation: Walking | 134 | 97 | 91 | 65 | 86 | 65 | .95 | 132 | .41 |
| Ambulation: Wheelchair | 34 | 14 | 89 | 14 | 86 | 14 | .92 | 34 | .49 |
| Anxiety Control | 65 | 8 | 93 | 15 | 67 | 15 | .92 | 44 | -.64 |
| Balance | 46 | 23 | 100 | 23 | 70 | 23 | .48 | 46 | .78 |
| Body Positioning: Self Initiated | 40 | 21 | 96 | 21 | 57 | 21 | .75 | 40 | .81 |
| Bowel Elimination | 55 | 27 | 90 | 27 | 67 | 27 | .80 | 42 | .51 |
| Breastfeeding Establishment: Infant | 50 | 14 | 94 | 14 | 52 | 14 | .76 | 49 | (.18) |
| Breastfeeding Establishment: Maternal | 82 | 28 | 91 | 23 | 57 | 23 | .49 | 73 | (.14) |
| Cardiac Pump Effectiveness | 73 | 56 | 87 | 43 | 62 | 43 | .73 | 51 | .46 |
| Caregiver Performance: Direct Care | 26 | 24 | 94 | 24 | 54 | 24 | .53 | 21 | (.37)[a] |
| Caregiver Performance: Direct Care | | | | | | | | 20 | (-.31)[b] |
| Circulation Status | 48 | 48 | 87 | 43 | 63 | 43 | .58 | 44 | .40 |
| Cognitive Ability | 29 | 23 | 93 | 19 | 71 | 19 | .54 | 20 | .58 |
| Cognitive Orientation | 45 | 43 | 92 | 38 | 71 | 38 | .92 | 36 | -.76 |
| Comfort Level | 156 | 124 | 91 | 49 | 65 | 49 | .68 | 147 | -.23 |
| Communication Ability | 52 | 43 | 94 | 41 | 63 | 41 | .77 | 43 | .35 |
| Communication: Expressive Ability | 31 | 19 | 95 | 18 | 61 | 18 | .84 | 20 | .53 |
| Communication: Receptive Ability | 25 | 14 | 98 | 13 | 77 | 13 | .90 | 18 | .47 |
| Compliance Behavior | 38 | 36 | 88 | 35 | 57 | 35 | .76 | 38 | .60 |
| Concentration | 31 | 31 | 94 | 31 | 74 | 31 | .84 | 31 | .53 |
| Coping | 86 | 50 | 84 | 43 | 88 | 43 | .89 | 71 | (.01) |
| Decision Making | 47 | 39 | 92 | 39 | 74 | 39 | .89 | 46 | .68 |
| Distorted Thought Control | 47 | 19 | 91 | 15 | 53 | 15 | .24 | 38 | (-.16) |
| Endurance | 72 | 47 | 91 | 43 | 49 | 43 | .60 | 66 | -.59 |
| Energy Conservation | 105 | 76 | 90 | 57 | 63 | 57 | .56 | 81 | -.43 |
| Fluid Balance | 27 | 22 | 90 | 18 | 78 | 18 | .85 | 25 | (.10) |
| Health Beliefs | 49 | 42 | 86 | 42 | 64 | 42 | .51 | 37 | .36[c] |
| Health Beliefs | | | | | | | | 37 | (-.11)[d] |
| Heath Beliefs: Perceived Threat | | | | | | | | 25 | (.28)[c] |
| Heath Beliefs: Perceived Threat | 40 | 40 | 85 | 40 | 60 | 40 | .52 | 33 | (.26)[d] |

| Outcome | | | | | | | | |
|---|---|---|---|---|---|---|---|---|
| Health Orientation | 36 | 22 | 84 | 21 | 38 | 21 | .70 | 33 | (.29) |
| Health Promoting Behavior | 66 | 42 | 83 | 38 | 74 | 38 | .82 | 59 | .58 |
| Health Seeking Behavior | 64 | 49 | 92 | 47 | 66 | 47 | .68 | 62 | .62 |
| Hope | 27 | 11 | 93 | 8 | 38 | 8 | .52 | 23 | (.27) |
| Hydration | 27 | 19 | 94 | 17 | 59 | 17 | .11 | 23 | (.20) |
| Immunization Behavior | 25 | 25 | 76 | 25 | 60 | 25 | .61 | 24 | (.26) |
| Impulse Control | 50 | 10 | 87 | 6 | 67 | 6 | .86 | 34 | (-.26) |
| Infection Status | 74 | 61 | 94 | 55 | 78 | 55 | .73 | 38 | .32 |
| Information Processing | 46 | 37 | 93 | 34 | 71 | 34 | .87 | 40 | .63 |
| Joint Movement: Active | 49 | 49 | 97 | 49 | 76 | 49 | .85 | 35 | .62 |
| Joint Movement: Passive | 64 | 56 | 99 | 72 | 89 | 72 | .97 | 57 | .51 |
| Knowledge: Breastfeeding | 35 | 3 | 88 | 2 | 50 | 2 | .00 | 31 | (.32) |
| Knowledge: Diet | 43 | 41 | 82 | 40 | 50 | 40 | .66 | 40 | .37 |
| Knowledge: Disease Process | 93 | 54 | 92 | 46 | 63 | 46 | .81 | 82 | .74 |
| Knowledge: Health Resources | 48 | 42 | 90 | 41 | 56 | 41 | .66 | 44 | .59 |
| Knowledge: Medication | 76 | 52 | 86 | 50 | 68 | 50 | .84 | 62 | .65 |
| Knowledge: Prescribed Activity | 25 | 24 | 90 | 22 | 73 | 22 | .68 | 25 | (.22) |
| Knowledge: Treatment Procedure(s) | 36 | 25 | 95 | 26 | 64 | 26 | .86 | 34 | .68 |
| Knowledge: Treatment Regimen | 44 | 36 | 90 | 35 | 46 | 35 | .65 | 41 | .54 |
| Leisure Participation | 39 | 33 | 86 | 32 | 52 | 32 | .58 | 33 | .52 |
| Mobility Level | 140 | 87 | 95 | 72 | 92 | 72 | .97 | 112 | -.28 |
| Mood Equilibrium | 64 | 35 | 90 | 25 | 88 | 25 | .51 | 45 | -.59 |
| Muscle Function | 50 | 13 | 92 | 12 | 67 | 12 | .16 | 52 | .63 |
| Neurological Status: Autonomic | 33 | 28 | 90 | 23 | 61 | 23 | .67 | 30 | (.23) |
| Nutritional Status | 74 | 45 | 88 | 37 | 65 | 37 | .80 | 64 | .64 |
| Nutritional Status: Biochemical Measures | 29 | 18 | 96 | 16 | 50 | 16 | .88 | 30 | (.14) |
| Nutritional Status: Body Mass | 26 | 14 | 97 | 14 | 57 | 14 | .35 | — | — |
| Nutritional Status: Energy | 25 | 13 | 91 | 13 | 69 | 13 | .45 | 26 | (-.33) |
| Nutritional Status: Food & Fluid Intake | 33 | 22 | 90 | 19 | 53 | 19 | .68 | 19 | (.42) |
| Nutritional Status: Nutrient Intake | 72 | 50 | 90 | 44 | 59 | 44 | .79 | 59 | .65 |
| Oral Health | 37 | 20 | 93 | 18 | 89 | 18 | .89 | 34 | -.71 |
| Pain Control | 121 | 86 | 87 | 66 | 61 | 66 | .37 | 71 | .31e |
| Pain Level | 166 | 130 | 92 | 82 | 70 | 82 | .78 | 129 | -.28f |
| Pain Level | | | | | | | | 37 | -.50g |
| Pain: Disruptive Effects | 67 | 52 | 89 | 43 | 70 | 43 | .82 | 57 | -.37 |
| Parent-Infant Attachment | 66 | 32 | 86 | 27 | 63 | 27 | .48 | 54 | (.22) |
| Participation: Health Care Decisions | 51 | 37 | 89 | 34 | 53 | 34 | .70 | 44 | (.04) |

*Continued*

| NOC Outcomes | Patient N | IRR* Near Agreement N | IRR* Near Agreement % | IRR Absolute Agreement N | IRR Absolute Agreement % | Intra-Class Correlation N | Intra-Class Correlation ICC | Validity N | Validity r |
|---|---|---|---|---|---|---|---|---|---|
| Psychosocial Adjustment: Life Change | 31 | 24 | 82 | 23 | 74 | 23 | .77 | 30 | .57 |
| Quality of Life | 61 | 49 | 89 | 42 | 64 | 42 | .80 | 56 | .65 |
| Respiratory Status: Gas Exchange | 71 | 60 | 86 | 42 | 81 | 42 | .81 | 48 | (.10) |
| Respiratory Status: Ventilation | 95 | 67 | 89 | 55 | 65 | 55 | .69 | 52 | .36 |
| Rest | 54 | 42 | 94 | 38 | 63 | 38 | .72 | 47 | -.44 |
| Risk Control | 47 | 45 | 88 | 45 | 78 | 45 | .85 | 47 | .39 |
| Risk Control: Alcohol Use | 28 | 18 | 87 | 18 | 72 | 18 | .88 | 23 | -.45 |
| Risk Control: Tobacco Use | 50 | 47 | 88 | 44 | 57 | 44 | .70 | 47 | (.009) |
| Risk Detection | 51 | 51 | 90 | 51 | 61 | 51 | .53 | 51 | (.16) |
| Role Performance | 26 | 18 | 86 | 16 | 50 | 16 | .52 | 20 | -.80 |
| Safety Behavior: Fall Prevention | 72 | 58 | 87 | 53 | 58 | 53 | .44 | 82 | (.07) |
| Safety Behavior: Home Physical Environment | 44 | 43 | 89 | 43 | 47 | 43 | .64 | 41 | .45 |
| Safety Behavior: Personal | 26 | 11 | 91 | 10 | 50 | 10 | .82 | 15 | .59 |
| Safety Status: Falls Occurrence | 40 | 17 | 100 | 16 | 94 | 16 | .78 | 39 | .58 |
| Safety Status: Physical Injury | 33 | 26 | 98 | 26 | 73 | 26 | .62 | 34 | (.09) |
| Self-Care: Activities of Daily Living (ADL) | 186 | 166 | 94 | 134 | 84 | 134 | .84 | 113 | -.58 |
| Self-Care: Bathing | 41 | 23 | 90 | 23 | 87 | 23 | .96 | 39 | .64 |
| Self-Care: Dressing | 41 | 14 | 92 | 14 | 100 | 14 | 1.00 | 40 | .66 |
| Self-Care: Hygiene | 33 | 27 | 93 | 25 | 88 | 25 | .95 | — | — |
| Self-Care: Instrumental Activities of Daily Living (IADL) | 32 | 32 | 86 | 32 | 78 | 32 | .94 | 32 | -.55 |
| Self-Care: Non-Parenteral Medication | 44 | 43 | 85 | 43 | 67 | 43 | .82 | 27 | .76 |
| Self-Care: Parenteral Medication | 28 | 28 | 84 | 28 | 75 | 28 | .90 | 22 | .80 |
| Self-Care: Toileting | 31 | 23 | 98 | 23 | 78 | 23 | .93 | 24 | -.77[h] |
| Self-Care: Toileting | | | | | | | | 28 | .76[i] |
| Sleep | 64 | 46 | 92 | 41 | 66 | 41 | .65 | 39 | -.51[j] |
| Sleep | | | | | | | | 15 | (.08)[k] |
| Social Interaction Skills | 27 | 18 | 88 | 17 | 65 | 17 | .74 | 24 | -.44 |
| Social Involvement | 41 | 33 | 87 | 33 | 52 | 33 | .68 | 16 | .61 |
| Social Support | 53 | 43 | 92 | 40 | 73 | 40 | .75 | 45 | .40 |
| Spiritual Well-Being | 42 | 30 | 91 | 30 | 57 | 30 | .52 | 41 | .50 |
| Suicide Self-Restraint | 71 | 21 | 89 | 10 | 80 | 10 | .92 | 55 | .35 |
| Symptom Control | 53 | 43 | 88 | 42 | 52 | 42 | .54 | 52 | -.30 |
| Symptom Severity | 51 | 42 | 86 | 41 | 59 | 41 | .50 | 49 | -.47 |

| Outcome | | | | | | | | | |
|---|---|---|---|---|---|---|---|---|---|
| Tissue Integrity: Skin & Mucous Membranes | 82 | 60 | 94 | 55 | 62 | 55 | .59 | 73 | .27 |
| Tissue Perfusion: Cardiac | 46 | 38 | 88 | 32 | 75 | 32 | .74 | 46 | (.09) |
| Tissue Perfusion: Peripheral | 81 | 49 | 91 | 45 | 69 | 45 | .67 | 68 | .45 |
| Tissue Perfusion: Pulmonary | 27 | 20 | 95 | 16 | 56 | 16 | .72 | 26 | (-.05) |
| Transfer Performance | 53 | 33 | 97 | 33 | 91 | 33 | .94 | 53 | .78 |
| Treatment Behavior: Illness or Injury | 43 | 42 | 90 | 42 | 57 | 42 | .64 | 28 | .68 |
| Urinary Continence | 47 | 43 | 89 | 41 | 53 | 41 | .48 | 43 | -.67[l] |
| Urinary Continence | | | | | | | | 36 | .56[m] |
| Urinary Elimination | 79 | 31 | 92 | 26 | 81 | 26 | .88 | 42 | (.28) |
| Vital Signs Status | 70 | 57 | 94 | 55 | 76 | 55 | .88 | 66 | .48 |
| Well-Being | 38 | 24 | 92 | 23 | 65 | 23 | .83 | 36 | .80 |
| Wound Healing; Primary Intention | 53 | 12 | 88 | 11 | 82 | 11 | .89 | 33 | (-.32) |
| Wound Healing; Secondary Intention | 40 | 36 | 86 | 35 | 79 | 35 | .89 | 39 | .45 |
| **Outcomes With an N of Less Than 25** | | | | | | | | | |
| Abuse Recovery: Emotional | 1 | 1 | 83 | 1 | 100 | 1 | — | — | — |
| Abuse Recovery: Physical | 1 | 1 | 55 | 1 | 100 | 1 | — | — | — |
| Abuse Recovery: Sexual | 1 | 1 | 65 | 1 | 100 | 1 | — | — | — |
| Blood Transfusion Reaction Control | 10 | 8 | 98 | 4 | 75 | 4 | .87 | 10 | (.16) |
| Body Image | 9 | 9 | 83 | 9 | 33 | 9 | .54 | 9 | (-.25) |
| Bone Healing | 12 | 10 | 96 | 9 | 78 | 9 | .87 | — | — |
| Bowel Continence | 16 | 12 | 92 | 12 | 50 | 12 | .83 | 16 | -.80 |
| Breastfeeding Maintenance | 6 | 6 | 91 | 6 | 100 | 6 | 1.00 | — | — |
| Caregiver Adaptation to Patient Institutionalization | 3 | 1 | 100 | 1 | 100 | 1 | — | 3 | 1.00[a] |
| Caregiver Emotional Health | 18 | 15 | 91 | 15 | 73 | 15 | .68 | 18 | (-.27) |
| Caregiver Home Care Readiness | 13 | 11 | 88 | 11 | 91 | 11 | .92 | 13 | (.08) |
| Caregiver Lifestyle Disruption | 16 | 10 | 90 | 10 | 40 | 10 | .57 | 16 | -.68 |
| Caregiver Performance: Indirect Care | 12 | 11 | 93 | 11 | 45 | 11 | .55 | 12 | -.65 |
| Caregiver Physical Health | 13 | — | — | 12 | 71 | 12 | .46 | 13 | (-.28) |
| Caregiver Stressors | 14 | — | 91 | 7 | 67 | 7 | .69 | 14 | -.77 |
| Caregiver Well-Being | 21 | 7 | 95 | 15 | 50 | 15 | .67 | 21 | (.06) |
| Caregiver-Patient Relationship | 20 | 15 | 92 | 14 | 75 | 14 | .41 | 20 | .49[a] |
| Caregiver-Patient Relationship | 20 | 14 | — | — | — | — | — | 20 | -.56[b] |
| Caregiving Endurance Potential | 6 | 4 | 87 | 4 | 56 | 4 | .87 | 6 | (.28) |
| Dignified Dying | 10 | 6 | 97 | 6 | 100 | 6 | 1.00 | 5 | (-.54) |
| Electrolyte & Acid/Base Balance | 19 | 20 | 88 | 18 | 78 | 18 | .71 | 19 | (.37) |
| Fear Control | 14 | 5 | 86 | 5 | 80 | 5 | .67 | 5 | (.16) |

*Continued*

| NOC Outcomes | Patient N | IRR* Near Agreement† N | % | IRR Absolute Agreement‡ N | % | Intra-Class Correlation N | ICC | Validity N | r |
|---|---|---|---|---|---|---|---|---|---|
| Grief Resolution | 15 | 8 | 80 | 8 | 75 | 8 | .85 | 10 | -.78 |
| Health Beliefs: Perceived Ability to Perform | 21 | 21 | 93 | 21 | 76 | 21 | .53 | 18 | (.32)c |
| Health Beliefs: Perceived Ability to Perform | | | | | | | | 20 | (.18)n |
| Health Beliefs: Perceived Control | 22 | 22 | 96 | 22 | 82 | 22 | .79 | 16 | .58c |
| Health Beliefs: Perceived Control | | | | | | | | 10 | -.76o |
| Health Beliefs: Perceived Resources | 21 | 21 | 82 | 21 | 76 | 21 | .72 | 14 | .82c |
| Health Beliefs: Perceived Resources | | | | | | | | 21 | -.56p |
| Identity | 1 | 1 | 93 | 1 | 100 | — | — | — | — |
| Immobility Consequences: Physiological | 20 | 19 | 92 | 18 | 61 | 18 | .77 | 10 | (.52) |
| Immobility Consequences: Psycho-Cognitive | 21 | 21 | 93 | 21 | 62 | 21 | .71 | 18 | .65 |
| Immune Hypersensitivity Control | 13 | 13 | 92 | 10 | 60 | 10 | .40 | 11 | (.23) |
| Immune Status | 24 | 12 | 90 | 11 | 36 | 11 | .49 | 15 | (.08) |
| Knowledge: Energy Conservation | 16 | 16 | 91 | 16 | 56 | 16 | .70 | 16 | .50 |
| Knowledge: Health Behaviors | 20 | 20 | 81 | 20 | 35 | 20 | .02 | 20 | (.34) |
| Knowledge: Infection Control | 14 | 14 | 88 | 13 | 69 | 13 | .70 | 9 | (.00) |
| Knowledge: Personal Safety | 9 | — | — | — | — | — | — | 8 | (.24) |
| Knowledge: Substance Use Control | 15 | 6 | 97 | 4 | 50 | 4 | .14 | 12 | .73 |
| Loneliness | 21 | 14 | 86 | 14 | 64 | 14 | .69 | 16 | (-.45) |
| Maternal Status: Postpartum | 10 | 15 | — | 10 | 60 | 10 | .23 | — | — |
| Memory | 22 | 18 | 90 | 16 | 75 | 16 | .89 | 14 | (-.63) |
| Neglect Recovery | 5 | 3 | 91 | 3 | 33 | 3 | .20 | — | — |
| Neurological Status | 12 | 8 | 91 | 5 | 100 | 5 | 1.00 | 9 | .94 |
| Neurological Status: Central Motor Control | 6 | 4 | 82 | 2 | 100 | 2 | 1.00 | 5 | .99 |
| Neurological Status: Consciousness | 17 | 10 | 95 | 10 | 40 | 10 | .88 | 13 | (.13) |
| Neurological Status: Cranial Sensory/Motor Function | 7 | 5 | 96 | 4 | 100 | 4 | 1.00 | 7 | (.42) |
| Neurological Status: Spinal Sensory/Motor Function | 7 | 5 | 84 | 4 | 75 | 4 | .73 | 6 | (.77) |
| Parenting | 15 | 9 | 91 | 9 | 67 | 9 | .61 | 11 | (.09) |
| Parenting: Social Safety | 3 | 3 | 93 | 3 | 67 | 3 | .75 | — | — |
| Physical Aging Status | 14 | 14 | 95 | 14 | 64 | 14 | .72 | — | — |
| Risk Control: Drug Use | 20 | 13 | 91 | 12 | 33 | 12 | .58 | 19 | (-.30) |
| Risk Control: Sexually Transmitted Diseases (STD) | 15 | 12 | 83 | 12 | 58 | 12 | .41 | — | — |
| Risk Control: Unintended Pregnancy | 3 | 3 | 92 | 3 | 100 | 3 | 1.00 | — | — |
| Self-Care: Eating | 18 | 11 | 94 | 11 | 73 | 11 | .82 | 18 | .59 |
| Self-Care: Grooming | 20 | 13 | 88 | 13 | 62 | 13 | .69 | 19 | .60 |

| | | | | | | | | | |
|---|---|---|---|---|---|---|---|---|---|
| Self-Care: Oral Hygiene | 20 | 13 | 84 | 13 | 62 | 13 | .83 | — | — |
| Self-Esteem | 19 | 11 | 88 | 9 | 78 | 9 | .77 | 18 | .88 |
| Self-Mutilation Restraint | 7 | — | — | — | — | — | — | 7 | (.30) |
| Substance Addiction Consequences | 16 | 10 | 87 | 7 | 43 | 7 | .53 | — | — |
| Thermoregulation | 14 | 14 | 89 | 10 | 60 | 10 | .87 | 14 | .75 |
| Tissue Perfusion: Abdominal Organs | 9 | 7 | 8 | 7 | 100 | 7 | 1.00 | 9 | .66 |
| Tissue Perfusion: Cerebral | 19 | 10 | 91 | 8 | 75 | 8 | .64 | 16 | .64 |
| Will to Live | 1 | — | — | — | — | — | — | — | — |

( ) not statistically significant (p≤ 0.05)

*IRR = Inter-rater reliability.

†Numerical ratings of 0-1 value difference on 5-point Likert scale for label and indicators.

‡Numerical ratings that are identical for both raters for outcome label.

Name of criterion tool for outcomes with more than one tool

a.  Picot's Caregiver Rewards Scale (2nd version)
b.  Sense of Competence Questionnaire (SCQ)
c.  Breast Self-Examination Health Belief Model Scale
d.  Osteoporosis Health Beliefs Scale
e.  Health Promoting Lifestyle Profile II
f.  Numeric Pain Intensity Scale
g.  Wong Baker Faces Rating Scale
h.  Katz Index of ADL

i.  Functional Independence Measure (FIM)
j.  Pittsburgh Sleep Quality Index (PSQI)
k.  Chart Review
l.  Incontinence Management Scale
m.  MDS Score Section F
n.  Perceived Health Competence Scale
o.  Multidimensional Health Locus of Control Scales: Form A
p.  Barriers Scale

774 Part Six   Appendixes

BASELINE, 2ND RATING AND AVERAGE DAYS BETWEEN RATINGS FOR 165 OUTCOMES

| NOC Outcomes | N | Avg Base Rating | Ave Follow Rating | Ave Change | Min Change | Max Change | SD | Count | Avg # Days Between | Min # Days Between | Max # Days Between | SD of Days Between |
|---|---|---|---|---|---|---|---|---|---|---|---|---|
| Abuse Recovery Emotional | 1 | 4.00 | 4.00 | 0.00 | 0 | 0 | | 1 | 32.00 | 32 | 32 | |
| Abuse Recovery: Physical | 1 | 4.00 | 4.00 | 0.00 | 0 | 0 | | 1 | 32.00 | 32 | 32 | |
| Abuse Recovery: Sexual | 1 | 4.00 | 4.00 | 0.00 | 0 | 0 | | 1 | 32.00 | 32 | 32 | |
| Abusive Behavior Self-Control | 5 | 2.00 | 3.60 | 1.60 | 1 | 3 | 0.89 | 5 | 4.00 | 1 | 8 | 3.67 |
| Acceptance: Health Status | 32 | 3.66 | 3.88 | 0.22 | -1 | 2 | 0.75 | 32 | 16.78 | 1 | 89 | 18.40 |
| Adherence Behavior | 20 | 2.50 | 3.20 | 0.70 | 0 | 4 | 0.92 | 20 | 39.45 | 1 | 171 | 59.12 |
| Aggression Control | 22 | 2.68 | 3.55 | 0.86 | -2 | 3 | 1.32 | 22 | 40.64 | 1 | 307 | 97.07 |
| Ambulation: Walking | 108 | 2.51 | 3.09 | 0.58 | -2 | 4 | 1.37 | 107 | 19.44 | 0 | 320 | 58.62 |
| Ambulation: Wheelchair | 10 | 3.90 | 3.70 | -0.20 | -1 | 1 | 0.63 | 10 | 44.30 | 1 | 301 | 91.43 |
| Anxiety Control | 20 | 2.20 | 2.95 | 0.75 | -1 | 3 | 0.91 | 20 | 32.95 | 1 | 313 | 90.65 |
| Balance | 19 | 3.53 | 3.53 | 0.00 | -1 | 1 | 0.47 | 19 | 7.89 | 2 | 21 | 5.98 |
| Blood Transfusion Reaction Control | 9 | 4.56 | 4.56 | 0.00 | -2 | 2 | 1.22 | 9 | 2.11 | 0 | 7 | 2.03 |
| Body Image | 3 | 3.67 | 3.00 | -0.67 | -2 | 0 | 1.15 | 3 | 46.00 | 8 | 67 | 32.97 |
| Body Positioning: Self-Initiated | 20 | 3.10 | 3.30 | 0.20 | -1 | 1 | 0.52 | 20 | 5.75 | 0 | 23 | 5.35 |
| Bone Healing | 2 | 2.00 | 2.50 | 0.50 | 0 | 1 | 0.71 | 2 | 2.00 | 2 | 2 | 0.00 |
| Bowel Continence | 9 | 3.22 | 3.00 | -0.22 | -1 | 0 | 0.44 | 9 | 5.44 | 2 | 14 | 4.13 |
| Bowel Elimination | 31 | 3.42 | 3.94 | 0.52 | -1 | 3 | 0.89 | 31 | 4.55 | 0 | 14 | 3.15 |
| Breastfeeding Establishment: Maternal | 55 | 3.22 | 4.07 | 0.85 | -1 | 3 | 0.83 | 55 | 1.36 | 0 | 4 | 0.82 |
| Breastfeeding Establishment: Infant | 46 | 3.07 | 3.78 | 0.72 | -1 | 3 | 0.91 | 46 | 1.13 | 0 | 3 | 0.72 |
| Breastfeeding Maintenance | 4 | 4.00 | 4.00 | 0.00 | -1 | 1 | 0.82 | 4 | 1.50 | 1 | 3 | 1.00 |
| Cardiac Pump Effectiveness | 43 | 3.35 | 3.93 | 0.58 | -1 | 4 | 0.96 | 43 | 34.07 | 0 | 344 | 94.21 |
| Caregiver Adaptation to Patient Institutionalization | 3 | 3.33 | 4.00 | 0.67 | 0 | 1 | 0.58 | 3 | 58.33 | 36 | 92 | 29.67 |
| Caregiver Emotional Health | 17 | 3.94 | 4.24 | 0.29 | 0 | 1 | 0.47 | 17 | 19.35 | 2 | 89 | 23.19 |
| Caregiver Home Care Readiness | 13 | 4.08 | 4.23 | 0.15 | -1 | 1 | 0.55 | 13 | 6.23 | 0 | 27 | 6.81 |
| Caregiver Lifestyle Disruption | 16 | 3.50 | 3.50 | 0.00 | -1 | 1 | 0.52 | 16 | 23.63 | 2 | 92 | 29.05 |
| Caregiver Performance: Direct Care | 23 | 3.91 | 4.13 | 0.22 | -1 | 1 | 0.52 | 23 | 9.35 | 1 | 47 | 10.70 |
| Caregiver Performance: Indirect Care | 11 | 3.55 | 4.00 | 0.45 | 0 | 1 | 0.52 | 11 | 15.91 | 2 | 47 | 13.12 |

| Outcome | | | | | | | | | | | | |
|---|---|---|---|---|---|---|---|---|---|---|---|---|
| Caregiver Physical Health | 12 | 4.33 | 4.67 | 0.33 | -1 | 1 | 0.65 | 12 | 11.75 | 3 | 47 | 13.08 |
| Caregiver Stressors | 13 | 3.15 | 3.38 | 0.23 | -1 | 1 | 0.60 | 13 | 26.46 | 1 | 116 | 37.84 |
| Caregiver Well-Being | 20 | 3.80 | 4.00 | 0.20 | -1 | 1 | 0.52 | 20 | 27.50 | 1 | 116 | 34.33 |
| Caregiver-Patient Relationship | 18 | 3.94 | 4.33 | 0.39 | -1 | 2 | 0.70 | 18 | 29.39 | 1 | 116 | 35.56 |
| Caregiving Endurance Potential | 6 | 3.33 | 3.33 | 0.00 | 0 | 0 | 0.00 | 6 | 16.17 | 4 | 47 | 17.36 |
| Circulation Status | 36 | 3.83 | 4.11 | 0.28 | -1 | 2 | 0.81 | 36 | 18.14 | 0 | 320 | 55.26 |
| Cognitive Ability | 25 | 2.84 | 3.28 | 0.44 | -1 | 3 | 1.00 | 25 | 92.20 | 0 | 331 | 140.02 |
| Cognitive Orientation | 36 | 3.72 | 3.75 | 0.03 | -3 | 2 | 1.00 | 36 | 118.75 | 1 | 383 | 147.88 |
| Comfort Level | 137 | 2.64 | 3.48 | 0.85 | -1 | 3 | 0.87 | 137 | 7.63 | 0 | 80 | 9.09 |
| Communication Ability | 30 | 3.20 | 4.13 | 0.93 | -1 | 4 | 1.41 | 30 | 15.37 | 1 | 171 | 36.07 |
| Communication: Expressive Ability | 12 | 3.00 | 3.00 | 0.00 | -1 | 1 | 0.43 | 12 | 78.58 | 4 | 330 | 132.27 |
| Communication: Receptive Ability | 8 | 3.38 | 3.13 | -0.25 | -2 | 1 | 1.04 | 7 | 97.86 | 2 | 364 | 157.15 |
| Compliance Behavior | 25 | 3.20 | 3.52 | 0.32 | -1 | 2 | 0.75 | 25 | 31.24 | 1 | 171 | 41.07 |
| Concentration | 16 | 3.81 | 4.00 | 0.19 | -1 | 1 | 0.54 | 16 | 46.31 | 4 | 172 | 59.09 |
| Coping | 41 | 2.80 | 3.22 | 0.41 | -1 | 2 | 0.87 | 41 | 28.59 | 0 | 316 | 66.37 |
| Decision Making | 28 | 3.29 | 3.46 | 0.18 | -1 | 2 | 0.72 | 28 | 19.07 | 0 | 114 | 26.07 |
| Distorted Thought Control | 33 | 2.27 | 3.58 | 1.30 | -3 | 4 | 1.33 | 33 | 32.27 | 0 | 322 | 80.38 |
| Electrolyte & Acid/Base Balance | 18 | 3.67 | 4.33 | 0.67 | -1 | 2 | 0.84 | 18 | 2.39 | 0 | 18 | 4.13 |
| Endurance | 50 | 2.98 | 3.72 | 0.74 | -2 | 3 | 0.96 | 49 | 16.71 | 0 | 288 | 47.56 |
| Energy Conservation | 58 | 3.14 | 3.62 | 0.48 | -2 | 2 | 0.71 | 58 | 11.07 | 1 | 118 | 23.09 |
| Fear Control | 3 | 2.33 | 3.33 | 1.00 | 0 | 2 | 1.00 | 3 | 4.00 | 1 | 9 | 4.36 |
| Fluid Balance | 21 | 3.62 | 4.00 | 0.38 | -2 | 3 | 0.92 | 21 | 14.52 | 0 | 267 | 57.88 |
| Grief Resolution | 6 | 4.00 | 3.83 | -0.17 | -2 | 1 | 1.17 | 6 | 18.33 | 0 | 42 | 15.49 |
| Health Beliefs | 16 | 3.50 | 4.00 | 0.50 | 0 | 2 | 0.63 | 16 | 85.81 | 15 | 270 | 78.01 |
| Health Beliefs: Perceived Ability to Perform | 5 | 3.80 | 3.40 | -0.40 | -1 | 0 | 0.55 | 5 | 88.20 | 63 | 114 | 18.29 |
| Health Beliefs: Perceived Control | 5 | 3.60 | 4.20 | 0.60 | 0 | 1 | 0.55 | 5 | 67.80 | 36 | 114 | 30.95 |
| Health Beliefs: Perceived Resources | 8 | 3.13 | 3.00 | -0.13 | -1 | 0 | 0.35 | 7 | 44.29 | 5 | 90 | 32.99 |
| Health Beliefs: Perceived Threat | 17 | 3.47 | 3.41 | -0.06 | -1 | 1 | 0.75 | 17 | 17.18 | 1 | 195 | 46.14 |
| Health Orientation | 24 | 3.58 | 3.79 | 0.21 | -2 | 2 | 0.93 | 24 | 58.38 | 0 | 207 | 52.59 |
| Health Promoting Behavior | 48 | 3.08 | 3.56 | 0.48 | -1 | 3 | 0.90 | 47 | 24.83 | 0 | 195 | 40.82 |
| Health Seeking Behavior | 37 | 3.27 | 3.86 | 0.59 | -1 | 2 | 0.69 | 37 | 36.54 | 1 | 206 | 43.90 |

*Continued*

**BASELINE, 2ND RATING AND AVERAGE DAYS BETWEEN RATINGS FOR 165 OUTCOMES**

| NOC Outcomes | N | Avg Base Rating | Ave Follow Rating | Ave Change | Min Change | Max Change | SD | Count | Avg # Days Between | Min # Days Between | Max # Days Between | SD of Days Between |
|---|---|---|---|---|---|---|---|---|---|---|---|---|
| Hope | 18 | 2.44 | 3.33 | 0.89 | −1 | 3 | 1.23 | 18 | 27.00 | 1 | 289 | 66.23 |
| Hydration | 20 | 4.00 | 4.55 | 0.55 | −1 | 2 | 0.76 | 20 | 19.60 | 0 | 327 | 72.42 |
| Immobility Consequences: Physiological | 14 | 3.36 | 3.57 | 0.21 | −1 | 1 | 0.58 | 14 | 5.36 | 1 | 18 | 5.11 |
| Immobility Consequences: Psycho-Cognitive | 18 | 3.22 | 3.44 | 0.22 | −1 | 1 | 0.65 | 18 | 5.83 | 0 | 27 | 6.84 |
| Immune Hypersensitivity Control | 11 | 3.27 | 3.91 | 0.64 | 0 | 2 | 0.67 | 11 | 6.36 | 2 | 18 | 6.12 |
| Immune Status | 12 | 3.75 | 4.17 | 0.42 | −1 | 3 | 1.00 | 12 | 3.83 | 0 | 14 | 4.24 |
| Immunization Behavior | 14 | 3.64 | 3.79 | 0.14 | −1 | 2 | 0.86 | 14 | 73.86 | 1 | 230 | 69.49 |
| Impulse Control | 32 | 1.94 | 3.41 | 1.47 | −1 | 3 | 1.08 | 32 | 12.19 | 0 | 293 | 51.31 |
| Infection Status | 50 | 4.08 | 4.28 | 0.20 | −1 | 3 | 0.93 | 50 | 9.82 | 0 | 216 | 30.80 |
| Information Processing | 34 | 3.59 | 3.88 | 0.29 | −1 | 3 | 0.97 | 34 | 43.82 | 0 | 327 | 88.10 |
| Joint Movement: Active | 36 | 3.58 | 3.56 | −0.03 | −1 | 2 | 0.51 | 36 | 13.36 | 0 | 206 | 33.86 |
| Joint Movement: Passive | 42 | 2.12 | 2.81 | 0.69 | −2 | 2 | 0.90 | 42 | 12.10 | 1 | 367 | 56.16 |
| Knowledge: Breastfeeding | 35 | 2.80 | 3.63 | 0.83 | 0 | 2 | 0.79 | 35 | 2.80 | 0 | 62 | 10.32 |
| Knowledge: Diet | 30 | 3.37 | 3.50 | 0.13 | −1 | 2 | 0.86 | 30 | 26.37 | 1 | 294 | 56.45 |
| Knowledge: Disease Process | 69 | 3.06 | 3.23 | 0.17 | −1 | 3 | 0.75 | 69 | 8.54 | 0 | 104 | 19.75 |
| Knowledge: Energy Conservation | 11 | 4.09 | 4.00 | −0.09 | −1 | 1 | 0.70 | 11 | 6.55 | 2 | 13 | 3.42 |
| Knowledge: Health Behaviors | 9 | 3.56 | 3.78 | 0.22 | 0 | 1 | 0.44 | 9 | 61.33 | 7 | 118 | 41.05 |
| Knowledge: Health Resources | 32 | 3.41 | 3.50 | 0.09 | −1 | 1 | 0.69 | 32 | 11.91 | 0 | 86 | 19.75 |
| Knowledge: Infection Control | 13 | 3.62 | 4.00 | 0.38 | 0 | 1 | 0.51 | 13 | 6.38 | 1 | 21 | 6.50 |
| Knowledge: Medication | 43 | 2.81 | 3.42 | 0.60 | −1 | 3 | 1.05 | 43 | 22.86 | 0 | 189 | 49.62 |
| Knowledge: Personal Safety | 9 | 1.89 | 3.67 | 1.78 | 1 | 3 | 0.83 | 9 | 4.56 | 0 | 13 | 3.71 |
| Knowledge: Prescribed Activity | 22 | 3.45 | 3.77 | 0.32 | −1 | 3 | 0.84 | 22 | 5.73 | 0 | 16 | 4.79 |
| Knowledge: Substance Use Control | 12 | 2.00 | 2.58 | 0.58 | −1 | 2 | 0.90 | 12 | 2.75 | 1 | 6 | 1.71 |
| Knowledge: Treatment Procedure(s) | 31 | 3.23 | 3.29 | 0.06 | −1 | 1 | 0.36 | 31 | 4.74 | 0 | 28 | 6.49 |
| Knowledge: Treatment Regimen | 32 | 3.41 | 3.47 | 0.06 | −1 | 1 | 0.56 | 32 | 12.81 | 0 | 161 | 29.21 |
| Leisure Participation | 16 | 4.00 | 4.00 | 0.00 | −2 | 2 | 1.03 | 15 | 156.60 | 2 | 344 | 139.65 |
| Loneliness | 9 | 4.67 | 4.33 | −0.33 | −1 | 1 | 0.71 | 9 | 27.11 | 5 | 53 | 12.54 |

| Outcome | | | | | | | | | | | | |
|---|---|---|---|---|---|---|---|---|---|---|---|---|
| Maternal Status: Postpartum | 10 | 3.50 | 4.50 | 1.00 | 0 | 3 | 1.15 | 10 | 2.20 | 2 | 4 | 0.63 |
| Memory | 18 | 3.61 | 3.44 | -0.17 | -2 | 2 | 0.86 | 18 | 94.06 | 1 | 344 | 135.99 |
| Mobility Level | 78 | 2.64 | 3.63 | 0.99 | -2 | 4 | 1.21 | 78 | 27.49 | 0 | 336 | 73.57 |
| Mood Equilibrium | 34 | 2.94 | 3.79 | 0.85 | -1 | 3 | 1.08 | 34 | 81.91 | 0 | 350 | 140.63 |
| Muscle Function | 22 | 4.09 | 3.36 | -0.73 | -3 | 1 | 1.03 | 22 | 282.91 | 36 | 332 | 56.38 |
| Neurological Status | 9 | 3.33 | 4.00 | 0.67 | 0 | 1 | 0.50 | 9 | 2.78 | 1 | 7 | 2.33 |
| Neurological Status: Central Motor Control | 5 | 4.40 | 4.20 | -0.20 | -1 | 0 | 0.45 | 5 | 1.80 | 1 | 3 | 0.84 |
| Neurological Status: Consciousness | 6 | 1.50 | 4.83 | 3.33 | 2 | 4 | 1.03 | 6 | 1.83 | 0 | 6 | 2.14 |
| Neurological Status: Cranial Sensory/Motor Function | 3 | 4.67 | 4.33 | -0.33 | -1 | 0 | 0.58 | 3 | 5.67 | 2 | 8 | 3.21 |
| Neurological Status: Spinal Sensory/Motor Function | 6 | 3.17 | 3.67 | 0.50 | 0 | 1 | 0.55 | 6 | 2.17 | 0 | 5 | 1.72 |
| Neurological Status: Autonomic | 26 | 3.73 | 4.23 | 0.50 | -1 | 3 | 0.95 | 26 | 3.31 | 0 | 20 | 4.23 |
| Nutritional Status | 31 | 3.32 | 3.55 | 0.23 | -1 | 2 | 0.62 | 31 | 31.90 | 0 | 342 | 71.73 |
| Nutritional Status: Biochemical Measures | 10 | 3.60 | 3.50 | -0.10 | -1 | 1 | 0.57 | 10 | 84.00 | 2 | 331 | 129.84 |
| Nutritional Status: Body Mass | 6 | 1.83 | 2.50 | 0.67 | 0 | 2 | 1.03 | 6 | 75.17 | 7 | 171 | 67.92 |
| Nutritional Status: Energy | 7 | 3.71 | 3.71 | 0.00 | -1 | 1 | 0.58 | 7 | 57.00 | 13 | 137 | 47.02 |
| Nutritional Status: Food & Fluid Intake | 28 | 2.64 | 3.54 | 0.89 | -2 | 4 | 1.45 | 27 | 109.41 | 0 | 385 | 155.38 |
| Nutritional Status: Nutrient Intake | 41 | 2.59 | 3.39 | 0.80 | -1 | 3 | 1.25 | 41 | 8.61 | 1 | 104 | 17.24 |
| Oral Health | 12 | 3.08 | 3.50 | 0.42 | -1 | 2 | 0.90 | 12 | 53.92 | 1 | 172 | 58.77 |
| Pain Control | 103 | 3.67 | 4.16 | 0.49 | -2 | 3 | 0.87 | 103 | 9.25 | 0 | 368 | 41.03 |
| Pain Level | 143 | 3.15 | 3.61 | 0.45 | -3 | 4 | 1.09 | 142 | 17.75 | -116 | 300 | 51.60 |
| Pain: Disruptive Effects | 48 | 3.29 | 3.65 | 0.35 | -1 | 3 | 0.81 | 48 | 11.92 | 0 | 149 | 30.02 |
| Parent-Infant Attachment | 36 | 3.92 | 4.14 | 0.22 | -2 | 2 | 0.87 | 36 | 1.86 | 0 | 7 | 1.53 |
| Parenting | 12 | 3.67 | 3.92 | 0.25 | -1 | 1 | 0.75 | 12 | 3.83 | 1 | 32 | 8.88 |
| Participation: Health Care Decisions | 33 | 2.97 | 3.61 | 0.64 | -1 | 4 | 1.19 | 33 | 18.24 | 0 | 189 | 43.82 |
| Physical Aging Status | 8 | 4.25 | 4.63 | 0.38 | 0 | 1 | 0.52 | 8 | 15.75 | 3 | 80 | 26.14 |
| Psychosocial Adjustment: Life Change | 15 | 3.27 | 4.07 | 0.80 | -1 | 3 | 1.08 | 15 | 52.13 | 3 | 320 | 82.73 |
| Quality of Life | 50 | 3.16 | 3.58 | 0.42 | -1 | 2 | 0.78 | 50 | 20.48 | 0 | 270 | 45.41 |
| Respiratory Status: Gas Exchange | 43 | 2.95 | 4.05 | 1.09 | -1 | 3 | 0.92 | 43 | 3.79 | 1 | 15 | 2.73 |

*Continued*

**BASELINE, 2ND RATING AND AVERAGE DAYS BETWEEN RATINGS FOR 165 OUTCOMES**

| NOC Outcomes | N | Avg Base Rating | Ave Follow Rating | Ave Change | Min Change | Max Change | SD | Count | Avg # Days Between | Min # Days Between | Max # Days Between | SD of Days Between |
|---|---|---|---|---|---|---|---|---|---|---|---|---|
| Respiratory Status: Ventilation | 49 | 3.31 | 4.12 | 0.82 | −1 | 3 | 0.91 | 49 | 11.53 | 0 | 101 | 24.70 |
| Rest | 35 | 3.20 | 3.66 | 0.46 | −1 | 2 | 0.78 | 35 | 10.46 | 0 | 137 | 25.76 |
| Risk Control | 23 | 3.39 | 3.52 | 0.13 | −1 | 2 | 0.76 | 23 | 48.78 | 0 | 207 | 50.25 |
| Risk Control: Alcohol Use | 14 | 1.86 | 2.79 | 0.93 | 0 | 2 | 0.83 | 14 | 16.43 | 1 | 100 | 29.89 |
| Risk Control: Drug Use | 11 | 1.82 | 2.73 | 0.91 | 0 | 2 | 0.70 | 11 | 32.91 | 1 | 230 | 73.51 |
| Risk Control: Sexually Transmitted Diseases (STD) | 6 | 3.00 | 3.17 | 0.17 | 0 | 1 | 0.41 | 6 | 15.33 | 1 | 56 | 20.84 |
| Risk Control: Tobacco Use | 18 | 2.50 | 2.67 | 0.17 | −1 | 2 | 0.71 | 18 | 55.61 | 1 | 195 | 66.95 |
| Risk Control: Unintended Pregnancy | 2 | 4.00 | 3.50 | −0.50 | −1 | 0 | 0.71 | 2 | 48.00 | 13 | 83 | 49.50 |
| Risk Detection | 12 | 3.75 | 3.83 | 0.08 | −1 | 1 | 0.67 | 12 | 101.92 | 6 | 230 | 75.36 |
| Role Performance | 11 | 2.27 | 3.27 | 1.00 | 0 | 2 | 0.89 | 11 | 29.91 | 1 | 207 | 60.90 |
| Safety Behavior: Home Physical Environment | 34 | 3.68 | 3.68 | 0.00 | −1 | 2 | 0.55 | 34 | 8.82 | 1 | 56 | 10.98 |
| Safety Behavior: Personal | 15 | 3.07 | 3.47 | 0.40 | −2 | 3 | 1.24 | 15 | 3.73 | 1 | 9 | 2.55 |
| Safety Behavior: Fall Prevention | 57 | 3.96 | 4.25 | 0.28 | −3 | 3 | 0.90 | 57 | 82.44 | 1 | 344 | 129.67 |
| Safety Status: Falls Occurrence | 19 | 4.16 | 4.47 | 0.32 | 0 | 1 | 0.48 | 19 | 4.74 | 0 | 21 | 4.85 |
| Safety Status: Physical Injury | 14 | 3.79 | 4.00 | 0.21 | 0 | 1 | 0.43 | 14 | 12.21 | 0 | 118 | 30.64 |
| Self-Care: Activities of Daily Living (ADL) | 134 | 3.28 | 3.54 | 0.26 | −2 | 4 | 1.16 | 133 | 89.21 | 0 | 346 | 133.91 |
| Self-Care: Bathing | 21 | 2.81 | 2.90 | 0.10 | −2 | 2 | 0.77 | 21 | 7.00 | 1 | 15 | 4.55 |
| Self-Care: Dressing | 11 | 3.09 | 3.18 | 0.09 | −1 | 1 | 0.54 | 11 | 6.27 | 2 | 14 | 3.80 |
| Self-Care: Eating | 8 | 3.25 | 3.63 | 0.38 | 0 | 2 | 0.74 | 8 | 4.50 | 2 | 12 | 3.55 |
| Self-Care: Grooming | 10 | 3.30 | 3.70 | 0.40 | 0 | 1 | 0.52 | 10 | 6.90 | 2 | 14 | 4.51 |
| Self-Care: Hygiene | 17 | 3.47 | 3.65 | 0.18 | −1 | 2 | 0.73 | 17 | 32.71 | 0 | 342 | 86.27 |
| Self-Care: Instrumental Activities of Daily Living (IADL) | 23 | 3.09 | 3.09 | 0.00 | −1 | 1 | 0.43 | 23 | 27.57 | 1 | 342 | 71.13 |
| Self-Care: Non-Parenteral Medication | 35 | 3.31 | 3.60 | 0.29 | −2 | 4 | 1.15 | 35 | 18.69 | 0 | 294 | 52.64 |
| Self-Care: Oral Hygiene | 10 | 3.80 | 3.60 | −0.20 | −2 | 1 | 1.03 | 10 | 7.40 | 1 | 28 | 8.19 |

| Outcome | | | | | | | | | | | | |
|---|---|---|---|---|---|---|---|---|---|---|---|---|
| Self-Care: Parenteral Medication | 16 | 3.50 | 4.00 | 0.50 | 0 | 2 | 0.82 | 16 | 6.44 | 0 | 28 | 7.45 |
| Self-Care: Toileting | 20 | 3.45 | 3.40 | -0.05 | -2 | 1 | 0.51 | 20 | 5.50 | 0 | 21 | 5.24 |
| Self-Esteem | 11 | 2.27 | 3.27 | 1.00 | 0 | 2 | 0.77 | 10 | 13.80 | 1 | 61 | 19.72 |
| Self-Mutilation Restraint | 7 | 2.14 | 4.14 | 2.00 | 1 | 4 | 1.15 | 7 | 2.43 | 1 | 5 | 1.62 |
| Sleep | 46 | 3.11 | 3.57 | 0.46 | -1 | 3 | 0.81 | 46 | 13.02 | 0 | 91 | 24.29 |
| Social Interaction Skills | 14 | 2.57 | 3.36 | 0.79 | 0 | 2 | 0.80 | 14 | 44.57 | 1 | 146 | 51.15 |
| Social Involvement | 30 | 3.20 | 3.20 | 0.00 | -1 | 2 | 0.69 | 30 | 30.17 | 0 | 230 | 48.92 |
| Social Support | 29 | 3.59 | 3.97 | 0.38 | -1 | 3 | 0.86 | 29 | 17.66 | 0 | 171 | 33.90 |
| Spiritual Well-Being | 26 | 4.35 | 4.50 | 0.15 | 0 | 1 | 0.37 | 26 | 39.12 | 3 | 134 | 33.17 |
| Substance Addiction Consequences | 11 | 2.73 | 3.55 | 0.82 | -1 | 3 | 1.25 | 11 | 25.27 | 1 | 230 | 68.01 |
| Suicide Self-Restraint | 42 | 2.40 | 3.86 | 1.45 | 0 | 4 | 1.02 | 42 | 2.40 | 0 | 11 | 2.27 |
| Symptom Control | 21 | 2.62 | 3.43 | 0.81 | -1 | 3 | 0.98 | 21 | 26.86 | 1 | 294 | 65.32 |
| Symptom Severity | 30 | 3.13 | 3.30 | 0.17 | -2 | 1 | 0.87 | 30 | 32.27 | 0 | 216 | 52.53 |
| Thermoregulation | 13 | 3.23 | 4.85 | 1.62 | 0 | 3 | 0.96 | 13 | 2.15 | 0 | 6 | 1.86 |
| Tissue Integrity: Skin & Mucous Membranes | 58 | 3.66 | 4.07 | 0.41 | -1 | 3 | 0.82 | 58 | 17.17 | 0 | 331 | 61.31 |
| Tissue Perfusion: Abdominal Organs | 9 | 3.89 | 4.11 | 0.22 | 0 | 1 | 0.44 | 9 | 1.67 | 1 | 4 | 1.12 |
| Tissue Perfusion: Cardiac | 43 | 3.84 | 4.56 | 0.72 | -1 | 4 | 0.96 | 43 | 1.77 | 0 | 14 | 2.24 |
| Tissue Perfusion: Cerebral | 9 | 4.56 | 4.67 | 0.11 | -1 | 1 | 0.60 | 9 | 6.00 | 1 | 20 | 5.87 |
| Tissue Perfusion: Peripheral | 48 | 3.92 | 4.42 | 0.50 | -1 | 2 | 0.74 | 48 | 3.29 | 0 | 12 | 2.64 |
| Tissue Perfusion: Pulmonary | 26 | 3.65 | 4.12 | 0.46 | -2 | 2 | 1.14 | 26 | 1.92 | 0 | 10 | 2.21 |
| Transfer Performance | 32 | 3.50 | 3.50 | 0.00 | -3 | 1 | 0.80 | 32 | 6.53 | 0 | 27 | 7.11 |
| Treatment Behavior: Illness or Injury | 21 | 3.48 | 3.62 | 0.14 | -1 | 2 | 0.73 | 21 | 35.43 | 1 | 129 | 37.19 |
| Urinary Continence | 37 | 3.43 | 3.41 | -0.03 | -2 | 2 | 0.87 | 36 | 143.08 | 1 | 378 | 156.87 |
| Urinary Elimination | 32 | 3.50 | 4.16 | 0.66 | -3 | 3 | 1.15 | 32 | 14.59 | 0 | 344 | 60.17 |
| Vital Signs Status | 52 | 3.98 | 4.42 | 0.44 | -1 | 3 | 0.92 | 52 | 14.10 | 0 | 216 | 36.30 |
| Well-Being | 31 | 3.35 | 3.81 | 0.45 | -1 | 4 | 1.34 | 31 | 38.13 | 0 | 316 | 62.62 |
| Wound Healing: Primary Intention | 12 | 3.08 | 4.17 | 1.08 | -1 | 4 | 1.24 | 12 | 3.17 | 1 | 15 | 3.90 |
| Wound Healing: Secondary Intention | 27 | 2.63 | 3.22 | 0.59 | 0 | 3 | 0.75 | 27 | 7.26 | 0 | 71 | 13.27 |

# Implementation Examples in Practice Settings

Four examples of how Nursing Outcomes Classification (NOC) is being implemented in practice settings are presented in this appendix. The first example describes the implementation of NOC in a 200-bed community hospital. The author addresses issues related to orientation and use of NOC in a commercial software application. The second example speaks to the implementation of NOC in a regional three-hospital system. The author describes some of the techniques used in orienting staff across three institutions and shares illustrations of the computerized care plans being used in these facilities. The third example describes the application of NOC for pediatric nurse specialists in a tertiary care center. The author outlines the planning that took place to implement the use of the paper form that is being piloted for use in an electronic record. The last application is in a parish nursing organization. The reader will note how the client is continually included in the application process. Examples of forms used in the organization and the rationale for their use are provided. Each of these examples provides valuable insights into problems and issues that arise with the implementation of NOC or any other standardized language in paper or electronic medical records.

# Implementation of NOC at Good Samaritan Hospital
## *Rosalind R. Willis, RN, C*

In 1999, because of Y2K, Good Samaritan Hospital administration purchased a number of Medical Information Technology, Inc. (Meditech, Westwood, MA) applications, including Patient Care Services (PCS), for bedside documentation. Good Samaritan Hospital is a 200-bed nonprofit community hospital in the city of Puyallup, Washington, that offers a full range of medical, surgical, obstetrical, and pediatric services including diagnostic cardiac catheterizations. The hospital has an average daily census of 150.

As part of our preparation for online documentation, the PCS assessments had to be customized. After reviewing the outcomes offered by Meditech, our 12-member core team decided that "met or not met" did not adequately reflect the real outcomes of our patients. The core team discussed the options and decided to use NOC outcomes for nursing documentation. As part of the core team's preparation for these changes, we asked Cindy A. Scherb, MS, RN, to come to Good Samaritan Hospital to educate us about Nursing Interventions Classification (NIC) and NOC.

Outcome documentation was a new concept for most of our nurses. A few of our plans of care included goal documentation, but they were nursing goals, not patient outcomes, and were documented as "met/not met." To reduce the learning curve for online documentation, we chose to implement paper care plans in which the NIC and NOC terminology was used before going to online documentation.

Our total education/implementation process took approximately 6 months. We used flyers attached to paychecks, posters, and our hospital newsletter to inform staff of the changes we were making to the plans of care and of upcoming classes. We kept our education department, as well as our nursing quality management department, informed of what we were doing.

The education began with a 1-hour class on NIC and NOC. We discussed the importance of standardized language and the difference between outcomes and goals. We explained the importance of outcomes as a means to evaluate our health care delivery system and as a means of providing cost-effective care with maximum benefit to the patient.

Classes were provided for all nursing units. We had two instructors per class with a class size of 8 to 12 students. We trained "super users" from each unit to field questions when we were not available. We made rounds daily to review the plans of care, answer questions, correct mistakes, and obtain feedback from the staff. For the first month, the plans of care were pilot only and were not being filed with the charts. Revisions were made based on the feedback we received from the staff.

Before we observed consistent, accurate scoring we had to help staff understand that we were scoring patient outcomes, not patient problems or nursing goals. We included the definition of the outcome to clarify the meaning on which the NOC score should be based. We also added a reminder to score the outcome definition.

Another question arose regarding discharge outcome documentation. If the patient did not reach the outcome goal that had been set on admission, how would we document the reason? The core team decided to include a means to document exceptions by using check boxes. If none of the exceptions apply, then staff members are expected to document the exception in the nursing progress notes.

The Likert scale was also problematic. Many of our staff members were used to rating scales that had 1 as most desirable and 5 as least desirable. Using test scores as an example helped: a 1 could be equated with an F, and a 5, with an A. To help us, our education department changed its evaluation forms to the Likert format. And of course, there were the questions of reliability of the scoring, since the scales have not been concretely defined.

Our intention was to implement at least one paper plan of care in the NIC/NOC language in every unit. We have actually only implemented two paper plans of care, a general surgical

*Text continued on p. 785*

# INITIATE APPROPRIATE PROBLEMS

## Surgical Plan of Care

| Date | Initials | Nursing Diagnosis | Patient Outcomes (For specific indicators see NOC.) | **NOTIFY PHYSICIAN IF ANY CHANGES IN PATIENT CONDITION** — Activities listed under NIC interventions are clinical guidelines only and do not replace nursing clinical judgement. For other activities see NIC.* | Start date | Stop Date |
|---|---|---|---|---|---|---|
| | | Pain | 1=Severe ⊗  2=Substantial  3=Moderate ☺  4=Slight  5=None ☺<br><br>**Pain Level 2102**<br>**Score Outcome Definition:** Amount of reported or demonstrated pain<br><br>ON INITIATION  1 2 3 4 5<br><br>PATIENT GOAL  1 2 3 4 5<br><br>AT RESOLUTION/ DISCHARGE  1 2 3 4 5<br><br>If Discharge Outcome at 3 or less, select all that apply.<br>☐ Chronic condition<br>☐ DC with services<br>☐ Compliance issues<br>☐ Transfer to other hosp<br>☐ Transfer to ECF<br>☐ AMA<br>☐ Expired<br>☐ Learning Barrier<br>☐ Physical Limitations<br>☐ Pt/Family Discussions<br>☐ If none apply make a note | **Pain Management: Pain Assessment**<br>1. Instruct pt to rate pain using 1 to 10 scale and determine realistic pain goals.<br>2. Assess pain level and document pain location, type, and intensity q 2-4h and PRN or per protocol<br>3. Intervene at onset of pain providing appropriate analgesic care<br>4. Assess VS prior to and after administration of medication<br>5. Monitor effectiveness of medication 20–60 min after administration or per protocol<br>6. Select and implement a variety of measures to facilitate pain relief, as appropriate<br><br>**Analgesic Administration-Intraspinal**<br>1. Check patency/function of catheter, port, or pump.<br>2. Monitor and record VS per protocol.<br>3. Monitor for adverse reactions: resp depression, urinary retention, undue somnolence, itching, seizures, nausea, and vomiting<br>4. Remove catheter according to agency protocol<br><br>**Medication Management: SAM Kit**<br>1. Determine patient's ability to self medicate<br>2. Teach pt and/or family expected action, side effects, administration method, interactions, as appropriate<br>3. Monitor for effectiveness, side effects, toxicity<br><br>**Patient-Controlled Analgesia (PCA) Assistance**<br>1. Teach pt and family how to use the PCA device<br>2. Teach patient/family the action and side effects of pain-relieving agents<br>3. Monitor and document effectiveness, side effects of medication<br>*Document care where you currently document i.e. flowsheet | | |
| | | Impaired Skin Integrity | **Wound Healing: Primary Intention 1102**<br>**Score Outcome Definition:** The extent to which cells and tissues have regenerated following intentional closure<br><br>1=None  2=Slight ⊗  3=Moderate ☺  4=Substantial  5=Complete ☺<br><br>ON INITIATION  1 2 3 4 5<br><br>PATIENT GOAL  1 2 3 4 5<br><br>AT RESOLUTION/ DISCHARGE  1 2 3 4 5<br><br>If Discharge Outcome at 3 or less, select all that apply.<br>☐ Chronic condition<br>☐ DC with services<br>☐ Compliance issues<br>☐ Transfer to other hosp<br>☐ Transfer to ECF<br>☐ AMA<br>☐ Expired<br>☐ Learning Barrier<br>☐ Physical Limitations<br>☐ Pt/Family Discussions<br>☐ If none apply make a note | **Incision Site Care**<br>1. Inspect incision for redness, swelling, or signs of dehiscence or evisceration<br>2. Note characteristics of any drainage<br>3. Monitor healing<br>4. Change or remove dressing as appropriate<br>5. Instruct patient/family in care of incision<br><br>**Tube Care**<br>1. Maintain patency of tube, monitoring drainage<br>2. Instruct patient/family in tube purpose and care<br>3. Administer skin/tube care as appropriate | | |
| Signature | | | | Addressograph | | |
| Initials | | | | | | |

* McCloskey, J.C., & Bulechek, G.M. (2000). Nursing interventions classifications (NIC) (3rd ed.). St. Louis: Mosby

Developed by Good Samaritan Hospital, Puyallup, WA, with special thanks to Rosalind Willis, RN, Joyce Mitchell, RN, Julie Clobes, RN, Kari Newman, RN, Karen Graybeal, RN, and the PCS Core Team. Used with permission.

# INITIATE APPROPRIATE PROBLEMS

| Date | Initials | Nursing Diagnosis | SURGICAL PLAN OF CARE<br>Patient Outcomes<br>For specific indicators see NOC. | **NOTIFY PHYSICIAN IF ANY CHANGES IN PATIENT CONDITION<br>Activities listed under NIC interventions are clinical guidelines only and do not replace nursing clinical judgement.<br>See NIC for other activities.* | Start date | Stop Date |
|---|---|---|---|---|---|---|
| | | Ineffective airway clearance | **Respiratory Status: Ventilation 0403**<br>**Score Outcome**<br>**Definition**<br>Definition: Movement of air in and out of lungs<br><br>ON INITIATION   1  2  3  4  5<br><br>PATIENT GOAL   1  2  3  4  5<br><br>AT RESOLUTION/ DISCHARGE   1  2  3  4  5<br><br>1=Extremely Compromised ☺  2=Substantially compromised ☺  3=Moderately compromised ☺  4=Mildly compromised  5= Not compromised ☺<br><br>If Discharge Outcome at 3 or less, select all that apply.<br>☐ Chronic condition<br>☐ DC with services<br>☐ Compliance issues<br>☐ Transfer to other hosp<br>☐ Transfer to ECF<br>☐ AMA<br>☐ Expired<br>☐ Learning Barrier<br>☐ Physical Limitations<br>☐ Pt/Family Discussions<br>☐ If none apply make a note | **Respiratory Monitoring: Respiratory Assessment**<br>1.  Assess resp. status q 4 h and PRN<br>2.  Turn, cough and deep breath q2h and PRN<br>3.  Obtain baseline O2 sat _____ %<br>4.  Administer O2 if sat 92% on RA or per MD order<br><br>Ventilation Assistance: IS<br>1.  Instruct and assist with IS as appropriate<br>2.  Encourage TCDB q2h and PRN<br>3.  Administer appropriate pain meds to prevent hypoventilation<br>4.  Teach breathing techniques as appropriate<br>5.  Administer O2 as appropriate | | |
| | | Impaired Physical Mobility | **Immobility Consequences: Physiological**<br>**Score Outcome**<br>**Definition**<br>Definition: Compromise in physiological functioning due to impaired physical mobility<br><br>ON INITIATION   1  2  3  4  5<br><br>PATIENT GOAL   1  2  3  4  5<br><br>AT RESOLUTION/ DISCHARGE   1  2  3  4  5<br><br>1=Severe ☺  2=Substantial 3=Moderate ☺  4=Slight  5=None ☺<br><br>If Discharge Outcome at 3 or less, select all that apply.<br>☐ Chronic condition<br>☐ DC with services<br>☐ Compliance issues<br>☐ Transfer to other hosp<br>☐ Transfer to ECF<br>☐ AMA<br>☐ Expired<br>☐ Learning Barrier<br>☐ Physical Limitations<br>☐ Pt/Family Discussions<br>☐ If none apply make a note | **Exercise Therapy-Ambulation:**<br>1.  Encourage to dangle or up in chair as tolerated<br>2.  Instruct and assist in transfer techniques as needed<br>3.  Encourage independent ambulation within safe limits<br>4.  Encourage to be up ad lib if appropriate<br>5.  Assess activity pattern daily _ Obtain Physical therapy consult if requires max assist of 2<br>6.  Consider OT consult<br>Positioning:<br>1.  Position of comfort with proper body alignment if immobile<br>2.  Position to promote ventilation/perfusion<br>3.  Turn per schedule while in bed | | |
| | | Risk of con-stipation | **Bowel Elimination 0501**<br>**Score Outcome**<br>**Definition**<br>Definition Ability of the GI tract to form and evacuate effectively<br><br>ON INITIATION   1  2  3  4  5<br><br>PATIENT GOAL   1  2  3  4  5<br><br>AT RESOLUTION/ DISCHARGE   1  2  3  4  5<br><br>1=Extremely comprised ☺  2=Substantially compromised ☺  3=Moderately compromised ☺  4=Mildly compromised  5=Not compromised ☺<br><br>If Discharge Outcome at 3 or less, select all that apply.<br>☐ Chronic condition<br>☐ DC with services<br>☐ Compliance issues<br>☐ Transfer to other hosp<br>☐ Transfer to ECF<br>☐ AMA<br>☐ Expired<br>☐ Learning Barrier<br>☐ Physical Limitations<br>☐ Pt/Family Discussions<br>☐ If none apply make a note | **Bowel Management:**<br>1.  Note date of last bowel movement.<br>2.  Monitor bowel movements including frequency, consistency, color<br>3.  Assess and record bowel sounds<br>4.  Monitor for S/S of diarrhea, constipation, and impaction<br>5.  Teach patient in a high fiber diet as appropriate<br>6.  Evaluate medications for GI side effects<br>7.  Administer bowel meds as appropriate and as ordered | | |

*McCloskey, J.C., & Bulechek, G.M. (2000). Nursing interventions classifications (NIC) (3rd ed.). St. Louis: Mosby.

*Continued*

# INITIATE APPROPRIATE PROBLEMS

## SURGICAL PLAN OF CARE

| Date | Initials | Nursing Diagnosis | Patient Outcomes | | **NOTIFY PHYSICIAN IF ANY CHANGES IN PATIENT CONDITION** Activities listed under NIC interventions are clinical guidelines only and do not replace nursing clinical judgement. For other activities see NIC.* | Start date | Stop Date |
|---|---|---|---|---|---|---|---|
| | | Anxiety | **1=Never demonstrated ☹ 2=Rarely Demonstrated 3=Sometimes demonstrated ☺ 4=Often demonstrated 5=Consistently demonstrated ☺**<br><br>Anxiety control 1402<br><br>**Score Outcome Definition:** Ability to eliminate or reduce feelings of apprehension and tension from an unidentifiable source<br><br>ON INITIATION   1 2 3 4 5<br><br>PATIENT GOAL   1 2 3 4 5<br><br>AT RESOLUTION/ DISCHARGE   1 2 3 4 5 | If Discharge Outcome at 3 or less, select all that apply.<br>☐ Chronic condition<br>☐ DC with services<br>☐ Compliance issues<br>☐ Transfer to other hosp<br>☐ Transfer to ECF<br>☐ AMA<br>☐ Expired<br>☐ Learning Barrier<br>☐ Physical Limitations<br>☐ Pt/Family Discussions<br>☐ If none apply make a note | Anxiety Reduction: Encourage verbalization of feelings<br>1. Use a calm, reassuring approach<br>2. Explain all procedures<br>3. Listen attentively<br>4. Support the use of appropriate defense mechanisms<br>5. Instruct patient on the use of relaxation techniques<br>6. Administer medications as appropriate | | |
| | | Know-ledge deficit | **1=None ☹ 2=Limited 3=Moderate ☺ 4=Substantial 5=Extensive ☺**<br><br>Knowledge: Illness Care 1824<br><br>**Score Outcome Definition:** Extent of understanding of illness-related information needed to achieve and maintain optimal health<br><br>ON INITIATION   1 2 3 4 5<br><br>PATIENT GOAL   1 2 3 4 5<br><br>AT RESOLUTION/ DISCHARGE   1 2 3 4 5 | If Discharge Outcome at 3 or less, select all that apply.<br>☐ Chronic condition<br>☐ DC with services<br>☐ Compliance issues<br>☐ Transfer to other hosp<br>☐ Transfer to ECF<br>☐ AMA<br>☐ Expired<br>☐ Learning Barrier<br>☐ Physical Limitations<br>☐ Pt/Family Discussions<br>☐ If none apply make a note | Teaching- Disease Process:<br>1. Evaluate patient understanding of disease process<br>2. Describe disease process<br>3. Provide information<br>   Video<br>   Handout<br>   Community Resources<br>   Verbal<br>4. Provide information re: patient progress<br>5. Refer to community agencies/support groups as indicated<br>6. Instruct on measures to prevent complications<br>7. Consider pharmacy consult for ≥ 5 discharge meds | | |

*McCloskey, J.C., & Bulechek, G.M. (2000). Nursing interventions classifications (NIC) (3rd ed.). St. Louis: Mosby.

plan of care and a general medical plan of care, which are being used in our medical and surgical units.

In part because of Good Samaritan's interest in using NOC in their online documentation, Meditech is in the process of revising the outcome portion of PCS to allow customers to choose scaled outcomes or "met or not met." Although we have not yet implemented online documentation, we will continue to use the paper plans of care with NOC outcomes.

# Implementation of NANDA, NIC, and NOC through a Regional Documentation Project

*Cindy A. Scherb, RN, PhD*

## OVERVIEW OF THE PROJECT

Three regional Mayo Health System organizations (Austin Medical Center [AMC-MHS] [80 beds], Albert Lea Medical Center [ALMC-MHS] [105 beds], and Immanuel St. Joseph's [ISJ-MHS] [272 beds]) embarked on implementation of North American Nursing Diagnosis Association (NANDA), NIC, and NOC terminology into their computerized clinical documentation system in 1997. These three Mayo Health System organizations did not have a prior working relationship but did have a common computer system. The project began by educating nursing leadership and garnering their support for the project.

Once this support was established, a project coordinator was hired, a regional documentation group was formed, and a mission statement was developed. The mission of the project was to optimize health across the care continuum with standardization of interventions and outcomes supported by an integrated, user-friendly electronic medical record that enhances communication for the achievement of the goals of the patient and family. The goals established for the project were (1) to improve patient care, (2) to perform benchmarking among the three facilities in the regional project, and (3) to perform benchmarking with all facilities that use NANDA, NIC, and NOC.

Each organization established or reorganized existing documentation teams. The regional project coordinator conducted educational programs for each of these groups. Additional education was offered at some of the institutions for the labor/management committees. The educational sessions included review of the background of NANDA, NIC, and NOC and stressed the importance of using standardized nursing languages. After these educational sessions, the members of the documentation teams were asked to take on the responsibility of assisting with the development of the system and to be cheerleaders for the project as it was implemented and refined.

Once the regional documentation group determined how NANDA, NIC, and NOC would fit into the computer system, the documentation teams began their work of converting existing care plans and critical paths to these languages. The committee members reviewed the three languages and decided which nursing diagnoses, interventions, and nurse-sensitive patient outcomes should be included in the system. These decisions were aided by (1) the NANDA, NIC, and NOC publications; (2) care plan books; (3) previous institutional care plans and critical pathways; and (4) patient care guidelines established by another facility. Content validity of the linkages among the three classifications for the purpose of developing the standard care plans was determined by the expert opinion of the documentation team members.

All care plans were reviewed by each organization for inclusiveness of content for the practice patterns of the organization and for the population for which it was intended. All NIC activities and NOC indicators were reviewed and refined for the acute care setting and the practice patterns of these facilities. Not all NIC activities or NOC indicators were pertinent for these organizations.

## EDUCATIONAL EFFORTS

There was a learning curve associated with accurate documentation in which the standardized language was used. Many different educational formats were used to teach the nursing staff about NANDA, NIC, and NOC. Education efforts consisted of short informational articles on standardized nursing language (i.e., NANDA, NIC, and NOC) in the monthly hospital newsletter. For the purpose of capturing the nursing staff's attention, the slogan "If you want to walk the walk and talk the talk, you have to know about NANDA, NIC, and NOC" was used throughout the education process.

The first formal education was a 2-hour mandatory class on NANDA, NIC, and NOC for all nursing staff engaged in the documentation process. This class was taught by staff nurses from the documentation teams. One of the staff nurses wrote a charming poem in which names of different types of candy were used. The poem was used at the beginning of the educational session, and candy was thrown out to the group as the poem was read. Our own version of "Jeopardy" was played at the conclusion of the presentation.

The e-mail system was used to send out "fun" quizzes on various aspects of these standardized languages. These quizzes were developed as nonthreatening educational tools, and candy bar prizes were awarded each week to five staff members who responded to the quizzes.

A self-learning packet containing an article on NIC, an article on NOC, quizzes highlighting pertinent information from the articles, a computer tutorial, and a computer competency evaluation was developed and distributed to all nursing staff involved in patient care documentation. The nursing staff completed the self-learning packet before the "live" date of the new documentation system.

Another educational endeavor before going "live" was a 4-hour class on the standardized nursing languages and actual computer training. An index of commonly used nursing terms mapped to the standardized languages and "help" sheets were developed to assist the nursing staff with the documentation process. These were available at all computer terminals.

All of this was time-intensive activity for each facility, but staff members were rewarded for their efforts when each facility went "live" (ISJ-MHS in November of 1998, ALMC-MHS in May of 1999, and AMC-MHS in June of 1999) with this new computer documentation. All inpatient units went "live" at the same time except for Labor and Delivery. There are still some paper forms used throughout the organizations, but these are constantly monitored to determine whether they can be computerized.

Education continued after implementation of the new documentation system. The documentation team members monitored the documentation process. They identified areas of the documentation process that the nursing staff had mastered and areas in which they needed further education. Positive feedback was given by means of one-to-one communication and through e-mail messages. Poster boards, e-mail messages, and e-mail quizzes were used as educational mechanisms to assist the staff in learning how to improve their documentation efforts. One facility conducted a follow-up 2-hour educational class approximately 3 months after implementation. Monitoring of the documentation system and follow-up education continues to this day.

## COMPUTER DESIGN AND OUTCOME DOCUMENTATION

One of our biggest challenges in this project was figuring out how we would use NOC within our computer system. The "goal" dictionary was developed to use "met and not met" as the evaluation criteria for a given goal or outcome, but there was not enough room for the NOC definition or indicators to be stored within the dictionary. In consulting with our computer vendor, we determined that using the goal dictionary was not going to be an option. Thus we built the NOC outcomes into the "intervention" dictionary and labeled them as "outcomes" (Figure E-1). This made the outcomes readily apparent to the staff. In the intervention dictionary there is a protocol section. The NOC definitions and indicators were placed in the protocol section. When entering a care plan, nurses are able to view the protocol if they do not know the meaning of an outcome (Figure E-2).

One feature of the computer software that is extremely helpful to the nursing staff is the display of the care plan each time a nurse documents the care provided (Figure E-3). The nursing diagnoses, nurse-sensitive patient outcomes, and nursing interventions appear on the screen.

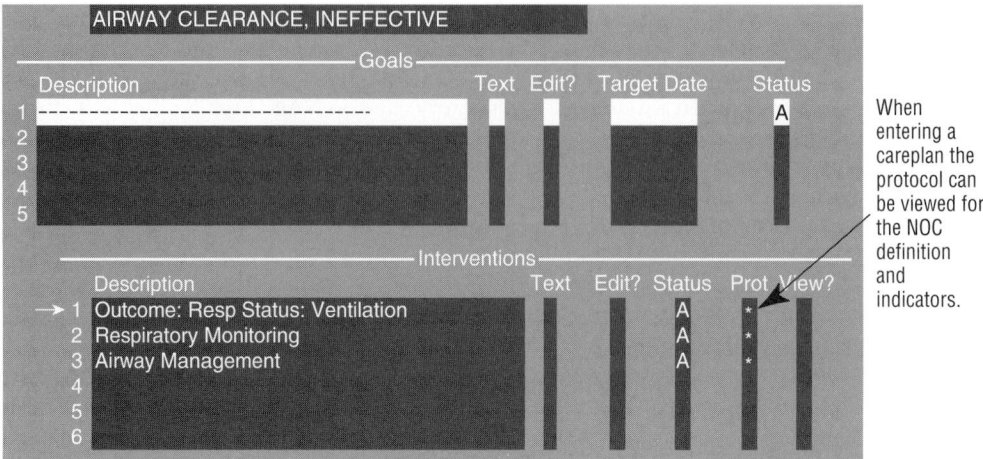

**Figure E-1** Screen print from the Clinical Documentation System. (Courtesy Immanuel St. Joseph's, Mayo Health System, Mankato, MN. Used with permission.)

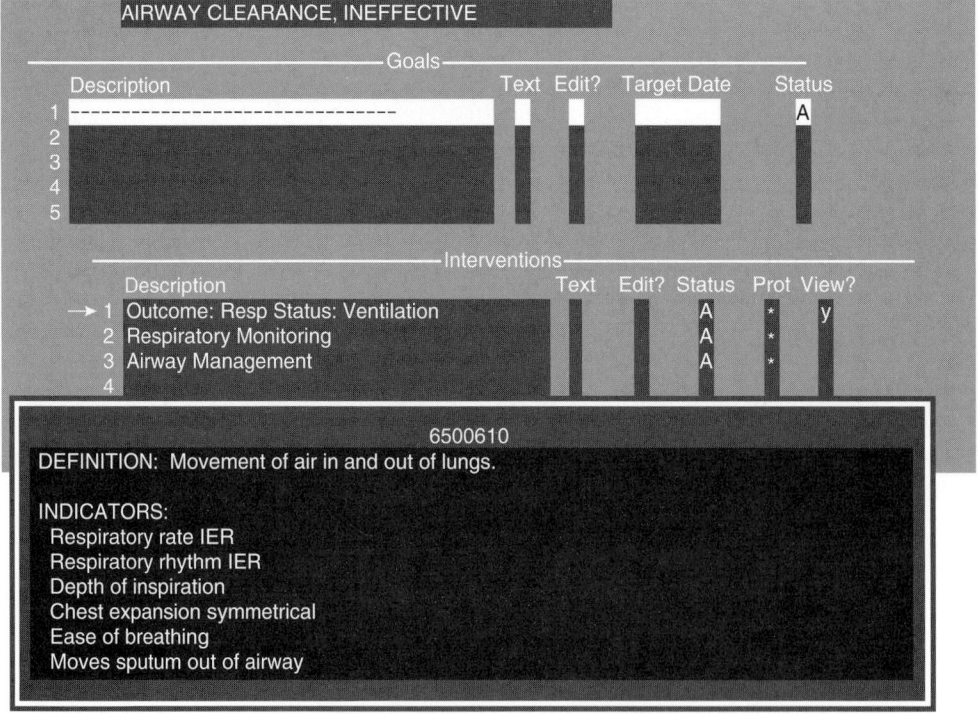

**Figure E-2** Viewing of NOC definition and indicators when entering a care plan. (Courtesy Immanuel St. Joseph's, Mayo Health System, Mankato, MN. Used with permission.)

When a nurse documents on an outcome, he or she uses a screen (Figure E-4) that displays the NOC definition and the indicators. A query is available to enter the overall outcome label rating of 1 to 5. The anchors for the scale are available in a lookup. Individual indicators are not rated.

The "Comment" query was requested by the nursing staff. The staff wanted to be able to note why a patient may have been discharged with a low outcome rating. This was viewed as being similar to completing a variance when an outcome is not achieved on a critical pathway. Thus if a patient is discharged with an outcome rating of 3 or below, the nurse will choose one of the responses shown in Figure E-5. This information is useful for quality improvement initiatives.

## CONCLUSION

We believe that we have been quite successful in developing a computerized documentation system that easily and comprehensively captures the outcomes achieved by the patients we serve. The process involved many dedicated nurses and months of hard work. It was through the vision and support of nursing leadership that we were able to accomplish the mission of our project.

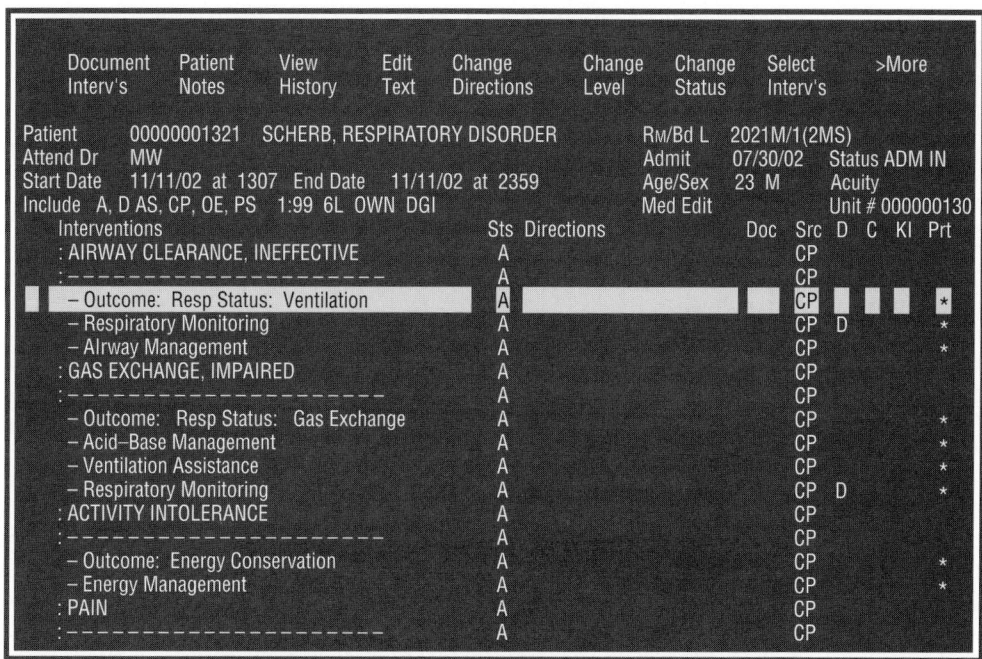

**Figure E-3**  Example of a care plan. (Courtesy Immanuel St. Joseph's, Mayo Health System, Mankato, MN. Used with permission.)

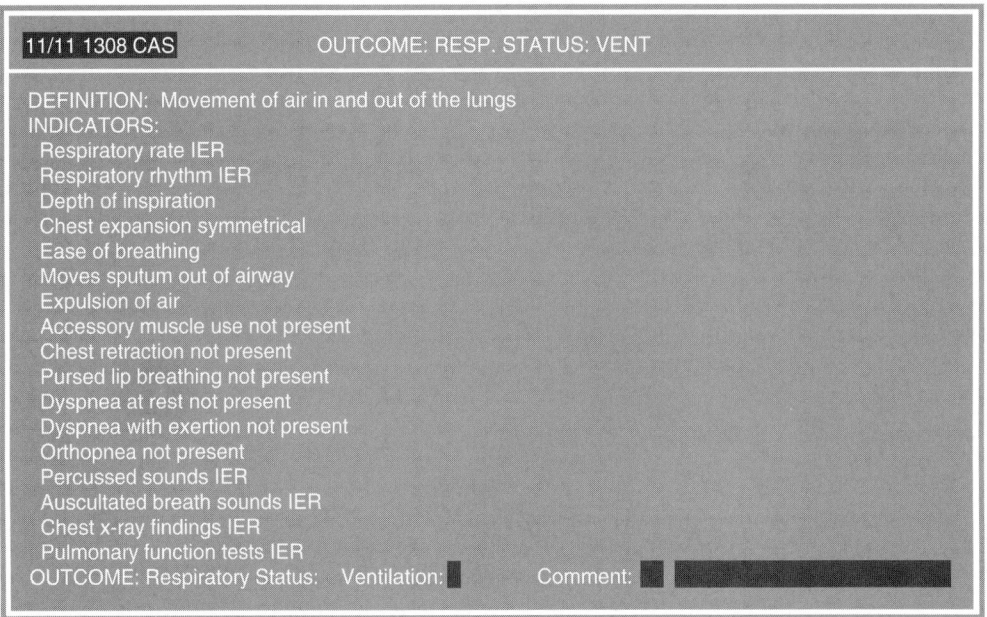

**Figure E-4** Example of NOC outcome documentation screen. (Courtesy Immanuel St. Joseph's, Mayo Health System, Mankato, MN. Used with permission.)

```
                    Outcome Comments Lookup

         Mnemonic            Responses

    1     01                 Chronic condition
    2     02                 Discharge with services
    3     03                 Discharge to Nursing Home
    4     04                 Learning barrier/limit
    5     05                 Compliance issues
    6     06                 Physical limitations
    7     07                 Pt/Family Decision
    8     08                 Transfer/Other acute care
    9     09                 AMA
    10    10                 Not Listed
```

**Figure E-5** Lookup responses for the "Comment" query on each outcome documentation screen. (Courtesy Immanuel St. Joseph's, Mayo Health System, Mankato, MN. Used with permission.)

# Implementing NANDA, NIC, and NOC for Pediatric Specialty Nurses

*Scott Chisholm Lamont, BSN, RN, CCRN, CFRN, ENC (C)*

Use of a paper charting system for patient care presents problematic issues of information accessibility (where is the chart?), delays in information appearing (when will the note be in the chart?), interdisciplinary information sharing (who looks at what sections of the chart?), and notification regarding critical information (how does one know when something important has been added to the chart?). In addition, nursing's unique contributions to patient care and patient outcomes may not appear in a visible and easily measurable format when narrative notes are used to document effectiveness of interventions (what method is used to report nursing outcomes in the chart?), which hampers improvement initiatives or attempts to bill directly for nursing care provided. However, it is possible to address the latter issue by using standardized nursing classification languages in paper charting. Creating a paper documentation system with such languages can, in turn, aid in the transition to electronic charting.

The University of New Mexico (UNM) Health Sciences Center is a tertiary academic health care campus that includes several patient care facilities, one of which is the UNM Children's Hospital. Nursing documentation at this center is generally performed by using traditional paper flow sheets and narrative notes. Although some aspects of the patient record are currently available in an electronic form, nursing documentation is not, and the complete patient chart remains in a paper format. The specialty nurses at the Children's Hospital recognized the limitations of documenting their care in a paper format and began a project to develop and carry out a trial of a new format of documentation. The goals of this project were to create a documentation process that was easy to use for specialty nurses in both the clinic and inpatient settings, would show up on the permanent chart in paper format and in the electronic format currently available, and would document potentially billable professional nursing services. This project was congruent with the Health Sciences Center's commitment to adopting an exclusively electronic chart in the near future. Several concurrent initiatives occurred with the beginning of this project, including revising outpatient flow sheets to support billing for nursing care provided in the clinic setting and initial planning to add nursing documentation to the electronic medical record (EMR).

The initial planning stages included a meeting with the pediatric specialty nurses to discuss documentation needs and potential formats. The group agreed that nursing classification languages would best serve the need to accurately reflect professional nursing practice and improve the visibility of nursing care provided to pediatric patients. The North American Nursing Diagnosis Association (NANDA) diagnostic language, the Nursing Interventions Classification (NIC), and the Nursing Outcomes Classification (NOC) were selected as the preferred languages for use in the documentation project. An additional critical element for documentation was identified by the group: time spent on each patient. It was believed that accurately tracking time would support measuring the workload of the specialty nurses, help to identify patient groups needing time-intensive interventions by nursing diagnostic group, and fit the billing system being developed by the outpatient clinics. A narrative format similar to that used for physician's notes was selected for development. This was due in part to the fact that these notes could be dictated into the centralized transcription system and thus, when completed, would appear on the current EMR as a patient note. These patient notes are available to all EMR users, addressing the accessibility and visibility issues of nursing documentation. In addition, users are notified when new notes are available on the EMR for any of their patients.

Templates of nursing notes with a NANDA/NIC/NOC format were developed and tested in two of the pediatric areas (see the sample notes that follow). The outcome measure is documented in two places on the general narrative note. First, it appears after the assessment and diagnosis and represents goal setting. Second, it appears at the end of the note to reflect assessed changes that can be compared with the goal set. When the patient interaction is brief or the outcome would not be expected immediately, an acceptable note for the second NOC measure is that no change was noted or anticipated at that point in time, and a follow-up assessment would be performed later.

After the refinement period, which took approximately 10 months, these templates were shared with the nursing administrator responsible for redesigning documentation for the eventual EMR. They were also shared with the transcription department for comment. Subsequent steps and implementation would include having each pediatric specialty area develop a list of their most commonly encountered nursing diagnoses, commonly used outcome measures, and frequently implemented interventions. These lists of labels would be used to populate the pulldown menus embedded in the narrative note templates in the transcription department. Familiarizing the nurses with dictation would also be a crucial step. Before implementation, additional review must be done by both the forms committee and the administrators responsible for informatics. This could take another 6 to 10 months to complete.

Both the transcription staff and the nursing staff require additional education on nursing classification languages. The nursing staff at UNM Hospitals are familiar with NANDA diagnostic language, which is currently an element of both the initial patient database and of the daily flow sheets used in the nursing units. The NIC format has been introduced to the nursing staff over the past several years and is currently used primarily to organize policies and procedures, which are listed with NIC labels and organized according to the NIC taxonomy. Students at the College of Nursing learn NIC and NANDA in the generic nursing program. NOC has only recently been introduced to the hospital nursing staff, mainly in the form of education lectures or nursing research rounds, but has not been formally included in the documentation system. NOC has been recently added to the College of Nursing curriculum. Adoption of all three languages into the formal documentation system would therefore take some time and effort but would not present an overwhelming obstacle to use of the documentation system piloted by the pediatric group. The nursing staff currently have enough knowledge to be able to use the dictated nursing notes when they appear on patient charts.

Complicating issues with making this documentation system billable include the reliance of the organization on the *Current Procedural Terminology* (*CPT*) coding system. The new outpatient clinic logs bill nursing time based on the acuity system found in the *CPT* codes, and interventions must be linked to *CPT* codes. Not all nursing interventions are reflected in the *CPT* system, making that linkage difficult. An additional issue is how to get the information found in the documentation into the billing system, which at this time would require filling out a billing form based on the narrative note and the time and intervention codes found therein. Because the system is a word processing system that is viewable on the patient EMR but does not populate a database or billing system, this would still need to be done by hand until such time as a transition to a full EMR occurred. It is hoped that demonstrating outcomes linked to nursing interventions will aid in the goal of billing for nursing care delivered, which makes the use of NOC potentially invaluable.

Although still in its very earliest stages, this pilot program demonstrates how a tertiary academic center is investigating methods of revamping its nursing documentation to better reflect care delivered by nurses while finding ways of integrating nursing documentation into an EMR.

**University of New Mexico Health Sciences Center**

2211 Lomas Blvd NE
Albuquerque, NM, 87106

**Last, First, MR# xxxxxxx**

**Date of Birth:** 08/15/xxxx

**Dictation Date and Time:** 02/01/2002 @ 1700

**Total Time Spent:** 60 minutes

**Assessment Data:**

Reason for visit, physical exam, psychosocial & family systems assessment, history and current medications and treatments.

**Primary Nursing Diagnosis:** Acute Pain (00132)

**Additional Nursing Diagnoses:** none

**Desired Outcome (NOC):** Pain Control (1605)

> **Selected Indicators:** 04 (score: 3, goal: 5); 05 (score: 4, goal: 5); 07 (score: 4, goal: 5); 11 (score: 2, goal: 4)

**Desired Outcome (NOC):** Pain: Disruptive Effects (2101)

> **Selected Indicators:** 03 (score: 2, goal: 5); 13 (score: 3, goal: 5)

---

**Nursing Note:**

I saw Xxxx in clinic today as a nurse visit, due to hxx complaint of ongoing leg pain, which has been worsening over time, limiting hxx mobility ......

**Intervention(s) Implemented or Utilized (NIC):**

1.  Pain Management (1400)
2.  Heat/Cold Application (1380)
3.  Teaching:  Prescribed Activity/Exercise (5612)
4.  Teaching:  Prescribed Medication (5616)
5.  Exercise Promotion:  Stretching (0202)
6.  Exercise Therapy:  Ambulation (0221)
7.  Telephone Follow-Up (8190)

**Actual Outcome (NOC):**  Pain Control (1605)

> **Selected Indicators:**   No changes expected or observed at this point, will follow-up with family by phone Monday to determine outcome scores

**Actual Outcome (NOC):**  Pain:  Disruptive Effects (2101)

> **Selected Indicators:**   No changes expected or observed at this point, will follow-up with family by phone Monday to determine outcome scores.

©The University of New Mexico Health Sciences Center, Albuquerque, NM, Submitted by Scott Lamont, BSN, RN, CCRN, CFRN, ENC(C), Specialty Nurse III, Pediatric Pain Team and Children's Heart Center. Used with permission.

**University of New Mexico Health Sciences Center**

2211 Lomas Blvd NE
Albuquerque, NM, 87106

**Last, First, MR# 4xxxxx**

**Date of Birth:** 11/29/xxxx

**Dictation Date and Time:** 6/15/200x @ xx00

**Total Time Spent:** xx minutes

**Assessment Data:**

xxxxxxxxxxxxxxxxxxxxxxxxxxxxxxxxx.

**Primary Nursing Diagnosis:** Xx (xxxxx)

**Additional Nursing Diagnoses:**

**Desired Outcome (NOC):** XX (xxxx)

　　**Selected Indicators:** xx (score: x, goal: y);

**Desired Outcome (NOC):** XX (xxxx)

　　**Selected Indicators:** xx (score: x, goal: y);

**Pediatric Cardiology Nursing Note:**

xxxxxxxxxxxxxxxxxxxxxxxxxxxx.

**Intervention(s) Implemented or Utilized (list NIC Labels & #s):**

**Actual Outcome (NOC):** XX (xxxx)

　　**Selected Indicators:** xx (score: y);

**Actual Outcome (NOC):** XX (xxxx)

　　**Selected Indicators:** xx (score: y);

# Integration: A Documentation System Reporting Whole-Person Care

*Lisa Burkhart, PhD, RN, MPH*

The Nursing Outcomes Classification (NOC), linked to the North American Nursing Diagnosis Association (NANDA) system and the Nursing Interventions Classification (NIC) system, has been embraced by the parish nursing community to reflect and measure the impact of the ministry of parish nursing practice. Parish nursing is a community-based nursing specialty ministering primarily to faith communities to provide health promotion and disease prevention care to individuals and aggregate populations. Parish nurses care for the whole person, integrating physical, psychological, and social dimensions—holding the spiritual dimension as central to the practice.

Used by parish nurses across the country, the *Integration Documentation System* embraces the use of nursing standardized languages to both simplify documentation in a check-off format and provide a method for statistically analyzing the impact of care. NOC, linked to the NANDA and NIC systems, is integral to this process. NANDA and NIC are used in a check-off format for day-to-day documentation, while NOC is used to measure changes in outcomes over a longer period. NOC offers the capability to measure spiritually focused outcomes, for example, Spiritual Well-Being, Grief Resolution, Loneliness, Acceptance: Health Status, and Hope. These outcomes can be linked to more traditional outcomes (e.g., infection rates, morbidity, and mortality rates) to better integrate spiritual issues with physical issues. The NANDA and NIC taxonomies offer the added benefit of providing a structure to summarize data into a statistical report that reflects whole-person care. The same statistical report communicates parish nursing in an understandable format to both health care stakeholders and faith communities (Figure E-6). The statistical report describes parish nursing from a health care perspective to health care stakeholders, while the same report describes parish nursing as a ministry of care to faith communities. The Integration Documentation System is a bridge between the health care system and faith communities.

## HOW IS NOC USED IN THE INTEGRATION DOCUMENTATION SYSTEM?

The Integration Documentation System uses NOC in several ways, depending on the needs of the institution, faith community, parish nurse, and client. Providing care within the spiritual dimension embraces the philosophy of empowering clients to improve their own health. This process is a journey. NOC is used to empower, guide, and measure that journey.

### Measuring Individual Care

When parish nurses provide individual, one-on-one care, clients can choose to begin using an Outcomes Tracking Form (Figure E-7). Outcomes are listed on the left side, organized by the appropriate scale. In this case, the Outcome Tracking Form is individualized to help each client measure health goals on the journey toward a healthier lifestyle. When the use of the form is initiated, both the parish nurse and client choose the outcomes to be listed. Using the definitions and indicators in this book, clients measure each chosen NOC and identify their goal measurement. Throughout the journey, clients decide when they want to re-measure the NOC. Each measurement is dated at the top of the column. The last two columns are used to re-establish a goal measurement. In this way, NOC is used as an empowering tool to help clients measure their own journey toward healthier lifestyles, while providing valuable outcome information for the parish nurse.

### Measuring the Effect of a Group Program

Parish nurses offer group programs, including educational programs (e.g., healthy eating), support groups (e.g., grief support), and spiritual retreats. NOC and indicator measurements can be

*Text continued on p. 810*

## Parish Nurse Program Report

| 2001 | August | Burkhart | N | % | | N | % |
|---|---|---|---|---|---|---|---|
| Individual Interactions: | | | | | | | |
| Number: | 6 | New Client | 2 | 33.3 | Age: 0-12 | 0 | 0 |
| | | | | | 13-17 | 0 | 0 |
| | | Previously Seen | 4 | 66.7 | 18-30 | 0 | 0 |
| Hours: | 5.5 | Male | 1 | 16.7 | 31-50 | 3 | 50 |
| | | | | | 51-60 | 1 | 16.6 |
| | | Female | 5 | 83.3 | 66-80 | 2 | 33.3 |
| | | Parishioner | 5 | 83.3 | Over 80 | 0 | 0 |
| | | | | | Unknown | 0 | 0 |
| | | Non-parishioner | 1 | 16.7 | Ethnic Heritage | | |
| | | Location | | | Caucasian | 6 | 100 |
| | | Church | 2 | 33 | Black | 0 | 0 |
| | | Nurse Office | 1 | 17 | Hispanic | 0 | 0 |
| | | Visit to HCP | 0 | 0 | Asian/Oriental | 0 | 0 |
| | | Hospital | 0 | 0 | Native American | 0 | 0 |
| | | Home Visit | 1 | 17 | Middle Eastern | 0 | 0 |
| | | Nursing home | 0 | 0 | Far East | 0 | 0 |
| | | Phone | 2 | 33 | Multi-cultural | 0 | 0 |
| | | Mail | 0 | 0 | Other | 0 | 0 |
| | | Pantry | 0 | 0 | Unknown | 0 | 0 |
| | | Other | 0 | 0 | | | |

**Figure E-6** Copyright Lisa Burkhart, MPH, PhD, RN, Marcella Niehoff School of Nursing, Loyola University, Chicago, IL. Used with Permission.

*Continued*

## Parish Nurse Program Report

| 2001 | August | Burkhart |
|---|---|---|

**Individual Interactions:**

| | N | % of Total Interactions | | Interventions | N | % of Total |
|---|---|---|---|---|---|---|
| Interdisciplinary Collaboration | | | | Physiological: Basic | 0 | 0 |
| Medical Categories | | | | Physiological: Complex | 0 | 0 |
| Cardiac/Vascular | 2 | 33.3 | | Behavior/Cognitive | 0 | 0 |
| Respiratory | 0 | 0 | | Communication Enhancement | 0 | 0 |
| Renal/Urinary | 0 | 0 | | Coping/Spiritual/Religious | 5 | 83.33 |
| GI/Hepatic/Biliary | 0 | 0 | | Client Education | 5 | 83 |
| Metabolic/Immune | 0 | 0 | | Psychological Comfort | 1 | 17 |
| Neuro/Sensory | 0 | 0 | | Safety | 2 | 33 |
| Muscular/Skeletal | 0 | 0 | | Family | 1 | 17 |
| Reproductive | 0 | 0 | | Health System | 2 | 33 |
| Drug Interactions | 0 | 0 | | | | |
| Psychological | 3 | 50 | | Source of Referral | N | % of New clients |
| Spiritual or Religious | 3 | 50 | | Client | 2 | 100 |
| | | | | Parishioner | 0 | 0 |
| Health Patterns (Concerns/Diagnoses) | | | | Non-parishioner | 0 | 0 |
| Health Promotion | 2 | 33 | | Pastoral staff | 0 | 0 |
| Nutrition | 0 | 0 | | Physician | 0 | 0 |
| Elimination | 0 | 0 | | Other Health Provider | 0 | 0 |
| Activity/Rest | 1 | 17 | | Media | 0 | 0 |
| Perception/Cognition | 3 | 50 | | Parish Nurse | 0 | 0 |
| Self/Perception | 0 | 0 | | Family | 0 | 0 |
| Role/Relationship | 1 | 17 | | | | |
| Sexuality/Reprod. | 0 | 0 | | Referral To: | | % of Total |
| Coping/Stress | 2 | 33 | | Pastoral staff | 0 | 0 |
| Life Principles | 2 | 33 | | Physician | 1 | 16.6 |
| Safety/Protection | 0 | 0 | | Other Health Provider | 0 | 0 |
| Comfort | 1 | 17 | | Church Resource | 0 | 0 |
| Growth/Development | 0 | 0 | | Community Resource | 0 | 0 |
| | | | | Total System Referrals | 1 | 16.6 |

**Fig. E-6** Copyright Lisa Burkhart, MPH, PhD, RN, Marcella Niehoff School of Nursing, Loyola University, Chicago, IL. Used with Permission.

## Parish Nurse Program Report

| 2001 | August | Burkhart |
|---|---|---|

**Group Activities**

Total Participants 65

Time (hours):  Plan 6  Program 4

| Screenings | Number | Participants | Abnormal | New |
|---|---|---|---|---|
| Blood Pressure | 2 | 65 | 9 | 1 |
| Cholesterol | 0 | 0 | 0 | 0 |
| Glucose | 0 | 0 | 0 | 0 |
| Lice | 0 | 0 | 0 | 0 |
| Health | 0 | 0 | 0 | 0 |
| Hearing/Vision | 0 | 0 | 0 | 0 |
| Ht/Wt | 0 | 0 | 0 | 0 |
| Other | 0 | 0 | 0 | 0 |

| Group Programs | Number | Participants |
|---|---|---|
| Education | 0 | 0 |
| Support | 0 | 0 |
| Spiritual | 0 | 0 |
| Environmental/Safety | 0 | 0 |
| Community Outreach | 0 | 0 |
| Other | 0 | 0 |

| Visual/Written Programs | |
|---|---|
| Newsletter/Bulletin | 1 |
| Health Display | 1 |

| Continuing Education | |
|---|---|
| Professional Development | 0 |
| Programs Attended | 1 |

| Meetings | # Times | Hrs. |
|---|---|---|
| Pastor/Staff | 4 | 4 |
| Health and Wellness | 0 | 0 |
| Other Church Committee | 0 | 0 |
| Community/Liaison/Networking | 1 | 1 |
| System/Liaison/Networking | 0 | 0 |
| Parish Nurse | 1 | 6 |
| Other | 0 | 0 |

| Attendance at Church Functions | | |
|---|---|---|
| Worship Services | 0 | 0 |
| Healing Services | 0 | 0 |
| Funerals | 1 | 2 |
| Wakes | 1 | 1 |
| Fellowship | 0 | 0 |
| Other | 0 | 0 |

| Office Work | | |
|---|---|---|
| Report Writing | | 0 |
| Resource Dev. | | 2 |
| Documentation | | 1.25 |
| Other | | 0 |
| Volunteer Coordination | | 2 |

| Total Hours | | 25 |
|---|---|---|
| Paid | | 20 |
| Unpaid | | 5 |

**Fig. E-6** Statistical Report. (Copyright Lisa Burkhart, MPH, PhD, RN, Marcella Niehoff School of Nursing, Loyola University, Chicago, IL. Used with permission.)

**Parish Nursing Services**
**Individual Client Outcome Tracking Form**

**Client Name:** XXXXX

| Nursing Outcome: | Measmt Date: 8/5/02 | Measmt Date: | Measmt Date: | Measmt Date: | Measmt Date: | Measmt Date: | Measmt Date: | Expected Goal | Goal (revised) | Goal (revised) |
|---|---|---|---|---|---|---|---|---|---|---|
| **Scale: 1=None, 2=Limited, 3=Moderate, 4=Substantial, 5=Extensive** | | | | | | | | | | |
| 1. Acceptance: Health Status | 2 LB | | | | | | | 4 LB | | |
| 2. Hope | 3 LB | | | | | | | 4 LB | | |
| **Scale: 1=Never demonstrated, 2=Rarely demonstrated, 3=Sometimes demonstrated, 4=Often demonstrated, 5=Consistently demonstrated** | | | | | | | | | | |
| 3. Anxiety Control | 3 LB | | | | | | | 5 LB | | |
| 4. Coping | 4 LB | | | | | | | 4 LB | | |
| 5. Symptom Control | 2 LB | | | | | | | 5 LB | | |
| **Scale: 1=Not at all, 2=To a slight extent, 3- To a moderate extent, 4=To a great extent, 5=To a very great extent** | | | | | | | | | | |
| 6. Blood Glucose Control | 2 LB | | | | | | | 5 LB | | |
| **Scale: 1=Extremely compromised, 2=Substantially compromised, 3=Moderately compromised, 4=Mildly compromised, 5=Not compromised** | | | | | | | | | | |
| 7. Quality of Life | 3 LB | | | | | | | 4 LB | | |
| 8. Rest | 2 LB | | | | | | | 5 LB | | |
| 9. Spiritual Well-being | 4 LB | | | | | | | 4 LB | | |

**Parish Nurse Signature/Initials:** *Lisa Burkhart, PhD, RN*

**Fig. E-7** Outcome tracking form. (Copyright Lisa Burkhart, MPH, PhD, RN, Marcella Niehoff School of Nursing, Loyola University, Chicago, IL. Used with permission.) *(NOC labels reprinted with permission from Mosby.)*

**Parish Nursing Services**

**Client Name:**

## Client Outcome Tracking Form:  Congestive Heart Failure

| Nursing Outcome: | Measmt Date: | Measmt Date: | Measmt Date: | Measmt Date: | Measmt Date: | Measmt Date: | Expected Goal | Goal (revised) | Goal (revised) | Goal (revised) |
|---|---|---|---|---|---|---|---|---|---|---|
| **Scale:   1=None, 2=Limited, 3=Moderate, 4=Substantial, 5=Extensive** | | | | | | | | | | |
| Acceptance: Health Status | | | | | | | | | | |
| Knowledge: Medication | | | | | | | | | | |
| Social Support | | | | | | | | | | |
| **Scale:   1=Never demonstrated, 2=Rarely demonstrated, 3=Sometimes demonstrated, 4=Often demonstrated, 5=Consistently demonstrated** | | | | | | | | | | |
| Compliance Behavior | | | | | | | | | | |
| Family Participation in Professional Care | | | | | | | | | | |
| **Scale:   1=Extremely compromised, 2=Substantially compromised, 3=Moderately compromised, 4=Mildly compromised, 5=Not compromised** | | | | | | | | | | |
| Activity Tolerance | | | | | | | | | | |
| Fluid Balance | | | | | | | | | | |
| Spiritual Well-being | | | | | | | | | | |
| Tissue Perfusion: Peripheral | | | | | | | | | | |
| **Scale:   1=Dependent, does not participate, 2=Requires assistive device, 3=Requires assistive person, 4=Independent with assistive device, 5=Completely independent** | | | | | | | | | | |
| Self Care: Activities of Daily Living | | | | | | | | | | |
| Self Care: Instrumental Activities of Daily Living | | | | | | | | | | |
| **Scale:   1=Severe, 2=Substantial, 3=Moderate, 4=Slight, 5=None** | | | | | | | | | | |
| Symptom Severity | | | | | | | | | | |

**Parish Nurse Signature/Initials:**

**Fig. E-8** Outcome tracking form for patients with congestive heart failure. Copyright Lisa Burkhart, MPH, PhD, RN, Marcella Niehoff School of Nursing, Loyola University, Chicago, IL. Used with permission.

used as pretests and posttests for these groups. For example, at both the first meeting and last meeting of a grief support group, participants can measure their level of grief using the Grief Resolution NOC. In this case, two copies of the Grief Resolution NOC are reproduced for each participant as it appears in the book—one for a pretest and one for a post-test. This process has many benefits. First, it empowers the client to help identify where he or she is on the journey. Second, it stimulates discussion by raising sensitive issues. Lastly, it helps the parish nurse measure the impact of the group program.

## Tracking Institutional Initiatives

All parish nurses are affiliated with a faith community. However, some parish nurses are also affiliated with a health care system. In the latter case, parish nurses can use NOC to integrate and communicate the ministry of parish nursing practice as part of the health care continuum. Many health institutions choose to target certain populations, track care provided to those populations, and measure the impact of care provided. A NOC template can be individualized for those populations. For example, an Outcome Tracking Form template can be generated for patients with congestive heart failure, as shown in Figure E-8. In this case, the parish nurse initiates this template for all clients who have congestive heart failure. When initiating the template, both the parish nurse and client measure current status and goals for each NOC outcome on the template. Additional measurements in subsequent columns can be made quarterly or at the end of an episode of care.

This format has several benefits. First, the parish nurse can integrate and measure spiritual outcomes along with physical outcomes. Second, parish nurses can identify trends in care for those targeted populations. Lastly, measurements from the Outcome Tracking Form templates can be aggregated and shared with health care system quality departments.

Faith communities can also create Outcome Tracking Form templates in a similar manner. However, these templates may include more spiritually focused outcomes. In addition, Outcome Tracking Form templates can be generated to measure outcomes associated with grants.

These techniques for using standardized vocabulary to reflect whole-person care are not limited to parish nursing. Other health care providers, including pastoral care and other community-based care providers, can use the Integration Documentation System to assist in documenting, integrating, and measuring physical, psychological, social, and spiritual dimensions of care. For more information about the Integration Documentation System, please e-mail Lisa Burkhart, RN, PhD, Assistant Professor, Loyola University, Chicago, at eburkha@luc.edu.

# Application Examples in Educational Settings

Four examples of how NOC has been applied in educational settings are included in this appendix. They demonstrate not only the application of NOC in the curriculum but also the methods used to assist students develop clinical decision-making skills. The first application illustrates the use of NOC in an associate degree program. Krenz describes how faculty used outcomes and indicators to set competency expectations for students. Examples of the competencies expected in extended care, oncology, and psychiatric nursing are included along with competencies expected in providing care for a childbearing family. The next three applications are in baccalaureate programs. All authors of the applications discuss the implementation process in a curriculum or course and provide examples of teaching materials used in the courses. Finesilver and Metzler provide examples used in adult nursing that are included in their monograph. Schoenfelder discusses the use of NOC in two practicum courses, one beginning core course and one gerontology course. Van de Castle provides a number of templates used in the curriculum and discusses the use of NOC codes by students and the rationale for including their use. Taken together, these examples provide ideas and materials that can be adapted for both associate and baccalaureate degree programs.

# The Use of the Nursing Outcome Classification to Direct a Competency-Based Curriculum

*Maryanne Krenz, RN*

Using the Nursing Outcome Classification (NOC) as a means of formulating a competency-based curriculum provides both clarity and direction. The transition from discrete specific learning objectives to broader, higher-level competency performances was a conceptual change that needed a roadmap. The curriculum redesign at Brookdale Community College, an associate degree program, occurred because of societal demands for increased accountability of graduates to be able to perform work-related competencies in a complex, rapidly changing environment.

The National League for Nursing defines *competency* as "the knowledge, attitudes, skills and behaviors that establish acceptable performance in a particular situation."[1] Inherent in this expectation is the need for a nurse with self-awareness, initiative, and the ability to appraise clinical situations to intervene in ways that will bring about positive outcomes. Critical thinking, the buzzword in education for the past 10 years, is essential to nursing judgment. Yet in the last decade, trying to meet this educational standard has been a difficult transition.

The struggle to develop a competency-based curriculum was intense and often frustrating because the faculty was asked to proceed in an endeavor that had multiple expectations, few guideposts, and a destination that was unclear. However, there was confidence that the direction in which we were being led was worthy of our efforts. The faculty was given the opportunity to experiment because the new design was considered "a work in progress, not a final product."

Change in any environment is a challenge, but there are two sayings, the sources of which are obscure, that apply specifically to nurses. One is "Trying to lead nurses is like trying to herd cats." The other states that changing a nursing curriculum is like trying to relocate a cemetery. Resistance and individuality exist in all efforts to enter an unfamiliar territory. Implementation strategies such as commitment, creativity, and cohesiveness among peers had to be generated.

Content-driven courses are burdensome for faculty and students because both struggle with "nice to know" versus "need to know" content. A study by Shell to identify barriers to critical thinking by nursing faculty isolated the perceived need to teach for content coverage as a variable that impeded critical thinking teaching strategies.[3] How can educators lead nursing into this century using methods enmeshed in outdated approaches for the acquisition of knowledge that may not be relevant in the future?

Using discipline-specific outcomes that are derived from research to write competency statements was appealing because the words reflect what the nurse is trying to achieve through the implementation of care. Words are very important according to biologist Francisco Varela who explains that we can only see what we talk about.[4] According to Peter Senge, "Reality is inseparable from our language and actions."[2] Is it not essential to help the novice see what the experts say can be achieved by their professional practice? Being explicit about what is expected of the learner enhances the application of knowledge. A syllabus is a reflection of performance expectations and a guide that reflects values. The use of NOC to write competencies empowers students and faculty by providing a beacon for both assessments and interventions.

The following are examples of competencies that reflect the language of the Nursing Outcomes Classification.

## EXTENDED CARE FACILITY

Evaluate the ability of purposeful movement and note deviations in joint movement, body alignment, muscle resistance, transfer, or ambulation performance.

Determine structural intactness of skin and mucous membranes and document temperature, color sensations, elasticity, texture, lesions, and devices that interrupt skin integrity.

Monitor airway patency, ventilation, and gas exchange by performing a respiratory assessment.

Prevent aspiration, maintain airway patency, enhance ventilation, and promote gas exchange by respiratory assessment, positioning, coughing enhancement, selection of foods according to swallowing ability, and appropriate consistency of liquids and foods.

Reinforce actions to monitor and compensate for hearing and vision loss such as positioning of self to advantage, use of assistive devices, and reports of deterioration.

Monitor and reinforce expressions of will to live, meaning of life, sense of belief in self and others, setting goals, and sense of inner peace.

Integrate Erikson's theory into the plan of care to enhance the developmental tasks of affiliation, accomplishment, generativity, and life review.

## ONCOLOGY ROTATION

Assess symptoms: onset, severity, frequency, and variation associated with the administration of chemotherapeutic agents and radiation therapy.

Monitor immune status through body temperature; presence of recurrent infections; positive cultures; white blood cell (WBC) counts; complaints of tissue integrity problems; gastrointestinal, respiratory, genitourinary changes; and evidence of malaise or fatigue.

Monitor and reinforce all client attempts to adjust to body image changes by using the following indicators:

- Congruence between body reality, body ideal, and body presentation
- Description of affected body part
- Willingness to look at and touch the affected body part
- Expression of satisfaction with body appearance and function
- Adjustment to changes in appearance and function
- Willingness to use strategies to enhance appearance and function
- Expression of feelings about self-worth and reaction of the significant other

Collect and analyze data to achieve balance of fluids and electrolytes as evidenced by the following:

- Food/fluid intake adequate
- Blood pressure, pulse, and respiratory rate normal
- Peripheral pulses palpable normal strength
- Orthostatic blood pressure not present
- 24-hour intake and output balanced
- Abnormal breath sounds not present
- Peripheral edema not present
- Confusion not present
- Skin/mucous membranes normal
- Ascites not present
- Osmolarity, hematocrit, and urine specific gravity normal
- Serum electrolytes normal
- Muscle strength normal
- Neuromuscular nonirritability
- Tingling in extremities not present
- Bowel elimination normal

Monitor and reinforce all behaviors that exhibit adjustments to the actual or impending loss such as the following:

- Expresses feelings, meaning of the loss, positive expectations about the future
- Verbalizes reality and acceptance of the loss and unresolved conflicts
- Participates in grooming, hygiene, social activities
- Reports adequate nutritional intake, sleep, usual sexual desire, and absence of somatic distress
- Seeks social and spiritual support and shares loss with significant others
- Discusses beliefs about death and participates in planning funeral
- Progresses through the stages of grief

## CHILDBEARING FAMILY

### Postpartum

Integrate teaching/learning principles in parent education related to the care of the neonate by using the following NOC guidelines:

- Description of normal infant characteristics
- Demonstration of proper way to hold the infant
- Demonstration of proper positioning of the infant
- Demonstration of bathing the infant
- Demonstration of umbilical cord care
- Description of infant stimulation methods

Plan care that incorporates the following NOC guidelines for successful breastfeeding:

- Description of benefits of breastfeeding
- Description of the physiology of lactation
- Description of breast milk composition, let-down process
- Demonstration of proper technique for attaching infant to the breast
- Demonstration of proper technique to break infant suction
- Demonstration of breast care and nipple evaluation

## PSYCHIATRIC ROTATION

### Schizophrenia

Monitor and reinforce all client attempts to do the following:

- Achieve control over distorted thoughts
- Meet developmental tasks
- Comply with prescribed treatment regimens
- Receive, interpret, and express messages appropriately
- Maintain social support

### Depression

Monitor and reinforce all client attempts to do the following:

- Concentrate on specific stimulus
- Maintain interests in life events
- Sustain social support
- Comply with prescribed treatment regimens
- Maintain role performance
- Adjust to prevailing emotional tone in response to circumstances

### Suicide Risk

Monitor and reinforce all client attempts to do the following:

- Identify personal health threats
- Refrain from gestures and attempts to kill self
- Make choices among alternatives
- Maintain social support

# References

1. National League for Nursing Accrediting Commission. (2001). *Accreditation manual and interpretive guidelines for associate degree programs in nursing*. New York: Author.
2. Senge, P. Retrieved http://www.deming.eng.clemson.edu/pub/tqmbbs/prin-pract/comcom.txt, MIT Center for Organizational Learning.
3. Shell, R. (2001). Perceived barriers to teaching for critical thinking by BSN nursing faculty. *Nursing and Health Care Perspectives, 22*, 286-291.
4. Varela, F. (1998). In J. Jaworski (Ed.), *Synchronicity: The inner path of leadership*. San Francisco: Berrett-Koehler.

# Implementation of NOC in an Undergraduate Curriculum

*Cynthia Finesilver, RN, MSN, CNRN, and Debbie Metzler, RN, C, MSN*

## OVERVIEW AND IMPLEMENTATION

During the past 7 years, the integration of the North American Nursing Diagnosis Association (NANDA), the Nursing Interventions Classification (NIC), and the Nursing Outcomes Classification (NOC) has been used as a framework for clinical decision making at Bellin College of Nursing. Although the NANDA taxonomy had been used to promote the critical thinking process in the classroom and clinical setting, a need to link the nursing diagnoses with client-centered goals and independent nursing activities was identified by the members of the curriculum committee. The decision was made to incorporate these languages at all levels of the curriculum, beginning with adult health, child health, and maternal health courses in the junior year. Over the next several semesters, the classification systems were used at all levels in the curriculum, including the acute care, long-term care, and community settings.

All members of the faculty at Bellin College of Nursing, an accredited baccalaureate program located in Green Bay, Wisconsin, are members of the nursing program curriculum committee. Course faculty are responsible for the development of criteria to ensure that course and program outcomes are achieved by the students through classroom and clinical experiences. Decisions about the use of NANDA, NOC, and NIC (NNN) are made by the course and department faculty to ensure that program outcomes related to critical thinking and knowledge synthesis are achieved as determined by student evaluation. Course and department faculty continue to evaluate and modify the use of the languages on a regular basis.

Some courses use NNN as criteria for ungraded course projects, such as clinical preparation tools, that students complete before and during their clinical experience. Other courses use NNN as criteria for graded course papers, such as nursing process papers that discuss the nursing process related to clients. Other faculty incorporate NNN into classroom content, postconference discussions, the laboratory learning setting, or community education.

## RATIONALE FOR USE OF NANDA, NOC, AND NIC IN A BACCALAUREATE CURRICULUM

NANDA, NOC, and NIC can be used as the organizing framework for the curriculum or can be easily incorporated into any theoretical framework. If faculty and students are already using NANDA to document the nursing process, it is easy to transition to NIC and NOC. NNN can be used at all levels of the curriculum, in multiple client care settings, and with varied populations. Because the language of NNN is general, it can be incorporated into all nursing courses and will assist the student develop critical thinking skills as they individualize the outcomes and activities.

Beginning nursing students have accepted NNN and have successfully used the classification system to plan nursing care for clients with common health alterations. The major advantages of NNN are that independent nursing activities are emphasized, the classifications are computer friendly, and use of the classifications does not entail a major curriculum change.

## IMPLEMENTATION OF NNN INTO AN UNDERGRADUATE CURRICULUM

Incorporation of NNN into a nursing curriculum does not require a major curriculum revision. NNN can be incorporated into the curriculum whenever the nursing process is introduced in classroom content or in the clinical setting. Typically, NNN is introduced in a beginning fundamentals nursing course (before or during the students' first clinical course).

A generic example for incorporating the nursing process and NNN into a nursing curriculum is as follows:

## Assessment

Data are collected, organized (according to whatever conceptual framework is used in the program), validated, and documented.

## Nursing Diagnosis

A judgment is formed based on the assessment data related to client's strengths and health concerns and documented in the NANDA format.

## Planning

Nurse-sensitive outcomes and client goals that are derived from the nursing diagnosis are identified. During this process, the student is instructed to find the NANDA diagnosis that is supported by their assessment data and then to identify the most appropriate NOC outcome to match the NANDA diagnosis and the client's identified problem. This is a great exercise in critical thinking. The student can then use the indicators from the NOC book for the selected outcome to aid in the development of the goals.

NOTE: Outcomes/goals are still written by using the same criteria that are included in the existing curriculum, such as client-centered, identified deadlines and the use of measurable terms that are realistic.

The second part of planning is the identification of the priority nursing interventions to meet the NOC goals. The student must choose the NIC interventions and associated activities that are appropriate to meet the client's goals. The student identifies the most appropriate activities for each intervention and individualizes these to meet the client's particular needs.

## Implementation

The student performs the identified NIC interventions. These may be independent and/or collaborative interventions.

## Evaluation

The student reviews the NOC outcomes/goals and determines whether the outcomes/goals have been met.

After the student learns the five steps of the nursing process in detail, it is important for him or her to have an opportunity to develop a plan of care for a client. One idea is to use a simple case study in class that describes a common health alteration familiar to the students. An example of a case study concerns an elderly client with constipation who has identified risk factors for constipation. Then the students could work in groups to write up a plan of care using the five steps of the nursing process and the incorporation of NNN. This format is useful for students who are beginning nursing courses and those have not begun clinical courses.

After the case study has been completed by the groups, it is interesting for the students to share their plans of care with the class while comparing and contrasting their plans with their classmates' plans.

The following is an example taken from Finesilver, C., & Metzler, D. (Eds.), *Curriculum guide for implementation of NANDA, NIC and NOC into an undergraduate nursing curriculum* (pp. 39-42). Iowa City: The University of Iowa, The Center for Nursing Classification & Clinical Effectiveness.

# 688-303 Nursing Care of Adults II
## *Cynthia Finesilver, RN, MSN, CNRN*
### *Assistant Professor*

This course provides students with the theoretical basis for the nursing care of young, middle-aged, and older adults and their families with alterations in health status. Students enhance critical thinking and problem-solving skills as they learn the roles of the nurse. Students develop competence in providing care to clients with alterations in oxygenation, fluid and electrolyte balance, urinary elimination, and the neurological systems. Clinical experiences occur in acute care settings, which are currently in neurology and cardiology units.

NNN is emphasized in the classroom, during clinical preparation by the student, during postconference discussion, and as a part of a written, graded paper. During the clinical component of this course, students are required to develop and submit a clinical preparation tool for each client. This tool includes assessment with the use of Roy's modes and subsystems, identification of a priority NANDA diagnosis, development of a NOC classification with long-term and short-term goals, selection of two appropriate NIC interventions, and evaluation of the client's progress toward the goals with modification as needed. In addition to this ungraded clinical preparation tool, students are required to submit a nursing process paper addressing a priority nursing diagnosis, one NOC classification with short-term and long-term goals, two NIC interventions with applicable activities, and evaluation/modification of the plan of care as needed (20% course grade).

One of the strengths of NNN use in this course is that the content related to NNN is threaded through the classroom content, into clinical preparation, into preconferences with individual students, and during group postconferences. The NOC classifications and NIC interventions are clinically useful with the populations studied during this course. Outcome and goal development is emphasized consistently, as well as the relationship between nursing diagnoses, outcomes, and interventions. Students are able to use the research-based NOC classification and NIC interventions to develop goals and activities for their clients. It is beneficial that the NOC classification and NIC interventions are applicable not only to the client but also to the family and community.

One concern about implementation is that students do not consistently develop individualized activities for clients and do not expand on the activities listed in the interventions. Students must be reminded to review pertinent literature and use additional references when using the NOC and NIC textbooks. In addition, students must be reminded to evaluate and modify client progress toward the stated goals and not evaluate the nursing activities.

The clinical preparation tool and nursing process paper have been used for approximately 5 years with minor modifications. The faculty does not anticipate any major changes in the course requirements at this time.

**688-303 Nursing Care of Adults II**
**Course Project: Applying the Nursing Process**

These criteria are designed to assist you as you develop your Nursing Process Case Study Paper for 688-303

<u>Directions:</u>  You may choose any client for this assignment but not on a client that you already did a complete clinical prep tool on.  This paper must be <u>typed</u>.  You also need to include a <u>brief</u> summary of the medical history.  Turn this form in with your paper, along with your client clinical prep tool.

Student Name _____   Client initials_____

<u>Key:</u>   1 - poor, 2 - fair, 3 - average, 4 - good, 5 - excellent

Criteria:

| | |
|---|---|
| 1. Professionally written:  (3 points)<br>    (spelling, grammar, sentence structure, medical terminology<br>    and reference page) | _____ points<br>Comments: |
| 2. <u>Nursing Diagnosis</u> (3 points) (Page number)<br>        Three-part statement that includes:<br>        1. Identify <u>one</u> priority problem (NANDA/label)<br>        2. Includes stimulus (etiology) (R/T) (pathophysiology)<br>        3. Defining characteristics (signs and symptoms,<br>            ineffective behaviors), match data (evidenced by) | _____ points<br>Comments: |
| 3. <u>Planning</u> (5 points)<br>        A. Identifies outcome label (NOC) (Page number)<br>            1. Label definition matches NANDA<br>            2. Include indicators<br>        B. Establishes client/family-centered goals<br>            1. Two-to-three short-term goals<br>            2. One long-term goal<br>            3. Written in measurable terms<br>            4. Timeline established<br>            5. Indicators | _____ points<br>Comments: |
| 4. <u>Interventions/Implementation</u> (10 points)<br>        A. Identifies two intervention categories (NIC) (Page numbers)<br>        B. Category matches (NANDA and NOC)<br>        C. Includes all appropriate bio-psycho-social-spiritual activities<br>        D. Use of additional resources related to NIC activities<br>        E. Activities must be individualized<br>        F. Must do separate activities for each selected NIC. | _____ points<br>Comments: |
| 5. <u>Evaluation</u> (4 points)<br>        A. State if goals were met or if progress toward client/family-<br>            centered goals was made (include indicators)<br>        B. Identifies modifications in the plan | _____ points<br>Comments: |

Total Points _____Average Points _____Letter Grade_____

Developed by Cynthia Finesilver, RN, MSN, CNRN, and Debbie Metzler, RN, C, MSN. Copyright, Bellin College of Nursing, Green Bay, WI. Used with permission.

**688-303 Nursing Care of Adults II**
**Example – Student Nursing Process Paper**

Krista Lukes (formerly Krista Hermus)
Bellin College of Nursing
Nursing Student

This is a 46-year-old male who presented to the emergency room with chest pain that had lasted for 13 hours. He was then admitted to an outlying hospital where heparin and nitroglycerin as well as thrombolytic therapy was started. After having been diagnosed as having an acute myocardial infarction, the patient was then transferred by ambulance to the hospital. On the way to hospital, the patient developed slurred speech and weakness of his right side. After admission to the hospital, the patient was diagnosed with a left hemorrhagic stroke that occurred in the left basal ganglia and the internal capsule leaving the patient with right-sided hemiplegia, hemisensory deficits, slurred speech, and expressive aphasia. The patient has a positive history of hypertension, coronary artery disease, coronary artery bypass surgery in 1991, noncompliance with diabetes treatment, and a 2–pack–per–day smoker for over 20 years.

**NURSING DIAGNOSIS**: *Impaired Verbal Communication* (p. 47) related to a left hemispheric bleed where blood is forced into the surrounding cerebral parenchyma thus creating a hematoma. This hematoma displaces and compresses the adjacent cerebral tissue causing ischemic processes and cerebral edema thus causing increased intracranial pressure which in turn affects motor and sensory functions as evidenced by slurred speech, expressive aphasia, frustration with responses, and short 1-2 word answers.

**PLANNING NOC:**

**Communication:** *Expressive Ability* (p. 130) #2 substantially compromised as indicated by slurred speech, frustration with speaking, and short 1-2 word answers.

**SHORT TERM GOAL:** Communication Expressive Ability improves to a #3 moderately compromised within 2 weeks as evidenced by:

- Patient using 2-3 word phrases when speaking to staff and family.
- A decrease in the patient's slurring of words.
- Patient stating needs and wants either verbally or with hand gestures that are understood by staff and family.
- Patient stating feeling less frustration with ability to speak.

**LONG-TERM GOAL:**

Communication: Expressive Ability improves to a #4 mildly compromised within 1 month as evidenced by:
- The patient using 4-5 word sentences when speaking to staff and family members.
- No slurring of words when patient speaks.

Courtesy Krista Lukes RN, BSN, graduate of Bellin College of Nursing, Green Bay, WI.

- Patient consistently stating his needs, wants, and feelings through verbal communication

## INTERVENTIONS:

**Communication Enhancement:** *Speech Deficit* (p. 180)

- Encourage the patient to use speech when doing nursing cares by asking him questions.
- Tape messages from family members for the patient to listen to every day to encourage the use of speech and make patient feel at ease.
- Keep eye contact with the patient while speaking to him.
- Use objects and printed words while asking the patient to identify them BID.
- Name objects used in daily cares such as names of procedures and names of the foods the patient is eating.
- Organize the patient's day with a schedule to make things more comfortable and familiar.
- Listen to the patient carefully in order to understand him and also to show interest.
- Treat the patient as an adult, making sure not to talk down to him.
- Include body contact when listening to the patient such as hand clutching or touching the patient's shoulder while listening to him speak.
- Question the patient if you cannot understand him.
- Verify your understanding of the patient when he speaks.

## EVALUATION:

Goal not met as indicated by the patient's continued use of 1-2 word statements, slurred speech, and frustration with verbal responses. I was not able to evaluate my patient at 2 weeks and 4 weeks in order to evaluate the outcomes after implementing my plan of care.

I think that this care plan would have been better if I had been able to evaluate my patient at 2 weeks and 4 weeks. One problem that I found with this care plan was the patient's speech problems could have also been due to his mood. This patient had a history of depression. The left hemorrhage could also be a major cause of his depression at this time, which could in turn cause him to be less cooperative with questions. When I was researching articles for my interventions, I came across an article that presented the correlation of stroke and depression. In this article by Janice L. Hinkle (1998), studies showed that patients who had left hemisphere damage (as my patient did) had a greater incidence of depression. After I found this information, I thought that my patient's lack of speech could actually be attributed to his lack of desire to speak because of depression. This could have led to a totally different nursing care plan based on my patient's depressed mood.

# Application in Practicum Courses
### *Deborah Perry Schoenfelder, PhD, RN*

Planning and implementing nursing care are central components of any undergraduate nursing practicum course. Students gain experience in choosing nursing diagnoses based on their clinical assessment and in selecting outcomes and interventions that target the nursing diagnoses. Teaching nursing students about the importance of outcome determination in the health care delivery system is a significant responsibility for nursing faculty.[2] This chapter describes my use of the Nursing Outcomes Classification (NOC) outcomes and indicators in two undergraduate practicum courses at the University of Iowa College of Nursing: Core Clinical Practicum and Gerontological Nursing Practicum. Nursing students used the NOC outcomes in group work, as well as in writing individual plans of care.

## DESCRIPTION OF THE COURSES

The course Core Clinical Practicum is a 4–semester hour course that focuses on the acute care of the hospitalized adult patient. Development of clinical decision-making skills that include evaluating patient outcomes is emphasized. During the three semesters I taught this course, we were located in a general medicine unit at The University of Iowa Hospitals and Clinics. Patients had a wide variety of acute and chronic health conditions.

The first written assignment that used the NOC was completed early in the semester during one postclinical conference time. Students, in groups of three to four, analyzed a brief case study in which they: (1) identified one priority nursing diagnosis, (2) selected one to two NOC outcome(s) and pertinent indicators, (3) rated the outcomes and indicators at baseline and projected a desired rating, (4) selected Nursing Intervention Classification (NIC) interventions and activities, giving rationale for their selection, and (5) discussed how they would evaluate the client, when they would next reevaluate the client, and any potential modifications to the plan of care. See case study.

At various times throughout the semester, students were required to list nursing diagnoses, NOC outcomes and indicators, and NIC interventions and activities for one patient cared for that particular week. The worksheet for these assignments is included in Figure F-1. In addition, we held a care plan conference twice during the semester in which students, in groups of three to four, developed a written care plan for one patient addressing the five points described in the previous paragraph for the case study. Refer to Figure F-2 for the form students completed for these assignments. My intention was to have students become familiar and comfortable with using standardized nursing language to define what it was they were doing as nurses and the effect their nursing care was having.

The course Gerontological Nursing Practicum is a 3–semester hour specialty course that focuses on applying the nursing process to promote, maintain, and restore the health of older adults. Opportunities to provide nursing care to healthy and acutely or chronically ill elderly persons are available in a variety of settings such as nursing homes, assisted living facilities, home health care agencies, hospital-based continuity of care clinics, senior centers, and community outreach health promotion programs for older adults. One of the course objectives is to evaluate the effectiveness of nursing interventions in the provision of care for older adults. As with the Core Clinical Practicum, I require students to use the NOC outcomes and indicators when evaluating the effectiveness of the nursing care they provide.

Each student spends a portion of his or her clinical time at a nursing home working with a registered nurse preceptor. During this clinical experience, one of the assignments is to collect health history and physical assessment data on an elderly nursing home resident and write a care plan on three selected nursing diagnoses. For each nursing diagnosis, the student must choose one to two NOC outcomes and relevant indicators. The student rates the outcomes and indicators at

CASE STUDY

Mrs. Hensen, hospitalized since yesterday, is an 89-year-old white widowed female sitting in a wheelchair with a blanket on her lap. In a calm mood and smiling. She describes her health as "Okay except that my family tells me I don't eat enough. I know I should eat more, but I just don't want to and don't feel hungry most of the time."

Current Medications:  Enteric-coated aspirin 650 mg po q 4h for arthritis pain
                                     MOM 30 cc po prn for constipation (uses this about once per month)

Height:  160.02 cm
Weight:  41.7 kg

Self-care abilities:  Able to feed herself, but requires encouragement from the nursing staff.

Nutrition history:
    24 hour recall—ate about half of each meal and snack provided
    No food intolerances
    Supplements—High protein drink 6 oz po TID
    Recent weight loss or gain—has lost 20 pounds in the past 3 months
    Appetite—"Poor. I rarely feel hungry."
    No alcohol or caffeine consumption

No history of heartburn, difficulty swallowing or chewing, N&V, diarrhea, or flatulence. Takes a laxative (MOM 30 cc po) about once per month for constipation.

PA:  Lips, mouth, gingivae, teeth all WNL.

baseline and projects desired ratings that are attainable for the resident. Then the outcomes and indicators are again rated at the end of the student's clinical experience with accompanying written comments about potential care plan modifications and the next evaluation date. The assignment form is the same as that used in the Core Clinical Practicum.

## TRAINING PROVIDED TO USE NOC

Nursing students at The University of Iowa are introduced to the NOC in two courses before they begin clinical experiences. The course Art and Science of Nursing includes a lecture on the NOC (and NANDA and Nursing Interventions Classification), followed by a written assignment in which students use standardized nursing language to develop a care plan. Use of the NOC is also practiced in a laboratory setting in the course Basic Concepts of Nursing. I draw on this prerequisite preparation, asking students in group discussion to tell me what they have learned about using the NOC and how they go about using the NOC outcomes and indicators to develop a care

Student Name _____

Date _____

Patient's Initials _____

Age _____

Gender _____

Medical diagnoses:




List the 2-part nursing diagnoses for this client:





Select 1-2 outcomes for this client and list relevant indicators for each of those outcomes:





Select 2-3 nursing interventions for this client and list relevant activities for each of those interventions:

**Fig. F-1**




plan. I then encourage students to review the introductory information in the NOC book,[3] highlighting particular portions that explain the process of using the NOC to develop a plan of care.

## CHALLENGES

As with any teaching endeavor, there are challenges to using the NOC in undergraduate clinical courses. Although it is a strength that all students come to the clinical courses with the previously mentioned didactic preparation and laboratory application practice, the amount of actual practice with the NOC differs among students. And as is typical with teaching, students come to courses with widely varying ability levels in using the NOC outcomes and indicators. This challenge is not particularly problematic. I encourage students to consult with me as they have questions when writing the assigned nursing care plans so that I can guide them in using the NOC correctly.

| DATE | NURSING DX's (NANDA) | NOC OUTCOMES & INDICATORS (Outcome #, page #) | Baseline rating | NIC INTERVENTIONS & ACTIVITIES (Intervention #, page #) | RATIONALE (for the intervention) | EVALUATION End ratings for Outcomes/Indicators |
|------|----------------------|-----------------------------------------------|-----------------|--------------------------------------------------------|----------------------------------|-----------------------------------------------|
|      | Write a 2-part ND: Subjective Data: Objective Data: |  |  |  |  |  |

Fig. F-2

A bigger obstacle is the fact that most practice sites do not currently use the NOC in their care planning or formal documentation, so students cannot readily compare the existing care plan with their own. Nevertheless, we are able to have discussions that compare the measurability and specificity of the selected NOC outcomes and indicators with the written goals in the practicum sites' care plans for the same individuals.

## RESULTS OF IMPLEMENTING NOC

I have found the NOC easy to use in teaching undergraduate practicum courses. Nursing students are typically taught, and rightly so, that outcome statements should be patient-specific, measurable, and reasonably attainable for clients.[1] The issues of being patient-specific and measurable immediately become nonissues when students use the NOC. Students' efforts are then concentrated on choosing and rating outcomes and indicators that are reasonable for the client. Another advantage of using the NOC along with the NIC is the elimination of students' confusion about what constitutes an outcome versus an intervention.

Group discussions are excellent, as I move among subgroups of three to four students developing care plans, hearing them decide what indicators are appropriate for the individual being discussed. Students, even those who are more reserved, become actively engaged in discussions and gain confidence as they see that they can select outcomes that are on target for the assessment data they have collected. In addition, there have been no instances in which students have been unable to find appropriate NOC outcomes and indicators for clients' identified health needs and problems. The NOC is comprehensive, addressing all possibilities that arise in clinical settings.

Another strength of using the NOC is the rating of indicators. Students are instructed to rate the indicators at baseline, indicate a projected rating, and then complete a final rating at the end of the clinical experience. When these ratings have been done, I have found that most students are able to follow through with evaluations that are well thought out and concise. They are able to discuss what modifications, if any, they recommend in a clear and focused manner that is based on their ratings of the indicators. Finally, having students use the NOC in both discussions and written assignments provides an excellent evaluation tool for me. I am able to follow students' line of thinking and provide feedback that helps students to mature in their decision-making abilities as professional nurses.

## CONCLUSION

Practicing clinical decision making in practicum courses is an essential part of the learning experience for nursing students. Standardized languages provide the tools for gaining experience in making sound professional judgments. Nursing students find the NOC outcomes and indicators comprehensive in scope and easy to select and rate for individuals. The NOC outcomes and indicators are invaluable tools in the education of future professional nurses.

## References

1. Chase, S. K. (1998). Teaching baccalaureate nursing students to project outcomes to nursing interventions. *Nursing Diagnosis, 9,* 62-70.
2. Denehy, J. (1998). Integrating nursing outcomes classification in nursing education. *Journal of Nursing Care Quality, 12,* 73-84.
3. Johnson, M., Maas, M., & Moorhead, S. (2000). *Nursing outcomes classification (NOC)* (2nd ed.). St. Louis: Mosby.

# The Integration of NIC and NOC into the Baccalaureate Curriculum

## *Barbara Van de Castle, APRN, BC*

Faculty in The Johns Hopkins University School of Nursing baccalaureate program have been using a NANDA/NIC/NOC (NNN) care plan format since 1997. A care plan design (see preliminary templates) was created by using the nursing process with NIC and NOC. When the design was conceptualized and sample templates were developed, the templates were presented to the baccalaureate curriculum committee. A pilot study involving two clinical groups from the adult medical-surgical nursing unit was conducted. The students, as well as the instructors, gave their approval of the design after the rotation, and this feedback was also presented to the curriculum committee. The care plan templates were then adopted throughout all clinical rotations in which care plans were used. The flow of information within the care plans was simple to follow, and the care plans provided a table format that the students could use in a word processing program. Templates were created in Microsoft Word and saved to the school's network for easy access by the students.

Several changes occurred as a result of integrating NOC into the student care plans; the plan now had an outcome term with a definition, the ability to create an *expected* outcome statement for the patient, and a measurement scale. The measurement scale was set up to measure the outcomes at different times during the care of the patient, which is more meaningful than just stating whether the patient's expected outcomes were met. The students are able to show how their care influenced the outcome for the patient by using the measurement scale. This gives each student a feeling of worth and transfers that feeling into concrete evidence when it appears on a care plan. The concept of assessing the patient over a period of time with NOC was appealing to both the students and faculty.

NOC is also important to use with NANDA and NIC because it helps to establish clinically appropriate linkages for the student's patients. These linkages among the diagnoses, interventions, and outcomes can be used by other staff members as they care for the same patients during follow-up care.

When the care planning form is created, it is important to use the codes provided for NIC, as well as NOC. We have found that when a student chooses activities and lists the codes, this helps him or her relate back to the specific intervention. Activities can be combined to form different interventions. This can give the instructor an idea as to how many activities were chosen from a given intervention and can also demonstrate a level of creativity that would be lost if the intervention codes were not added to the activity. In the second edition of NOC, the individual indicators were coded, and the students started to include the indicator codes, as well as the NOC codes. This added coding is helpful to faculty who may be tracking the individual indicators that students are choosing.

The whole idea behind having the students use the codes within their care plans is to reinforce the importance of tracking what it is that an individual nurse does for a patient. A quote that nurses in informatics have often cited is "If we cannot name it, we cannot control it, finance it, teach it, research it, or put it into public policy."[1] This quote always gets the students thinking about how nursing is viewed as a profession and how nursing information can be retrieved from clinical information systems. By using nursing terminologies with codes attached, we can start to pull from a computer system specific nursing data that can be studied and developed into nursing standards and guidelines.

Our first template begins with a brief description of the patient and is followed by a table that gives the reader a means for pairing nursing diagnoses with a problem list. Many of our clinical areas use multidisciplinary problem lists, which provide the student with the ability to match a problem on the list to a NANDA diagnosis.

We then have a data sheet that allows for subjective and objective (S & O) information to be displayed with corresponding scientific rationale. In the students' first rotation, they are required to categorize the S & O data into the NIC domains and identify the specific NIC class they are using. In all other rotations, the students will need to combine similar S & O data, independent of the domain. This helps combine the data into a comprehensive source for decision making.

The third template describes the expected outcome; lists the scale descriptors where each indicator chosen has its provided scale individualized to meet the patient's needs; and presents a table that provides for the measurement of the indicator over a period of time. Also included is a free text area where the students can state whether they would continue this plan after discharge, how frequently they would measure for this outcome, and any additional comments they would like to provide to the instructor.

The fourth template has an area where the domain, class, and interventions can be identified. Then the specific activities chosen are described and individualized to meet the patient's needs. There is a corresponding column with the activities where the student can state the rationale/research base for each activity. The student then needs to follow up with appropriate references for each care plan.

Built into the curriculum is a Microsoft Word care plan class where the steps of working in tables and inserting templates into a file are covered in detail so that students feel confident in using the files. The students are able to copy the templates for home use. In recent years the students have taken to e-mailing the care plans to their instructor, which has worked to the benefit of everyone.

Overall, students are able to implement the nursing process while using three of the American Nurses Association approved nursing languages. This experience will provide the students with the background they need in applying the nursing process and an awareness of nursing languages that is lacking in many baccalaureate nursing programs. These languages will help begin to define nursing as a profession in the twenty-first century.

## Reference

1. Clark, J., & Lang, N. (1992). Nursing's next advance: An international classification for nursing practice. *International Nursing Review, 39,* 109-111, 128.

# Care Plan

**Resident/Patient Profile:** Mrs. C. is a 64-year-old, widowed female of Italian descent. Recently admitted to an assisted living facility because of ambulating and incontinence problems. She has a daughter who visits frequently. Speaks English fluently but with a heavy accent.

| Problem List | Nursing Diagnosis |
|---|---|
| 1. Incontinent of urine | 1. Alteration in urinary elimination: stress incontinence RT weak pelvic muscles secondary to multiple childbirth as evidenced by complaining of frequent leakage with coughing and/or standing. |
| 2. Prolapsed urinary bladder | 2. |

Courtesy Johns Hopkins University School of Nursing, Baltimore, MD.

| Johns Hopkins University School of Nursing Care Plan | | |
|---|---|---|
| **Subjective Data**<br>**Domain:** Physiologic Basic<br>**Class:** Elimination<br>Management | **Objective Data** | **Analysis of Data** |
| 1. "I have a lot of problems . . . . Whenever I cough or stand up, I pee myself. It really smells up my clothes. The other people stare at me." | 1. Smells of urine and her clothes are wet. Wearing a housecoat and slippers. | 1. At least 15% to 30% of the American population over age 60 and 50% of those individuals who live in extended-care facilities or receive home care are incontinent (Taylor, Lillis, LeMone, 1997, p. 1230). Incontinence can be transient (Carpenito, 1997, p. 907). Although incontinence is not normal, Mrs. C.'s incontinence is a common problem for her age group. |
| 2. "I been having it for a long time, but I just can't stand it any longer. Maybe 2 years is when it started . . . . Nothing I do seems to help. I stopped drinking iced tea during my evening TV shows." | 2. Skin is pinkish, warm, and moist. Walks alone to bathroom and around room with cane. On a soft diet and eats all of food. | 2. Skin should be warm and the temperature should be equal bilaterally (Jarvis, 1996, p. 227). Mobility is fine for her age. "Lifelong eating habits are developed out of tradition, ethnicity, and religion" (Ebersole, Hess, 1998, p. 160). |
| 3. "No, I haven't had any fevers, and my urine smells normal." | 3. Vital signs are T = po 98.6° F, R = 24, P = 78/ min, B/P = 128/76 (R arm, sitting). Skin is warm and dry to touch. Voided 50 cc into a cup, urine is yellow and clear with no foul odor or sediment. | 3. Normal range of temperature for adults is 96.8° to 100.4° F (Potter, Perry, 1997, p. 595). Mrs. C. has no signs of fever. Normal R rate is 12-20, normal P 60-100/min, and normal B/P is 120/80. Mrs. C. is in the normal range (Jarvis, 1996, p. 204). In healthy persons, urine is amber-colored with a slightly acid reaction, has a peculiar odor. Mrs. C.'s urine meets these requirements (Thomas, Tabers, 1997 CD-ROM). |

| Johns Hopkins University School of Nursing<br>Care Plan—cont'd | | |
|---|---|---|
| **Subjective Data**<br>**Domain:** Physiologic Basic<br>**Class:** Elimination<br>Management | **Objective Data** | **Analysis of Data** |
| 4. "I only take one pill a day. It is a water pill." | 4. The medication bottle reads 20 mg Lasix po qd. | Lasix is a loop diuretic that inhibits sodium and potassium reabsorption in the ascending limb of the loop of Henle. This drug can be used to control hypertension. Major side effects can be ↓ sodium, ↓ potassium, and ↓ chloride. The usual oral dosage for adults is 20-80 mg/dose, bid. Mrs. C. is within the normal range (Mathewson-Kuhn, 1994, p. 797). |

**Nursing Diagnosis:** Impaired urinary elimination: stress incontinence RT weak pelvic muscles secondary to multiple childbirth as evidenced by complaining of frequent leakage with coughing and/or standing.

**Expected Outcome:** The patient will have *urinary continence* (p. 302) at a level of 3 by Friday.

**Scale Descriptors:**
*Urge (050201):* 1 = *Never demonstrated*, never recognizes urge; 2 = *Rarely demonstrated*, recognizes the urge once a week; 3 = *Sometimes demonstrated*, recognizes the urge three times a week; 4 = *Often demonstrated*, recognizes the urge twice a day; 5 = *Consistently demonstrated*, always recognizes the urge to void.
*Pattern (050202):* 1 = *Never demonstrated*, never records pattern in notebook; 2 = *Rarely demonstrated*, records in notebook once a week; 3 = *Sometimes demonstrated*, records in notebook three times a week; 4 = *Often demonstrated*, records in notebook twice a day; 5 = *Consistently demonstrated*, records in notebook for each voiding episode.
*Responds (050203):* 1 = Never demonstrated, *is always incontinent*; 2 = Rarely demonstrated, *voids in the bathroom once a week*; 3 = Sometimes demonstrated, *voids in the bathroom three times a week*; 4 = Often demonstrated, *voids in the bathroom twice a day*; 5 = Consistently demonstrated, *always voids in bathroom.*

| Name of Outcome:<br><br>*Urinary<br>Continence*<br><br>*Indicators* | Date: | 1 | 2 | 3 | 4 | 5 |
|---|---|---|---|---|---|---|
| Recognizes urge to void | Friday, June 28 | | × | | | |
| Predictable pattern to passage of urine | Friday, June 28 | | × | | | |
| Responds in timely manner to urge | Friday, June 28 | | × | | | |

**Continue at discharge?** (Yes/No) Yes, this patient will need continued work to achieve continence.

**Frequency of measurement:** She should continue to keep a log of when she is incontinent and her fluid intake. She should do her documentation daily and should continue with health care follow up with this issue weekly. Will measure at next visit.

**Additional comments:** Mrs. C. was enthusiastic about keeping a log because she said she didn't know how often she really went to the bathroom or became incontinent herself! She is willing to follow the interventions, but during the visit, Mrs. C. was incontinent twice. Also, she said it never occurred to her that drinking a lot of liquid before bed made her pee during the night! She was very appreciative of the interventions and promised she would continue with the follow-up from the health care provider.

**Interventions Template**

| Domain | Physiological: Basic | |
|---|---|---|
| Class | Elimination Management | |
| Interventions | Urinary Incontinence Care (0610)<br>Urinary Bladder Training (0570) | |
| Activity | | Rationale/Research Base |
| | 1. Identify multifactorial causes of incontinence (0610). Discuss with patient the problems she may have had with labor and voiding after giving birth. Confirm history of surgical procedures or any medications that might influence urination. Assess for areas of skin breakdown | 1. In women, diminution of muscle tone associated with normal aging, childbirth, or surgical procedures can cause weakness of the pelvic floor muscles and can result in stress incontinence (Porth, 1998, p. 695). |
| | 2. Determine ability to recognize urge to void (0570). Assess if patient "senses" the fullness of her bladder. When she senses it, is it too late to get to the bathroom? | 2. If patient is unable to sense fullness of the bladder, she may have neurological damage that would require different intervention. May need to consult an M.D. or a urologist (Thomas, Tabers, 1997, p. 227). |
| | 3. Keep a continence record for 3 days to establish voiding pattern (0570). Use a notebook to track the time of each void and the amount and type of fluid she drinks. | 3. A regular voiding pattern can prevent incontinent episodes (Carpenito, 1997, p. 921). For a "bladder drill" the patient is to note time, amount, and interval between voiding so that gradually the time is increased between voidings (Thomas, Tabers, 1997, p. 228). |

## References

Carpenito, L.J., (1997). *Nursing diagnosis: Application to clinical practice* (7th ed.). Philadelphia: Lippincott.

Ebersole, P., & Hess, P. (1998). *Toward healthy aging: Human needs and nursing response.* St. Louis, MO: Mosby.

Jarvis, C. (1996). *Student laboratory manual for physical examination and health assessment.* Philadelphia: W.B. Saunders.

Mathewson-Kuhn, M. (1994). *Parmacotherapeutics: A nursing process approach: Instructor's guide.* Philadelphia: F.A. Davis Company.

Porth, CM (1998). *Pathophysiology: Concepts of Altered Health States* (5th ed.). Philadelphia: Lippincott-Raven.

Potter, P., & Perry, A. (1997). *Fundamentals of nursing* (4th ed.). St. Louis: Mosby.

Taylor, C., Lillis, C., & LeMone, P. (1997). *Fundamentals of nursing: The art and science of nursing care.* Philadelphia: Lippincott-Raven Publishers.

Thomas, C.L. (1997). *Taber's cyclopedic medical dictionary* (18th ed.). Philadelphia: F.A. Davis Company.

Thomas, C.L. (1997). *Taber's cyclopedic medical dictionary* (18th ed. CD-ROM). Philadelphia: F.A. Davis Company.

# Guidelines for Submission of a New or Revised Outcome

## NURSING-SENSITIVE OUTCOMES CLASSIFICATION REVIEW FORM

The Nursing-Sensitive Outcomes Classification (NOC) research team is interested in feedback and submission of outcomes for review and potential addition to the NOC.

## A. GENERAL COMMENTS ABOUT THE CLASSIFICATION

Comments about the classification in general are welcome as are suggestions for outcomes that need to be developed. The outcome suggestions for development can be at the individual, family, or community level.

## B. FEEDBACK ON AN OUTCOME

If the submission is a revision of an existing NOC outcome, provide a paragraph briefly describing the rationale for changes, and note the changes on a copy of the existing outcome. Suggestions can include changes in the definition, indicators, or scale. Additional indicators and references can be suggested.

## C. FEEDBACK ON A MEASUREMENT SCALE(S)

Comments on a particular scale are encouraged. Please briefly explain your suggestion and provide background on your experience in using the scale. Identify the outcome and provide a brief description of the patient populations(s) you are using the outcome with.

## D. GUIDELINES FOR OUTCOME SUBMISSION

Each submission of a proposed outcome must include a label, a definition, indicators, and a short list of references that support the outcome and indicators. You also may suggest a scale to use with the outcomes. A brief paragraph describing the rationale for adding the outcome to the NOC should be included. The rationale should note how the proposed outcome is different from outcomes already included in the NOC.

### General Principles for Developing Outcomes

1. Define the outcome as a variable patient or client state, behavior, or perception that is responsive to nursing intervention(s).
2. Labels should be concise, stated in five or fewer words.
3. Colons can be used to make broader concepts more specific.
4. Labels should describe concepts that can be measured along a continuum.
5. Labels should be neutral and not stated as goals.
6. A group of indicators, more specific than the outcome, must be listed that are used to determine the status of the outcome.
7. The definition should be a brief phrase that defines the concept and encompasses the indicators.

## E. FEEDBACK ON LINKAGES TO NANDA INTERNATIONAL NURSING DIAGNOSES

Comments on linkages to nursing diagnoses are welcome. Please suggest additions or revisions with a brief rationale. For additions to the linkage list for a specific diagnosis, identify whether the NOC outcome should be listed as suggested or as an additional associated outcome.

## F. FEEDBACK ON CORE OUTCOMES BY SPECIALTY

Comments on core specialty outcomes are welcome. The new outcomes added to the 3rd edition are not in current list of outcomes. Please send suggestions for additional outcomes as well as any deletions you think are needed.

Comments and suggestions can be sent to:

Sue Moorhead
458 NB, College of Nursing
The University of Iowa
Iowa City, Iowa 52242
E-mail: sue-moorhead@uiowa.edu
Phone: (319) 335-7110
FAX: (319) 335-6820

# Selected Publications

Maas, M., & Delaney, C. (In press). Nursing process outcome linkages: An assessment of literature and issues. *Medical Care.*

Caldwell, C., Dixon, L., Wasson, D., Brighton, V., & Anderson. M.A. (in review). *Personal autonomy: Development of a nursing outcome (NOC) label.*

Wasson, D., Dixon, L., Grighton, V., Caldwell, C., & Anderson, M.A. (in review). Hyperactivity control: Development of a nursing outcome (NOC) label.

*2002*

Johnson, M.R. (2002). Tools and systems for improved outcomes. Outcomes for an outcomes information system. *Outcomes Management, 6*(4), 143-145.

Johnson, M.R. (2002). Tools and systems for improved outcomes.Variables for outcome analysis. *Outcomes Management, 6*(3), 95-98.

Johnson, M.R. (2002). Tools and systems for improved outcomes. Institute of Medicine report on healthcare quality. *Outcomes Management, 6*(2), 45-48.

Johnson, M.R. (2002). Tools and systems for improved outcomes. Criteria for standardized languages. *Outcomes Management, 6*(1), 1-3.

Maas, M., Reed, D., Reeder, K.M., Kerr, P., Specht, J., Johnson, M., & Moorhead, S. (2002). Nursing outcomes classification: A preliminary report of field testing. *Outcomes Management, 6*(3), 112-119.

Scherb, C.A. (2002). Outcomes research: Making a difference in practice. *Outcomes Management, 6*(1), 22-26.

*2001*

Cavendish, R., Lunney, M., Kraynyak-Luise, B., & Richardson, K. (2001). The nursing outcomes classification: Its relevance to school nursing. *The Journal of School Nursing, 17*(4), 189-197.

Frederick, J., Scherb, C.A., Smith-Foreman, K., Witt, S., Quiram, J., Wagenaar, J., Slama, C., Bottema, K., Muilenburg, J., & Evans, K. (2001). Speaking a common language: Standardized nursing languages have increased the visibility of nursing practice at three facilities. *American Journal of Nursing, 101*(3), 2400-2403.

Head, B. (2001). Impaired home maintenance management. In M. Maas, K. Buckwalter, M. Hardy, T. Tripp-Reimer, M. Titler, & J.P. Specht, (Eds.). *Nursing care of older adults: Diagnoses, outcomes and interventions* (pp. 64-74). St. Louis: Mosby.

Johnson, M., Bulechek, G., Dochterman-McCloskey, J. Maas, M., & Moorhead, S. (2001). *Nursing diagnoses, interventions, and outcomes: NANDA, NIC, and NOC linkages.* St. Louis: Mosby.

Legge, L. (2001). Measure of success: Southern Minnesota project documents nursing's effectiveness. *Nursing Minnesota, 6*(3), 8-13.

Maas, M.L., Buckwalter, K.C., Hardy, M D., Tripp-Reimer, T., Titler, M., & Specht, J. (Eds.). (2001). *Nursing care of older adults: Diagnoses, outcomes and interventions.* St. Louis: Mosby.

Maas, M., & Specht, J. (2001). Bowel incontinence. In M. Maas, K. Buckwalter, M. Hardy, T. Tripp-Reimer, M. Titler, & J.P. Specht, (Eds.). *Nursing care of older adults: Diagnoses, outcomes and interventions* (pp. 238-251). St. Louis: Mosby.

Maas, M., & Specht, J. (2001). Impaired physical mobility. In M. Maas, K. Buckwalter, M. Hardy, T. Tripp-Reimer, M. Titler, & J.P. Specht, (Eds.). *Nursing care of older adults: Diagnoses, outcomes and interventions* (pp. 337-365). St. Louis: Mosby.

Mastal, P. (2001). Ambulatory nursing outcomes. *AACN Viewpoint 23(4),* 6-7.

Moorhead, S., & V. Brighton. (2001). Anxiety and fear. In M. Maas, K. Buckwalter, M. Hardy, T. Tripp-Reimer, M. Titler, & J.P. Specht, (Eds.). *Nursing care of older adults: Diagnoses, outcomes and interventions* (pp. 571-592). St. Louis: Mosby.

Schoenfelder, D.P., & Culp, K. (2001). Sleep pattern disturbance. In M. Maas, K. Buckwalter, M. Hardy, T. Tripp-Reimer, M. Titler, & J.P. Specht, (Eds.). *Nursing care of older adults: Diagnoses, outcomes and interventions* (pp. 401-413). St. Louis: Mosby.

Specht, J., & Maas, M. (2001). Urinary incontinence: Functional, iatrogenic, overflow, reflex, stress, total and urge. In M. Maas, K. Buckwalter, M. Hardy, T. Tripp-Reimer, M. Titler, & J.P. Specht, (Eds.). *Nursing care of older adults: Diagnoses, outcomes and interventions* (pp. 252-278). St. Louis: Mosby.

Swanson, E., & Drury, J. (2001). Sensory/Perceptual alteration. In M. Maas, K. Buckwalter, M. Hardy, T. Tripp-Reimer, M. Titler, & J.P. Specht, (Eds.). *Nursing care of older adults: Diagnoses, outcomes and interventions* (pp. 476-491). St. Louis: Mosby.

Wakefield, B. (2001). Altered nutrition: less than body requirements. In M. Maas, K. Buckwalter, M. Hardy, T. Tripp-Reimer, M. Titler, & J.P. Specht, (Eds.). *Nursing care of older adults: Diagnoses, outcomes and interventions* (pp. 145-157). St. Louis: Mosby.

Wakefield, B. (2001). Ineffective breathing pattern. In M. Maas, K. Buckwalter, M. Hardy, T. Tripp-Reimer, M. Titler, & J.P. Specht, (Eds.). *Nursing care of older adults: Diagnoses, outcomes and interventions* (pp. 313-323). St. Louis: Mosby.

Wakefield, B., Mentes, J., et al. (2001). Acute confusion. In M. Maas, K. Buckwalter, M. Hardy, T. Tripp-Reimer, M. Titler, & J.P. Specht, (Eds.). *Nursing care of older adults: Diagnoses, outcomes and interventions* (pp. 442-454). St. Louis: Mosby.

Weiler, K., & Moorhead, S. (2001). Self determination. In M. Maas, K. Buckwalter, M. Hardy, T. Tripp-Reimer, M. Titler, & J.P. Specht, (Eds.). *Nursing care of older adults: Diagnoses, outcomes and interventions* (pp. 706-718). St. Louis: Mosby.

Williams, J., Skirton, H., Reed, D., Johnson, M., Mass, M., & Daack-Hirsch, S. (2001). Genetic counseling outcomes validation by genetics nurses in the UK and US. *Journal of Nursing Scholarship, 33*(4), 369-374.

## 2000

Aquilino, M., & Keenan, G. (2000). Having our say: Nursing's standardized nomenclatures. *American Journal of Nursing,* 100(7), 33-38.

Daly, J. (2000). Bowel elimination. In H. Harkreader (Ed.), *Fundamentals of nursing: Caring and clinical judgment* (pp. 846-883). Philadelphia: W. B. Saunders.

Daly, J. (2000). Planning for intervention. In H. Harkreader (Ed.), *Fundamentals of nursing: Caring and clinical judgment* (pp. 237-261). Philadelphia: W. B. Saunders.

Denehy, J. (2000). Measuring the outcomes of school nursing practice: Showing that school nurses do make a difference. *Journal of School Nursing,* 16(1), 2-4.

Dorr, G.G., Prophet, C.M., Gibbs, T.D., Porcella, A.A., & Clemons, D.K. (2000). *Implementation and evaluation of Standardized Nursing Languages (SNLs) in a Clinical Information System (CIS)* (183-189). Proceedings at the Nursing Informatics: One Step Beyond: The Evolution of Technology and Nursing. Auckland, New Zealand: Adis International.

Iowa Outcomes Project. M. Johnson, M. Maas & S. Moorhead (Eds.). (2000). *Nursing Outcomes Classification (NOC)* (2nd ed.). St. Louis: Mosby.

Kerr, P. (2000). Comparing two nursing outcomes reporting initiatives. *Outcomes Management for Nursing Practice, 4*(3), 144-149.

Maas, M., Moorhead, S., Specht, J., Schoenfelder, D., Swanson, E.A., Johnson, M., & Westra, B.L. (2000). Concept development of nursing-sensitive patient outcomes. In B. Rogers & K. Knafl (Eds.). *Concept analysis in nursing research*, (pp. 387-400). New York: Springer Publishing.

McBeth, A.J., Weydt, A.P., Frederick, J.A., Scherb, C.A., & Foreman, K.M. (2000). Staffing challenges and opportunities in the rural setting. In. M.F. Fralic (Ed.), *Staffing management and methods: Tools and techniques for nurse leaders* (AONE Management Series) San Francisco: Jossey-Bass.

Morrison, R. (2000). Evaluation of NOC instruments with chronically ill patients. *Southern Online Journal of Nursing Research 1*(1), 1-11.

Peters, R.M. (2000). Using NOC outcomes of risk control in prevention, early detection, and control of hypertension. *Outcomes Management for Nursing Practice, 4*(1), 39-45.

Prophet, C.M. (2000). The evolution of a clinical database: From local to standardized clinical languages. *Proceedings of the Annual Symposium of the American Medical Informatics Association (AMIA)*(660-664), Hanley & Belfus, Inc..

Scherb, C.A. (2000). Measuring nursing effectiveness using standardized nursing languages. *Nursing Minnesota, 5*(9), 12.

Scherb, C.A., Frederick, J. (2000). Standardized nursing language: A necessity for computer information systems. *Clinical Data Management, 7*(1), 4-7, 12.

Scherb, C.A. (2000). Outcomes research: Making a difference in patient care. *Network News, 2*(5), 14.

Schoenfelder, D.P., Swanson, E.A., Specht, J.K.P., Johnson, M., & Maas, M. (2000). Outcome indicators for direct and indirect caregiving. *Clinical Nursing Research: An International Journal, 9*(1), 47-69.

Specht, J., Maas, M., Willit, S., & Meyers, N. (2000). Intermittent catheterization. In G. Bulechek, G. & J. McCloskey (Eds.). *Nursing interventions: Treatments for nursing diagnoses*, (3rd edition). Philadelphia: Saunders.

## 1999

Denehy, J., & Poulton, S. (1999). The use of standardized language in individualized healthcare plans. *The Journal of School Nursing, 15*(1), 38-45.

Heller, C., & Vlasses, F. (Eds.). (1999) Models of care for Asthma 2(2). Chicago: Athena Healthcare Communications, pp. 2, 32.

Johnson, M., & Maas, M. (1999). Nursing-sensitive patient outcomes: Development and importance for use in assessing health care effectiveness. In E. Cohen & V. DeBack (Eds.). *The outcomes mandate, case management in health care today,* (pp. 37-48). St. Louis: Mosby.

Kinnaird, L. (1999). Patient education management: For nurse managers, education directors, case managers, discharge planners. *American Health Consultants, 6*(12), 133-135.

Maas, M., & Kerr, P. (1999). Risk adjustment in nursing effectiveness research. *Outcomes Management for Nursing Practice, 3*(2), 50-52.

Maas, M., & Specht, J.P. (1999). Context and patient outcomes in nursing homes. In A.S. Hinshaw & F. Feetham (Eds.), *State of the science in nursing research* (pp.655-663). New York: Springer Publishing.

Poulton, S., & Denehy, J. (1999). Standardized languages in nursing: Integrating NANDA, NIC, and NOC into IHPs. In M.J. Arnold & C.K. Silkworth, *The school nurse's source book of individualized healthcare plans,* Volume II. (pp. 25-40). North Branch, MN: Sunrise River Press.

## 1998

Cox, R. (1998). Implementing nurse-sensitive outcomes into care planning at a long-term care facility. *Journal of Nursing Care Quality, 12*(5), 41-51.

Denehy, J. (1998). Integrating Nursing Outcomes Classification in nursing education. *Journal of Nursing Care Quality, 12*(5), 73-84.

Donahue, M.P., & Brighton, V. (1998). Nursing Outcomes Classification: Development and implementation. *Journal of Nursing Care Quality, 12*(5), vii-viii.

Garand, L., Gerdner, L.A., Buckwalter, K.C., & Wakefield, B. (1998). Neuropsychiatric disorders. In M.A. Boyd & M.A. Nihart (Eds.), *Psychiatric mental health nursing* (pp. 612-666). Philadelphia: Lippincott.

Goode, C. (1998). About identifying nurse-specific cardiac outcomes. *Nursing Management, 29*(11), 72.

Hayewski, C., Maupin, J., Rapp, D., Sitterding, M., & Pappas, J (1998). Implementation of Nursing Intervention Classification and Nursing Outcome Classification in a patient education plan. *Journal of Nursing Care Quality, 12*(5), 30-40.

Johnson, M., & Maas, M. (1998). The Nursing Outcomes Classification. *Journal of Nursing Care Quality, 12*(5), 9-20.

Johnson, M. (1998). Overview of the Nursing Outcomes Classification (NOC). *On-line Journal of Nursing Informatics, 2*(2). [On-line]. Available: *http://www.eaa-knowledge.com/ojni/ni/dm/v2n2.html*

Johnson, M., & Maas, M. (1998). Nursing Outcomes Classification. In J.J. Fitzpatrick (Ed.), *Encyclopedia of nursing research* (pp. 378-379). New York: Springer.

Johnson, M., & Maas, M. (1998). Implementing the Nursing Outcomes Classification in a practice setting. *Outcomes Management for Nursing Practice, 2*(3), 99-104.

Keenan, G., & Aquilino, M. (1998). Standardized nomenclatures: Keys to continuity of care, nursing accountability and nursing effectiveness. *Outcomes Management for Nursing Practice, 2*(2), 81-86.

Maas, M., Delaney, C., & Huber, D. (1998). Contextual variables and assessment of the outcome effects of nursing interventions. *Outcomes Management for Nursing Practice, 3*(1), 4-6.

Maas, M., & Head, B. (1998). Moving to measurement. *Outcomes Management for Nursing Practice, 2*(4), 139-142.

Maas, M. (1998). Structure and process constraints on nursing accountability. *Outcomes Management for Nursing Practice, 2*(2), 51-53.

Maas, M. (1998). Outcome data accountability. *Outcomes Management for Nursing Practice, 2*(1), 3-5.

Maas, M. (1998). Nursing's role in interdisciplinary accountability for patient outcomes. *Outcomes Management for Nursing Practice, 2*(3), 92-94.

McCloskey, J.C., & Maas, M. (1998). Interdisciplinary team: The nursing perspective is essential. *Nursing Outlook, 46,* 157-163.

Moorhead, S., Head, B., Johnson, M., & Maas, M. (1998). The nursing outcomes taxonomy: Development and coding. *Journal of Nursing Care Quality, 12*(6), 56-63.

Moorhead, S., Clarke, M., Willits, M., & Tomsha, K. (1998). Nursing Outcomes Classification implementation projects across the care continuum. *Journal of Nursing Care Quality, 12*(5), 52-63.

Prophet, C., & Delaney, C. (1998). Nursing Outcomes Classification: Implications for nursing information systems and the computer-based patient record. *Journal of Nursing Care Quality, 12*(5), 21-29.

Rankin, M., Donahue, P., Davis, K., Katseres, J., Wedig, J.A., Johnson, M., & Maas, M. (1998). Dignified dying as a nursing outcome. *Outcomes Management for Nursing Practice, 2*(3),105-110.

Scherb, C.A., Rapp, C.G., Johnson, M., & Maas, M. (1998). The Nursing Outcomes Classification (NOC): Validation by rehabilitation nurses. *Journal of Rehabilitation Nursing 23*(4), 174-191.

Timm, J., & Behrenbeck, J. (1998). Implementing the Nursing Outcomes Classification in a clinical information system in a tertiary care setting. *Journal of Nursing Care Quality, 12*(5), 64-72.

## 1997

Daly, J., Maas, M., & Johnson, M. (1997). Development of play and leisure nursing-sensitive patient outcomes. *Journal of Clinical Geropsychology, 3*(4), 267-273.

Daly, J., Maas, M., & Johnson, M. (1997). Nursing-sensitive Outcomes Classification (NOC): An essential element in data sets for nursing and health care effectiveness. *Computers in Nursing, 15(2)* Suppl., S82-S86.

Head, B., Maas, M., & Johnson, M. (1997). Outcomes for home and community nursing in integrated delivery systems. *Caring Magazine, 16*(1), 50-56.

Iowa Outcomes Project. (1997). M. Johnson & M. Maas (Eds.). *Nursing Outcomes Classification (NOC)*. St. Louis: Mosby.

Maas, M., & Johnson, M. (1997). Advancing nursing's accountability for outcomes. *Outcomes Management for Nursing Practice, 2*(1), 3-4.

Maas, M. (1997). Nursing-sensitive Outcomes Classification (NOC): Completing the essential comprehensive languages for nursing. Classification of Nursing Diagnosis: *Proceedings of the 12th Conference North American Nursing Diagnosis Association (NANDA)*, Pittsburgh, PA, 40-47.

Prophet, C., Dorr, G.G., Gibbs, T.D., & Porcella, A.A. (1997). Implementation of standardized nursing languages (NIC, NOC) in on-line care planning and documentation (pp. 395-400). *Informatics: The Impact of Nursing Knowledge on Health Care Informatics*. Amsterdam: IOS Press.

Swanson, E., Jensen, D.P., Specht, J., Saylor, D., Johnson, M., & Maas, M. (1997). Caregiving: Concept analysis and outcomes. *Scholarly Inquiry for Nursing Practice: An International Journal, 11*(1), 65-76.

### *1996*

Johnson, S.L., Brady-Schluttner, K., Ellenbecker, S., Johnson, M., Lassengard, E., Maas, M., Stone, J., & Westra, B.L. (1996). Evaluating physical functional outcomes: One category of the system. *MEDSURG Journal of Nursing, 5*, 157-162.

Maas, M., Johnson, M., & Kraus, V. (1996). Nursing-sensitive patient Outcomes Classification. In K. Kelly (Ed.), *Series on nursing administration: Outcomes of effective management practices (Vol. 8*, pp. 20-35). Thousand Oaks, CA: Sage Publications.

Maas, M., Johnson, M., & Moorhead, S. (1996). Classifying nursing-sensitive patient outcomes. *Image—Journal of Nursing Scholarship, 28* (4), 295-301.

### *1995–1992*

Johnson, M., & Maas, M. (1995). Classification of nursing-sensitive patient outcomes. In N.M. Lang (Ed.). *Nursing Data Systems: The emerging framework,* (pp. 177-183). Washington, DC: The American Nurses Association.

Delaney, C., Mehmert, M., Prophet, C., & Crossley, J. (1994). Establishment of the research value of nursing minimum data sets. *Nursing informatics: An international overview for nursing in a technological era, June 17-22, Amsterdam: Elsevier*, 169-173.

Johnson, M., & Maas, M. (1994). Nursing-focused patient outcomes: Challenge for the nineties. In J.C. McCloskey & H. Grace (Eds.), *Current issues in nursing* (4th ed., pp. 136-142). St. Louis: Mosby.

Prophet, C. (1994). Nurses' orders in manual and computerized systems. In S.J. Grobe & E.S.P. Pluyter-Wenting (Eds.), *Nursing informatics: An international overview for nursing in a technological era* (pp. 286-289). Amsterdam: Elsevier.

Prophet, C.M., & Walker, K.P. (1993). Integration of systems applications: Computerized documentation of the patient discharge referral (pp.185-196). *Proceedings of the 1993 annual Healthcare Information and Management Systems Society (HIMSS) conference, San Diego, CA.*

Prophet, C. (1993). Patient problem/nursing diagnosis form: A computer-generated chart document (pp.326-330). *Proceedings of the Seventeenth Annual Symposium on Computer Applications in Medical Care (SCAMC).* Washington DC: McGraw-Hill.

Delaney, C., Mehmert, P., Prophet, C., Bellinger, S., Gardner-Huber, D., & Ellerbe, S. (1992). Standardized nursing language for healthcare information systems. *Journal of Medical Systems, 16*(4), 145-159.

# Index